VOLUME TWO **Pathology**

VOLUME TWO **Pathology**

Edited by

W. A. D. Anderson
M.A., M.D., F.A.C.P., F.C.A.P.

Professor of Pathology and Chairman of the
Department of Pathology, University of Miami School
of Medicine, Miami, Fla.; Director of the Pathology
Laboratories, Jackson Memorial Hospital, Miami, Fla.

SIXTH EDITION (two volumes)

With 1566 figures
and 6 color plates

THE C. V. MOSBY COMPANY

ST. LOUIS   1971

Contributors

Lester Adelson, M.D.

Associate Professor of Forensic Pathology, Department of Pathology, Case Western Reserve University School of Medicine, Cleveland, Ohio; Chief Pathologist and Chief Deputy Coroner, Cuyahoga County Coroner's Office, Cleveland, Ohio.

Arthur C. Allen, M.D.

Director of Laboratories, The Jewish Hospital and Medical Center of Brooklyn, Brooklyn, N. Y.; Clinical Professor of Pathology, State University of New York Down State Medical Center, Brooklyn, N. Y.; Consultant, Hunterdon Medical Center, Flemington, N. J.; Consultant, Fort Hamilton Veterans Administration Hospital, Brooklyn, N. Y.

W. A. D. Anderson, M.A., M.D., F.A.C.P., F.C.A.P.

Professor of Pathology and Chairman of the Department of Pathology, University of Miami School of Medicine, Miami, Fla.; Director of the Pathology Laboratories, Jackson Memorial Hospital, Miami, Fla.

Roger Denio Baker, M.D.

Professor of Pathology, The State University Rutgers Medical School, New Brunswick, N. J.

Granville A. Bennett, B.S., M.D.

Professor of Pathology Emeritus and former Dean, University of Illinois College of Medicine, Chicago, Ill.

Chapman H. Binford, A.B., M.D.

Chief, Special Mycobacterial Diseases Branch, and Research Pathologist, Leonard Wood Memorial (American Leprosy Foundation), Armed Forces Institute of Pathology, Washington, D. C.; Medical Director, Leonard Wood Memorial, Washington, D. C.

Jacob L. Chason, M.D.

Professor of Pathology (Neuropathology) and Chairman of the Department of Pathology, Wayne State University School of Medicine, Detroit, Mich.

E. V. Cowdry, Ph.D.

Emeritus Professor of Anatomy, Washington University School of Medicine, St. Louis, Mo.

A. R. Currie, B.Sc., M.D., F.R.C.P.(Edinburgh and Glasgow), F.C.Path., F.R.S.(Edinburgh)

Regius Professor of Pathology, University of Aberdeen, Aberdeen, Scotland; Honorary Consultant Pathologist and Regional Advisor in Pathology, North-Eastern Regional Hospital Board, Aberdeen, Scotland.

Charles E. Dunlap, A.B., M.D.

Professor of Pathology, Tulane University School of Medicine, New Orleans, La.

Hugh A. Edmondson, M.D.

Professor of Pathology and Chairman of the Department of Pathology, University of Southern California School of Medicine, Los Angeles, Calif.; Director of Laboratories and Pathology, Los Angeles County–University of Southern California Medical Center, Los Angeles, Calif.

John C. Finerty, Ph.D.

Professor of Anatomy and Vice Chancellor, Louisiana State University Medical Center, New Orleans, La.

Hazel Gore, M.B., B.S.

Professor of Pathology and Associate Professor of Obstetrics and Gynecology, University of Alabama School of Medicine, Birmingham, Ala.

Ira Gore, M.D.

Professor of Pathology, University of Alabama School of Medicine, Birmingham, Ala.

Robert J. Gorlin, A.B., D.D.S., M.S.

Professor and Chairman of the Division of Oral Pathology, University of Minnesota School of Dentistry, Minneapolis, Minn.

Emmerich von Haam, M.D.

Professor of Pathology, The Ohio State University College of Medicine, Columbus, Ohio.

Béla Halpert, M.D.

Emeritus Professor of Pathology, Baylor University College of Medicine, Houston, Texas.

Gordon R. Hennigar, M.D.

Professor of Pathology and Chairman of the Department of Pathology, Medical University of South Carolina, Charleston, S. C.

Arthur T. Hertig, M.D.

Shattuck Professor of Pathological Anatomy, Harvard Medical School, Boston, Mass.; Consultant in Pathology, Boston Lying-in Hospital, Boston, Mass.; Consultant in Pathology, Free Hospital for Women, Brookline, Mass.; Chief of Division of Pathobiology, New England Regional Primate Research Center, Southborough, Mass.

Howard C. Hopps, M.D., Ph.D.

Curators' Professor, Department of Pathology, University of Missouri School of Medicine, Columbia, Mo.

Robert C. Horn, Jr., M.D.

Chairman, Department of Pathology, Henry Ford Hospital, Detroit, Mich.

David B. Jones, M.D.

Professor of Pathology, State University of New York Upstate Medical Center, Syracuse, N. Y.

John M. Kissane, M.D.

Professor of Pathology and of Pathology in Pediatrics, Washington University School of Medicine, St. Louis, Mo.

Joseph F. Kuzma, B.S., M.D., M.S.

Professor of Pathology, Medical College of Wisconsin (formerly Marquette University School of Medicine), Milwaukee, Wis.; Consultant, Veterans Administration Center, Wood, Wis.

Paul E. Lacy, M.D.

Mallinckrodt Professor and Chairman of the Department of Pathology, Washington University School of Medicine, St. Louis, Mo.

Jan E. Leestma, M.D.

Major, United States Air Force Medical Corps, Genitourinary Pathology Branch, Armed Forces Institute of Pathology, Washington, D. C.

Maurice Lev, M.D.

Director, Congenital Heart Disease Research and Training Center, Hektoen Institute for Medical Research, Chicago, Ill.; Professor of Pathology, Northwestern University Medical School, Chicago, Ill.; Professorial Lecturer, Pritzker School of Medicine of The University of Chicago, Chicago, Ill.; Lecturer in the Departments of Pathology at the University of Illinois College of Medicine and at the Chicago Medical School, University of Health Sciences, Chicago, Ill., and at the Loyola University Stritch School of Medicine, Maywood, Ill.; Career Investigator, Chicago Heart Association, Chicago, Ill.

Raúl A. Marcial-Rojas, M.D.

Professor and Chairman, Department of Pathology and Legal Medicine, University of Puerto Rico School of Medicine, San Juan, Puerto Rico; Chief of Pathology, Puerto Rico Medical Center and Dr. I. González-Martínez Oncologic Hospital, San Juan, Puerto Rico; Director, Institute of Legal Medicine of Puerto Rico.

William A. Meissner, M.D.

Clinical Professor of Pathology, Harvard Medical School, Boston, Mass.; Chairman of Departments of Pathology, New England Deaconess and New England Baptist Hospitals, Boston, Mass.

John B. Miale, M.D.

Professor of Pathology and Associate Chairman of the Department of Pathology, University of Miami School of Medicine, Miami, Fla.; Director of Clinical Pathology, Jackson Memorial Hospital, Miami, Fla.

Max Millard, M.A., M.B.(Dublin), F.R.C.P.(Ireland), F.R.C.Path.(England), D.C.P.(London)

Associate Professor of Pathology, University of Miami School of Medicine, Miami, Fla.; Director of Pathologic Anatomy, Pathology Laboratories, Jackson Memorial Hospital, Miami, Fla.

Alan R. Moritz, M.D.

Professor of Pathology, Case Western Reserve University School of Medicine, Cleveland, Ohio.

Fathollah K. Mostofi, A.B., B.Sc., M.D.

Chief, General and Special Pathology Division and Genitourinary Branch, Armed Forces Institute of Pathology, Washington, D. C.; Registrar, Urologic Registries, and Head, World Health Organization International Reference Center on Tumors of Male Genitourinary Tract at the Armed Forces Institute of Pathology and Veterans Administration Special Reference Laboratory for Pathology at the Armed Forces Institute of Pathology, Washington, D. C.; Clinical Professor of Pathology, Georgetown University Medical Center, Washington, D. C.; Assistant Professor of Pathology, Johns Hopkins University Medical School, Baltimore, Md.

James E. Oertel, M.D.

Chief of Endocrine Pathology Branch, Armed Forces Institute of Pathology, and the Veterans Administration Special Reference Laboratory for Anatomic Pathology at the Armed Forces Institute of Pathology, Washington, D. C.

Robert L. Peters, M.D.

Professor of Pathology, University of Southern California School of Medicine, Los Angeles, Calif.; Director of Pathology and Laboratory, John Wesley County Hospital, Los Angeles, Calif.

Henry Pinkerton, B.S., M.D.

Emeritus Professor of Pathology, St. Louis University School of Medicine, St. Louis, Mo.

Thomas M. Scotti, A.B., M.D.

Professor of Pathology, University of Miami School of Medicine, Miami, Fla.; Attending Pathologist, Jackson Memorial Hospital, Miami, Fla.; Consultant in Pathology, Veterans Administration Hospital, Miami, Fla.

Richard Shuman, B.S., M.D.

Professor of Pathology, Medical College of Pennsylvania, Philadelphia, Pa.; Consultant in Pathology, Veterans Administration Hospital, Philadelphia, Pa.; formerly Chief of Soft Tissue Section, Pathology Division, Armed Forces Institute of Pathology, Washington, D. C.; formerly Head of International Center for Soft Tissue Tumors, World Health Organization, Washington, D. C.

Stanley B. Smith, M.D.

Asssistant Professor of Pathology, University of Miami School of Medicine, Miami, Fla.; Attending Pathologist, Jackson Memorial Hospital, Miami, Fla.

Sheldon C. Sommers, M.D.

Director of Laboratories, Lenox Hill Hospital, New York, N. Y.; Clinical Professor of Pathology, Columbia University College of Physicians and Surgeons, New York, N. Y.; Clinical Professor of Pathology, University of Southern California School of Medicine, Los Angeles, Calif.

Robert A. Vickers, D.D.S., M.S.D.

Professor of Oral Pathology, University of Minnesota School of Dentistry, Minneapolis, Minn.

Shields Warren, M.D., D.Sc., LL.D.

Emeritus Professor of Pathology, Harvard Medical School at the New England Deaconess Hospital, Boston, Mass.; formerly United States Delegate to United Nations Scientific Committee on Effect of Atomic Radiation.

D. L. Wilhelm, M.D., Ph.D.

Professor of and Head of School of Pathology, University of New South Wales, Sydney, Australia; Director of Pathology, The Prince Henry Hospital and The Prince of Wales Hospital, Sydney, Australia.

J. Daniel Wilkes, M.D.

Pathologist, Suburban Hospital Association, Bethesda, Md.

Lorenz E. Zimmerman, M.D.

Chief, Ophthalmic Pathology Branch, Armed Forces Institute of Pathology, and Clinical Professor of Ophthalmic Pathology, The George Washington University School of Medicine, Washington, D. C.

Preface

TO SIXTH EDITION

In this new edition of *Pathology,* much of the content has been modified to include new knowledge and concepts in medical sciences. Significant progress in the fields of ultrastructure, cytology, genetics, immunopathology, and biochemistry has led to a merging of the medical sciences—among themselves and with biology. The borderland of pathology has always been both varying and ill-defined, but never more so than now. Thus, the choice of inclusion or exclusion of many subjects must be somewhat arbitrary, although based on subjective judgment aimed at correlating pathology with the total field of medical education and clinical practice.

The entire book has undergone revision. The chapters on inflammation and healing, drug and chemical injury, ophthalmic pathology, upper respiratory tract and ear, lower urinary tract, prostate, and male genitalia, hemopoietic system (reticuloendothelium, spleen, lymph nodes, blood, and bone marrow), thymus, pituitary gland, thyroid gland, parathyroid glands, adrenal glands, and nervous system and skeletal muscle have been completely rewritten. In addition, major changes have been made in the discussions of hypersensitivity diseases and immunopathology, mycotic infections, viral diseases, neoplasms, and diseases of kidney, lung, liver, and pancreas.

The basic nature of disease, and of medical practice, does not change. However, the extent and depth of our knowledge and understanding and of our conceptual and practical approaches are changing rapidly and no doubt will continue to do so. In the life of a student of medicine and a physician, the study of disease must be a continuing program. In these times of core curricula in medical schools, the continuing study and correlation of basic subjects with clinical experience is a necessity. It is hoped that these volumes will continue to be useful in the study of medicine, not only during but also after formal courses, and will assist in the practice of pathology or of other disciplines of medicine.

I am grateful for the patient and helpful cooperation of the contributors to this book and am deeply appreciative of the interest and assistance of my secretaries, Miss Edna Mae Everitt and Mrs. Louise Rhodes.

W. A. D. ANDERSON

Preface

TO FIRST EDITION

Pathology should form the basis of every physician's thinking about his patients. The study of the nature of disease, which constitutes pathology in the broad sense, has many facets. Any science or technique which contributes to our knowledge of the nature and constitution of disease belongs in the broad realm of pathology. Different aspects of a disease may be stressed by the geneticist, the cytologist, the biochemist, the clinical diagnostician, etc., and it is the difficult function of the pathologist to attempt to bring about a synthesis, and to present disease in as whole or as true an aspect as can be done with present knowledge. Pathologists often have been accused, and sometimes justly, of stressing the morphologic changes in disease to the neglect of functional effects. Nevertheless, pathologic anatomy and histology remain as an essential foundation of knowledge about disease, without which basis the concepts of many diseases are easily distorted.

In this volume is brought together the specialized knowledge of a number of pathologists in particular aspects or fields of pathology. A time-tested order of presentation is maintained, both because it has been found logical and effective in teaching medical students and because it facilitates study and reference by graduates. While presented in an order and form to serve as a textbook, yet it is intended also to have sufficient comprehensiveness and completeness to be useful to the practicing or graduate physician. It is hoped that this book will be both a foundation and a useful tool for those who deal with the problems of disease.

For obvious reasons, the nature and effects of radiation have been given unusual relative prominence. The changing order of things, with increase of rapid, world-wide travel and communication, necessitates increased attention to certain viral, protozoal, parasitic, and other conditions often dismissed as "tropical,"
to bring them nearer their true relative importance. Also, given more than usual attention are diseases of the skin, of the organs of special senses, of the nervous system, and of the skeletal system. These are fields which often have not been given sufficient consideration in accordance with their true relative importance among diseases.

The Editor is highly appreciative of the spirit of the various contributors to this book. They are busy people, who, at the sacrifice of other duties and of leisure, freely cooperated in its production, uncomplainingly tolerated delays and difficulties, and were understanding in their willingness to work together for the good of the book as a whole. Particular thanks are due the directors of the Army Institute of Pathology and the American Registry of Pathology, for making available many illustrations. Dr. G. L. Duff, Strathcona Professor of Pathology, McGill University, Dr. H. A. Edmondson, Department of Pathology of the University of Southern California School of Medicine, Dr. J. S. Hirschboeck, Dean, and Dr. Harry Beckman, Professor of Pharmacology, Marquette University School of Medicine, all generously gave advice and assistance with certain parts.

To the members of the Department of Pathology and Bacteriology at Marquette University, the Editor wishes to express gratitude, both for tolerance and for assistance. Especially valuable has been the help of Dr. R. S. Haukohl, Dr. J. F. Kuzma, Dr. S. B. Pessin, and Dr. H. Everett. A large burden was assumed by the Editor's secretaries, Miss Charlotte Skacel and Miss Ann Cassady. Miss Patricia Blakeslee also assisted at various stages and with the index. To all of these the Editor's thanks, and also to the many others who at some time assisted by helpful and kindly acts, or by words of encouragement or interest.

W. A. D. Anderson

Contents

VOLUME TWO

COLOR PLATES

VOLUME TWO **Pathology**

Chapter 23

Lung, pleura, and mediastinum

Max Millard

■ Lung

PULMONARY STRUCTURE AND FUNCTION

The gross and microscopic morphology of the lung as shown by standard methods is altered, so that the true details of pulmonary structure are not always clear. The anatomy of pleurae and of pulmonary lobes and segments is left to specialized texts and the consideration here commences with the branching of the bronchi.[12]

Bronchial branching occurs dichotomously up to twenty-five times, starting from the main bronchus at the hilus of the lung and ending with the terminal bronchiole near the periphery. Between these two points, the airways function as afferent and efferent air-conditioning tubes and play no active role in respiratory exchange. The latter role belongs to the alveoli.

Walls of the *bronchi* consist of mucosa, glands, muscle, and fibrous tissue with cartilage. The mucosa is mainly lined by a pseudostratified ciliated columnar epithelium, with some intervening goblet cells and undifferentiated basal cells. From the latter, the other types are regenerated. The cilia beat rapidly against the undersurface of the covering mucus, moving it upward. The epithelium rests on a prominent continuous, thick, eosinophilic basement membrane, a feature easily seen in large bronchi, although still present in a much thinner form in the small ones. Beneath the mucosa are seromucinous glands, decreasing in number and becoming purely mucous as the bronchi branch. Glands disappear altogether at the level of the terminal bronchioles.

Bronchial muscle, surrounding the mucosa, is not circular but is in the form of a right and a left spiral of smooth muscle that extends up to the level of and into the alveolar ducts. This aids contraction and shortening, or dilatation and lengthening. A loose fibrous tissue sheath surrounds the muscle and allows the bronchial lengths and diameters to alter without affecting tensions in the neighboring alveoli. The hyaline cartilage plates extend, in diminishing size, into the small bronchi.

In large bronchi, the entire circumference is supported by cartilage, whereas in small bronchi, this support is only partial, so that chance section may include no cartilage. Hence, large bronchi have rigidity and can stay patent if there is massive collapse of the lung, in which condition small bronchi also will collapse.

Bronchioles, originally defined as those passages with a diameter of 1 mm or less, are now considered to be those airways distal to the last plate of cartilage and having no mucous glands and few goblet cells. Thus, the mucosa, lined by cuboidal epithelium with few or no cilia, is surrounded by smooth muscle and scanty fibrous tissue. It is important to realize how poor is their ability to drain themselves. There are no glands to secrete and wash away impurities and no cilia to move surface material, but only the few lymphatics and the macrophages of the alveoli and connective tissue.

Investigations of an unusual type of cell described by von Hayek[11] subsequently was recognized as being one of two types of non-ciliated bronchiolar epithelial cells called Clara cells. Recognizable only by electron miscroscopy, it is possible that they may secrete surfactant.[5a, 8a, 13a, 17a]

At the end of the bronchiolar tree are the *terminal bronchioles,* the most peripheral bronchioles to have a complete epithelial lining. They come in a cluster of three or five from a final division, the preterminal bronchiole.

Terminal bronchioles give rise to *respiratory bronchioles* of similar caliber to their parent; the maintenance of the original diameter after branching serves to reduce the velocity of the air. Nevertheless, they differ in that a number of alveoli open directly into their muscular walls. In addition, some respiratory bronchioles follow a recurrent path, bringing them back and parallel to their parent terminal bronchiole, with which their alveoli communicate by a narrow channel (Fig. 23-1). This bronchiolar-alveolar anastomosis becomes an important bypass in the event of bronchiolar obstruction. Between the openings of the alveoli, the respiratory bronchiole still has cuboidal epithelium and smooth muscle, the latter surrounding the openings of the alveoli. A respiratory bronchiole will branch several times into further respiratory bronchioles.

The next division is into the *alveolar ducts.* These are elongated passageways that really do not have walls but only the framework of the continuous chain of alveoli opening from them. They therefore have no epithelial lining,

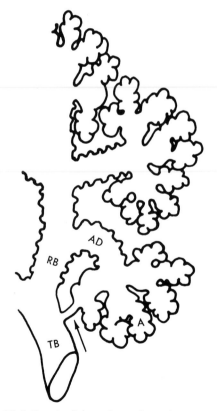

Fig. 23-1 Terminal branches of respiratory tree. **TB,** Terminal bronchiole. **RB,** First-order respiratory bronchiole. **AD,** Alveolar duct. **A,** Atrium with alveoli. Arrow points to bronchiolar-alveolar anastomosis.

but a ring of muscle surrounds the alveolar openings as in the respiratory bronchioles. The knobs of muscle are easily seen where the alveolar septa join the ducts.

Finally, from the alveolar ducts come about four air sacs or *atria*—structures in which muscle fibers end and the greatest number of *alveoli* are formed (Fig. 23-1).

The electron microscope has settled the controversy about *alveolar structure* (Fig. 23-2). It shows a continuous alveolar surface (septal) epithelium, providing a covering to the septal capillary network, only 0.2 μm* thick. This is the type I, or membranous pneumonocyte. It cannot be seen in ordinary sections, but occasional attenuated nuclei are visible (Fig. 23-30). These cells are extremely elastic to conform with respiration. Lying under the epithelium are the alveolar cells. Some drop off to be alveolar macrophages and are replaced by differentiation of alveolar septal fibroblasts.[6] Others, with large nucleus and granular cytoplasm, are thought to secrete pulmonary surfactant (dipalmitoyl lecithin).[9] These are the type II, or granular, pneumonocytes. Hardly recognizable under the light microscope, they are cuboidal with, as seen under the electron microscope, characteristic osmophilic lamellated bodies (Fig. 23-2) which, although associated with surfactant, have not been proved to produce it. In fact, some argue that these cells are phagocytic and that the bronchiolar Clara cells are the source of surfactant.[8a] A filmy surface layer of surfactant lipoprotein covers the alveoli. It helps the elastic recoil of the lung after expansion, and it maintains the alveoli open in expiration. Surfactant is needed throughout life and constantly needs to be replaced (it lasts about three days).[8] Morgan reviews the role played by loss of surfactant in many diseases, drowning, and surgery on the lung.[13a]

The alveolar epithelium has its own basement membrane, continuous with that of the bronchioles, separated from that of the capillaries by an important tissue space containing reticulin and elastic fibers. A thickness of 0.5 μm to 2.5 μm has to be traversed by the respiratory gases.

Preparations of the alveolar septal capillary network indicate that the vessels branch so much that they almost touch each other. An

*In this chapter, the new nomenclature for a unit of length, micrometer (μm), is used instead of the micron (μ).

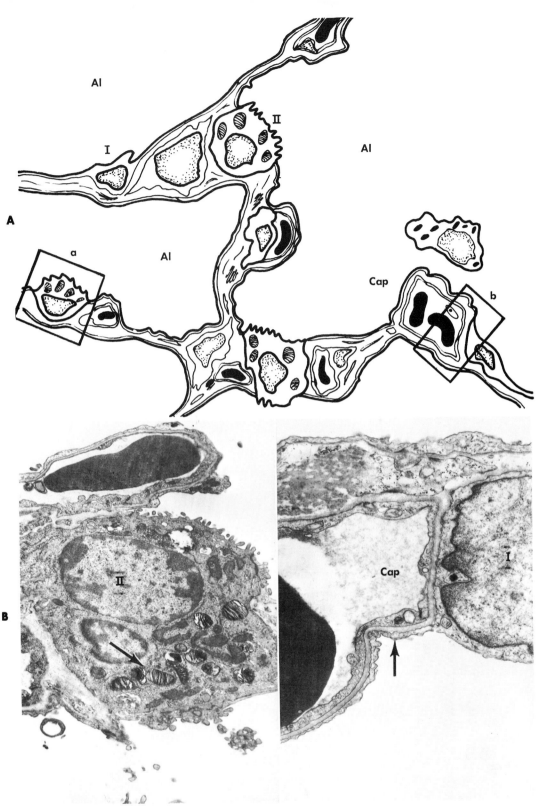

Fig. 23-2 A, Normal alveolar wall with type I and type II pneumonocytes. Wall includes capillaries **(Cap)**, fibroblasts, collagen, and elastin. Macrophage may be seen free in alveolar space, **Al,** to right. **B,** Type II pneumonocyte as seen at **a** in **A.** Cell has few irregular processes on its free alveolar edge and lamellated bodies (arrow) in its cytoplasm. **C,** Blood-gas barrier, as seen at **b** in **A,** includes epithelial cell and endothelial cell. To right is nucleus of type I cell with thin cytoplasmic flange (at arrow) covering capillary and separated from endothelial cell by their respective basement membranes. Above, space between endothelium and epithelium is wider, since it includes collagen and elastin. (**B,** ×7500; **C,** ×11,000; **A** to **C,** courtesy Miss Barbara Meyrick.)

elastic and reticular fiber network supports them. In it are mesenchymal cells and phagocytes. The interalveolar septa have numerous pores of Kohn, 10 μm in diameter, which allow free intercommunication between alveoli —even those from different alveolar ducts or lobules. These are seen easily in organizing pneumonia, when young fibrous tissue grows through them, linking solidified alveoli (Fig. 23-34). Otherwise, the pores become an effective bypass if a bronchiole is blocked.

Functional units. Although the concept of the *lobule* as a functional unit is no longer favored, it will be defined so that the reader can understand older writings. The primary lobule, the respiratory tissue arising from one alveolar duct, has been abandoned as a unit because it is too small. "Lobule" is now synonymous with the secondary lobule. The latter is much larger and refers to the lung supplied by the three to five terminal bronchioles arising from a preterminal bronchiole.

Most practical of all is the concept of the *acinus,* which is the lung distal to one terminal bronchiole. It is a readily visible unit on the cut surface of a lung perfused with formalin. One lobule is composed of three to five acini. Acini are most easily recognized when black dust is deposited around their central bronchiole (Fig. 23-32). Near the sharp margins of the lungs, septa run a short way in from the pleura, often demarcating the sides of acini. These septa are inconstant and unreliable markers. Even where they are absent (which is the case farther within the lung), a more trustworthy lateral boundary to the acinus can be found—a thin line, which is the acinar vein, a vessel which is always here, never in the center where the bronchiole and artery run.

One tends to assume that the whole lung is in uniform action at all times. Contrary evidence has been presented by Towers[16] that there are functional units that roughly correspond to present-day lobules and which he calls "pneumons" (a poor choice, since this is the Greek word for "lung"). Reserve pneumons are brought into use when needed by relaxation of bronchiolar and alveolar duct muscle.

Supporting structures. Although ordinary microscopic sections do not reveal the mechanism, the lung remains expanded as atmospheric pressure stretches the supporting pulmonary framework of closely linked collagenous and elastic fibers.[12] Reticular fibers have a lesser function in this respect. When air enters the pleural cavity, the intrapulmonary and extrapulmonary pressures become equal, and the collagenous and elastic fibers pull the lung close to its root (collapse).

The collagenous and elastic fibers encircle and support the openings of all alveoli, just as they support the terminal air passages. They run from one alveolar duct to another, sending branch filaments to neighboring alveoli and vessels. Other fibers originate in vessel walls and then run out to alveoli. In this way, all the passages and vessels are linked to neighboring structures, allowing changing tensions to be spread evenly throughout. In routine sections, the elastic fibers are best demonstrated in the tips of the interalveolar septa, where the alveoli open into the air passages. When the collagenous and elastic fibers are fragmented by disease, the reticular fibers maintain the integrity of the alveolar capillary network.

The interlobular connective tissue septa in the adult lung are mostly concentrated in the subpleural zone, particularly at the sharp edges and angles of the lungs.[14, 15] They are relatively scarce over the costal surfaces and absent over the fissural surface and in the deeper parts of the lung. It is fundamental to the operation of collateral air drift in the human lung that these septa are incomplete, not enclosing lobules. The mosaic pattern of subpleural lymphatics bears no constant relationship to the septa, although the two may overlap.[15]

Fetal and neonatal lung. In utero, the lung contains much fluid, but otherwise the alveolar surfaces are generally apposed. Introduction of air by the first breath requires relatively great force to overcome the surface tension in the bronchioles and alveoli and also to move away the fluid.[5] Once the first airways open, their original surface tensions fall, and they tend to stay open. The next breath will open air spaces farther out in the lung and so on in a series (the "pop-pop-pop" mechanism).

From the beginning of their development, the lungs are covered by pleura. In the five-week fetus, the two main bronchi grow out from the trachea, which is, in turn, a bud off the foregut. They subdivide (Fig. 23-3) until, by the sixteenth week, all the airways down to the ends of the terminal bronchioles are created, and no more will be formed. Interlobar septa form very early. A lung in this *"glandular"* or *"bronchial" phase* is recognized by the cuboidal cells lining the airways, which

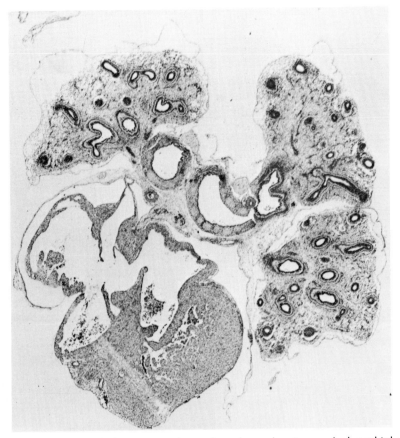

Fig. 23-3 Heart and both lungs in eight-week embryo showing early bronchial tree in undeveloped mesenchyme. (×24.)

are surrounded by mesenchyme. Pulmonary arteries are now in position. The *"canalicular" phase* occupies the sixteenth to twenty-fourth weeks. Rapid proliferation of capillaries between groups of epithelial cells of the air passages converts the epithelium into channels, on the surface of which lie networks of capillaries. A hasty glance at the lungs of a fetus of this age might lead one to believe that these are primitive vascular alveoli lined by cuboidal cells. During this phase, the formation of surfactant commences, and attenuation of the epithelium of the channels begins, allowing the blood to approach closer to the alveolar lumen. Extrauterine life cannot be maintained prior to these events. While this vital opening of the distal airways is proceeding, the mesenchyme is contributing the bronchial cartilage and elastic and collagen fibers.

Not until the twenty-fourth week does the *"alveolar" phase* begin. Fetal alveoli are very shallow evaginations of the primitive bronchiolar walls. Boyden's important wax reconstructions have shown that, from now on, functional lung tissue grows centripetally by the conversion of peripheral terminal bronchioles into respiratory bronchioles.[7] No further airways develop after the sixteenth week.

At birth the full-term infant has twenty million alveoli. They are so small that they barely resemble normal adult alveoli, which are formed only after birth. Boyden prefers to call them saccules.[7] The number increases (with the growth of the thorax) to the adult total of three hundred million by the eighth year, after which they further increase in size.[1] The original plump alveolar lining cell of the alveolar phase very slowly becomes attenuated. Even in an infant, many of them remain visible. Alveolar septa of a newborn infant are thick-walled structures because of the prominent capillaries.

Throughout fetal life, the lower respiratory tract produces a highly complex lung fluid that is held under pressure during later fetal life by sphincterlike contraction of the laryngeal muscles. The resultant positive pressure is considered to be a factor in the expansion and growth of the lung. From time to time, the larynx relaxes and some fluid is released, to be promptly swallowed. Paralysis of the laryngeal muscles by damage to the vagus will be followed by atelectasis, a condition also found when there is a wide tracheo-esophageal fistula.[16]

As the fetus grows older, the amount of phospholipid in the lung fluid increases. The fluid in the upper trachea and larynx is mainly a highly viscous mucus, secreted locally by glands. It seems probable that this must be squeezed out of the infant (i.e., by vaginal delivery) rather than inspired. Absence of squeezing, as in cesarean section, may explain why babies delivered in this fashion are more prone to respiratory distress.[16] So it seems that the fetal lung functions like an exocrine gland, secreting fluid and the surface-tension-lowering lipoprotein, and that the bronchioles act as the excretory ducts. At birth, the fluid is removed via pulmonary vascular and lymphatic channels.

The viable fetus (i.e., over 1,000 gm) is able to remain alive without true alveoli because the bronchiolar capillaries are so well developed as to be able themselves to permit gaseous exchange.

Pulmonary blood and lymphatic vessels. The ultimate destination of the pulmonary arteries is the capillary network of the interalveolar septa. The return is into the *pulmonary venous system,* which also picks up blood from the bronchial arterial flow and from veins originating from larger bronchi. Other bronchial veins drain the pleural surfaces and the largest bronchi, entering the azygos vein on the right and the hemiazygos or innominate vein on the left.

In the adult, the ill-defined adventitia being omitted from the measurement, elastic *arteries* are said to have an external diameter greater than 1 mm, smaller vessels being muscular arteries. In turn, the transition between these and arterioles is at 0.1 mm.

Orthodox for many years, the foregoing concept is inaccurate because it is based on lungs in which the arteries have not been standardized by injection to their true size.[1] Reid's careful investigations should be consulted to gain understanding of the mechanisms of the pulmonary arterial system.[1] Pulmonary arteries have an internal and an external elastic lamina, whereas in bronchial arteries only the internal elastica is well developed. Even more noticeable in bronchial arteries is an additional muscular layer in the intima, the fibers appearing longitudinal, although most of them follow a spiral course.

It is difficult to tell an arteriole from a venule (unless the former can be traced to an artery), because neither vessel normally has any muscle. In other words, pulmonary arterioles are really precapillaries and do not resemble arterioles of other organs.[17]

At the moment of birth, the full-term infant has pulmonary arteries with thick-walled and muscular small branches. This creates a narrow lumen to cut down the pulmonary blood flow, for which there is little need in utero. Within a few days, the walls become thin, and, before the end of a year, they are of adult type. The elastic arteries are recognized in the lung of the newborn infant by the loose layers of connective tissue that surround them as well as by their predominantly elastic media.

The *bronchial arteries* exist to nourish the bronchi, in whose walls they ramify as far as the terminal bronchioles. Normally, they do not have significant anastomoses with pulmonary arterial branches but can be an important source of collateral circulation when the pulmonary arterial circulation is blocked or in emphysema or diffuse fibrosis.

The *lymphatic vascular system* provides a pleural plexus of capillaries that may outline the lobules. The pleural plexus drains to the hilar lymph nodes but also communicates with the pulmonary lymph vessels, which begin at the respiratory bronchioles.[13] These drain the tissue spaces of the interalveolar septa and the bronchial and vascular trees into the hilar lymph nodes. From here, drainage is to tracheobronchial nodes and eventually to the right lymphatic duct and, on the left, to the thoracic duct. Some lymph also passes to scalene and retroperitoneal lymph nodes.

Lymphoid nodules occur at the bifurcation of bronchi, as far down as the respiratory bronchioles, so that collections of lymphocytes in the muscle coat are not necessarily proof of the presence of chronic inflammation.

CONGENITAL ANOMALIES

Total absence of lungs may occur in anencephalic monsters. Unilateral *atresia,* the absence of a lung, does not endanger life, but serious malformations often accompany it.[28] Usually, there is no trace of the missing lung's bronchus or vessels. Sometimes one lobe or a whole lung is *hypoplastic.* This may be primary or be secondary to the pressure of a large tumor or cyst or to abdominal organs entering the thorax. *Potter's syndrome* is deformity of the ears, widely set eyes, prominent epicanthic fold, receding chin, and pulmonary hypoplasia accompanying severe renal hypoplasia or cystic disease.

It is not uncommon to find an *excessive or diminished number of pulmonary lobes* in the absence of any functional effect. An *accessory lobe* (which may become infected) is an independent pulmonary structure, invested by its own pleura and supplied by an accessory bronchus. The *azygos lobe* is produced by a low-arching azygos vein pulling down into the right apex, rendering it bifid because the vein drags down with it a fold of pleura.

Bronchopulmonary sequestration

A sequestered pulmonary segment is one totally or partly separated from the normal lung. More often it is intralobar, meaning within a pulmonary lobe, but there is an extralobar variety.

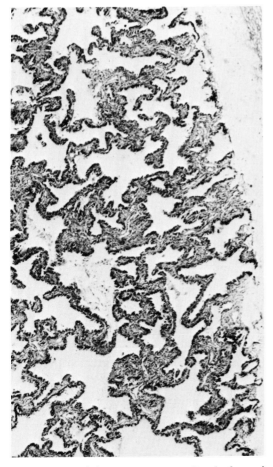

Fig. 23-4 Extralobar sequestration. Poorly formed distal pulmonary tissue under its pleura. No recognizable bronchioles. (×56.)

Intralobar sequestration. Intralobar sequestration is observed in young adults in whom a large mass is found, generally in the left lower lobe. There is no communication with the bronchial tree, and blood is supplied from a large artery from the aorta, arising just above or below the diaphragm.[17] Venous return is pulmonary. As Borrie et al.[21] report, the mass turns out to be a single large cyst, a cluster of small ones in firm fibrotic lung, or mainly solid lung tissue with abscesses.[21] In the cysts is pus or viscid material. Infection can be severe enough to spread to the pleura.

Extralobar sequestration. At first glance, extralobar sequestration is merely an accessory lobe but nearly always is basal and left-sided and shows no communication with the bronchial tree. It has a variable blood supply from the aorta, and its veins drain to the azygos system. Unlike the intralobar variety, it is covered by its own pleura (Fig. 23-4), and often is found in infancy.

Sequestration communicating with eosphagus or stomach. On rare occasions, a sequestration of either type is served by a bronchus growing directly out of the midesophagus, lower esophagus, or gastric fundus.[24] This gives us an important clue to the possibility that sequestrations are closely related to one another and to accessory bronchopulmonary tissues, all of which may well be termed bronchopulmonary-foregut malformations.

Cystic disease

Pulmonary cysts in older children and adults frequently are so altered by inflammation and fibrosis that forms of bronchial distention distal to an occlusion, bronchiectasis, or honeycomb lungs cannot be distinguished from congenital cysts by any combination of clinical findings and microscopy. Findings in favor of cystic bronchiectasis are as follows:

1 Situation in a lower lobe
2 Earlier stages of bronchiectasis in other bronchi
3 Easy demonstration of a bronchus directly entering the cavity

Bronchogenic (bronchial) cyst. Close to the hilum, there may arise a tracheobronchogenous cyst, attached to the trachea near the bifurcation or to a main bronchus. This is really an accessory bronchial bud, although it rarely communicates with the lumen. It is a unilocular sphere containing watery fluid and having an attenuated wall of bronchial type, including surface epithelium, glands, muscle, and cartilage (which causes trabecula-tion of the lining). Such a cyst, if detached from its parent bronchus, appears as a mediastinal bronchogenic cyst. Other cysts, in exactly the same position, are found to be enterogenous—cysts of foregut origin lined by gastric or intestinal epithelium. Some bronchial cysts are paraesophageal or even within the esophageal wall.

A solitary bronchial cyst within the lung has a very similar appearance. Infection may convert its fluid content into an abscess.

Multiple cysts. Small cysts up to 1 cm in diameter may be clustered in the peripheral portions of one or more lobes. They are congenital anomalies of the more distal bronchi, and hence their linings are simpler than those of bronchogenic cysts. The lining of these peripheral cysts is of columnar cells, sometimes ciliated, covering elastic and fibrous connective tissue with a little muscle. The cysts may or may not communicate with bronchi or with each other. Those entering a bronchus are originally filled with air. The blind ones contain fluid. When a lung is anthracotic, a region associated with an atretic or long-stenosed bronchus can be recognized by its lack of pigment.

There is the possibility that some of these peripheral cysts are derivatives of the visceral pleura.[29] Folds of the latter may dip into clefts in the lung in the region of interlobular septa and, becoming separated, form into cysts. Possibly, too, pouches of mesothelium are nipped off between growing lung buds. In either case, the cyst lining resembles the structure of the pleura. There will be no muscle coat.

Multiple lung cysts may be present in patients with Marfan's syndrome or tuberous sclerosis.

Congenital cystic adenomatoid malformation. A rare form of diffuse hamartoma found in the newborn infant (especially the premature infant), congenital cystic adenomatoid malformation endangers life.[18] Generally confined to one lobe, it can be diagnosed radiographically by the presence of an enlarged lung with a mass containing cystic cavities. *Grossly,* the lobe, which requires surgical removal, is so large that it displaces the mediastinum, partly compresses normal lung, and interferes with the hemodynamics of the heart (Fig. 23-5). Cysts of up to 2 cm or 3 cm bulge under the pleura and are found on the cut surface. They have one or more cavities containing air, since they communicate with the bronchial tree, but there is not a

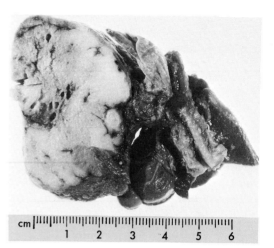

Fig. 23-5 Diffuse hamartoma (congenital cystic adenomatoid malformation of lung). Most of right lung replaced by firm white tissue containing tiny cysts. Left lung compressed and partly hidden by turned-down trachea.

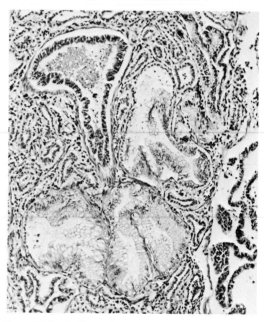

Fig. 23-6 Diffuse hamartoma. Mucinous and cuboidal epithelium are present. (×165.)

normal bronchial system. Around them is collapsed and indurated white lung.

Microscopically, the cysts and the remnants of the alveoli have two possible linings. One is a bronchial type (without underlying cartilage) sometimes thrown into a polypoid configuration—hence the name "adenomatoid." The second is a tall columnar cell with a small basal nucleus and a bounteous cytoplasm full of mucin. Around the epithelium

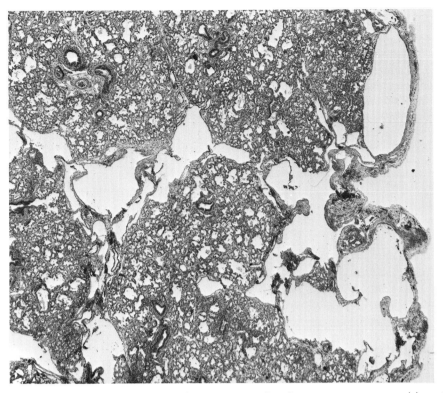

Fig. 23-7 Congenital pulmonary lymphangiectasis. Dilated spaces are not around bronchi and arteries, thereby distinguishing condition from interstitial emphysema. (×21.)

is a thin layer of connective tissue and smooth muscle (Fig. 23-6). Inflammation is not a primary feature of the condition but may complicate it.

Congenital pulmonary lymphangiectasis. A cystic disease, congenital pulmonary lymphangiectasis is due to a bilateral, diffuse but irregular, dilatation of pulmonary lymphatic vessels and is found only in the newborn infant. These vessels, mainly under the pleura and in the interlobular septa, are distended with clear fluid to a diameter of several millimeters (Fig. 23-7). The cysts are lined by an endothelium resting on a little fibrous tissue.[27]

The fully developed condition is incompatible with life. A number of the cases have been associated with malformations of the left side of the heart.[31] Some investigators consider the disease to be analagous to lymphangiomatosis elsewhere in the body.

Vascular anomalies

Arterial anomalies. The main pulmonary trunk or its right or left branch may be lacking, in which case the arterial supply is from a patent ductus, with contributions from the bronchial arteries and accessory branches.

Congenital stenosis of the pulmonary artery branches may be single or multiple, local or diffuse. There is right ventricular hypertrophy, and one can easily see dilatation distal to each arterial narrowing.[23]

Venous anomalies. There may be a totally *anomalous venous drainage* of the lungs in that the four main veins converge behind the left atrium. They form a chamber of their own (cor triatriatum). From it emerges a single vein that runs into the left innominate vein, the coronary sinus, the right atrium, the inferior vena cava below the diaphragm, or the portal vein. Patients with such anomalies are cyanotic, but those in whom some of the veins drain normally can be quite asymptomatic. When drainage is totally anomalous, 75% of infants will die or require operation before their first birthday.[20]

An anomaly well known to radiologists is the "scimitar sign." A broad, curving paracardiac shadow is produced by abnormal right pulmonary venous drainage into the inferior vena cava at or below the diaphragm. Symptoms produced by this partial shunt from the left to the right side of the heart depend on the amount of blood involved. Some time after this condition was first described, it was realized that two other ab-normalities accompany it—a hyparterial right upper lobe bronchus (the right tracheobron-chial tree is a mirror image of the left) and systemic pulmonary arteries to the right lung. Accordingly, we now speak of the *scimitar syndrome.*[26] Conditions associated with this are bronchiectasis, anomalous right hemidia-phragm, atrial or ventricular septal defects, patent ductus arteriosus, aortic coarctation, and arteriovenous anomalies of the right lung.

One or more of the pulmonary veins may be *stenotic.*[25]

Arteriovenous fistula (aneurysm). Arterio-venous fistula is a tumorlike malformation that enlarges over the years. Many of the pa-tients have hereditary hemorrhagic telangiec-tasia. Multiple lesions are more common than single ones, and the usual site is immediately beneath the pleura (Fig. 23-8). Each lesion is an interweaving complex of arteries and very thin-walled veins, with one large vessel entering and one leaving. This abnormal com-munication is usually between a pulmonary arterial branch and a vein (occasionally a bronchial or an intercostal artery). If the shunt is large enough, the patient is polycy-

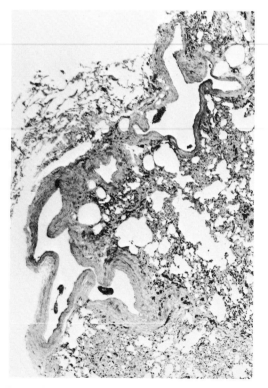

Fig. 23-8 Arteriovenous fistula. Large, misshapen, thick-walled vessels run aimlessly just below pleura. (×24.)

themic and cyanotic. Fatal rupture may occur into the lung or pleural space.

ACQUIRED VASCULAR DISEASE
Acquired arteriovenous fistula

Some patients with cirrhosis (portal or due to schistosomiasis) have a decrease in arterial oxygen saturation. A smaller number are cy-anotic and have clubbed fingers. This is due to the development of multiple, tiny, arterio-venous anastomoses in the lung.[35] If the pul-monary vessels are specially injected, many more such cases of pulmonary spider nevi will be uncovered, and it is speculated that they result from the same mechanism that pro-duces them in the skin.

Hyperemia and congestion

Active hyperemia. Active hyperemia is the result of an acute infective condition of the lung or of the presence of a gaseous, liquid, or particulate irritant. The term implies active dilatation of pulmonary vessels, and hence edema is likely to appear soon after, marked microscopically by the presence of fibrin strands and leukoctyes.

Passive hyperemia. Passive hyperemia is usually called *congestion,* the result of left-sided heart failure, which interferes with pul-monary venous drainage. The lungs are dark blue and heavy, with diminished air con-tent. Edema is a frequent sequela that is evident from the bloody, frothy fluid that pours from the cut surface. This occurs be-cause the alveolar capillaries are not only overdistended, but also because they suffer from hypoxia and increased pressure, which promote escape of fluid across the vascular endothelium. The normal resorptive powers of the alveoli are overwhelmed.

Initially, a pale eosinophilic amorphous or granular material is seen in the alveoli, with erythrocytes and macrophages. The inter-alveolar septa are widened by the prominent, hitherto inconspicuous, capillaries. Edematous thickening of the interlobular septa is ap-parent, and the lymph channels within them and around vessels and bronchi are dilated. Veins in the walls of the bronchi also are congested.

Chronic passive congestion. In chronic pas-sive congestion, seen classically in mitral steno-sis, the lungs are firmer and drier, with a faint brown tinge (brown induration). The larger vessels seen on the cut surface are wider and thicker than usual. The alveoli con-tain many macrophages stuffed with brown hemosiderin granules (heart failure cells) (Fig. 23-9). Tortuous alveolar capillaries are expanded to the width of several red cells, and the interalveolar septa undergo fibrosis. When this has developed, the alveolar surface cells become much more prominent. Fibrosis also thickens the interlobular septa and the perivascular and peribronchial tissues and ultimately may obliterate alveolar capillaries. In the most severe instances, the alveolar material becomes ossified, neighboring areas combining to form particles of bone several millimeters in diameter, large enough to be recognized radiographically (Fig. 23-50).

The microscopic changes include medial and intimal thickening of the small muscular pulmonary arteries. Uncommonly, there is necrotizing arteritis.[38]

Iron in alveolar macrophages may not necessarily be the result of bleeding into the lung. As the cells take up plasma protein in edema fluid, this will include acid mucopolysaccharide. The latter has the property of impregnating the mucin with iron, presumably from plasma transferrin.[36]

Simple brown induration should be differentiated from three conditions. The first is *idiopathic pulmonary hemosiderosis.* Nearly all the patients have been male children. Repeated sudden attacks of intra-alveolar bleeding cause severe anemia with dyspnea and jaundice. Death ensues after a few years.

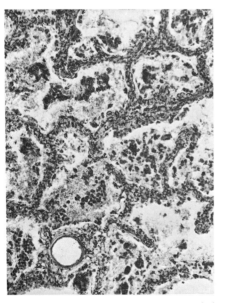

Fig. 23-9 Chronic passive congestion of lung. Alveolar septa are thickened because they are hypervascular. Alveoli contain pigment-laden macrophages and protein.

The changes in the lungs resemble those of severe brown induration, and the hilar nodes also are brown. In the bleeding phase, the alveoli are filled with fresh blood with a marked phagocytic reaction. Dilated capillaries may appear to be devoid of covering alveolar epithelium. Later, macrophages carry hemosiderin to the interalveolar septa, which become fibrotic, and to the interlobular, subpleural, peribronchial, and perivascular connective tissues. In all of these sites, nodular fibrosis forms in reaction to the hemosiderin. The elastic fibers in the alveolar septa, pulmonary stroma, and small and medium-sized pulmonary arteries are hemosiderin-encrusted. The vascular elastica may be degenerate. The alveolar surface cells are crowded, swollen, and occasionally multinucleated. Soergel and Sommers[37] have collected a total of about 100 reported cases. A total of nearly fifty cases in adults has been published. Attempts to understand the disease by electron microscopic examination of lung biopsies have produced conflicting findings.[34a] Alveolar capillary endothelium is swollen, and there are dense protein deposits on the underlying basement membrane.

The second disease to be distinguished from simple brown induration is *Goodpasture's syndrome.* This is a lethal combination of an initial disease closely resembling (both clinically and pathologically) idiopathic pulmonary hemosiderosis but soon followed by a severe proliferative glomerulonephritis. Some have suggested the designation *lung purpura with glomerulonephritis,* especially since Goodpasture did not recognize the syndrome named for him. Immunofluorescence investigations of the patients indicate that their alveoli and glomeruli share some common antigens to which antibodies are formed, creating pulmonary and renal lesions in which immunoglobulins can be detected.[34] Perhaps the kidney is the source of the immunizing agent, especially since bilateral nephrectomy followed by renal homotransplantation appears to cure the disease.[36a]

A third, rare, condition to be distinguished from brown induration is *mechanical obstruction of the pulmonary veins,* in which an interstitial (septal) pulmonary fibrosis develops, with some deposition of hemosiderin.[33]

Hypostatic congestion. Hypostatic congestion is a gravitational congestion and edema of the lungs in persons with weakening cardiac and respiratory action. Such areas are ideal breeding grounds for bacteria, which bring about hypostatic bronchopneumonia in the immobile patient.

Massive pulmonary hemorrhage in newborn infants

Infants thought clinically to have died from hyaline membrane disease sometimes are found to have massive hemorrhage into the whole of two or more lobes. Most die by the end of their second postnatal day. Many resemblances are noted to hyaline membrane disease both in the patients at risk and in the course of the disease, but the condition also occurs in stillborn infants and may cause respiratory distress from the moment of birth. Massive hemorrhage and hyaline membrane disease often coexist. Avery[5] cannot explain the bleeding and notes that there is no specific treatment. Adamson et al.,[32] having analyzed the bloody fluid aspirated from the trachea of two living infants, believe that the condition is really one of hemorrhagic pulmonary edema.

Edema and shock

Pulmonary edema, alone or with minimal congestion, is caused by administration of too much intravenous fluid, by conditions of increased intracranial pressure (via a reflex pathway), or by exposure to chemical or physical irritants (including irradiation, p. 258) or may occur in fulminating bacterial or viral infection, anaphylactic shock, and angioneurotic edema. Severe acute pulmonary edema may develop in unacclimatized persons who ascend to an altitude of 10,000 ft or more. Two young men who were natives of the mountains were reported to have died after returning from a visit of a month or two to lower altitudes.[39]

The lungs are large, pallid and wet, pit on finger pressure, and pour out copious frothy fluid when cut. When associated with fatal intracranial conditions, edema frequently is confined to one or both upper lobes.[40] Microscopically, the alveolar vessels are inconspicuous, and the interlobular septa, air spaces, and bronchi are filled by the pale-staining, protein-containing fluid (Fig. 23-10).

The two high-altitude victims mentioned previously also had hyaline membranes, thrombosis of the precapillaries, and wide dilatation of the pulmonary venous system, including the capillaries. It would be important to know if they had a hemoglobinopathy, but, as has been pointed out,[42] most of the patients have been accustomed previously to high altitude. The obscure mechanism is considered by Friedberg[43a] to revolve around increased pressure or permeability (or both) of the pulmonary capillaries.

Radiologists recognize edema by the appearance of Kerley's lines, which are produced by edema of various interlobular septa and distended lymphatics within them.

Acute pulmonary edema. Acute pulmonary edema[40] has manifold causes. It is particularly likely to involve the pulmonary medulla.[43] As much as 2 or 3 liters of foamy fluid can appear within one or two hours and a fulminating variety can be fatal in ten or twenty minutes. Among the causes are myocardial infarction, pulmonary embolism, mitral stenosis, and disorders of cardiac rhythm. One must also consider the *shock-lung syndrome* seen in patients treated for prolonged shock who die of acute respiratory insufficiency one to several days following recovery from the shock.[44] Microscopically, not only are there the changes of pulmonary edema, but also widespread intravascular thrombosis affecting the capillaries.[42a] Bacterial toxic shock is another cause of these changes.[40] A cause of fulminating, often fatal and still unexplained, pulmonary edema is heroin overdosage.[46]

Fibrinous pulmonary edema. In the past, attempts have been made to distinguish at least two types of fibrinous pulmonary edema—that occurring in uremia ("uremic lung or pneumonitis") and that occurring in acute rheumatic fever ("rheumatic lung or pneumonitis"). For years, radiologists have

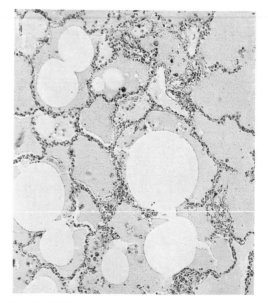

Fig. 23-10 Pulmonary edema.

recognized the butterfly or bat's wing hilar shadows produced by the protein-rich fluid that is concentrated around the roots (medullae) of both lungs. Uremia is one of the commonest causes and may produce the radiologic picture in a few days. Chronic left ventricular failure in essential hypertension is another important cause.[45]

The lung is dark purple, with a very soft, rubbery consistency. The edema fluid gives the lung around the hilum, particularly the lower lobes, an increase in consistency. Because it is so rich in fibrin, the cut surface is wet and glassy.[41] "Solid edema" had been observed by pathologists for years prior to this distinction.

The fluid does not pour away easily because of the coagulation of the fibrin; firm pressure will release the fluid.

What damages the capillary walls so as to allow fibrinogen to pass through is not known. There is evidence that in conditions of anoxia or increased pulmonary venous pressure, the blood flow is much diminished in the outer parts of the lungs, thereby encouraging the central distribution of the uremic change. This is merely a manifestation of the division of the normal lung into two zones: (1) medulla, comprising large bronchi and vessels

and the lobules in the angles of their bifurcations and (2) cortex, the outer third, composed of most of the alveoli and of the small bronchi and vessels.[43]

Microscopically, the difference between the uremic lung and ordinary edema is the greater eosinophilia of the alveolar fluid in the former. Moreover, a hyaline membrane is very common. The fluid also will be found in the alveolar ducts, and edema of the interlobular septa will be noticed. Any cellular infiltrate is scanty—mostly neutrophilic (Fig. 23-11). Given chronicity, it is possible for the fibrin to undergo organization in both alveoli and bronchioles (Fig. 23-12). These changes are not specific for uremia but can be seen in any case of high-protein edema, especially in left ventricular failure.[45] Undoubtedly in the past, the changes have been confused with organizing pneumonia. The young fibrous tissue contains hemosiderin macrophages and may be covered by proliferating alveolar epithelium, which also grows over the alveolar septa.

A similar condition has been observed in patients given antihypertensive drugs such as

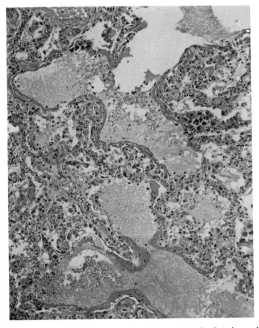

Fig. 23-11 Lung in uremia. Protein-rich fluid and erythrocytes fill alveoli, and hyaline membranes line septa, which are edematous and contain some macrophages. (×115.)

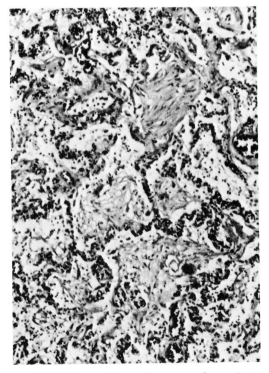

Fig. 23-12 Organizing pulmonary edema. Intra-alveolar fibrin with some erythrocytes is being organized into solid masses by young fibroblasts. No inflammatory reaction is present. Dark cells in alveolar capillaries are erythrocytes. (×24.)

hexamethonium, if the drugs prolong life. Chronic pulmonary edema appears, with proliferation of alveolar surface cells and, sometimes, hyaline membranes. Finally, there is fibrosis of the interalveolar septa and the alveoli without inflammatory reaction. The patients develop dyspnea and may die of respiratory failure.

Postperfusion lung syndrome is a term applied to a form of severe respiratory insufficiency occurring in some patients undergoing operations in which cardiopulmonary bypass is used. There are no characteristic naked-eye changes, but microscopically there is marked pulmonary edema, with much fibrin and hyaline membranes, and perivascular and alveolar hemorrhage.[48a] The cause is unknown, but one is struck by the resemblance to oxygen toxicity, shock-lung, and fibrinous edema.

Lung in rheumatic fever. Grossly and microscopically, the lung in rheumatic fever has the picture of pulmonary edema plus hemorrhagic areas. Added to this are many large mononuclear cells, both septal and intra-alveolar, which may compress the alveolar capillaries. Hemorrhage into alveoli is common, and rarely there is fibrinoid necrosis of the capillaries. Small pulmonary arteries may contain thrombi and show fibrinoid mural changes. Aschoff bodies do not appear, but perivascular lymphocytes, histiocytes, and fibroblasts can be observed. Proliferation of the septal cells creates multinucleated giant cells.

Finally, there is organization of the alveolar exudate and septal fibrosis. Moolten[47] has described eighty-eight of 166 cases of rheumatic heart disease in which autopsy disclosed interstitial fibrosis of the lung. A number of these cases could be shown not to be due to chronic passive congestion but to "rheumatic pneumonia."

Thromboembolism and infarction

General remarks on the nature of thrombi, emboli, and pulmonary infarctions will be found in Chapter 4.

Incidence. Pulmonary embolism has been found in up to 25% of autopsies performed in general hospitals. Embolism is not synonymous with infarction, which is seen in about half the cases. The majority of the patients are on the medical (particularly cardiac) rather than surgical wards and are at least 40 years of age. The noncardiac medical patients are likely to have pleural effusions, pneumonia, or other lung disease. Pulmonary embolism may be a cause of unexpected death in supposedly normal persons.[49, 52, 56a] Phlebothrombosis may be demonstrated in such patients. About 150 cases have been reported in children. There is also an association with childbirth, obesity, severe trauma, and thrombophlebitis (including that due to intravenous therapy).

The risk of venous thrombosis is increased fourfold in women taking contraceptive pills. Persons with carcinoma, (for some reason, most commonly of the stomach and pancreas) have an unexplained tendency to venous (even arterial) thrombosis. Some have noted what they call pulmonary microembolism as a cause of morbidity and death after major vascular surgery; what they consider to be fibrin emboli in the lung are, in fact, a manifestation of the shock-lung syndrome (p. 886).

Sites of origin. The sites of origin of thrombi are the deep or superficial veins of the lower limb, the iliac, prostatic, or utero-ovarian veins, and the right side of the heart (atrial fibrillation, or endocardial damage by myocardial infarction). Frequently, search for the origin is in vain because the embolus is the whole thrombus. Less common sources are the mesenteric-portal veins and those of the neck and arms.

Gross appearance of embolus. A thrombus more than a few days old is readily distinguished from a postmortem clot. The latter is soft, moist, and red, with perhaps sedimentation into a dark lower layer of cells and an upper yellow layer of plasma. The typical thrombus is much drier and paler, is brittle, and has on its surface parallel wavy thin lines of Zahn. If it has been in situ for a few days or more, it may be partly adherent to the arterial intima. A thrombus only a day old on arriving in the lung may be indistinguishable from a postmortem clot. It should be noted whether it has the shape of a systemic vein or bears imprints of its valves. Otherwise one can never be sure. Present criteria for diagnosis of antemortem thrombus (i.e., embolus) may be too narrow. A newly formed thrombus at the advancing head of an older one is loosely attached and so can break free.[51]

Obstructive effect. The largest emboli cannot pass the major pulmonary arteries unless they fragment, immediately or later. Smaller emboli also may block a major vessel or even the main bifurcation if they become coiled upon themselves. Obstruction of a main artery can be relieved by a change in shape of a soft, loose embolus. Smaller emboli most commonly travel to the vessels of the lower lobes.

Massive emboli in the main pulmonary trunk or straddling the bifurcation commonly cause death instantly or in ten to fifteen minutes. This is too quick for the vascular changes of infarction to supervene. The patients die in shock with acute right atrial dilatation that spreads to the right ventricle if the patient survives longer. Usually, marked bulging of the main pulmonary artery will be observed before it is opened. The lung may appear quite normal or may have suffered some collapse and edema. There is a good chance that it will show several small older infarcts, since multiple infarctions are so common.

Effect of embolism. Why patients with embolism die is not known. Some patients with large emboli have survived, the vessels having distended around almost completely occlusive thrombi.[55] The collateral circulation gives aid, and the patient may have few symptoms.[56] One must always consider the possibility that these were emboli that stimulated later thrombosis which extended retrogradely. Alternatively, they may simply be thrombi (p. 892).

Emboli that reach lobar or smaller arteries are those commonly causing infarction, but they may produce only "incipient infarction." In the latter condition, the territory of supply of the occluded vessel is congested by an inflow of blood from bronchial arteries in surrounding lung. The area is red and microscopically is edematous, with greatly congested alveolar capillaries. The tissues are not necrotic and presumably can recover.

Embolization to small pulmonary arteries (miliary emboli) can have profound physiologic effects. Innocuous at first sight, they may be fatal or build up a cor pulmonale as new showers of emboli fall. Their effect is aggravated by superimposed thrombosis. Why a series of small infarcts in congestive heart failure brings about death is not known. The matter is discussed by Gorham.[53] Pulmonary angiography has demonstrated that the affected area is well aerated but is not perfused with blood. It is possible that oxygen desaturation brought about by thromboembolism leads to vasoconstriction and increasing pulmonary hypertension.[50] Release of serotonin, fibrinopeptides, and kinins also is suspected of playing a part.

Appearance of infarct. The classic sterile infarct is a wedge-shaped area up to 5 cm in greatest dimension. Some infarcts are irregular or quadrilateral. The base of the infarct rests on the pleura, and often the blocked vessel

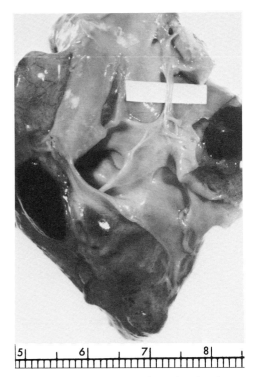

Fig. 23-13 Webs in major branch of pulmonary artery, which are residues of organized thrombi.

can be found on cutting into the lung just proximal to the apex of the infarct. After the first day, there is a covering fibrinous pleuritis, and the area bulges slightly. In addition, it is indurated and the cut surface is ill defined, moist, and dark purple. One or two days later, the pleural surface is depressed, and the cut surface is dry, granular, and pale red, becoming brown; the margins are sharp. Organization and retraction leave a well-concealed thin scar at right angles to the pleura, which may have undergone local thickening. The thrombus is organized into a fibrous band or net.[17] (Fig. 23-13).

Microscopically, intense alveolar capillary congestion and alveoli filled with blood are seen in the first twenty-four to forty-eight hours. After this time, the interalveolar septa undergo coagulative necrosis (Fig. 23-14), nuclear detail is lost, and the erythrocytes become pale discs. Their hemoglobin is converted into hemosiderin, taken up by phagocytes. During the second week, fibroblasts grow in from the periphery. Organization takes weeks or months, depending on how big the infarct is.

The microscopic structure of the embolus is described in Chapter 4.

Septic emboli produce infarcts in which suppuration and abscess formation commence

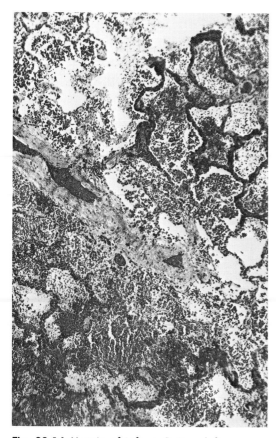

Fig. 23-14 Margin of infarct. Bottom left, masses of erythrocytes and extensive necrosis of intra-alveolar septa. Top right, earlier stage. Top left, congestion only. (×63.)

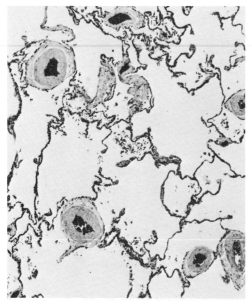

Fig. 23-15 Idiopathic pulmonary hypertension. Marked muscular thickening of minor pulmonary arteries. (×75.)

in the center. As the process spreads outward, the original similarity to a bland infarct is lost. Instead of a fibrinous pleurisy, there is a fibrinopurulent one.

Only the earlier infarcts will be recognized for what they are, both grossly and microscopically, because of the peripheral tissue necrosis and central suppuration.

The emboli are small, coming as they do from brittle fragments released from veins or cerebral sinuses with purulent thrombophlebitis or from bacterial endocarditis on the right side of the heart. Consequently the infarcts are not massive.

Noninfected cavitation can occur as a rarity in pulmonary infarcts larger than 4 cm in diameter.[54]

Nonthrombotic embolism

Embolism by fat globules, air, etc. is discussed in Chapter 4.

Pulmonary arteriosclerosis

Pulmonary arteriosclerosis, no matter how advanced, is never so severe as that in the aorta. The plaques are smooth and only slightly raised. Heaped-up or ulcerated deposits rarely are seen, but secondary thrombosis does occur. The condition may be merely due to old age, but it is also an accompaniment of pulmonary hypertension.

Primary (unexplained) pulmonary hypertension

Pulmonary hypertension of unknown cause is an uncommon condition. Pulmonary hypertension coexisting with Raynaud's phenomenon in patients suffering from a generalized "collagen-vascular" disease or disordered protein (cryoglobulin) should not be considered as primary.

Most patients have been young women, although even children have been affected. The principal complaint is worsening exertional dyspnea. Syncopal attacks and chest pain are experienced by about half of the patients. Right ventricular hypertrophy is marked, and the pulmonary arteriogram resembles a pruned leafless shrub in autumn instead of the normal leafy bush of springtime.[57] Death comes in a few years from right-sided heart failure, sometimes quite suddenly or after cardiac catheterization or angiocardiography.

The Wagenvoorts have been able to study the lung vessels in 156 clinically diagnosed cases, the largest series yet recorded.[59a]

The pulmonary arteries and their lobar branches are dilated and atherosclerotic. Under the microscope, the elastic arteries show some medial hypertrophy and intimal fibrosis (uniform, not eccentric). Intimal changes begin as a cellular proliferation narrowing or occluding the lumen of smaller pulmonary arteries. Later, fibrous tissue may appear, the intima becoming less and less cellular. Finally, the process may extend centrally to involve larger arteries. Functionally, the important changes are those in the muscular arteries. These undergo progressive medial hypertrophy until there is virtually no lumen (Fig. 23-15). The unusual finding of an outer longitudinal muscle coat is seen, and the elastic laminae are prominent. Accompanying this are three dilatation lesions[17]:

1 Dilatation causes thinning of some muscular arteries so that they resemble large veins.

2 Dilated thin vessels surround a parent muscular artery in an angiomatous fashion (angiomatoid lesion) and then join alveolar capillaries.

3 A dilatation filled with narrow tortuous vessels links its parent artery to thin wide vessels that join alveolar capillaries (plexiform lesion or glomus) (Fig. 23-16). Proximally, the parent small muscular pulmonary artery shows medial hypertrophy and intimal fibrosis. Then comes the dilated segment whose lumen is filled with the plexus of tortuous capillaries. Beyond this again, the blood enters the distal dilated artery. Plexiform lesions occur probably only in pulmonary hypertension due to congenital heart disease with a shunt, in pulmonary schistosomiasis, and in primary pulmonary hypertension.[59a]

Primary hypertension may be complicated by thrombosis in the affected vessels or by acute necrotizing, hypertensive arteritis. These complications also may be seen in forms of secondary hypertension, such as that of mitral stenosis.

Secondary pulmonary hypertension

The following outline, based on Wood's simple approach,* lists the principal causes of secondary pulmonary hypertension, most of which are discussed in the relevant sections of this book. All of these must be excluded be-

---

*Based on Wood, P.: Mod. Conc. Cardiovasc. Dis. 28:513-518, 1959.

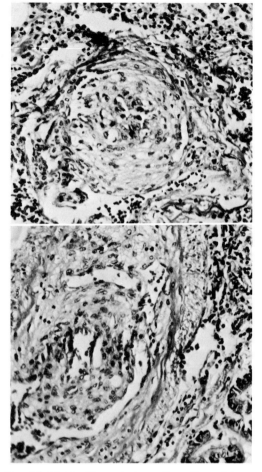

Fig. 23-16 Plexiform lesions. Complicated intertwining mass of tiny vessels with plump endothelial cells arises in relation to wall of larger pulmonary artery. (×196.)

fore the primary variety is diagnosed. There are four basic mechanisms, but, in general, the condition begins as pulmonary venous hypertension, which gives rise to vasoconstriction and induces pulmonary arterial hypertension.

1 Passive type—produced by diseases raising pulmonary venous pressure
  a Mitral stenosis
  b Chronic left ventricular failure (mostly in aortic stenosis, severe myocardial fibrosis, and essential hypertension)
  c Myxoma of left atrium
  d Ball valve thrombus, mitral orifice
  e Totally anomalous pulmonary venous drainage
2 Reactive or hyperkinetic type—produced by congenital heart defects that cause increased blood flow through pulmonary vasculature
  a Patent ductus arteriosus
  b Atrial or ventricular septal defect
  c Eisenmenger's complex

3 Vaso-occlusive type
  a Obstructive
    1 Multiple emboli or thrombosis
    2 Sickle cell disease
    3 Miliary carcinomatosis
    4 Polyarteritis nodosa
    5 Amniotic fluid embolism
    6 Schistosomiasis
    7 Congenital pulmonary artery stenosis
  b Vasoconstrictive—usually transient and related to hypoxia due to alveolar hypoventilation; also high altitude
  c Obliterative—due to reduction of vascular bed by chronic parenchymal disease
    1 Emphysema
    2 Advanced fibrosis, all types
    3 Pneumoconiosis
    4 Granulomatosis
4 Kyphoscoliosis—chest deformity which leads to hypoventilation, pulmonary hypertension, and cor pulmonale with hypercapnea[57a]

Vascular changes in secondary pulmonary hypertension are similar to those in the primary form, although muscular artery hyperplasia is not so advanced and plexiform dilatation lesions are seen only in certain types.

Pulmonary artery thrombosis in the major arteries has been well authenticated (e.g., by Schein et al.[59]). Several hundred cases are on record. It is fatal only when the cor pulmonale it produces becomes decompensated. Thrombosis of the smaller muscular branches alone is uncommon, seen mainly in pulmonary stenosis, according to Spencer.[4] Ring and Bakke[58] have noted that:

1 75% of the pulmonary artery cross section may be occluded before systolic blood pressure falls.
2 90% must be occluded before death occurs.
3 There is a reserve of readily distensible small vessels, and bronchial artery anastomosis will appear.
4 Much blood may still flow around the thrombus.

Rezek and Millard have discussed the difficulty of determining at autopsy whether an older thrombus originated from an earlier embolus or arose autochthonously.[2]

The most common variety of pulmonary artery thrombosis is secondary to the impaction of multiple emboli. Microscopically, thrombi and emboli will be found in most of the small arteries and arterioles, in all stages from fresh to organizing and recanalizing thrombi.

ATELECTASIS AND COLLAPSE

It seems useful to maintain a distinction between the terms *atelectasis* and *collapse,* atelectasis meaning incomplete expansion of the newborn infant's lung and collapse meaning reduction in lung size due to loss of air.

Atelectasis

Atelectasis is a neonatal condition resulting from weak respiratory action. It tends to occur in premature infants and in infants with various forms of cerebral birth injury, central nervous system malformation, and intrauterine hypoxia. Total atelectasis is found in stillborn infants. In these infants, the lungs are dark blue and fleshy and devoid of crepi-

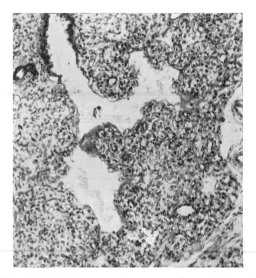

Fig. 23-17 Atelectasis. Respiratory bronchiole and alveolar ducts are expanded, whereas alveoli are entirely unexpanded.

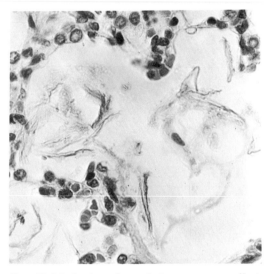

Fig. 23-18 Aspirated amniotic squamous cells in alveolus. One cell is nucleated. (×564.)

tation. They are so small that they occupy only the posterior-central portions of the pleural cavities. No pleural lobular markings are visible. In microscopic slides, thick and vascular interalveolar septa and small alveolar spaces are seen (Fig. 23-17). The latter contain granular amniotic debris and nucleated squamous cells aspirated in utero under the stimulus of hypoxia (Fig. 23-18). Distended respiratory bronchioles also may be seen.

An infant who survives atelectasis for some hours must have some aerated lung. This will be mainly in the upper lobe, where scattered pinker areas are to be found. In these cases, pneumothorax or interstitial emphysema is an indication of the infant's own violent efforts to breathe or of overstrenuous attempts at artificial respiration.

Frequently, it is not possible to say why an infant did not survive. To blame atelectasis is to beg the question of the cause of atelectasis in a healthy-looking child. Further discussion is to be found in the text by Rezek and Millard.[2]

Perinatal pneumonia and *intrauterine pneumonia* are grossly indistinguishable from atelectasis and should always be looked for, since they are rather common. Langley and Smith's investigation[61] disclosed three types: (1) fetal, occurring near full term, (2) early perinatal, with death occurring on the first day, and (3) late perinatal, with death occurring in the first week but after the first day. The percentages of autopsies in which they were found were 10%, 25%, and 30%, respectively. The pneumonia sometimes is the result of inspiration of infected or irritant amniotic fluid. Neutrophils are found in the alveolar septa and the alveoli, which also contain recognizable amniotic fluid material. Often, the diagnosis is difficult to prove because, in spite of thickened septa, the inflammatory cells are scanty. Every effort must be made to obtain bacterial cultures. For further consideration of the significance of atelectasis and of the importance of pleural petechiae and of cultures, see the discussion by Rezek and Millard.[2] In addition, I am sympathetic to the view that the leukocytes in the alveoli may have been inhaled with infected amniotic fluid, causing either "drowning in pus" or first setting up bacterial pneumonia.[62] Furthermore, the presence of polymorphonuclear leukocytes is no proof of bacterial infection but may be a reaction to tissue degeneration or, in the fetal lung, a reaction to hypoxia.[62]

Hyaline membrane disease. Hyaline membrane disease may be regarded as a special form of pulmonary atelectasis or collapse occurring a few hours after birth and sometimes after apparently full expansion of the lungs. The lungs become solid and airless. The body is edematous. Microscopically, interalveolar septa are apposed, but bronchioles are distended. Many of the terminal and respiratory bronchioles are internally coated with thick "hyaline membranes" of a homogeneous eosinophilic material (Fig. 23-19). The material has the staining characteristics of fibrin, a finding confirmed by the use of fluorescein-labeled fibrin antibody and by electron microscopy. The membranes take a little time to develop and are not found in infants who have never breathed.

Lauweryns[67] considers widespread distention of pulmonary lymphatics and impaired perfusion of small muscular pulmonary arteries and of pulmonary arterioles to be of pathogenetic importance. Membranes appear to form in situ after necrosis of the epithelial cells lining the affected bronchioles.[64] In the late stages of the disease, phagocytosis of the lining membrane and reformation of the epithelium are noted.

Those most susceptible to the disease are the premature infants (the greater the prematurity, the worse the disease) and full-term infants of mothers who have diabetes mellitus or who require cesarean section. Minutes or hours after birth, the infants progress to

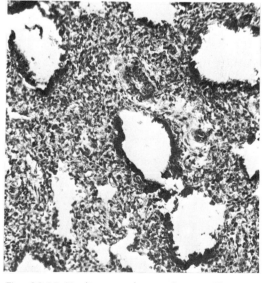

Fig. 23-19 Hyaline membrane disease. Homogeneous dark material lining air spaces is eosinophilic membrane. (×152.)

desperate anoxia, but if they survive the first two days, they seem to recover completely. (Seventy infants were followed for two to five years after recovering from the disease; six had radiologic evidence suggestive of pulmonary fibrosis, confirmed by biopsy in two.[70]) The membranes are found in 20% to 40% of liveborn infants dying in the first few days of life, or in up to 70% of infants dying in the early neonatal period in whom no other major abnormality is encountered.[66] This amounts to 25,000 deaths annually in the United States.

The evidence is strong that these striking membranes do not cause the atelectasis and that atelectasis produces the membranes. Avery and Mead's demonstration[63] of the absence of the surface tension–lowering alveolar surface film does everything but explain its absence. The consequent inability of the infant to force open the alveoli (p. 876) leads to congestive failure. Protein-containing fluid transudes from pulmonary capillaries into the alveoli, which become lined with fibrin. Lieberman[68] suggests, in addition, a deficiency of plasminogen activator so that the fibrin cannot be broken down by fibrinolysin. Under such circumstances, premature infants are forced to attempt respiration by means of the alveolar ducts, in which hyaline membranes then form.

In recognition of the secondary role of the hyaline membrane, not present in every case, the alternative name of *respiratory distress syndrome* is employed.

A most interesting observation is that commonly there are pressure ulcers on the true and false vocal cords.[69] These are considered to be caused by laryngeal dysfunction producing abnormal closure of the larynx.

There are *other causes of hyaline membrane* formation. It has been seen in children dying from kerosene poisoning and is common in adults with viral pneumonia, chemical pneumonitis, severe uremia, rheumatic involvement of the lung, severe pulmonary edema, bacterial pneumonia, and after irradiation. Of 156 adult patients at autopsy, seven had hyaline membranes. They also had a fibrinolytic defect.[65]

Collapse

Two main types of collapse of the lung exist—compressive and obstructive, two important variants of the latter being acute massive collapse and middle lobe syndrome.

Compressive collapse. The mechanism in compressive collapse is external pressure, gen-

erally by pleural fluid and less often by air (pneumothorax), intrathoracic tumor (including a large heart), high diaphragm, or spinal deformity. The subpleural regions undergo greater collapse than the central areas, and the lower lobes are affected most often. The effect tends to spread throughout the lung unless pleural fibrosis or adhesions help keep the lung expanded.

Collapsed lungs are dark red or blue, poorly crepitant, and smaller than normal, and they exhibit slightly wrinkled pleura. For a long time, they remain capable of reexpansion, but, if this does not happen, low-grade inflammation will set in, to be followed by extensive fibrosis.

At first, the microscopic picture mirrors the gross condition. Alveolar septa are close together, and their vessels are prominent. The larger bronchi remain open. Later, the interlobular, perivascular, and peribronchial tissue increases, alveolar capillaries become increasingly bloodless, and arteriolar walls are thickened. Eventually, a condition resembling organizing pneumonia may be seen.

Obstructive (absorptive) collapse. The term *obstructive collapse* refers to the cutting off of air to a group of lobules or even a whole lobe by obstruction of many bronchioles or a large bronchus. Possible causes are pressure by enlarged lymph nodes, intrabronchial tumor, foreign body, or an especially viscid mucous secretion. The last results from acute bronchiolitis (especially in young children), suppression of the cough reflex (including neurologic diseases and anesthesia), severe bronchial asthma, cystic fibrosis of the pancreas, dehydration, and tracheotomy.

Obstructive collapse is less severe than the compressive variety because the absorbed air is largely replaced by edema fluid and bronchial secretion. The collapse is likely to be patchy, creating dark blue depressions in between apparently raised, normal pink areas over the lung surface (Fig. 23-20). If bronchial drainage is not restored, chronic or organizing pneumonia is likely, with areas of endogenous lipid pneumonia.

Acute massive collapse is a widespread loss of air space occurring occasionally in adults after surgery. It is thought that depressed cough reflex, immobile abdomen, and oversecretion of bronchial mucus combine to diminish the airway. It has also occurred in patients who have undergone open chest surgery or bronchography or have suffered a chest wall injury. Spencer[4] believes that the

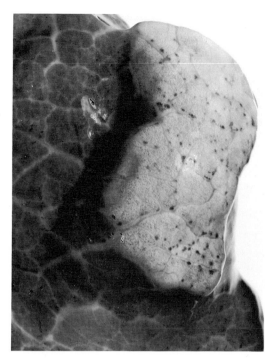

Fig. 23-20 Obstructive collapse. There is clear contrast between pale, still-aerated lung and dark depressed lung beside it. Normal pleural lymphatic network is easily seen.

original injury is severe acute pulmonary edema, with severe secondary bronchospasm that attempts to overcome it. Raffensperger et al.[72] have observed that, while air is slowly absorbed distal to blocked bronchi, oxygen and anesthetic gases disappear quickly, allowing prompt collapse. The difference lies in the absence of nitrogen in anesthesia.

Middle lobe syndrome is a consequence of enlargement of the lymph nodes in the angle between the middle and lower lobar bronchi of the right lung. The middle bronchus is thereby kinked and obstructed, cutting off the air to the middle lobe and resulting in obstructive collapse. Just as in lobar emphysema of infants (see below), exception has been taken to a purely mechanical explanation for middle lobe syndrome. In none of a series of nine patients was there obstruction of the lobar bronchus and its segmental bifurcation (as investigated by bronchoscopy and/or bronchography).[71]

EMPHYSEMA

Emphysema has passed beyond the simple concept of hyperinflation of alveoli called "diffuse vesicular emphysema." Erroneous views were engendered by the examination of unfixed collapsed lungs. The inflation technique advocated by Laennec was ignored for over a century.

Classification

Emphysema may mean something different to the pathologist, to the clinician, and to the radiologist. Its meaning differs on either side of the Atlantic. In the United States, it means an increase in size of air spaces distal to the terminal bronchioles, with destruction of their walls and minimal fibrosis. In Britain, the term is taken to include the combination of the effects of both chronic bronchitis (chronic productive cough and dyspnea) and emphysema and includes simple distention. Acceptance of these concepts permits four mechanisms of production of emphysema[1]:

1 *Atrophy* (emphysema of aging, coal miner's pneumoconiosis, bronchitis and bronchiolitis, and scar and paraseptal emphysema)
2 *Hypoplasia* during the postnatal phase of alveolar development (bronchitis and bronchiolitis of childhood and most cases of unilateral hyperlucent lung)
3 *Overinflation* (so-called compensatory emphysema, ball-valve obstruction, and infantile lobar emphysema)
4 *Destruction* (as when alveolar destruction is associated with chronic bronchitis or with scars)

A simple classification of emphysema, both anatomic and descriptive, would be as follows:

1 Localized
  a Acute
  b Chronic
  c Paraseptal
  d Lobar
  e "Compensatory"
2 Generalized
  a Centriacinar ("focal")
  b Diffuse
    1 Panacinar ("vesicular")
    2 Acute obstructive
  c Multiple focal
3 Aging lung ("senile")
4 Interstitial
5 "Bronchiolar"

More helpful to understanding is the classification shown in Fig. 23-21, in which the various mechanisms are displayed. Three concepts are vital to its understanding: (1) the alveoli are distended beyond the size normal in deep inspiration, (2) the unit involved in emphysema is the anatomic acinus (p. 878), and (3) emphysema is either associated with

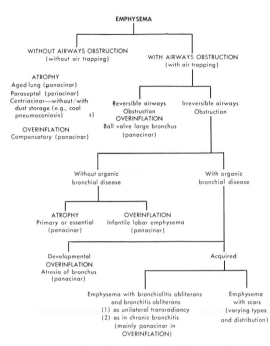

Fig. 23-21 Classification of emphysema by morphology and pathogenesis (see text). (Modified from Reid, L.: The pathology of emphysema, Lloyd-Luke [Medical Books] Ltd.)

airways obstruction (trapping) or it is not. When air is trapped, that lobe or lung will not deflate when removed from the body. Most clinically significant types of emphysema fall into the category of *irreversible airways obstruction.*

In this text, *emphysema is defined as* a condition of the lung characterized by permanent increase beyond normal in the size of the air spaces distal to the terminal bronchioles. This may arise from destruction, dilatation, hypoplasia, or atrophy, but the functionally significant varieties will have at least the factor of destruction.

Localized emphysema
Acute localized emphysema

Acute localized emphysema is most often seen in association with bronchopneumonia or with bronchiolitis of children. Many pulmonary lobules are affected by alternating areas of collapse and reversible overdistention. It is now correct to term such conditions *hyperinflation* so as to stress the preservation of intact architecture.

Chronic localized emphysema

Chronic localized (irregular) emphysema is found in relation to chronic local inflammation and fibrosis, or to calcified foci, especially

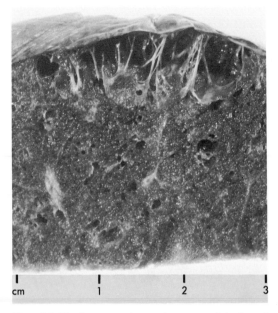

Fig. 23-22 Paraseptal emphysema. Subpleural distended air spaces are traversed by fibrotic strands of vessels, bronchioles, and septa.

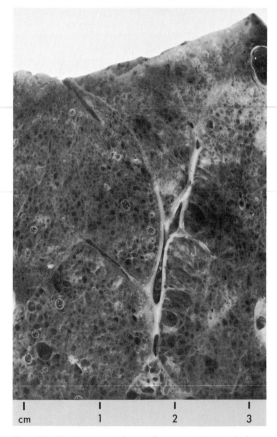

Fig. 23-23 Paraseptal emphysema. Distended air spaces are to right of vertically running blood vessel. Grade I panacinar emphysema also may be seen.

around apical scars. Frequently, the large empty spaces render the scar insignificant. Microscopically, in a central fibrous area, cuboidal cells line residual terminal bronchioles and alveoli. Opening off these are fibrous, stretched-out septa that are poorly vascular, contain some dust, and enclose irregular giant air spaces.

Paraseptal emphysema

Paraseptal emphysema has a distribution all of its own, whether subpleural (Fig. 23-22) or within the lung. In the first instance, it is along the sharp edges of the lung or on the mediastinal or diaphragmatic surfaces. When internal, it is found against connective tissue septa, against larger vessels or bronchi (Fig. 23-23), or even within the angle of bronchial divisions. Even in lungs perfused with formalin, lesser degrees of paraseptal emphysema are readily overlooked. There is a beadlike row of uniform holes, each gently bending outward the apposed pleura. At first measured in millimeters, some eventually progress in size to be measured in centimeters. They are bounded by the subpleural connective tissue septa that eventually tear and allow confluence so that bullous emphysema is born (Figs. 23-24 and 23-29). The cavities of the internal variety do not attain great size.

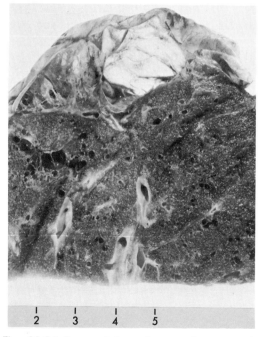

Fig. 23-24 Paraseptal emphysema in more advanced state than that shown in Fig. 23-23 displaying how condition can develop into bullous emphysema.

Atrophy appears to be the cause of paraseptal emphysema. Remember two important facts: (1) it has nothing to do with centriacinar or panacinar emphysema (which could be present by coincidence) and (2) it rarely causes impaired respiratory function, unless a bulla ruptures (pneumothorax) or is big enough to compress neighboring lung.

Lobar emphysema of infants

Lobar emphysema of infants arises in the first few months of life. An upper or middle lobe of the lung is blown up with air so suddenly and severely that surrounding lung is collapsed and a marked mediastinal shift ensues. The diaphragm on that side is forced down. Without surgery the child may die quickly. Further, surgery also prevents permanent damage.

There are several causes: (1) partial intrabronchial obstruction by a congenital web, foreign body, or infection, (2) extrabronchial compression by an abnormally large or anomalous vessel, and (3) absence or hypoplasia of bronchial cartilages, permitting collapse of the walls during expiration. In spite of this impressive list, Reid[1] is strongly of the opinion that most of the cases have no organic block and that the obstruction is functional, probably within the alveoli. The concept of an anomaly of cartilage has erroneously been seized upon because the variability of the state of development and maturity of bronchial cartilage in early life is not widely known, and neither is the fallacy of the random sectioning of a bronchus (p. 875).

The disease is not to be confused with tension cyst (p. 908).

The affected lobe is tense and hugely swollen. The alveoli give the cut surface a honeycomb pattern, and microscopically they have the look of large, unruptured, adult-sized air sacs.

Compensatory emphysema

Compensatory emphysema is a misleading term used for the expansion of remaining normal lung that occurs after another portion has been removed or damaged by fibrosis or collapse. The lung is airy, and its alveoli are distended until they may give way, but there is no increase in functional activity—rather a decrease. The compensation is to fill the extra space that has been created. Liebow[83] has suggested the term "traction emphysema."

Unilateral hyperlucent lung. A discussion of localized emphysema appears to be the appropriate place to mention a newer entity, unilateral hyperlucent lung. Named also the Swyer-James syndrome and the MacLeod syndrome, it refers to a lung with unilateral radiologic transradiancy, without collapse, with little ventilation, and with little pulmonary artery blood flowing through it. The lung is smaller than normal but airy. Reid et al.[91] have observed distortion or obliteration of many bronchi or bronchioles, hypoplasia of the pulmonary arteries, and emphysema. They believe the condition is the result of infective damage to the airways in childhood, the small lung with its small arteries being secondary to this. These authors derive strong evidence for the noncongenital nature of the condition from three children who began with radiologically normal pulmonary vasculature and developed secondary hypoplasia (retarded development) of alveoli and vessels after severe pneumonia.[91] Abnormally large alveoli in a small or normal-sized lung is a sign of pulmonary hypoplasia, since a lower than normal number of alveoli have to expand to fill the thorax.

Generalized emphysema

The discussion of generalized emphysema considers those varieties commonly implied by the word emphysema (chronic obstructive pulmonary emphysema).

Etiology. Etiologic theories about emphysema related to primary vascular disease or destruction of alveolar elastic tissue have been virtually abandoned. Suspicions of the danger of blowing wind instruments have been replaced by those of the dangers of coughing cigarette smoke. Emphysema is considered by McLean[84] to be the consequence of prolonged inflammation and obstruction of the respiratory bronchioles. Permanent damage leads to bronchiolar obliteration. In spite of collateral ventilation via the pores of Kohn, the incomplete interlobular septa and the bronchioloalveolar anastomoses, air trapping is claimed to result. This may distend and even disrupt air passages distal to the obstructed bronchioles. If the pressure of the trapped air is high, as with coughing, so much the worse. Unfortunately, these obstructive bronchiolar lesions may not be seen, although it is inferred that the bronchioles have been destroyed from evidence of their numerical reduction.[84] The concept of selective bronchiolar inflammation also has been challenged.

The view of Leopold and Gough[81] is that chronic inflammation damages the walls of the most distal respiratory bronchioles, which dilate more and more (centriacinar emphysema). Affected third-order respiratory bronchioles fuse into a dilatation (the "common pool") at the level of the second-order bronchiole. The process may come to involve the interalveolar septa also (panacinar emphysema) if there is inflammatory damage to alveolar ducts and the air sacs distal to these.

According to Spain and Kaufman,[94] the essence of emphysema is chronic inflammation within the walls of and around the terminal bronchioles. These become thickened, rigid, and narrowed, causing trapping of air in expiration, with distention of the alveoli.

These three leading theories share a belief in the role of chronic bronchiolitis. It is probably a mistake to assume that there is only *one* cause of emphysema. Although it is stated that pigment deposits occur only secondarily,[88] it is difficult to escape the observation that in some city dwellers there are focal areas of centriacinar or panacinar emphysema associated with anthracosis. Coal dust alone has been considered to cause centriacinar emphysema in miners.[79] The assumption that the black particles in the lungs are necessarily carbon is false. Clinical and fine structural studies have demonstrated a mixture of inorganic silicates and aluminates, some trace metals, elemental carbon, and a highly soluble, probably organic pigment not yet identified.[87] Ferritin also is often present in patients with congestive heart failure.

What we are considering, therefore, is not just coal dust (itself not pure carbon), not just tobacco derivatives, not just pollutants of our air. What we have done is to equate blackness with badness. We have assumed that the blackness of coal workers' lungs is to be equated with functional impairment. In fact, dust and centriacinar emphysema may coexist and, equally, may exist independently (p. 929). Gough[10] seems to add confusion by confining the term focal dust emphysema to the centriacinar emphysema of coal and other industrial workers and by regarding the morphologically similar condition of nonindustrial workers as having an inflammatory origin. More recently, he has (with Ryder et al.[91a]) reported on the findings in autopsies on 247 miners who had suffered from coal worker's pneumoconiosis. This painstaking study, using a matching series of nonminers, showed that there was much more emphysema among miners and that it was of the focal dust type. Only a minority had what Gough would recognize as centriacinar or panacinar emphysema, and it was seen in areas with little or no dust.

The reader is referred also to the work of Heard[77, 78] and that of Reid,[89] who believe that the disease commences with inflammatory destruction of the walls in the junctional region between the terminal and respiratory bronchioles, and to a review by Thurlbeck.[96]

Since the last edition of this book, no basic discovery has been made as to the cause of disabling emphysema. We do not even know why air is trapped. Clinicians experience extraordinary difficulty in distinguishing chronic bronchitis from emphysema. This is expressed (and hidden) in the invention of the term "chronic obstructive pulmonary disease." Against this ignorance must be weighed a new observation. Familial cases of panacinar or bullous emphysema are being uncovered (as many as fifteen members in one family[96a]). Common factors to all of them are onset in early adult life, equal sex incidence, reduction of patient's serum alpha$_1$-antitrypsin to 10% of normal (hence, serum protein electrophoresis will show no appreciable amount of alpha$_1$-globulin in these persons). Other members of the family may be homozygous or heterozygous for the deficiency (40% to 80% of normal antitrypsin.[86] Heterozygotes develop less severe disease, and at a later age, than do homozygotes.

The inhibitor is not specific for trypsin. It also will inhibit proteolytic enzymes of leukocytes and bacterial elastases. Therefore, in its absence, inflammatory reactions in the lung may proceed much further than normal. Trypsin-inhibitory capacity of serum in sixty-six patients hospitalized with emphysema was found deficient in 26%, and most of these were heterozygotes; 48% of those patients under the age of 50 years were deficient.[82]

Another discovery of less relevance to man is that long-term inhalation of nitrogen dioxide in moderate concentrations can produce emphysema in rats.[75]

Incidence. Only in the last decade has an attempt been made to study the frequency of emphysema in the United States. Figures are incomplete, but the new interest has revealed many more cases than were previously reported. In Great Britain, emphysema causes twice as many deaths in men as does carcinoma of the lung and is responsible for nine-tenths of all cor pulmonale, which, in turn, accounts for 5% to 10% of all cases of cardiac disease.[74] In series of random autopsies, at least half of the patients have been found to have emphysema, not necessarily severe or symptomatic during life.

Centriacinar emphysema

The term *centriacinar* emphysema refers to emphysema confined to the central portion of the acinus, its distribution being segmental, lobar, or generalized.

Lungs fixed by formalin perfusion. Simply by crudely perfusing the bronchial tree for three days with formalin under moderate pressure, one can recognize the condition of the cut surfaces. The more refined methods of Heard[77, 78] are recommended, and his illustrations show what can be achieved.

Special care allows one to see earlier phases, to grade severity of emphysema, and to recognize two important centriacinar types (atrophic and destructive[1]). In atrophy, the central hole in the acinus is composed of a group of widened air spaces crossed by tenuous strands of tissue (Fig. 23-25). Microscopically, the architecture is more or less preserved, although alveolar walls are flimsy. In destruction, much the rarer of the two types, there is a completely empty central hole of 1 cm diameter or more. Its wall appears smooth and is composed of interrupted alveolar walls that have retracted and flattened. No evidence is available that atrophy progresses to destruction, and they are not usually found together. Even widespread and well-developed atrophic centriacinar emphysema gives no symptoms because great numbers of peripheral and perfect alveoli are available and because there is no air trapping. Nor is the condition a usual sequel of chronic bronchitis.

When centriacinar emphysema is so advanced that the periphery of the lobule is being destroyed, the condition will be indistinguishable from panacinar emphysema of similar severity, and the degree of respiratory impairment will depend on the volume of lung destroyed. A few persisting normal alveoli at the periphery indicate centriacinar emphysema (Fig. 23-26).

One gets a better impression of emphysema from looking at the whole lung, perhaps with a hand lens, than from microscopic slides. It is the detailed work of Snider et al.,[93] Reid,[1] and Pratt et al.[88] that has developed the concept of centriacinar emphysema as usually symptomless and as separate from deposits of dust. Therefore, when a mild to moderate degree of the condition is found at autopsy in a patient who had respiratory disability,

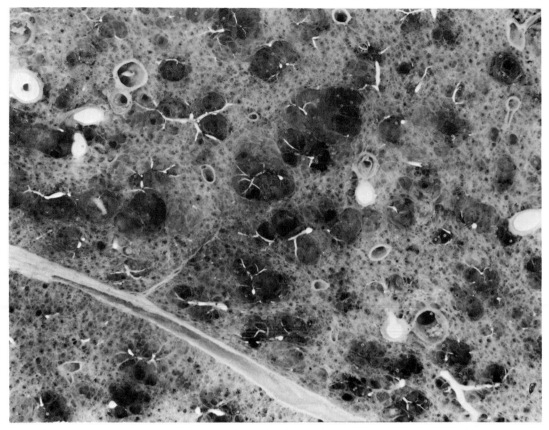

Fig. 23-25 Centriacinar emphysema. Lung fixed with formalin under pressure. Pulmonary arteries have been injected with barium-gelatin mixture. Dark spaces are centriacinar areas of destruction. Around these, alveoli of normal size have been preserved. (×3; from Heard, B. E.: Thorax **13**:136-149, 1958.)

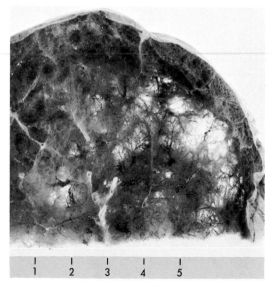

Fig. 23-26 Centriacinar emphysema—severe. Residues of normal lung tissue at periphery of acini situated beneath pleura are clue to naming this particular case centriacinar rather than severe panacinar.

chronic bronchitis is likely to have been responsible.

In London, centriacinar emphysema is found in one of five fluid-fixed lungs of persons with normal chest x-ray films and no clinical lung disease. We do not know if it contributes to disability when obstructive lung disease also is present. It is not a constant factor in disabled coal miners.

According to the severity of the disease, the lesions expand or even become confluent. They are more advanced in the upper parts of the lobes, particularly the upper lobes. These impressions have been confirmed microscopically.[97] Black pigment is concentrated along the course of the dilated bronchioles. Their walls appear to have undergone fibrous thickening. An intramural and perimural infiltrate of lymphocytes is present. The damaged interalveolar septa are thinned and fractured. In the unfixed lung, there will be seen only a focal or generalized disruption of septa, again thinned and with diminished vascularity.

Panacinar ("vesicular") emphysema

It is not settled whether panacinar emphysema is the late stage of centriacinar emphysema or is a distinct entity. It is that form of the disease that comes to the average physician's mind when "emphysema" is mentioned, with the connotation of chronic bronchitis, cigarette smoking, and atmospheric pollution. The disease is nearly as common as the centriacinar form. Mixed forms also occur.

"Panacinar" means that all alveoli of the acinus are uniformly distended. Localized forms occur in compensatory overinflation, in ball-valve obstruction of a large bronchus, in infantile lobar emphysema, and in unilateral hyperlucent lung. Involvement of most of both lungs will be seen in the aging lung, in association with chronic bronchitis or as idiopathic disease. Whereas centriacinar emphysema favors the upper two-thirds of the lungs and is much commoner in men, the panacinar emphysema of the aging and idiopathic types involves all of the lungs and has an equal sex incidence. Panacinar emphysema occurring in α_1-antitrypsin deficiency is distinctive in that it preferentially damages the lower lobes.

Panacinar emphysema of lowest grade is seen in the perfused lung as innumerable 1 mm holes that are individual enlarged alveoli (Fig. 23-27). When of medium severity, the holes are several millimeters in size, and re-traction of the damaged alveoli causes the vessels, bronchi, and septa to stand up. The most severe panacinar emphysema has confluent large holes occupying all of the acinus. It is to such advanced disease that the following description applies.

The patients have a barrel-shaped chest of increased anteroposterior diameter, with widened, nearly horizontal, intercostal spaces. There is moderate kyphosis, and the costal cartilages may be calcified. Most of the patients are men 40 to 60 years of age.

The lungs are so full of air that they depress the diaphragm and hide the heart. The pleura is dry and smooth and the surface corrugated by identations by the ribs, alternating with expansions representing the intercostal spaces. The lungs are pale gray, with carbon deposits that tend to follow the rib markings. Finger pressure creates permanent depressions. Dryness is the outstanding feature of the airy, spongy, cut surface, which discloses innumerable empty spaces 1 mm or 2 mm in diameter (Fig. 23-28). (Normal alve-

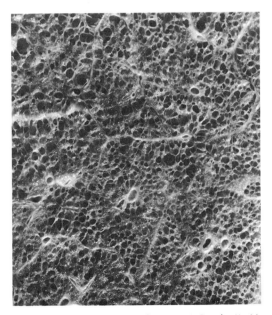

Fig. 23-27 Panacinar emphysema—Grade II. No part of acinus is spared.

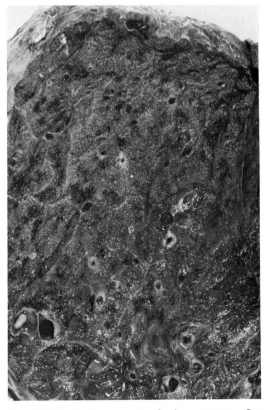

Fig. 23-28 Emphysema in fresh specimen. Cut surface is spongy, with tiny spaces surrounded by tissue that can easily be torn.

oli in middle age are about 120 μm to 140 μm in diameter and thus cannot be appreciated by the unaided eye.)

In ordinary microscopic sections, alveoli appear enlarged or, their walls having ruptured, are fused into spaces of irregular size and shape into which the broken ends of the original septa project as spurs. All the septa are very thin, and their vessels are barely evident. An occasional dilated respiratory bronchiole may be recognized.

Special preparations reveal that alveoli are replaced by larger thick-walled empty spaces.[98] These represent fused alveoli crossed by strands of obliterated vessels. All of the acinus is involved, and not only are alveolar pores dilated, but also lobules may communicate with one another, indicating formation of bullae. The most advanced lesions are in the basal segments of the lower lobes and the lower part of the lingula and middle lobe.

The great reduction of the number of alveolar capillaries is followed by muscular hypertrophy and hyperplasia of their parent vessels, which may have little lumen left. There is great expansion of the venous collateral circulation, whereby desaturated blood may be shunted from the systemic into the pulmonary veins when the right side of the heart fails.[83] This will aggravate the anoxia and hypercapnia. In contrast, the bronchial arteries take on additional function. They enlarge and anastomose into the pulmonary arteriolar system.

The bronchi are likely to show the glandular hyperplasia so characteristic of bronchitis. They may be dilated and thin-walled.

Radiologic correlation. It has been shown that even large air spaces in centriacinar emphysema do not produce radiologic changes of widespread emphysema. Such changes are produced only by the more severe grades of panacinar emphysema, but only if widespread.[1] Hence, if clinical aspects are taken into consideration, a normal x-ray film will almost exclude gross widespread panacinar emphysema with air trapping.[92] Shadows seen in chest x-ray films of persons with heavy dust deposits are due to the dust alone, not to any disease caused by the deposits.

Clinical correlation. If one takes a group of adults suffering from dyspnea of pulmonary origin, there will be an association with idiopathic emphysema in 10% and with chronic bronchitis in the rest. Only 50% of patients with bronchitis who are short of breath have significant emphysema, 20% have normal lungs, 20% have panacinar emphyse-

ma of a degree expected at their age, and 10% have centriacinar emphysema (Reid[90]).

Idiopathic (primary) emphysema. Having established that idiopathic emphysema is a form of panacinar emphysema that is not too common, it remains to say that when widespread it can be fatal. It occurs equally in both sexes and often appears in the third decade. Bullae are common, and there is marked air trapping. The emphysema is of a severe degree. Nothing is known of the cause except that the basic change is atrophy of the alveolar wall and capillary bed.[1]

Emphysema with chronic bronchitis. Two circumstances have to be considered: (1) emphysema caused by chronic bronchitis, when infection damages and scars small airways and alveoli, and (2) emphysema associated with, but not caused by, chronic bronchitis, a circumstance in which the bronchitis is much more serious and the emphysema benign.

Chronic bronchitis causes destruction, overinflation, and atrophy, processes extending from bronchioli to alveoli. The emphysema is panacinar.

Bullous emphysema and blebs. Whereas bullae have been described as possible components of advanced panacinar emphysema, occasionally extremely large bullae are found (often in younger adults) in the absence of a history of chronic lung disease and without emphysema elsewhere in the lung. A distinction is made by some who call these cysts "blebs," meaning the result of rupture of alveoli directly into the subpleural interstitial tissue plane. Such blebs cannot be demarcated laterally by interlobular septa and may compress much of a lobe. They are a common cause of spontaneous pneumothorax. A bulla is a manifestation of emphysema, whereby progressive dilatation and destruction of alveolar walls form a large subpleural air space, contained laterally by lobular septa. At the apices, along the anterior margin, and along free edges of the bases, the distended alveoli often expand into bullae several centimeters in diameter (Fig. 23-29). Such large air cysts have smooth, tissue paper–thin walls, which are reticulated if there are clinging remnants of alveolar and tissue septa. The space may be crossed by strands of tissue, vessels, or bronchi. It is thought that bullae are found at the sites mentioned because here lobular septa are complete, and collateral air flow is therefore inadequate to dissipate the high pressure.

During life, a bulla cannot project from the lung as it so dramatically does in the pathol-

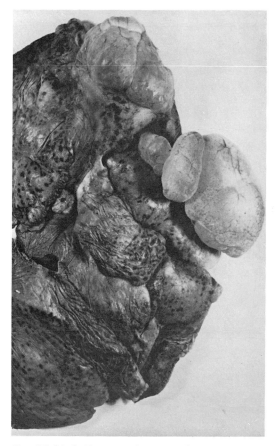

Fig. 23-29 Bullous emphysema of anterior margin of lung.

ogist's specimen. The thoracic cage is unyielding, and a bulla has to bulge into the lung. If large, it will compress a considerable volume of normal lung.

Various types of bullae occur.[1] Among them should be included "tension pneumatocele" or "vanishing lung" (pp. 908 and 962).

Complications of severe chronic emphysema

Complications of severe chronic emphysema are as follows:

1 Right-sided heart failure (cor pulmonale)
2 Respiratory acidosis, causing fatal coma (due to carbon dioxide retention, which depresses respiration; aggravating factors such as infection, sedatives, narcotics, and administration of pure oxygen, all cause further depression)
3 Acute and chronic peptic ulceration (found in up to 20% of emphysematous patients at autopsy)
4 Simulation of brain tumor in small proportion of severe cases (hypercapnia ap-

pears to cause cerebral vasodilatation, which increases cerebrospinal fluid pressure[73])
5 Pneumothorax

Cor pulmonale is defined here as right ventricular hypertrophy secondary to pulmonary disease (the term has been misused in many variants). The index of hypertrophy is usually taken as a right ventricular thickness greater than 4 mm, a measurement reliable only when that ventricle is not dilated. Only by weighing the right ventricle can hypertrophy accurately be determined. Using Fulton's method, by which a weight of 80 gm is abnormal,[76] Millard showed that electrocardiography is not a reliable guide to the presence of right ventricular hypertrophy and that it is almost useless for quantitating the degree of hypertrophy.[85]

Diffuse acute obstructive emphysema

In diffuse acute obstructive emphysema, the obstruction is widespread rather than complete and is the result of severe acute bronchiolitis, asthma, pertussis, anaphylaxis, war gases, or suffocation. It is more correct to consider the condition an acute overdistention. The lungs are so full of air that they cover the front of the heart, yet they can be quite readily compressed manually. Such force probably overcomes many points of bronchial obstruction due to thick mucus, pus, or aspirated material.

Microscopic examination confirms that this is not a true emphysema, since the air spaces are overinflated without destructive changes.

Multiple focal emphysema

The term multiple focal emphysema applies to honeycomb lung and pneumoconiosis in which interstitial fibrosis appears to pull on the surviving lung tissue, causing what has been called a *paracicatricial emphysema* or, in the latter disease, *focal dust emphysema*.[10]

Aging lung (so-called senile emphysema)

It used to be thought that "senile emphysema" was a lung disorder secondary to the development of a barrel chest. In fact, it is the result of an aging atrophy of the alveolar walls, unassociated with air trapping. A still incomplete survey in my department already has shown it to be by far the commonest type of emphysema to be seen, and it commences at about the age of 40 years. It is always a low-grade panacinar emphysema, similar to the early stages of the severe idiopathic emphysema, yet inexplicably never known to progress to become clinically significant. The whole of each lung is affected.

At autopsy, the lungs are airy, fluffy, and small, for they lose air when the thorax is opened. Microscopically, although the alveoli are enlarged and their walls very thin with reduced numbers of capillaries, the most telling changes are the reduction in number of alveoli and their simpler outline, which is due to the loss of some of the angles in their walls.

Interstitial emphysema

When air escapes into the connective tissue framework of the lung, it travels in the form of silvery bubbles 1 mm or 2 mm in diameter, occasionally a little larger.

The bubbles will first be noted beneath the pleura, especially where it fuses with the interlobular septa. On the cut surface, bubbles travel along the perivascular sheaths to the hilum. From here, air can spread into the mediastinum, neck, and trunk.

The air is best seen after formalin fixation. The largest bubbles are at the hilum and may have compressed the pulmonary vessels. Sometimes the pressure will tear a small vein, leading to air embolism. Rupture of a pleural bleb sets up a pneumothorax.

The condition is seen in newborn infants as a result of too powerful artificial respiration or positive pressure oxygenation. Other infants produce it themselves in a desperate effort to overcome bronchial obstruction by mucus or meconium or because of pneumonia, aspiration, atelectasis, intrapulmonary hemorrhage, or hyaline membrane disease.[80]

In older patients, the cause is acute generalized emphysema, brought about by the raised intra-alveolar pressure of coughing in pertussis, penetrating trauma and rib fracture, air embolism, blast injury, intratracheal anesthesia, straining against a closed glottis, or introduction of the point of a needle through the chest wall into the lung.

Microscopically, there are distended alveoli (particularly noticeable in newborn infants), and there may be an alveolus communicating with a pleural bleb. Clear spaces running outside the bronchi and blood vessels and in connective tissue septa are evidences of the passage of air. This is not true emphysema, for alveoli are not damaged.

"Bronchiolar" emphysema

Bronchiolar emphysema is a misconceived concept, named here to dispel the notion that

it might have anything to do with emphysema. It is a form of honeycomb lung (p. 937).

VIRAL AND RICKETTSIAL DISEASES

The pulmonary manifestations of viral and rickettsial diseases are described in Chapter 11.

FUNGAL DISEASES

For a discussion of pulmonary manifestations of fungal diseases, see Chapter 12.

PROTOZOAL AND HELMINTHIC DISEASES

The effects of protozoal and helminthic diseases on the lung are discussed in Chapter 13. For *Pneumocystis carinii* pneumonia, see p. 914.

PNEUMONIA
Bacterial pneumonia

Anthrax, pertussis, plague, glanders, melioidosis, *Klebsiella-Aerobacter* infection, and tularemia have important pulmonary manifestations. A discussion of these is found in Chapter 8, with an account of the general nature of the organisms causing the pneumonias discussed below. Leprosy is considered

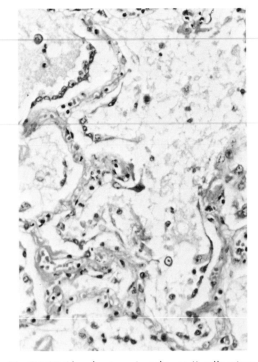

Fig. 23-30 Alveolar type I and type II cells stimulated in case of viral pneumonia. Only in such types of irritation are these cells seen clearly under light microscope. Elongated cytoplasm of type I cell readily apparent, while type II is cuboidal. (×215.)

in Chapter 9, and spirochetal diseases are discussed in Chapter 10.

Lobar pneumonia

Pneumococcal pneumonia, the classic lobar variety, has become a rarity. Now it is seen mainly in persons who lie ill and unattended at home, those in whom chest injuries cause pulmonary congestion and edema, and those who recently have undergone general anesthesia or in alcoholics exposed to cold.

The route of the infection is the bronchial tree itself. When the cocci reach the alveoli, there is a hyperemic response, with migration of macrophages and leukocytes to the area. The organisms multiply in the protein-containing fluid of the inflammatory reaction, which spreads through the lobe.

Phases. Untreated pneumococcal pneumonia follows a series of phases. The onset is in the hilar region, usually in a lower lobe, sometimes bilaterally. A whole lobe is not necessarily affected.

Initial phase. The initial phase (one to two days) is one of acute congestion and edema, unlikely to be met with alone but commonly found as the advancing edge of a central consolidation. The region is gray-red, and frothy bloody fluid can be squeezed from it. Pneumococci are present in large numbers in smears made from the cut surface. Tiny fibrin plugs adhere to a knife edge scraped over the cut surface.

Microscopically, prominent alveolar capillaries can be seen. Nuclei of septal cells are prominent (Fig. 23-30), and neutrophils are migrating into the alveoli (Fig. 23-31, *A*). These are filled with eosinophilic fluid, and Gram stains will divulge the many cocci.

Early consolidation (red hepatization). In

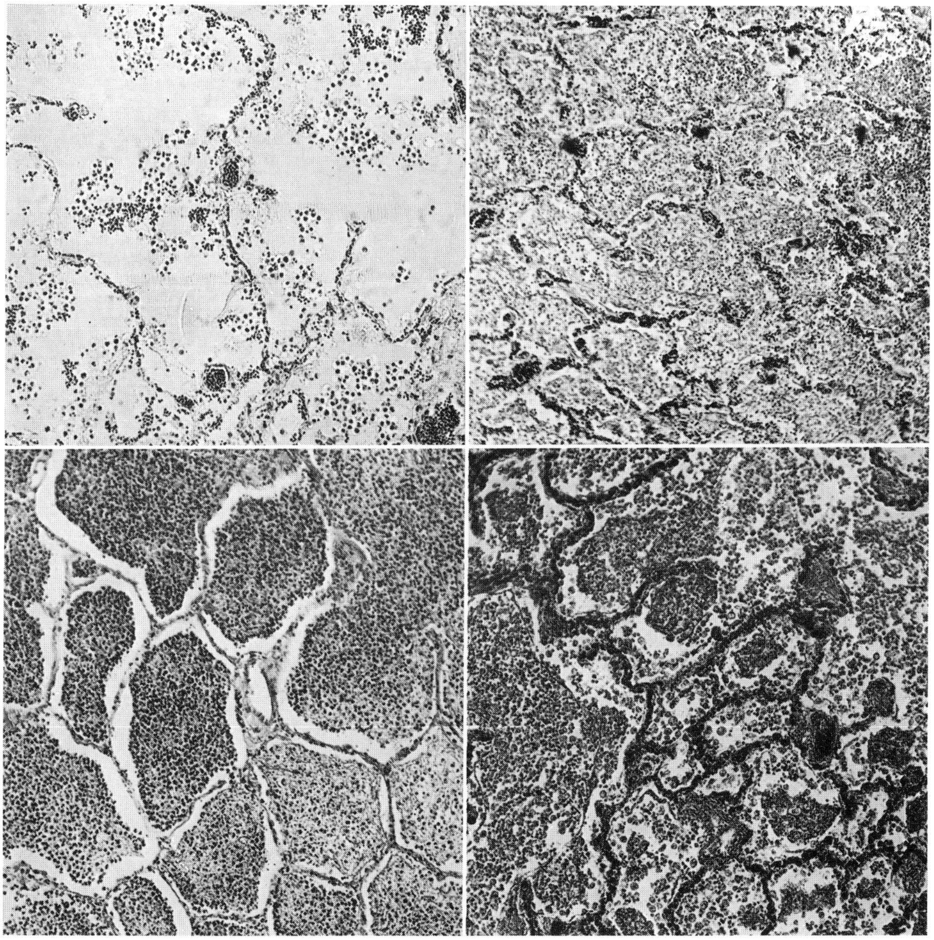

Fig. 23-31 Stages of lobar pneumonia. **A,** Edema in early leukocytic infiltration. **B,** Leukocytic stage. Engorgement persists. Fibrin is scanty. **C,** Late fibrinous stage. Beginning of contraction of alveolar exudate. Alveolar walls ischemic. **D,** Resolution. Macrophages predominate. Masses of fibrin free in alveolar spaces and alveolar capillaries engorged.

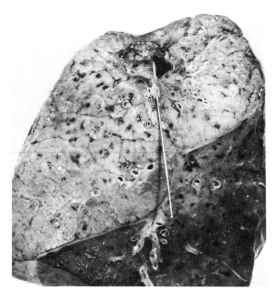

Fig. 23-32 Pneumonia of entire upper lobe in stage of gray hepatization. Disease stops sharply at interlobar septum and is in marked contrast with congested lower lobe. Abscess cavity has formed near apex and can be seen to drain into bronchus. (From Rezek, P. R., and Millard, M.: Autopsy pathology, Charles C Thomas, Publisher.)

the phase of early consolidation (two to four days), the oldest (central) area becomes voluminous and consolidated. Cellular exudation replaces edema. The cut surface is dry, very friable, dull red, and granular (as a result of fibrin in the individual alveoli, the cut walls of which retract below the exudate). Although the color is traditionally red, because of persisting engorgement, it may be no darker than pink. If the pleura has been reached, it has an easily removed coat of fibrin.

The main microscopic feature in this phase is replacement of alveolar fluid by densely packed neutrophils, thin strands of fibrin, and a few erythrocytes. Because engorgement is diminishing, the alveolar septa are much less prominent than in the first stage (Fig. 23-31, *B*).

Late consolidation (gray hepatization). In the late consolidation phase (four to eight days), one lung may weigh as much as 1,500 gm. The cut surface is dry, granular, and gray (Fig. 23-32). The area is quite airless, with the consistency of liver, and slices of it retain straight, sharp edges. The lobe may have the marks of ribs and intercostal spaces. Fibrinous pleurisy is easily seen, and the bronchial mucosa is red.

During this stage, the fluid portion of the exudate has been removed, and a large amount of fibrin has been left behind. There are no organisms. Neutrophils in the alveolar exudate are reduced in number, and many are disintegrating, as their pyknotic nuclei indicate. The remaining exudate is often separated from the septa by a thin clear space (Fig. 23-31, *C*).

Resolution. In the resolution stage (eight days), healing or cure will occur. Exudate is liquefied by enzymatic action, and blood circulation becomes very active once again. Consistency is not so firm as in earlier phases, and the tissue is friable. Some areas, generally the older central ones, are already softened. In fact, resolution may start in such regions while consolidation is still spreading at the periphery. The cut surface is mottled and is gray, red, or dirty brown. It is smooth and moist. A large amount of frothy, yellow, creamy fluid can be squeezed out.

Microscopically, one sees large numbers of macrophages, some coming out of the septal walls into the shrunken fibrin masses and engulfing neutrophils and debris. Alveolar capillaries are congested (Fig. 23-31, *D*).

Resolution and reaeration of the lung require one to three weeks. Antibiotic therapy induces resolution on about the third day.

Complications. The principal complications of pneumococcal pneumonia are as follows:

1 Organization of exudate (see following discussion)
2 Pleural effusion—5% of treated cases
3 Empyema—less than 1% of treated cases; pus is thick and green with clumps of fibrin; can either be free or be encysted in the pleural cavity or in an interlobar fissure; organization of such empyema creates a thick fibrous pleural casing in which fluid locules may be buried
4 Lung abscess—very rare complication that may actually indicate secondary infection by another organism
5 Mediastinitis
6 Cardiac complications—purulent pericarditis, acute bacterial endocarditis, and myocarditis
7 Meningitis
8 Acute otitis media and mastoiditis
9 Purulent arthritis—mainly in infants
10 Paralytic ileus

Organizing (nonresolving) pneumonia. Although resolution appears to depend on fibrinolysins, we do not know the full mechanism and cannot explain the few occasions when it does not work. The lobe is at first fleshy (carnification) and light brown–pink. Pleu-

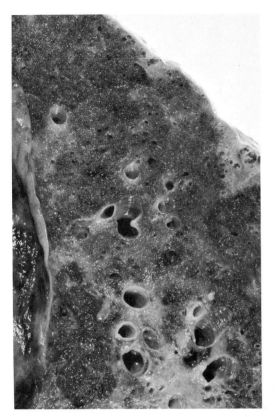

Fig. 23-33 Late stage of organizing pneumonia. Paler, solid areas are fibrous.

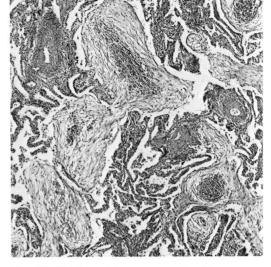

Fig. 23-34 Organizing pneumonia. Young connective tissue fills and distends alveoli and travels from one alveolus to another via pore of Kohn. (×54.)

ral adhesions form, and later the affected area becomes tough, airless, leathery, and gray (Fig. 23-33). At the margins, there may be focal emphysema. Bronchiectasis may follow. Seen microscopically, the fibrinous exudate undergoes organization into fibrous tissue. Interalveolar septa are preserved, but the fibroblasts can easily be seen growing through the pores of Kohn, linking one solidified alveolus with its neighbor (Fig. 23-34). The fibrous tissue matures into poorly cellular scar tissue, and cuboidal metaplasia coats the alveoli (Fig. 23-35).

Organizing pneumonia also is seen in the neighborhood of chronic suppuration, distal to bronchial obstruction or bronchiectasis, around a carcinoma, and in relation to granulomatous disease. There is an impression that organizing pneumonia has increased since the use of antibiotics.[99] Possibly the drugs cut down the inflammatory response, thereby reducing the quantity of fibrinolysin.

Pneumococcus type III pneumonia

Pneumococci of type III have an abundant capsular mucopolysaccharide that imparts a slimy quality to the exudate and thus to the cut surface of the lung. Pneumococcal pneumonia with abscess formation is most likely to be caused by this organism.

Klebsiella pneumonia

Pneumonia caused by *Klebsiella pneumoniae* (Friedländer's bacillus) is particularly destructive. Older men, particularly alcoholics or those with diabetes or severe oral sepsis, most often are afflicted. Spencer[4] makes the point that the preference for the posterior segment of the right upper lobe indicates an inhalational type of infection. *Klebsiella pneumoniae* is a large gram-negative organism with plentiful capsular material recognized in the sticky mucoid exudate.

Infected lobules create red-gray consolidated nodules that, in confluence, become lobar. The infection is destructive, terminating by forming extensive abscesses, a point of distinction from pneumococcus type III pneumonia.

Microscopically, in the early stages the condition is distinguished (even with hematoxylin and eosin stain) by the bacteria in the alveolar exudate. Neutrophilic outpouring is accompanied by destruction of the interalveolar septa. Marked edema is seen in interlobular septa and around vessels and bronchi. Soon the abscesses form, with the breaking down of inflammatory cells and total loss of alveolar structure. A chronic state can supervene as granulation tissue turns to fibrosis and ab-

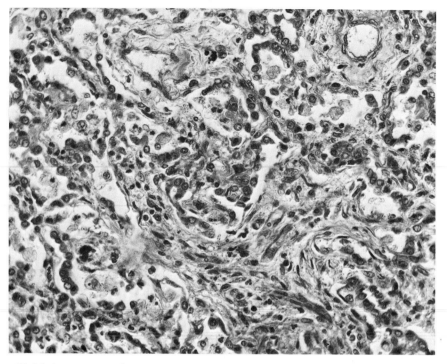

Fig. 23-35 Late stage of organizing pneumonia. Alveoli are contracted and lined by cuboidal cells. (×246.)

scesses become simple cavities. The latter are fibrous walled, and the inflammatory cells are now lymphocytic.

Since the abscesses are usually apical, one's first impression is tuberculosis, although other bacteria, such as staphylococci, have to be considered. Our experience has confirmed reports[110] that the tribe Mimeae can cause a pneumonia that, in the Miami cases at least, is destructive and produces sticky pus (the organisms are encapsulated). The important members of the tribe, are *Herellea vaginicola* and *Mima polymorpha*. These are gram-negative pleomorphic aerobic rods and cocci, resistant to penicillin. Methods for their identification are indicated by Robinson et al.[110]

Staphylococcal pneumonia

Up to 5% of bacterial pneumonias are caused by *Staphylococcus pyogenes*, but the incidence rises during epidemics of influenza, pertussis, and measles. The infection may terminate the course of leukemia or of cystic fibrosis of the pancreas. Apart from these special cases, the mortality rate is around 20% and is even higher in young infants. A chronic state may precede death.

A thick fibrinous or fibrinopurulent pleuritis coats the affected lung in nearly all cases. Infants, especially those infected in nursery epidemics, frequently develop empyema and bronchopleural fistula. They die in a few days. Those who die soonest appear to have only hemorrhagic consolidation of the lungs, with little pleuritis. The bronchial mucosa is red if not covered by a shaggy yellow membrane. Even when examined under the microscope, the inflammatory element is not impressive in the beginning. Alveoli are filled with eosinophilic fluid, erythrocytes, a few neutrophils, and many cocci.

A similar acute variety is common in adults. Hemorrhagic edema fluid is present in copious amounts, making the lung heavy, bulky, and dark purple but not necessarily consolidated.

In older infants and adults, the condition tends to pass from this phase into one of multiple foci of gray-yellow consolidation. In a few days, these become irregular, small, yellow abscesses (Fig. 23-36). They tend to unite into a honeycomb or into a small number of large abscess cavities. In either case, bronchial communications are to be expected, and, if there is an empyema, it will turn into a pyopneumothorax. Infection can spill into other bronchi, setting up new infections. A check-valve obstruction at the junction of the bronchus and abscess results in a rapidly expanding air-filled *tension cyst (tension pneumatocele)*. The surrounding inflammation in-

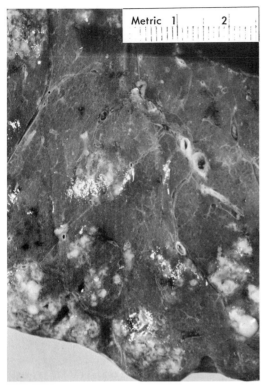

Fig. 23-36 Staphylococcal pneumonia. Numerous 1 mm to 2 mm areas are becoming confluent.

terferes with the normal collateral ventilation. A tension cyst may rupture and cause a simple or tension pneumothorax, with or without empyema.

Tension cysts (so-called "vanishing lung") also are seen in drug-treated tuberculosis but seem otherwise to be a peculiarity of staphylococcal pneumonia in infants. The cyst is spherical, can be centimeters in diameter, and has a thin wall. This is necrotic and ragged at first but later becomes fibrotic and smooth. Usually, the air is absorbed after infection is cured.

Microscopically, abscess-forming staphylococcal pneumonia exhibits alveolar septa and air spaces packed with neutrophils. Often, the septa have been destroyed, and bronchioles are caught up in the same neutrophilic outpouring. There may be edema and neutrophilic filling of pulmonary septal lymphatics. The first pleural changes are congestion and fibrin exudation. Neutrophils pour into the fibrin, which rapidly thickens and, later on, fibroblasts grow into it. The wall of a pneumatocele is at first such inflamed and necrotic lung tissue, surrounded by a zone of compressed lung. Later, a thin wall of fibrous connective tissue forms.

Less common is the fulminating staphylococcal pneumonia of adults, which is fatal in one to two days. The lungs are heavy and watery but without consolidation. The patients are most likely to have had staphylococcal septicemia. The diagnosis will be missed if cultures are not taken from lung and blood, because only moderate neutrophilic activity is seen in the congested alveoli.

Streptococcal pneumonia

Most instances of streptococcal pneumonia (due to β-hemolytic *Streptococcus pyogenes*) are secondary to influenza, measles, or other childhood viral infections. Formerly, the disease comprised 3% to 5% of all childhood pneumonias, and 20% of the patients developed empyema. Others had abscesses, bronchopleural fistulas, or pericarditis, and the mortality rate was high. The organism was the main cause of death in the 1918-1919 influenza pandemic, with *Haemophilus influenzae* less frequently the causative organism.

Today the disease is rare, even as an accompaniment of influenza but Welch et al.[115] have documented a small primary epidemic in previously healthy young men. Seven of eleven children with streptococcal pneumonia in one report had had preceding viral disease.[109]

The heavy, blue-purple lungs are covered by a fibrinous pleurisy. Streptococcal empyema is at first watery with fibrin flakes, turning thick and purulent with loculation of the fluid.

The mucosa of the entire respiratory tract is red and swollen and may be coated by a membrane. Ulcers may be found in the larynx, trachea, and bronchi, whose lumina are filled with bloody fluid. Streptococcal pneumonia is extensive, bilateral, interstitial, and bronchiolar. The most acute form resembles acute staphylococcal pneumonia, both grossly and microscopically. Later, the soggy lungs develop ill-defined, moist, consolidated areas that will become confluent or turn into abscesses. Smaller bronchi and the bronchioles are prominent because they are filled with pus and because their pale yellow walls are thickened by inflammation.

Microscopically, the airways are extensively denuded of epithelium and are stuffed with neutrophils and debris. Neutrophils, fibrin, and some lymphocytes infiltrate the hyperemic walls of the airways and pour into the surrounding alveoli. Lymphatic vessels are engorged with neutrophils. Pulmonary necrosis or abscess, bronchiectasis, mediastinitis, or pericarditis may be present. In nonfatal cases, the severe destruction can be repaired only by fibrosis.

Haemophilus influenzae pneumonia

Haemophilus influenzae was at first thought to be the cause of influenza, but the great pandemic made clear the primary role of a virus. The combination of this organism and a virus is serious, because it produces a bronchopneumonia in which the walls of smaller bronchi and bronchioles are damaged or destroyed. Pure hemophilus pneumonia has complicated chronic lung disease in adults.[114] The gross appearance of this rare pulmonary infection is similar to that of streptococcal pneumonia.

Bronchopneumonia

Bronchopneumonia is an inflammation that originates in bronchioles and extends into the surrounding alveoli. The causes are as follows:

1 Inhalation of noxious gases and dusts
2 Aspiration of fluid and solid contents of the alimentary tract
3 Bacterial infection, either primary or complicating viral infections such as influenza or ornithosis, rickettsial diseases, congestive heart failure, bronchiectasis, bronchial obstruction, or pulmonary mycoses

Bacterial infection or aspiration tends to occur in weak or debilitated individuals such as premature and full-term newborn infants and in bedridden or comatose patients with hypostatic congestion.

The organisms commonly responsible are species of *Staphylococcus, Streptococcus, Klebsiella, Haemophilus,* and *Pneumococcus.* Tillotson and Lerner[113] have recorded the various pneumonias caused by gram-negative bacilli. Specific features are observed in pseudomonal pneumonia in the form of well-demarcated, firm, necrotic nodules. These are composed of a necrotic coagulum, particularly situated around blood vessels and containing large numbers of the bacteria and a minimal inflammatory response of lymphocytes. Vascular thrombosis is inconstant.[104] There is also a tuberculous bronchopneumonia (p. 955).

Terminal or hypostatic bronchopneumonia is very hard to recognize grossly, since it is hidden by the preexisting basal and posterior congestion and edema. The other types are classically patchy. Focal red or gray areas of consolidation (often centered on small bron-

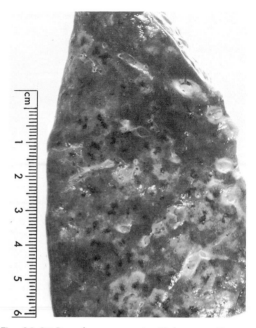

Fig. 23-37 Bronchopneumonia. Lighter small areas are groups of alveoli filled with inflammatory exudate.

chi) lie beside raised, pink, aerated normal areas and dark blue, sunken, collapsed areas (Fig. 23-37). This patchwork of 1 cm contrasting zones is, however, not so common. It often takes the passage of the fingertips over the cut surface to pick up the areas of differing consistency. The bronchial mucosa is frequently bright red. Another variety is peribronchial pneumonia, in which infection picks out peribronchiolar alveoli only, and the consolidation parallels the bronchial tree. If progressive, bronchopneumonia will become confluent, imitating a lobar pneumonia. Careful inspection is likely to disclose a residual patchwork rather than a smooth homogeneity.

The complications of bronchopneumonia are generally those of lobar pneumonia, with a greater tendency for bronchopneumonia to cause permanent damage. Bronchiolar fibrosis and narrowing, with organization of exudate, may lead to bronchiectasis.

The microscopic lesions of bronchopneumonia are alveoli filled with neutrophils and fibrin, the septa being thickened by the congested capillaries which contain leukocytes (Fig. 23-38). Acute bronchitis and bronchiolitis also will be seen.

Inhalation (aspiration) pneumonia

Inhalation pneumonia results from inhaling food, gastric contents, or a foreign body, which may occur when anesthesia has been

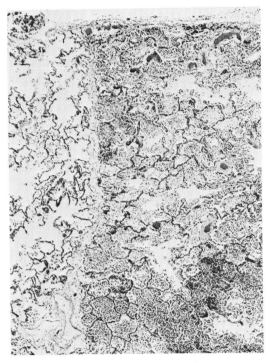

Fig. 23-38 Bronchopneumonia. Inflammation is contained by vertically running septum. (×33.)

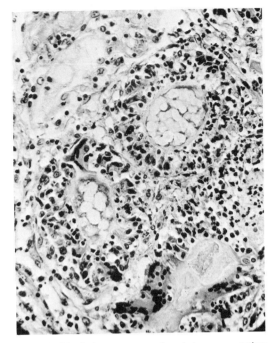

Fig. 23-39 Pulse pneumonia. Intense reaction around partly digested cotyledons of beans. (Approximately ×300.)

induced on a full stomach because of obstetric or other emergency. Other predisposing conditions are drunkenness, epileptic or other convulsions, coma, and neurologic disorders interfering with the swallowing, coughing, and breathing mechanisms. Feeble infants or those with a tracheoesophageal fistula may aspirate their feedings. In addition, aspiration may occur in patients with necrotic oropharyngeal tumors and those vomiting copiously with intestinal obstruction.

Some die quickly from asphyxiation or laryngospasm, without pneumonia. The large airways are filled with the foreign material, and the mucosa may be reddened by irritation.

If smaller amounts are aspirated, the foreign material may trickle into narrower air passages, and often it is inhaled into alveoli; therefore, no foreign material may be visible to the naked eye.

Sterile foreign matter sets up a chemical pneumonitis. The lung undergoes severe congestion and edema, confirmed microscopically by alveoli filled with hemorrhagic fluid and neutrophils. Particles are readily found in bronchioles. Secondary bacterial infection is likely to follow. A few hours after aspiration, patients with chemical pneumonitis dramatically develop cyanosis, dyspnea, shock, and frothy, bloody sputum. They appear to be suf-

fering from pulmonary edema and are likely to die of cardiac failure.

A nonsterile aspirate rapidly causes widespread bronchopneumonia, which becomes confluent with multiple necrotic areas. These are yellow, green, or a dirty gray-green or brown, and they are poorly defined and foul smelling. The odor may be recognized in the bronchi. Putrefactive anaerobes induce a friable gangrenous destruction of the lung, as opposed to the abscesses of pyogenic aerobes. Gangrenous cavities are more irregular and ragged.

The microscopic appearance is of tissue necrosis surrounded by alveoli filled with many erythroctyes and macrophages, a few neutrophils, and, above all, debris that may be recognizable as altered food or may be crystalline or amorphous. Readily recognizable are the starch-containing cotyledons of the pulses (lentils, peas, beans, and peanuts), which cause local pneumonic infiltrates that may pass on to granulomas with giant cells (Fig. 23-39). Disintegration of the pulse may leave an apparently inexplicable giant cell pneumonia.

Frequently, very ill or postsurgical patients given food (marked with barium) aspirate some of it.[106] Also, barium introduced into the stomach immediately after death has been

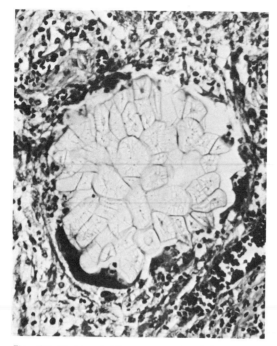

Fig. 23-40 Vegetable pneumonia. Inflammatory and foreign body reaction around undigested vegetable cells in bronchus. (×222.)

shown in the lungs, sometimes reaching even to the alveoli. It appears that moving the body and the force exerted in removing the lungs are responsible.[106] Therefore, gastric contents in bronchi or alveoli cannot be taken as evidence of antemortem aspiration unless the trachea is closed off immediately after death and before the body has been moved. Microscopic signs of aspiration may be otherwise unexplained diffluent hemorrhage in dependent parts of the lungs, perhaps with interstitial emphysema. Some cellular response can be found even in patients dying quickly from aspiration. The cellular reaction continues in the lungs after clinical death.

Lipid pneumonia

Inflammatory and even fibrous reactions associated with the presence of intra-alveolar lipid have long been known. The lipid is not necessarily inhaled from an external source but may be liberated within the lung.

Exogenous lipid pneumonia

The exogenous variety of lipid pneumonia is associated with the long-continued use of oily nosedrops or sprays taken for rhinitis, sinusitis, or similar chronic conditions. The oily base is mineral oil (liquid paraffin). This oil is taken regularly at bedtime and during sleep is quite easily aspirated in small amounts, which accumulate. There is a similar danger for young children who are forcibly given oily vitamins or other medicine. If they splutter over feedings, milk and its fats are readily inhaled. Similarly, an enfeebled elderly person may not even know that food has trickled into his bronchi. By no means does tube feeding protect against this accident, for there is regurgitation and the cardiac sphincter is lax.

A related condition is the occasional reaction to radiopaque contrast media instilled for bronchography. Practically all the patients eventually dispose of the medium by expectoration and phagocytosis, but in a few it remains as an irritant with a resulting lipid pneumonia.[101, 105]

Nature of irritants. Least irritant are olive oil and the neutral vegetable oils used as contrast media. They stimulate slight fibrosis and can be slowly absorbed. Much more irritative is mineral oil, in spite of its being chemically inert. It is emulsified and engulfed by phagocytes, but the residue slowly induces fibrosis. Duration of action and amount of the oil are important factors. Animal oils (cod-liver, halibut, and milk) tend to decompose and are converted by human lipases into irritating fatty acids that stimulate a rather severe inflammation and more rapid fibrosis. The three types are distinguishable only histochemically (see following discussion). It is postulated that in some cases of cot death, the inhalation of milk into an infant's lungs leads to a fatal type I or type III reaction in the lungs.[132, 140] Most of the deaths, however, are due to fulminant viral infections of the respiratory tract or are never explained.[103a]

Clinical picture. Lipid pneumonia often is unsuspected until revealed by radiographic examination or autopsy. It tends to be symptomless, unless a secondary bacterial infection ensues. Radiographic diagnosis of lipid pneumonia must be followed by lung biopsy. Neither presence nor absence of fat droplets in sputum is diagnostic.

Gross appearance. In more active patients, the lesions are mostly in the right middle and lower lobes and the left lower lobe. In those confined to bed, the lesions are found in the upper lobes. There are two possible findings. The commoner lesion is a diffuse process, commencing as scattered foci that subsequently fuse. By then, much or all of a lobe is indurated and noncrepitant, with a pale yellow, solid cut surface. The other finding is the oil granuloma, a well-localized rounded

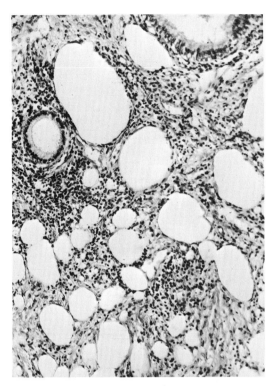

Fig. 23-41 Exogenous lipid pneumonia. Late stage with almost complete replacement of lung structure by fat and fibrous tissue. (×105.)

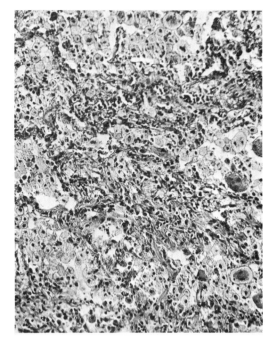

Fig. 23-42 Endogenous lipid pneumonia. Foamy macrophages fill alveoli. (×109.)

area, sometimes with scalloped margins. The firm tumorlike mass can be mistaken for a carcinoma. Neighboring lung may be slightly collapsed or show marked inflammatory changes in the bronchi.

Microscopic appearance. The important characteristic of exogenous lipid is its existence, either free or in macrophages, as clear droplets. In the early stages, these are in the alveoli, accompanied by neutrophils. Macrophages become so numerous that the air spaces are filled. Alveolar phagocytes become cuboidal, merge into giant cells, and rest on a fibrous framework. The inflammatory reaction becomes lymphocytic. Lung structure in the involved area is rendered totally abnormal (Fig. 23-41). Terminal bronchioles are dilated. Small arteries have undergone obliteration by intimal proliferation and medial fibrosis. Fat droplets are released from the macrophages. Foreign body giant cells and Langhans' giant cells, aided by the presence of epithelioid cells, create a resemblance to an infectious granuloma. If some of the lipid is present as cholesterol, it gives the macrophages a foam instead of a bubbly cytoplasm, but cholesterol needles are not seen. Within a few hours of cod-liver oil entering alveoli,

a hyaline membrane forms around the oil, and well-marked foreign body giant cell reaction is stimulated. This oil can be resorbed with minimal fibrosis if the dose is small.

The Liebermann-Burchardt reaction demonstrates cholesterol in sections. Cod-liver oil is stained by scarlet red and Nile blue sulfate and forms a black precipitate with osmic acid. Mineral oil is stained by scarlet red and is nonreactive with osmic acid.

Endogenous lipid pneumonia

The endogenous variety of lipid pneumonia, of which cholesterol pneumonitis is an example, is the result of metabolic, allergic, neoplastic, or inflammatory processes that release lipid by causing tissue breakdown. The commonest causes are nonresolving pneumonia, carcinoma, and abscesses[112] (Fig. 23-96). Naked-eye differentiation from the exogenous form is impossible. Of course, there is no gravitational distribution, but instead there is a relationship to the primary condition. The lipid tends to be finely dispersed in the cytoplasm of macrophages, changing them into foamy macrophages (Fig. 23-42), whereas large intracytoplasmic droplets (vacuoles) in macrophages or giant cells characterize exogenous lipid pneumonia. The interalveolar fibrosis and later replacement of lung tissue are the same as seen with exogenous lipid.

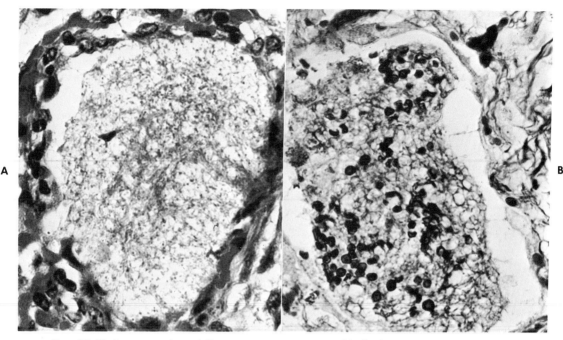

Fig. 23-43 *Pneumocystis carinii* pneumonia. **A,** Minute black dots are individual nuclei. **B,** Alveolus shown in **A** stained with methenamine silver. Dark spheres are capsules of individual organisms. (**A,** Hematoxylin and eosin; ×600; **B,** ×600.)

The lipid results from hyperactivity of type II pneumonocytes whose laminated cytosomes are extruded in excessive numbers into the alveolar spaces, which may reflect excessive surfactant production. Free in the alveoli, the type II inclusion bodies are taken into pulmonary macrophages, which feast on them until bloated and inactive. Lipid is released on the death of these cells and is sufficiently irritative to induce interstitial fibrosis.[102]

Pneumocystis carinii pneumonia

Also known as plasma cell pneumonia, *Pneumocystis carinii* pneumonia is a rare disease in the United States but is common in central Europe. Large numbers of the protozoon *Pneumocystis carinii* are present in the alveoli and are presumed to be responsible for the disease, the occurrence of which is mainly confined to the first few months of life. The infantile cases usually arise in epidemic form, but in some cases the children affected have been debilitated or have had abnormalities of gamma globulin. Many of the cases in adults and some in children are associated with leukemia, lymphoma, or cytomegalic inclusion disease. There are three clinical varieties and a subclinical form.[111]

Up to 30% or 40% of the infants die and are found to have voluminous, gray-pink, firm, airless lungs. There is no pleuritis. The cut surface reveals confluent or completely homogeneous, firm, dry, gray tissue. The regional lymph nodes are unaltered, and the bronchi are empty.

Microscopically, the alveoli are filled with a foamy, pale, eosinophilic substance. In it are faintly staining dotlike bodies surrounded by a little clear space and a capsule, each no more than 1 μm in diameter (Fig. 23-43, *A*). As many as eight of these may be gathered within a cyst of 8 μm to 12 μm in diameter. Lymphocytes, monocytes, and plasma cells distend the interalveolar septa in typical cases. The plasma cells are often predominant but in a number of reports have been totally absent, particularly in cases secondary to hematologic diseases. Hematoxylin does not always stain the individual organisms, which are seen much better with the periodic acid–Schiff method. Gomori's silver methenamine staining brings out the cysts very well (Fig. 23-43, *B*).

Variants of the disease are beginning to appear. Occasionally, typical granulomas containing parasites have appeared in the lung, sometimes progressing to fibrosis and calcification. More surprising are the reports of patients who not only have pneumocystosis of

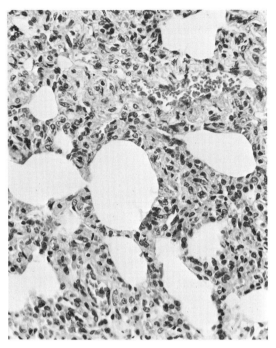

Fig. 23-44 Advanced interstitial viral pneumonia. (×288.)

the lung but also of the spleen, liver, lymph nodes, and bone marrow.[100]

Interstitial pneumonia

Although viral pneumonia is discussed elsewhere, it is necessary to mention the microscopic findings here to distinguish them from the pneumonias just described.[103, 107, 108, 116] At least some cases of organizing pneumonia are a combination of chronic interstitial pneumonia and superimposed acute pneumonia.[108] Many of these cases also may merge with diffuse interstitial pulmonary fibrosis.

In uncomplicated interstitial pneumonia, the exudate is in the interalveolar septa. These are greatly thickened by increased numbers of reticulin fibers and a gathering of lymphocytes, plasma cells, and histiocyes (Fig. 23-44). Cuboidal metaplasia may occur in the alveolar lining. Some alveoli are greatly reduced in size, while nearby there may be focal emphysema. It is Gross' concept that not only may connective tissue be laid down in the septa but that also fibrosis may be initiated by alveolar cell proliferation on the alveolar surface.[107, 108] Only in the latter case will the air space be compromised.

PULMONARY ABSCESS AND GANGRENE

Causes. The flood of antibiotics has barely dampened the fires of abscesses in the lungs.

The most common cause is inhalation of foreign material. This may be food, decaying teeth, gastric contents, or necrotic tissue dislodged during surgery on the mouth, upper respiratory tract, or nasopharynx. Severely infected gingivae and teeth can be the source of pus draining into the lungs during sleep. When a bronchus has become obstructed an abscess may form distally; this may the first sign of a bronchial carcinoma or an impacted foreign body. Necrosis within a tumor, followed by bacterial infection, leads to an abscess. Severely infected cystic disease of the lung, or bronchiectasis, can develop into an abscess. Another important group of abscesses includes those arising during bacterial pneumonia. The organisms are most likely to be type III pneumococci, *Klebsiella pneumoniae*, staphylococci, and hemolytic streptococci. Only in a minority of cases is an abscess due to septicemia or a septic infarct, as in acute osteomyelitis or bacterial endocarditis. Rare causes are trauma to the lung, and direct extension from a suppurating focus in the esophagus or mediastinum, subphrenic area, or vertebral column.

Distribution. Abscesses of inhalational origin are likely to be in the right upper lobe or in the apex of the right lower lobe. The more vertical course of the right bronchus puts it more in line with the trachea, thus rendering it more receptive to inhaled material. The center of the abscess is the bronchus where the foreign body lodges. Suppuration also begins in a bronchus in bronchiectasis and in bronchial obstruction. It spreads distally in the air passages and is likely to destroy the bronchial wall and spread into the surrounding lung. Tiny foreign particles will set up inflammation in the alveoli and are therefore more likely to approach the pleura. An abscess complicating pneumonia will have no primary relationship to a bronchus. Abscesses in septicemia, usually staphylococcal or streptococcal, are scattered throughout the lungs but are likely to be small and subpleural. Septic infarcts are described on p. 889.

Appearance. Sympneumonic abscesses are described in the discussion of pneumonia under each organism. As to the other varieties, an early abscess is yellow or white and firm. Septicemic abscesses have a thin red rim. Soon the center undergoes liquefaction and cavity formation. The lining is ragged, yellow, and necrotic. Odor may be absent or extremely unpleasant, the latter indicating the need for anaerobic as well as aerobic cultures. With time, the pus is likely to become gray or green and to undergo complete liquefaction. Around it is a wall of granulation tissue, which has been erroneously called a pyogenic membrane. An abscess in pneumonia will be surrounded by a wide zone of consolidation, and an abscess in a tumor will be surrounded by tumor tissue. The chronic abscess has a thin, firm, fibrous wall and a greater amount of organizing pneumonia external to it. If originally there was communication with a bronchus, it may have persisted.

Course. Complete healing of a small abscess is possible. Resolution may leave a fibrous scar with a small central sterile cavity. An abscess close to the pleura induces a fibrinous or purulent pleurisy, in turn to be followed by empyema. An abscess can perforate into a bronchus (bronchopulmonary fistula) or into the mediastinum. The fistula promotes further spread through the lung, and a series of small intercommunicating abscesses may appear. Pulmonary septa form no barrier to the inflammation, which can even cross an interlobar fissure if the two surfaces have first been united by adhesions. Serious bleeding will be produced by erosion of a vessel in the abscess wall. A distant complication of pulmonary abscess is dissemination to the brain, which occurs in 5% to 10% of cases. No antibiotics can be expected to repair the damage wrought by larger abscesses. However, the lining is converted into a smooth fibrous wall on which a single layer of squamous or columnar cells can be demonstrated microscopically. The nature of a tension pneumatocele is described on p. 908.

Microscopic appearance. Destruction of alveoli or bronchial tissue is readily recognized, and masses of neutrophils fill the area. The center is likely to be necrotic and, peripherally, individual inflammatory cells are pyknotic. Hypervascularity will be observed at the edges, where plump young fibroblasts are proliferating to form a capsule. Bacterial colonies may be recognized without special stains. Around the abscess, alveoli are likely to be filled with organizing exudate.

Gangrene. The term gangrene is not accurately used with reference to the lung, since there is no massive ischemic necrosis followed by putrefaction. The lesion is, in fact, a rather rapidly progressive abscess in which, in addition to aerobes, anaerobic organisms such as bacteroides, streptococci, clostridia, fusiform bacilli, and spirochetes play an active role. Characteristically, the abscess is not walled off, and therefore destruction is very extensive. There are irregular cavities surrounded by soft, airless, moist, green or black tissue. It is hardly possible to touch this tissue without its breaking, and strands of it float in the foul-smelling pus.

NONNEOPLASTIC ACQUIRED DISEASES OF BRONCHI
Acute bronchitis and bronchiolitis

In adults, acute bronchitis may be restricted to large and medium-sized bronchi. Infection may have descended from the upper respiratory tract or may be airborne. The mucosa is edematous and dark red from congestion. It produces a plentiful mucin that may become purulent and yellow. More severe

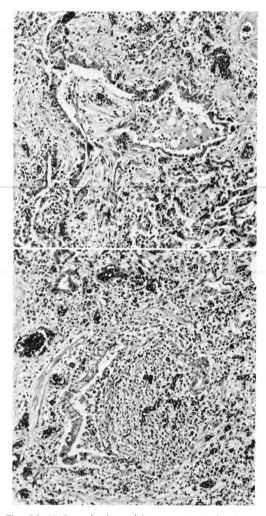

Fig. 23-45 Bronchiolitis obliterans. **A,** Early stage. **B,** Later stage. Young vascular fibrous tissue is growing into lumen of bronchus, organizing exudate and obliterating lumen. (**A** and **B,** ×165.)

inflammation leads to mucosal ulceration. Diphtheria and severe pyogenic infection form a fibrinous membrane covering the mucosa. Necrotizing bronchitis and hemorrhagic bronchitis are the most severe forms, generally occurring in influenza with secondary infection.

This progression is mirrored microscopically. Increased secretion is observed in the glands and goblet cells. Then neutrophils appear in the bronchial wall and migrate into the lumen. Hypervascularity is apparent, and some mucosal cells are cast off, sometimes still in strips. Once the wall is exposed, the inflammatory reaction is heightened. A covering membrane is recognized as a mesh of fibrin with entrapped necrotic leukocytes and epithelial cells.

Acute bronchitis in children[118] *and elderly persons*[117] is important because of accompanying bronchiolitis. In severe cases, there is a laryngotracheobronchitis, which may be associated with acute generalized or interstitial emphysema. Bronchioles are plugged with yellow, mucinous droplets. In acute inflammation, numerous goblet cells are rapidly formed by metaplasia in bronchioles that usually have none. Inflammation follows as in acute bronchitis, and there is bronchopneumonia around the terminal and respiratory bronchioles. The major danger is respiratory failure from blockage of so many bronchioles. There is the risk of obliteration of the bronchioles by fibrous organization of the highly fibrinous exudate (bronchiolitis obliterans fibrosa) (Fig. 23-45). Such a process is akin to what happens to alveolar exudate in organizing pneumonia. Most adult cases have been exposed to poisonous gases. Bronchiolitis obliterans is otherwise rare as a widespread condition.

Chronic bronchitis

The only satisfactory definition of chronic bronchitis is a clinical one, that of the British Medical Research Council, accepted by the American Thoracic Society. It reads: "Chronic bronchitis is characterized by the production of sputum in the absence of cardiac or other pulmonary disease. The sputum must be produced on most days for at least three months of the year and for at least two years." Therefore, if one sees many lymphocytes in a bronchial wall, this is an abnormality that cannot be called chronic bronchitis. I suggest "lymphocytic bronchitis,"

which represents a true inflammatory reaction. In fact, "chronic bronchitis" is a most unsuitable name for the disease we are discussing.

The sputum is produced by an increased number of mucous cells throughout the bronchial tree. The fact that the glands are hypertrophied can be seen (and measured). The Reid index is the ratio of the depth of the glands to the thickness of the mucosa (the

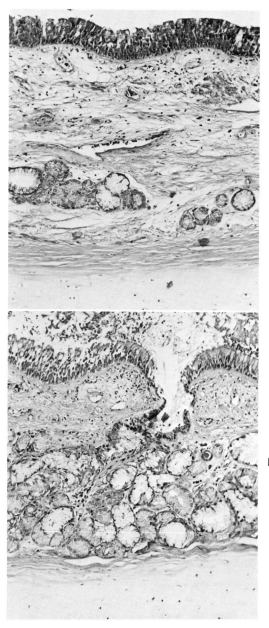

Fig. 23-46 A, Bronchus with normal glands. **B,** Marked hypertrophy and hyperplasia of bronchial glands in chronic bronchitis (gland/wall ratio, about 0.6). (**A** and **B,** ×145.)

gland/wall ratio—0.14 to 0.36 normally but 0.41 to 0.79 in chronic bronchitis)[1] (Fig. 23-46). In bronchioles, where glands are not present, goblet cells are present in large numbers, replacing the ciliated epithelium. Simple histochemical techniques have shown that there are changes in the proportion of different cell types of the bronchial glands, thereby resulting in a change in the components of the bronchial secretion.[1]

The disease has its highest incidence and is most severe in Great Britain, where it causes nearly 10% of all deaths. There is reason to believe that its incidence in the United States is much underrated, mainly due to its being confused with emphysema, an error made even by workers in the field of respiratory disease.[119, 120]

Chronic bronchitis often is provoked by nasal sinusitis, is perpetuated by repeated respiratory infections, and often leads to emphysema and cor pulmonale. Chronic passive congestion of the lungs in heart failure is a common precursor of chronic bronchitis. Climate, air pollution, and cigarette smoking are important external factors, but why it commences and becomes a long-continuing disease is unknown. Evidence from England strongly suggests that *Haemophilus influenzae* and pneumococci are the most common pathogens in chronic bronchitis.

At first, there is mucosal edema with hypersecretion. Later, bacterial infection creates a purulent fluid. This is thought to be the most important factor in causing permanent destruction of the bronchi and bronchioles.[124] Later, the mucosa of larger bronchi is purple, velvety, or granular (hypertrophic) or thin, pale, and smooth, with longitudinal and transverse gray ridges (atrophic). In either case, the wall is thickened, and eventually inflammation spreads into peribronchial tissues, causing patchy pneumonia and a thin investment of fibrous tissue. Here, too, from involvement of terminal bronchioles, lies the origin of some cases of emphysema. Chronic suppuration can cause bronchiectasis.

Microscopically, hyperplasia of the mucous glands and goblet cells of the bronchi occurs at the expense of serous cells and of cilia, so that the increased secretion is removed poorly or not at all, with a consequent risk of bacterial infection. Only during attacks of acute infection is there infiltration by inflammatory cells, with damage to the epithelium. Many patients undergo squamous metaplasia of the mucosa. Large numbers of goblet cells

make their appearance in the bronchiolar epithelium.

Clinical correlation. Chronic bronchitis should be considered in conjunction with the discussion of emphysema, where it is stressed that in life the airways obstruction that both diseases can cause may make them indistinguishable. Further confusion arises from those cases in which chronic bronchitis causes emphysema. Sputum is a manifestation of mucous hypersecretion, but the degree of hypersecretion has little correlation with the patient's disability. That is due to obstruction of small airways, which may be blocked by pus or mucopus and damaged by fibrosis. Careful bronchographic study in severe chronic bronchitis often will disclose a variety of structural and obstructive abnormalities in the peripheral bronchial tree.[125]

It is extremely difficult to recognize wherein lies the airway obstruction which is so serious in chronic bronchitis. Hogg et al.[123a] have proved that in normal persons the resistance to air flow in distal airways is only 25% of the total, the other 75% being provided by the proximal airways. In bronchitis, bronchiectasis, and emphysema, this peripheral resistance is increased at least four times. This is due to mucous plugging and narrowing and obliteration of the small airways.[123a] Accordingly, this group of investigators now uses the term "chronic obstructive disease of small airways."[123b]

Disability can be present in patients who deny habitual expectoration but who have "morning catarrh" or "throat clearing." Most of the excess secretion comes from the glands, but it is the hypersecretion in the peripheral small airways that is mainly responsible for the disturbance of respiratory function.

Infection has not been demonstrated to be a prime cause of the damage, and recent prospective studies by Gregg in London have cast further doubt upon the role of infection.[122, 123] Trials of prophylactic chemotherapy have not reduced the number of exacerbations but have lessened the severity and duration of each episode. Retained secretions are the key factor in the onset of respiratory failure.

"Blue bloaters and pink puffers" is the colorful phrase crystallizing the opposite mechanisms at work in chronic bronchitis and emphysema. Some patients with obstructive pulmonary disease tend to hypoventilate and their Pco₂ rises. They suffer recurrent episodes of CO_2 retention, cyanosis, and

edema, usually in association with a purulent exacerbation of chronic bronchitis. These "blue bloaters" have little emphysema, and oxygen therapy must be carefully controlled so as to avoid CO_2 narcosis. Other patients maintain a normal Pco_2 and remain pink in spite of their difficulty in maintaining ventilation. These emphysematous "pink puffers" have little bronchitis. Their disease is grave, and little can be done to help it, although it is usually safe to give them oxygen.

Bronchiectasis

Bronchiectasis is the persistent dilatation of, and fibrosis around, bronchi resulting from inflammatory damage to their walls. About one-half of the patients give a history of previous pneumonia or bronchopneumonia, particularly during the infectious diseases of childhood. Infection during the course of tuberculosis and cystic fibrosis of the pancreas also belongs in this group. Bronchial obstruction is the other important cause and, in turn, may be due to bronchial tumor, inhaled foreign body, or bronchial compression by diseased hilar nodes or aortic aneurysm. A third group of cases is associated with pulmonary fibrosis, such as the pneumoconioses. What is described as *congenital bronchiectasis* of children and young adults usually is confined to one lobe. It is probably a form of congenital cystic disease in which normal alveolar tissue does not form, but the proximal bronchial tree develops chronic inflammation.

Patients with bronchiectasis cough up great volumes of foul sputum. In some, this is blood stained, and a minority suffer massive hemoptysis. Finger clubbing, chest pain, and exertional dyspnea are fairly common.

Bronchial inflammation leads to hypersecretion of mucus, which becomes infected and viscous. Infection advances into the wall, and its destruction begins. When obstruction comes first, it is followed by hypersecretion and then by infection. In either case, the lung adjoining the involved bronchus participates in the inflammation. The normal expansile forces in the lung can pull on the damaged bronchi, causing them to be widened. There is sufficient cartilage in the first four divisions of lobar bronchi to protect them from dilatation.

Bronchiectasis involves bronchi running more or less vertically, usually in the lower lobes. When found in an upper lobe, it is likely to be secondary to destructive tuberculous lesions. A single site of bronchiectasis is most likely to be due to a relatively large obstruction.

The dilatation is most often cylindrical, a uniform widening of considerable length. Bronchi of a diameter of several millimeters can be found right down to the pleura. No scissors will normally reach as far. Sometimes the widening is fusiform, increasing to a maximum and then diminishing. In the saccular variety, in which the bronchiectasis has changed into a spherical abscess, there are beadlike bulges along the course of the bronchi. These remain even if the inflammatory process is cured.

The early mucosal change is a soft, hyperemic, velvety thickening. Later, there is ulceration, and, with mucosal atrophy, a transverse, linear rope-ladder pattern is produced in which the mucosa is folded over prominent bands of circular muscle. The normal longitudinal mucosal folds provide the vertical lines. In the presence of suppuration, the lining is necrotic with underlying granulation tissue. Small bronchi or bronchioles distal to these areas may have suffered fibrous obliteration. Lung tissue close by the affected bronchi undergoes pneumonitis. Widening of the bronchial arteries and an increase in their communications with the pulmonary arteries are demonstrable. Eventually, the pleura is involved with chronic inflammation and fibrosis. In the end stages, affected bronchi are thickened by mural and peribronchial fibrosis, a reaction diminished by adequate antibiotic therapy (Fig. 23-47, *A*).

Microscopically, the mucosa becomes edematous, ulcerated, and converted into granulation tissue. Loss of epithelium, or conversion of ciliated cells to goblet cells or metaplastic stratified squamous epithelium, is an important aggravating change in nonobstructive cases, for it causes retention of secretion. The wall is extensively infiltrated by lymphocytes and plasma cells. Sometimes, these are collected into submucous lymphoid nodules large enough to raise the mucosa into folds (Fig. 23-47, *B*).

Later, all components of the normal wall are replaced, allowing dilatation. The lining is now very similar to an abscess wall. The end result is a fibrous wall lined by a single atrophic epithelial layer or stratified squamous epithelium.

Complications of bronchiectasis are localized pleurisy, empyema, bronchopleural fistula, lung abscess, acute and chronic pneumonia, cerebral abscess, meningitis, and right

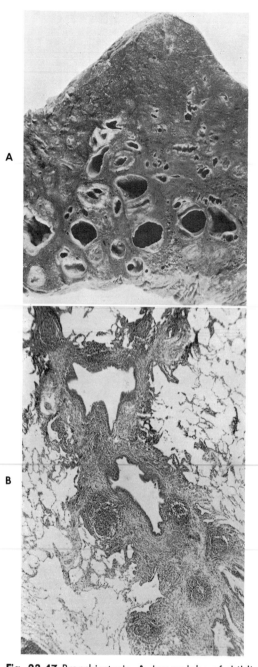

A

B

Fig. 23-47 Bronchiectasis. **A,** Lower lobe of child's lung removed surgically. At lower left is bronchiectatic abscess. **B,** Dilatation and fibrous thickening of wall of bronchiole. Mucosal lining is preserved. Nodular and diffuse lymphocytic infiltration. (**B,** ×40.)

ventricular hypertrophy. Some bronchiectatic cavities have given rise to squamous cell carcinoma and tumorlets.

Foreign bodies in bronchi

Most of the patients who inhale foreign bodies into the bronchi are children. In adults,

aspiration under anesthesia or a sudden gasp while holding something in the mouth is the usual cause. The object tends to enter the more vertical right main bronchus. On becoming lodged, it causes edema and inflammation, which serve to impact it more tightly. Complete obstruction, or a ball-valve action, lets air out only, so that the supplied segment collapses. A check-valve effect, letting air in only, causes hyperinflation. Local pressure is followed by inflammation, ulceration, and suppuration. From this can result bronchial stenosis, bronchiectasis, pneumonia, lung abscesses, or gangrene. In addition, the foreign body may act as a chemical irritant.

Broncholithiasis. Broncholithiasis is the presence of stony bodies in the bronchial lumen. These bodies consist of portions of calcified hilar lymph nodes that have eroded their way into the air passage. Rarely do they come from an intrapulmonary granuloma. The usual site is the left middle lobe bronchus, because a node lies in the acute angle between it and the lower lobe bronchus.

Quite large stony bodies have been recorded. They are calcareous, cartilaginous, or osseous and generally follow tuberculosis or histoplasmosis.

Bronchial fistulas

Three types of abnormal tracts originate in bronchi: bronchopleural, bronchoesophageal, and bronchodiaphragmatic fistulas.

Bronchopleural fistula is the commonest and is a complication of tuberculosis, pneumonia caused by staphylococci, streptococci, and klebsiella, bronchiectasis, lung abscess, and pulmonary mycosis. Complications are tension pneumothorax and empyema.

Bronchoesophageal fistula is less common and is most often the result of an esophageal carcinoma, perforation by foreign bodies, and trauma. Food is inhaled into the lungs.

Bronchodiaphragmatic fistula is least common. Subphrenic and hepatic abscesses, whether pyogenic, amebic, or echinococcal, may cause obliteration of the pleura. The abscess can then penetrate the diaphragm and break into the lung, with eventual communication with a bronchus.

CYSTIC FIBROSIS OF PANCREAS

Cystic fibrosis of the pancreas, a disease still lacking a suitable name, causes the majority of cases of chronic nontuberculous pulmonary disease in children in the United States. The cause is the abnormal and inspissated mucin secreted by the bronchial glands.

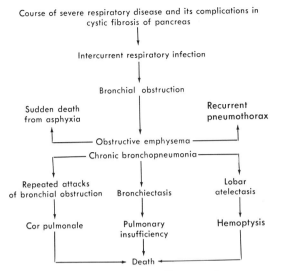

Course of severe respiratory disease and its complications in cystic fibrosis of pancreas

↓

Intercurrent respiratory infection

↓

Bronchial obstruction

Sudden death from asphyxia

Recurrent pneumothorax

—— Obstructive emphysema ——

—— Chronic bronchopneumonia ——

Repeated attacks of bronchial obstruction

Bronchiectasis

Lobar atelectasis

Cor pulmonale

Pulmonary insufficiency

Hemoptysis

→ Death ←

Fig. 23-48 Effects of cystic fibrosis of pancreas on lung. (Slightly modified from di Sant'Agnese, P. A.: Amer. J. Med. **21**:406-422, 1956.)

For a discussion of the subsequent course of events, see p. 1280.

UNUSUAL CAUSES OF PULMONARY CONSOLIDATION
Pulmonary alveolar microlithiasis

The descriptive name pulmonary alveolar microlithiasis is given to a diffuse bilateral filling of the majority of alveoli by calcific concretions called calcospherites. So numerous are they that radiologically they mimic miliary tuberculosis, and yet the disease is asymptomatic for many years. Its existence may be disclosed only by routine chest x-ray examination. Eventually, there is a decrease in vital capacity, leading to pulmonary insufficiency and right ventricular hypertrophy. Sex incidence is about equal, and most patients have been middle-aged, although childhood cases are reported. Familial cases are known, but the cause of the disease is a mystery.

The lungs are very heavy, together weighing 2 kg to 4 kg. Except for some adhesions, the pleura is not affected. Beneath it, gritty particles can be felt, and the lungs are solid and uncollapsed. The basal regions are the most severely involved. If it is possible to cut the lungs with a knife, a grittiness creates much resistance; a saw may be needed to slice the lung. The concretions on the dry, bloodless cut surface glisten in reflected light and may be picked out with the fingernails. Other tissues, including the regional lymph nodes, are not involved.

Microscopic examination shows concentrically laminated calcified bodies in one-fourth

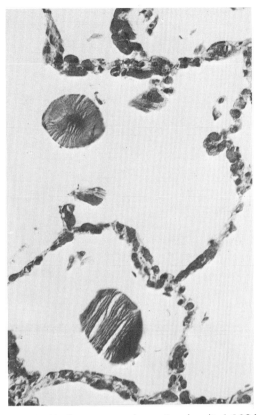

Fig. 23-49 Corpora amylacea in alveoli. (×108.)

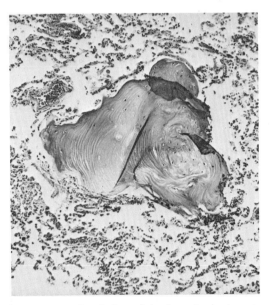

Fig. 23-50 Ossified nodule in mitral stenosis. (×66.)

to three-fourths of the alveoli. Their number depends on the duration and severity of the disease, and their size averages 50 μm to 200 μm. The centers stain more darkly, and they resemble the noncalcified eosinophilic corpora

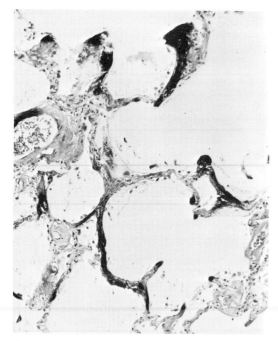

Fig. 23-51 Metastatic calcification. (×105.)

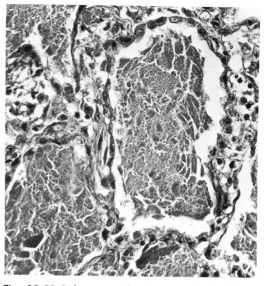

Fig. 23-52 Pulmonary alveolar proteinosis. Prominent alveolar lining cells. (Hematoxylin and eosin; ×330.)

amylacea commonly and incidentally found in the pulmonary alveoli of aged individuals[126] (Fig. 23-49). Ossification is sometimes seen around the calcospherites, but this is not to be confused with the ossified nodules of mitral stenosis (Fig. 23-50). The alveolar walls may be unaltered, but many areas have undergone marked fibrous thickening.

Metastatic and dystrophic calcification bear no relationship to alveolar microlithiasis. Metastatic calcification is by far the commoner in the lung, where it appears in routine stains as a blue line marking the alveolar and bronchiolar basement membranes (Fig. 23-51).

Pulmonary alveolar proteinosis

Pulmonary alveolar proteinosis appears to be a rare example of a "new" disease entity. Its microscopic appearance is so characteristic that it can hardly have been overlooked in the past. The first published report, citing twenty-seven cases, appeared in 1958.[130] The total reported number now is over 150 cases.

The disease affects adults, preponderantly men, and is manifested by dyspnea, cough (often with yellow sputum), increasing fatigue, and loss of weight. About one-third of the patients have died after a chronic course. Over the years, cor pulmonale builds up. Although the cause is unknown, exposure to chemicals has been suspected, as has an abnormality of protein formation. Some of the patients also have suffered from thrombocythemia, aplastic anemia, or pneumocystis pneumonia. In approximately 10% of the cases reported to date, patients also have had nocardiosis (not always pulmonary).

Only the lungs are involved. Confluent gray nodules of consolidation appear under the pleura, each as large as 2 cm in diameter. The intervening lung is likely to be affected. In the late stages, no normal lung is recognizable, and a little milky or yellow fluid may be squeezed from the cut surface. Each lung weighs between 1 kg and 2 kg.

The microscopic features are a filling of many alveoli with a finely and coarsely granular eosinophilic material. Within it are fine needle-shaped spaces, deeper eosinophilic, rounded, structureless bodies, desquamated and degenerating septal cells, and other rounded laminated bodies the size of large cells. The alveolar septal cells proliferate in great number and project into the alveoli (Fig. 23-52). They may form multinucleated cells. Their cytoplasm is plentiful and gives the same staining reactions (e.g., periodic acid–Schiff positive and alcian blue negative), as does the material in the alveoli. Vacuolated cytoplasm indicates the presence of lipid. It is possible to see septal cells becoming detached, the nuclei being fragmented or pyknotic and the cytoplasm becoming granular like the alveolar material. As the cells degenerate further, the nucleus disappears and the cytoplasm is transformed into the laminated or round bodies already mentioned.

The alveolar septa are devoid of inflammation or abnormal deposits, and their capillaries appear normal. In some patients, there has been some interstitial fibrosis, but this is not the rule. The proteinaceous content of the alveoli is also to be found in bronchioles, which are otherwise unchanged. It has sometimes been possible to diagnose the disease during life by recognizing the peculiar eosinophilic content of the sputum.

In patients who have recovered, biopsies taken from areas previously shown radiologically to be involved have revealed alveoli that have regressed almost to normal.

Attempts to explain the nature and origin of the alveolar material have been only partly successful. It appears to be palmitoyl lecithin of alveolar lining origin but devoid of surface tension–lowering activity. Such a complex structure militates against its being a passive transudate. Since it is not foreign to the alveolus, this may explain the lack of cellular reaction to it. Possibly it is a metabolic by-product of surfactant.[129]

It is quite likely that there is more than one pathway to proteinosis. One of my patients was a young man who died after a lifetime of repeated pulmonary and dermal infections. A chest x-ray film of good quality, taken a week before death, was normal, yet at autopsy there was extensive bilateral proteinosis. Corrin and King have produced an identical condition by exposing rats to crystabolite, quartz, aluminum, and other dusts. They also showed that the alveolar material originated from type II pneumonocytes.[102] Four young sandblasters have had a rapidly fatal illness characteristic of acute silicosis but were all found to have a combination of interstitial fibrosis and alveolar proteinosis.[127] In a study of thirteen fatal cases of thymic alymphoplasia in infancy, six were found to have a condition microscopically indistinguishable from pulmonary alveolar proteinosis. It is not yet possible to say whether the latter condition is related to hypogammaglobulinemia.[128]

ALLERGIC GRANULOMAS AND RELATED CONDITIONS

To be considered in this discussion are bronchial asthma, Löffler's syndrome, tropical eosinophilia, eosinophilic pneumonias, drug reactions, hypersensitivity pneumonitis due to inhaled organic antigens, Wegener's granulomatosis, lethal midline granuloma, allergic granulomatosis, and angiitis.

Bronchial asthma

It has been suggested that asthma should be defined as obstruction to the airway that changes in severity over short periods of time, either spontaneously or in response to treatment. It appears to be a hypersensitivity reaction related either to allergy or infection, particularly bronchitis.

Few people die directly from asthma. Among sixty-eight fatal cases, asthma was primary in fifty-two and secondary to bronchitis in sixteen. Infection and psychologic factors were most important in precipitating attacks, often of the status asthmaticus variety.[131] Anaphylactic accidents also were important.

Impacted viscid mucous plugs are a significant factor in causing death, but right ventricular failure sometimes plays a role. Bronchospasm is not considered to be a major factor. Estimates have been made of a fatality rate of 1.5 per 1,000 asthmatic patients per year.[135]

The lungs are pale and distended, but not emphysematous. The cut surface reveals thick-walled large and small bronchi. Those of medium and small size are plugged by thick, viscid mucus (Fig. 23-53).

Microscopically, the lumina of all bronchi contain eosinophilic mucin, in which are many eosinophils and shed epithelial cells. The glands are enlarged and hyperactive, their wide mouths filled with mucin. Many goblet cells are present in the mucosa, the basement membrane of which is thickened many times over into a broad, homogeneous, bright pink, wavy band. The mucosa is thrown into folds by contraction of the greatly hypertrophied muscle coat. This does not necessarily reflect the degree of contraction (spasm) during life (Fig. 23-54). Shedding of the ciliated mucosal cells is prominent, and this is attributed to a transudation of edema fluid from the submucosa.[132] This will greatly impair clearance of the bronchi. The even mingling of the cells and of eosinophils in the bronchial mucus is evidence against the shedding being due to autolysis. Furthermore, bronchial epithelium in some areas displays regenerative activity, including mitoses. There is no satisfactory explanation for the thickening of the basement membrane.

Recent work has disclosed additional antigens causing asthma. Among them in atopic subjects in Britain and the United States are the spores of *Aspergillus fumigatus,* which grow within their lungs, although not causing the disease aspergillosis.[134a] This demonstrates type I of the four different types of allergic reaction in man.[134] The reaction is in the bronchi, whereas in nonatopic subjects the invasive and destructive form of aspergillosis occurs. Dutch workers have uncovered the role of acarine mites of species of the genus *Dermatophagoides* as the antigen of house dust, bedding, and human dander.[133]

Löffler's syndrome; tropical eosinophilia

In 1932, Löffler described a group of patients with an infiltrate seen radiologically to consist of transient, irregular, small opacities throughout the lung. Many of the patients appear to have asthma, and all have respiratory symptoms. There is a peripheral blood eosinophilia of up to 50% or 60%. No specific infecting or infesting agent has even been demonstrated, and the condition is benign.

Accordingly, there has been little material for pathologists to study. The salient features are massive filling of alveoli with eosinophils, some macrophages and giant cells, and eosinophilic infiltration of bronchial walls, which have thick hyaline basement membranes.

An allied condition is *tropical eosinophilia.* Seen widely in India, Malaysia, China, the Philippines, Polynesia, Africa, and the Caribbean, persons suffering from it have roentgenographic findings resembling those in Löffler's syndrome. They are sicker, with fever, severe, persistent coughing, and a prolonged illness with blood eosinophilia. Use of a filarial complement fixation test[138] shows that in many the condition is a hypersensitivity reaction to circulating microfilariae. These are still unidentified and are considered to be of a type infecting animals and incapable of a complete cycle in human beings. This work does not exclude alternative causes such as ascariasis, fungi, mites, and molds.

The lung is covered by a fibrotic pleura. Its cut surface is a blend of small hemorrhages and gray-white nodules up to 1 cm in size. Microscopically, many eosinophils are found in the alveoli and interstitium, with smaller

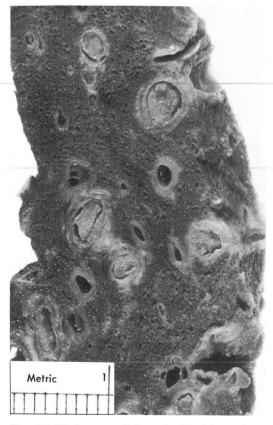

Metric   1

Fig. 23-53 Portion of formalin-fixed lung from patient dying in status asthmaticus. (From Rezek, P. R., and Millard, M.: Autopsy pathology, Charles C Thomas, Publisher.)

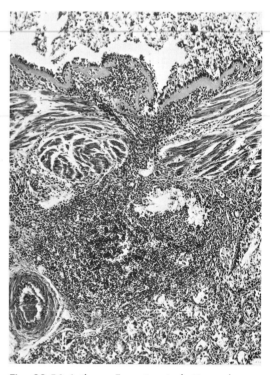

Fig. 23-54 Asthma. From top to bottom: desquamated epithelium, thickened basement membrane, muscular hyperplasia, dense infiltration by eosinophils, and glandular hyperplasia. (×75.)

numbers of lymphocytes and plasma cells. Eosinophils also are present in the secretion filling the bronchi. Foreign body–type granulomas are present in the inflammatory foci. Elsewhere there is interstitial fibrosis.

Eosinophilic pneumonias

Liebow and Carrington[151] discuss all the varieties of pulmonary disease with eosinophilia. They then present a number of cases of eosinophilic pneumonia, a chronic severe illness with fever, night sweats, weight loss, and dyspnea. Only some of the patients had asthma. X-ray films showed rapidly progressive, dense, peripheral infiltrates. In biopsy material, alveoli are filled with eosinophils and vacuolated mononuclear cells. The former may be so packed as to resemble abscesses with necrotic centers and granulomatous response. Eosinophils, with a smaller number of plasma cells and lymphocytes, infiltrate the interstitial tissues and the walls of small bronchi and bronchioles. Although the cause is unknown, the prognosis is generally good, particularly if the patient responds to steroids.

This disease bears some resemblance to infection by *Aspergillus fumigatus* in which growth in the medium-sized bronchi of atopic individuals causes a mixed type I and type III reaction. It is more severe because the reaction is around, as well as in, the bronchi, with alveolitis in addition. Superimposed on asthma are repeated, transient pulmonary infiltrations, eosinophilic pneumonia, and thick bronchial mucous plugs at the site of which there is an irregular bronchiectasis, possibly due to a type III reaction focally in the wall.[137]

Drug reactions

Detailed consideration of the allergic types of drug-induced lung disease is not possible here. Davies has presented an extensive review.[139] Some examples are asthma induced by many antibiotics, radiopaque organic iodides, antisera, vaccines, pituitary snuff (see below); pulmonary eosinophilia due to nitrofurantoin; hydralazine-induced systemic lupus erythematosus. What appears to be an allergic lung disease in drug addicts is, in fact, cumulative pulmonary vascular obstruction due to insoluble particulate contaminants in the intravenously administered drugs (see Chapter 6).

Hypersensitivity pneumonitis due to inhaled organic antigens

Certain conditions hitherto regarded in isolation can now be gathered under the heading hypersensitivity pneumonitis due to inhaled organic antigens. Their symptoms and pathologic manifestations are similar but their origins diverse.

Group I—Antigenic molds (thermophilic actinomycetes, genus *Micropolyspora*)
Moldy hay
  Farmer's lung (p. 935)
  Fog fever in cattle
Moldy residue of sugar cane
  Bagassosis (p. 935)
Compost for growing mushrooms
  Mushroom worker's disease
Contamination of air-conditioning and heating systems[140a]

Group II—Antigenic bird droppings
Bird-breeder's lung (pigeons; budgerigars)

Group III—Antigenic fungus in dead wood
Maple bark–stripper's disease (*Cryptostroma corticale,* which may persist in the human lesion and be mistaken for *Histoplasma*)[140]
Sequoiosis (redwood sawdust; fungus)
Suberosis (oak and cork dust; fungus not identified)

Group IV—Antigen in wheat flour (*Sitophilus granarius;* wheat weevil)

Group V—Antigen porcine and bovine posterior pituitary
Pituitary snuff-taker's disease

Bird-breeder's (fancier's) lung. All of the foregoing groups of conditions represent a type III (Arthus) allergic reaction. Manifestations are directly related to the intensity of exposure. Intermittent exposure results in attacks coming on acutely after five or six hours, the patient having fever, malaise, and muscle pains followed by cough and dyspnea. Regular, frequent exposure results in the insidious development of the disease, concealing the causal relationship. The morphologic responses are mainly in the alveolar tissues, and x-ray films show miliary infiltrations either basally or widespread. There is weight loss.

Only biopsy material is available as yet from bird-breeder's lungs. Alveolar septa are thickened by an infiltrate of lymphocytes, plasma cells, and histiocytes. In the acute phases, many large foamy macrophages are seen in the alveolar septa and lumina, intermingled with the other inflammatory cells or massed together. Foci of lymphocytes, without germinal centers, are common, especially beside bronchioles. Foreign body giant cells and sarcoidlike granulomas are common (Fig. 23-55). Eosinophils, vasculitis, and necrosis are not found.

When the disease becomes chronic, the characteristic foam cells of the early phase are diminished but, as shown in Fig. 23-56, obliterative and fibrotic changes ensue, and the basic lesion becomes chronic interstitial pneu-

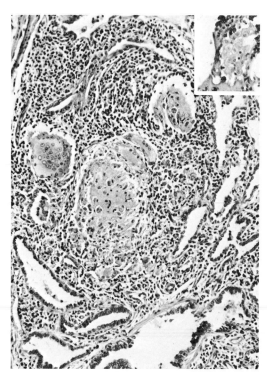

Fig. 23-55 Hypersensitivity pneumonitis. Small sarcoidlike granulomas have formed in relation to several bronchioles and are accompanied by leukocytic and plasmacellular reaction. Inset, Foam cells that were found in another part of same slide. Allergen was not identified in this case. (×177.)

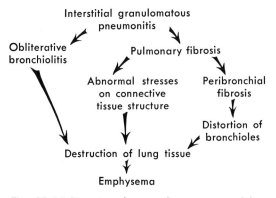

Fig. 23-56 Diagram showing how interstitial hypersensitivity (granulomatous) pneumonitis can lead to permanent pulmonary damage. (From Schlueter, D. P., Fink, J. N., and Sosman, A. J.: Ann. Intern. Med. **70:** 457-470, 1969.)

monia with fibrosis.[141] This variant of the condition is now called "extrinsic allergic alveolitis"[139a] (p. 943).

We see, then, that cases of hypersensitivity pneumonitis have microscopic features in common with sarcoidosis and diffuse interstitial pneumonia. It may be that the latter two diseases also may be related to pulmonary hypersensitivity. The reader must remember the following maxim when evaluating lung biopsies—if a dyspneic nontubercular patient has widespread miliary or nodular opacities on radiologic examination, consider first hypersensitivity pneumonitis. Of all the forms so far known, the most severe is farmer's lung (p. 935), but there must be many so-far unrecognized causes of interstitial inflammation with sarcoidlike granulomas. New sources of environmental contamination are constantly being found (in malt workers, furriers, coffee workers), often allergenic fungal spores.

Wegener's granulomatosis

Klinger described this condition as a form of polyarteritis nodosa, but Wegener is credited

with separating the two processes. Using Rössle's definition of pathergy as "the totality of the morbid phenomena which can be produced by a state of altered reactivity," Fienberg[149] prefers the term "pathergic granulomatosis" for this condition. The disease is a pathologic triad consisting of (1) necrotizing granulomas in the nose, the paranasal sinuses, and the lung, (2) vasculitis of small arteries and veins, and (3) glomerulitis. Clinically, there is a corresponding triad of intractable rhinitis and sinusitis, nodular pulmonary lesions with cough and hemoptysis, and terminal uremia.

As of 1969, at least 150 cases have been reported. All have been fatal, usually within six months, with a few patients lingering up to four and one-half years.

It is important to me to preserve the "sanctity of the syndrome." Unless an error by earlier writers can be demonstrated or new information added that must modify earlier opinion, one cannot include cases satisfying only two of the three criteria. Carrington and Liebow have recognized this in reporting cases of necrotizing pulmonary granulomatosis under the title "limited forms of angiitis and granulomatosis of Wegener type."[146] Some of these patients have had multiple, bilateral, round masses in the lungs which have been classified microscopically as a lymphomatoid variant of "limited Wegener." On the other hand, some patients with the triad have additional evidence of vasculitis in the spleen, synovia, central nervous system,[145, 148] orbit, breast, and skin, so that the patient may be first in the care of a dermatologist, a neurologist, an ear, nose, and throat specialist, or a general physician.

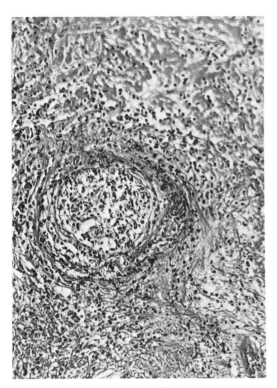

Fig. 23-57 Wegener's granulomatosis. Remnants of artery destroyed by vasculitis and surrounded by inflammatory and necrotic tissue. (×150.)

The paranasal sinuses are filled with thick pus and lined by thickened mucosa. There are ulceration and partial destruction of the bony walls of the sinuses, so that the disease may encroach upon the central nervous system. Many patients have ulceration of the lips, tongue, nasopharynx, larynx, and trachea. Microscopic examination of all such mucosal lesions reveals, apart from shallow or deep ulcers, a heavy infiltration by lymphocytes and plasma cells. This also involves walls of small vessels. In their walls and in the tissues are giant cells, necrosis, and fibroblastic reaction.[150]

The kidneys are slightly enlarged and may be pale or have petechiae on the surface. Small infarcts also may be seen. The microscopic findings include focal necrotizing glomerulitis of 10% to 70% of the glomeruli. It is a fibrinoid type of necrosis that usually affects only one or a few tufts. Later stages ("healing") of such lesions are represented by hyalinization, proliferation of capsular epithelium, or fibrous crescent formation, and by capsular adhesions. Necrosis also will be seen in the afferent arterioles and small renal arteries. Similar granulomatous and arteritic changes will be observed in the other sites previously mentioned.

Our present interest is in the lungs. In advanced cases, these are large and nodular. Over such nodules is a fibrinous pleuritis. When the lung is cut, several well-circumscribed firm areas are disclosed. Their centers tend to be softer than the rubbery periphery and are yellow or red-brown compared with the gray of the edges. There may be central cavitation. Some reach a diameter of 5 cm, but 3 cm is average. Infarcts of various sizes also are present. Small ulcers of the bronchial mucosa are common.

The key to the diagnosis is the microscopic demonstration of arteritis and phlebitis away from large areas of necrosis. Unlike polyarteritis nodosa and hypersensitivity angiitis, fibrinoid necrosis and eosinophilic infiltration of vascular walls are almost never seen. Most of the involved vessels are 2 mm or less in diameter. All their layers are infiltrated by lymphocytes and plasma cells, with some histiocytes and rare giant cells. A simple (nonfibrinoid) necrosis and abundant granulation tissue replaces much of the wall and narrows the lumen. Similar changes are seen in nearby small bronchi and bronchioles. Initial lung biopsies have been mistakenly diagnosed as rheumatoid lung disease, because Wegener's lesions sometimes closely mimic rheumatoid granulomas.

It can be difficult to prove the diagnosis microscopically because necrosis may destroy the evidence of vasculitis. Necrotic areas tend to be confluent. They may show no residue of structure or have a hazy stromal pattern in which there is cellular debris. Beyond the necrosis is a zone of granulation tissue with lymphocytes, plasma cells, and neutrophils. Eosinophils are not part of the typical picture of Wegener's granulomatosis in the tissues or in the blood. Giant cells of foreign body type and Langhans' type are numerous. Epithelioid cells, so much a part of tuberculoid granulomas, do not appear. At the periphery is a well-formed zone of fibroblasts.

Lethal midline granuloma

The title lethal midline granuloma fits the pathologic findings in a small group of patients suffering from a mutilating, progressive, ulcerating condition of the nose, sinuses, face, palate, and upper respiratory tract, including neighboring bone. Pulmonary, renal, or generalized vascular granulomas have been reported. The disease proves fatal, after a course of one or two years, from hemorrhage, meningitis, or cachexia. The disease's identity has been discussed by Spear and Walker.[144] It has been considered by some to be just one form of vasculitis and by others to be related to Wegener's granulomatosis.[143]

Allergic granulomatosis

Patients with allergic granulomatosis resemble those with Wegener's granulomatosis. They differ in having a definite allergic history, asthma, and blood eosinophilia. There is no upper respiratory tract necrosis, and there is a Löffler type of pneumonia.[152]

Angiitis

The several conditions mentioned here are discussed in detail in Chapter 20.

The variety of *hypersensitivity angiitis* that is rapidly fatal after the administration of a

drug is a necrotizing process very similar to polyarteritis nodosa but, unlike the latter, is prone to affect the lungs, where small infarcts are the result. Heart and kidney are also subject to damage. *Rheumatic arteritis* is not an important differential diagnosis even when it involves the lung.

Polyarteritis nodosa is uncommon in the lungs. There are important contrasts between Löffler's syndrome and polyarteritis nodosa with pulmonary infiltration and eosinophilia.[147]

Unifying remarks

Most pathologists accept the concept of "lymphoma" as referring to definite histologic types having corresponding clinical courses. They also recognize that one type may convert into another or terminate as leukemia. To me, the just-described granulomas of the respiratory tract are analogous to the lymphomas. Certain pathologic types are associated with a certain course, but transformation and borderline cases are known to occur. An attempt to demonstrate this point is shown in Fig. 23-58.

PNEUMOCONIOSIS

A century ago Zenker coined the etymologically correct term "pneumonokoniosis," meaning "dust retained in the lungs." Modern definitions stating that the dust must stimulate fibrosis are incorrect. Pneumoconiosis is the focal deposition in the lungs of dusts that may be inert or may be fibrogenic. "Massive fibrosis" is induced in any pneumoconiosis by an infection, usually tuberculous. The inert dusts are gypsum, cement, and the oxides of tin, iron, and barium. Pure coal dust is almost inert. The harmful dusts are silica, asbestos, bauxite, and beryllium.

All the dusts or fibers inhaled and deposited in the lungs are the result of industrial activity. Anthracosis is imposed upon the inhabitants of a smoky city, and it is fortunate that it is so rarely a significant condition.

What makes a dust dangerous remains a problem that is only partly solved. The usual factors of dose and individual susceptibility are in evidence. Some dusts are more irritant than others. Their solubility is most important, and there is often a significance in size of particle. These points will be amplified in the consideration of the individual dust diseases. At least for a while, the lungs have a powerful defense against dusts in the phagocytes and the blanket of mucin that the cilia constantly move upward.

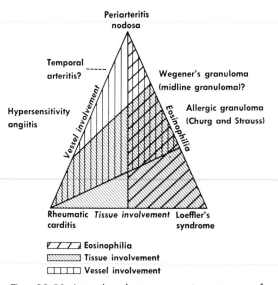

Fig. 23-58 Interplay between various types of vasculitis and granulomatosis in lung. At base are two conditions in which tissue involvement predominates and vascular involvement is negligible. Löffler's syndrome is a benign, transitory eosinophilic infiltration. Proceeding along right side of triangle, there is increasing vascular involvement as we reach allergic granuloma, which combines vasculitis and eosinophilia. Wegener's granulomatosis is closer to periarteritis nodosa, in which eosinophilia is a minor finding; tissue granulomas and vasculitis are prominent. Periarteritis nodosa is antithesis of Löffler's syndrome in that vasculitis is major feature and tissue involvement negligible. Passing down left side of triangle, we encounter conditions with vasculitis and no eosinophilia. In temporal arteritis, tissue involvement is not a feature, nor is it in hypersensitivity angiitis. Finally, we reach rheumatic carditis with its high incidence of tissue changes (Aschoff bodes). (From Sokolov, R. A., Rachmaninoff, N., and Kaine, H. D.: Amer. J. Med. **32:**131-141, 1962.)

Anthracosis and simple coal worker's pneumoconiosis

Anthracosis, a condition closely related to simple coal worker's pneumoconiosis, is the deposition in the lungs of coal dust and soot particles inhaled from the open air. Much of the carbon will be expectorated, but some is taken by macrophages from the alveoli into the pulmonary lymphatic vessels, ending up as fixed cells beneath the pleura, in septa, around vessels and bronchioles, and in the periphery of scars of the lung. This is the well-known blackening seen in virtually every adult lung.

Simple coal worker's pneumoconiosis is seen in those who handle soft bituminous coal—either in the mines or by shoveling it in large quantities. No silicosis is involved. Those coal particles in the dusty air that are not coughed up fill the alveoli and are taken into phagocytes.

The dust penetrates the epithelium of the respiratory bronchioles and then enters the lymphatic vessels as free particles, some traveling to the hilar nodes and others farther, particularly to abdominal lymph nodes. Still others enter the bloodstream and are carried to the liver and spleen.

Some of the dust-filled macrophages return to the interstitium of the interalveolar septa and are prone to collect in alveoli in such relatively fixed areas as the septa and subpleura and around arteries and bronchioles. Because alveoli in such situations have a limited ventilatory excursion, clearance of dust from them is limited.

Coal particles that reach the alveoli are no larger than 5 μm in diameter. They reach all parts of the lungs, but their concentration is greatest in the upper lobes. Carbon is considered to be harmless, and the focal centriacinar emphysema found in coal miners may well be coincidental, similar to that sometimes found in the rest of the population, or else is due to silica contamination in the dust.[4] There is no impairment of health or of ability to work. Some of the dust is carried not to the hilar nodes but to the normal small lymphoid collections. Here, the macrophages are held up indefinitely, and some die, releasing the dust. Grossly visible black nodules and streaks are the result. If these lymphatic vessels are destroyed, the buildup of dust will be greater. Connective tissue response to the particles is irregularly arranged bundles of fibers but not a functionally significant fibrosis.

I have seen an upper lobe totally blackened by carbon and centrally cavitated. Others have reported similar cases with progressive massive fibrosis after prolonged exposure to nonsiliceous carbon dust, probably in areas with previous tuberculosis.[164]

Silicosis and coal worker's pneumoconiosis

Silica (silicon dioxide) and silicates occur all over the world. Wherever rock is to be cut, whether to gain granite, coal, gold, copper, or tin, silica dust is likely to fill the air. In the case of coal, it is the hard or anthracite variety that is accompanied by large amounts of silica. Other workers face the hazard—particularly stonemasons, sandblasters, boiler scalers, and those preparing clay for the manufacture of pottery.

Radiologically, there is a wide network through the lung fields, known as reticulation. At this time, the patient suffers no symptoms. Only with the onset of complications and conglomeration does dyspnea appear.

Role of silica. It has long been believed that were silica totally unsoluble, it would not cause serious disease. It is, in fact, poorly and weakly soluble, but the products of its solution are not the direct cause of disease. Only those particles less than 5 μm in diameter are significant. The apparent importance of particles less than 1 μm and even of ultramicroscopic size (less than 0.2 μm) is now being studied. The nature of the reactive surface area and the total weight of dust present are vital factors. Many more factors are discussed in detail in the publication of American Medical Association's Council on Occupational Health.[153] Current opinion is that silica particles, in conjunction with or coated by the patient's plasma proteins, form an antigen the response to which leads to fibrosis.

Some of the inhaled silica particles will never get past an alveolar lumen. Others will adhere to the alveolar wall, damage the membranous pneumonocyte, and enter the interalveolar space, where they will be taken up by macrophages. A macrophage dies because the ingested particle damages the wall of the phagosome in which it lies, releasing lysosomal enzymes. Chemical substances released from the dead cell are fibrogenic, not the silica itself, and the greater the extent of destruction of macrophages, the greater the fibrosis.[4]

Still more silica particles penetrate the alveolar wall in the free state and can pass in this way to the hilar nodes, where at last they are trapped. When the particles are fine,

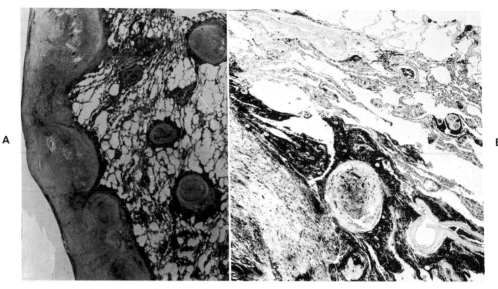

Fig. 23-59 Silicosis. **A,** Silicotic nodules in lung and pleura. **B,** Dense fibrosis with entrapped carbon. In center, silicotic nodule with parallel collagenous fibers. Normal lung above. (**A,** Low power; **B,** ×22.)

some will enter the bloodstream, to be taken up by the liver and spleen.

It takes ten to fifteen years for the disease to develop except in the acute or rapid variety. The earliest symptoms are dyspnea and dry cough. Chest pain, night sweats, and hemoptysis occur later.

Gross appearance. The particles in lymphatic vessels are carried to the pulmonary lymphoid nodules at the bifurcations of major vessels and airways. Dying macrophages begin their irritative reaction in these sites, and the earliest lesions are only 1 mm or 2 mm in size, mostly in the upper lobes. It is nodularity that gives silicosis its unique appearance among the pneumoconioses. The nodules are fibrous and slowly increase in size until they can be recognized on roentgenographic examination. As nodules reach the surface of the lung, pleural adhesions are formed. Whatever anthracotic pigment is inhaled tends to be caught in the nodules, blackening them. By the time the patient dies of the disease, all parts of the lung are affected, the pleural cavities may be obliterated, and the nodules are readily palpated. They are black or gray-white and hard and grate when cut. In an advanced case, the lungs may be almost completely solid. The hilar nodes are much enlarged, and their cut surface resembles the nodules. Important complications are emphysema, bronchiectasis, and cor pulmonale. Any cavities found should be considered to be a complicating tuberculosis until proved otherwise (see following discussion).

Microscopic appearance. The silica indirectly provokes connective tissue proliferation, and this becomes collagenous and densely hyalinized. The fibers are arranged in concentric bands that may interweave—a pattern seen much better with a reticulin stain. (Fig. 23-59). No inflammatory reaction is present, but there may be some central necrosis. The periphery usually is quite sharply demarcated, although strands may weave into the neighboring interstitium of alveolar septa. Most of the trapped carbon will be at the periphery, where the silica mainly lies. Silica crystals can be seen only with polarized light. The nodule may obliterate perivascular lymphatic vessels or destroy an arterial or bronchial wall.

Variants of silicosis

Silicosis with tuberculosis. In some countries, two-thirds of the men with silicosis also have pulmonary tuberculosis. According to other reports, it occurs in 10%—still a high incidence. Large nontuberculous cavities occur in a minority of patients with silicosis as a result of ischemia and necrosis.[165] There appears to be a synergism between silica and tubercle bacilli. In a number of patients, the disease advances fast and is fatal. It has been shown experimentally that the bacilli reproduce more rapidly in tissues in the presence of silica and that strains not normally virulent lead to progressive tuberculosis in guinea pigs made to inhale quartz dust.

This type of tuberculosis is a central caseation of silicotic nodules with a peripheral reaction of tuberculous inflammation. The usual tubercles will be found in the nonsilicotic areas of the lung.

Progressive massive fibrosis. Progressive massive fibrosis (tuberculosilicosis; conglomeration) also is known as complicated pneumoconiosis. Following the onset of tuberculosis or a nonspecific infection in a patient with preexisting silicosis, conglomerate areas of fibrosis will develop (Fig. 23-60). These masses are irregular and slowly enlarge. There is occasionally central cavitation due either to caseation or to ischemia. Ischemic cavities tend to be small and slitlike and contain nonpurulent black fluid. They are caused by the vascular obliteration induced by the fibrosis. Small branches of the pulmonary artery are compressed and often totally fibrosed. The tuberculosis is not typical of tuberculosis in a nonsilicotic lung, and tubercles may not be seen. Mycobacteria may be hard to isolate from the lesions, and in some patients there is no demonstrable cause of massive fibrosis.

Bronchitis and emphysema become superimposed upon the pneumoconiosis. Emphysema and cor pulmonale are now much more important causes of death in silicosis than any other complication.

A black lung with the features of silicosis is found in *graphite* miners and those who work with the dust. Once again, silica is the fibrogenic agent.

Diatomite fibrosis. Diatomaceous earth contains fossil diatoms of almost pure silica less than 1 μm in diameter. The disease produced in those who mine or work with it appears in one to three years. It causes not a nodular but a linear fibrosis of the pulmonary stroma. This is similar to the effects of pneumoconiosis due to fuller's earth, a complex silicate.[167]

Rapid silicosis. Rarely, in men suffering heavy exposure to silica, typical silicosis will appear in two years. One reported case is that of a sandblaster who developed silicosis in seventeen months and died two years after starting his occupation.[163] The authors who reported the case quote the estimate that this would require exposure to 100 million particles of pure silica per cubic foot of air. The patient's lungs weighed 3,750 gm, and the right ventricular myocardium was 1 cm thick.

Rheumatoid pneumoconiosis. A modification in the pattern of silicosis has been ob-

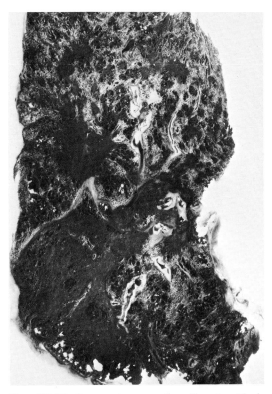

Fig. 23-60 Progressive massive fibrosis. Black areas were almost stony hard, due not to calcification, but to dense collagenization. Small dark areas are nodular lesions of silicosis.

served in coal miners who develop rheumatoid arthritis.[154] It is a superimposition of the typical rheumatoid nodule upon silicotic lesions of a rather massive and extensive nature. This may occur quite early in the disease. Calcification, rare in progressive massive fibrosis, is seen in rheumatoid pneumoconiosis. The disease has been seen not only in coal workers, but also in sandblasters, potters, persons working with asbestos, and those working in foundries. Not all patients with pneumoconiosis and extrapulmonary rheumatoid disease develop rheumatoid lung lesions. A good account of rheumatoid pneumoconiosis is found in the article by Rickards and Barrett.[166]

Asbestosis

Asbestosis differs from the other dust diseases in that the irritant particles are relatively large, occurring in the form of fibers up to 50 μm by 0.5 μm. These are derived by crushing the rock in which the fibers are up to 2 cm long. Asbestos dust contains the microscopic fibers of this silicate. There is danger, therefore, to the miners, to the crushers, and to workers in the many industries employing asbestos (fire-resistant materials, paper, plastics, brake linings, acoustical tiles, etc.). The products are ubiquitous. Usually, the disease develops about fifteen years after exposure commenced, but occasionally this time is very much shorter. Breathlessness and cough appear relatively early, even when radiologic changes are minimal or absent.

Of the different types of asbestos, chrysotile is the commonest used. Compound silicates are formed in such a way that the crystals are fibrous.[155] Certain aspects of the disease have altered in recent years. Pulmonary fibrosis in factory workers due to exposure to the dust has become uncommon, and when it does occur is less severe than it used to be.[160] This is a reflection of better protective measures. Other workers are now being affected (e.g., builders and insulators). The whole atmosphere of a town having an asbestos factory can be polluted, and even in a clean city like Miami in 1965, asbestos bodies were found at autopsy in the lungs of 20% of women and 30% of men.[169] (Gross and Thomson have taken opposing sides in the controversy as to whether all ferruginous bodies are to be considered asbestos bodies.[157] The point is critical with regard to the potential dangers of our urban air. Gross insists that any number of artificially produced materials in the form of transparent fibers of respirable size can cause the development of "typical" ferruginous bodies undistinguishable from asbestos bodies. A preliminary study of ferruginous bodies in residents of Pittsburgh has shown that their unidentified cores were not chrysotile.[158])

Pathogenesis. The flexible, sharp-pointed fibers at first lie in the respiratory bronchioles, where they act as physical rather than chemical irritants. Nearly all of them are in the lower lobes. In time, a number pass into alveolar ducts and alveoli. The response is proliferation of connective tissue (later to be hyalinized) around the respiratory bronchioles and in the interalveolar septa, interlobular septa, and visceral pleura. The functional effect is an alveolocapillary block that causes symptoms to appear early. British workers noted an increased incidence of tuberculosis in these patients. This was in the 1940's, when the level of dust exposure was far greater than it is now; concomitant tuberculosis has virtually disappeared. Those who have had lengthy industrial exposure (twenty years or so) have at least a tenfold risk of developing lung carcinoma in the affected lobe. Furthermore,

there is a heightened susceptibility to pleural mesothelioma (p. 986) or, through the diaphragm, peritoneal mesothelioma.[156, 168] A patient seen by me developed mesothelioma thirty years after six months of exposure to asbestos. Asbestos could still be found in the lung sections. Although the risk of carcinoma is greatest in those exposed to asbestos for more than twenty years (whether or not they develop fibrosis), mesothelioma can arise earlier and from smaller doses.[161]

Gross appearance. An immediately noticeable change is great pleural fibrosis, frequently sufficient to obliterate the pleural space around the lower lobes. The pleura is so thick that it becomes rigid. Such a change is most characteristically seen as wide hyaline plaques of a cartilaginous consistency. They are composed of dense laminated acellular collagen, presumed to be a reaction to asbestos. In advanced disease, the lung is firm and small, the lower lobe being more severely damaged. The cut surface of the lung is a sponge of alveoli and bronchioles surrounded by a fibrous network. Eventually, the fibrosis obliterates much lung tissue. Cor pulmonale and bronchiectasis are common. Because the asbestos fibers are too large to enter lymphatic vessels, there is no significant change in the hilar nodes.

Microscopic appearance. There is the interstitial fibrosis that the foregoing considerations would lead one to expect. Fibrosis begins around bronchioles, slowly extending into and obliterating alveoli. Many alveolar cells have undergone cuboidal metaplasia. Later, alveolar lumina are filled by fibrous tissue, although special stains will reveal an intact elastic framework. The fibrosis will envelop and destroy many lymphatic vessels, bronchioles, and small vessels. It is erroneous to regard the well-known asbestos bodies as pathognomonic. First, lungs commonly contain asbestos bodies without the disease asbestosis being present. Second, patients with talc pneumoconiosis have in their lesions material very similar to asbestos bodies. Third, formation of bodies resembling asbestos bodies is not to be confused with pathogenicity. Although apparently identical, the central fiber may not be asbestos, a fact leading Gross to propose the term "ferruginous body." He was able to produce them in hamsters given fibrous aluminum silicate, silicon carbide whiskers, cosmetic talc, and glass fibers.[159]

The appearance of an asbestos body is not that of a simple fiber. This is hidden beneath a yellow or golden-brown encrustation of iron salts and protein. Uneven deposition of this coat is responsible for the beaded shape with drumstick ends. By this stage of the disease, it is probably not possible for the bodies to move farther. They lie where alveolar spaces used to be and are enveloped in fibrous tissue. Sometimes foreign body giant cells are close by (Fig. 23-61).

Berylliosis

Beryllium and a number of its salts can cause both a chronic and an acute respiratory disease. Miners and handlers of crude beryl and related ores do not suffer from berylliosis. This affects those who extract beryllium from the ores or who handle it in industry, as in the making of alloys. Beryllium is no longer used in the manufacture of fluorescent lamp tubes because of the danger to personnel.

Acute berylliosis is a chemical pneumonitis (bronchoalveolitis) induced by breathing fumes of beryllium oxide during the extraction process. Some patients die in two weeks. Others recover and appear to be well, although their chest x-ray films are abnormal. A third group of patients develop the chronic pulmonary form.

In the acute phase, the lungs are extremely heavy because of great edema. Alveoli are filled with fluid in which are macrophages, erythrocytes, fibrin, and some neutrophils.

To diagnose *chronic berylliosis*, the risk of exposure must be known because of the close resemblance to sarcoidosis. Differential points are the absence, in berylliosis, of ocular involvement, uveoparotid fever, cystic bone changes, or hilar node enlargement without lung disease. Also, sarcoidosis is noted for its change in reactivity to tuberculin. There is also similarity to farmer's lung, in which, again, the occupational history is vitally important. It is now possible to demonstrate minute amounts of beryllium in tissue sections by use of microemission spectrography.[178]

Chronic berylliosis is of insidious onset, with lassitude, shortness of breath, loss of weight, and bilateral pulmonary infiltration shown in x-ray films.

Eventually, the lungs become bulky with emphysema, yet are rubbery from the changes within. There is pleural fibrosis, and the cut surface discloses streaks and nodules of fibrous tissue. The intra-alveolar granulomatous reaction of the early stage spreads to interstitial tissue. Initial lesions coalesce, forming focal, small, gray-white fibrous areas. Small cystic spaces with fibrous walls are also present.

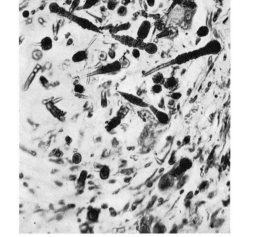

Fig. 23-61 Asbestos bodies. (Approximately ×400.)

Later, the fibrosis increases irregularly, and small nodular fibrotic areas are present in the pleural and hilar nodes. All parts of the lungs are affected. Granulomas also will be found in the skin, liver, kidney, skeletal muscle, and extrathoracic lymph nodes.

Microscopically, the basic lesion is the noncaseating granuloma, formed in vast numbers in the interstitial tissue beneath the pleura, in the septa, and around vessels and bronchi.[170] The earliest lesion is a loose collection of epithelioid cells surrounded by an ill-defined zone of lymphocytes, plasma cells, and Langhans' giant cells. In the latter, and sometimes lying free, may be seen any of three types of foreign body, which also are to be found in sarcoidosis. First is a sharp-edged birefringent, 3 μm to 10 μm crystal, occurring singly or in clumps. It is calcium carbonate in the form of calcite, and it forms the nidus of the second type. Next is the conchoidal (Schaumann) body, so called because of its scalloped margin (Fig. 23-62). It may be as large as 50 μm, it has a concentric, laminated, deeply basophilic structure, and in the very center there may be a refractile crystal. The laminations appear to be successive depositions of calcium and iron upon a beryllium–plasma protein compound.[162] Further investigations suggest that they originate

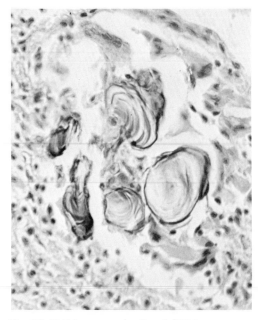

Fig. 23-62 Schaumann bodies. (×390.)

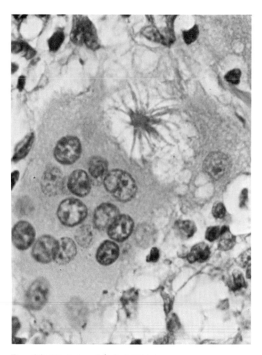

Fig. 23-63 Asteroid. (×1,026.)

from aggregation of residual bodies (end products of activated lysosomes).[171] The third foreign body is the asteroid, which has a delicate, acidophilic, star-shaped cytoplasmic structure (Fig. 23-63). Its occurrence is quite infrequent compared with the 46% incidence of birefringent crystals and 42% incidence of conchoidal bodies in Williams' series.[170] Histochemical methods have failed to establish the composition of asteroids.

The granuloma ultimately undergoes fibrosis, which entraps the surrounding cells (Fig. 23-64). Later still, there is final replacement by hyalinized tissue. Meanwhile, lymphocytes and plasma cells advance into the interalveolar septa, which also become fibrotic, setting up a diffusion barrier to the blood gases. Damage to the alveolar septa results in the cyst formation seen grossly. Granulomas similar to those in the lung are to be found in the hilar nodes and follow the same changes.

Siderosilicosis

Iron oxide appears to be almost innocuous, but frequently a quantity of silica accompanies it. The result is a modified silicosis, seen in hematite miners, welders, boiler scalers and other iron workers, and silver polishers.

The lungs of a miner of pure hematite may be the color of brick but free of fibrosis. When silica also has been present, changes similar to those of coal worker's pneumoconiosis are produced. Some patients have small fibrous nod-

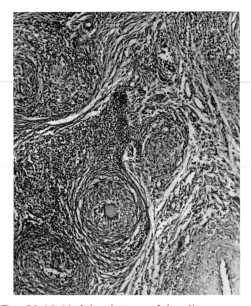

Fig. 23-64 Nodular lesions of beryllium granuloma in subcutaneous tissue. There is lamination of collagenous fibers around central giant cell.

ules in the upper lobes, centrally red and whorled and peripherally dark red-brown. Variable amounts of anthracosis can be present, and pleural fibrosis is marked. Another variety is marked by widespread centriacinar emphysema and a diffuse brick-red fibrosis. Finally, tuberculosis or ischemic necrosis may induce progressive massive fibrosis with cavitation.

All these may be summarized as silicosis with a hematite hue, and the microscopy need not be repeated. It should be pointed out, however, that hematite is orange in polarized light, in contrast to the white of silica, and that tissue reactions around the nodules liberate iron from hematite, so that a Prussian blue stain is positive.

The lungs of silver polishers and arc welders may be blackened by iron oxide dust and fumes, respectively. It is deposited in vessel walls and alveolar septa and fills some alveolar spaces. Once within macrophages, it can give a Prussian blue reaction. Accompanying silica may induce fibrosis in some arc welders.

Talcosis

Workers who prepare hydrated magnesium silicate (talc) or use it in factories may succumb to the fibrogenic impurities that accompany it. Among these is tremolite, which is one mineral form of asbestos. It causes a disease characterized by small fibrous nodules in the lower lobes. The nodes are gray and may coalesce to produce larger fibrous areas that are likely to undergo central cavitation. The absence of carbon distinguishes talcosis from coal miner's pneumoconiosis. Talc particles are taken into macrophages in alveolar septa, around small, but not large, vessels, and under the pleura. They are doubly refractile, irregular, and 1 μm or 2 μm in size. Tremolite fibers will form asbestos-like bodies and will induce further interstitial fibrosis.

INDUSTRIAL LUNG DISEASES

In this section are discussed those inhalational lung diseases in which the noxious agents are molds or fumes.

Bagassosis

Bagasse (from an old word referring to the waste skin left after the oil is pressed out of olives) is the fibrous cellulose part of sugar cane, the residue after the juice has been crushed out. Bagasse still has use—e.g., in the manufacture of insulating materials. When men take it in a dry state from storage, they develop symptoms of hypersensitivity pneumonia, particularly in the upper lobes. This condition results only after several weeks or months of exposure. In some patients, it progresses to interstitial fibrosis with bronchiectasis and emphysema.

The cause is thermophilic actinomycetes, but, whereas the disease was thought to be peculiar to New Orleans in the United States, it has been seen in other countries in which sugar cane is grown and in those to which bagasse is exported.[174, 177]

Farmer's lung

Persons who come into close contact with grain or hay in silage or spoiled by dampness may suddenly become very ill, with dry cough, severe dyspnea, and fever. This disease, known as farmer's lung, is due to sensitization to *Thermopolyspora polyspora* (p. 925) in the moldy grain. In the United States, Wisconsin has had the most cases. Patients require several months to recover, and, if they return to the same work, their illness will recur more severely.

There is an early granulomatous reaction with nodules of poorly defined epithelioid cells and tubercle formation. Langhans' giant cells are found in all cases, but there is no caseation. There is a similarity to sarcoidosis.[180] Distinction from berylliosis may require careful clinical investigation. The inflammation is both interstitial and alveolar, with bronchiolar involvement (Fig. 23-55). The participating cells are lymphocytes and plasma cells. Large clear fibers are sometimes seen in the cytoplasm of foreign body giant cells. Some of the patients have developed interstitial fibrosis, for collagen fibers are deposited around the granulomas and in the alveolar septa.

Farmer's lung is recognized in Britain as an industrial (occupational) disease. By 1968, in a chest clinic serving a population of 90,000 in a rural area of Wales, 245 cases of the disease had been registered.[181] It is most incapacitating when chronic, rather than when acute, and is then productive of airways obstruction. Five autopsies in the Welsh series have shown diffuse interstitial pulmonary fibrosis, honeycombing, histologic changes of pulmonary hypertension, and cor pulmonale. From a neighboring area in England comes an account of the first fatal acute case, a farmer's son who died after a few weeks of illness.[172]

Byssinosis

A nonfatal but disabling disease, byssinosis (Greek *bussos*, an ancient fine textile fiber) occurs in persons who work with cotton, flax, and hemp. It is characterized by its asthmalike symptoms, with severe chronic bronchitis that is never present on Sunday and worse on return to work on Monday. Byssinosis is a nonfibrogenic disease. Round or oval dust bodies are present in the lungs. They may be as large as 10 μm, with a black center surrounded by yellow. It appears that cotton dust contains a substance that releases endogenous histamine from lung tissue, causing bronchiolar contraction. The source is the bract rather than the fibers.

Byssinosis is an interesting disease because it gives the false impression of being due to antigens released in textile dust or from cotton, hemp, or flax and because its existence is so often denied or its eradication falsely claimed.[175]

Diseases due to industrial fumes

Mention already has been made of arc welder's disease and acute berylliosis. The fumes of cadmium and bauxite also are dangerous.

The risk from *cadmium* arises in atomic reactors, electroplating, and the production of alloys. About one in five men exposed to the fumes of cadmium oxide dies. Within the day, the affected person develops dyspnea, cough, and fever—an acute chemical pneumonitis. After a week, there is marked swelling and hyperplasia of the alveolar and bronchiolar lining cells (Fig. 23-65). The condition passes into a chronic pneumonitis with little fibrosis

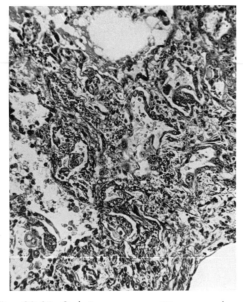

Fig. 23-65 Cadmium pneumonitis, example of chemical pneumonitis. Deformed alveoli lined by hyperplastic septal cells. Air spaces largely occupied by masses of similar cells, including bizarre giant cells.

(mainly peribronchial and perivascular) and without specific findings.

Abrasives are manufactured from calcined *bauxite* at a high temperature, which releases fumes of submicron-sized silica and alumina (corundum). Although the lungs of those who work with these chemicals contain much silica, they do not have silicotic nodules, and the responsible component of bauxite fumes is not known. Aluminium is suspected, for it is no longer considered harmless. Dust of aluminum metal has caused lung disease.

The chemical pneumonitis leads to a diffuse interstitial fibrosis that is followed by pronounced peripheral emphysema with bullae. Spontaneous pneumothorax is extremely common. The hilar nodes undergo a simple enlargement.

Silo filler's disease has sometimes been confused with farmer's lung because of the relationship to grain and farmers. A silo is a large, airtight chamber in which green crops are pressed and kept for fodder. In it, nitrogen dioxide is released by fermentation. The gas is present in greatest amount in the first seven to ten days after the silo is filled. Anyone entering may become unconscious in minutes and never recover. Other patients have had a latent period of several days or weeks.

The oxides of nitrogen are readily soluble in water, forming nitrous and nitric acids. *Nitrous fumes* are a potential hazard in many industries and cause a disease identical to that suffered by silo fillers.[4] Those most severely affected die in a few days from pulmonary edema and chemical bronchopneumonia, with shedding of bronchiolar and alveolar lining cells. Patients with subacute and chronic disease develop severe congestion, and bronchioles and alveoli are filled with blood, macrophages, and fibrin. There may be a hyaline membrane. Cuboidal cells line many alveoli. Later, the exudate organizes, typically resulting in bronchiolitis fibrosa obliterans. Fibrosis occurs widely through the lungs and extends into the alveoli.[179]

PULMONARY FIBROSIS

While the various industrial diseases are causes of pulmonary fibrosis, the term tends to be used in reference to other diseases such as organizing pneumonia (p. 906), lipid pneumonia (p. 912), and brown induration (p. 884). In the section that follows are discussed pulmonary fibrosis as found in several connective tissue diseases, sarcoidosis, and eosinophilic granuloma, diffuse interstitial fibrosis, and fibrosis due to drugs.

First, some general information about alveolocapillary block and honeycomb lung is pertinent. *Alveolocapillary block* is a term coined in 1951 to encompass certain clinical, physiologic, and pathologic changes. There is progressive dyspnea, tachypnea at rest, cyanosis (eventually even at rest), basal rales, and absence of wheezing or evidence of bronchial obstruction. Later, there is right-sided heart failure, and there may be clubbing of digits. There is a reduction of diffusing capacity of the lung and reduced lung volume.[183] The underlying pathologic process is a diffuse and widespread fibrosis of the interalveolar septa, or septal thickening also by fluid, collagen, and proliferated cells of other than connective tissue origin. The usual causes include the following: sarcoidosis, irradiation, the pneumoconioses, carcinomatous lymphangiosis, miliary tuberculosis, eosinophilic granuloma, progressive systemic sclerosis, rheumatoid lung, diffuse interstitial pneumonia, and other granulomas and fibroses of uncertain cause.

Honeycomb lung is an excellent description of a widespread acquired disease in which large numbers of small cysts are formed in fibrotic lungs (Fig. 23-66), the causes being those of alveolocapillary block. The essential change is obliteration, by fibrosis or granulo-

ma, of some of the bronchioles and their subdivisions.[185] Neighboring unaffected bronchioles undergo compensatory dilatation, forming cysts next to consolidated or fibrotic areas. Associated with this is alveolar septal fibrosis, often abetted by chronic pneumonitis or the specific pathologic process in the particular case. Some cysts become lined by flat or cuboidal epithelium, which may be ciliated and mucin secreting (Fig. 23-67). Squamous metaplasia is common, and there is a risk of scar carcinoma (p. 966). The interstitial and pericystic tissue is composed of young fibroblasts, with lymphocytes, plasma cells, histiocytes, some giant cells, and smooth muscle in bundles and single fibers. The last is a form of muscular hyperplasia from air passages and blood vessels. There is much elastic tissue from similar sources.

In a careful study of the musculature of the lungs in chronic pulmonary disease, it has been shown that considerable masses of smooth muscle may proliferate from bronchi, bronchioles, arteries, veins, and lymphatic vessels[186] (Fig. 23-68). The muscle bundles run in various directions in relation to the channels from which they originated. Since these channels tend to become obliterated, both by the primary disease and by the proliferating muscle, muscle seems to arise directly out of interstitial fibrous tissue, the pulmonary septa, or the visceral pleura. To name this process, as some have done, "muscular cirrhosis" is an

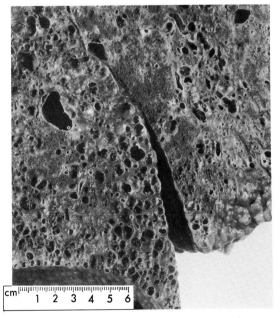

Fig. 23-66 Honeycomb lung showing at bottom right nodularity of pleural surface that has misled some to call condition "muscular cirrhosis."

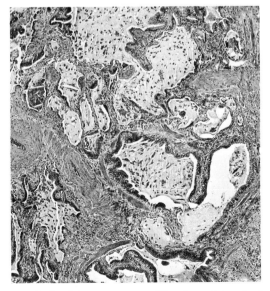

Fig. 23-67 Adenomatous proliferation of terminal bronchiolar cells in fibrous area of lung. (×67.)

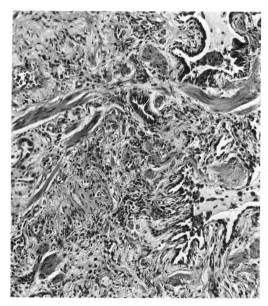

Fig. 23-68 Smooth muscle hyperplasia in fibrotic area of lung. (×102.)

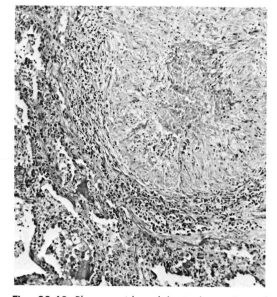

Fig. 23-69 Rheumatoid nodule in lung. Central necrosis with peripheral palisading of reactive cells and outer inflammatory exudate. (×165.)

insensitive misuse of the word "cirrhosis" (Fig. 23-66).

Connective tissue diseases
Rheumatoid lung

The recognition of extra-articular manifestations of rheumatoid diseases has been especially centered on the cardiovascular system, central nervous system, and lungs. The pulmonary lesions differ in that there is a male predominance instead of a female preponderance, as in simple rheumatoid arthritis.

In some patients, pleurisy with effusion accompanies exacerbations of rheumatoid arthritis. In others, it precedes joint disease. A constantly noted characteristic of the pleural fluid is a very low glucose level (less than 10 mg to 15 mg per 100 ml). The common findings in the pleura are nonspecific adhesions and dense fibrosis. Only in a minority of patients have pleural biopsies revealed granulomas similar to those in the subcutaneous tissue.

In addition, there can be interstitial pneumonia, fibrosis, or honeycombing. The earliest change is a nonspecific interstitial pneumonia that can resolve. This is seen as edema and congestion of interalveolar septa. Lymphocytes infiltrate the septa and the area around vessels and bronchioles. Fibrin and some macrophages are in the alveoli.[182]

Should this condition persist, alveolar septa undergo progressive fibrosis. Germinal centers appear in some of the collections of lympho-

cysts, and this is an important clue to the possibility of rheumatoid disease. Nodules form and may be 1 cm in diameter (Fig. 23-69). These are areas of fibrosing interstitial pneumonia, rarely containing small granulomas of the rheumatoid type (central necrosis with infiltrating neutrophils and a wavy palisade of radially arranged macrophages and, beyond this, scanty giant cells and a zone of lymphocytes and plasma cells). The granulomatous reaction is not always so specific, for there may just be the inflammatory cells with small collections of macrophages and areas of fibrosis. Rheumatoid nodules are much commoner in miners with rheumatoid arthritis than in other persons with that disease. In some, the joint lesions appear several years after the pulmonary nodule is recognized.

The next stage is bronchiolectasis, consequent upon fibrosis. Many of the small and medium-sized arteries undergo fibrosis, beginning in the intima, extending into the media, and causing great luminal narrowing. The dilated bronchioles have no cartilage but retain a muscle coat. Their epithelial lining is a single layer of flat or cuboidal cells. Dilatation is eventually great enough to lead to a honeycomb appearance apparent to the naked eye, bronchioles now being surrounded by thick fibrous tissue containing many lymphocytes and plasma cells with occasional macrophages. Septal fibrosis is still apparent, and some alveoli are dilated.

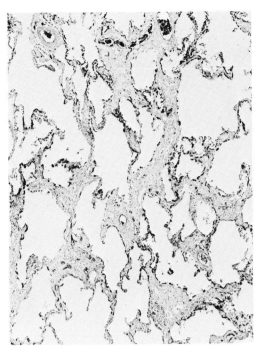

Fig. 23-70 Progressive systemic sclerosis. Severe interstitial fibrosis. (×52.)

A distinct variety of rheumatoid lung disease, Caplan's syndrome or rheumatoid pneumoconiosis, is discussed on p. 931. Rheumatoid lung bears a relationship to some cases of fibrosing alveolitis (p. 942) although Scadding[187] is more cautious about accepting it than is Spencer.[4]

Systemic lupus erythematosus

In systemic lupus erythematosus, pleurisy (with or without effusion) is common and may cause the first symptoms. The patient frequently appears to have nonspecific patchy bronchopneumonia or interstitial pneumonia, with repeated attacks in different areas of the lungs. No diagnostic microscopic features are known, there being eventual fibrosis. In a few lungs, there is arteritis with fibrinoid degeneration.

Progressive systemic sclerosis (scleroderma)

Pulmonary involvement by scleroderma was recognized in the latter part of the nineteenth century. The patients are likely to be women in later life. Localizing symptoms are a dry or productive cough and increasing dyspnea. These may precede the cutaneous findings, and a pulmonary component is rather common. There is an increased collagen-like deposition in the basement membranes of the small pulmonary vessels. In turn, there is fibrosis of the alveolar septa and interstitial tissue (Fig. 23-70). As the arteriolar lumina become narrowed, the alveolar tissues become necrotic, and microcysts are formed. At this stage, the patients have an alveolocapillary block. Fibrosis is progressive, and the lung loses its elasticity. In the end, even the bronchi undergo fibrosis, with areas of constriction and sacculation.

Grossly, the lower lobes suffer most. The pleura is fibrotic. On the cut surface, a network of interstitial fibrosis encloses cystic spaces no bigger than 1 cm in diameter. There are also fibrous nodules of 1 mm to 15 mm in diameter. The cysts are frequently peripheral, and the dense, fibrous, airless areas are central.[184] In the latter, the vascular and alveolar structures are replaced. Bronchiectasis is common. As might be expected, in such far-advanced cases there are pulmonary hypertension and right ventricular hypertrophy.

Microscopically, in the earlier stage the alveolar septa are thickened by cellular proliferation and prominent capillaries. As they are smothered by ever-increasing collagen deposition, the septa undergo disruption and now surround spaces larger than alveoli. Lymphocytes in moderate numbers infiltrate this tissue, and the alveolar lining cells proliferate. Arterioles are obliterated, and slowly, over some years, the fibrosis progresses until in many areas alveoli cannot be recognized. Meanwhile, the inflammatory reaction has abated.

Sarcoidosis

For all its wide geographic range, sarcoidosis (sarcoid, fleshlike) remains a mystery. Its characteristic lesion closely resembles that of any granuloma in a nonnecrotic or noncaseous stage, whether fungal or tuberculous, and it is indistinguishable from berylliosis and certain lesions of leprosy and histoplasmosis. Histologic reactions identical to it are well known in the regional lymph nodes draining a carcinoma.[190] I have seen such lesions develop within a couple of months in a wound resulting from a child falling against a stone step and have been informed of the same results in a person who fell upon a seashell, suggesting the reaction to a siliceous substance. Many patients with sarcoidosis live in pine forest regions (Scandinavia, as well as the northern and southern United States). Pine pollen is an acid-fast substance and, when injected into guinea pigs, produces localized sarcoidlike lesions. In Scotland, Switzerland, and

Japan (among a number of countries), the incidence of sarcoidosis is higher in the non-piney rather than the piney areas. Users of deodorant containing zirconium develop local sarcoidlike reactions.

In Britain, it is thought, in part because of the persistent teachings of Scadding,[196] that sarcoidosis is a manifestation of tuberculosis. In his series of 230 cases, tubercle bacilli were isolated from eighteen patients in the sarcoid phase, from eleven during overt caseating tuberculosis that preceded sarcoidosis, and from five when sarcoidosis was followed by caseating tuberculosis. Bacilli were of the human strain and were virulent for guinea pigs, and the organisms were sometimes first isolated when the disease passed from the clinical picture of sarcoidosis to one of caseating tuberculosis. This coincided with a change from the state of tuberculin negativity to that of positivity. In a study similar[191] to Scadding's, there were fourteen black adults, five of whom developed sarcoidosis following well-documented tuberculosis. Six started with sarcoidosis, developed tuberculosis, and then reverted to the sarcoid state. In three patients, the two diseases coexisted.

Scadding suggests that there is an immunologic abnormality that precedes the occurrence of sarcoidosis and that this results in tuberculous infection being associated with sarcoidosis instead of tuberculosis. Whether this explains the failure of sarcoidosis to respond to antituberculosis drugs is doubtful, but it is possible that some of the organisms are of the nonsusceptible anonymous mycobacterium group. The lesions are modified by steroids.

Further evidence of a relationship to tuberculosis is as follows:

1 The prevalence of sarcoidosis changes in the same direction as tuberculosis in several ethnic groups.[197]

2 A prospective study of 360 sarcoidosis patients in Philadelphia disclosed the subsequent development of tuberculosis in thirteen (3.6%).[193]

3 A joint study from Cincinnati and Czechoslovakia has demonstrated acid-fast bacilli in 100 patients with sarcoidosis.[200]

4 A more speculative argument is based on the demonstration that, while patients with tuberculosis or sarcoidosis often also are infected with mycobacteriophages, only in those with sarcoidosis is there an absence of antibody to the phage; perhaps this makes the difference between their developing tuberculosis or sarcoidosis.[195] Phage-infected mycobacteria lose their acid-fastness and hence are difficult to identify. Lack of phage-neutralizing antibodies may account for the lack of caseation in sarcoidosis and the relative anergy to tuberculin. It may be that patients who already have sarcoidosis have increased vulnerability to mycobacterial infection.[199]

The Kveim test is nearly always negative in tuberculosis and leprosy. There are well-documented cases of sarcoidlike lesions following BCG vaccination, and even clinical sarcoidosis has occurred.[192] Others merely become Kveim positive. These findings accentuate the complex interrelationship of sarcoidosis, tuberculosis, and Kveim antigen.

Many have suggested that the worldwide sarcoidosis with identical clinical, radiologic, and pathologic findings is a syndrome of many causes, so that one might speak of tuberculous sarcoidosis, beryllium sarcoidosis, or, in the case of the injuries mentioned previously, quartz or silica sarcoidosis. What we are now discussing may be "idiopathic sarcoidosis." Waksman's hypothesis is attractive: "that all lesions of sarcoid type are immunologic reactions to more or less widely disseminated antigens which are either of low solubility or unmetabolisable."* Scadding's admittedly fanciful conclusion is that, if most sarcoidosis is mycobacterial and since tuberculosis is declining, the controversy around the etiology of sarcoidosis may not be resolved before the disease disappears![197]

Clinical picture and diagnosis. Sarcoidosis spares practically no organ and may be widely spread throughout the body. Epithelial and endothelial surfaces, and the adrenal glands, are strange exceptions to this. Although its manifestations are protean, its course may be so silent that only a routine chest x-ray examination discloses its presence. A joint study from London and New York indicates that symptomatic sarcoidosis (respiratory, dermatologic, and lymph node) is balanced by an equal amount of silent disease.[194] Many cases have been unexpected findings at autopsy, and many others undergo spontaneous regression. There is a significant female predominance, and the highest incidence of the disease is among blacks and Scandinavians. The majority of the blacks are young women.

---

*From Waksman, B. H.: Medicine (Balt.) **41**:93-141, 1962; copyrighted by The Williams & Wilkins Co.

Most of the childhood cases in the United States have been in blacks. The lung is a common site of involvement, usually with an initial hilar lymphadenopathy. Rarely, this may incite a middle lobe syndrome by bronchial compression. Otherwise, the complaints are vague and slight—persistent cough, sometimes loss of weight, and occasionally fever and sweating. Pulmonary insufficiency is rare and indicates extensive fibrosis. Among the few persons who die from sarcoidosis, the commonest cause of death is heart failure associated with severe pulmonary damage. Others have succumbed to direct cardiac or cerebral involvement.

Serum protein levels often are abnormal, with reduced albumin and globulin of 3.5 or more grams per 100 ml. In 10% to 20% of patients, there is a serum calcium of 11 mg to 15 mg per 100 ml, with normal phosphorus levels.

The *Kveim test* involves the use of a saline extract of known human sarcoid tissue that, when injected intradermally into persons with sarcoidosis, will slowly produce a local sarcoid granuloma in 60% to 90% of cases. This must be identified by biopsy four to seven weeks later. The reaction is weaker or negative in quiescent stages and becomes positive again with recurrences.[188] The Kveim test is positive in 84% of those with histologic sarcoidosis and in many without it who later develop such lesions.[198] The rate of false positivity is 1% to 2%.[198]

The reliability of the Kveim test has been questioned. It has been found to be positive in many patients with Crohn's disease, and in a recent study of patients with sarcoidosis, it was positive only when there was marked lymphadenopathy. Furthermore, it was positive in patients with chronic lymphocytic leukemia, tuberculosis, infectious mononucleosis, and nonspecific cervical adenitis.[192a]

A valuable differential point for clinical diagnosis is a biopsy from the gastrocnemius, which is not likely to be affected by tuberculosis but may reveal sarcoid granulomas. Scalene node and liver biopsies are also fruitful.

Gross appearance. The hilar and mediastinal lymph node enlargement is sometimes so great that the designation "potato nodes" has been applied. This is only in the early stages, because later on there is healing that ranges from restoration of the normal state to fibrosis without calcification. In the lung, there are disseminated miliary or nodular

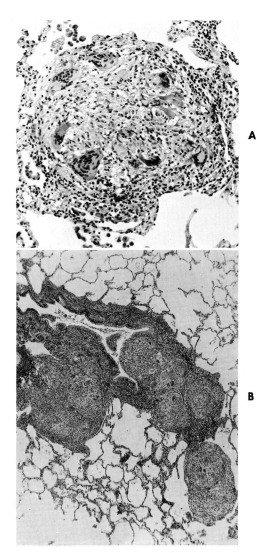

Fig. 23-71 Sarcoidosis. **A,** Single noncaseating granuloma. **B,** Nodular granulomas surround bronchiole and small vein. (**A,** ×153; **B,** ×40.)

fibrous foci with diffuse linear infiltrations. They extend out from the hila in a bilaterally symmetric fashion, tending to become broader and more extensive. Interstitial fibrosis and transformation of alveoli into enlarging cysts create the rare examples of sarcoid honeycomb lung. The nodular variety of sarcoidosis produces lesions measured in a few millimeters, but they may reach 1 cm or 2 cm in diameter. Cavitation is very rare.

Microscopic appearance. The characteristic appearance has been mentioned in the discussion of berylliosis. There is a small, sharply delimited collection of epithelioid cells. Among them are foreign body giant cells, Langhans' giant cells, and the Schaumann and asteroid bodies, which have little value in diagnosis

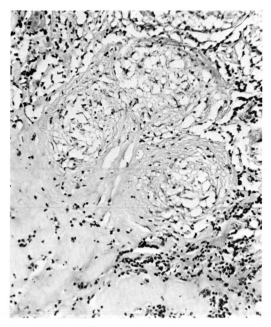

Fig. 23-72 Collagenization of sarcoid lesion. (×165.)

since they are nonspecific. Peripherally, there is a small zone of lymphocytes and plasma cells (Fig. 23-71, *A*). These discrete nodules appear in clusters and, by partial coalescence, form larger complexes (Fig. 23-71, *B*).

It is incorrect to believe that central coagulative necrosis, or even apparent caseation, rules out the diagnosis of sarcoidosis. Small zones of eosinophilic granular necrosis may occur (but with intact reticulin), and acid-fast stains will be negative. If regression is taking place, fibroblasts grow in and lay down a dense collagen between the epithelioid cells (Fig. 23-72). This is the tissue that produces pulmonary fibrosis. The lesions are in alveolar walls but are also perivascular and peribronchial. In fact, the diagnosis of sarcoidosis can often be confirmed by random biopsy of the bronchial mucosa. Fibrosis in such situations can lead to stenosis of bronchi or bronchioles.

In conclusion, it must be said that microscopic evidence does not prove a diagnosis of sarcoidosis. The report must be in such terms as "tuberculoid granuloma compatible with sarcoidosis" if such is the clinical impression.

Diffuse interstitial pulmonary fibrosis (fibrosing alveolitis)

Many diseases fulfill the descriptive designation "diffuse interstitial pulmonary fibrosis." Hamman and Rich thought they were describing a new and relatively acute entity.[202]

Their definition of an acute disease observed in four patients is now unacceptable. We now recognize an acute disease becoming chronic, "characterized by an inflammatory process in the lung beyond the terminal bronchiole having as its essential features (1) cellular thickening of the alveolar walls showing a tendency to fibrosis, and (2) the presence of large mononuclear cells, presumably of alveolar origin, within the alveolar spaces."* This is a broad general category of disease and inflammation. To define the Hamman-Rich syndrome requires inclusion of the clinical concept and a recognition that there may be several causes. In the first cases described, the patients survived six weeks to six months. We now know that most patients live for a number of years, and ten-year survival has occurred. Death from the disease is not inevitable.

Liebow and associates[202a, 203, 204] call the disease under discussion "usual interstitial pneumonia" in order to distinguish it from "desquamative interstitial pneumonia" and from "lymphoid interstitial pneumonia."

Most patients have been adults 30 to 50 years of age, with a slight predominance of males. They have progressive dyspnea, unproductive cough, cyanosis, and weight loss. Tachypnea, fever, and cyanosis at rest are common in the later stages. Respiratory studies indicate alveolocapillary block.[205]

Grossly, the lungs in earlier cases already suspected clinically have increased consistency. Microscopic changes are already well under way. Eventually, the lung becomes rather solid, often with pleural fibrosis. Typically, there is the widespread bilateral, but not uniform, appearance of honeycomb lung. In some lungs, the surface is nodular, the raised areas being up to 1 cm and corresponding to projecting cysts. The depressions between them are of fibrous tissue. Such changes are greatest in the lower and outer zones and resemble the exterior of a hobnailed liver.

Microscopically, the initial changes are edema and increased vascularity of the interalveolar septa. Then mononuclear and histiocytic infiltration of the septa appears with fibrous exudate in the alveoli. Reticulin fibers are being laid down. Alveolar lining cells become cuboidal, and relatively few erythrocytes and leukocytes are seen in the alveolar space. A hyaline membrane is sometimes seen. Retic-

*From Scadding, J. G., and Hinson, K. F. W.: Thorax 22:291-304, 1967.

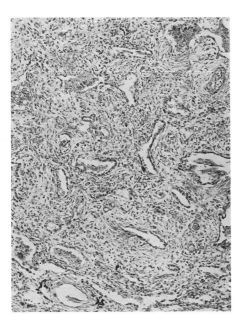

Fig. 23-73 Acute diffuse interstitial fibrosis of lung. (Section courtesy Dr. A. R. Rich.)

ulin becomes collagen, and alveolar capillaries gradually are replaced, whereas in other places they undergo a remarkable hyperplasia in the midst of young fibrous tissue (Fig. 23-73). The disease is also active around terminal bronchioles and alveolar ducts. As interstitial fibrosis advances, many alveoli and bronchioles are converted by metaplasia of their lining into a pseudoglandular pattern. The small pulmonary arteries undergo intimal thickening. Intra-alveolar fibrosis follows, and alveoli are squeezed out of existence. Smooth muscle hyperplasia is apparent in the fibrous tissue. Small cysts are created.[187, 209] The normal tiny lymph follicles of the lungs become hyperplastic. An interesting observation is that, even in a late stage of the disease, coexisting early lesions can be found nearby.

The foregoing are not specific findings, but the absence of bacteria and the minor role of inflammation are significant. With the knowledge from the roentgenogram that the condition is diffuse and bilateral, that the known causes of honeycomb lung have been excluded, and that the patient suffered a (usually) chronic course, the pathologist can diagnose idiopathic diffuse interstitial pulmonary fibrosis. This means the exclusion of late stages of hypersensitivity pneumonias (p. 925), sarcoidosis, berylliosis, connective tissue disorders, silo filler's disease, mercury vapor inhalation, irradiation damage, and rheumatoid disease. Cases of fibrosis known to

be due to inhaled allergens are now known as "extrinsic allergic alveolitis"; the others as "cryptogenic fibrosing alveolitis."[139a] Fifteen families are now known in which many members (starting sometimes in early childhood) have diffuse interstitial pulmonary fibrosis, transmitted as an autosomal dominant.[210] In 27% of one series of cases, rheumatoid factor was present in the patients' sera. In another series, 14% of the patients had rheumatoid arthritis. Furthermore, deposits of IgM and rheumatoid factor have been demonstrated along the alveolar walls.[187]

Desquamative interstitial pneumonia

A disease of unknown cause, desquamative interstitial pneumonia causes dyspnea, dry cough, fatigue, and weight loss without fever. About fifty cases are reported. Radiologic changes include a ground glass opacity in the bases of each lobe. This corresponds to patchy, firm, airless, yellow-gray areas. Striking microscopic findings are the uniform diffuse masses of intact desquamated granular pneumonocytes and macrophages filling many alveoli. They are large, with plentiful PAS-positive, brown, granular cytoplasm that is free of lipid and contains little iron. Lined up along the alveolar septa, they continue to divide after desquamation. Hyperplastic lymphoid follicles are prominent. In spite of the name of the disease, interstitial inflammatory activity is slight and fibrosis usually insignificant. Consequently, the patients do quite well and are helped by steroids.

Giant cell interstitial pneumonia is a very rare disease, possibly related to desquamative interstitial pneumonia. Bilaterally, there is a lymphocytic interstitial infiltrate, and bizarre multinucleated giant cells fill the alveoli.[207b]

Lymphoid interstitial pneumonia

Lymphoid interstitial pneumonia appears to be an immunoproliferative disorder not related to interstitial fibrosis. Many of the patients have hypergammaglobulinemia without a monoclonal peak, but the latter also is recorded.[207] Clinically, this is a slowly progressing disease with increasing dyspnea. In sections, one sees alveolar septa distended by masses of mature lymphocytes with some intermingled large mononuclears and plasma cells. The infiltrate extends into interlobular septa and encloses bronchioles and vessels (Fig. 23-74). Differentiation from lymphoma

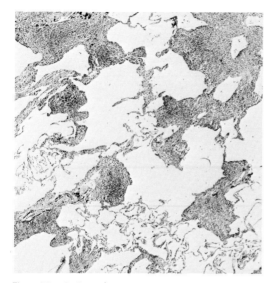

Fig. 23-74 Lymphocytic interstitial pneumonia. (×50.)

depends on the mixture of mature cells and the absence of lymph node involvement.

Whereas lymphoid interstitial pneumonia is probably an entity, it is possible that desquamative interstitial pneumonia is merely a densely cellular, lightly fibrous type of fibrosing alveolitis,[208] and several more cases are now reported suggesting this.[207a]

Eosinophilic granuloma and related conditions

All three members of the histiocytosis X triad, when disseminated, also may affect the lung, but *eosinophilic granuloma* may be solely pulmonary. Eosinophilic granuloma may be defined as a chronic inflammatory disease of unknown etiology characterized primarily by the presence of histiocytes, eosinophils, and fibroblasts. With wider recognition of the entity, many cases confined to the lung have been described. To date, electron microscopic studies have failed to elucidate the nature of the disease in the lung.[212a]

Most of the patients have been young men. A number of cases are symptomless and are discovered by routine chest x-ray examination, which discloses increasing diffuse, bilateral reticulonodular densities. Some patients remain well for as long as fifteen years.[212] Others suffer progressively worsening cough and dyspnea, which may be totally disabling as the disease advances. Corticosteroids have aided these patients. Because of the formation of bullae, pneumothorax is a common complication.

Detailed gross descriptions of the earlier

stages are lacking, but the few open thoracotomies performed have allowed observation of many nodules up to 1 cm in diameter. In advanced cases, there are extensive fibrosis, emphysema, and honeycomb lung, more marked in the upper lobes.

Knowledge of the microscopic pattern of the disease comes from pulmonary biopsies. These reveal fairly well-demarcated, nodular, interstitial lesions composed of eosinophils and histiocytes, with some lymphocytes and plasma cells. They may have some resemblance to noncaseating tubercles. Alveoli are filled with histiocytes, and the septa are thickened by proliferation of fibroblasts. Some of the histiocytes contain hemosiderin. Later, eosinophils become scanty, interstitial fibrosis is predominant, and many distal air spaces are lined by cuboidal or low columnar epithelium. Diagnosis at this stage is difficult, and one should look for the iron-containing histiocytes and make multiple sections, for one of the characteristics of eosinophilic granuloma is its variability of development from one area to another. A helpful point is that the elastic fibrils and laminae of alveolar septa, bronchioles, and vessels become progressively more disrupted and scanty and finally they disappear.[211] Although this also is observed in sarcoidosis and viral pneumonia, it is not seen in usual interstitial pneumonia.

Hand-Schüller-Christian disease and Letterer-Siwe disease are discussed elsewhere (p. 1321). They are not primarily pulmonary diseases. Another condition of more generalized nature is *chronic granulomatous disease*. This syndrome consists of chronic suppurative lymphadenitis, hepatosplenomegaly, eczematoid dermatitis, and pulmonary infiltrations associated with hypergammaglobulinemia. These lesions resemble those of cat-scratch disease, with numerous pigmented histiocytes. In the classic form, confined to boys, death comes in the first decade. The basic anomaly is the failure of the patient's neutrophils to kill bacteria after ingesting them. There are other familial and nonfamilial variants, some in girls, some with defective immunoglobulins.[213]

Fibrosis due to drugs

A number of drugs have been reported to cause interstitial pulmonary fibrosis. Among them are busulfan (Myleran), nitrofurantoin (Furadantin), hexamethonium, methysergide, and oxygen. It is always difficult to prove that a particular drug is responsible, but at least there is an association.[216] Heard and Cooke[214]

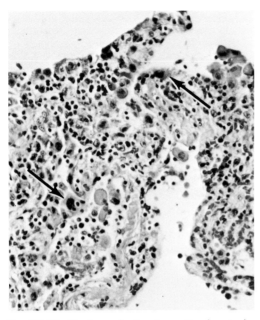

Fig. 23-75 Atypism of alveolar cells due to busulfan therapy. (×223.)

have shown that the alleged interstitial fibrosis of busulfan and hexamethonium is intraalveolar due to organization of fibrinous edema presumably caused by the drugs. Busulfan also stimulates epithelial cells in various parts of the body to enlarge, including the alveolar lining cells, which reach up to 40 μm by 20 μm in size (Fig. 23-75).

That *oxygen* in high concentration is poisonous to animals has been known for many years. Pratt drew attention to the human manifestations in 1958, but not until 1967, when Nash et al.[215] reported on seventy cases, was there wide acceptance of the danger of mechanical respirators. Damage is related to the concentration of oxygen and the duration of exposure. It begins to appear in about four days, and concentrations greater than 80% are the most damaging (see also p. 193).

Experiments on monkeys show that the alveolar lining epithelium is almost completely destroyed in four days and that the type I cells are replaced by type II cells, which, with interstitial fibers and cells, greatly thicken the alveolar septa. Initially, however, the injury is

to the alveolar capillary endothelial cells. In these experiments, complete return to normal function was possible.[214a]

The damage caused by oxygen has complicated interpretation of manifestations of a number of diseases, especially hyaline membrane disease and postperfusion lung.

A striking appearance is seen when the lungs are sliced. They are heavy, relatively

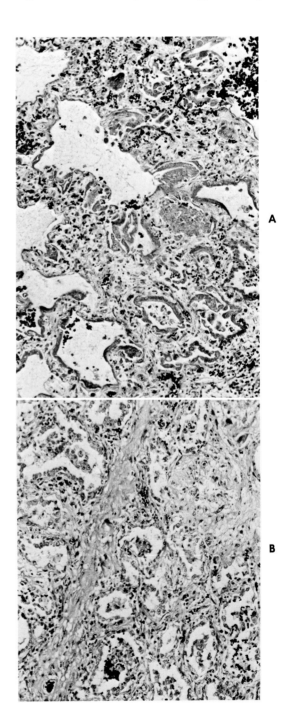

Fig. 23-76 Oxygen toxicity. **A,** Early stage— about sixth day. Hyaline membrane, reactive alveolar cells, and marked interstitial edema and congestion without inflammatory reaction. **B,** Later stage—about fourteenth day. Progression to early interstitial fibrosis, still without significant inflammation. (**A** and **B,** ×165.)

dry, and beefy. In the early phases, there is congestion, edema, and hemorrhage in the alveoli. A fibrin exudate is turned into a hyaline membrane. No inflammation is seen. Later, edema is marked in the alveolar and interlobular septa. Alveolar lining cells are prominent and hyperplastic, and beneath them fibroblasts begin to proliferate (Fig. 23-76). By now damage is severe and alveolar-capillary block has started. The dilemma is there—oxygen is needed and "the brain softens before the lung hardens."

TUBERCULOSIS

Tuberculosis is the infectious disease caused by several different species of mycobacteria. Originally only *Mycobacterium tuberculosis* var. *hominis* and *Mycobacterium tuberculosis* var. *bovis* were identified as pathogenic for man. In recent years, the unclassified (anonymous, atypical) mycobacteria have become important.

Prevalence

The high infectivity of pulmonary tuberculosis and the extent of disease in cows have caused this to be one of the most common and lethal infectious diseases throughout the world. In North America and Western Europe, improved hygiene and living standards have greatly diminished the prevalence of tuberculosis, with pasteurization of milk and control of herds playing an important role. Earlier diagnosis and more effective treatment also play their part. In the United States in 1965, about 52,000 new cases of pulmonary tuberculosis were reported. This dropped to 44,000 in 1967, still an enormous number of cases of a largely preventable disease.

In the United States, the *death rate* from tuberculosis dropped from 200 per 100,000 population in 1900 to 5.9 per 100,000 in 1960. The *case rate* in 1960 was 30.8 per 100,000. That there can be wide differences between the two rates is shown by the 1959 figures from Japan—death rate, 35.4; case rate, 537.7. Moreover, these data represent the prevalence of *tuberculous disease,* whereas if the entire population was given skin tests, there would be a third, even higher figure—the prevalence of *tuberculous infection.*[245] This includes active disease and disease overcome in the past, but with skin allergy persisting. Unfortunately, even in the Western world, the sharp decline in the death rate has not been accompanied by a proportionate fall in the number of new cases. At present, the death rate in Africa and

Asia stands at about 300 per 100,000. The world's lowest incidence rates are in Holland, Denmark, New Zealand, and Australia (in order of increasing figures). The total of world deaths from the disease per year is five million.

Organism

Mycobacterium tuberculosis is a slender, straight, or slightly curved rod. Its length varies from 1 μm to 4 μm, with occasional longer filamentous forms. It is either homogeneous or beaded in the Ziehl-Neelsen stain or the Fite-Feraco stain, superior because it shows more acid-fast bacilli.

No attempt is made here to detail information that belongs in textbooks of microbiology. It is stressed, however, that there is no way of identifying microscopically which species of mycobacterium has caused the disease.

The organism is aerophilic but can multiply slowly at fairly low oxygen tensions, as would be found near the center of a caseous lesion or when a lung is collapsed or the blood supply to the center of a lesion is cut off. Bacilli do not proliferate in the center of closed caseous areas, yet often multiply at an enormous rate if aeration is reestablished, as by a bronchus or blood vessel opening into the lesion.[226] It is also likely that this will alter the pH of the region in favor of more rapid growth. Fatty acids released in caseous areas inhibit their growth. A single organism is potentially infective, but there must be one million bacilli or clumps of bacilli per milliliter of bacterial suspension before microscopic examination reveals more than one organism per ten oil immersion fields. Therefore, the report of "absent or scanty organisms" can be extraordinarily misleading.

Chemistry of tubercle bacillus

The tubercle bacillus does not have exotoxins or endotoxins to explain its virulence, but there are important chemical components in its body that produce far-reaching effects in the human being. Fifty percent of the organism is lipid, which, although no longer thought to form a waxy coat, is, in some way, responsible for acid-fastness. The more virulent the organism, the more lipid it contains. Lipids also seem to stimulate monocytes and macrophages to become epithelioid cells or to divide into multinucleated Langhans' cells.

The protein fraction, "tuberculoprotein," is principally important for inducing sensitization in the patient, but it also stimulates formation of Langhans' cells and epithelioid cells. The carbohydrate, in the form of polysaccharides, provokes a neutrophilic reaction locally and an outpouring of young neutrophils from the bone marrow.

Tuberculin test

Products derived from the tuberculoprotein can be injected intracutaneously for the Mantoux test. These include old tuberculin (OT) and purified protein derivative (PPD). A positive test indicates that a person now has, or had in the past, active tuberculosis. Therefore, it is mainly of exclusionary value except in "conversion"—when a patient previously known to be negative becomes positive to a later test.

Unclassified (atypical) mycobacteria

Pinner[247] in 1935 was among the first to suggest a possible cause-effect relationship between what were then considered to be saprophytic acid-fast bacilli and human disease. About 1948, confirmed infections by what were called "yellow" or "atypical" acid-fast bacilli were being reported. Today, in the United States, subject to geographic variations, 1% to 10% of persons thought to have tuberculosis have *mycobacterial pseudotuberculosis* (nontuberculous mycobacteriosis) caused by what are now called anonymous or unclassified mycobacteria. They differ vastly from *Mycobacterium tuberculosis* in that their cultural characteristics are distinct, they do not cause progressive disease in guinea pigs but sometimes do so in mice, and they are resistant to streptomycin, isoniazid, and para-aminosalicylic acid. Some newer drugs have been effective, and the Group II organisms have been found particularly susceptible to chemotherapy.

The term "unclassified" means that characteristics are not yet sufficiently established to allow designation of species. The grouping that follows is not classification in the biologic sense. These organisms are atypical in many of their growth characteristics, and a major feature of all of them is the lack of communicability of the disease from an infected person to other persons. We do know that these organisms are not mutants produced by drugs.

Four groupings of these organisms have been made. Full details may be found in articles dealing with this subject.[221, 253] Group I, the photochromogens, is probably a homogeneous group, *Mycobacterium kansasii*. About

two-thirds of mycobacterial infections in Britain are due to Group I. In the United States, the organisms of this group cause mainly pulmonary disease in older white males, particularly in Kansas, Illinois, and Texas. In one study,[237] the group was found to be the cause of 9% of mycobacterial disease in Dallas. Also, these organisms are a cause of cervical lymph node infection in children.[254] Among ninety-nine patients in Dallas having *Mycobacterium kansasii* infection of the lungs, there were eighty-five with cavitary disease. Interestingly, thirty-eight of the whole group previously had normal lungs, the rest having had signs or symptoms of "chronic pulmonary disease."[233]

Groups, II, III, and IV are composed of diverse strains. Group II, the scotochromogens (*Mycobacterium scrofulaceum*), is reported to be an important cause of acute or subacute lymphadenitis in children.[263] Members of this group very rarely cause pulmonary disease. The organisms can be isolated from the sputum and saliva of many healthy people. Group III, the nonphotochromogens, includes the important Battey type, the chief cause of pulmonary mycobacteriosis of white men in Georgia, Alabama, and Florida.[224] Cervical lymphadenitis in children also has been caused by organisms of Group III. The Battey organism has been named *Mycobacterium intracellulare*. Nine cases of disseminated tuberculosis caused by this organism are now on record.[236] A minor member of the group is *Mycobacterium avium*, which causes less than 0.1% of mycobacterial infections. Group IV, the rapid growers, includes *Mycobacterium fortuitum*, a rare cause of pulmonary disease, sometimes fatal. Also in Group IV is *Mycobacterium marinum (balnei)* found in the slime of fresh and salt water swimming pools. They grow in skin scraped by the rough pool walls, causing "swimming pool granulomas." The organism also grows in fish tanks.

Some unusual mycobacteria are *classified*, because even though they are photochromogens, they have clearly defined characteristics. One is worth mentioning. *Mycobacterium ulcerans* has been found to be the cause of the extensive superficial ulcers of the skin of children and young adults in the Buruli district of Uganda. An associated fat necrosis can extend down to muscle or bone, producing gigantic "Buruli ulcers," never causing systemic tuberculosis.

Tendon sheaths, joints, and bursae or soft tissues may be infected by unclassified mycobacteria.[235] Osteomyelitis has been caused by a nonphotochromogen. Such cases are important because they indicate hematogenous infection.

Nontuberculous mycobacteriosis of lymph nodes tends to be more suppurative than tuberculosis, but in the lungs the two generally are considered to be indistinguishable pathologically.[242] Among a group of thirty-six children with atypical mycobacterial lymphadenitis, seven had a pattern of suppurative and granulomatous inflammation, alone or with typical tuberculous reaction, and four had a nonspecific diffuse granulomatous or chronic inflammatory reaction.[250] This was not considered characteristic enough to be diagnostic. Others have commented on finding longer, wider and more heavily beaded acid-fast organisms in mycobacteriosis. One is led to speculate that at least some cases of clinical cat-scratch disease may be due to mycobacteriosis.

Therefore, only the bacteriologist or special skin tests can demonstrate the difference between the two types of mycobacterial disease. Patients suffering from pulmonary mycobacteriosis mistakenly treated in tuberculosis sanatoria are in danger of a superinfection by tuberculosis. The primary disease in such patients will not respond to standard antituberculous chemotherapy, so that surgery may be the only cure.

Special purified protein derivatives have been prepared. There is one for each important group, and their use has demonstrated widespread reactivity (e.g., 70% with PPD-Battey in some southeastern areas). More blacks than whites react, whereas most of the patients with actual disease are white. Only about half of the patients react to standard PPD.

The noncontagious nature of pulmonary mycobacteriosis has been demonstrated.[224] Not one case was discovered among 500 contacts (including 151 spouses) of 158 patients infected by nonphotochromogens. Isolation is therefore quite unnecessary. The organisms are, in the view of Prather et al.,[248] opportunists capable of producing serious repiratory disease only after resistance has been lowered by other disease. Most of their patients were from rural areas and of low social and economic status. We do not know how these persons become infected or where the organisms reside. Soil is considered a possibility. I believe that a number of sarcoidlike lesions may be linked to mycobacteriosis.

In conclusion, an uncommon variant de-

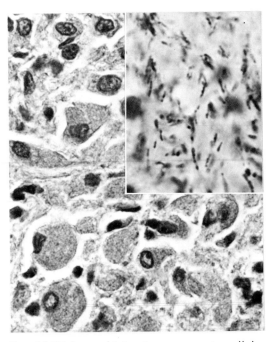

Fig. 23-77 Large histiocytes were main cellular reaction in fatal case of widely disseminated mycobacterial pseudotuberculosis. Cytoplasmic granularity is due to large numbers of organisms. Inset, Ziehl-Neelsen stain of these cells. (×837; inset, ×1,620.)

serves comment. Occasionally a child presents with an enlarged spleen and enlarged lymph nodes. Bone marrow smears contain numerous cells of the Gaucher type. They are also in the spleen and lymph nodes and are found to be histiocytes packed with acid-fast bacilli that create the foamy appearance (Fig. 23-77). Caseating granulomas do not appear, but there are "hard" tubercles among the histiocytes. Such cases may be related to variants of miliary tuberculosis in elderly persons (p. 957) and to nonreactive tuberculosis (p. 960).

Transmission

The main routes of tuberculous infection are (1) pulmonary, (2) intestinal, (3) tonsillar, (4) cutaneous, and (5) placental (congenital). The disease usually is spread by droplets from a patient with a cavitary lesion that opens into a bronchus. Coughing, sneezing, and spitting emit a potent spray to which members of the same family frequently are exposed. Infection in a child is too often the first indication that grandpa's cough is not due to smoking. The organisms are quite resistant to drying and persist as infective agents in dust. According to one illustrative report,[246] infected dust particles in the crew's quarters lingered after four sailors with pulmonary tuberculosis were removed from a ship. The particles appeared to be responsible for a high rate of tuberculin conversion among the remaining members of the crew for a period of several months.

Occupational hazards exist for all hospital personnel, and the risk for British laboratory workers is two to nine times the national rate.

In some parts of the world, infected milk causes up to 10% of cases of tuberculosis, whereas in countries with a well-supervised dairy industry, this is unknown. Organisms swallowed from outside the body (usually the bovine variety) may infect the tonsils and cervical lymph nodes. The tonsillar disease may pass unnoticed, whereas the cervical node enlargement is prominent. Similarly, the first intestinal lesion is mucosal ulceration, which tends to heal readily, leaving the impression that disease commenced in the mesenteric lymph nodes. After the catastrophe at Lübeck resulting from the accidental oral administration of BCG contaminated by living tubercle bacilli to 251 newborn infants, advanced pulmonary lesions of progressive primary type were found in fifteen of the seventy-two who died. These were due to direct aspiration of bacilli. Primary lesions were found in the alimentary tract in every case. The investigation established that primary tuberculosis in the lung is not caused by alimentary tract infection.

Inoculation of tubercle bacilli into the skin is among the lesser dangers faced by pathologists and rarely leads to infection of the internal organs. Butchers may be infected by handling contaminated meat.

Congenital tuberculosis is rare, there being only 158 cases accepted by one group of investigators[225] up until 1960. For this diagnosis to be accepted, lesions must have been present at birth or must have appeared within a few days, the child having been immediately separated from all infectious persons. The primary complex is found in the liver and portal lymph nodes, since infection has been blood borne through the placenta. Less often, infection is from swallowing tuberculous amniotic fluid (leading to intestinal and mesenteric disease) or inhalation (causing pulmonary lesions).

Factors determining course of infection

Native resistance. Native resistance occurs among the different species. Rats are highly resistant to tuberculosis, although the organisms readily multiply within their bodies. Rabbits are susceptible to the bovine organism, but by virtue of developing an acquired resistance to infection by the human species of mycobacteria, they appear to have native resistance. Lurie has observed that "the natural resistance of human beings to tuberculosis bears a certain relationship to the resistance of the rabbit to the human tubercle bacillus. The vast majority of civilized mankind completely recovers from its primary infection just like the rabbit. There is no race of human beings which is completely immune to tuberculosis."* The guinea pig has virtually no resistance to tuberculosis. Studies from the United States Army, where whites and blacks are housed and fed together, indicate that black soldiers have a somewhat higher incidence of the disease and a four times greater mortality than white soldiers. Tuberculosis in American blacks follows a course intermediate between generalized rapidly progressive primary disease and the localized (pulmonary) chronic ulcerative disease of white adults. It is believed that black adults react to tuberculous infection strikingly differently from white adults.[251] When influences such as dosage, previous infection, and environment are equalized, blacks are found to have a lower degree of racial resistance.

Age and sex. Age and sex have an influence on the incidence of the disease. There are considerably more male than female patients after 25 years of age. Tuberculosis during infancy is at its lowest incidence but has a high death rate. Many healthy persons pick up resistance from subclinical infection. At the beginning of this century, probably the entire population up to 20 years of age was tuberculin positive. Now, less than 20% of young American adults have a positive reaction, confirming the statistics which show that, in countries with low case rates, tuberculosis is a disease of older people.

Economic status. Economic status plays an important role in the impoverished areas of the world. It is difficult to assess the importance of racial differences when poverty alone can explain much of the higher incidence, as in the Orient. The great increase in numbers of cases of tuberculosis during famine and war points to the importance of diet and housing conditions. Debilitating diseases may predis-

---

*From Lurie, M. B.: Native and acquired resistance to tuberculosis, Amer. J. Med. 9:591-610, 1950.

pose a person to tuberculosis, and the combination aggravates the tuberculosis, increasing the death rate. The high incidence of tuberculosis in silicosis is well known.

Hormonal influences. Hormonal influences have been established. Whether diabetes has a direct effect on tuberculosis has not been decided. Hyperthyroidism exerts a favorable effect on the course of tuberculosis, and hypothyroidism acts in the opposite way. Cortisone and ACTH will worsen active disease and light up the inactive, a dangerous effect that does not arise when antituberculous drugs are given at the same time. It is not certain that pregnancy (as a hormonal effect) has a deleterious effect on the tuberculous mother. Any worsening of the disease could be due merely to defective nutrition, inadequate rest, and excessive physical work.[251]

Tissue susceptibility. Tissue susceptibility is as noticeable in this disease as in any other. In children, the lymph nodes are particularly heavily attacked, and the meninges, lungs, and spleen often are involved. Among adults, the lungs bear most of the disease. Second place is shared roughly by the adrenal glands, kidneys, fallopian tubes, epididymides, meninges, and serous membranes. The liver, spleen, bone, red bone marrow, and lymphoid tissue come next. The mucosae of the upper respiratory tract and intestine of adults are rather resistant unless the dose is massive. Rarely infected are cardiac and skeletal muscle, stomach, thyroid gland, pancreas, testis, and breast.

Reactions of tissues to infection

Following introduction of tubercle bacilli into animals, the more virulent the strain and the more vulnerable the organ, the greater the extent of the immediate reaction: edema, hyperemia, and neutrophilic infiltration.[239] Having taken up bacilli, the neutrophils die and, in turn, are ingested by phagocytes. At first the bacilli continue to multiply within the cells. More mononuclear phagocytes collect at the periphery of the nodule that is being formed. What happens at the very beginning in man is unknown. We cannot explain why tubercle bacilli inspired throughout the lungs usually produce a lesion in only one area. Infection is by very small clumps of bacilli or even by single ones. In a special search among 1,000 persons who died suddenly, not a single prenecrotic focus of macroscopic size attributable to airborne infection could be found, although there was evidence of tuberculosis in three-fourths of the bodies examined.[241]

With equal infecting doses, the quantity of exudate in the early lesions is greater in hypersensitive tissues than in nonsensitized. From this observation has come the concept of the exudative and the proliferative lesions.

Exudative reaction. The exudative reaction is an expression of poorer host resistance than is met with in the proliferative reaction and is most often seen in the lungs in rapidly progressive tuberculosis. There is exudation of fibrinous fluid into the alveoli, with outpouring of neutrophils. It may progress to massive caseation that is poorly localized. Numerous organisms are present in acute exudative tuberculosis. However, if the lesion becomes caseous, few organisms can be found in the cheesy matter. If it later softens further so as to become semiliquid, the organisms usually multiply at a great rate.[220] Different reticulin patterns are present in the proliferative, softening, and healing phases.[258]

Proliferative reaction. The end of the proliferative reaction is the hard tubercle, a nonspecific granuloma also seen in sarcoidosis, deep mycoses, syphilis, and berylliosis and in some forms of leprosy. The term "hard" signifies merely that there is no necrosis. Tubercle bacilli are much fewer than in the exudative phase.

The tubercle is a compact collection of a score or so of a special form of mononuclear phagocyte. These have a plentiful, palely eosinophilic cytoplasm and an oval vesicular nucleus. Although the cells have only the faintest resemblance to epithelial cells, they were long ago called "epithelioid cells." Their peculiarity is the bacterial lipoprotein in the cytoplasm. Among the cells, or at their periphery, there is often a giant cell with a plentiful pink cytoplasm and as many as twenty to forty round or oval nuclei (Fig. 23-78). When the nuclei are arranged in a complete or partial marginal ring, the cell is described as a Langhans' giant cell. If the nuclei are uniformly scattered, the cell resembles a common foreign body giant cell. Both types of giant cell originate from phagocytes. An acid-fast bacillus must be seen to identify the hard tubercle as mycobacterial. It is very unusual to find organisms in Langhans' cells. The few that are demonstrable in the tubercle are free or in epithelioid cells.

The tubercle enlarges by migration of more macrophages from blood and tissues, and its periphery is cuffed by a zone of lymphocytes. Numbers of tubercles exist side by side and may fuse with one another (Fig. 23-79). This

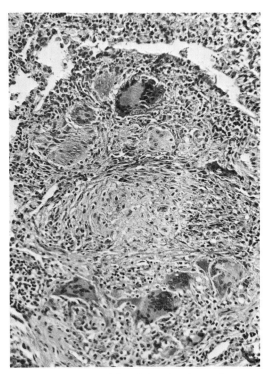

Fig. 23-78 Young ("hard") tubercle with prominent epithelioid cells. (×120.)

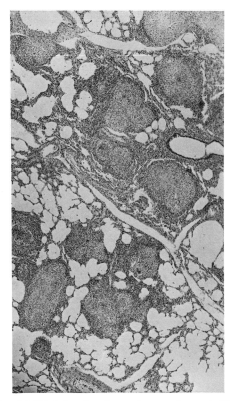

Fig. 23-79 Tubercles becoming confluent (miliary tuberculosis).

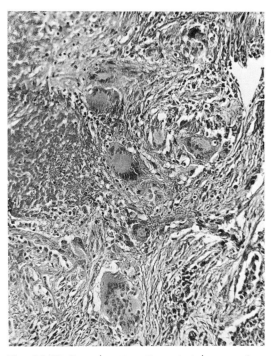

Fig. 23-80 Granular necrotic material appearing in center of tubercle. (×168.)

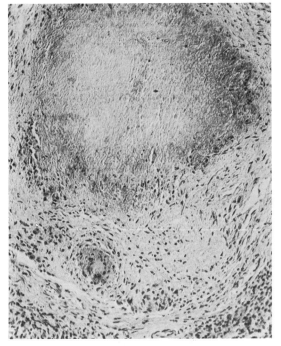

Fig. 23-81 Soft tubercle. Caseous center and early formation of fibrous capsule.

will render them grossly visible for the first time. Tubercles in the livers of guinea pigs killed six weeks after inoculation with tuberculous material can be readily studied.

The next stage is the conversion to the soft tubercle. Starting in the center of the tubercles, the tissue and the epithelioid cells become necrotic and are replaced by an eosinophilic substance at first coarsely granular and dotted with nuclear remnants (Fig. 23-80). Once it becomes homogeneous and quite structureless, it is termed caseous (cheesy), having the naked-eye appearance of a thick, pasty, pale yellow-white substance in the 1 mm or 2 mm miliary tubercle. In turn, "miliary" implies a resemblance to the millet seed, an object seen by few occidental pathologists. This total obliteration of structure (Fig. 23-81) is what distinguishes caseation from coagulation necrosis because even the interstitial fibrous tissue has gone. The dead tissue is rich in lipids, and it may persist for a very long time, apparently because the lipids inhibit proteolytic enzymes.

Bacilli are variable in distribution in necrotic tissue.[241] They range from numerous to totally absent. They may be found only in the center in some cases, even in colony formation, whereas in other lesions they are near the periphery of the area of necrosis. A known long-standing necrotic lesion with a peripheral fibrous zone can never be assumed to be innocuous.

Since chemotherapy has become the principal treatment, the presence of tubercle bacilli in the tissues is affected. In a proportion of treated patients, resected lung specimens may show readily stainable nonculturable bacilli.[262] The significance of these bacteria is uncertain. The assumption that the bacilli are dead is questionable, although varied techniques fail to "revive" them.[261] Nevertheless, the visible persistence of the organism may be an indication for surgery. The lowest yield of positive cultures from resected lungs is obtained in those patients whose sputum has become negative within three months of chemotherapy or has been negative for more than six months before surgery.[238]

There is much evidence that caseation does not occur before hypersensitivity has been established. It begins to appear about two weeks after injection of large doses of virulent bacilli into relatively resistant animals. Caseation is progressive as long as tubercle bacilli can proliferate in the tissues, allowing the process to extend. When the macrophages can destroy bacilli as rapidly as they are reproduced, effective fibrous encapsulation can occur. Such fibrous capsules can protect against progressive caseation only if they are complete. The danger is the lingering survival of a minority of organisms that lie dormant almost as if they were spores. They can immediately be reactivated by oxygen brought in by rupture of the capsule or bleeding into the caseous center. Fresh tuberculoprotein now released may induce further caseation and obliteration of the fibrous barrier. Langhans' giant cells are completely nonspecific.

The potential development of the tubercle has been fully described. Even on reaching this stage, the tubercle is not histologically diagnostic. It is a "caseating tuberculoid granuloma," awaiting a positive Ziehl-Neelsen stain or successful culture.

What happens next is either further spread or healing, depending on the host-bacillus relationship. "Healing" as used in pathology lacks the connotation of restitution to normal. In tuberculosis it refers to increasing fibrosis creeping into the diseased area, creating a scar. Very common also is calcification, in no sense a protective process. Calcium carried in blood plasma to caseous areas is deposited as relatively insoluble compounds, possibly influenced by the high concentration of lipids.

Among the infants in the Lübeck series, calcification was first seen at fifty-eight days. Reportedly, calcification can appear in primary lesions after two months, whereas in postprimary infection six months are required.[229] Calcium must accumulate for about a year to be seen radiologically. After about three years, the lesion attains a chalky character. Stony foci are at least five years old and may be ossified. At first, the calcium is seen in routine sections as irregular pale blue clouds. With time, the color intensifies, particularly at the periphery. Viable bacilli may still be present in noncalcified areas.

Calcification in tuberculosis, therefore, merely indicates that caseous necrosis has taken place but is not evidence of cure or sterilization. Identical pulmonary calcification can be produced by histoplasmosis.

Pathogenicity of tubercle bacilli

To be infectious, tubercle bacilli must be inhaled with particles no larger than 15 μm in order to reach the alveoli. Bigger clumps will be returned by cilia to the sputum.

Tubercle bacilli are readily phagocytosed. It is believed that within these phagocytes the most effective processes of immunity take place.[226] The overcoming of infection probably depends on the power of the host's monocytes to kill the engulfed bacilli. For some days they multiply freely as if harmless cellular parasites. Similar multiplication is seen in lepromatous leprosy and Johne's disease of cattle. It also occurs in the human infection by anonymous mycobacteria referred to on p. 947 and in Fig. 23-77. At about fifteen days, the peaceful relationship between mycobacteria and host cells is suddenly altered by the appearance of sensitization to tuberculoprotein. Tubercle bacilli begin to act with virulence. During the relatively slow disintegration of the organisms within the phagocytes, complex antigens are released. This happens only in vivo.

Nature of hypersensitivity and immunity

Around tuberculoprotein and the nature of Koch's phenomenon appears to revolve the complicated reaction to tuberculous infection. The nature of *Koch's phenomenon* is this. When a healthy guinea pig is injected with live tubercle bacilli, a nodule appears at this site in ten to fourteen days. It enlarges and becomes an ulcer that persists until the animal dies of generalized tuberculosis. The regional lymph nodes also become tuberculous. Living tubercle bacilli or their breakdown products injected in already tuberculous guinea pigs immediately elicit, at the new site of injection, an acute exudative response that, within two to four days, advances to shallow ulceration that heals. Regional lymph nodes do not react. This is the simplest expression of the complex hypersensitivity to tuberculoprotein. The animal has reacted hypersensitively but has localized the infection and disposed of it.

It has been much disputed whether this hypersensitivity or allergy is also the mechanism of the patient's *acquired immunity*. It is more likely that they are responses to different antigenic agents. Tuberculin sensitivity cannot be induced by the injection of tuberculin. Injection of tuberculoprotein may sensitize normal animals to the tuberculoprotein but not to tuberculin. Heat-killed tubercle bacilli produce typical tuberculous lesions, but these regress and are absorbed. Only tuberculoprotein associated with tubercle bacilli induces sensitivity to tuberculin. Animals have been successfully desensitized to tuberculoprotein and then have been shown still to have greater immunity than a normal animal. The chief mechanism of immunity is the increased

capacity of mononuclear phagocytes to inhibit the growth of tubercle bacilli. Nevertheless, it is thought that under certain conditions the reaction of hypersensitivity may aid in protection.[239] Although various antibodies are found in sera of tuberculous patients, they confer no immunity on susceptible animals. Sera of highly immunized animals have no in vitro bactericidal effect on tubercle bacilli.

As hypersensitivity appears, the macrophages become epithelioid cells, and all but the most virulent organisms are killed. The more epithelioid cells, the more quickly this phase progresses. The change in the appearance of the cells is due to the fine, intracytoplasmic dispersion of lipid from the bacilli. Thus, the appearance of epithelioid cells is associated with death of the bacilli. In reinfection tuberculosis, the bacilli cannot multiply as they can in primary infection, and formation of nodules and epithelioid cells is accelerated. Under these conditions, the mononuclear cells have a directly augmented activity independent of any contribution from the patient's serum. They are not only phagocytic, but also bacteriostatic.

In one study, silk bags containing collodion and tubercle bacilli were placed in the peritoneal cavities of normal and immune rabbits. These bags allow body fluids to enter but bar the animals' cells. The fluids of immune animals inhibited growth of the bacilli in vivo.[239] Hence, there must be a humoral component of acquired resistance. This also means that the reinfected animal has greater resistance to infection.

All these sequences in animals apply equally to man. Whether or not hypersensitivity can be equated with immunity, the inflammatory process in the reinfected patient develops more quickly and is more destructive in the form of caseation. Yet, these lesions are more effectively localized by fibrous tissue, and regional lymph node inflammation is not so prominent a feature as it is in primary disease. In this sense, hypersensitivity is associated with better defenses. Therefore, hypersensitivity may be said to work with the increased monocytic function that is the major activity of immunity. On the other hand, hypersensitivity has an unfavorable action in that it is responsible for serious tissue destruction, even though this will also decrease the local multiplication of tubercle bacilli.

A few organisms usually survive in the primary site and years later can start a new bout of progressive disease (p. 955). Under these circumstances, the host-parasite relationship is an unstable equilibrium. Over a long time, the ascendancy can pass to either one in a cycle of progressive and quiescent disease. In the same organ, there can simultaneously be healing and progressing lesions.

There is no immunity without hypersensitivity. Patients with either primary or reinfection tuberculosis are hypersensitive, the state being more pronounced in children than in adults. It is not known why this difference exists. The *bacille Calmette-Guérin (BCG)* is a permanently attenuated living bovine organism[227] that almost invariably causes harmless infection. Blattner has reviewed a dozen instances of death in children from disseminated "BCG tuberculosis" within some months of vaccination.[219] Many had hypogammaglobulinemia, and others suffered repeated infections or were debilitated prior to vaccination. These conditions, therefore, are contraindications to giving BCG, as is a positive tuberculin reaction. BCG is injected to immunize human beings, but there is no way to measure the immunizing potency of any particular batch. Considerable variation occurs. Vaccination is offered to tuberculin-negative persons in areas with a high risk of infection.

The Medical Research Council in England has conducted follow-up studies of over 50,000 tuberculin-negative children for seven to ten years. They were vaccinated with BCG or another nonpathogenic organism, the vole bacillus *(Mycobacterium tuberculosis* var. *muris)*. The incidence of tuberculosis in the vaccinated group was only one-fifth that of a similar but unvaccinated group, and the protection appeared to be long-lasting.[228, 240]

In regard to the histopathology of BCG vaccination, of particular interest is the frequent occurrence of Schaumann bodies in the tuberculoid granulomas. They are probably formed from fatty acids. It has been speculated that the bodies are part of the morphologic expression of the development of the antigenic response to the bacilli.[260]

Populations with a low rate of tuberculosis are not vaccinated because other methods of control of the disease have been successful. In these people, tuberculin conversion is a valuable sign to disclose a new case that could readily be treated by chemotherapy. BCG vaccination can always be given if a high incidence of tuberculin positivity appears in a group exposed to a special risk.

Tuberculosis of lung
Primary tuberculosis and primary complex

When tuberculosis was a very common disease in the western world, "primary" tuberculosis and "childhood" tuberculosis were synonymous. Now, a person may be unexposed to the risk until adult life, so the term "primary" is used. Most often, primary tuberculous infection is overcome without signs or symptoms or with only slight fever, cough, or chest pain. Only skin testing discloses that it has occurred.

The *primary complex* is a focal lung lesion with a beady chain of miliary tubercles running in the lymphatic vessels to the third component, the enlarged hilar lymph nodes (Fig. 23-82).

The *pulmonary component* is the primary (Ghon) focus. It occurs with equal frequency on either side and tends to be subpleural, in the midportion of a lobe rather than apical. Rare multiple primary complexes may be the result of exposure to a source of heavy infection. One lesion can be in the lung and the other extrapulmonary.

The true early lesion rarely is seen. It resembles nontuberculous bronchopneumonia, passing through red and gray stages of consolidation. Around it is an extremely wide, red, less firm perifocal reaction. The latter is an alveolar filling with serum, phagocytes, and erythrocytes but without inflammatory cells.[218] This is rapidly converted into a quite well-demarcated area of consolidation 1 cm to 2 cm in diameter. Its cut surface is a rather dry or crumbling, gray or white caseous tissue surrounded, during the most active phase, by a red zone of tuberculous granulation tissue. Rarely does it undergo complete resolution. More often, the area becomes caseous, encapsulated by fibrous tissue (which has formed from the granulation tissue), and it is sometimes calcified. Such a calcified (even ossified) residue may be only a few millimeters in diameter. In other patients, the remnant is a small, puckered, pleural scar.

The early histologic response has been described on p. 950. This passes on to caseation and, in patients with good resistance, to creation of a fibrous capsule.

The *lymphatic vessel component* may not be seen at all in a random slice made into the lung. It heals with complete resolution.

The *lymph node component* is a massive enlargement of hilar and tracheobronchial nodes that in children is much greater than

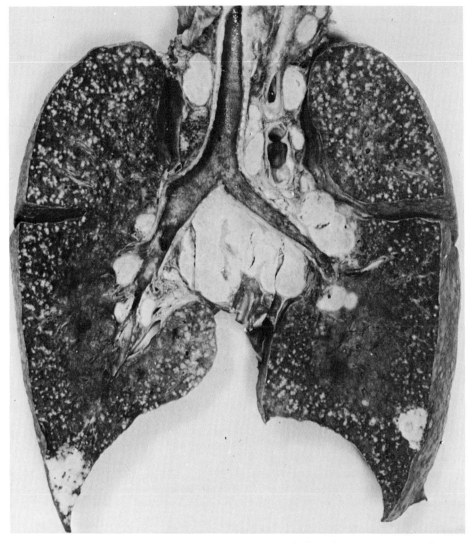

Fig. 23-82 Bilateral tuberculous primary complexes. Subpleural caseous primary focus in each lower lobe. Hilar and tracheobronchial nodes have undergone massive enlargement and caseation. In addition, advanced miliary dissemination can be seen. (From Giese, W.: In Kaufmann, E., and Staemmler, M., editors: Lehrbuch der speziellen pathologischen Anatomie, vol. II, Berlin, 1959-1960, Walter De Gruyter & Co.)

the area drained. In some adults, the reverse is the case. Generally, all the nodes in the group are necrotic and matted into a yellow-white conglomeration with spots of calcification. The greatest enlargement and most caseation occur in the hilar nodes. Encapsulation and extensive calcification follow, but not before the anterior mediastinal, and sometimes even cervical and abdominal, lymph nodes have been involved. Nodal lesions take longer to regress than those in the lung, often years, and they remain a potential source of reinfection. Much later, these lymph nodes shrink to normal size but are largely calcified. Microscopic examination of the lymph nodes

discloses the extensive caseation, with peripheral tubercles and fibrosis.

Progressive
primary infection

Instead of regression of the primary complex, there is progression of the lesions in a small number of persons—especially in susceptible individuals or those subjected to very heavy infection. Most often affected are black infants or children.

The process is a tuberculous bronchopneumonia with caseation (Fig. 23-83). It spreads in three ways: (1) by direct extension, (2) into bronchi, and (3) into the bloodstream. The

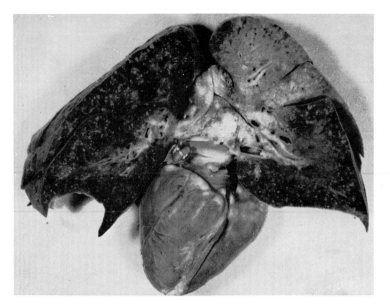

Fig. 23-83 Progressive primary tuberculosis (posterior view) in 18-month-old infant. Coalescent tuberculous bronchopneumonia of right upper and middle lobes. Acinar-nodose tuberculosis in remainder of lungs. Caseation of hilar nodes.

periphery is irregular and poorly defined, and there is no limiting zone of granulation tissue.

Bronchial dissemination arises by one of two methods. First, caseous matter erodes into the lumen of a small bronchus and, with its organisms, is distributed along the ramifications of the bronchus into previously healthy lung. This creates a pyramid with its base on the pleura. Second is a similar infection of a much larger bronchus by caseous material from one of the massive hilar nodes. The resultant bronchopneumonia can be so extensive and progressive that it is fatal. If a cavity forms, its wall is shaggy and its outer wall is ill defined, without a capsule. Spillage of infection into a medium-sized bronchus sets up cone-shaped areas of bronchopneumonia that caseate and are likely to be confluent.

Rupture of the tuberculous lesion into a blood vessel may result in hematogenous dissemination—i.e., generalized miliary tuberculosis (see following discussion).

Progressive primary tuberculosis is not inevitably fatal and may be arrested at any stage. Exudative lesions can be resolved, and caseous areas can be encapsulated and calcified. Eventually, the lung will have multiple, relatively large calcified and fibrous areas. The microscopic appearance of these lesions has been described previously. Tuberculous caseous pneumonia is described later in this chapter (p. 959).

Reactivated primary tuberculosis

Local reactivation of a subsided primary focus is a rare phenomenon (about 0.2% of cases) seen in young patients years after the patient has become healthy. The lesion often has become calcified. There is a distinct predilection for children. The reactivation, which is unexplained, always begins with liquefaction and cavitation at the periphery of the old focus. Tubercle bacilli are usually demonstrable and often viable.[255]

Miliary tuberculosis

Tubercle bacilli may spill into the blood, directly or via lymphatic vessels. Penetration of a pulmonary vein is likely to infect all of the body, whereas entrance of bacilli into a pulmonary artery is likely to restrict them to its territory within the lung. Mycobacteria entering a major lymphatic vessel will be returned by the right ventricle to both lungs. Cells of the reticuloendothelial system destroy many of them, often by forming small noncaseating tubercles that disappear after they have performed their task. A harmless infection leaves a residue of tiny calcified dots in the liver, spleen, apices of the lungs, meninges, or skeletal system. For a while, it is possible for one of these to light up as active disease. If so, the condition of miliary tuberculosis is set up. However, there is reason to believe that organisms, in spite of their lodging in susceptible tissues, can be promptly killed. This is more likely in adults than in infants.

Infection may come from a primary focus or from a later stage of tuberculosis, in which the miliary disease may be merely a terminal event. In the adult, miliary tuberculosis is more likely to be of extrapulmonary origin, even though the lung is seen to be infected the most heavily and even though it contains chronic lesions that initiated extrapulmonary disease. More and more cases of miliary tuberculosis are being reported in elderly persons, with half of the cases in those past the age 60 years being "cryptic." This means that the usual clinical and radiologic features are absent. A typical patient is an elderly woman with pyrexia, pancytopenia, or leukemoid reaction. Many such patients have been fruitlessly investigated for blood dyscrasia, and sometimes lymphocytic leukemia has been erroneously diagnosed. Therapeutic trial has been advocated as a method of diagnosis.[249]

In children, miliary tuberculosis may be more or less confined to the lungs. More often, in addition, liver, spleen, and kidneys bear a great number of tubercles, followed by meninges, bone marrow, lymph nodes, and thyroid gland. Only muscle tissue is spared.

The pleura generally shows little reaction. The cut surface of the lung is studded with firm white tubercles 1 mm in diameter or caseating tubercles several millimeters in diameter (Fig. 23-82). Tubercles in the upper lobes are the largest, but the distribution of tubercles is even throughout. The heavier the infection, the closer and more numerous they will be. Tubercles grow smaller as the infection is resisted. Specific chemotherapy will allow scar formation and disappearance of the lesions after only a few weeks, as opposed to several months in untreated patients. The latter may develop interstitial fibrosis or perifocal emphysema. Childhood miliary tuberculosis can heal without trace, but the adult variety rarely does.

The tubercles are chiefly within alveolar septa where the bacterial emboli lodge. They are of the hard variety at first but enlarge and caseate. Fibrous capsules are formed in those patients who survive a longer time. *Chronic and recurrent types of pulmonary miliary tuberculosis* occasionally are found in adults. Giese[229] refers to Gujer's 176 cases of miliary tuberculosis, 54 of which were subacute or chronic. The lungs are heavy, and the pleura is fibrotic. On the cut surface, tubercles are seen to have coalesced into small nodules with central caseation and eventual cavitation. In other patients, there is extensive fibrosis around the nodules. Chronic disseminated tuberculosis involving several organs also has been described.[222]

Reinfection (reactivation) tuberculosis

Reinfection can be endogenous, resulting from reactivation of a primary focus, or exogenous, caused by organisms received from an external source. These events usually occur in adults, those over 40 years of age being particularly prone to exogenous disease. One series of postmortem studies[241] incriminated exogenous infection in 73% of cases of reactivated disease in patients past the age of 40 years. Numerous authorities in many countries reject such views, although they also are widely held. Stead[257] presents persuasive evidence that exogenous reinfection is uncommon and that nearly all chronic pulmonary tuberculosis develops from reactivation of dormant foci implanted during primary infection. In Medlar's series,[241] 91% of the progressive pulmonary lesions in patients under 40 years of age were due to continuation and endogenous reactivation of primary disease.

Reinfection favors the subapical region of any lobe, especially the right, some 2 cm to 4 cm below the apex. The reason for this site of predilection, which is characteristic of reinfection tuberculosis, is not known. The lesion is a small area of dry, confluent, tuberculous bronchopneumonia that tends to fan out to the apical pleura. Regional lymph node involvement is minor.

Healing leaves a small scar around which, as around any pulmonary scar, carbon pigment tends to collect in blocked lymphatic vessels. Such scars are restricted almost entirely to the pleura, which is thick, hyalinized, calcified or, rarely, ossified. The pleural surface is uneven, often puckered, and slaty blue or black, and pleural adhesion is common. Often, the scar has an area of several square centimeters but little depth. Sometimes one finds a 5 mm calcified nodule or a zone no more than 1 cm deep in which the lung is black and airless or contains a tiny cavity with a smooth inner lining. Focal emphysema may surround the scar. At this stage, the entire process is spoken of as *arrested tuberculosis*.

The microscopic lesions begin with an exudative reaction that passes into tubercle formation, caseation, and peripheral fibrosis.

Further caseation and tissue destruction produce the gross lesion. "Arrest" is recognized by the reduced amount of caseous matter, with a marked fibrocalcific reaction. The lesions of arrested tuberculosis lack Langhans' cells and stainable acid-fast bacilli, but may still be infectious for the guinea pig.

Progressive reinfection (reactivation) tuberculosis. An advancing lesion occupies much of the upper lobe, undergoes massive central caseation, and, if it breaks into a bronchus, will form a cavity. The latter type is "chronic ulcerative tuberculosis," and the noncavitary variety is "chronic fibrocaseous tuberculosis." No matter how soft the center, a cavity cannot form without drainage into a bronchus or bronchiole.

Some patients develop *acute cavities,* usually during caseous pneumonia. The out-

line of such a lesion is irregular or branching, corresponding to the fusion of lobular areas. The lining is shaggy and necrotic and may contain remnants of septa, vessels, and bronchi. It may break through the pleura, setting up a tuberculous pyopneumothorax. Other specimens disclose tubular cavities, which indicate a destructive caseous bronchitis. Progression of the cavity is rapid, with little likelihood of its becoming chronic.

A newly formed *chronic cavity* has necrotic, ragged walls, with adherent, pale yellow, cheesy material. No odor is present. Active cavities have three definite linings. Innermost is the caseous tissue with debris, many bacilli, and, in places, epithelioid cells and some fibroblasts. Beyond this is a red zone of tuberculous granulation tissue composed of many dilated capillaries, epithelioid and Langhans' cells, and fibroblasts. The external layer is a thin gray zone of loose connective tissue, which has arisen from organization of the perifocal zone. This merges indefinitely into consolidated or normal lung. The opening into the bronchus may be very small.

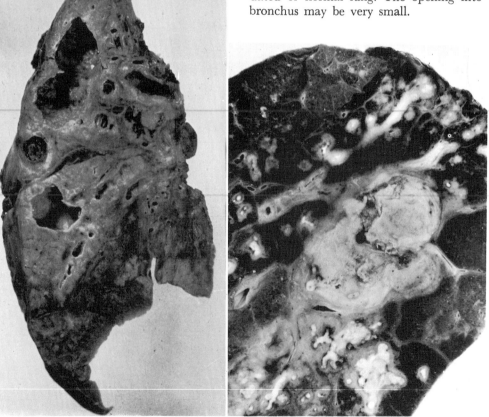

Fig. 23-84 Fibrocaseous tuberculosis. **A,** Advanced lesion with cavitation. Cavities have thick walls and communicate with larger bronchi by wide openings. **B,** Large areas of caseation with attempts at fibrous encapsulation. There is also extensive tuberculous bronchitis. (From Giese, W.: In Kaufmann, E., and Staemmler, M., editors: Lehrbuch der speziellen pathologischen Anatomie, vol. II, Berlin, 1959-1960, Walter De Gruyter & Co.)

Chronicity is indicated by a fibrous outer wall, which forms from organization of the perifocal reaction and is 1 mm or 2 mm thick. The outline tends to be markedly irregular because of uneven breakdown of the tissues. Several cavities may intercommunicate, and the bronchus of each may be identified (Fig. 23-84, *A*).

The lining of older cavities is gray or pink and shaggy. A smooth fibrous lining replaces this granulation tissue as the infection is overcome. Around it are foci of tuberculous bronchopneumonia, caseation, fibrosis, and bronchiectasis. Overlying pleura is fibrotic. The pleural space may develop an empyema or be totally obliterated by adhesions. The pleural fibrosis is protective against bronchopleural fistula, empyema, and transpleural dissemination of infection into neighboring lung. However, it cannot prevent the tuberculous cavity from enlarging, and new fibrous tissue is laid down as the older is destroyed from within. Little change is to be found in the regional nodes.

All of these changes, except cavitation, occur in fibrocaseous tuberculosis (Fig. 23-84, *B*).

Cavities of 5 cm or more may be crossed by strands of connective tissue, blood vessels, or bronchi. The vessels usually have been obliterated by thrombosis. If not, the tuberculous process may weaken their walls, permitting aneurysm formation or massive, often fatal, bleeding. Bleeding is more likely to come from a vessel in the cavity wall. The incidence of fatal hemoptysis has not been decreased by chemotherapy.

Cavities enlarge either by constant destruction of their lining or by neighboring areas of caseation breaking into the cavity. The oldest lesions are in the upper posterior portion of the lung, for extension is toward the base. Usually, the anterior portion of the lung is spared. The entrance of air and drainage away of inhibiting fatty acids greatly favor accelerated growth of the tubercle bacilli. Most of a lobe may be converted into large coalescing cavities surrounded by solid lung tissue altered by tuberculosis in different stages. Fibrosis may obliterate many vessels and induce pulmonary hypertension.

In the mechanism of closed healing of cavities, the bronchus is obliterated at its entry to the cavity. This may be mediated by collapse of the lung, endobronchitis, a caseous plug in the bronchial lumen, or a gradual pinching off of the bronchus by contraction of surrounding granulation tissue. The cavity fills with necrotic material, air and fluid are absorbed, calcification follows, and either nothing is left but a radial scar or, in the case of larger cavities, there is marked contraction and a walling off.[217] Closing off occurs more readily in the smaller, more pliable and collapsible bronchi of children. This may explain why children suffer less frequently than adults from chronic cavities.

Early, small cavities that are emptied of their contents have walls thin and pliable enough to become apposed and adherent. Healing will leave only a minimal scar. The effects of chemotherapy are discussed on p. 962.

Complications of reinfective tuberculosis. Cavitation, pleurisy, and empyema have just been discussed. From cavities comes the danger of bronchogenic dissemination of bacilli. An upper lobe cavity tends to infect other parts of that lobe and the apex of the lower lobe, less often its posterobasal region. Infection also can spread to the opposite lung, usually its lower lobe. Tubercle bacilli in sputum may set up ulcerative tracheal or laryngeal tuberculosis or, in late stages of the disease, infect the tongue and mucosal lymphoid tissue of the small and large intestines. Hematogenous miliary dissemination has already been described, but there is also danger of active disease in a single site—particularly meninges, kidney, bone, epididymis, and fallopian tube. Infection of the regional lymph nodes in the mediastinum is usually not significant. Patients with extensive chronic tuberculosis are in considerable hazard of developing amyloidosis.

The microscopic appearance of reinfection tuberculosis can be judged from the general remarks about tuberculosis, for it has a limited repertoire of histologic reaction. The essential point is to prove the diagnosis by culture and acid-fast stains.

Tuberculous caseous pneumonia

Tuberculous caseous pneumonia is a rapidly progressive bronchogenic disease. It occurs in children, when a caseous hilar node erodes a bronchial wall, and in unusually hypersensitive adults when there is perforation of a tuberculous cavity into a bronchus. A great amount of infected material is spilled over, and the condition is analogous to Koch's phenomenon in guinea pigs. The affected area at first includes one or two lobules, which are solid, dry, gray, and granular. Enough lung tissue remains to cause confusion with a diffusely infiltrating bronchial carcinoma, adenocarcinoma, or gray hepatization.

Large quantities of tuberculoprotein reach uninfected tissue of an already hypersensitive individual, provoking a vigorous exudative response in the alveoli, with many bacilli. Tissue necrosis follows rapidly, and adjacent foci enlarge and coalesce. Microscopic tubercles are uncommon. Soon the gray turns to yellow or gray-red, and the whole lobe is felt to be firm. A whole lung, or most of both lungs, can be affected, and those parts not massively consolidated may show patchy bronchopneumonia centered around caseous bronchi. The peripheral zones may be moist, translucent, shiny, smooth, and somewhat gelatinous (gelatinous pneumonia, a term that should not be applied to the entire tuberculous lesion). Gelatinous pneumonia is seen microscopically as filling of intact thick-walled alveoli by much fluid and fibrin with many macrophages. Other inflammatory cells are much fewer.

The larger the diseased areas, the more likely is it that caseation and cavitation will occur in the center of the older areas, beginning around the bronchi. The cut surface is a firm, dry, opaque, yellow-white substance with whatever anthracotic markings were already there. Tubercles are found in and around the bronchi, which are ulcerated and may be destroyed. Tuberculous pleurisy and caseous hilar nodes are very frequently present. Eventually, an opening will be forced into a large bronchus. Miliary dissemination is common. The most severe cases used to be called "galloping consumption."

If such widespread disease can be arrested, the eventual fibrosis is most extensive. Resolution of the exudate is possible only before necrosis occurs.

Nonreactive tuberculosis

Since 1882, persons have been reported with marked hypersensitivity and low resistance, and who have developed widespread pulmonary tuberculosis lacking the characteristic histologic response.[243] Disease of the hematopoietic system often is present (primary or secondary). Should the tuberculosis be unsuspected and the patient be given steroids, this variant of the disease may advance rapidly. Some such lungs have contained a number of yellow miliary to nodular areas,

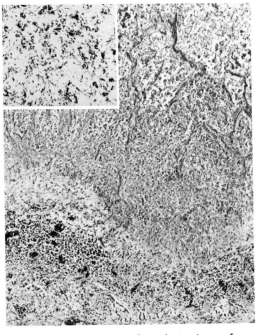

Fig. 23-85 Nonreactive tuberculosis. Area of central cavitary necrosis (top right), vascular zone with cellular necrosis (middle), and hypervascular and early fibrous area (bottom). No cellular reaction typical of tuberculosis. Inset shows masses of tubercle bacilli found in vascular zone. (×75; inset, ×460.)

but in others the lesion resembles an ill-defined bacterial pneumonia, sometimes with abscess cavities. Nodular areas are seen under the microscope to be fairly well-defined eosinophilic necroses with some nuclear debris, mostly from inflammatory cells. Caseation is not common and is early and limited in area. Peripherally, the usual granulation tissue, epithelioid cells, and Langhans' cells are lacking. In lungs that appear pneumonic, there is widespread hyperemia, hemorrhagic alveolitis with edema, or widespread necrosis like that of an ischemic infarct. Whichever type is present, there will be an enormous number of tubercle bacilli (Fig. 23-85). Regional nodes, liver, spleen, and bone marrow may contain similar lesions.

Acinar (acinonodose) tuberculosis

In both cavitary and fibrocaseous tuberculosis, an entire lobe or lung may be riddled by what appears to be magnified miliary disease. This is acinar tuberculosis, caused by infection of respiratory bronchioles and their alveoli by aspiration of infected material from chronic tuberculosis higher up in the lung. These small units undergo caseation with a clover-

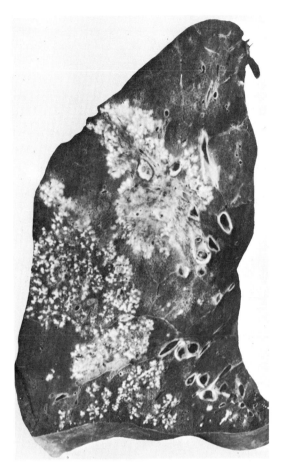

Fig. 23-86 In upper lobe is large, chronic, fibro-caseous area with small central cavity. Condition is spreading peripherally. In lower lobe is typical, partly confluent, acinar tuberculosis. (From Giese, W.: In Kaufmann, E., and Staemmler, M., editors: Lehrbuch der speziellen pathologischen Anatomie, vol. II, Berlin, 1959-1960, Walter De Gruyter & Co.)

leaf pattern, followed later by fibrosis. Close inspection always discloses a small, central, thick-walled bronchus in each area. Cavitation does not occur. Individual areas may fuse and reach a size of 1 cm to 2 cm (Fig. 23-86).

Acinar lesions are a hallmark of reinfection tuberculosis when resistance is good. Healing by fibrosis is possible, leaving only gray-black bands of connective tissue. Should the lesions progress, lobular pneumonia is the result. Microscopically, there is an initial alveolar exudation of fibrin and neutrophils, rapidly overshadowed by tubercle formation.

Tuberculous bronchitis

Tuberculous bronchitis is commoner with lower lobe disease and with cavitation. Its incidence increases with the severity of the pulmonary disease.[234] A search among 197

autopsies in a mental hospital disclosed scars of large bronchi in 27%,[230] a figure similar to those in a number of European reports. The scars formed depressed troughs and rings covered by mucosa. They were interpreted as representing healed perforations by tuberculous lymph nodes.

The earliest lesion is the submucosal tubercle. As tubercles increase and caseation appears, the mucosa becomes ulcerated. Finally, segments of the bronchus are lined by tuberculous granulation tissue. The latter tends to heal with fibrosis, a complication compounded by fibrous tissue laid down in concomitant inflammatory processes around the bronchus. The lumen is narrowed for a variable distance. It may even be closed, either by fibrosis or by caseous material. Distal to this there may bronchiectasis. Patchy collapse of the lung follows bronchial obliteration.

Dissemination of tuberculosis within peribronchial lymphatic vessels eventually infects the bronchial walls. The affected bronchi fan out from the hilum. They look like thick-walled white tubes from which caseous material can be squeezed, clearing the lumen, which may have been invisible. Normal lung lies between the bronchi.

In children in whom primary tuberculosis leads to pulmonary collapse, bronchiectasis frequently develops, most often in infants.[231] Less often, bronchial strictures occur, and only one-third of such children have normal bronchi.

Tuberculoma

A tuberculoma is a nodular, conglomerate area of caseous necrosis with a well-formed fibrous capsule. It occurs in adults with reinfection tuberculosis. Usually, tuberculomas vary in size from 0.5 cm to 4 cm.[256] Most are solitary and occur in an upper lobe. The cut surface shows a uniform or lamellated, dry, caseous matter with areas of calcification (Fig. 23-87) or a cavity. The capsule is 1 mm to 3 mm thick, and the surrounding lung is normal or has minimal tuberculosis (Fig. 23-88). Although tuberculomas are thought of as inactive, they may break down and discharge their contents into the bronchial tree, indicating reactivation.[252]

Pathology of treated pulmonary tuberculosis

Surgical procedures that aim at physical collapse of the diseased lung are followed by marked fibrosis of the pleura and the tuberculous foci of the lung. "Closed healing" of small cavities is described on p. 959. Large cavities leave a residuum of inspissated necrotic tissue within a thick capsule surrounded by looser fibrous tissue.

The general effect of *specific chemotherapy* is to accelerate healing. Cavities follow a process of "open healing." They are converted

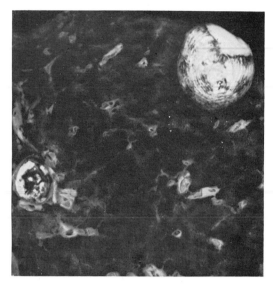

Fig. 23-87 Lamellated tuberculoma formed from Ghon tubercle in adult.

to a spherical cyst filled with air under tension, with a fibrous wall 1 mm to 2 mm thick. The cyst may be 10 cm or 15 cm across, occupying much of a lobe. An active cavity is distinguished by its irregular and frankly tuberculous inner surface.

The cyst, also called a tension cavity, has a smooth or slightly wrinkled gray or gray-pink glistening lining, on which a small amount of pink granulation tissue may rest. In some surgically removed specimens, small foci of caseation remain at the periphery. A bronchus will nearly always be found entering the cyst, which probably exists because of patency of the bronchocavitary junction.

The cyst generally is bigger than the original cavity because of a check-valve action at the bronchocavitary junction by tuberculous granulation tissue in the early stages. During the response to treatment, the valve effect is lost and the cavity decreases. Any fluid remaining becomes inspissated and calcified.

The outstanding feature of drug therapy in tuberculosis is regression of perifocal lesions and the healing of tuberculous ulcers with regeneration of epithelium, which may be flat or stratified squamous.[217] This permits drainage and inactivation of the infection of the cavitary wall, and hence only a thin, fibrous,

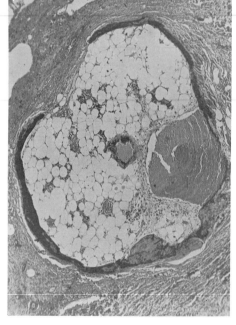

Fig. 23-88 Ossified tuberculoma. Shell of bone almost completely envelops lesion, most of which has been converted to fatty bone marrow with lingering nodule of caseous substance at right.

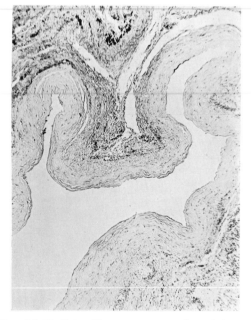

Fig. 23-89 Thin, fibrous cavity wall in lobe removed after one year of chemotherapy.

outer zone appears because of the accelerated course. Usually, no tubercle bacilli can be isolated. A patient so "healed" is still in danger of aspergilloma, perforation, suppuration, bleeding, or reactivation. Therefore, surgical removal often is performed.

Reported incidence of open healing varies from 6%[223] to a figure closer to 10%. In the days before chemotherapy, open healing was very uncommon in patients with chronic pulmonary tuberculosis.[217]

Microscopically, the healed part of the wall is concentric lamellae of hyalinized connective tissue, with scanty capillaries and a few lymphocytes. Scattered calcium deposits are present (Fig. 23-89). There is sharp demarcation from adjacent lung. On the inner surface, there are flattened connective tissue cells, not an epithelium, although cells may grow in from the entering bronchus for a very short way. Any active areas are recognized by tubercle formation. If they contain granulation tissue, this can be so vascular as to form a source of bleeding.

Chemotherapeutic agents also can cause closed healing, a hyalinization and calcification brought about in a few months instead of one or two years.. Healing is always more rapid if the necrotic tissue has not undergone liquefaction.

Noncavitary caseous disease responds to chemotherapy by rapid disappearance of the peripheral lesions and by forming a thin fibrous capsule. There is a much lower incidence of fibrosis in the lung.

Causes of death from tuberculosis

Murasawa and Altmann[244] analyzed in 1958 the causes of death in 570 autopsies performed at a hospital for tuberculosis. In 52%, pulmonary tuberculosis was considered the main cause. After this came arteriosclerotic heart disease, malignancy, and surgery on the lung. A 1963 report[232] reviews 295 autopsies performed on tuberculous patients in the period from 1950 to 1960. In 1950, progressive tuberculosis was listed as the principal cause of death in 74% of cases. In 1959 and 1960, this was the cause of death in only 15%. Conditions unrelated to tuberculosis, such as carcinoma, myocardial infarction, and cerebral hemorrhage, rose from 6% to 64% as causes of death. Conditions related to tuberculosis, but not necessarily associated with active disease, increased from 20% in 1950 to 31% in 1959 and 1960. These were pulmonary hemorrhage, pulmonary insufficiency, spontaneous pneumothorax, death during thoracic surgery, cor pulmonale, and amyloid disease. One-third of the autopsied patients were considered to have healed tuberculosis.

CARCINOMA

The commonest tumor of the lung is *metastatic carcinoma,* the lungs being involved in 20% to 45% of all cases of carcinoma. Most often, the tumor cells arrive in the pulmonary arteries. Less often, they come retrogradedly in lymphatics, by direct invasion, or in the bronchial arteries.

No fixed pattern is observed. There may be one or innumerable secondary tumors, ranging in size from a millimeter to many centimeters. They are nearly always spherical, often with a finely or deeply scalloped edge. Metastatic renal carcinoma, seminoma, and sarcoma are particularly well rounded, producing the radiologic "cannonball lesions." It is not often possible even to guess at the source of a metastasis, although the brown of melanoma and the pink and red of chorioepithelioma are characteristic, as is the moist fish-flesh appearance of many sarcomas.

Primary carcinoma

The overwhelming majority of primary tumors of the lung are carcinomas.

Classification

Many pathologists have not followed the World Health Organization's classification of lung tumors. Both Spencer[4] and Melamed[297] have found need to modify it. A major objection is its largely artificial separation of adenocarcinoma from alveolobronchiolar carcinoma (p. 976). In this discussion are considered most of the following tumors, classified by their origin:

Bronchial epithelium

Squamous cell (epidermoid) carcinoma (with variants spindled and papillary)
Oat (small) cell carcinoma
Undifferentiated large cell carcinoma
Melanoma

Bronchial epithelium and/or glands

Adenocarcinoma (with variant giant cell carcinoma)
Carcinoid
Adenoid cystic carcinoma
Mucoepidermoid carcinoma
Clear cell carcinoma
True adenoma
Benign clear cell tumor (origin unknown)

Bronchiolar and alveolar epithelium

Peripheral adenocarcinoma (bronchioloalveolar carcinoma)
Scar carcinoma (glandular or squamous)
Tumorlet
Peripheral carcinoid

Mesenchymal

Connective tissue tumors (benign and malignant)
Granular cell myoblastoma of bronchus
Chemodectoma
Lymphoma

Mixed

Hamartoma
Blastoma
Teratoma

Pleural

Mesothelioma

Pseudotumor

Plasma cell granuloma
Sclerosing angioma
Pseudolymphoma

Incidence

Although the incidence of some malignances is slowly rising, carcinoma of the lung stands out by an increase too great to explain by blaming errors in diagnosis in earlier years. By 1955, the lung cancer death rate for males in England and Wales was 69.3 per 100,000 population, and in the United States it was 33.0. The figures for females were 10.6 and 6.7, respectively. The actual number of deaths from carcinoma of the lung in the United States rose from 27,000 in 1955 to 55,000 in 1968, with an estimate of 64,000 in 1971. Over the preceding thirty-five years in the United States, male deaths from lung cancer have increased fifteen times and female deaths have been roughly doubled. At the beginning of this century (before cigarettes became popular), the sex incidence was roughly equal. About 85% of patients are men. In Britain, the disease accounts for more than 10% of all deaths in persons between 45 and 64 years of age.

Etiology

The close relationship between certain types of lung carcinomas and *cigarette smoking* has been made well known, as has the lesser relationship to cigar and pipe smoking. Whether or not a cause-and-effect relationship has been proved is a blend of logical, statistical, and emotional argument. It is impossible adequately to summarize the issue here. Opinion prevails in Britain that cigarettes are an etiologic factor, based particularly on Doll and Hill's study of over 40,000 doctors.[282] The 1964 United States Surgeon General's Advisory Committee report concluded that cigarette smoking is causally related to lung carcinoma in men and that its effect far outweighs all other factors. Risk increases with the duration of smoking and the amount smoked daily. A heavy cigarette smoker has at least a twenty times greater risk of having lung carcinoma than a nonsmoker. There are less extensive data for women, but they point to the same conclusion.[306] A study has been made of 163 cases of lung cancer in women compared with 1,192 cases in men attending the same hospital during the same period.[313] In the women, the ratio of cigarette-associated carcinoma (squamous and oat cell) to the other varieties was 0.34:1, compared to 3.05:1 in the men. When lung cancer was surveyed during a three-year period at Memorial Hospital, eight nonsmokers out of 401 (2%) men and twenty-six nonsmokers out of sixty-four (41%) women were found. Adenocarcinoma was present in five of the men and most of the women.[318]

A very careful constructive criticism of these interpretations of the available data has been made by Berkson,[274] physician and statistician, who believes particularly that the population samples of some large studies have been unrepresentative and that the conclusions are too sweeping.

The presumably chemical agent that acts as a carcinogen has not been identified, nor is it known whether or not this agent might be only one link in a chain of causality, having an effect, for example, on an enzyme or oxidation-reduction reaction. Various hydrocarbons have been extracted from burning cigarettes and polluted atmosphere. Most carcinogenic to the skin of mice and rats are the benzopyrenes, but one cannot accurately assess their significance in relation to the mucosa of human lungs. Carcinoma of the lung has not been reproduced in animals by products extracted from burning tobacco. Anderson reviews experiments that succeeded in producing carcinoma in animals exposed for long periods to nitro-olefins—products which are possibly found in automobile engine exhausts.[264]

In mining and textile manufacturing areas of England and Wales, an inverse ratio has been discovered between the incidence of chronic bronchitis and of lung cancer. Coal miners, for instance, have less lung cancer than expected statistically if they have chronic bronchitis.[265] Another statistical study shows the reverse. In Manchester, Rimington observed that smokers have a greater risk of developing chronic bronchitis than nonsmokers and that those who do develop chronic bronchitis are more likely to have lung cancer.[306a]

Associated factors may or may not be of importance—atmospheric pollution, the cigarette paper, different tobaccos favored in different countries, simultaneous pulmonary disease such as chronic bronchitis and emphysema, contaminants, length of the discarded butt (filter action), etc.

Atmospheric pollution from industrial and automobile exhausts has long been considered a significant factor in lung carcinoma. The air in many cities contains some of the carcinogens isolated from tobacco smoke.

While one is impressed by the fact that the place with the world's highest per capita consumption of cigarettes (the Channel Islands) has the highest incidence of lung carcinoma, one is puzzled by the much lower incidence in heavy smokers in the rural areas of any country as compared with their urban counterparts. It may be because the countryman's carcinogens are received only from cigarettes—not from the air as well.

Several occupational lung cancers occur. In uranium mines at Jachymov (Joachimstal), Czechoslovakia, half of all miners' deaths were due to lung carcinoma. In cobalt mines at Schneeberg, Saxony, three-fourths of deaths were caused by carcinoma of the lung. The common factor was radioactive ore and radon gas. Many hundreds of men died before safety measures were employed. Mortality from lung carcinoma in uranium miners in Colorado is four times greater than expected.[314]

Increased risk is recognized among those working in the preparation of chromates, nickel, arsenic, and iron dust, ore, or fumes.[274a, 281] Asbestos workers with continuous exposure of the order of twenty years have an increased risk of developing lung carcinoma.

Changes in the mucosa of large bronchi are commonly found away from the region of the tumor. They range from basal cell hyperplasia with or without atypism, to stratification (flattening of the superfical cells), to squamous metaplasia, and, finally, to carcinoma in situ (Fig. 23-90). These changes have been found in 98.8% of multiple sections of the tracheobronchial tree of men who died with pulmonary carcinoma.[269] Almost as many sections from smokers who died with other diseases had the changes. Only 16.8% of the sections

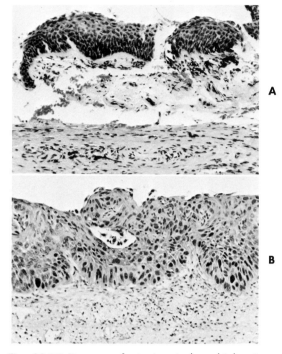

Fig. 23-90 Degrees of atypism in bronchial epithelium. **A,** Moderate dysplasia. **B,** Squamous cell carcinoma in situ. (**A** and **B,** ×300.)

from nonsmokers exhibited mucosal abnormality, which rarely exceeded basal cell hyperplasia. Repeating the study in children, the changes were found in 16.6% of sections, chiefly squamous metaplasia and stratification (14.6%) and basal cell hyperplasia (2.4%).[268] In children, there is a frequent association between the epithelial lesion and healing of mucosal ulcers.

The foregoing changes also are found in the trachea, where carcinoma is rare. Practical experience, not analyzed statistically, appears to show that smokers "cured" of laryngeal carcinoma have an increased incidence of carcinoma of the lung.

Chronic inflammation progressing to fibrosis is associated with lung tumors of two varieties, the *tumorlet* and the *scar carcinoma*. The initial stage appears to be an *atypical bronchiolar proliferation*. Observations of atypical areas in diseased portions of lungs have been made for thirty or forty years. When fibrous tissue surrounds and replaces alveoli, the surviving alveoli are lined by uniform small cuboidal cells (cuboidal metaplasia from alveolar epithelium). This may be seen in tuberculosis, nonresolving pneumonia, chronic pneumonitis, bronchiectasis, lipid pneumonia, chronic abscess, in and around infarcts,

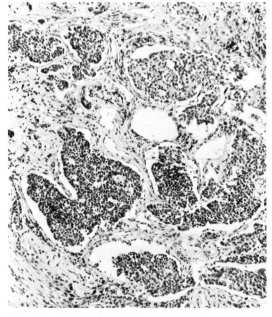

Fig. 23-91 Tumorlet. Cells appear to be in endothelial-lined spaces. (×109.)

anthracosis, and in the group of honeycomb lungs.[298] The nuclei are usually dark but are regular. In other cases, adenomatous proliferation of cells of the terminal bronchioles is apparent. Dilated spaces are lined by a single layer of uniform low or tall columnar cells with small basal nuclei and pale cytoplasm (Fig. 23-67). When such areas are large, the problem of adenomatosis versus carcinoma arises, a problem amplified on p. 975.

Basal cell hyperplasia, basal atypism, or squamous metaplasia of the bronchiolar epithelium is often visible in addition. It is not known what induces metaplasia to pass on to neoplasia, but time appears to be a factor in allowing the formation of a tumor.

Tumorlet is the name chosen by Whitwell[317] for the next stage, which others have considered to be minute carcinomas ranging from microscopic size up to 3 mm in diameter.[310] In one or more fibrous areas of the lung, in the mucosa or walls of bronchi or bronchioles, or in the wall of a chronic abscess, there are isolated groups of small hyperchromatic cells of spindled or oat cell type (Fig. 23-91). Often, there is a suggestion of a palisade layer. Cytoplasm is usually scanty, and the nuclei are quite uniform, with very rare mitoses. In some slides, the cell clusters are observed directly arising from metaplastic cuboidal epithelium of alveoli or bronchioles. The more pulmonary scars are examined microscopically, the more tumorlets will be found. Confusion

with the rather similar small peripheral carcinoids (p. 979) and chemodectomas (p. 983) should be avoided.

Tumorlets are often within spaces resembling lymphatic vessels. In one published report of ninety tumorlets,[299] lymph nodes contained metastases of the cells in five cases. Survival in perfect health is recorded as long as twelve years after removal of many tumorlets.[296] This is certainly not the course expected of oat cell carcinoma. What would have happened if the tumor had not been removed? Criteria for the diagnosis of atypia are not rigid. In summary, tumorlets appear to be nearly always benign. When they do metastasize, it is not known how dangerously malignant they are. Primary lung carcinomas of the same tiny size often are associated with fatal metastases.

Lung scar carcinoma was brought into prominence about 1940 by Friedrich and by Rössle, and a number of cases have been described since. Tumorlets do not appear to turn into scar cancers which, as the name implies, are always malignant. Because pathologists prior to the 1960's often did not recognize the nature of scar adenocarcinoma, a review of the literature is pointless. The true incidence of these tumors is much higher than recorded. About two-thirds of the tumors are less than 3 cm in diameter. Most are subpleural and appear as puckered scars. The cell type is usually adenocarcinomatous[272a] (Fig. 23-92) but is sometimes squamous or undifferentiated.[319] Not enough reports have been made to state the incidence of lung scar carcinoma. An important point is that these small tumors can set up massive, early metastases in the lymphatic vessels and nodes around the large bronchi, creating the false impression that the hilar mass is the site of origin. A change in the radiologic appearance of a long-stable pulmonary scar should promptly raise the suspicion of carcinoma.

Types of carcinoma

If the term "bronchial carcinoma" is considered to refer to tumors arising from mucosa, this group comprises squamous cell carcinoma, oat cell carcinoma, pleomorphic and giant cell types, and undifferentiated carcinoma. To these could be added bronchial adenocarcinoma. Arising from the mucous glands are carcinoid, adenoid cystic carcinoma, and mucoepidermoid carcinoma. Since bronchial epithelium of the respiratory bronchioles pos-

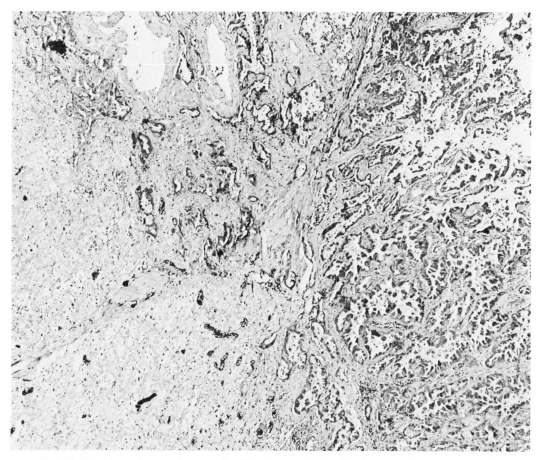

Fig. 23-92 Scar adenocarcinoma. Proliferating atypical glands trapped in scar on left, progressing to rather poorly differentiated adenocarcinoma on right. (×52.)

sibly gives rise to bronchiolar carcinoma, one becomes aware of the deficiencies of the term "bronchial" carcinoma, so that "carcinoma of the lung" has an appealing simplicity.

To this confusion must be added variation in diagnostic criteria, which renders numerous large series of cases incapable of comparison. I believe some carcinoids have been misdiagnosed oat cell or poorly differentiated squamous cell carcinomas. Some will diagnose squamous cell carcinoma only if intercellular bridges, epithelial pearls, or keratinization is present. Other tumors will be called undifferentiated. In the absence of these findings, other pathologists, using their experience of squamous cell carcinoma elsewhere, feel justified in diagnosing poorly differentiated squamous cell carcinoma. Different opinions about adenocarcinoma and bronchiolar carcinoma create further difficulties. Finally, there is the common experience that the more sections one cuts, the likelier one is to observe a combination of cellular patterns, such as squamous and

glandular. Willis has quite emphatically asserted that there is only one carcinoma of the lung. The incidence of mixed glandular and squamous carcinoma of the lung in the literature ranges from 3% to 19%, a figure of about 7% of lung cancers being common.

Bronchial carcinoma

In the group referred to as bronchial carcinoma will be discussed squamous cell, oat cell, and undifferentiated large cell carcinomas. This group has its peak incidence between the ages of 40 and 65 years. Only a few dozen cases are reported before 20 years of age.[279]

Gross appearance

About 60% to 75% of carcinomas involve a main bronchus (Fig. 23-93) or its bifurcation or even extend to the carina. Two-thirds of the tumors in a large series of resected specimens were at the periphery.[286] This may reflect the selection of operable cases. About

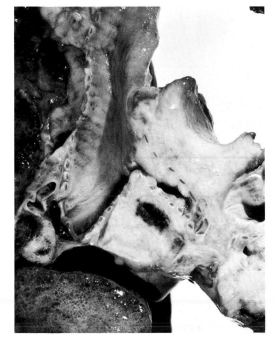

Fig. 23-93 Carcinoma of left main bronchus almost completely occluding its lumen and growing along bronchial tree. Note preservation of cartilage in main bronchus. (From Rezek, P. R., and Millard, M.: Autopsy pathology, Charles C Thomas, Publisher.)

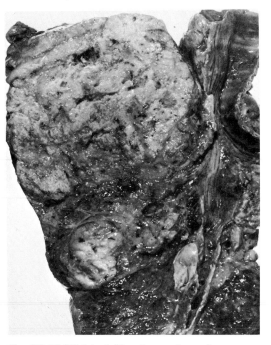

Fig. 23-94 Widely infiltrating variety of squamous cell carcinoma simulating lobar pneumonia or tuberculosis. (From Rezek, P. R., and Millard, M.: Autopsy pathology, Charles C Thomas, Publisher.)

one-third of squamous cell carcinomas, three-quarters of adenocarcinomas, and one-fifth of oat cell carcinomas arise in the periphery of the lung.[4] Hence, a hilar tumor is likely to be squamous or oat cell. Of the two, the oat cell variety is smaller, has much less chance of central necrosis, and is particularly likely to metastasize early.

Beginning as a firm roughening of the mucosa that becomes warty, growth continues into the lumen, filling it with white tissue that becomes yellow, soft, and friable. Growth also occurs through the bronchial wall into contiguous lung, initially sparing bronchial cartilages. Later, the neoplasm may become fused with its metastases in the hilar nodes. Although any large tumor will be necrotic, yellow, granular, cheesy material usually is associated with squamous cell carcinoma (Fig. 23-94). Otherwise, gross morphology does not assist much in the recognition of the type of tumor present.[267, 276]

In the lung, as on the pleura and pericardium, and in lymph nodes, necrotic squamous cell carcinoma closely resembles caseating tuberculosis. An extensive carcinoma, when partially necrotic, often presents as a broad, gray, ill-defined area resembling lobar or tubercu-lous pneumonia or the diffuse type of bronchiolar carcinoma.

Given time, the tumor will grow along the branches of the stem bronchus, removing any chance of deciding the point of origin. In the 250 cases described in one series,[276] the tumor crossed the carina in seven cases. In an investigation of the bronchial stump in 100 surgical cases, there was direct extension of the tumor in the bronchus proximal to the tumor in twelve, submucosal lymphatic spread in six, and significant epithelial metaplasia in fifteen.[280] The stump must be examined microscopically in every case in order to evaluate the chance of recurrence.

A more limited spread is along a medium-sized bronchus and its smaller branches (Fig. 23-95). Their walls are thickened by white tumor tissue. A similar "pipestem" pattern may be seen in metastatic tumors, especially from the breast and stomach. Carcinoma arising some distance from the hilum is inclined to invade the lung so as to create a fairly well-demarcated, peripherally firm, and centrally friable gray-white sphere (Fig. 23-96). It is often difficult to demonstrate its bronchial origin.[276]

An uncommon type of tumor is shown in

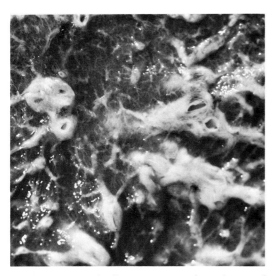

Fig. 23-95 Bronchial carcinoma with widespread peribronchial dissemination. (From Rezek, P. R., and Millard, M.: Autopsy pathology, Charles C Thomas, Publisher.)

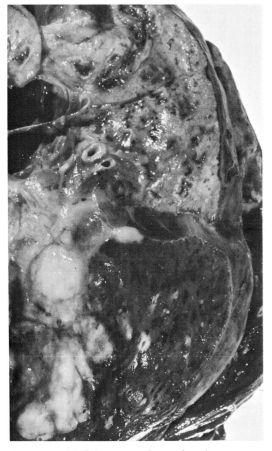

Fig. 23-96 Nodular type of peripheral squamous cell carcinoma. In upper portion of lung is paler area of endogenous lipid pneumonia (see Fig. 23-94).

Fig. 23-97. This has been called exophytic endobronchial carcinoma.[308] The carcinoma is polypoid or papillomatous, with superficial invasion of the bronchial wall. The prognosis appears to be much better than for more invasive types, perhaps because symptoms of bronchial obstruction arise early. The tragedy of lung cancer is that a pathologist may only once in his life get the chance to diagnose early invasive or *in situ* bronchial carcinoma in a living patient. Only the cytology of sputum can achieve this. Multiple mass radiography has failed.[305]

Multiple primary bronchial carcinomas

Painstaking studies have been made of the tracheobronchial trees of 255 patients who died of bronchial carcinoma. Using strictest criteria, nine patients (3.5%) had two or more bronchial primary lesions. With less rigid criteria, such multiplicity could be found in up to 12.5%.[270]

Local effects

Obstruction of the lumen is caused either by intraluminal growth or by a stenosing tumor encircling the wall. If the bronchial lumen is partly blocked, a valve effect may induce obstructive overinflation in the distribution of the bronchus. Usually obstruction will

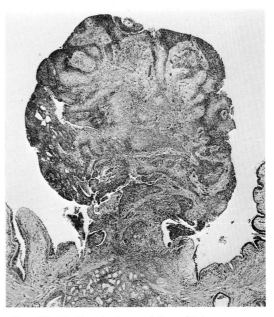

Fig. 23-97 Exophytic endobronchial squamous cell carcinoma with superficial submucosal invasion. (×19.)

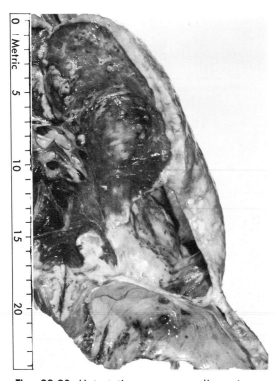

Fig. 23-98 Metastatic squamous cell carcinoma encasing entire lung. Without demonstrating primary lung tumor, this appearance also would be compatible with mesothelioma or sometimes even with fibrous end stage of pyogenic or tuberculous empyema.

side of the trachea. It may extend into the pericardium. If the tumor reaches the pleura, as it commonly does, it sets up a serous or sanguinous effusion, and, if cavitated, its rupture may be responsible for empyema. Seeding of the pleura can thickly coat the entire lung, like a mesothelioma (Fig. 23-98). Growth can continue into the chest wall or into a neighboring lobe. An apical tumor can destroy the neighboring ribs and brachial plexus. Invasion of the cervical sympathetic trunk brings about Horner's syndrome (ptosis of the upper eyelid, constricted pupil, and decreased sweating on the same side of the face). All primary neoplasms of the lung and practically all metastases are fed by systemic arteries.

Microscopic appearance

The largest series of cases in which a realistic classification of lung carcinomas was used is the 5,000 cases from Memorial Hospital under the aegis of William Watson.[297] It should form the basis of comparison for future series from other large centers. The series was divided as follows: squamous, 40%; large cell anaplastic, 33%; combined adenocarcinoma and bronchiolar, 16%; oat cell, 11%. The reader must understand that these figures will be different in a surgical series (biased toward resectable and peripheral tumors) and an autopsy series (including hopelessly inoperable central tumors).

Squamous cell carcinoma. A well differentiated keratinizing tumor of the squamous cell variety is uncommon in the lung. More often, one can recognize epithelial pearl formation, intracellular bridges, or a whorling of cells within true pearls. There may be only an occasional deeply eosinophilic, individually keratinized cell.

The cells are in sheets, cords, and bundles separated by varying amounts of vascular connective tissue. Cellular pleomorphism usually is marked, but mitoses are not necessarily numerous. Often, the outer cell layer has a palisade effect, and this, when cut at a particular angle, can give a pseudoglandular appearance. At times, some of the larger tumor cells are of the signet type (Fig. 23-99), but mucin stains will be negative. This imitation of adenocarcinoma is seen in tissues where there is no possibility of two cell types being present, particularly in cervical metastases from carcinoma of the oral cavity. In about 7% of lung tumors, there is a mixture of true glandular and squamous types (p. 967).

later become complete, and the air is then absorbed. The collapsed area is usually the site of organizing pneumonia. Obstruction also can lead to infection of retained secretions, bronchiectasis, abscess, or gangrene. Chronic pneumonitis or an abscess is a common first sign of a carcinoma and may even be the cause of death. Necrotic tumor tissue can be evacuated through the originating bronchus. The cavity is lined by firm necrotic tumor tissue and does not have the dirty gray or pink softer lining of an uncomplicated lung abscess.

Further invasion by tumor produces significant clinical effects. The primary tumor or its metastases can compress a pulmonary artery or vein or grow around and into the superior vena cava. The latter happens most often when the tumor is in the right main bronchus. The effect is great venous distention of the head, neck, and upper arms, with edema and cyanosis of these areas. Erosion of a large vessel in the wall of a bronchus or cavitated carcinoma can cause fatal bleeding. Hilar tumor may destroy the recurrent laryngeal and phrenic nerves as they run down the

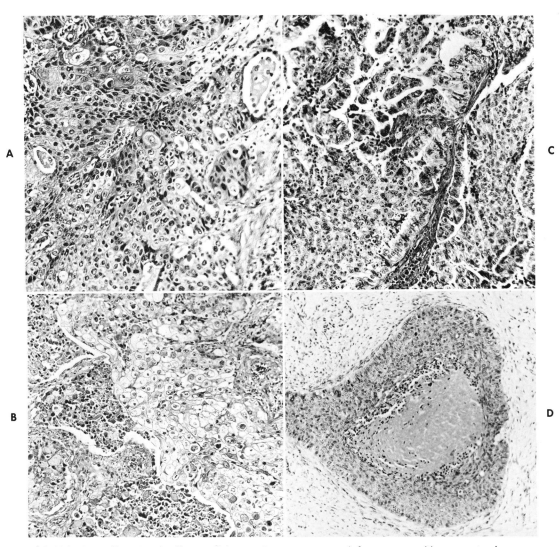

Fig. 23-99 Squamous cell carcinoma. **A,** Lesion in upper left corner readily recognized as squamous cell carcinoma. In remainder of photomicrograph, tumor is poorly differentiated and forms pseudoglands, which appear to contain secretion that is actually degenerating material. **B,** Formation of large clear cells that look as though they might contain mucin but do not react with mucin stains. This clarity of cytoplasm is probably due to hydropic degeneration. Same tumor as shown in **A. C,** Area with mixture of undifferentiated and tall columnar glandular cells. **D,** Necrotic form of squamous cell carcinoma, form more often seen in upper respiratory tract but also resembling comedocarcinoma of breast. (**A,** ×150; **B,** ×109; **C,** ×132; **D,** ×141.)

Another variety of the endobronchial squamous carcinoma (Fig. 23-100) is the *papillary carcinoma,* sometimes multiple and sometimes built up of neoplastic transitional-type epithelium rather than squamous.

Oat cell carcinoma (small cell carcinoma). The name oat cell carcinoma applies to a specific tumor that appears to develop beneath the columnar mucosal layer. Mitoses are common, and, in lighter-staining nuclei, prominent nucleoli are present. The tumor usually is characterized by diffuse sheets of closely

packed cells about 8 μm in diameter, somewhat larger than a lymphocyte in formalin-fixed tissue. There is little or no cytoplasm—merely very hyperchromatic round, oval, or spindle-shaped nuclei in which little structural detail is visible (Fig. 23-101). Metastases of these cells in lymph nodes often can only be appreciated initially because they replace normal structure. Careful search will always disclose the elongated forms and set aside the diagnosis of lymphosarcoma. In 84% of one series of cases,[316] the nuclei of lymph node metastases were larger and paler, and there was more cytoplasm, resembling cells of anaplastic squamous cell carcinoma. Some definite structural pattern has been noted.[271] The cells may be arranged in "streams" (i.e., clumps of cells with a parallel orientation of their long axes). Another variant is the "ribbon," one to several cells in width, often running in festoons (Fig. 23-102). Pseudorosettes, rosettes, tubules, and ductules also can be seen. Ductules sometimes contain epithelial mucin, but there is no resemblance to poorly differentiated adenocarcinoma.

Serious misconceptions have been held for many years about the nature of oat cell carcinoma. For a long time it was thought to be a mediastinal lymphosarcoma and then, till recently, an anaplastic (possibly epidermoid) carcinoma. The fallacy of the latter was demolished in three stages: (1) Azzopardi's demonstration of the structural pattern,[271] (2) the recognition of endocrine activity in some of these tumors (p. 974), and (3) the electron microscopic delineation of the close relationship of oat cell carcinoma to carcinoid.

Rarely in pathology is orthodoxy so profoundly demolished and reconstructed as in the work of Bensch et al.[273] They have confirmed that in normal bronchial epithelium (especially in the first year of life) occasional argyrophilic cells are present. In fact, they are Kulchitsky cells—not surprising in view of the foregut origin of the respiratory bud.[294] Electron microscopy disclosed neurosecretory-type granules in their cytoplasm. Similar granules are present in the cytoplasm of oat cell carcinomas and of bronchial carcinoids. Here lies the explanation of the difficulty we sometimes experience in deciding whether we are

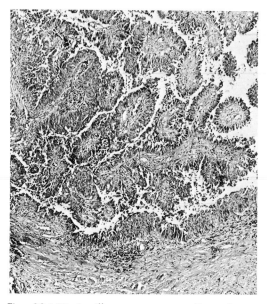

Fig. 23-100 Papillary squamous cell carcinoma of bronchus, type sometimes called transitional carcinoma. (×90.)

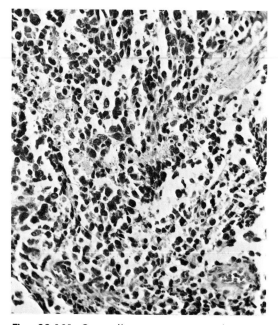

Fig. 23-101 Oat cell carcinoma, "usual" type. (×234.)

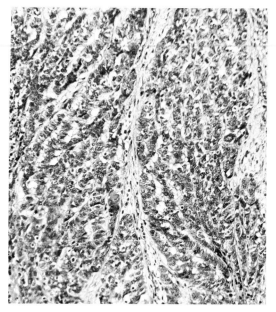

Fig. 23-102 Oat cell carcinoma. Variant with cells arranged in ribbons. (×152.)

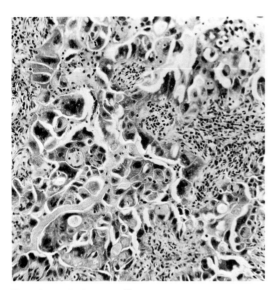

Fig. 23-103 Giant cell carcinoma. (×168.)

looking at an oat cell carcinoma or a carcinoid. Perhaps this is a clue as to why most endocrine syndromes caused by lung cancer are associated with the oat cell variety.

Undifferentiated large cell carcinoma. Undifferentiated large cell carcinomas lack differentiation into epidermoid or glandular character but have cells of varying types. The diagnosis begins by exclusion of recognizable features of squamous cells, oat cells, or glandular cells. With differing criteria, this group swells and diminishes in various studies. The cells are close together in a medullary or solid alveolar arrangement. Invasion of small blood vessels and lymphatic vessels is common. Individual cells are oval, spindled, angular, or polyhedral. Results of nuclear and cytoplasmic staining are very variable, but the nuclei tend to be large, with prominent nucleoli.

The variant known as *giant cell carcinoma* is uncommon, invades blood vessels, is more widely metastasizing, and is the most rapidly fatal of all lung carcinomas. The cells are loosely set in a stroma, scanty even when subjected to reticulin stains. Cells are nearly all of the multinucleated giant cell type, frequently extremely bizarre and hyperchromatic (Fig. 23-103). Occasionally, one tumor cell is seen ingesting another. Smaller single-nucleated pleomorphic cells are present, and there are areas with spindled and strap cells, suggesting rhabdomyosarcoma but without cross striations.[302] Ozzello and Stout[304] showed by tissue culture that the cells are epithelial. Melamed[297] considers that this is just one form of undifferentiated large cell carcinoma.

There is reason for believing that most, if not all, giant cell carcinomas may be anaplastic adenocarcinoma.[288] Earlier impressions that the tumor arises earlier than the common carcinomas have turned out false.

Spindle cell carcinoma. Spindle cell carcinoma frequently has been mistaken for carcinosarcoma, which probably accounts for the excessive number of case reports of the latter. In sites such as the esophagus, urinary bladder, and oral mucosa, squamous cell carcinoma is well known to undergo transition to a spindled form, as can malignant melanoma. In breast carcinoma, cartilaginous and osseous metaplasia is recognized. Therefore, the diagnosis of carcinosarcoma of the lung is difficult to uphold.

Pattern of metastases

Lymphatic spread. Spread to hilar lymph nodes is seen in the great majority of cases, particularly when the tumor is in a large bronchus. Extension then occurs to the mediastinal and paratracheal groups. When the hilar lymph nodes have been destroyed, retrograde flow in the pulmonary lymphatic vessels reaches the subpleural plexus. The condition of carcinomatous lymphangiosis is the delicate white lacework produced when vessels of the plexus are totally permeated (Fig. 23-104). This condition is often also secondary to numerous small arterial emboli of tumor cells. Tumor cells may travel into the chest wall via lymphatic vessels in pleural adhesions. By retrograde extension through the diaphragm, lymph nodes along the abdominal aorta are colonized. Of great prognostic importance is the group of small nodes on the scalenus anterior muscle. These nodes are frequently biopsied, for their involvement renders the disease incurable. Invasion and obstruction of the thoracic duct cause chylothorax.

Hematogenous spread. Carcinoma of the lung can spread in the blood to any part of the body. Collier et al.[278] examined resected lungs for blood vessel invasion. They found that in patients with such invasion the five-year survival rate was 6%, whereas 72% of the few patients without vascular invasion lived for five years.

Extrathoracic metastases are usual, partly because the pulmonary veins are so often invaded. In one large series of autopsied cases, no metastases were present in 10.5%, most of which were squamous cell tumors.[312] Studies of other large groups of cases indicate that

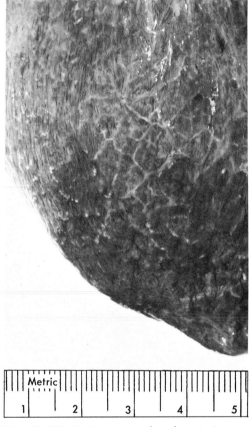

Fig. 23-104 Carcinomatous lymphangiosis.

metastases are found in the liver in about one-third, in the adrenal glands in 20% to 33%, in the skeletal system in 15% to 21%, in the brain in about 18%, in the kidneys in 14% to 17%, and in the spleen in about 5%.[4] Involvement of the liver can be massive at an early stage and may cause both jaundice and seeding back to the lungs. Frequently, the metastases from carcinoma of the lung present clinically as primary brain tumors. Extensive meningeal involvement can simulate meningitis or encephalitis.

Skin, pancreas, myocardium, and intestine occasionally are invaded. The pituitary gland, particularly the posterior lobe, often has metastases, and these rarely cause deficiency syndromes.

Extrapulmonary manifestations of bronchial carcinoma

A remarkable property of some bronchial carcinomas is their ability to produce hormones or effects on the neuromuscular system. To date, the following have been recorded: adrenocorticotropin, glucagon, sero-tonin or related substances, antidiuretic hormones, parathormone-like and insulin-like substances, and gonadotropin.

The clue to *gonadotropin* is the appearance of gynecomastia, which was seen in four men, all of whom had large anaplastic carcinomas of the bronchus.[323]

Nearly all the endocrine syndromes are associated with oat cell carcinoma, and the commonest is *Cushing's syndrome,* 115 examples of which had been collected by 1965.[320] (Note that islet cell carcinomas and thymomas sometimes also have this association.) It is typical that Cushing's syndrome secondary to lung carcinoma comes on rapidly and may be fulminant. The tumor either produces ACTH or a corticotropin-like substance that stimulates the adrenal glands and depresses ACTH secretion by the pituitary gland. In fact, sixteen of twenty patients with oat cell carcinoma (and without Cushing's syndrome) had increased numbers of pituitary hyaline basophils (Crooke's cells).[325] This is the hallmark of increased circulating cortisone-type hormones. In the Cushing cases, the adrenal glands are hyperplastic (two to three times normal weight) but, even without the syndrome, autopsies on patients who had oat cell carcinoma frequently disclose lesser degrees of adrenocortical hyperplasia. The latter is taken to indicate that there are two types of adrenocorticopin, one relating to adrenal weight and the other (in Cushing's syndrome) to steroid production. Finally, Cushing's syndrome may be associated with bronchial carcinoid.[329] Again, we see a relationship between the latter and oat cell carcinoma.

Inappropriate antidiuretic hormone activity has been reported about twenty-six times, nearly all the tumors being oat cell carcinoma, with occasional adenocarcinoma.[320] The hormone may be produced directly by the tumor. The clinical effects include hyponatremia and urinary sodium wastage, absence of edema, and renal and adrenal malfunction, these leading to lethargy, confusion, and coma. The last three are the symptoms of hypercalcemia of malignancy and of the *parathyroid-like activity.* Myers[301] discusses twenty-eight cases of hypercalcemia in various cellular types of lung cancer. Squamous cell carcinoma is the commonest associated tumor.

Another mysterious combination, and the commonest, is the group of neuromuscular abnormalities that may be associated with carcinoma of the lung.[321] *Cortical cerebellar degeneration* produces loss of cerebellar function. *Peripheral neuropathy,* usually purely sensory, is associated with degeneration of neurons in the posterior root ganglia. In some patients, *mental changes* are prominent. They are considered a metabolic effect of the tumor, since they occur in the absence of metastases. The effects range from impaired mental acuity to severe dementia. All three neuromuscular disorders may be combined in a mixed form. A fourth abnormality, a muscle weakness termed *carcinomatous myopathy,* is recognized. There are degenerative changes in the muscles of the limb girdle and trunk. These variants were found in 16% of the 250 patients examined in one study.[322] By 1966 a review had collected 165 cases, and oat cell carcinoma comprised 54% of the lung tumors in the patients.[327] Some patients with oat cell carcinoma developed a myasthenic syndrome with a relatively poor response to neostigmine.[324] This may be seen in as many as 6% of cases.[326]

Prognosis

Analysis of the results of surgical therapy in 2,156 patients suffering from bronchial carcinoma has revealed that in only 464 was resection possible, and 347 of these survived the operative phase. The five-year survival of the 347 patients was 28%, or slightly under 5% for the whole group.[287]

A better prognosis can be expected in cases of solitary nodular carcinomas of lung. When these are no bigger than 4 cm in diameter, the resection-for-cure rate is as high as 94%, and in persons surviving the operation for curative resection, the five-year survival is 51%. In a series of 193 such tumors, 58% were adenocarcinoma and alveolar cell carcinoma, 39% squamous and large cell carcinoma, and 3% oat cell carcinoma.[292]

A review[303] of fifty-one patients living five years after surgical therapy disclosed no special factors, such as early diagnosis, that would explain this survival. Of 2,540 patients, fifty-six survived ten years, but some still developed recurrences or new primary tumors. Prognosis is closely related to cell type. Survival is poor in all types, but least in oat cell carcinoma and best in adenocarcinoma, with squamous cell carcinoma coming next.[277, 285, 293, 312] In one series, of those patients who survived surgery, the five-year survival in those with oat cell carcinoma was 9%; large anaplastic carcinoma, 30%; squamous cell carcinoma, 42%; and adenocarcinoma, 54%.[293] Characteristic of this series, as of all others, is

the overall survival. That is to say, there were 767 patients, of whom only 184 could be offered surgery with a hope of cure (24%). Out of the 767, only 8% lived five years.

From the foregoing discussion, the value of accurate histologic typing becomes apparent. It is one factor in the evalution of prognosis. There is a close association between smoking and the oat, squamous, and large undifferentiated carcinomas. Certain cell types are associated with extrapulmonary manifestations.

Feinstein has written extensively as a biostatistician on the importance of a scientific methodology in clinical medicine. In particular, his considerations of the clinical and intellectual causes of defective statistics for the prognosis (and treatment) of cancer should be read.[283]

The *causes of death* from bronchial carcinoma are various combinations of pneumonia, lung abscess, bronchiectasis, asphyxia, bleeding, fistulas to the pleura or esophagus, and the effects of the various metastases. Adrenal cortical insufficiency is rare, even when the glands are extensively replaced.

Pulmonary adenomastosis, bronchiolar carcinoma, and adenocarcinoma

Clear distinctions between pulmonary adenomatosis, bronchiolar carcinoma, and some cases of adenocarcinoma of the lung often are difficult and perhaps unnecessary. **Adenomatosis** was referred to in the discussion of scar tumors and of changes in areas of chronic inflammation and fibrosis. Another variety is seen in the absence of fibrosis, when a single layer of well-differentiated tall columnar cells lines the alveoli in one or more areas. The cells have basal nuclei and copious pale cytoplasm that sometimes contains mucin. Cilia are rare. Sometimes, the cells are separated slightly from one another, creating a peglike appearance. Although usual histologic criteria of malignancy are lacking, the description may be the same in many cases of metastasizing **bronchiolar carcinoma.** It is impossible to distinguish the forms except by behavior, and one might infer that all such lesions are malignant.[4]

Several cases have been described in which carcinoma of the pancreas and a few from the stomach, ovary, or breast metastasized to the lung, exactly imitating bronchiolar carcinoma microscopically.[290] The frequency of peripancreatic node involvement at autopsy aggravates this problem of deciding which involved area is primary.

The third form, **adenocarcinoma,** remains for consideration. Like the other two, it is usually in the periphery of the lung. The only way to recognize it as an entity is to see it arising grossly as a roughening of the mucosa of a bronchus, with microscopic origin from the mucosa or the submucosal glands. It is uncommon in this form.

The preceding discussion gives reasons leading some to the view that all three lesions are only variants of one type of neoplasm. Shinton[309] considers bronchiolar carcinoma to be "a form of spread" of adenocarcinoma "rather than a histologic type." Liebow has not been able to distinguish the two unless by noting origin of a poorly differentiated adenocarcinoma from a small bronchus and by being aware of its rapid growth and early bloodborne metastases.[295]

It would seem best to consider that adenocarcinoma may be well or poorly differentiated, rarely arises from bronchi, often commences in scars (in half of one series of 100 cases[272a]), and is usually peripheral. Ultrastructural studies tend to show that it is a tumor of type II pneumonocytes.

Nature of disease

Adenocarcinoma occurs with equal frequency in men and women. However, it is proportionately a more frequent carcinoma of the lung in women because they have only one-sixth the number of bronchial carcinomas suffered by men. The incidence of the tumor appears to be increasing. Cases have been noted arising in relation to chronic pneumonitis and pulmonary scars.[272] Some of these have been in cases of honeycomb lung or diffuse interstitial fibrosis[298] and others in cases of progressive systemic sclerosis.[284] Three cases were complications of chronic mineral oil pneumonia.[275] Although an infectious disease of similar microscopic appearance is quite common in sheep ("jaagsiekte") and in horses, guinea pigs, and rats, this does not unravel the mystery. Disagreement remains about origin from bronchiolar or alveolar cells. Hence, this adenocarcinoma is variously named "alveolar cell," "bronchiolar," and "bronchioloalveolar." Discord arises as to whether or not multiple lesions in the lung indicate multicentricity. The majority view is that there is one origin with prolific airborne

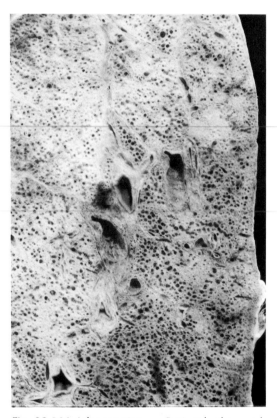

Fig. 23-106 Adenocarcinoma. Patient had no nodules of tumor, but most alveoli in both lungs were lined by single layer of well-differentiated cells like those shown in Fig. 108, A. Patient died of alveolocapillary block without metastases, and by some this would be regarded as an example of pulmonary adenomatosis.

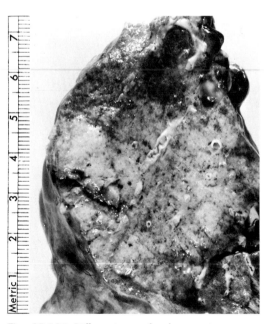

Fig. 23-105 Diffuse type of adenocarcinoma resembling diffuse type of squamous cell carcinoma (see Fig. 23-94).

dissemination along alveolar septa and the bronchial tree.[289]

Gross appearance

In the unusual instance of an adenocarcinoma arising from bronchial mucosa, the lesion will be close to the hilum and will resemble the other hilar tumors. Microscopically, there are small, quite well-formed but irregular glands lying in a connective tissue stroma and lined by a single or pseudostratified layer of tall columnar cells. These have large hyperchromatic nuclei and pale cytoplasm and may be ciliated.

Adenomatosis and bronchiolar carcinoma cannot be distinguished grossly even by those who regard them as separate conditions. About half of the cases are of nodular type, one-third diffuse (lobular or lobar) (Fig. 23-105), and the remainder mixed. In about two-thirds, both lungs are ultimately affected to a significant degree, in striking contrast to the bronchial group.

The nodules are gray-white consolidated areas averaging 3 cm to 5 cm and are fairly well demarcated. Very often they are multiple and present in some or all lobes. The diffuse variety is so extensive that it mimics a gray area of pneumonia (Fig. 23-106) or the yellow-white of organizing or lipid pneumonia. Central necrosis is common. Often, mucin secreted by the tumor cells makes the cut surface resemble that of klebsiella or pneumococcus type III pneumonia (Fig. 23-107). Efforts to demonstrate an origin from a bronchus will nearly always fail.

In a report on 205 cases of bronchiolar carcinoma, metastases were found to be present in 54% (19% local only, 16% distant only, and 20% local and distant). Mediastinal nodes were affected in 26%, liver in 13%, and the following sites (listed in descending order) each involved in less than 10%: abdominal nodes, bones, adrenal glands, brain, pleura, kidneys, pericardium, cervical nodes, spleen, heart, and diaphragm.[311] Note that the first five sites in this list have a high incidence of metastases in bronchial carcinoma.

Microscopic appearance

In the best-differentiated adenocarcinoma, a single layer of tall columnar cells lines alveolar septa (Fig. 23-108, *A*). Nuclei are small, basal, hyperchromatic, and fairly uniform, and the cytoplasm is pale or full of mucin. Mucin may distend some alveoli and even flatten the tumor cells lining them. Slender papillae of the cells may project into the alveoli. When respiratory bronchioles are recognized, tumor cells will be seen growing along the mucosal surface, and, proximally, a transition to the more cuboidal normal respiratory lining cells may be seen. However, just because cells line a fine membrane and enclose spaces the size and shape of alveoli, it does not mean that they are alveoli. Very likely, the membranes are often just fine stromal strands. Characteristically, at the periphery of the lesions it is easy to find tumor cells along some alveolar septa. Many cells, apparently viable, are free in the alveoli. A few cells lining septa rarely are ciliated, a feature not seen in any other tumor of the lung. In less-differentiated forms, the nuclear characteristics of malignancy appear—hyperchromasia, irregularity and pleomorphism, and mitoses. There is a sclerotic form in which the tumorous "acini" are separated from one another by connective tissue. Of still lower differentiation are the varieties with irregular glands no longer the shape and size of alveoli (Fig. 23-108, *B*) or with a cribriform pattern as if a duct were crossed by interlacing strands of tumor cells.

What is called *clear cell carcinoma* (Fig. 23-109) has been considered by some as a poorly differentiated adenocarcinoma.[300] There

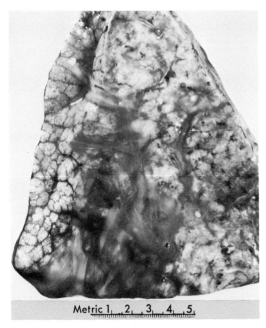

Fig. 23-107 Mucoid adenocarcinoma. Most of lung replaced by white soft tumor. Lower two-thirds of cut surface covered by tenaceous mucin, so that specimen resembles that of very mucinous pneumococcal or klebsiella pneumonia.

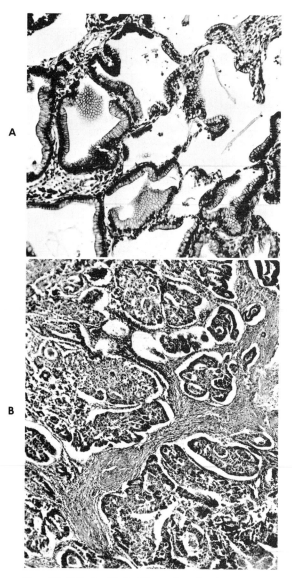

Fig. 23-108 A, Well-differentiated adenocarcinoma growing along interalveolar septa. **B,** Poorly differentiated adenocarcinoma with little resemblance to alveolar pattern. (**A,** ×124; **B,** ×111.)

are sheets and alveolar clumps of large rounded cells with clear nonstaining cytoplasm that often reacts with mucin stains. Others have identified glycogen in some of the cells. Some examples appear to be variants of squamous cell carcinoma with hydropic cytoplasm. The main problem is to exclude the presence of a primary carcinoma in the kidney.

"Bronchial adenoma"

The term "bronchial adenoma" should mean a benign glandlike proliferation of bronchial mucosa, but only eleven cases had been collected by 1967, all apparently in larger

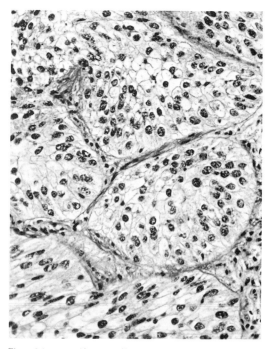

Fig. 23-109 Clear cell carcinoma. (×189.)

bronchi.[334] In practice, the term "bronchial adenoma" is used to designate a group of malignant or potentially malignant tumors: carcinoid, adenoid cystic carcinoma, and mucoepidermoid carcinoma. Some use the description "relatively benign primary epithelial tumors of bronchi." In a collection of 162 of these tumors, 89.5% were carcinoids, 8% were adenoid cystic carcinoma, and 2.5% (four cases) were mucoepidermoid carcinoma.[336]

"Bronchial adenomas" appear some years earlier on the average than carcinomas of the lung, and the sex distribution is equal. The three types cannot be distinguished grossly, although adenoid cystic carcinoma tends to be closer to the carina and may be in the trachea. The tumors are polypoid or sessile, but although they extend into the lumen, they are very likely to grow into the bronchial wall and expand into neighboring lung as a dumbbell shape, so that removal by bronchoscope is impossible. The surface of the endobronchial part is covered by intact mucosa and is smooth or lobulated. Gross examination gives no clue as to malignancy. Some carcinoids are partly ossified.

The microscopic appearance is the same as described for these tumors in the salivary gland and gastrointestinal tract (Fig. 23-110). *Carcinoids* of the lung have a number of microscopic variants. Osseous metaplasia may

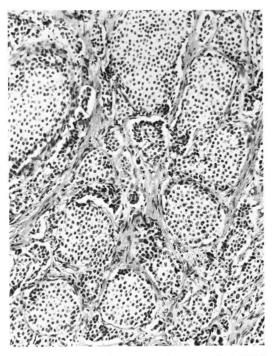

Fig. 23-110 Typical pattern of carcinoid. (×153.)

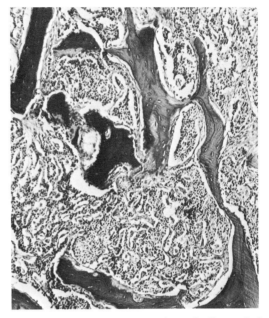

Fig. 23-111 Bronchial carcinoid. Markedly ossified stroma. (×96.)

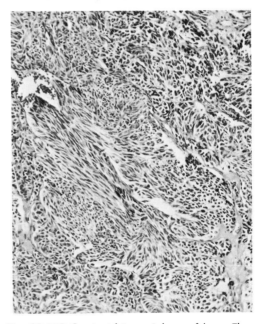

Fig. 23-112 Carcinoid in periphery of lung. There is marked spindled pattern. This tumor was malignant, although cellular pattern is not indicative of this. (×165.)

occur between the tumor cells (Fig. 23-111). A few carcinoids have pink granular cells of the oncocytic type. Glandular differentiation and mucin secretion are quite common in carcinoids and in no way rule out that diagnosis.[333] Also, a carcinoid is quite often poorly differentiated and can have a hardly recognizable organized pattern with extreme nuclear irregularity. Such cases may be mistaken for undifferentiated bronchial carcinoma. A distorted bronchial biopsy specimen makes this an even more difficult decision. Spindle-celled carcinoids also have to be recognized (Fig. 23-112). They are especially to be found peripherally, where carcinoids with granular cytoplasm also occur. Both types tend to be small, probably arising from small bronchi or bronchioles.[331] It would be easy to confuse such variants with tumorlets. The presence of bronchial mucosa to one side of the poorly defined tumor and the absence of a scar would point to a peripheral carcinoid.

In difficult cases, where the pattern is only suspicious for carcinoid, one cannot rely on argyrophil or argentaffin stains for cytoplasmic granules, since these are hard to see in any bronchial carcinoid. Dr. Victor Pardo has helped me by demonstrating the granules in electron microscopic studies of formalin-fixed tumor tissue.

Malignancy of carcinoids in the lung can be as difficult to determine as it is in the intestine.[337] With the recognition of the relationship to oat cell carcinoma (p. 972), some tumors that might in the past have been wrongly classed as oat cell carcinoma will now be recognized as malignant carcinoids.

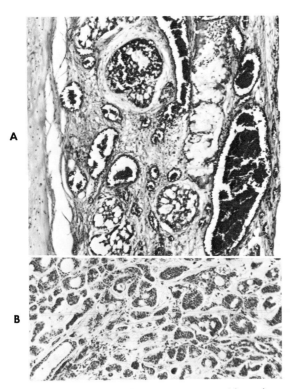

A

B

Fig. 23-113 Adenoid cystic carcinoma of bronchus. **A,** Its origin from mucosal glands. **B,** Deeper infiltrating portion. (**A,** ×84; **B,** ×119.)

About one dozen examples of carcinoid syndrome in association with a metastasizing bronchial carcinoid are now on record.[332] Carcinoids of different embryonic parts of the gut have differing carcinoid syndromes. That of the bronchi (foregut) is remarkable for severe and prolonged episodes of flushing, apparently because carcinoids have produced histamine and 5-OH tryptophan instead of serotonin. Such variation is marked ultrastructurally by recognizable differences in the morphology of carcinoids in different sites.[330] Bronchial carcinoids are argyrophilic but not argentaffin.

As of 1968, there were twenty-one cases of "bronchial adenoma" in children under the age of 16 years. Of those that were microscopically identified, nine were carcinoids, three adenoid cystic, and two mucoepidermoid.[339] A handful of cases of mediastinal carcinoids has been seen. Their origin is thought to be mediastinal remnants of bronchial anlagen.

Prognosis

In one reported series, only 57% of twenty-one patients with bronchial *carcinoid* tumor survived five years, and 44% of twenty-seven patients with such tumors had metastases.[333] In another series, *adenoid cystic carcinoma* was a slowly growing, infiltrating malignancy, invading adjacent structures, destroying cartilage, and eventually producing distant metastases[336] (Fig. 23-113). Most of the two dozen or so reported cases of *mucoepidermoid carcinoma* of the bronchus have been low grade (Fig. 23-114), and the three metastasizing cases cited in one study[335] are unusual.

RARE PULMONARY TUMORS
Bronchial chondroma

Bronchial chondroma is a smooth-surfaced but lobulated, pedunculated, or sessile tumor projecting into the lumen. Grossly, its cartilaginous nature is recognized on the cut surface, and it is seen microscopically to be well-formed hyaline cartilage. It is not to be confused with hamartoma (below).

Bronchial papillomatosis

The commoner laryngeal papillomatosis rarely extends down the trachea into the bronchial tree. Most of the patients are children, but occasionally adults are affected.[345] Death in such cases is from obstruction, aspiration, and pulmonary infection. The innumerable bronchial lesions are warty, with a microscopic structure of acanthotic stratified squamous epithelium covering the papillary and branching connective tissue core. There may be epithelial atypism or even malignant change.

Lipoma

One-fifth of pulmonary lipomas arise in fat normally present beneath the pleura. The remaining tumors are in the normal fat of the bronchial submucosa. When symptomatic, they mimic carcinoma. Histologically, they resemble lipomas seen in any part of the body.[348] By 1968, only thirty-three bronchial lipomas had been recorded.[342]

Bronchial hamartoma

Albrecht's original definition of hamartomas is "tumorlike malformations in which occur only an abnormal mixture of the normal constituents of the organ in which they are found. These malformations may consist of a change in the quantity, arrangement, degree of differentiation or any combination of these."*

---

*Translated from Albrecht, E.: Verh. Deutsch. Path. Ges. 7:153-157, 1904.

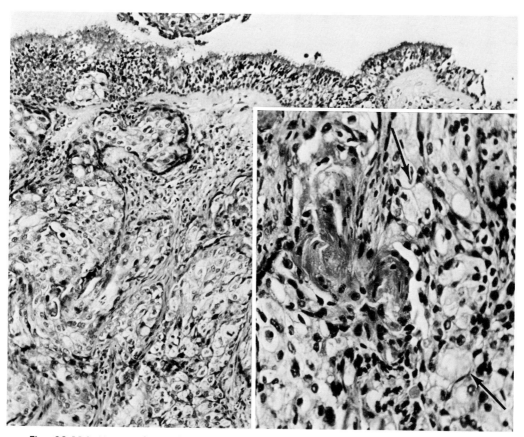

Fig. 23-114 Mucoepidermoid tumor of bronchus showing submucosal nature of tumor. Arrows in inset point to mucin-containing cells, to left of which is well-developed keratinization of other cells. (×177; inset, ×330.)

Bateson believes this is a tumor of undifferentiated mesenchyme in the bronchial submucosa and that it may grow into or away from the lumen.[340a] This relieves us of the embarrassment of trying to explain why no cases have been seen in childhood.

Although a case is recorded in a premature infant, nearly all the several hundred reported hamartomas of the lung have been in adults, with a preference for men. Most of the tumors are close to the pleura. They are usually 1 cm to 4 cm in diameter and spherical or ovoid, with lobulation. They shell out easily and have a cartilaginous appearance, often with foci of calcification (Fig. 16-23 and Fig. 23-115). Those with much fat are yellow. Usually, the principal microscopic component is hyaline cartilage, but some of Hodges' cases had elastic cartilage.[344] In the typical cases, between the masses of cartilage are clefts lined by bronchial epithelium, beneath which are fat and smooth muscle fibers (Fig. 23-116). Sometimes, the cartilage is replaced by fibromyxomatous tissue. About 1% of pulmonary hamartomas are endobronchial. Up to 1965, only fifty-three cases of the latter were recorded in the English literature.[346]

Lymphoma and leukemia

Lymphoma frequently is found to have spread to the lungs.[349] Primary lymphoma in the lungs is difficult to prove once the disease has become disseminated,[352] whereas many cases labeled lymphosarcoma are undoubtedly "pseudolymphoma."[350] Over ninety cases of primary lymphoma of the lung, most of which were lymphosarcoma, were collected by Saltzstein.[361] Pulmonary involvement in leukemia is commonest in the pleura and subpleura, but leukemic infiltration also is found in the interalveolar septa and around vessels and bronchi.[343] It may cause symptoms of alveolocapillary block, especially in lymphocytic leukemia.

Diffuse hamartoma

For a discussion of diffuse hamartoma, see p. 882.

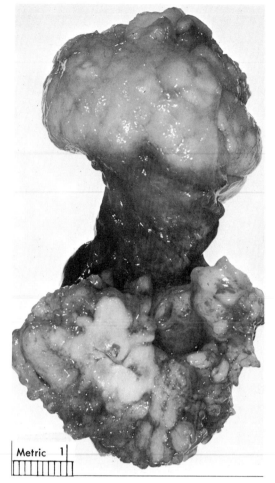

Fig. 23-115 Surgically removed hamartoma of lung. Some of cut surface can be seen in lower portion.

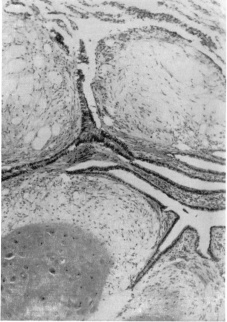

Fig. 23-116 Bronchial hamartoma. Hyaline cartilage, lower left, surrounded by loose connective tissue and fat and covered in turn by bronchial epithelium. Beneath this in places are smooth muscle fibers.

Pulmonary blastoma and carcinosarcoma

A *blastoma* is a tumor arising from a pluripotential cell of one germ layer that can undergo progressive and unlimited expansion. In the lung, it has appeared at any age between adolescence and late adult life, manifested as a well-demarcated white mass. Microscopically, there are solid tubelike cords of epithelial cells and irregular glandlike structures resting in an immature stroma of spindled or stellate cells (Fig. 23-117). Some consider this to be a replication of fetal lung. Metastases of such tumors occur.

Carcinosarcoma may be related to or even be a more malignant form of blastoma. It is grossly similar, has a similar age incidence, metastasizes more often, and may be either multiple or endobronchial.[351] Microscopically, there are various types of adenocarcinoma intermingled with fibrosarcoma, sometimes with osteosarcoma or chondrosarcoma.

No explanation has been made that is satisfactory to all authorities. Spencer[4] firmly believes that it is a counterpart of Wilms' tumor (a mesoblastic tumor) and does not explain the absence of childhood cases. Barson et al.[340] are convinced that the similarity to fetal lung is fortuitous and that all the tumors must be carcinosarcomas of varying degrees of malignancy. Stackhouse et al.[351] quote Willis' point that adult mesenchymal tissue may contain undifferentiated cells that could revert to their pluripotential embryonic state. Viewing the available evidence, I incline to the carcinosarcoma theory, keeping in mind the analogy not of Wilms' tumor but of cystosarcoma phyllodes of the breast. The latter is a lesion, benign or malignant, that appears late in adolescence and later.

Other tumors

Chemodectoma, benign clear cell tumor, fibroma, leiomyoma, neurofibroma, granular cell myoblastoma, and sarcoma of the lower respiratory tract are great rarities.[4]

Of this group, *sarcomas* of muscle are among the least rare. Over forty leiomyosarcomas have been reported.[347] They should not be

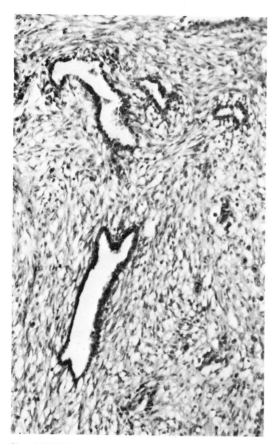

Fig. 23-117 Pulmonary blastoma. Poorly formed tubular pattern in abundant mesenchymal stroma. (×165.)

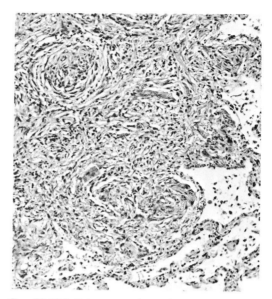

Fig. 23-118 Pulmonary chemodectoma from case with pulmonary hypertension. (×147.)

confused with spindle-celled carcinoma (p. 973) and fibrous histiocytoma (bottom of opposite column). Many are bronchial rather than pulmonary.[4] Only nine rhabdomyosarcomas are known to have occurred in the lung.[341] These should not be confused with giant cell carcinoma (p. 973).

Chemodectoma is probably a functional hyperplasia of normal nonchromaffin paraganglionic tissue in relation to pulmonary venules that supply them with blood (Fig. 23-118). Perhaps the cells "sample" the blood before it returns to the heart. The lesion is infrequent and usually multiple. It is to be distinguished from tumorlet and the angiomatoid lesion of pulmonary hypertension.

Benign clear cell tumor is rare but important, since it may be confused with metastatic renal cell carcinoma and sclerosing hemangioma. It appears as a coin lesion chiefly in middle-aged persons. Microscopically, it is composed of uniform, large, pale clear cells, rich in cytoplasmic glycogen, and has a sinusoidal blood supply.[346a]

SOLITARY PULMONARY NODULES

One of the most important clinical problems is evidence of a single radiopaque nodule, often discovered by chance. In one reported study[354] of resected solitary pulmonary nodules from 887 men in seventy-eight hospitals, in 316 cases the nodules were malignant (280 primary, twenty-six metastatic, seven "adenoma," and three miscellaneous). There were sixty-five cases of hamartoma and 474 of granuloma. Most of the latter were histoplasmosis (164), tuberculosis (122), and coccidioidomycosis (98). A miscellaneous group of twenty-three comprised entities such as infarct, bronchial cyst, pneumonitis, and vascular disorder. There were nine cases of tumor of pleura or chest wall. In patients over 50 years of age, 56% of the nodules were malignant.

These represent the findings in surgical series of cases. In public health surveys, the yield of primary malignancies is 5% or less of persons found to have solitary nodules by x-ray examination.[353] One important lesson is that calcification does not necessarily exclude the diagnosis of malignancy.

PSEUDOTUMORS
Histiocytoma

In the soft tissues of the body, we have become aware of the large family of *fibrous histiocytoma* (fibrous xanthoma), some members of which are malignant, and which takes its protean nature from the ability of the

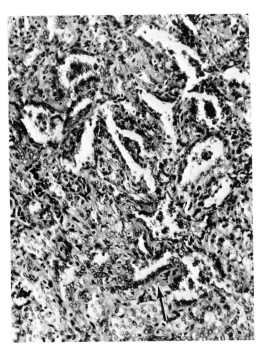

Fig. 23-119 Sclerosing hemangioma. Pale or clear cells among dilated small vessels. Arrow points to cuboidal change in trapped alveoli. (×195.)

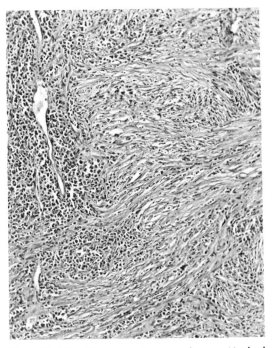

Fig. 23-120 Plasma cell granuloma. Marked fibroblastic reaction (fibers arranged in parallel bundles) is heavily infiltrated by plasma cells. (×165.)

tissue histiocyte to convert into a fibroblast. Two members of the family seem to have settled in the lung, sclerosing hemangioma and plasma cell granuloma. Here, virtually none has been reported as malignant, and excision is curative.

Sclerosing hemangioma

Sclerosing hemangioma (Fig. 23-119) takes the form of a benign solitary nodule in the lung, sometimes involving a bronchus. It is oval or spherical and well encapsulated, usually ranging in diameter from 1.5 cm to 8 cm.[358] Most have been in the lower lobes and in women. The cut surface is gray-pink and fleshy, with yellow and hemorrhagic areas. Microscopically, there is vascular proliferation, the channels varying from large and thin-walled vessels with flat lining cells to those with small lumina and thick hyaline walls. In some areas, proliferation of hyalinized connective tissue appears to replace the vessels. In places, vessels project in papillary fashion into alveoli, the cells of which react with marked cuboidal metaplasia. As the collagenous areas fuse and alveoli disappear, this throttling of vessels causes bleeding (in fact, Spencer[4] believes the process is not primarily

a proliferation of vessels). Many areas of old and recent hemorrhage are present, with numerous large histiocytes filled with lipid or hemosiderin.[355, 362]

Plasma cell granuloma

Plasma cell granuloma is another rare cause of a large solitary nodule, especially in younger persons. The alternative name, *inflammatory pseudotumor*, hints at the possible etiology. Grossly, it resembles sclerosing hemangioma. Some have been well-demarcated nodules of 2 cm to 4 cm, but larger ones, occupying much of a lobe, have been seen. When hard, they have a streaky gray-white cut surface. Softer forms are yellow. Microscopically, there are masses of plasma cells, both mature and immature. Many contain Russell bodies. Lymphocytes and even lymphoid follicles may be present.[359] Often, parallel bands of cellular fibrous tissue make up the bulk of the tumor (Fig. 23-120), sometimes with foamy histiocytes in the interstices. This tumor is no form of myeloma or plasmacytoma,[359] although true myeloma of the lung does occur (6.9% of the Mayo Clinic cases of myeloma, in which admittedly nearly all the cases were examples of direct invasion of the lung from ribs or vertebrae).[357] It is not likely that *tumoral amyloidosis* of the lung[356] is a later stage in which masses of amyloid are laid down.

Pseudolymphoma

Sometimes, unexplained accumulations of lymphoid tissue are found in the lung. Although unencapsulated and frequently very large, the lesions do not become disseminated and have histologic features that further distinguish them from lymphomas. An individual pseudolymphoma may be several centimeters in diameter or may replace most of a lobe. The cut surface is gray-white and homogeneous. Microscopically, the important finding is a mixed cellular infiltrate, predominantly of mature lymphocytes, with some reticulum cells, plasma cells, and neutrophils. Of great significance is the presence of true germinal centers, not found in lymphomas, and the noninvolvement of the hilar lymph nodes. Sometimes, these distinctive features are lacking, and only time will tell if a true lymphoma is present.[361] The condition is similar to that seen in the mediastinum (p. 988) and must bear a close relationship to lymphoid interstitial pneumonia[360] (p. 943).

■ Pleura
PNEUMOTHORAX

Air or gas may enter the pleural cavity in the following conditions, usually as a result of "spontaneous" rupture: trauma, emphysema, cystic disease of lung, tuberculosis, bronchopleural fistula, abscess, septic infarct, pneumonia, bronchiectasis, perforation of the esophagus or stomach, honeycomb lung, berylliosis, diffuse interstitial fibrosis, influenza, and without demonstrable cause.

In most cases, pneumothroax is not dangerous, but sometimes the air collects under pressure because of valve action. The lung on the involved side will be totally collapsed, and the mediastinal structures will be displaced to the opposite side. The air in a pneumothorax usually is slowly resorbed. Complications are effusion, hemorrhage, infection, interstitial emphysema, and rapid death.

PLEURAL FLUID

Three classes of pleural fluid can be present: transudates, exudates, and a miscellaneous group.

A *transudate* or hydrothorax is the result of passage of fluid brought about by increased hydrodynamic pressure or decreased colloid-osmotic pressure of the blood or lymph in the vascular bed of the visceral or parietal pleura. Most commonly, this is the circulatory disturbance of cardiac failure. It also may be due to mechanical obstruction, as when a hilar tumor blocks lymphatic drainage or when the superior vena cava or azygos vein is obstructed. Changes in plasma osmotic pressure occurring in hypoproteinemia or sodium retention also will allow fluid to escape into the pleural cavity. The cause of the hydrothorax accompanying ovarian fibroma (Meig's syndrome) is unknown.

An *exudate* is the result of pleural inflammation—either primary, or secondary to bacterial infection in the underlying lung, viral and rickettsial disease, fungal infection, or parasitic infestation (amebiasis, trichinosis, paragonimiasis). Noninfective irritant causes include tumors of the lung and pleura, pulmonary infarction, rheumatic fever, collagen disease, and pneumothorax.

Transudates are watery, straw-colored fluids of low specific gravity and low protein content, none of which features are constant enough to be reliable.[2] Exudates, apart from their possible cellular or microbial content, have more protein. It is usual to classify transudates as serofibrinous, purulent, or sanguineous. The serofibrinous fluid of early tuberculosis is pale yellow and either contains small rounded fibrin balls when removed or else clots in vitro. Shaggy fibrin coats the pleural surfaces to varying degrees and, if present a long time, may organize into a fibrous mantle or obliterate the pleural cavity. Most chest physicians believe that the term "idiopathic pleural effusion" should not be used and that the condition should be assumed to be tuberculosis until strenuous diagnostic efforts have been made to exclude this diagnosis (roentgenography, culture of the fluid, skin testing, and pleural biopsy).

Polyserositis (Concato's disease) is characterized by effusions in pleural, pericardial, and peritoneal cavities, terminating in constrictive pericarditis, "sugar icing" of the liver and spleen, and fibrous thickening of the linings of all these cavities.

Hemorrhagic exudates always raise the suspicion of tuberculosis, cancer, or pulmonary infarction.

The collection of purulent exudate in the pleural space is called *empyema* or pyothorax. It is the result of pyogenic or tuberculous inflammation of the lung, necrotic infected tumor, lung abscess, fistula, infection introduced at surgery, systemic mycosis, blood-borne infection, subdiaphragmatic abscess, bronchopleural fistula, trauma, or mediastinitis. Any organism may be responsible, but the three commonest are pneumococci, staphylococci, and hemolytic streptococci. The appearance of the pus varies to some extent with the different organisms. At first, a thick shaggy fibrin layer covers the pleurae, the surfaces being separated by pus. Very commonly, the empyema becomes walled off, or encysted, either in the main pleural cavity, at the base of the lung, against the mediastinum, or in an interlobar fissure. In the final stage, organization of this material so encases the lung that it cannot expand. The effect is even worse in childhood because there is retarded growth of the thoracic cage on the affected side. At any age, the organized tissue may become calcified.

Tuberculous empyema varies between a thin, watery, yellow-white fluid and a thick, creamy, or caseous yellow fluid. Either variety may be blood-stained.

The chief member of the *miscellaneous group* of fluids is *chylothorax*. This means the presence of chyle in the pleural cavity due to obstruction of, or injury to, the thoracic duct or its tributaries. Obstruction is most often due to pressure by enlarged mediastinal lymph nodes, while the trauma can be either accidental or a complication of intrathoracic surgery. There is also a rare congenital chylothorax, which may be fatal. The fluid is an emulsion of fat globules that give it an opalescent creamy appearance, and there is separation into an upper fatty layer on standing. It is odorless and alkaline and can be cleared by adding fat solvents or stained with dyes such as scarlet red. This distinguishes chylothorax from a *pseudochylous effusion,* a fluid that is turbid or milky from cholesterol and lecithin or albuminous particles in fine suspension. There are no fat droplets. Lipoid nephrosis, subacute glomerulonephritis, and tuberculous pleurisy are the causes. *Chyliform effusion* appears creamy because of its content of breaking-down inflammatory or neoplastic cells.

PLEURAL TUMORS

Very rarely, there are benign or malignant tumors of the subpleural connective tissues. Except for these, and subpleural tumors of the lung, the only pleural tumor to consider is the *mesothelioma.* A firm diagnosis of mesothelioma cannot be made without proof that there is no carcinoma in the body, for metastases of adenocarcinoma with marked desmoplasia can mimic mesothelioma. A primary tumor in the stomach, colon, pancreas, ovary, or adrenal gland must first be ruled out. The relationship to asbestosis[363] is discussed on p. 932. A survey of fifty-two cases of pleural mesothelioma revealed a history of industrial association with asbestos in 80% of the series.[366a] Mesothelial cells can form phagocytes, fibroblasts, and epithelial cells. Recognition of this fact removes intellectual qualms about the varied pictures of these tumors, and tissue cultures appear to have proved the mesothelial origin of the tumor. There are two arbitrary groups—localized mesothelioma and diffuse spreading mesothelioma.

Localized mesothelioma occurs in late middle age in either sex and can be benign or, rarely, malignant. It creates an encapsulated, pedunculated, or sessile firm mass on the surface of the lung, in a fissure, or buried within the lung. Size ranges from a few to many centimeters. The cut surface is yellow or gray-white, sometimes with a pink tinge or with cystic areas containing pale yellow fluid. The microscopic picture is of a fibroma, with interweaving bundles of fibroblasts lying in a collagenous tissue. In this may be small clefts lined by a single layer of flat or cuboidal cells (Fig. 23-121). Other varieties have a

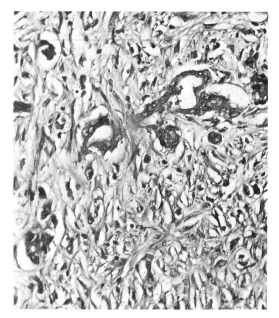

Fig. 23-121 Mesothelioma. (×228.)

predominantly papillary pattern, with or without tubular structures. The fibrous component may be very cellular or may, in places, be hyalinized.

Benignancy is shown by the lack of recurrence or metastasis and by a very slow course.[364] Blood-stained pleural fluid is common even in the benign varieties, and mitoses can be found in the connective tissue component of even clinically benign solitary mesotheliomas. Only recurrence with intrathoracic spread or invasion of the chest wall indicates malignancy, for metastasis of this variety is not reported.[366]

Diffuse spreading mesothelioma is always malignant. A thick white or pink tissue ensheathes part or all of a lung, particularly the basal portion. It may involve the visceral pleura, and the pleural space contains watery or bloody fluid until the tumor becomes so thick that the space is obliterated. Underlying lung is collapsed but not otherwise involved. The tumors spread by direct extension, invasion of neighboring tissues and organs, pleural implantation, and lymphatic and hematogenous metastases.[365] Microscopically, both epithelial and connective tissue elements resemble those of the solitary form, although the degree of atypism may be greater. The epithelial cells may be in a cordlike, tubular, glandular, or papillary carcinomatous pattern. The connective tissue ranges from quite well-differentiated to fibrosarcomatous types.

■ Mediastinum

The mediastinum is the median connective tissue in which are slung the heart and the hila of the lungs, while posteriorly the aorta, thoracic duct, and esophagus run through it. The *superior mediastinum* lies above the pericardium and contains the aortic arch, great vessels, thymus, trachea, esophagus, and thoracic duct. The *inferior mediastinum* has three compartments: anterior, middle, and posterior. The *anterior mediastinum* is the shallow space between the pericardium and body of the sternum, containing some lymph nodes. The *middle mediastinum* contains the heart and pericardium, the tracheal bifurcation, and the pulmonary arteries and veins. The *posterior mediastinum* is behind the trachea, pericardium, and posterior surface of the diaphragm. It is the space in front of the vertebral column containing the thoracic aorta, azygos and hemiazygos veins, esophagus, and thoracic duct.

INFLAMMATORY DISEASES

Mediastinal emphysema. Mediastinal emphysema is the escape of air into the interstitial tissue. It usually comes from the lungs, but sometimes escapes from the esophagus in certain kinds of trauma.[381]

Mediastinitis. Mediastinitis is a serious acute inflammation most often caused by trauma, external or internal. The latter includes rupture of the esophagus by swallowed foreign bodies or incoordinated vomiting. Perforation of the trachea or esophagus by carcinoma is an important cause. Mediastinal infection can be set up from the local lymph nodes, pleural cavity, pericardium, subdiaphragmatic abscess, and osteomyelitis of the thoracic cage. In some patients, there is widespread mediastinal cellulitis, whereas others develop an abscess.

Chronic fibrous mediastinitis. Chronic fibrous mediastinitis is a manifestation of granulomatous disease such as histoplasmosis and tuberculosis. Sometimes, patients have fibrocaseous granulomatous disease from which organisms cannot be cultured.[368, 389] The commonest effect is constriction of the superior vena cava, but obstruction may be apparent in the tracheobronchial tree, pulmonary veins, and esophagus. In presenting a case in which both pulmonary arteries were seriously impinged on, Nelson suggests that cases without granulomas may be variants of idiopathic mediastinal fibrosis (below) more often than is suspected.[383]

Idiopathic mediastinal fibrosis. Idiopathic mediastinal fibrosis is an abnormal proliferation of fibrous tissue in the superior mediastinum.[369] It surrounds the great veins at the formation of the superior vena cava and thus sets up venous hypertension in its catchment area. The patient is saved from serious consequences by a slowly developing collateral circulation. This disease resembles idiopathic retroperitoneal fibrosis, an opinion shared by Lattes and Pachter,[380] who prefer the term "fibromatosis." In a reported series of twenty cases,[376] there was partial or complete caval obstruction in twelve, involvement of the tracheobronchial tree in four, esophageal obstruction in two, and one death due to stenosis of the pulmonary vein.

TUMORS AND CYSTS

Diseases of the thymus are considered in Chapter 32. There remain the following categories: (1) enlargement of lymph nodes, (2) mesenchymal tumors, (3) nerve tissue tumors, (4) intrathoracic thyroid and parathyroid glands, (5) cysts, and (6) teratomas. These are arranged in order of incidence and site of relative frequency in the following list*:

Superior mediastinum

Goiter
Bronchogenic cyst
Parathyroid adenoma
Myxoma
Lymphoma

Anterior mediastinum

Thymoma
Teratoma
Goiter
Parathyroid adenoma
Lymphoma
Lipoma
Fibroma
Lymphangioma
Hemangioma
Chondroma
Giant lymph node hyperplasia
Thymic cyst
Rhabdomyosarcoma

Middle mediastinum

Bronchogenic cyst
Lymphoma
Pericardial cyst
Plasma cell myeloma

Posterior mediastinum

Neurilemoma
Neurofibroma
Ganglioneuroblastoma
Malignant schwannoma
Fibrosarcoma
Lymphoma
Goiter
Xanthofibroma
Gastroenteric cyst
Chondroma
Myxoma
Heterotopia of bone marrow
Meningocele
Paraganglioma

In one series of forty-two cysts and tumors of the mediastinum in patients under 16 years of age, one-third of the lesions were malignant.[377]

Enlargement of lymph nodes

In this group are the lymphomas and leukemias, metastases, infections, and granulomas. They may press upon the trachea, esophagus, large veins, hilar structures, or thoracic duct. Two additional entities require discussion.

Mediastinal lymph node hyperplasia pro-

duces single or multinodular masses 5 cm to 15 cm in diameter, mainly in the posterior mediastinum. The cut surface is soft and homogeneously gray-red. In the past, such masses have been diagnosed as misplaced thymomas, but most now consider this condition to be a chronic nonspecific inflammatory process in lymph nodes. The masses sometimes are considered to be hamartomas, since the lesions have occurred in regions in which lymph nodes are not found, including soft tissues of the neck and shoulder and within skeletal muscle.[380] Later authors have drawn attention to a distinctive, large systemic arterial supply to the mass. No longer is there the normal vascular supply to a lymph node but proliferation (with endothelial cell mitoses) of stromal vessels originating from the capsular region. When vessels enter a lymphoid follicle in these cases, they frequently become hyalinized, creating a resemblance to a Hassall's corpuscle. If the lesion is a vascular hamartoma modifying lymphoid tissue, then the alternative term *angiomatous lymphoid hamartoma* is preferable.[391] Usually, they are

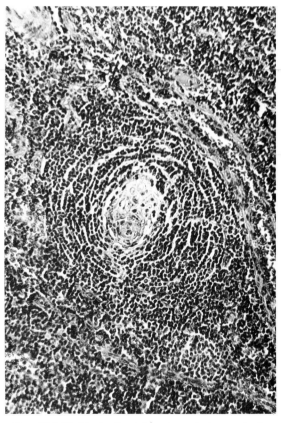

Fig. 23-122 Mediastinal lymph node hyperplasia with pseudo-Hassall's corpuscles. (×150.)

---

*Modified from Schlumberger, H. C.: Tumors of the mediastinum. In Atlas of tumor pathology, Sect. V, Fasc. 18, Armed Forces Institute of Pathology.

detected accidentally and have to be removed for diagnostic purposes. Microscopically, the tissue does not have the structure of true lymph nodes, because there is no cortico-medullary pattern, medullary cords, hilum, or subcapsular sinuses.[379] A predominant feature is the exceedingly rich vascularization to which are added marked proliferation of lymphoid tissue, including hyperplasia of lymphoid follicles with and without germinal centers. In the center of follicles is a marked endothelial proliferation of small vessels. They are responsible for the mistaken diagnosis of thymoma because they have hyperplastic endothelium and thick hyalinized walls, often concentrically arranged, resembling Hassall's corpuscles[370] (Fig. 23-122). When the lumina become obliterated, the deception is complete.

Massive intrathoracic hematopoiesis appears in some persons with chronic hemolytic anemia or hereditary spherocytosis. Single or multiple masses of bone marrow, up to 6 cm or 7 cm in diameter, are found paraspinally in the posterior mediastinum.[371]

Mesenchymal tumors

Of the mesenchymal tumors, lipoma is the commonest, but it is in itself a rarity.[385]

Nerve tissue tumors

The commonest tumors of the mediastinum are nerve tissue tumors, teratoma and thymoma coming next. They are found in the paravertebral region, since they arise from sympathetic nerve trunks or intercostal nerves. They occur at all ages, but the more malignant ones appear in the young, who are more likely to have tumors arising from ganglion cells. The tumors of nerve sheaths, in descending order of frequency, are neurile-moma, neurofibroma, and malignant schwan-noma (neurofibrosarcoma). Tumors of ganglion cells are ganglioneuroma, ganglioneuro-blastoma, and neuroblastoma (sympathico-blastoma).

The benign tumors may reach 10 cm to 20 cm in diameter and are generally firm and well encapsulated.[384, 386] They are rounded, lobulated, or, if growing intraspinally into the mediastinum, dumbbell shaped. Neurile-moma is encapsulated and often centrally necrotic. Neurofibroma may be mistaken for a malignant tumor because it has no capsule. Ganglioneuroma can form the largest of all mediastinal tumors. Attachment to the sympathetic trunk or an intercostal nerve is frequently demonstrable.

Intrathoracic thyroid and parathyroid glands

When thyroid and parathyroid glands are displaced into the mediastinum, they are subject to their usual diseases. A large mediastinal goiter can compress the trachea. Parathyroid glands enjoy a variety of positions, including the anterior mediastinum, behind the esophagus, or within the thymus.

Cysts

All mediastinal cysts are rare. The most frequent are bronchogenic, pericardial, lymphatic, gastric and enterogenous, and nonspecific cysts.[367, 378, 382] *Bronchogenic cysts* are described on p. 881. When mediastinal, they may cause obstruction of the tracheobronchial tree of children.[375]

Pericardial cysts lie in one of the cardiophrenic angles. They rarely communicate with the pericardial cavity but are attached to the anterior pericardium directly or by a pedicle. Microscopically, there is a thin connective tissue wall lined by one layer of flat or cuboidal cells.

Lymphatic cysts vary from unilocular through multilocular to cavernous lymph-angioma. Sometimes, they undertake an infiltrative character and are then called *cystic hygroma.* Large lymphangiomas often are associated with chylothorax and apparent obliteration of the thoracic duct. It may be that the ductal changes are primary and the "lymphangioma" secondary.[372]

Gastroenterogenous cysts are most likely to be found posteriorly near the hila on either side of the midline and are, in infants, the commonest cause, after neuroblastoma, of a posterior mediastinal mass. They arise from a diverticulum of the developing foregut that becomes adherent to the notochord. This explains their close attachment or relationship to the vertebrae and the frequency of accompanying vertebral malformations. The cyst may be lined by gastric epithelium or small or large intestinal epithelium. A related cyst is the *esophageal cyst,* attached to the esophagus and lined by noncornifying stratified squamous epithelium and sometimes by ciliated cells. About 100 cases of esophageal and gastroenterogenous cysts have been recorded.

Nonspecific cysts are considered to be the result of inflammation and hemorrhage in the various types just described.[382]

To this group of mediastinal cysts can be added the *intrathoracic meningocele,* which arises by extension of dura and subarachnoid through a spinal nerve foramen, creating a large cystic dilatation beneath the pleura. The wall is of delicate vascular connective tissue resembling arachnoid.

Teratomas

The anterior mediastinum is the third commonest site of teratoma after the ovary and testis. How these tumors start in the mediastinum is caught up in the mystery of the nature of all teratomas. The *benign cystic teratoma* (dermoid cyst) is as described in the ovary and is two or three times commoner than the malignant variety.

Malignant teratoma is predominantly solid and may have recognizable pieces of bone or cartilage. There may be extension into the pericardium or lung. Nineteen of the twenty recorded[390] cases occurred in men, and survival after diagnosis is usually less than one year.[387] The malignant component is squamous or glandular carcinoma, rarely sarcoma.

Chorioepithelioma is a particular variety of highly malignant teratoma that is friable and very hemorrhagic. Since it is found only in men, a primary tumor in the testis should be excluded.[388] Some authorities will not accept a case as arising extratesticularly if there is even a scar or cyst in the testis.

Seminoma of the mediastinum is a very rare tumor, probably a variant of teratoma. Thirty-one seminomas were collected in a 1968 review.[374]

REFERENCES
General

1 Reid, L.: The pathology of emphysema, London, 1967, Lloyd-Luke (Medical Books) Ltd.
2 Rezek, P. R., and Millard, M.: Autopsy pathology, Springfield, Ill., 1963, Charles C Thomas, Publisher.
3 Saphir, O., editor: A text on systemic pathology, vols. I and II, New York, 1958, Grune & Stratton, Inc.
4 Spencer, H.: Pathology of the lung (excluding pulmonary tuberculosis), ed. 2, London/New York, 1968, Pergamon Press, Inc.

Pulmonary structure and function

5 Avery, M. E.: The lung and its disorders in the newborn infant, ed. 2, Philadelphia, 1968, W. B. Saunders Co.
5a Azzopardi, A., and Thurlbeck, W. M.: Amer. Rev. Resp. Dis. 99:516-525, 1969.
6 Bertalanffy, F. D.: Amer. Rev. Resp. Dis. 91:605-609, 1965.
7 Boyden, E. A.: Amer. J. Anat. 121:749-761, 1967.
8 Clements, J. A.: In Liebow, A. A., and Smith, D. E., editors: The lung, Baltimore, 1968, The Williams & Wilkins Co., (surface active materials in lungs).
8a Clements, J. A.: Amer. Rev. Resp. Dis. 101:984-990, 1970.
9 Divertie, M. B., and Brown, A. L., Jr.: Med. Clin. N. Amer. 48:1049-1054, 1964.
10 Gough, J.: Postgrad. Med. J. 41:392-400, 1965.
11 von Hayek, H.: In Ciba Foundation Symposium on Pulmonary structure and function, Boston, 1962, Little, Brown and Co.
12 Krahl, V. E.: Amer. Rev. Resp. Dis. 80:(July suppl.):24-44, 1959.
13 Lauweryns, J. M.: Amer. Rev. Resp. Dis. 102:877-885, 1970.
13a Morgan, T. E.: New Eng. J. Med. 284:1185-1193, 1971.
14 Reid, L.: Thorax 13:110-115, 1958.
15 Reid, L.: Thorax 14:138-145, 1959.
16 Towers, B.: In Assali, N., editor: Biology of gestation, 1969, Academic Press, Inc., (fetal and neonatal lung).
17 Wagenvoort, C. A., Heath, D., and Edwards, J. E.: The pathology of the pulmonary vasculature, Springfield, Ill., 1964, Charles C Thomas, Publisher.
17a Wang, N. S., Huang, S. N., Sheldon, H., and Thurlbeck, W. M.: Amer. J. Path. 62:237-246, 1971.

Congenital anomalies

18 Belanger, R., LaFlèche, L. R., and Picard, J-L.: Thorax 19:1-11, 1964.
19 Bessolo, R. J., and Maddison, F. E.: Amer. J. Roentgen. 103:572-576, 1968.
20 Bonham Carter, R. E., Capriles, M., and Noe, Y.: Brit. Heart J. 31:45-51, 1969.
21 Borrie, J., Lichter, I., and Rodda, R. A.: Brit. J. Surg. 50:623-633, 1963.
22 Edwards, J. E.: Lab. Invest. 9:46-66, 1960.
23 Franch, R. H., and Gay, B. B.: Amer. J. Med. 35:512-529, 1963.
24 Gerle, R. D., Jaretzki, A., III, Ashley, C. A., and Berrie, A. S.: New Eng. J. Med. 278:1413-1419, 1968.
25 Good, C. A.: Amer. J. Roentgen. 85:1009-1024, 1961.
26 Kittle, C. F., and Crockett, J. E.: Ann. Surg. 156:222-233, 1962.
27 Laurence, K. M.: J. Clin. Path. 12:62-69, 1959.
28 Maltz, D. L., and Nadas, A. S.: Pediatrics 42:175-188, 1968.
29 Moffat, A. D.: J. Path. Bact. 70:361-372, 1960.
30 Moncrieff, M. W., Cameron, A. H., Astley, R., Roberts, K. D., Abrams, L. D., and Mann, J. R.: Thorax, 24:476-487, 1969.
31 Rywlin, A. M., and Fojaco, R. M.: Pediatrics 41:931-934, 1968.

Acquired vascular disease
Hyperemia and congestion

32 Adamson, T. M., Boyd, R. D. H., Normand, I. C. S., Reynolds, E. O. R., and Shaw, J. L.: Lancet 1:494-495, 1969.
33 Andrews, E. C., Jr.: Bull. Johns Hopkins Hosp. 100:28-42, 1957.
34 Beirne, G. J., Octaviano, G. N., Kopp, W. L., and Burns, R. O.: Ann. Intern. Med. 69:1207-1212, 1968.

34a Elliott, M. L., and Kuhn, C.: Amer. Rev. Resp. Dis. **102:**895-904, 1970.

35 Hutchinson, D. C. S., Sapru, R. P., Sumerling, M. D., Donaldson, G. W. K., and Richmond, J.: Amer. J. Med. **45:**139-151, 1968.

36 McCarthy, C., Reid, L., and Gibbons, R. A.: J. Path. Bact. **87:**39-47, 1964.

36a Siegel, R. R.: Amer. J. Med. Sci. **259:**201-213, 1970.

37 Soergel, K. H., and Sommers, S. C.: Amer. Rev. Resp. Dis. **85:**540-552, 1962.

38 Spain, D. M.: Arch. Path. (Chicago) **62:**489-493, 1956.

Edema and shock

39 Arias-Stella, J., and Kruger, H.: Arch. Path. (Chicago) **76:**147-157, 1963.

40 Dalldorf, F. G., Carney, C. N., Rackley, C. E., and Raney, R. B., Jr.: J.A.M.A. **206:**583-586, 1968.

41 Doniach, I.: Amer. J. Roentgen. **58:**620-628, 1947.

42 Editorial: Lancet **1:**309, 1962.

42a Editorial: Brit. Med. J. **4:**5, 1970.

43 Fleischner, F. G.: Amer. J. Cardiol. **20:**39-46, 1967.

43a Friedberg, C. K.: Diseases of the heart, ed. 3, Philadelphia, 1966, W. B. Saunders Co.

44 Hardaway, R. M., James, P. M., Jr., Anderson, R. W., Bredenberg, C. E., and West, R. L.: J.A.M.A. **199:**779-790, 1967.

45 Heard, B. E., Steiner, R. E., Herdan, A., and Gleason, D.: Brit. J. Radiol. **41:**161-171, 1968.

46 Karliner, J. S., Steinberg, A. D., and Williams, M. H., Jr.: Arch. Intern. Med. (Chicago) **124:**350-353, 1969.

47 Moolten, S. E.: Amer. J. Med. **33:**421-441, 1962.

48 Richards, P.: Brit. Med. J. **2:**83-86, 1963.

48a Weedn, R. J., Coalson, J. J., and Greenfield, L. J.: Amer. J. Surg. **120:**584-590, 1970.

Thromboembolism and infarction

49 Breckenridge, R. T., and Ratnoff, O. D.: New Eng. J. Med. **270:**298-299, 1964.

50 Editorial: Lancet **1:**91-92, 1964.

51 Evans, W. E. D.: J. Forensic Med. **6:**5-14, 1959.

52 Fleming, H. A., and Bailey, S. M.: Brit. Med. J. **1:**1322-1327, 1966.

53 Gorham, L. W.: Arch. Intern. Med. (Chicago) **108:**8-22, 189-207, 418-426, 1961.

54 Grieco, M. H., and Ryan, S. F.: Amer. J. Med. **45:**811-816, 1968.

55 Hampton, A. O., and Castleman, B.: Amer. J. Roentgen. **43:**305-326, 1940.

56 Leinassar, J. M., and Niles, N. R.: Circulation **17:**60-64, 1958.

56a Zimmerman, T. S., Adelson, L., and Ratnoff, O. D.: New Eng. J. Med. **283:**1504-1505, 1970.

Pulmonary hypertension

57 Evans, W., Short, D. S., and Bedford, D. E.: Brit. Heart. J. **19:**93-116, 1957.

57a Fishman, A. P.: In Zorab, P. A., editor: Proceedings of a symposium on scoliosis, London, 1965, National Fund for Research into Poliomyelitis and Other Crippling Diseases.

58 Ring, A., and Bakke, J. R.: Ann. Intern. Med. **43:**781-806, 1955.

59 Schein, C. J., Rifkin, H., Hurwitt, E. S., and Lebendiger, A.: Arch. Intern. Med. (Chicago) **101:**592-605, 1958.

59a Wagenvoort, C. A., and Wagenvoort, N.: Circulation **42:**1163-1184, 1970.

60 Wood, P.: Mod. Conc. Cardiovasc. Dis. **28:**513-518, 1959.

Atelectasis

61 Langley, F. A., and Smith, J. A. M.: J. Obstet. Gynaec. Brit. Emp. **66:**12-25, 1959.

62 Osborn, G. R.: Lancet **1:**275, 1962.

Hyaline membrane disease

63 Avery, M. E., and Mead, J.: Amer. J. Dis. Child. **97:**517-523, 1959.

64 Barter, R. A., Byrne, M. J., and Carter, R. F.: Arch. Dis. Child. **41:**489-495, 1966.

65 Capers, T. H., and Minden, B.: Amer. J. Med. **36:**377-381, 1964.

66 Gregg, R. H., and Bernstein, J.: Amer. J. Dis. Child. **102:**871-890, 1961.

67 Lauweryns, J. M.: Hum. Path. **1:**175-204, 1970.

68 Lieberman, J.: Amer. J. Med. **35:**443-449, 1963.

69 Osborn, G. R., and Flett, R. L.: J. Clin. Path. **15:**527-541, 1962.

70 Shepard, F. M., Johnston, R. B., Jr., Klatte, E. C., Burko, H., and Stahlman, M.: New Eng. J. Med. **279:**1063-1071, 1968.

Collapse

71 Culiner, M. M.: Dis. Chest. **50:**57-66, 1966.

72 Raffensperger, J. G., Diffenbaugh, W. G., and Strohl, E. L.: J.A.M.A. **174:**1386-1388, 1960.

Emphysema

73 Editorial: Brit. Med. J. **1:**272-273, 1958.

74 Editorial: Brit. Med. J. **2:**229-231, 1959.

75 Freeman, G., and Haydon, G. B.: Arch. Environ. Health. (Chicago) **8:**125-128, 1964.

76 Fulton, R. M.: Quart. J. Med. **22:**43-58, 1953.

77 Heard, B. E.: Thorax **13:**136-149, 1958.

78 Heard, B. E.: Thorax **14:**58-70, 1959.

79 Hepplestone, A. G., and Leopold, J. G.: Amer. J. Med. **31:**279-291, 1961.

80 Kirschner, P. A., and Strauss, L.: Dis. Chest **46:**417-426, 1964.

81 Leopold, J. G., and Gough, J.: Thorax **12:**219-235, 1957.

82 Lieberman, J.: New Eng. J. Med. **281:**279-284, 1969.

83 Liebow, A. A.: Amer. Rev. Resp. Dis. **80**(July suppl.)**:**67-93, 1959.

84 McLean, K. H.: Amer. J. Med. **25:**62-74, 1958.

85 Millard, F. J. C.: Brit. Heart J. **29:**43-50, 1967.

86 Miller, F., and Kuschner, M.: Amer. J. Med. **46:**615-623, 1969.

87 Newman, J. K., Vatter, A. E., and Reiss, O. K.: Arch. Environ. Health (Chicago) **15:**420-429, 1967.

88 Pratt, P. C., Jutabha, P., and Klugh, G. A.: Amer. Rev. Resp. Dis. **87:**245-256, 1963.

89 Reid, L.: Brit. J. Radiol. **32:**294-295, 1959.

90 Reid, L.: Personal communication, 1968.

91 Reid, L., Simon, G., Zorab, P. A., and

Seidelin, R.: Brit. J. Dis. Chest **61**:190-192, 1967.

91a Ryder, R., Lyons, J. P., Campbell, H., and Gough, J.: Brit. Med. J. **3**:481-487, 1970.

92 Simon, G.: Clin. Radiol. **15**:293-306, 1964.

93 Snider, G. L., Brody, J. S., and Doctor, L.: Amer. Rev. Resp. Dis. **85**:666-683, 1962.

94 Spain, D. M., and Kaufman, G.: Amer. Rev. Tuberc. **68**:24-30, 1953.

95 Stovin, P. G. I.: Thorax **14**:254-262, 1959.

96 Thurlbeck, W. M.: Amer. J. Med. Sci. **246**:332-353, 1963.

96a Townley, R. G., Ryning, F., Lynch, H., and Brody, A. W.: J.A.M.A. **214**:325-331, 1970.

97 Wyatt, J. P., Fischer, V. W., and Sweet, H. C.: Lab. Invest. **10**:159-177, 1961.

98 Wyatt, J. P., Fischer, V. W., and Sweet, H. C.: Dis. Chest **41**:239-259, 1962.

Pneumonia

99 Auerbach, S. H., Mims, O. M., and Good-pasture, E. W.: Amer. J. Path. **28**:69-87, 1952.

100 Barnett, R. N., Hull, J. G., Vortel, V., and Schwarz, J.: Arch. Path. (Chicago) **88**:175-180, 1969.

101 Cabrera, A., Pickren, J. W., and Sheehan, R.: Amer. J. Clin. Path. **47**:154-159, 1967.

102 Corrin, B., and King, E.: Thorax **25**:230-236, 1970.

103 Cross, K. R.: Arch. Path. (Chicago) **63**:132-148, 1957.

103a Editorial: Lancet **2**:1021-1022, 1970.

104 Fetzer, A. E., Werner, A. S., and Hagstrom, J. W. C.: Amer. Rev. Resp. Dis. **96**:1121-1130, 1967.

105 Friedell, G. H., Kaufman, S. A., Laforet, E. G., and Strieder, J. W.: Amer. J. Roengen. **87**:847-852, 1962.

106 Gardner, A. M. N.: Quart. J. Med. **27**:227-242, 1958.

107 Gross, P.: Arch. Path. (Chicago) **69**:706-715, 1960.

108 Gross, P.: Arch. Path. (Chicago) **72**:607-619, 1961.

109 Kevy, S. V., and Lowe, B. A.: New Eng. J. Med. **264**:738-743, 1961.

110 Robinson, R. G., Garrison, R. G., and Brown, R. W.: Ann. Intern. Med. **60**:19-27, 1964.

111 Sheldon, W. H.: J. Pediat. **61**:780-791, 1962.

112 Sundberg, R. H., Kirschner, K. E., and Brown, M. J.: Dis. Chest **36**:594-601, 1959.

113 Tillotson, J. R., and Lerner, A. M.: Medicine (Balt.) **45**:65-76, 1966.

114 Tillotson, J. R., and Lerner, A. M.: Arch. Intern. Med. (Chicago) **121**:428-432, 1968.

115 Welch, C. C., Tombridge, T. L., Baker, W. J., and Kinney, R. J.: Amer. J. Med. Sci. **242**:157-165, 1961.

116 Wolman, M., and Goldberg, M. G.: Arch. Path. (Chicago) **65**:272-278, 1958.

Nonneoplastic acquired diseases of bronchi
Acute bronchitis and bronchiolitis

117 Ham, J. C.: Ann. Intern. Med. **60**:47-60, 1964 (adults).

118 Wittig, H. J., and Chang, C. H.: Pediat. Clin. N. Amer. **16**:55-66, 1969 (children).

Chronic bronchitis

119 Bates, D. V.: New Eng. J. Med. **278**:546-551, 600-605, 1968.

120 Fletcher, C. M., Jones, N. L., Burrows, B., and Niden, A. H.: Amer. Rev. Resp. Dis. **90**:1-13, 1964.

121 Garston, B.: Dis. Chest **40**:530-538, 1961.

122 Gregg, I.: Respiration **26**(suppl.):123-130, 1969.

123 Gregg, I.: Aspen Emphysema Conf. **11**:235-248, 1968.

123a Hogg, J. C., Macklem, P. T., and Thurlbeck, W. M.: New Eng. J. Med. **278**:1335-1360, 1968.

123b Macklem, P. T., Thurlbeck, W. M., and Fraser, R. G.: Ann. Intern. Med. **74**:167-177, 1971.

124 Reid, L:. Brit. J. Radiol. **32**:291-292, 1959.

125 Simon, G.: Brit. J. Radiol. **32**:292-294, 1959.

Unusual causes of pulmonary consolidation
Pulmonary alveolar microlithiasis

126 Baar, H. S., and Ferguson, F. F.: Arch. Path. (Chicago) **76**:659-666, 1963.

Pulmonary alveolar proteinosis

127 Buechner, H. A., and Ansari, A.: Dis. Chest **55**:274-278, 1969.

128 Haworth, J. C., Hoogstraten, J., and Taylor, H.: Arch. Dis. Child. **42**:40-54, 1967.

129 Ramirez, J., and Harlan, W. R., Jr.: Amer. J. Med. **45**:502-512, 1968.

130 Rosen, S. H., Castleman, B., and Liebow, A. A.: New Eng. J. Med. **258**:1123-1142, 1958.

Allergic granulomas and related conditions
Bronchial asthma

131 Cardell, B. S., and Pearson, R. S. B.: Thorax **14**:341-352, 1959.

132 Dunnill, M. S.: J. Clin. Path. **13**:27-33, 1960.

133 Editorial: Lancet **1**:1295-1296, 1968.

134 Gell, P. G. H., and Coombs, R. R. A.: Clinical aspects of immunology, ed. 2, Oxford, 1968, Blackwell Scientific Publications.

134a Golbert, T. M., and Patterson, R.: Ann. Intern. Med. **72**:395-403, 1970.

135 Gottlieb, P. M.: J.A.M.A. **187**:276-280, 1964.

136 Pepys, J.: J. Roy. Coll. Physicians London **2**:42-48, 1967.

137 Scadding, J. G.: J. Roy. Coll. Physicians London **2**:35-41, 1967.

Eosinophilic pneumonias

138 Danaraj, T. J.: Arch. Path. (Chicago) **67**:515-524, 1959.

Drug reactions

139 Davies, P. D. B.: Brit. J. Dis. Chest **63**:59-70, 1969.

Hypersensitivity pneumonitis due to inhaled organic antigens

139a Editorial: Lancet **1**:999-1000, 1971.

140 Emanuel, D. A., Wenzel, F. J., and Lawton, B. R.: New Eng. J. Med. **274**:1413-1418, 1966.

140a Fink, J. N., Banaszak, E. F., Thiede, W. H., and Barboriak, J. J.: Ann. Intern. Med. **74**:80-83, 1971.

141 Hensley, G. T., Garancis, J. C., Cherayil, G. D., and Fink, J. N.: Arch. Path. (Chicago) **87**:572-579, 1969.

142 Schlueter, D. P., Fink, J. N., and Sosman, A. J.: Ann. Intern. Med. **70**:457-470, 1969.

Lethal midline granuloma

143 Friedmann, I.: Proc. Roy. Soc. Med. **57:**289-297, 1964.
144 Spear, G. S., and Walker, W. G., Jr.: Bull. Johns Hopkins Hosp. **99:**313-332, 1956.

Allergic granulomatosis; angiitis

145 Åström, K. E., and Lidholm, S. O.: J. Clin. Path. **16:**137-143, 1963.
146 Carrington, C. B., and Liebow, A. A.: Amer. J. Med. **41:**497-527, 1966.
147 Divertie, M. B., and Olsen, A. M.: Dis. Chest **37:**340-349, 1960.
148 Drachman, D. A.: Arch. Neurol. (Chicago) **8:**145-155, 1963.
149 Fienberg, R.: Amer. J. Med. **19:**829-831, 1955.
150 Godman, G. C., and Churg, J.: Arch. Path. (Chicago) **58:**533-553, 1954.
151 Liebow, A. A., and Carrington, C. B.: Medicine (Balt.) **48:**251-285, 1969.
152 Sokolov, R. A., Rachmaninoff, N., and Kaine, H. D.: Amer. J. Med. **32:**131-141, 1962.

Pneumoconiosis

153 American Medical Association Council on Occupational Health: Arch. Environ. Health (Chicago) **7:**130-171, 1963.
154 Caplan, A., Payne, R. B., and Withey, G. L.: Thorax **17:**205-212, 1962.
155 Elmes, P. C.: Postgrad. Med. J. **42:**623-635, 1966.
156 Enticknap, J. B., and Smither, W. J.: Brit. J. Industr. Med. **21:**20-31, 1964.
157 Gross, P., and Thomson, J. G.: Arch. Path. (Chicago) **82:**195-196, 1966.
158 Gross, P., deTreville, R. T. P., and Haller, M. N.: Arch. Environ. Health (Chicago) **19:**186-188, 1969.
159 Gross, P., deTreville, R. T. P., Cralley L. J., and Davis, J. M. G.: Arch. Path. (Chicago) **85:**539-546, 1968.
160 Hourihane, D. O., and McCaughey, W. T. E.: Postgrad. Med. J. **42:**613-622, 1966.
161 Knox, J. F., Holmes, S., Doll, R., and Hill, I. D.: Brit. J. Industr. Med. **25:**293-303, 1968.
162 McCallum, R. I., Rannie, E., and Verity, C.: Brit. J. Industr. Med. **18:**133-142, 1961.
163 Michel, R. D., and Morris, J. F.: Arch. Intern. Med. (Chicago) **113:**850-855, 1964.
164 Miller, A. A., and Ramsden, F.: Brit. J. Industr. Med. **18:**103-113, 1961.
165 Morrow, C. S., and Armen, R. N.: Ann. Intern. Med. **46:**598-613, 1956.
166 Rickards, A. G., and Barrett, G. M.: Thorax **13:**185-193, 1958.
167 Sakula, A.: Thorax **16:**176-179, 1961.
168 Selikoff, I. J., Churg, J., and Hammond, E. C.: J.A.M.A. **188:**22-26, 1964.
169 Thomson, J. G., and Graves, W. M., Jr.: Arch. Path. (Chicago) **81:**458-464, 1966.
170 Williams, W. J.: Brit. J. Industr. Med. **15:**84-91, 1958.
171 Williams, W. J., and Williams, D.: J. Path. Bact. **96:**491-496, 1968.

Industrial lung diseases

172 Barrowcliff, D. F., and Arblaster, P. G.: Thorax **23:**490-500, 1968.
173 Bouhuys, A., Barbero, A., Lindell, S.-E., Roach, S. A., and Schilling, R. S. F.: Arch. Environ. Health (Chicago) **14:**533-544, 1967.

174 Buechner, H. A.: J.A.M.A. **174:**1237-1241, 1960.
175 Editorial: New Eng. J. Med. **277:**209-210, 1967.
176 Hapke, E. J., Seal, R. M. E., and Thomas, G. O.: Thorax **23:**451-468, 1968.
177 Hearn, C. E. D., and Holford-Strevens, V.: Brit. J. Industr. Med. **25:**267-282, 283-292, 1968.
178 Prine, J. R., Brokeshoulder, S. F., McVean, D. E., and Robinson, F. R.: Amer. J. Clin. Path. **45:**448-454, 1966.
179 Rafii, S., and Godwin, M. C.: Arch. Path. (Chicago) **72:**424-433, 1961.
180 Rankin, J., Jaeschke, W. H., Callies, Q. C., and Dickie, H. A.: Ann. Intern. Med. **57:**606-626, 1962.
181 Seal, R. M. E., Hapke, E. J., and Thomas, G. O.: Thorax **23:**469-489, 1968.

Pulmonary fibrosis

182 Cruickshank, B.: J. Dis. Chest **53:**226-236, 1959.
183 Eldridge, F.: Arch. Intern. Med. (Chicago) **105:**665-667, 1960.
184 Getzowa, S.: Arch. Path. (Chicago) **40:**99-106, 1945.
185 Heppleston, A. G.: Thorax **11:**77-93, 1956.
186 Liebow, A. A., Loring, W. E., and Felton, W. L., II: Amer. J. Path. **29:**885-911, 1953.
187 Scadding, J. G.: Proc. Roy. Soc. Med. **62:**227-238, 1969.

Sarcoidosis

188 Danbolt, N.: Acta dermatovener. (Stockholm) **42:**355-362, 1962.
189 Editorial: Brit. Med. J. **2:**1657-1658, 1960.
190 Gregorie, H. B., Othersen, H. B., Jr., and Moore, M. P., Jr.: Amer. J. Surg. **104:**577-586, 1962.
191 Haroutunian, L. M., Fisher, A. M., and Smith, E. W.: Bull. Johns Hopkins Hosp. **115:**1-28, 1964.
192 Hart, P. D., Mitchell, D. N., and Sutherland, I.: Brit. Med. J. **1:**795-804, 1964.
192a Israel, H. L., and Goldstein, R. A.: New Eng. J. Med. **284:**345-349, 1971.
193 Israel, H. L., and Sones, M.: Amer. Rev. Resp. Dis. **94:**887-895, 1966.
194 James, D. G., Siltzbach, L. E., Sharma, O. P., and Carstairs, L. S.: Arch. Intern. Med. (Chicago) **123:**187-191, 1969.
195 Mankiewicz, E.: Acta Med. Scand. suppl. 425, pp. 68-73, 1964.
196 Scadding, J. G.: Brit. Med. J. **2:**1617-1623, 1960.
197 Scadding, J. G.: Sarcoidosis, London, 1967, Eyre & Spottiswoode (Publishers) Ltd.
198 Siltzbach, L. E.: J.A.M.A. **178:**476-482, 1961.
199 Siltzbach, L. E.: Practitioner **202:**613-618, 1969.
200 Vaněk, J., and Schwarz, J.: Amer. Rev. Resp. Dis. **101:**395-400, 1970.
201 Waksman, B. H.: Medicine (Balt.) **41:**93-141, 1962.

Diffuse interstitial pulmonary fibrosis (fibrosing alveolitis) and variants

202 Hamman, L., and Rich, A. R.: Bull. Johns Hopkins Hosp. **74:**177-212, 1944.
202a Liebow, A. A.: In Liebow, A. A., and Smith,

D. E., editors: The lung, Baltimore, 1968, The Williams & Wilkins Co.

203 Liebow, A. A., and Carrington, C. B.: In Simon, M., editor: Frontiers of pulmonary radiology, New York, 1969, Grune & Stratton, Inc.

204 Liebow, A. A., Steer, A., and Billingsley, J. G.: Amer. J. Med. 39:369-404, 1965.

205 Livingstone, J. L., Lewis, J. G., Reid, L., and Jefferson, K. E.: Quart. J. Med. 33:71-103, 1964.

206 Mackay, I. R., and Ritchie, B.: Thorax 20:200-205, 1965.

207 Montes, M., Tomasi, T. B., Jr., Noehren, T. H., and Culver, G. J.: Amer. Rev. Resp. Dis. 98:277-280, 1968.

207a Patchefsky, A. S., Banner, M., and Freundlich, I. M.: Ann. Intern. Med. 74:322-327, 1971.

207b Reddy, P. A., Gorelick, D. F., and Christianson, C. S.: Chest 58:319-325, 1970.

208 Scadding, J. G., and Hinson, K. F. W.: Thorax 22:291-304, 1967.

209 Sheridan, L. A., Harrison, E. G., Jr., and Divertie, M. B.: Med. Clin. N. Amer. 48:993-1010, 1964.

210 Swaye, P., Van Ordstrand, H. S., McCormack, L. J., and Wolpaw, S. E.: Dis. Chest. 55:7-12, 1969.

Eosinophilic granuloma and related conditions

211 Anderson, A. E., and Foraker, A. G.: Arch. Intern. Med. (Chicago) 103:966-973, 1959.

212 Bickers, J. N., Buechner, H. A., and Ekman, P. J.: Amer. Rev. Resp. Dis. 85:211-219, 1962.

212a Gracey, D. R., Divertie, M. B., and Brown, A. L.: Chest 59:5-8, 1971.

Chronic granulomatous disease

213 Holland, M. E., Hardy, R., and Dunlap, C. E.: Bull. Tulane Univ. Fac. 27:251-262, 1968.

Fibrosis due to drugs

214 Heard, B. E., and Cooke, R. A.: Thorax 23:187-193, 1968.

214a Kapanci, Y., Weibel, E. R., Kaplan, H. P., and Robinson, F. R.: Lab. Invest. 20:101-118, 1969.

215 Nash, G., Blennerhassett, J. B., and Pontoppidan, H.: New Eng. J. Med. 276:368-374, 1967.

216 Rosenow, E. C., III, DeRemee, R. A., and Dines, D. E.: New Eng. J. Med. 279:1258-1262, 1968.

Tuberculosis

217 Auerbach, O.: Amer. J. Surg. 89:627-636, 1955.

218 Auerbach, O.: Med. Clin. N. Amer. 43:239-251, 1959.

219 Blattner, R. J.: J. Pediat. 65:311-314, 1964.

220 Canetti, G.: The tubercle bacillus in the pulmonary lesion of man, New York, 1955, Springer Publishing Co., Inc.

221 Chapman, J. S.: Med. Clin. N. Amer. 51:503-517, 1967.

222 Cleve, E. A., Young, R. V., and Vicente-Mastellari, A.: Dis. Chest 32:671-677, 1957.

223 Corpe, R. F., and Stergus, I:. Amer. Rev. Tuberc. 75:223-241, 1957.

224 Crow, H. E., Corpe, R. F., and Smith, C. E.: Dis. Chest 39:372-381, 1961.

225 Davis, S. F., Finley, S. C., and Hare, W. K.: J. Pediat. 57:221-224, 1960.

226 Dubos, R. J.: Amer. J. Med. 9:573-590, 1950.

227 Dubos, R.: Amer. Rev. Resp. Dis. 90:505-515, 1964.

228 Editorial: Brit. Med. J. 1:966-967, 1963.

229 Giese, W.: In Kaufmann, E., and Staemmler, M., editors: Lehrbuch der speziellen pathologischen Anatomie, vol. II, Berlin, 1959-1960, Walter de Gruyter & Co.

230 Grosz, H. J.: Dis. Chest 36:514-520, 1959.

231 Hill, L. E., and Pearson, J. E. G.: Brit. J. Dis. Chest 53:278-295, 1959.

232 Jenney, F. S., and Cohen, A. C.: Dis. Chest 43:62-67, 1963.

233 Johanson, W. G., Jr., and Nicholson, D. P.: Amer. Rev. Resp. Dis. 99:73-85, 1969.

234 Jones, R. S., and Alley, F. H.: Amer. Rev. Tuberc. 63:381-398, 1951.

235 Kelly, P. J., Weed, L. A., and Lipscomb, P.: R.: J. Bone Joint Surg. 45-A:327-336, 1963.

236 Koenig, M. G., Collins, R. D., and Heyssel, R. M.: Ann. Intern. Med. 64:145-154, 1966.

237 LeMaistre, C.: Ann. N. Y. Acad. Sci. 106:62-66, 1963.

238 Lester, W., Colton, R., and Kent, G.: Amer. Rev. Resp. Dis. 85:847-857, 1962.

239 Lurie, M. B.: Amer. J. Med. 9:591-610, 1950.

240 Medical Research Council: Brit. Med. J. 1:973-978, 1963.

241 Medler, E. M.: Amer. J. Med. 9:611-622, 1950.

242 Merckx, J. J., Soule, E. H., and Karlson, A. G.: Amer. J. Clin. Path. 41:244-255, 1964.

243 Montes, M., and Phillips, C.: Amer. Rev. Tuberc. 79:362-370, 1959.

244 Murasawa, K., and Altmann, V.: Sea View Hosp. Bull. 17:85-94, 1958-1959.

245 Muschenheim, C.: In Beeson, P. B., and McDermott, W., editors: Cecil-Loeb Textbook of medicine, ed. 11, Philadelphia, 1963, W. B. Saunders Co.

246 Ochs, C. W.: J.A.M.A. 179:247-252, 1962.

247 Pinner, M.: Amer. Rev. Tuberc. 32:424-439, 1935.

248 Prather, E. C., Bond, J. O., Hartwig, E. C., and Dunbar, F. P.: Dis. Chest 39:129-139, 1961.

249 Proudfoot, A. T., Akhtar, A. J., Douglas, A. C., and Horne, N. W.: Brit. Med. J. 2:273-276, 1969.

250 Reid, J. D., and Wolinsky, E.: Amer. Rev. Resp. Dis. 99:8-12, 1969.

251 Rich, A. R.: The pathogenesis of tuberculosis, ed. 2, Springfield, Ill., 1950, Charles C Thomas, Publisher.

252 Rüttimann, A., and Suter, F.: Schweiz. Med. Wschr. 83:591-600, 1953.

253 Runyon, E. H.: Amer. Rev. Resp. Dis. 95:861-865, 1957.

254 Salyer, K. E., Votteler, T. P., and Dorman, G. W.: J.A.M.A. 204:1037-1040, 1968.

255 Snijder, J., and Vossenaar, T.: Amer. Rev. Tuberc. 78:547-562, 1958.

256 Sochocky, S.: Amer. Rev. Tuberc. 78:403-410, 1958.

257 Stead, W. M.: Amer. Rev. Resp. Dis. 95:729-745, 1967.

258 Steer, A.: Amer. Rev. Resp. Dis. **95:**200-208, 1967.
259 Terplan, K.: Amer. Rev. Tuberc. **42**(suppl.): 1-176, 1940.
260 Vortel, V.: Amer. Rev. Resp. Dis. **86:**336-349, 1962.
261 Wayne, L. G.: Amer. Rev. Resp. Dis. **82:**370-377, 1960.
262 Wayne, L. G., and Salkin, D.: Amer. Rev. Tuberc. **74:**376-387, 1956.
263 Wolinsky, E.: Ann. N. Y. Acad. Sci. **106:**67-71, 1963.

Carcinoma

264 Anderson, W. A. D.: Amer. J. Clin. Path. **46:** 1-26, 1966.
265 Ashley, D. J. B.: Brit. J. Cancer **21:**243-259, 1967.
266 Ashley, D. J. B., and Davies, H. D.: Thorax **22:**431-436, 1967.
267 Auerbach, O.: In Spain, D. M., editor: Diagnosis and treatment of tumors of the chest, New York, 1960, Grune & Stratton, Inc., chap. 4.
268 Auerbach, O., Stout, A. P., Hammond, E. C., and Garfinkel, L.: Amer. Rev. Resp. Dis. **82:** 640-648, 1960.
269 Auerbach, O., Stout, A. P., Hammond, E. C., and Garfinkel, L.: New Eng. J. Med. **265:**253-267, 1961.
270 Auerbach, O., Stout, A. P., Hammond, E. C., and Garfinkel, L.: Cancer **20:**699-705, 1967.
271 Azzopardi, J. G.: J. Path. Bact. **78:**513-519, 1959.
272 Beaver, D. L., and Shapiro, J. L.: Amer. J. Med. **21:**879-887, 1956.
272a Bennett, D. E., Sasser, W. F., and Ferguson, T. B.: Cancer **23:**431-439, 1969.
273 Bensch, K. G., Corrin, B., Pariente, R., and Spencer, H.: Cancer **22:**1163-1172, 1968.
274 Berkson, J.: Proc. Staff Meet. Mayo Clin. **35:** 367-385, 1960.
274a Boyd, J. T., Doll, R., Faulds, J. S., and Leiper, J.: Brit. J. Industr. Med. **27:**97-105, 1970.
275 Bryan, C. S., and Boitnott, J. K.: Amer. Rev. Resp. Dis. **99:**272-274, 1969.
276 Budinger, J. M.: Cancer **11:**106-116, 1958.
277 Burford, T. H., Center, S., Ferguson, T. B., and Spjut, H. J.: J. Thorac. Surg. **36:**316-328, 1958.
278 Collier, F. C., Enterline, H. T., Kyle, R. H., Tristan, T. T., and Greening, R.: Arch. Path. (Chicago) **66:**594-603, 1958.
279 Compton, H. L., and Kittle, C. F.: Amer. Surg. **29:**26-32, 1963.
280 Cotton, R. E.: Brit. J. Dis. Chest **53:**142-150, 1959.
281 Doll, R.: Brit. J. Industr. Med. **16:**181-190, 1959.
282 Doll, R., and Hill, A. B.: Brit. Med. J. **2:** 1071-1081, 1956.
283 Feinstein, A. R.: Med. Clin. N. Amer. **51:**549-562, 1967.
284 Fox, B., and Risdon, R. A.: J. Clin. Path. **21:** 486-491, 1968.
285 Galofré, M., Payne, W. S., Woolner, L. B., Clagett, O. T., and Gage, R. P.: Surg. Gynec. Obstet. **119:**51-61, 1964.
286 Garland, L. H., Beier, R. L., Coulson, W.,

Heald, J. H., and Stein, R. L.: Radiology **78:** 1-11, 1962.
287 Gifford, J. H., and Waddington, J. K. B.: Brit. Med. J. **1:**723-730, 1957.
288 Hathaway, B. M., Copeland, K., and Gurley, J.: Arch. Surg. (Chicago) **98:**24-30, 1969.
289 Hawkins, J. A., Hansen, J. E., and Howbert, J.: Amer. Rev. Resp. Dis. **88:**1-5, 1963.
290 Hewer, T. F.: J. Path. Bact. **81:**323-330, 1961.
291 Hukill, P. B., and Stern, H.: Cancer **15:**504-514, 1962.
292 Jackman, R. J., Good, C. A., Clagett, O. T., and Woolner, L. B.: J. Thorac. Cardiovasc. Surg. **57:**1-8, 1969.
293 Kirklin, J. W., McDonald, J. R., Clagett, O. T., Moersch, H. J., and Gage, R. P.: Surg. Gynec. Obstet. **100:**429-438, 1955.
294 Lauweryns, J. M., and Peuskens, J. C.: Life Sci. **8:**577-585, 1969.
295 Liebow, A. A.: Advances Intern. Med. **10:** 329-358, 1960.
296 MacMahon, H. E., Werch, J., and Sorger, K.: Arch. Path. (Chicago) **83:**359-363, 1967.
297 Melamed, M. R.: In Watson, W. L., editor: Lung cancer, St. Louis, 1968, The C. V. Mosby Co.
298 Meyer, E. C., and Liebow, A. A.: Cancer **18:** 322-351, 1965.
299 Mikail, M., and Sender, B.: Amer. J. Clin. Path. **37:**515-520, 1962.
300 Morgan, A. D., and Mackenzie, D. H.: J. Path. Bact. **87:**25-27, 1964.
301 Myers, W. P. L.: In Watson, W. L., editor: Lung cancer, St. Louis, 1968, The C. V. Mosby Co.
302 Nash, A. D., and Stout, A. P.: Cancer **11:** 369-376, 1958.
303 Overholt, R. H., and Bougas, J. A.: J.A.M.A. **161:**961-963, 1956.
304 Ozzello, L., and Stout, A. P.: Cancer **14:**1052-1056, 1961.
305 Pearson, F. G., and Thompson, D. W.: Canad. Med. Ass. J. **94:**825-833, 1966 (need for cytology, failure of radiography).
306 Report of Advisory Committee to Surgeon General: Smoking and health, Washington, D. C., 1964, U. S. Government Printing Office.
306a Rimington, J.: Brit. Med. J. **2:**373-375, 1971.
307 Rosenblatt, M. B., Lisa, J. R., and Trinidad, S.: Dis. Chest **49:**396-404, 1966 (metastases to bronchi).
308 Sherwin, R. P., Laforet, J. W., and Streider, E. G.: J. Thorac. Cardiovasc. Surg. **43:**716-730, 1962.
309 Shinton, N. K.: Brit. J. Cancer **17:**213-221, 1963.
310 Spain, D. W., and Parsonnet, V.: Cancer **4:** 277-285, 1951.
311 Storey, C. F. S., Knudtson, K. P. K., and Lawrence, B. J. L.: J. Thorac. Surg. **26:**331-406, 1953.
312 Strauss, B., and Weller, C. V.: Arch. Path. (Chicago) **63:**602-611, 1957.
313 Vincent, T. N., Satterfield, J. V., and Ackerman, L. V.: Cancer **18:**559-570, 1965.
314 Wagoner, J. K., Archer, V. E., Lundin, F. E., Jr., Holaday, D. A., and Lloyd, J. W.: New Eng. J. Med. **273:**181-188, 1965.
315 Watson, W. L.: Cancer **18:**133-135, 1965.

316 Watson, W. L., and Berg, J. W.: Cancer **15:** 759-768, 1962.
317 Whitwell, F.: J. Path. Bact. **70:**529-541, 1955.
318 Wynder, E. L., and Berg, J. W.: Cancer **20:** 1161-1172, 1967.
319 Yokoo, H., and Suckow, E. E.: Cancer **14:** 1205-1215, 1961.

Extrapulmonary manifestations of bronchial carcinoma

320 Bower, B. F., and Gordan, G. S.: Ann. Rev. Med. **16:**83-118, 1965.
321 Brain, Lord: Lancet **1:**179-184, 1963.
322 Croft, P. B., and Wilkinson, M.: Lancet **1:** 184-188, 1963.
323 Fusco, F. D., and Rosen, S. W.: New Eng. J. Med. **275:**507-515, 1966.
324 Greene, J. G., Divertie, M. B., Brown, A. L., and Lambert, E. H.: Arch. Intern. Med. (Chicago) **122:**333-339, 1968.
325 Kennedy, J. H., Williams, M. J., and Sommers, S. C.: Ann. Surg. **160:**90-94, 1964.
326 Kennedy, W. R., and Jimenez-Pabon, E.: Neurology (Minneap.) **18:**757-766, 1968.
327 Morton, D. L., Itabashi, H. H., and Grimes, O. F.: J. Thorac. Cardiovasc. Surg. **51:**14-29, 1966.
328 Nichols, J., and Gourley, W.: J.A.M.A. **185:** 696-698, 1963.
329 Riley, C. J., and Lécutier, M. A.: Brit. Med. J. **2:**291-292, 1969.

"Bronchial adenoma"

330 Black, W. C., III.: Lab. Invest. **19:**473-486, 1968.
331 Felton, W. L., Liebow, A. A., and Lindskog, G. E.: Cancer **6:**555-567, 1953.
332 Frank, H. D., and Lieberthal, M. M.: Arch. Intern. Med. (Chicago) **111:**791-798, 1963.
333 Goodner, J. T., Berg, J. W., and Watson, W. L.: Cancer **14:**539-546, 1961.
334 Kroe, D. J., and Pitcock, J. A.: Arch. Path. (Chicago) **84:**539-542, 1967 (true adenoma).
335 Ozlu, C., Christopherson, W. M., and Allen, J. D., Jr.: J. Thorac. Cardiovasc. Surg. **42:** 24-31, 1961.
336 Payne, W. S., Ellis, F. H., Woolner, L. B., and Moersch, H. J.: J. Thorac. Cardiovasc. Surg. **38:**709-726, 1959.
337 Smith, R. A.: Thorax **24:**43-50, 1969.
338 Tauxe, W. N., McDonald, J. R., and Devine, K. D.: Arch. Otolaryng. (Chicago) **75:**364-376, 1962.
339 Verska, J. J., and Connolly, J. E.: J. Thorac. Cardiovasc. Surg. **55:**411-417, 1968.

Rare pulmonary tumors

340 Barson, A. J., Jones, A. W., and Lodge, K. V.: J. Clin. Path. **21:**480-485, 1968.
340a Bateson, E. M.: J. Path. **101:**77-83, 1970.
341 Conquest, H. F., Thornton, J. L., Massie, J. R., and Coxe, J. W., III: Ann. Surg. **161:** 688-692, 1965.
342 Crutcher, R. R., Waltuch, T. L., and Ghosh, A. K.: J. Thorac. Cardiovasc. Surg. **55:**422-425, 1968.
343 Green, R. A., and Nichols, N. J.: Amer. Rev. Resp. Dis. **80:**833-844, 1959.
344 Hodges, F. V.: Dis. Chest **33:**43-51, 1958.

345 Kaufman, G., and Klopstock, R.: Amer. Rev. Resp. Dis. **88:**839-846, 1963.
346 Kurrus, F. D., and Conn, J. H.: J. Thorac. Cardiovasc. Surg. **50:**138-140, 1965.
346a Liebow, A. A., and Castleman, B.: Yale J. Biol. Med. **43:**213-222, 1971.
347 McNamara, J. J., Paulson, D. L., Kingsley, W. B., Salinas-Izaquirre, S. F., and Urschel, H. C., Jr.: J. Thorac. Cardiovasc. Surg. **57:** 635-641, 1969.
348 Plachta, A., and Hershey, H.: Amer. Rev. Resp. Dis. **86:**912-916, 1962.
349 Robbins, L. L.: Cancer **6:**80-88, 1953.
350 Saltzstein, S. L.: Cancer **16:**928-955, 1963.
351 Stackhouse, E. M., Harrison, E. G., Jr., and Ellis, F. H.: J. Thorac. Cardiovasc. Surg. **57:** 385-399, 1969.
352 Sternberg, W. H., Sidransky, H., and Ochsner, S.: Cancer **12:**806-819, 1959.

Solitary pulmonary nodules

353 McClure, C. D., Boucot, K. R., Shipman, G. A., Gilliam, A. G., Milmore, B. K., and Lloyd, J. W.: Arch. Environ. Health (Chicago) **3:** 127-139, 1961.
354 Steele, J. D.: J. Thorac. Cardiovasc. Surg. **46:** 21-39, 1963.

Pseudotumors

355 Arean, V. M., and Wheat, M. W., Jr.: Amer. Rev. Resp. Dis. **85:**261-271, 1962.
356 Duke, M.: Arch. Path. (Chicago) **67:**110-117, 1959.
357 Herskovic, T., Andersen, H. A., and Bayrd, E. D.: Dis. Chest **47:**1-6, 1965.
358 Liebow, A. A., and Hubbell, D. S.: Cancer **9:** 53-75, 1956.
359 Romanoff, H., and Milwidsky, H.: Brit. J. Dis. Chest **56:**139-143, 1962.
360 al-Saleem, T., and Peale, A. R.: Amer. Rev. Resp. Dis. **99:**767-772, 1969.
361 Saltzstein, S. L.: Cancer **16:**928-955, 1963.
362 Titus, J. L., Harrison, E. G., Clagget, O. T., Anderson, M. W., and Knaff, L. J.: Cancer **15:**522-538, 1962.

Pleura
Pleural tumors

363 Editorial: Brit. Med. J. **2:**202-203, 1964.
364 Foster, E. A., and Ackerman, L. V.: Amer. J. Clin. Path. **34:**349-364, 1960.
365 Godwin, M. C.: Cancer **10:**298-319, 1957.
366 Manguikian, B., and Prior, J. T.: Arch. Path. (Chicago) **75:**236-249, 1963.
366a Whitwell, F., and Rawcliffe, R. M.: Thorax **26:**6-22, 1971.

Mediastinum

367 Abell, M. R.: Arch. Path. (Chicago) **61:**360-379, 1956.
368 Aronstam, E. M., and Thomas, P. A., Jr.: Dis. Chest **41:**547-552, 1962.
369 Barrett, N. R.: Brit. J. Surg. **46:**207-218, 1958.
370 Castleman, B., Iverson, L., and Pardo Menendez, V.: Cancer **9:**822-830, 1956.
371 Coventry, W. D., and LaBree, R. H.: Ann. Intern. Med. **53:**1042-1052, 1960.
372 Dische, M. R.: Amer. J. Clin. Path. **49:**392-397, 1968.

373 Editorial: Brit. Med. J. **2:**135-136, 1969.

374 El-Domeiri, A. A., Hutter, R. V. P., Pool, J. L., and Foote, F. W., Jr.: Ann. Thorac. Surg. **6:**513-521, 1968.

375 Grafe, W. R., Goldsmith, E. I., and Redo, S. F.: J. Pediat. Surg. **1:**384-393, 1966.

376 Hache, L., Woolner, L. B., and Bernatz, P. E.: Dis. Chest **41:**9-25, 1962.

377 Heimburger, I. L., and Battersby, J. S.: J. Thorac. Cardiovasc. Surg. **50:**92-103, 1965.

378 Herlìtzka, A. J., and Gale, J. W.: Arch. Surg. (Chicago) **76:**697-706, 1958.

379 Krasznai, G., and Juhász, I.: J. Path. **97:**148-151, 1969.

380 Lattes, R., and Pachter, M. R.: Cancer **15:**197-214, 1962.

381 Medelman, J. P.: Minn. Med. **40:**410-417, 421, 1957.

382 Morrison, I. M.: Thorax **13:**294-307, 1958.

383 Nelson, W. P., Lundberg, G. D., and Dickerson, R. B.: Amer. J. Med. **38:**279-285, 1965.

384 Oberman, H. A., and Abell, M. R.: Cancer **13:**882-898, 1960.

385 Pachter, M. R., and Lattes, R.: Cancer **16:**74-94, 95-107, 108-117, 1963.

386 Pachter, M. R., and Lattes, R.: Dis. Chest **44:**79-87, 1963.

387 Pachter, M. R., and Lattes, R.: Dis. Chest **45:**301-310, 1964.

388 Schlumberger, H. C.: Tumors of the mediastinum. In Atlas of tumor pathology, Sect. V, Fasc. 18, Washington, D. C., 1951, Armed Forces Institute of Pathology.

389 Silver, C. P., and Steel, S. J.: Lancet **1:**1254-1256, 1961.

390 Spock, A., Schneider, S., and Baylin, G. J.: Amer. Rev. Resp. Dis. **94:**97-103, 1966.

391 Tung, K. S. K., and McCormack, L. J.: Cancer **20:**525-536, 1967.

Chapter 24

Ophthalmic pathology

Lorenz E. Zimmerman

This chapter is concerned not only with pathologic processes affecting the eyeball, but also with alterations in the eyelids, conjunctiva, and orbital tissues.

EYELIDS

The eyelids are covered externally by epidermis and internally by the palpebral conjunctiva (Fig. 24-1), between which are the corium, subcutaneous tissues, layer of skeletal and smooth muscles, and the tarsal plate with its contained meibomian glands. In general, pathologic processes affecting the eyelids are not sufficiently different from those observed elsewhere to warrant separate discussion, even though the eyelids are sites of predilection for many dermatologic entities such as basal cell carcinoma, nevi, the melanotic freckle of Hutchinson, extrasacral mongolian spots, cavernous hemangioma, neurofibroma, senile and sebaceous keratosis, xeroderma pigmentosum, verruca filiformis, xanthomas (xanthelesma and juvenile xanthogranuloma), lipid proteinosis, mulluscum contagiosum, keratoacanthoma, pseudoepitheliomatous hyperplasia, trichoepithelioma, and syringoma. These are described in the chapter on the skin. A few conditions, however, should be considered here.

Dermoid and epidermoid cysts

Dermoid cyst is a developmental anomaly usually encountered in the upper eyelid, most often temporally, and sometimes involving the orbit as well as the eyelid. Its wall is composed of epidermal and dermal tissues, including such adnexal structures as hair follicles, sebaceous glands, and sweat glands, all of which typically contribute their products to the contents of the cyst, the principal ingredient of which is desquamated keratin (Fig. 24-2).

Epidermoid cysts also are encountered in the eyelids. These differ from dermoid cysts

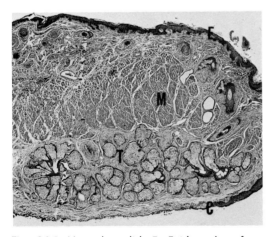

Fig. 24-1 Normal eyelid. **E,** Epidermal surface. **C,** Conjunctival surface. **M,** Muscular plane. **T,** Tarsal plate with meibomian glands. (×19; AFIP 61-3230; from Boniuk, M.: Int. Ophthal. Clin. **2:** 239-317, 1962; Little, Brown and Co.)

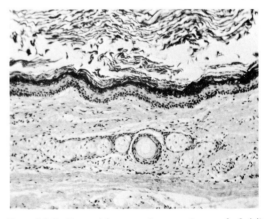

Fig. 24-2 Dermoid cyst. Lumen (top of field) filled with desquamated keratin and lined by epidermis. Hair follicles and sebaceous glands present in its wall. (×125; AFIP 72852-24102; from Hogan, M. J., and Zimmerman, L. E.: Ophthalmic pathology, ed. 2, W. B. Saunders Co.)

in that they are lined by epidermal tissue without adnexal structures and the lumen contains only keratin.

Following trauma, the contents of dermoid and epidermoid cysts may escape into the adjacent tissues, provoking a severe foreign body granulomatous reaction and presenting a clinical picture suggestive of a rapidly growing malignant neoplasm.

Sty

Sty, or external hordeolum, is an acute suppurative inflammation of one of the specialized glandular structures associated with the eyelash follicles. Frequently a complication of a staphylococcal blepharitis, the infection involves the sebaceous glands of Zeis, the apocrine glands of Moll, and the eyelash follicles. Much less frequently encountered is an acute

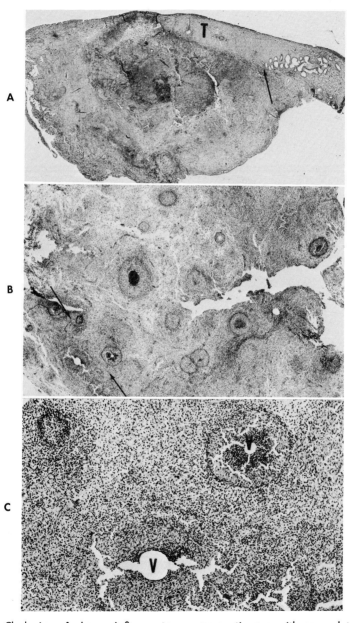

Fig. 24-3 Chalazion. **A,** Large inflammatory mass continuous with scarred tarsus, **T,** occupies most of eyelid. Arrow indicates juncture of chalazion with residual meibomian gland. **B,** Biopsy specimen revealing multiple discrete granulomatous lesions and abscesses. Area between arrows shown at greater magnification in **C. C,** Lipoidal vacuoles, **V,** in center of two granulomas. (**A,** ×9; AFIP 56-10004; **B,** ×15; AFIP 56-22051; **C,** ×63; AFIP 56-22049; **B** and **C,** from Hogan, M. J., and Zimmerman, L. E.: Ophthalmic pathology, ed. 2, W. B. Saunders Co.)

suppurative inflammation of the meibomian gland called an internal hordeolum.

Chalazion

Chalazion is the name given to a chronic inflammatory process involving the meibomian glands. Pathogenetically, it is believed to develop as a consequence of obstruction to the drainage of secretions. It is, therefore, often seen as a complication of various tumors and other disease processes at the eyelid margin. In the course of its slowly progressive evolution, the inflammatory process leads to a destruction of the walls of some of the meibomian glands and ducts and a consequent escape of secretions and inflammatory products into the tarsal plate. The process may then spread within the tarsus to involve adjacent glands, or it may perforate through to either the conjunctival surface posteriorly or the muscular plane and subcutaneous tissues anteriorly. Clinically, the resultant indurated mass may be mistaken for a deeply situated neoplasm. An important problem in clinical diagnosis here is differentiating a chalazion from a carcinoma of the meibomian glands, because both develop within the tarsus and because a tumor of the meibomian glands actually may produce a chalazion.

Microscopically, the chalazion is a great imitator, for the resultant histopathologic picture may resemble that of tuberculosis, sarcoidosis, cat-scratch disease, lipogranulomas, foreign body granulomas, or even plasmacytomas (Fig. 24-3). Although there is nothing highly specific about the microscopic picture, the diagnosis is based on two main features: (1) location in the tarsus and (2) presence of globules of fat in the center of some of the granulomas and abscesses. The lipid deposits, of course, appear as empty spaces in paraffin sections, but their histochemical characteristics can be demonstrated with frozen sections and stains for fat.

Sebaceous carcinoma

Sebaceous carcinoma is an exceedingly rare tumor elsewhere in the body, but in the eyelids it is second in frequency among malignant tumors only to basal cell carcinoma. In my experience, it is observed more frequently than either squamous cell carcinoma or malignant melanoma. While basal cell carcinomas have a predilection for the lower eyelid, sebaceous carcinomas arise more frequently in the upper eyelid, perhaps because the meibomian glands are larger and more numerous

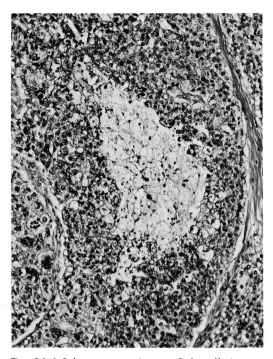

Fig. 24-4 Sebaceous carcinoma. Pale cells in center of lobule are swollen with cytoplasmic lipid. (×130; AFIP 58-13416; from Hogan, M. J., and Zimmerman, L. E.: Ophthalmic pathology, ed. 2, W. B. Saunders Co.)

in the upper than in the lower lids. While sebaceous carcinomas are generally believed to arise mainly from the meibomian glands within the tarsal plate, we have observed a number of cases in which the sebaceous glands of Zeis, which are associated with the lash follicles, were either solely responsible or participated along with the meibomian glands in giving rise to the tumor. Clinically, these tumors may produce a localized or a diffuse thickening of the tarsus, an ulcerated or a papillomatous tumor at the eyelid margin, or the picture of an inflammatory process variously resembling a chalazion, a chronic blepharitis, or a keratoconjunctivitis.

Microscopically, most sebaceous carcinomas show sufficient maturation to permit easy differentiation from basal cell carcinoma and squamous carcinoma. Areas usually can be found in which the tumor produces lobules showing progressive sebaceous differentiation of the constituent cells as they pass from the basaloid reserve cells peripherally toward the large sebaceous cells with abundant foamy cytoplasm centrally (Fig. 24-4). The ducts of the meibomian glands normally produce some keratin as they approach the eyelid margin, and one should therefore not be surprised

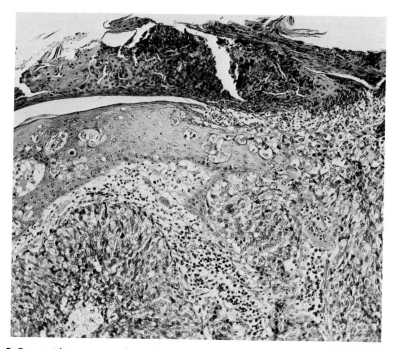

Fig. 24-5 Pagetoid invasion of epidermal surface of eyelid by sebaceous carcinoma of meibomian gland derivation. (×115; AFIP 58-13414; from Hogan, M. J., and Zimmerman, L. E.: Ophthalmic pathology, ed. 2, W. B. Saunders Co.)

if some production of keratin is occasionally observed. Diagnosis may be difficult when one has only small biopsy fragments to examine, but if the possibility of sebaceous carcinoma has been considered, frozen sections and stains for fat should be used to help establish the correct diagnosis. When one has, in addition to the tumor itself, enough of the adjacent normal eyelid to permit orientation, demonstration that the tumor has arisen within the tarsal glands or in the vicinity of the eyelash follicles where the glands of Zeis are located will greatly facilitate correct histopathologic interpretation. These points are emphasized because it has been my impression that in the past many pathologists have mistakenly interpreted sebaceous carcinomas of the eyelid as either basal cell or squamous cell carcinoma. Correct diagnosis is not merely of academic interest, for sebaceous carcinomas are among tumors of the eyelid second only to malignant melanoma in their capacity to metastasize.

Extramammary Paget's disease

Extramammary Paget's disease has been observed rather frequently in association with sebaceous carcinoma of the eyelids. This is the only important exception to the usual experience that mucus-secreting, apocrine-type carcinomas are those that are typically responsible

for the invasion of the overlying epidermis by individual neoplastic cells and the consequent development of a chronic eczematoid inflammatory process that often accounts for long delays in arriving at a correct diagnosis.

In the eyelids, we have often observed this phenomenon secondary to carcinomas arising in the meibomian and/or Zeis glands. Individual neoplastic cells containing sebaceous secretions in their cytoplasm may be observed in both the epidermal and conjunctival surfaces along the eyelid margin (Fig. 24-5). Sometimes, these cells also may be observed at a remarkable distance away from the underlying tumor in the tarsal glands. We have seen several cases in which even the bulbar conjunctiva and cornea were so affected. In such cases, the patients had presented clinically with the picture of a chronic unilateral keratoconjunctivitis that was unresponsive to all forms of medical therapy. Whether the neoplastic cells observed in the cornea and bulbar conjunctiva have actually migrated there from the eyelid margin or have undergone a peculiar neoplastic metaplasia in situ remains to be determined. The affected epidermal and conjunctival tissues are typically acanthotic and exhibit varying degrees of hyperkeratosis and parakeratosis as well as subacute inflammation.

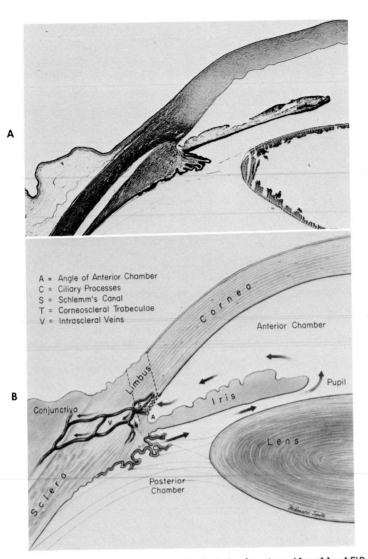

A = Angle of Anterior Chamber
C = Ciliary Processes
S = Schlemm's Canal
T = Corneoscleral Trabeculae
V = Intrascleral Veins

Fig. 24-6 Normal eye. **A,** Actual section. **B,** Artist's drawing. (**A,** ×11; AFIP 56-11490; **B,** AFIP 57-18073; from Zimmerman, L. E.: In Saphir, O., editor: A text on systemic pathology, Grune & Stratton, Inc.; by permission.)

CONJUNCTIVA AND CORNEA

The conjunctiva and cornea are discussed together here because so many of the more common pathologic processes affect them together, either concurrently or sequentially.

The conjunctiva covers the inner surface of the eyelids, where it is very firmly attached to the tarsal plates. This portion is called the tarsal or palpebral conjunctiva. At the upper end of the upper eyelid and at the lower end of the lower eyelid, the conjunctiva is redundant and loosely attached to the underlying tissues as it is reflected onto the surface of the globe, where it is called the bulbar conjunctiva. Most of the bulbar conjunctiva is rather loosely attached to the underlying

sclera, but it becomes more firmly attached as it merges with the cornea (Fig. 24-6).

The transitional zone between the bulbar conjunctiva and the cornea is called the limbus. The corneal margin of the limbus is easily defined and recognized by the fact that the stratified squamous epithelium of the cornea and its basement membrane are very intimately and firmly adherent to Bowman's membrane, the most superficial portion of the corneal stroma. Bowman's membrane terminates abruptly at the limbus, where a loose connective tissue (the substantia propria) containing capillaries begins to make its appearance between the epithelium and the sclera. In the limbal area, the conjunctival epithe-

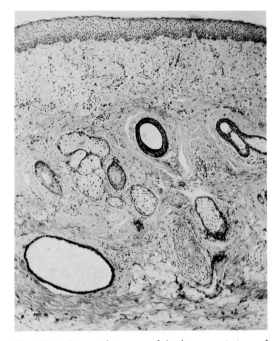

Fig. 24-7 Dermoid tumor of limbus consisting of choristomatous mass of cutaneous and adnexal tissues. (×75; AFIP 203027-24101; from Hogan, M. J., and Zimmerman, L. E.: Ophthalmic pathology, ed. 2, W. B. Saunders Co.)

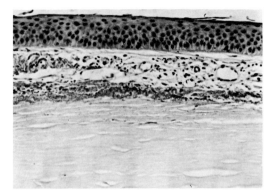

Fig. 24-8 Inflammatory pannus. Thick layer of vascularized connective tissue infiltrated by inflammatory cells has replaced Bowman's membrane and some superficial lamellae of corneal stroma. (AFIP 47564; from Hogan, M. J., and Zimmerman, L. E.: Ophthalmic pathology, ed. 2, W. B. Saunders Co.)

lium is nonkeratinizing stratified squamous with very few goblet cells. Peripherally goblet cells become more numerous, and the conjunctival epithelium becomes progressively more stratified columnar in type.

Dermoid tumors

Dermoid tumors are solid choristomatous malformations that are seen most frequently in the limbal area temporally. They are typically covered with keratinized epidermal tissue beneath which are masses of dermal collagen and adipose tissue containing various adnexal structures, including hair follicles (Fig. 24-7). A related choristoma, the **dermolipoma**, is typically devoid of skin appendages and contains more adipose tissue. It usually is encountered in the bulbar conjunctiva near the outer canthus.

Conjunctivitis and keratoconjunctivitis

Conjunctivitis and keratoconjunctivitis are very common, for the conjunctiva and cornea are exposed to a broad spectrum of chemical, physical, microbial, and allergenic stimuli capable of evoking the full gamut of humoral, cellular, and tissue responses that are observed in acute, subacute, and chronic forms of inflammation. In addition to the general aspects of inflammation that are important

wherever the processes develop, there are certain special aspects of ocular inflammations.

The eye is an exceptionally sensitive organ in many ways, including hypersensitivity to pain and light. Thus, the acutely inflamed eye is typically very painful and photophobic. Relatively trivial lesions that affect the cornea may not only be exquisitely painful but also may cause a marked reduction in vision by affecting corneal transparency in a variety of ways. In the acute stages of inflammation, corneal edema and infiltration by inflammatory cells may have a profound effect on corneal transparency. In more chronic forms of inflammation, blood vessels invade the normally avascular cornea. In the late stages of the interstitial keratitis of congenital syphilis, for example, the main clinical and histopathologic alteration is the deep stromal vascularization.

Pannus formation is another important corneal complication of keratoconjunctivitis. The inflammatory pannus is a wedge of vascularized connective tissue infiltrated by lymphocytes and plasma cells that invades the superficial layers of the cornea from the limbus, after destroying portions of Bowman's membrane and some of the most superficial stromal lamellae (Fig. 24-8).

Among the tissue responses that characterize the conjunctival reaction to chronic inflammation, two deserve special comment: **follicular hyperplasia** and **papillary hypertrophy**. Although the conjunctiva does not normally contain lymph nodes, it does have an amazing capacity to respond to chronic irritation, especially to such chronic infections

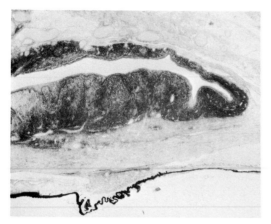

Fig. 24-9 Massive lymphoid hyperplasia of bulbar and fornical conjunctiva in trachoma, with formation of lymph follicles. (×39; AFIP 67237; from Hogan, M. J., and Zimmerman, L. E.: Ophthalmic pathology, ed. 2, W. B. Saunders Co.)

as trachoma, by the proliferation of an abundance of lymphoid tissue with the formation of lymph follicles that contain prominent germinal centers (Fig. 24-9). The follicular hyperplasia of lymphoid tissue may become so prominent that it is readily recognizable by the clinician, especially on slit-lamp examination. The lymph follicles produce avascular grayish white granular elevations in the normally smooth transparent conjunctiva. Papillary hypertrophy is the result of a proliferation of blood vessels and connective tissue elements in the substantia propria in multiple foci, causing irregular elevations of the overlying epithelium (Fig. 24-10). Between the papillae, cryptlike proliferations of mucus-secreting conjunctival epithelium are formed. Since the papillae contain a prominent core of blood vessels and the lymph follicles in follicular hyperplasia are avascular, the ophthalmologist usually has no difficulty in distinguishing these two types of tissue response.

Infectious causes of conjunctivitis and keratitis include bacteria (e.g., the gonococcus, pneumococcus, streptococcus, staphylococcus, Koch-Weeks bacillus, diplobacillus of Morax-Axenfeld, tubercle bacilli, leprosy bacilli, *Pasteurella* tularensis, etc.), fungi (opportunistic pathogens such as various species of *Aspergillus*, *Cephalosporium*, and *Fusarium* as well as some of the better known pathogens such as *Coccidioides immitis*, *Nocardia asteroides*, *Sporotichum schenkii*, and *Rhinosporidium seeberi*), parasites (one of which, *Oncocerca volvulus*, is responsible for a great deal of blindness in Africa and in Central America),

and several groups of viruses (especially the adenoviruses, *Chlamydia,** herpesviruses, and poxviruses). Viral infections are especially important because of their prevalence and high degree of contagiousness and, in some cases, because of their chronicity (e.g., trachoma) or tendency to recur (e.g., herpes simplex) coupled with their potential for producing severe corneal opacification leading to blindness.

Trachoma and **inclusion conjunctivitis** are caused by very closely related agents that have been placed in the genus *Chlamydozoon: Chlamydozoon trachomatis* and *Chlamydozoon oculogenitalis*, respectively. Collectively, they are commonly called the TRIC agents. The agent causing trachoma under natural conditions appears to be infectious only for the conjunctival epithelium of man. The disease is extremely prevalent in many countries in which poverty and poor personal hygiene are widespread. It is estimated that about 400 million people are infected and that about one in twenty have been blinded by the disease.

Early in the course of infection, the trachoma agent proliferates in the conjunctival epithelium, where it can be recognized in the form of basophilic cytoplasmic inclusion bodies (of Halberstaedter and Prowazek). The conjunctival epithelium becomes hyperplastic and infiltrated by mononuclear inflammatory cells. Lymph follicles develop in the substantia propria (Fig. 24-9). As the disease progresses, degeneration and necrosis of epithelial cells stimulate a more intense inflammatory reaction. Macrophages containing phagocytosed cellular debris (Leber cells) appear and papillary hypertrophy becomes pronounced. The stroma is markedly thickened and heavily infiltrated by plasma cells as well as lymphocytes. An inflammatory pannus invades the cornea. Scarring and vascularization of the cornea account for the blindness that is so common a complication of trachoma.

Inclusion conjunctivitis, although caused by an agent that is morphologically indistinguishable from that causing trachoma, is a much

---

*Although it is still common practice as well as convenient to consider the Chlamydia that cause trachoma, inclusion conjunctivitis, psittacosis, and lymphogranuloma venereum as viruses because they pass through Berkefeld filters, are obligate intracellular parasites, and produce inclusion bodies resembling those of poxviruses, they have now been placed in a separate taxonomic family, the *Chlamydozoaceae*.

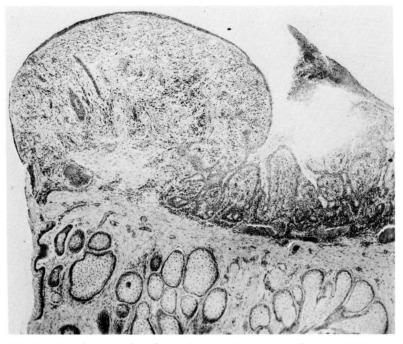

Fig. 24-10 Papillary hypertrophy of tarsal conjunctiva in vernal conjunctivitis. (×50; AFIP 60-5084; from Hogan, M. J., and Zimmerman, L. E.: Ophthalmic pathology, ed. 2, W. B. Saunders Co.)

less severe disease. Two main forms of infection are recognized, both attributable to a genital reservoir. Inclusion blennorrhea is an acute, purulent conjunctivitis of the newborn infant resembling gonorrhea neonatorum epidemiologically in that the infection is acquired from the mother's genital tract during birth. Inclusion conjunctivitis in the adult is a less acute follicular conjunctivitis that may occur in epidemic form when large numbers of people are exposed as, for example, when swimming in nonchlorinated pools—hence the name "swimming pool conjunctivitis." Both in infants and in adults, the disease tends to be self-limiting and the cornea is spared.

Vernal conjunctivitis is a chronic recurring type of inflammation involving mainly the upper tarsal conjunctiva of boys in the spring. Marked papillary hypertrophy dominates the picture (Fig. 24-10). The large papillae, which develop broad flat tops, contain a stroma that is heavily infiltrated by chronic inflammatory cells and eosinophils.

Metabolic disorders

Metabolic disorders may affect the cornea and/or conjunctiva, sometimes producing lesions that are very helpful in clinical diagnosis.

In **Wilson's hepatolenticular degeneration,** for example, there is a curious deposit of a copper compound in Descemet's membrane of the peripheral cornea (Fig. 24-11). This gives rise to a peculiar ruby red to greenish brown opacification, the Kayser-Fleischer ring, that is pathognomonic of the disease (see p. 1208).

In **cystinosis,** fine scintillating polychromatic cystine crystals are deposited in the substantia propria of the conjunctiva and in the corneal stroma, where they can be readily observed with the slit lamp and obtained for microscopic examination by biopsy.

In **ochronosis,** brownish discoloration occurs in the outermost scleral and episcleral connective tissues (Fig. 24-12) and in the peripheral cornea of the interpalpebral zone, where these tissues are exposed to air and light.

In **hypercalcemia,** regardless of the specific cause, calcium salts may be deposited in Bowman's membrane.

In **familial hypercholesterolemia** and in certain other forms of **disturbed lipid metabolism,** arcus senilis becomes prominent at an early age, and the corneal disturbance is appropriately called arcus juvenilis. Clinically, this is a milky opacification of the corneal stroma in a ring-shaped band peripherally, with a thin clear zone between it and the limbus. In ordinary paraffin sections of the cornea, no abnormalities are noted, even though clinically the arcus may have been

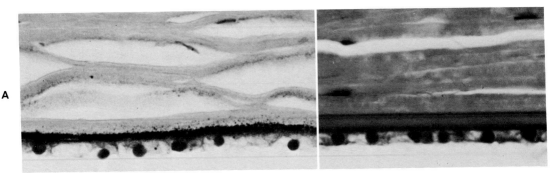

Fig. 24-11 A, Kayser-Fleischer ring. Dark band is copper compound that has been deposited in Descemet's membrane close to endothelium. **B,** Normal cornea for comparison. (**A,** ×600; AFIP 264768; **B,** ×600; AFIP 64-1883; **A,** from Hogan, M. J., and Zimmerman, L. E.: Ophthalmic pathology, ed. 2, W. B. Saunders Co.)

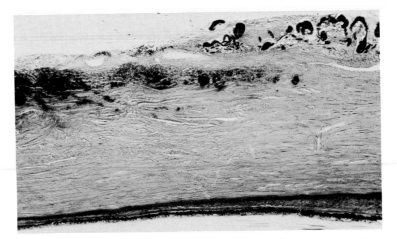

Fig. 24-12 Ochronosis. Marked pigmentation in degenerated elastic and collagenous tissues of sclera and episclera. (×70; AFIP 59-699; from Rones, B.: Amer. J. Ophthal. **49:** 440-446, 1960.)

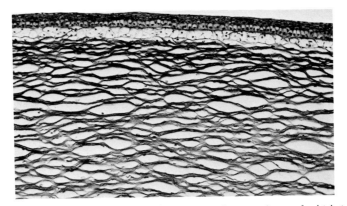

Fig. 24-13 Hurler's disease. Collection of histiocytic cells, cytoplasm of which is filled with acid mucopolysaccharide, is present in superficial layers of corneal stroma. (×90; AFIP 68-4418.)

very pronounced. Frozen sections and stains for fat are required to demonstrate the large amount of lipid present in Bowman's and Descemet's membranes and in the corneal stroma.

In **Hurler's disease** (gargoylism), there is a definite clouding of the cornea that may be present at birth but often begins near the end of the first year and severely interferes with vision. It is the result of an accumulation of abnormal mucopolysaccharides in the stromal and endothelial cells of the cornea and in histiocytic cells that may accumulate in large numbers, replacing Bowman's membrane (Fig. 24-13). Similar changes are observed in the Morquio, Scheie, and Maroteaux-Lamy syndromes, which are also the result of disturbances in mucopolysaccharide metabolism. Highly characteristic changes also are found in **Fabry's disease.** There is a diffuse haziness in the corneal epithelium and denser opacities that radiate out toward the periphery in wavy lines and bands from a focus near the center. Histologically, the basal cell layer of the corneal epithelium is swollen by an accumulation of glycolipids.

Pinguecula

Pinguecula is a common degenerative process believed to be a consequence of excessive

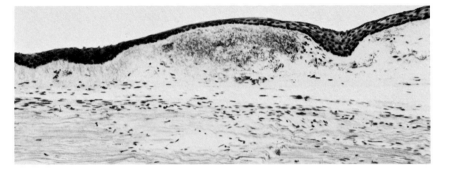

Fig. 24-14 Pinguecula. Marked elastosis of collagen in substantia propria. (×120; AFIP 86530; from Hogan, M. J., and Zimmerman, L. E.: Ophthalmic pathology, ed. 2, W .B. Saunders Co.)

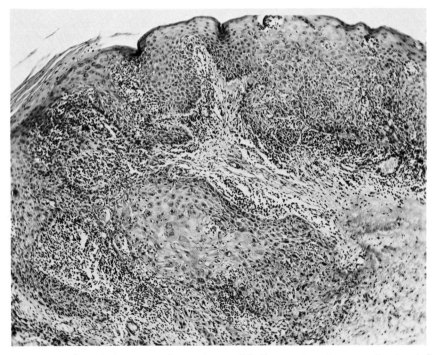

Fig. 24-15 Pseudoepitheliomatous hyperplasia of bulbar conjunctiva complicating inflammation of pinguecula. (×75; AFIP 55-16489.)

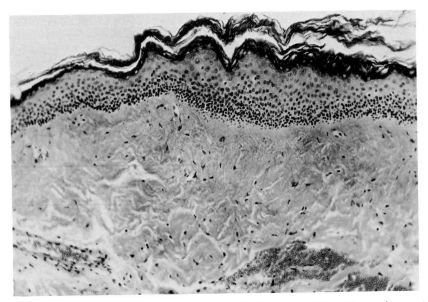

Fig. 24-16 Epidermidalization of conjunctiva. Well-developed keratin and prominent granular layer are present. These are not normally seen in conjunctiva. (×125; AFIP 338247-13081; from Hogan, M. J., and Zimmerman, L. E.: Ophthalmic pathology, ed. 2, W. B. Saunders Co.)

actinic damage to the collagen in the substantia propria of the bulbar conjunctiva. It occurs most frequently in the interpalpebral region, where the tissues are most exposed, and appears clinically as a yellowish thickened area. Histologically, it is characterized by senile elastosis between the often atrophic overlying epithelium and the unaffected underlying sclera (Fig. 24-14). When a pinguecula becomes large, it may become secondarily irritated and inflamed. As a result, pseudoepitheliomatous hyperplasia of the overlying epithelium may develop and give rise to concern about cancer (Fig. 24-15). In some individuals, the actinic stimulation affects the epithelium as well as the substantia propria, giving rise to dyskeratotic lesions similar to those of the epidermis in senile keratosis. Only rarely, however, do these acanthotic lesions progress to squamous carcinoma. When they do, however, they are typically very low-grade, well-differentiated, nonmetastasizing tumors.

Pterygium

Pterygium is believed to be a lesion very closely related to the pinguecula. The essential difference is that the pterygium arises at the limbus and typically progresses into the cornea, forming a wedge of vascularized connective tissue that dissects the epithelium away from Bowman's membrane. It is a more important lesion than the pinguecula because it is potentially sight-impairing as it progresses toward the center of the cornea, diminishing the transparency of the latter, because it is cosmetically much more objectionable and because it is more difficult to excise permanently since it has a greater tendency to recur. Secondary epithelial changes (pseudoepitheliomatous hyperplasia and dyskeratotic processes) may complicate the picture just as with the pinguecula.

Epidermidalization

Epidermidalization is a nonspecific descriptive term used to designate metaplasia of the normally thin, transparent, nonkeratinized conjunctiva into a thicker, acanthotic, keratinizing squamous epithelium that may have a striking resemblance microscopically to epidermis (Fig. 24-16). Clinically, the affected tissue appears pearly white and when localized to a placoid area, the descriptive term leukoplakia is appropriate (Fig. 24-17). This term, however, implies nothing etiologically or prognostically, nor does it indicate what the histopathologic picture might be, for other processes besides epidermidalization can produce leukoplakic lesions. Leukoplakia should, therefore, be used only for clinical description. A variety of factors may lead to epidermidalization, including an insufficiency of tears, excessive drying when the eyeball is chronically exposed as a result of neuroparalytic disorders or pathologic processes affecting

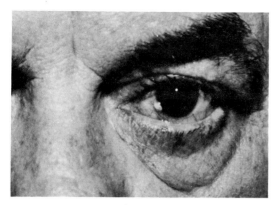

Fig. 24-17 Leukoplakia of limbus. (AFIP 60-5604; from Zimmerman, L. E.: In Boniuk, M., editor: Ocular and adnexal tumors, The C. V. Mosby Co.)

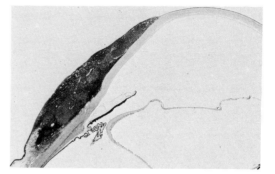

Fig. 24-18 Malignant melanoma of limbus that arose in compound nevus of conjunctiva. (×7; AFIP 57-16759; from Hogan, M. J., and Zimmerman, L. E.: Ophthalmic pathology, ed. 2, W. B. Saunders Co.)

closure of the eyelids (e.g., severe exophthalmos), vitamin A deficiency, etc. Bitot's spots are foci of keratinization in which xerosis bacilli proliferate saprophytically in the keratin layer, producing a foamy substance that can be wiped away.

Tumors
Benign tumors

Benign tumors of the conjunctiva include papillomas, nevi, angiomatous malformations, neurofibromas, and lymphomas. All others are too rare to mention, and only the so-called *lymphoma* requires comment here.

Most of the massive proliferations of lymphoid tissue that present clinically as epibulbar tumors prove to be benign, both on histopathologic examination and upon long-term follow-up study. When follicle formation is evident and when a significant admixture of other inflammatory cells besides the lymphocytes can be seen, the lesion can rather easily be recognized as a reactive lymphoid hyperplasia. However, when lymphocytes without formation of follicles are seen almost exclusively, then the possibility of a well-differentiated lymphosarcoma or a lymphocytic leukemia must be given serious consideration and appropriate clinical and hematologic studies undertaken. It is only very rarely, however, that an epibulbar tumor is the initial clinical manifestation of a malignant lymphoma or leukemia.

Malignant tumors

Malignant tumors of the conjunctiva are rare and only two, malignant melanoma and squamous cell carcinoma, will be considered here. Both arise much more frequently on the bulbar conjunctiva than on the palpebral conjunctiva or in the fornices, and both are observed most frequently in the limbal area of the interpalpebral zone.

Malignant melanomas. Malignant melanomas of the conjunctiva may arise from pre-existing nevi, within an area of acquired melanosis, or de novo in apparently normal conjunctiva. Malignant melanomas arising in conjunctival nevi are very similar histopathologically to those of the skin (Fig. 24-18).

Clinically, the patient, who is often a young or middle-aged adult, usually is able to give a very meaningful history. A pigmented spot is known to have been present in the exposed part of the bulbar conjunctiva since early childhood. For years, it did not change in appearance and then began to grow larger, typically as an exophytic epibulbar mass. Patients with malignant melanomas arising in areas of acquired melanosis give a different history. They tend to be older and deny the presence of any conjunctival lesion during childhood or during the early adult years. During middle age, they become aware of a slowly progressive brownish discoloration of the conjunctival epithelium of one eye. There is a great deal of variability in the degree and extent of this acquired melanosis. In some patients almost the entire conjunctiva and much of the corneal epithelium may be affected, whereas in others only a relatively small area may be involved. After a period of years, during which time the pigmentary disturbance may have progressed steadily, waxed and waned, or remained stationary, about one-fifth of the patients develop one or more nodules within the area of melanosis. These may or may not be pigmented. Such a change is always a cause for alarm, because

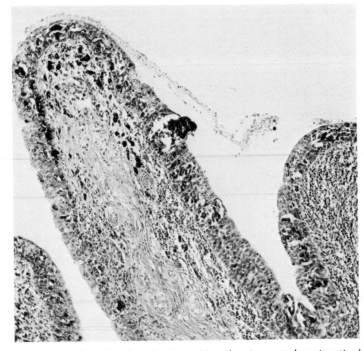

Fig. 24-19 Acquired melanosis of conjunctiva. Heavily pigmented conjunctival epithelium contains many large prominent nests of nevoid cells, and there is dense infiltrate of chronic inflammatory cells in substantia propria. (×115; AFIP 59-90; from Zimmerman, L. E., Paul, E. V., and Smith, M. E.: In Ackerman, L. V. [in collaboration with Butcher, H. R., Jr.]: Surgical pathology, The C. V. Mosby Co.)

it usually is an indication that a malignant melanoma has arisen and calls for excision or biopsy.

When feasible, the entire area of pigmentary disturbance should be excised for histopathologic study, but when considered too extensive, one or more of the nodules alone may be excised for microscopic examination. With only the malignant melanoma itself available for histopathologic study, the pathologist usually cannot determine whether the tumor arose from a nevus, in acquired melanosis, or de novo. This distinction is best made by the clinician, but if the pathologist has a sufficiently generous sample of the surrounding conjunctiva available for examination, as is the case when the orbital contents have been exenterated, he often can make the differential diagnosis microscopically. When the adjacent tissues contain clusters of benign nevoid cells and cystic inclusions of conjunctival epithelium in the substantia propria, these are features typical of a preexisting compound nevus. If, on the other hand, no nevoid clusters are present in the substantia propria but the conjunctival epithelium exhibits intense melanotic pigmentation, activated clear cells, and intraepithelial nests of large atypical melanocytes, these features are characteristic of acquired melanosis (Fig. 24-19).

Acquired melanosis often has been called "precancerous" melanosis in the ophthalmic literature, but because the development of a malignant melanoma in the affected tissues is the exception rather than the rule, occurring in only 15% to 20% of cases, this term gives a false impression as to the neoplastic potential of the pigmentary disturbance. The condition is believed to be the conjunctival equivalent of the melanotic freckle of Hutchinson.

Malignant melanomas of the conjunctiva, regardless of their histogenetic derivation, carry a guarded prognosis. Although less frequently lethal than melanomas of the skin, they do have the capacity for invasion of lymphatic and vascular channels. Those that are still quite localized and confined to the limbal zone often can be controlled by simple excision, whereas those that involve the conjunctiva more diffusely with spread onto the eyelids, caruncle, or canthi usually must be treated by a more radical procedure such as exenteration of the orbital contents.

Squamous cell carcinoma. Squamous cell carcinoma of the conjunctiva presents most often as a very well-differentiated exophytic

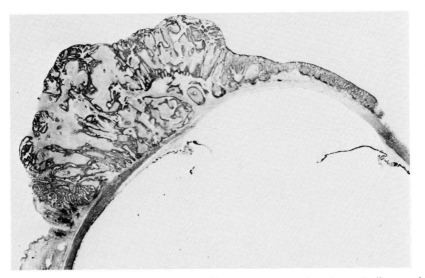

Fig. 24-20 Well-differentiated squamous cell carcinoma growing in typically exophytic manner from bulbar conjunctiva. (×10; AFIP 72108; from Hogan, M. J., and Zimmerman, L. E.: Ophthalmic pathology, ed. 2, W. B. Saunders Co.)

mass at the limbus on the nasal or temporal side (Fig. 24-20). It is rather rare in the United States and in Europe, but there is evidence that it is encountered more frequently in the Middle East, Africa, and India. Most squamous cell carcinomas seem to arise at sites of actinic keratosis. This fact, coupled with the unavailability of adequate medical care to permit removal of all cosmetic blemishes on the conjunctiva, probably offers the best explanation for the apparent geographic variation in the occurrence of these tumors. Other factors, such as racial susceptibility, tribal customs, etc., also may play a role.

Although actinic keratosis is probably the most important precursor lesion responsible for the development of squamous cell carcinomas, there is another group of epithelial changes that seem to play a role. They seem to be analogous to the spectrum of intraepithelial changes observed in such other mucous membranes as the uterine cervix, ranging from dysplasia through carcinoma in situ to invasive carcinoma (Fig. 24-21). In the ophthalmic literature, these intraepithelial lesions have often been called collectively "Bowen's disease." Although convenient, this is an inappropriate designation because there is only a superficial similarity of these conjunctival lesions to the distinctive cutaneous tumor that Bowen described.

Clinically, the dysplasia–carcinoma in situ group often can be differentiated from the actinic keratosis group. The latter almost always are confined to the exposed conjunctival and limbal tissues in the interpalpebral area and have a leukoplakic appearance because of the marked tendency of the acanthotic epithelium to develop a keratotic crust over its surface. Dysplasia and carcinoma in situ develop in portions of the conjunctiva covered by the eyelids as well as in the exposed areas, spread more frequently into the cornea, and are characterized by a grayish opalescent or gelatinous appearance of the affected epithelium that is less acanthotic and seldom covered by a keratotic crust.

Regardless of their histogenesis, squamous cell carcinomas of the conjunctiva carry a very favorable prognosis and should be treated by the most conservative excisional methods feasible. If permitted to grow large, they may invade the eye or the orbit, but metastasis is very rare.

ORBIT

In addition to the eyeball and optic nerve, the orbit contains the extraocular muscles, many blood vessels and peripheral nerves, and one important epithelial structure, the lacrimal gland—all embedded in a matrix of adipose tissue. Although these orbital tissues may be involved in a broad spectrum of systemic as well as localized disease processes, the single most important aspect of orbital pathology is the formation of a space-occupying mass that displaces the eyeball, usually with protrusion forward (proptosis or exophthalmos). These orbital tumors include be-

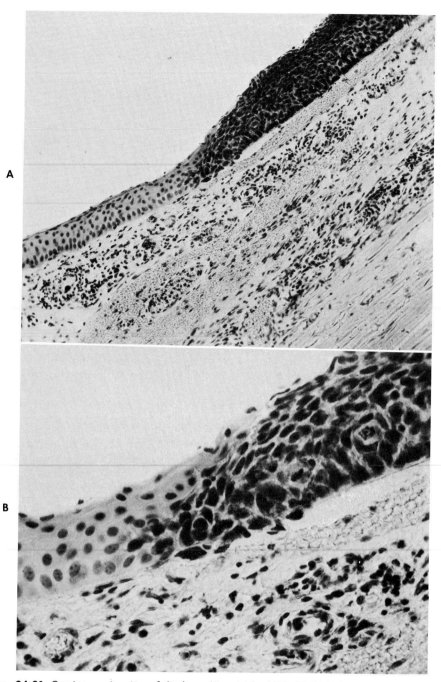

Fig. 24-21 Carcinoma in situ of limbus. (**A,** ×160; AFIP 53-21692; **B,** ×570; AFIP 53-21693; **B,** from Hogan, M. J., and Zimmerman, L. E.: Ophthalmic pathology, ed. 2, W. B. Saunders Co.)

nign and malignant neoplasms, hamartomatous and choristomatous growths, and inflammatory masses that are commonly (although inappropriately!) called inflammatory pseudotumors. In addition, the orbital tissues may become diffusely involved in pathologic processes related to systemic diseases.

Endocrinopathic exophthalmos

Endocrinopathic exophthalmos is a convenient term under which the main ophthalmic manifestations of Graves' disease can be grouped collectively. Graves' disease usually is divided into two types: mild, often referred

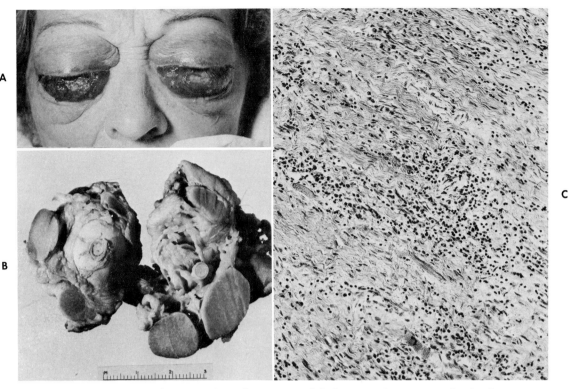

Fig. 24-22 Graves' disease with malignant exophthalmos. **A,** Severe periorbital edema and chemosis as well as proptosis. **B,** Massively enlarged extraocular muscles. **C,** Markedly degenerated extraocular muscles scarred and infiltrated by mononuclear inflammatory cells. (**A,** AFIP 55-3860; **B,** AFIP 55-10706; **C,** ×145; AFIP 58-13128; from Zimmerman, L. E.: In Ackerman, L. V. [in collaboration with Butcher, H. R., Jr.]: Surgical pathology, The C. V. Mosby Co.)

to as thyrotoxic or benign exophthalmos, and severe, also called thyrotropic, malignant, or infiltrative exophthalmos.

Although eyelid retraction and an apparent exophthalmos are characteristic features of Graves' disease, in its classic form one rarely sees evidence of more than a minimal effect on the orbital tissues, and severe secondary damage to the eyeball is not observed. In thyrotropic exophthalmos, on the other hand, the orbital tissues and extraocular muscles may become so massively involved that an extreme degree of rapidly progressive exophthalmos develops (Fig. 24-22, *A*). This may so seriously threaten the eye that the eyelids must be sutured together to prevent exposure keratitis. This form of endocrinopathic exophthalmos often is called "malignant exophthalmos" because of its severity, difficulty to control, and damaging sequelae. It is typically a bilateral disorder, but unilateral involvement occurs with sufficient frequency that it is considered by many ophthalmologists to be the leading cause of unilateral proptosis in adults. The pathologic changes include an accumula-

tion of water-binding mucopolysaccharides throughout the orbital tissues, severe degeneration of extraocular muscles that may become massively enlarged (Fig. 24-22, *B*) and eventually scarred (Fig. 24-22, *C*), and diffuse lymphocytic infiltration.

Anderson[21] has recently reviewed a large amount of the very abundant current literature on the mechanisms involved in the pathogenesis of Graves' disease and endocrine exophthalmos and has prepared an admirable summary. Because the old terms thyrotoxic and thyrotropic exophthalmos give an erroneous oversimplified concept of the pathologic physiology involved and because the many descriptive terms that have been used for various clinical manifestations of Graves' disease are equally objectionable, Werner[33] has recently proposed a new objective classification: Class 0, no signs or symptoms; Class 1, only signs, no symptoms; Class 2, symptoms and signs; Class 3, proptosis; Class 4, extraocular muscle involvement; Class 5, corneal involvement; Class 6, optic nerve involvement with loss of sight.

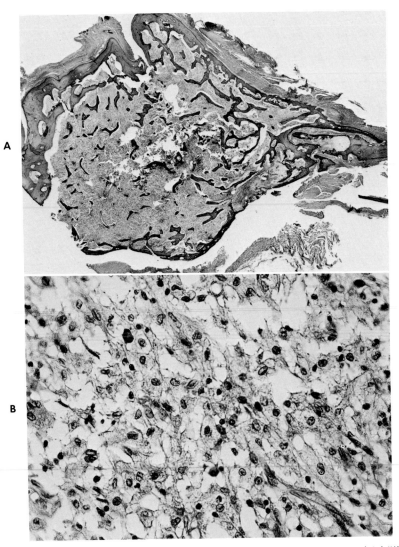

Fig. 24-23 Massive thickening and destruction of bony roof of orbit in Hand-Schüller-Christian disease. (**A,** ×6; AFIP 58-5349; **B,** ×305; AFIP 58-4501; **A** and **B,** from Hogan, M. J., and Zimmerman, L. E.: Ophthalmic pathology, ed. 2, W. B. Saunders Co.)

Histiocytosis X

Histiocytosis X, a group of related disorders that includes Hand-Schüller-Christian disease, eosinophilic granuloma of bone, and Letterer-Siwe disease, may have unilateral or bilateral proptosis as an important, sometimes presenting, clinical manifestation.

In Hand-Schüller-Christian disease, massive thickening and destruction of the bony walls of the orbit by the xanthogranulomatous process, with infiltration also into the soft tissues, occur so frequently that proptosis is considered one of the cardinal signs of the disease (Fig. 24-23). In eosinophilic granuloma of bone, there is often only a single focus of bone destruction, but this may be located in the orbit, most often in the upper temporal region, where thickening of the soft tissues of the eyebrow and eyelid may be a prominent clinical sign. Orbital involvement is rare in Letterer-Siwe disease.

Phycomycosis

Phycomycosis (often called mucormycosis) is described here because it is typically encountered as a most impressive complication of uncontrolled acidosis, especially in diabetic patients. It is a mycotic infection that is described more fully in Chapter 12, but because of its frequently devastating ocular and orbital complications, it must be mentioned here.

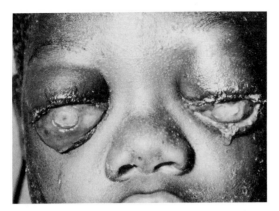

Fig. 24-24 Bilateral orbital involvement in Burkitt's African lymphoma. (AFIP 68-7157-5; from Karp, L. A., Zimmerman, L. E., and Payne, T.: Arch. Ophthal. [Chicago] **85:**295-298, 1971.)

Pathogenetically, it has been shown that some of the saprophytic fungi belonging to the *Phycomycetes* become extremely virulent when the host is acidotic. Clinically insignificant infections involving the nose and paranasal sinuses may then lead to rapidly spreading orbital cellulitis with frequent vascular complications (occlusive arteritis as well as thrombophlebitis). Gangrenous areas rapidly appear about the orbit, nose, and palate, and ischemic infarction involving the optic nerve and retina produce a rapidly progressive blindness. If not recognized early in its development and if the underlying disorder (diabetic acidosis, etc.) is not corrected promptly, the infection and its vascular complications spread back into the brain, resulting in a fatal outcome, often within a week of onset of symptoms.

Leukemia and malignant lymphoma

Leukemia and malignant lymphoma may involve any of the orbital tissues, but only rarely is the orbital lesion the initial manifestation of the disease. In some patients (especially in children) destined to develop acute granulocytic leukemia, a mass of very immature cells of the granulocytic series, often resembling the cells of reticulum cell sarcoma, may appear in the orbit long before any hematologic evidence of leukemia is found. Primary reticulum cell sarcomas of the orbit are extremely rare. Whenever a tumor suggestive of a reticulum cell sarcoma is encountered in the orbit, the pathologist should investigate the possibility that the lesion is, in actuality, a granulocytic sarcoma (also called

chloroma), an undifferentiated or transitional carcinoma that has spread into the orbit from an asymptomatic primary lesion in the nasopharynx or paranasal sinuses, or an inflammatory pseudotumor in which an exuberant reactive hyperplasia of reticulum cells has dominated the picture.

There is only one form of malignant lymphoma that involves the orbital tissues frequently—*Burkitt's African lymphoma.* This peculiar, highly undifferentiated malignant lymphoma has a curious predilection for the bones of the face and jaws. There is often bilateral involvement of the maxillae with spread into the soft tissues of the orbit. Consequently, proptosis with upward displacement of the eyeball is not an unusual presenting manifestation (Fig. 24-24).

Macroglobulinemia and other dysproteinemias

Macroglobulinemia and other dysproteinemias may be accompanied by massive proliferation of lymphoid tissue in extralymph nodal sites. We have seen several cases in which a mass in the orbit, with or without lacrimal gland involvement, was the initial clinical manifestation.

Microscopic examination typically shows a mixed population of cells, including lymphocytes, plasma cells, and reticulum cells, but particularly impressive are those that seem to represent intermediate stages of plasmacytoid differentiation. The demonstration of plasmacytoid cells in which eosinophilic intranuclear inclusions staining positively with periodic acid–Schiff are conspicuously present (Fig. 24-25) should always suggest the possibility of a dysproteinemia and call for appropriate studies of the serum proteins.

Sjögren's syndrome

Sjögren's syndrome, characterized ophthalmologically by the occurrence of keratoconjunctivitis sicca in middle-aged arthritic women, may lead to either shrinkage or enlargement of the lacrimal and salivary glands.

Microscopically, the changes observed include nonspecific atrophy with disappearance of variable amounts of the glandular parenchyma and replacement by an infiltrate of lymphocytes, plasma cells, and reticulum cells with or without fibrosis. In some cases, Godwin's benign lymphoepithelial lesion is strikingly obvious. Whenever this alteration is observed in an enlarged lacrimal or salivary gland, the pathologist should investigate the

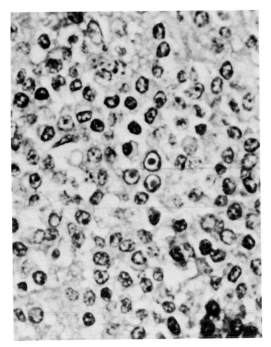

Fig. 24-25 Three cells in center of field contain intranuclear inclusions that stain positively with periodic acid–Schiff reaction in lymphoid pseudotumor in patient with macroglobulinemia. (Periodic acid–Schiff; ×750; AFIP 69-4960.)

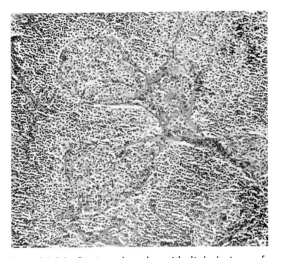

Fig. 24-26 Benign lymphoepithelial lesion of lacrimal gland. Epimyoepithelial islands such as one shown are all that remain of lacrimal gland, which is massively replaced by lymphoid cells. (×115; AFIP 63-1260.)

possibility that the patient may have clinical manifestations of Sjögren's syndrome. The benign lymphoepithelial lesion is characterized by a peculiar proliferation of both the epithelial and the myoepithelial cells of the larger ducts of the lacrimal and/or salivary glands and a virtually complete disappearance of all other glandular structures in the immediately adjacent areas. Thus one sees the epimyoepithelial islands in a sea of lymphoid cells (Fig. 24-26). Frequently, the lumens of the affected ducts are obliterated and some lymphocytes also are observed among the proliferated epimyoepithelial cells. In some cases of Sjögren's syndrome, the affected glands show a striking plasmacytoid reaction, and the PAS-positive inclusions that are always so suggestive of a dysproteinemia may be conspicuously present.

Mikulicz's syndrome

Mikulicz's syndrome is characterized by enlargement of multiple lacrimal and salivary glands. It may be observed in patients with Sjögren's syndrome, but it also may be observed in those with various other conditions (e.g., sarcoidosis, macroglobulinemia, leukemia, malignant lymphoma, etc.).

The term "Mikulicz's disease" always has been confusing because nobody really knows what disease process Mikulicz's patient had. Most writers today seem to be in agreement that this term therefore should be dropped and that the term "Mikulicz's syndrome" should be used only clinically for descriptive purposes.

Recklinghausen's neurofibromatosis

Recklinghausens' neurofibromatosis is another example of a very different type of systemic disease in which the orbit often is involved. In addition to having localized plexiform neurofibromas in the orbit or eyelids, patients with neurofibromatosis may exhibit gross disfigurement of the orbit (usually unilaterally) as a consequence of severe maldevelopment of both the osseous and soft tissues of the orbit. The eye also is often involved, and it may become either grossly enlarged, usually from an associated glaucoma, or shrunken from complications leading to phthisis bulbi.

Tumors

The following is a practical classification of tumors of the orbit.

Primary orbital tumors

A Choristomatous (examples, dermoid cysts and teratomas)
B Hamartomatous (examples, hemangiomas and lymphangiomas)
C Mesenchymal
    1 Adipose

2 Fibrous
3 Myomatous
4 Cartilaginous
5 Osseous
6 Vascular
D Neural
  1 Peripheral nerves
  2 Optic nerves
E Melanomatous (in association with nevus of Ota)
  1 Cellular blue nevus
  2 Malignant melanoma
F Epithelial
  1 Lacrimal gland
  2 Ectopic lacrimal gland
G Inflammatory "pseudotumors"
  1 Lymphoid
  2 Plasmacytoid
  3 Sclerosing nongranulomatous
  4 Granulomatous
  5 Lipogranulomatous

Secondary orbital tumors—from primary sites in adjacent tissues

A Intraocular
  1 Malignant melanoma
  2 Retinoblastoma
B Epibulbar
  1 Carcinoma
  2 Malignant melanoma
C Eyelids and skin of face
  1 Basal cell carcinoma
  2 Sebaceous carcinoma
  3 Malignant melanoma
  4 Squamous cell carcinoma
D Upper respiratory tract
  1 Carcinoma of various types
  2 Malignant melanoma
  3 Mucocele
E Intracranial
  1 Meningioma
  2 Pituitary adenoma

Metastatic

A Carcinoma
B Malignant melanoma
C Sarcoma
D Neuroblastoma

As with all classifications, there are lesions that would seem to fit into more than one category and there are others that do not seem to fit well into any. In the orbit, a good example is the fibrous xanthoma, a lesion that we are recognizing with increasing frequency. Is it a neoplasm or a peculiar form of inflammatory pseudotumor? If it is a neoplasm, is it basically fibrous, vascular, or histiocytic? At the present time, these questions cannot be answered satisfactorily.

It is difficult to comment on the relative frequency of orbital tumors because there is so much variation depending on the nature of one's particular experience. The pathologist who practices in a pediatric hospital will see many examples of orbital involvement late in the course of such conditions as neuroblastoma, leukemia, and Hand-Schüller-Christian's disease, but the ophthalmic pathologist rarely sees such cases. He and the clinical ophthalmologist, who deal primarily with those conditions whose initial manifestations are ocular or orbital, are much more likely to see hemangiomas, rhabdomyosarcomas, and gliomas of the optic nerve in their pediatric patients. One of the most common orbital tumors in the experience of radiologists is the mucocele of the paranasal sinuses, yet the ophthalmic pathologist rarely sees these lesions. In geriatric practice, one sees secondary and metastatic tumors of the orbit much more frequently than primary tumors. In equatorial Africa, primary malignant lymphoma involving the orbital bones is relatively common, whereas this is a very rare orbital neoplasm everywhere else in the world.

Whereas the foregoing comments indicate that it is difficult to generalize about orbital tumors, there does seem to be general agreement that endocrinopathic endophthalmos, hemangiomas, and inflammatory pseudotumors are the most frequent causes of proptosis in adults. Hemangiomas also are frequent in childhood. Of especial importance in childhood are rhabdomyosarcomas, gliomas of the optic nerve, leukemia, and lymphoma.

Rhabdomyosarcomas. Rhabdomyosarcomas of the orbit are usually of the embryonal type (Fig. 24-27) and are seen almost exclusively in the first fifteen years of life. They arise diffusely in the orbital tissues (only rarely in the substance of one of the extraocular muscles) and have a predilection for the upper inner portion, producing a downward and temporal displacement of the globe.

Typically sudden in appearance, the tumor often grows with alarming rapidity and frequently has spread diffusely by the time the orbit is explored. It is not only highly invasive, with a distinct tendency to invade the cranium, but it is also capable of metastasizing widely via the bloodstream. Its prognosis is very poor, although the treatment of orbital rhabdomyosarcomas has been more successful than has that of other embryonal rhabdomyosarcomas. This tumor does not generally affect visual acuity, although the displacement of the globe may cause diplopia. With severe proptosis, exposure keratitis eventually may complicate the picture.

Glioma of optic nerve. Glioma of the optic nerve is another orbital tumor encountered almost exclusively in the pediatric age group,

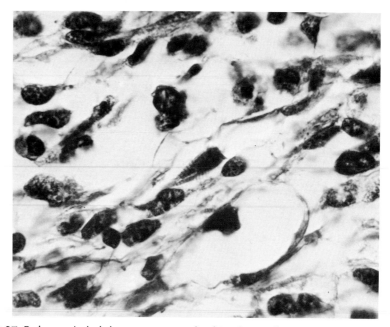

Fig. 24-27 Embryonal rhabdomyosarcoma of orbit. One cell in center of field has well-formed cross striations, whereas all others appear to be undifferentiated mesenchymal cells. (×720; AFIP 65-3236.)

about half of the cases being recognized by the age of 5 years. It is typically a very low-grade, well-differentiated, fibrillary type of astrocytoma that grows slowly within the parenchyma of the nerve (Fig. 24-28), gradually destroying the latter's axons as it displaces the eye forward. Those tumors that arise anteriorly in the nerve, close to the globe where the central retinal artery and vein pass through the nerve to enter the eye, are likely to compress and occlude these vessels. Thus, the child with a glioma of the optic nerve often shows a number of important ocular complications not often seen in patients with rhabdomyosarcomas of the orbit, including severe loss of vision, optic atrophy, papilledema, retinal hemorrhages and exudates, and even infarction of the retina.

Although prognosis for vision in the affected eye is very poor, prognosis for life is good. After a period of growth during childhood, the tumors seem to become quiescent. Spread from the optic nerve back into the brain is unusual, orbital recurrence is very rare, and hematogenous spread unknown, even though the tumor may have been untreated or incompletely resected.

Gliomas of the optic nerve occur more frequently in patients with Recklinghausen's neurofibromatosis than in otherwise normal individuals, and in such patients they may be bilateral, but less than 15% of patients with

these tumors show evidence of neurofibromatosis.

Meningiomas. Meningiomas, in contrast with gliomas, occur more frequently in adults than in children. There are three possible histogenetic explanations for the occurrence of orbital meningiomas.

One group arises from the leptomeningeal coverings of the optic nerve (Fig. 24-29). This type is almost always of the meningothelial variety, and psammoma bodies are usually demonstrable. The tumor often compresses and/or infiltrates the parenchyma of the optic nerve, producing optic atrophy and visual loss as well as proptosis.

Meningiomas of the second major group have an intracranial site of origin which clinically may be silent and difficult to detect. These tumors reach the orbit by infiltrating directly into the orbital bones or along the vessels and nerves that pass through the various foramina. They usually do not affect the optic nerve itself, and visual loss is therefore not characteristic.

The third group of mengingiomas is mainly of theoretical interest. It is postulated that meningiomas may arise from meningeal rests in the orbit. We know that ectopic neuroglial and meningeal tissue may be encountered in the orbit, giving rise to space-occupying choristomatous cysts and tumors (encephaloceles and meningoceles), but proof of the origin

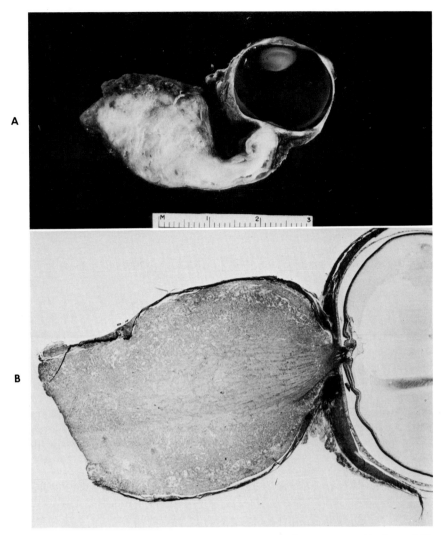

Fig. 24-28 Gliomas of optic nerve. (**A,** AFIP 57-890-3; from Hogan, M. J., and Zimmerman, L. E.: Ophthalmic pathology, ed. 2, W. B. Saunders Co.; **B,** AFIP 55-17314; from Zimmerman, L. E.: In Saphir, O., editor: A text on systemic pathology, Grune & Stratton, Inc.; by permission.)

of meningiomas from such rests is most difficult to establish. It is possible that some of the fibroblastic and fibroxanthomatous tumors encountered in the orbit may have taken origin from such ectopic meningeal tissue, but the great majority of unequivocal meningothelial and psammomatous meningiomas in the orbit either are of optic nerve origin or are secondary from an intracranial site of origin.

Leukemia and lymphoma. Leukemia and lymphoma have been mentioned earlier in this chapter (p. 1015). As an initial manifestation of a previously undetected leukemia, the child more likely than the adult may be seen with an apparently isolated tumor in the orbit, eyelids, or periorbital tissues. Thus, in the dif-

ferential diagnosis of any undifferentiated neoplasm encountered in the orbital tissues of a child, leukemia must be considered and appropriate hematologic investigations undertaken. Burkitt's African lymphoma is the most important malignant lymphoma that affects the orbit (p. 1354).

Postirradiation sarcomas and carcinomas. Postirradiation sarcomas and carcinomas were once of great importance in children who had received intensive radiation therapy for retinoblastoma. There was a period when 7,500-10,000 rads were being delivered through one or two portals in an effort to save at least one eye in selected patients with bilateral retinoblastoma. This treatment was frequently successful in controlling the retinoblastoma,

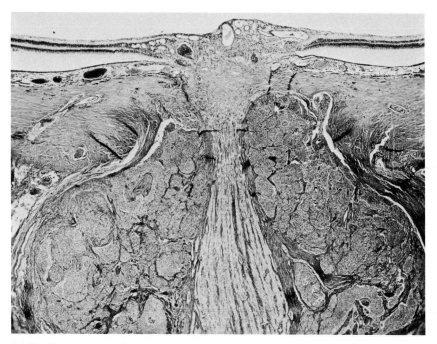

Fig. 24-29 Meningioma of optic nerve. (×22; AFIP 54-21636; from Zimmerman, L. E.: In Ackerman, L. V. [in collaboration with Butcher, H. R., Jr.]: Surgical pathology, The C. V. Mosby Co.)

but intraocular complications leading to eventual enucleation of the eye were common, and occasionally a second tumor appeared in the irradiated tissues five to twenty years later. Most of these were sarcomas and, of these, osteogenic and chondromatous sarcomas were seen most often. This is of pathogenetic significance because in nonirradiated orbital tissues malignant bone tumors are exceedingly rare neoplasms (except in adults who have Paget's disease of bone).

In recent years, with the availability of better methods of radiation therapy, it has been learned that much smaller doses of radiation in selected patients can control the retinoblastoma without adversely affecting the eye or adjacent orbital tissues, and it is hoped that postradiation cancers will no longer be encountered in this area.

Other primary malignant orbital tumors in children. Other primary malignant tumors of the orbit in children such as embryonal carcinoma, meningeal sarcoma, and alveolar soft part sarcoma are encountered too rarely to warrant further comment here.

Metastatic neuroblastoma. Metastatic neuroblastoma is the only important metastatic tumor of the orbit in children. It generally is encountered late in the clinical course, long after the child has been recognized as having a malignant retroperitoneal tumor. Thus, it rarely presents a diagnostic problem for either the ophthalmologist or the ophthalmic pathologist. Typically, the orbits are affected bilaterally, and there is often a hemorrhagic appearance to the affected eyelids and orbital tissues.

Benign orbital tumors. Benign orbital tumors in children are numerous. They include the relatively common dermoid cysts, the rare teratomas, which often are already huge at birth (Fig. 24-30), ectopic masses of neurogenic and/or meningeal tissues (encephaloceles and meningoencephaloceles), hemangiomas, lymphangiomas, and neurofibromas, and even such lesions that are more typically seen in adults such as meningiomas, lacrimal glands tumors, and inflammatory pseudotumors.

Lacrimal gland tumors. Lacrimal gland tumors include, in addition to the primary epithelial neoplasms, enlargements resulting from a variety of other pathologic processes. When a patient is seen with a mass in the position of the lacrimal gland, there is about a 50-50 chance that the cause will be found to be an epithelial neoplasm.

Enlargements not the result of epithelial neoplasms are most frequently caused by nonspecific inflammatory processes ("pseudotu-

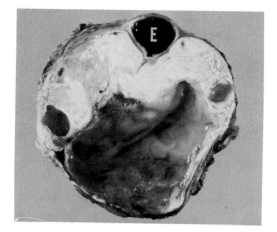

Fig. 24-30 Teratoma that massively enlarged orbit of newborn infant. Note size of eye, **E**, for comparison. (From Casanovas, R.: Arch. Ophthal. [Chicago] 77:795-797, 1967; AFIP 66-7224.)

mors"), but they also may be observed when the gland is involved in such specific granulomatous diseases as sarcoidosis, tuberculosis, and leprosy or when it is invaded by neoplasms that have arisen elsewhere. As was indicated in the discussion of Mikulicz's syndrome, the lacrimal glands may be enlarged along with one or more salivary glands in leukemia, malignant lymphoma, macroglobulinemia, Sjögren's syndrome, and a variety of other conditions. If both lacrimal glands are enlarged, one can be relatively certain that the cause is not an epithelial neoplasm because these are, almost without exception, always unilateral.

Epithelial neoplasms. Epithelial neoplasms of the lacrimal gland are very similar to those of the salivary glands, but one does not see such a great variety of tumor types in the lacrimal gland, and certain tumors (e.g., Warthin's tumor) that are relatively common in the salivary glands are either very rare or nonexistent in the lacrimal gland. For practical purposes, a very simple classification may be used. There are two major groups: the mixed tumors and carcinomas that are unrelated to mixed tumors.

The mixed tumors of the lacrimal gland are virtually identical to those of the salivary glands (p. 1101). Most of the mixed tumors are benign, but about one-third are malignant. The median age of patients with benign mixed tumors is 35 years, whereas patients with malignant mixed tumors tend to be about fifteen years older. The malignant mixed tumor by definition is one that contains areas of benign mixed tumor but, in addition, areas

exhibiting histologic features of malignancy. The latter are usually adenocarcinomatous, sometimes squamous, and very rarely sarcomatous. The malignant change may be evident when the tumor is first removed, or it may be observed only some years after a benign mixed tumor has been incompletely removed and then allowed to recur.

Adenocarcinomas that are unrelated to mixed tumors exhibit considerable architectural variation microscopically, but one type is of particular importance. This is the adenoid cystic or cylindromatous variety, which is comparatively more frequent in the lacrimal than in the major salivary glands. It is a tumor that in the past often has been confused with benign mixed tumors (and vice versa). Benign mixed tumors carry a favorable prognosis, whereas adenoid cystic carcinomas are extremely infiltrative, with a remarkable tendency to spread into and along nerves and through the bony wall of the orbit. Although the cure rate for benign mixed tumors is high, it is most unusual to be able to save a patient who has an adenoid cystic carcinoma of the lacrimal gland. Thus, the histopathologic delineation of adenoid cystic carcinoma from benign mixed tumor has been a major contribution to the study and prognosis of lacrimal gland tumors.

Pseudotumor. Pseudotumor is a term that has variable connotations. It is perhaps most precisely used when surgical exploration of the orbit fails to reveal any evidence of a mass in a patient who clinically was thought to have an orbital tumor. It is most frequently used, however, together with the adjective "inflammatory," to designate a mass composed of inflammatory tissue that clinically had been suspected of being a neoplasm. Microscopically, some of these can be placed in well-established categorical groups (e.g., sarcoidosis, tuberculosis, echinococcosis, foreign body granulomas, sclerosing lipogranulomas, etc.), but the majority are very nonspecific in their histopathologic appearance. They tend to be characterized by the production of variable proportions of dense fibrous connective tissue and lymphoid aggregates, the latter often exhibiting prominent reactive centers. In other instances, one may see a conspicuous vasculitis with eosinophilia, suggesting the possibility of an allergic process. In still other cases, the mass involves mainly skeletal muscle, suggesting a primary myositis of obscure cause.

Collectively, these inflamamtory pseudotumors constitute a large and important segment of the orbital tumor problem in adults because of their relative frequency, their obscure etiology, and their ineffectual therapy.

INFLAMMATIONS

Inflammations of the eye are named after the tissues that are principally affected. Since the uveal tract is the most highly vascular tissue of the eye, it tends to be the site of the major inflammatory response in most cases, and the term "uveitis" often is used in ophthalmology as an all-inclusive synonym for the more appropriate heading ocular inflammation. Both the clinician and the pathologist, however, should try to identify the main sites of involvement and use more appropriate terminology:

Sites of inflammation	Term
Entire uveal tract	Panuveitis
Iris	Iritis
Ciliary body	Cyclitis
Choroid	Choroiditis
Retina	Retinitis
Retina and choroid	Chorioretinitis or retino-choroiditis
Sclera	Scleritis
Sclera and uvea	Sclerouveitis
Cornea	Keratitis
Cornea and sclera	Sclerokeratitis
Exudate in anterior chamber	Hypopyon
Interior of eye	Endophthalmitis
Interior plus all tunics	Panophthalmitis
Optic nerve	Optic neuritis
Optic nerve head	Papillitis
Retina and optic nerve	Neuroretinitis

The terms provide no information as to specific cause or pathogenesis, nor do they indicate the type of pathologic process that is involved. For descriptive purposes and to facilitate a consideration of pathogenesis, it is convenient to classify intraocular inflammations as follows:

Acute suppurative
    Exogenous
    Endogenous
Chronic nongranulomatous
    Exogenous
    Endogenous
Chronic granulomatous
    Exogenous
    Endogenous

Acute suppurative inflammations

Acute suppurative inflammations are most often exogenous, following penetrating or perforating wounds of the globe with or without the introduction of foreign bodies. Bacteria, fungi, certain chemicals, including acids and

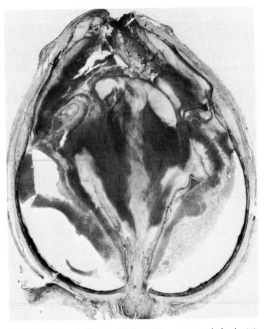

Fig. 24-31 Acute suppurative panophthalmitis secondary to perforation of corneal ulcer. (AFIP 28817; from Hogan, M. J., and Zimmerman, L. E.: Ophthalmic pathology, ed. 2, W. B. Saunders Co.)

alkalis, and all sorts of organic matter are potent irritants. When introduced into the eye, they tend to provoke a massive polymorphonuclear response leading to endophthalmitis or panophthalmitis. Much less frequently, acute suppurative inflammation develops after intraocular surgery, following perforation of a corneal ulcer (Fig. 24-31), or as a result of spread from an orbital cellulitis.

Endogenous suppurative inflammation is much less common. It is almost always the result of hematogenous infection of the eye from a primary bacterial or mycotic focus elsewhere in the body (Fig. 24-32), but extension to the eye via the optic nerve or subarachnoid fluid from an intracranial infection is also possible. Demonstration of the causative bacteria or fungi in cases of suppurative endophthalmitis or panophthalmitis usually requires a careful search of sections that have been appropriately stained for these organisms.

Mycotic infections deserve special comment not because they are more frequent or more devastating than the bacterial but because the eye is vulnerable to many organisms that are so lowly virulent that they are generally regarded as nonpathogenic saprophytes. The cornea and vitreous, being without an intrinsic blood supply and much slower to react to inflammatory stimuli, seem to permit saprophytic organisms to proliferate and establish themselves before an effective suppurative response can be developed to eradicate them. These fungi may be introduced from the soil or from vegetation when the cornea is scratched or the vitreous body penetrated. Prophylactic antibiotic therapy used in the management of ocular injuries has greatly reduced the frequency of serious bacterial infection, but at present no satisfactory drugs are available to protect the eye against infection by species of *Aspergillus, Cephalosporium, Fusarium,* and other fungi that may be introduced at the time of injury or surgery (Fig. 24-33).

Chronic nongranulomatous inflammations

Chronic nongranulomatous inflammations stand in sharp contrast with the acute suppurative inflammations. They are seldom exogenous and rarely are attributable to a specific infectious agent. The inflammatory reaction is most frequently restricted to the uvea, often to the iris and ciliary body (Fig. 24-34).

Because the tissues are infiltrated by lymphocytes and plasma cells, often with many Russell bodies being present, it is generally assumed that an immunopathologic mechanism is involved. Neither the clinician nor the histopathologist has enjoyed much success in the etiologic classification of nongranulomatous uveitis, although certain systemic diseases such as ankylosing spondylitis and Still's disease often are complicated by this type of uveitis.

Chronic granulomatous inflammations

Granulomatous inflammations are of special interest to the pathologist because they fre-

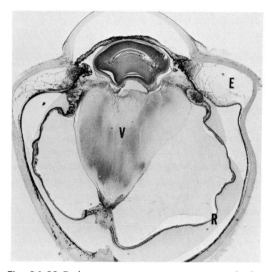

Fig. 24-32 Endogenous acute suppurative endophthalmitis, complication of meningococcemia in patient who also had meningitis. Purulent exudate in vitreous body, **V,** which has become detached from retina, **R,** which also is detached. Serous exudate present in preretinal, subretinal, and epichoroidal spaces, **E.** (×5.5; AFIP 56-9989; from Zimmerman, L. E.: In Saphir, O., editor: A text on systemic pathology, Grune & Stratton, Inc.; by permission.)

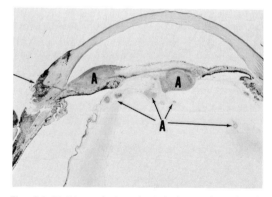

Fig. 24-33 Nocardial endophthalmitis that developed after cataract extraction. Arrows indicate surgical wound. Multiple abscesses, **A,** present in iris, posterior chamber, and vitreous. (×6; AFIP 68-2841; slightly modified from Meyer, S. L., Font, R. L., and Shaver, R. P.: Arch. Ophthal. [Chicago] **83:**536-541, 1970.)

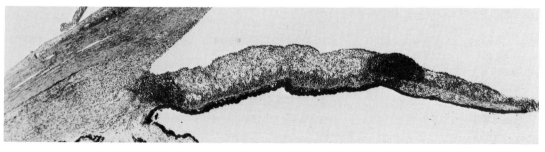

Fig. 24-34 Chronic nongranulomatous iridocyclitis. (×40; AFIP 60392.)

quently present patterns of tissue reaction that fall into meaningful pathogenetic groups, even though a specific causative agent is not demonstrable in the tissue. Important examples of both posttraumatic and purely endogenous granulomatous inflammation must be considered. In the first category are sympathetic ophthalmia, phacoanaphylaxis (described in the discussion on cataracts), and foreign body granulomas. Of these, however, only the latter can be considered entirely exogenous because systemic autosensitivity is believed to play an important role in the pathogenesis of the other two.

Sympathetic ophthalmia. Sympathetic ophthalmia is a diffuse granulomatous uveitis that affects both eyes after a penetrating injury to one eye. It is fortunately a rare complication because it often leads to very severe visual loss in both eyes, but it does occur periodically after intraocular surgery as well as following accidental wounds. A prolapse or loss of uveal tissue seems to be an important predisposing factor.

The condition is believed to develop as a result of an autosensitivity reaction to uveal tissue that has become altered in some mysterious way after the injury. The entire uveal tract becomes thickened by an infiltrate of lymphocytes and epithelioid cells (Fig. 24-

35). There is no necrosis, and virtually no polymorphonuclear leukocytes or plasma cells are observed.

Endogenous granulomatous inflammation. Endogenous granulomatous inflammation includes a large infectious group and a miscellaneous group of unknown cause. Many of the important systemic infectious diseases that characteristically produce a granulomatous response may involve the eye. Examples are tuberculosis, leprosy, syphilis, blastomycosis, cryptococcosis, coccidioidomycosis, sporotrichosis, cysticercosis, toxoplasmosis, visceral larva migrans, and cytomegalovirus infection. Since the ocular complications of most of these infections and their histopathologic characteristics are not particularly noteworthy, only the two especially important examples will be described here—toxoplasmosis and toxocariasis.

Toxoplasma chorioretinitis occurs in two main forms: congenital and acquired. In those cases in which congenital toxoplasmosis results in a stillborn baby or a neonatal death, there is a very high incidence of severe chorioretinitis. Less overwhelming congenital infections may be characterized by nonfatal damage to the brain and areas of chorioretinitis. There is also evidence that unilateral or bilateral chorioretinitis may be the only recognizable clinical manifestation of congenital toxoplasmosis. The intraocular inflammation in such cases often leads to chorioretinal scarring, but the infection may or may not be eradicated. The causative protozoan parasite may remain viable in an encysted form for long periods, giving rise periodically to bouts of renewed activity. The other form of the disease is

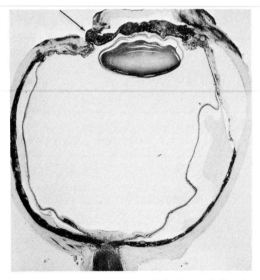

Fig. 24-35 Sympathetic ophthalmia following penetrating wound of limbus with prolapse of iris and ciliary body (arrow). Almost all of uvea thickened by infiltrate of lymphocytes and epithelioid cells. (×4; AFIP 53904-17111; from Friedenwald, J. S., Wilder, H. C., Maumenee, A. E., Sanders, T. E., Keyes, J. E., Hogan, M. J., Owens, W. C., and Owens, E. U.: Ophthalmic pathology, W. B. Saunders Co.)

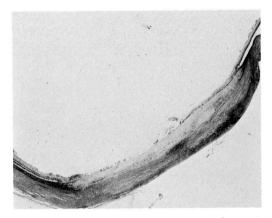

Fig. 24-36 Chorioretinitis due to toxoplasmosis. (×7; AFIP 57-1180; from Zimmerman, L. E.: In Ackerman, L. V. [in collaboration with Butcher, H. R., Jr.]: Surgical pathology, The C. V. Mosby Co.)

acquired toxoplasmosis occurring in adults, usually without any other associated clinical manifestations of systemic disease such as fever, malaise, skin rash, or lymphadenopathy. In these cases, the retina seems to be particularly vulnerable to infection by *Toxoplasma gondii,* providing the only focus where the parasite establishes itself in a pathogenetically significant manner.

What one sees microscopically in both the congenital and the acquired forms is a discrete area of coagulative necrosis in the retina (Fig. 24-36). Usually, the pigment epithelium and occasionally variable amounts of the adjacent choroid and sclera also exhibit coagulative necrosis. Surrounding the areas of coagulative necrosis, there is a diffuse granulomatous reaction affecting the choroid, sclera, and episclera. Away from this discrete focus of chorioretinitis, the picture is more variable and nondiagnostic. Often, there is a panuveitis that may be purely nongranulomatous or distinctly granulomatous. Usually, it is only in the area of coagulative necrosis that the free bow-shaped protozoans or their encysted forms can be seen (Fig. 24-37), although sometimes the encysted forms can be identified in the adjacent viable retina.

Ocular larva migrans is a nematodal endophthalmitis caused by larvae of *Toxocara canis* that wander into the eye via the uveal or retinal circulation. This, then, is the ocular equivalent of visceral larva migrans. *Toxocara canis* is a common inhabitant of the dog's intestinal tract, and its eggs contaminate the soil everywhere dogs are present. Young children who put dirty objects in their mouths or who actually eat soil (pica) are the ones who are most likely to become infected.

In the eye, the nematode larvae seem to have a predilection for the retina and vitreous body, producing a chronic, sclerosing inflammatory reaction in the vitreous and retina, usually without external signs and symptoms of ocular inflammation. Eosinophils often are present in large numbers in the vitreous. Eosinophilic abscesses and small granulomas often develop about the disintegrating larvae (Fig. 24-38). The vitreal reaction eventually produces a massive retinal detachment and a leukokoria that often leads to a clinical diagnosis of retinoblastoma.

Less frequently, the parasite may become localized in the choroid or between the choroid and retina, producing a focal chorioretinal mass in the vicinity of the macula or

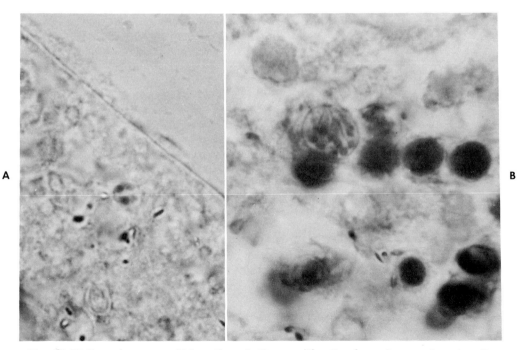

Fig. 24-37 *Toxoplasma gondii* in retina. **A,** Two proliferative forms in necrotic retina. **B,** Encysted forms in necrotic retina. (**A,** ×1800; AFIP 211318-21011; from Wilder, H. C.: Arch. Ophthal. [Chicago] **48**:127-136, 1952; **B,** ×1920; AFIP 57-1172; from Zimmerman, L. E.: In Ackerman, L. V. [in collaboration with Butcher, H. R., Jr.]: Surgical pathology, The C. V. Mosby Co.)

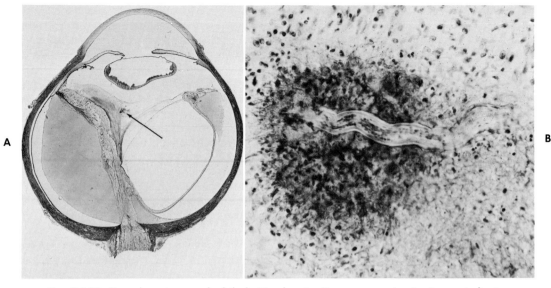

Fig. 24-38 Granulomatous endophthalmitis due to *Toxocara canis*. **A,** Arrow indicates site of granuloma containing larva shown in **B.** Preretinal inflammatory membrane has led to total detachment of retina. **B,** Nematode larva in granuloma in vitreous. (**A,** ×3; **B,** ×400; **A** and **B,** from Wilder, H. C.: Trans. Amer. Acad. Ophthal. Otolaryng. **55**:99-109, 1950; AFIP 198761.)

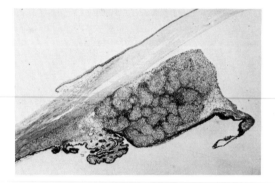

Fig. 24-39 Granulomatous iridocyclitis in sarcoidosis. (×20; AFIP 71412-08121; from Hogan, M. J., and Zimmerman, L. E.: Ophthalmic pathology, ed. 2, W. B. Saunders Co.)

optic disc. Ocular larva migrans is almost always a unilateral condition that is not accompanied by systemic manifestations, except perhaps for a mild eosinophilia. Why children with visceral manifestations of larva migrans should not have ocular complications and why those with ocular larva migrans should not have systemic manifestations are unexplained.

Noninfectious granulomatous disease. Noninfectious granulomatous disease of various types may affect the eye. Three examples that are particularly striking will be discussed: sarcoidosis, rheumatoid sclerouveitis, and juvenile xanthogranuloma.

Sarcoidosis frequently is complicated by the development of a granulomatous iridocyclitis (Fig. 24-39) and less often by a retinitis or chorioretinitis. The intraocular lesions, like those of other affected tissues, are typically noncaseating epithelioid tubercles. The granulomatous lesions of the iris and ciliary body often erupt into the anterior or posterior chambers, producing various complications (e.g., cataract, glaucoma, hypotony, corneal damage, etc.) that seriously affect vision and may lead to blindness. The retinal lesions are usually much less massive than those occurring in the anterior segment and tend to be distributed along the major vessels (Fig. 24-40), producing an ophthalmoscopic picture that has been described as resembling drippings of candle wax. Involvement of the central nervous system is said to occur with great frequency among those patients who are found to have this curious retinal form of sarcoidosis.

Rheumatoid sclerouveitis is characterized by the formation of patchy areas of coagulative necrosis of collagen in the sclera, usually anteriorly between the limbus and the equator of the globe. These areas are surrounded by a palisade of epithelioid cells, so that the lesions are reminiscent of the rheumatoid nodules that develop in the subcutaneous tissues, tendons, or other collagenous structures such as the dura in patients who have rheumatoid arthritis. When only a discrete focus

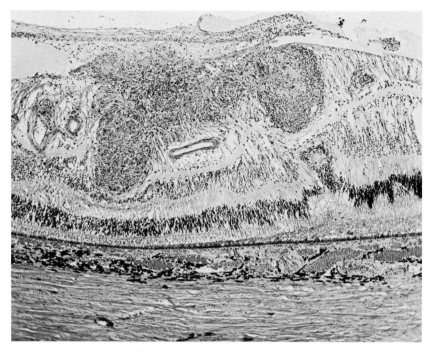

Fig. 24-40 Perivascular distribution of tubercles in patient with sarcoidosis who died as consequence of involvement of central nervous system. (×50; AFIP 63-1450.)

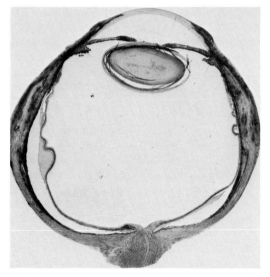

Fig. 24-41 Brawny scleritis. Sclera anteriorly is massively thickened by chronic granulomatous inflammatory reaction. (×5; AFIP 67159; from DeCoursey, E., and Ash, J. E.: Atlas of ophthalmic pathology, American Academy of Ophthalmology and Otolaryngology.)

of involvement is present, the lesion often is called a "rheumatoid nodule" of the sclera. Often, however, there are extensive areas of diffuse thickening and induration resulting from a massive infiltration by lymphocytes,

plasma cells, and histiocytes (Fig. 24-41). Clinically, this gives rise to a picture that has usually been called "brawny scleritis." In some patients, the same basic disorder seems to lead to a marked dissolution of the sclera with minimal inflammatory thickening. In such cases, the uvea may herniate through defects in the sclera, and the globe becomes vulnerable to rupture from minimal trauma. This form of the disease is called "scleromalacia perforans." In only about half of the patients who present with these various forms of sclerouveitis is there a well-established clinical history of rheumatoid arthritis or some other related systemic disease.

Juvenile xanthogranuloma is typically a benign, spontaneously regressing, granulomatous dermatosis of infants and young children who have no important visceral lesions. The only important exception to this generalization is observed in the rare child who develops lesions in the iris and ciliary body (Fig. 24-42). This uveal involvement frequently leads to one or both of two serious complications: spontaneous hemorrhage into the anterior chamber and secondary glaucoma resulting from an accumulation of histiocytic cells in the anterior chamber angle. The iris and ciliary body are infiltrated by lipid-laden histiocytes similar to those found

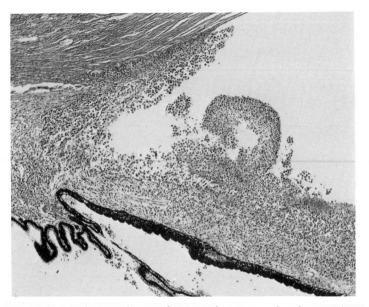

Fig. 24-42 Juvenile xanthogranuloma of iris and anterior chamber angle. (×50; AFIP 60-2778; from Hogan, M. J., and Zimmerman, L. E.: Ophthalmic pathology, ed. 2, W. B. Saunders Co.)

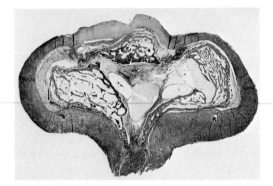

Fig. 24-43 Phthisis bulbi. (×3; AFIP 112917-07091; from Friedenwald, J. S., Wilder, H. C., Maumenee, A. E., Sanders, T. E., Keyes, J. E., Hogan, M. J., Owens, W. C., and Owens, E. U.: Ophthalmic pathology, W. B. Saunders Co.)

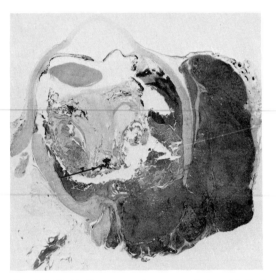

Fig. 24-44 Malignant melanoma of choroid that arose in phthisic eye that had been blind for twenty-two years following missile injury. Arrow points to retained metallic foreign body in scarred vitreous body. Note massive extraocular extension of tumor. (×2; AFIP 57-14185; from Hogan, M. J., and Zimmerman, L. E.: Ophthalmic pathology, ed. 2, W. B. Saunders Co.)

in the skin lesions, and Touton giant cells are often present. Ocular involvement is virtually always unilateral.

Complications

Complications of ocular inflammation may be very serious, leading to blindness. In the acute suppurative and granulomatous forms, necrosis of the retina and choroid leads to permanent scarring and loss of function of these tissues. If the macula or all of the retina is affected, severe visual loss is inevitable. When there has been more widespread destruction of intraocular tissues, severe scarring and gliosis are observed and the internal

architecture of the globe becomes markedly disorganized. The production of aqueous humor may be so greatly reduced that the eye becomes soft, atrophic, and shrunken. This state of advanced degeneration and disorganization of the entire eyeball is called phthisis bulbi (Fig. 24-43). Phthisical eyes pre-

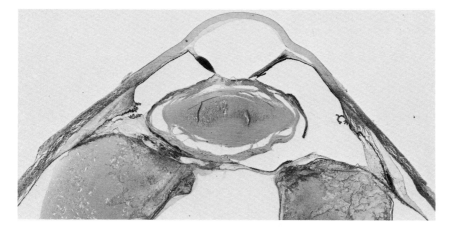

Fig. 24-45 Several complications of chronic iridocyclitis are present: broad peripheral anterior synechias, seclusion of pupil by posterior synechias, occlusion of pupil by fibrovascular membrane, iris bombé, and formation of cataract. (×5; AFIP 66-13055.)

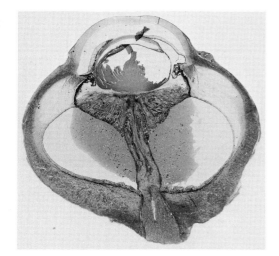

Fig. 24-46 Atrophia bulbi. (×4; AFIP 54885-07091; from Friedenwald, J. S., Wilder, H. C., Maumenee, A. E., Sanders, T. E., Keyes, J. E., Hogan, M. J., Owens, W. C., and Owens, E. U.: Ophthalmic pathology, W. B. Saunders Co.)

sent not only a cosmetic problem but are often irritable. Malignant melanoma may arise in such blind, phthisical eyes, and, because it is invisible, owing to opacification of the ocular media, the tumor often spreads out of the eye before it is detected (Fig. 24-44). For all these reasons, phthisical eyes often are enucleated.

More limited inflammatory processes, including those of the chronic nongranulomatous variety, also may produce a variety of significant complications, including leakage of plasma proteins and an accumulation of inflammatory cells in the aqueous humor and vitreous, adherence of the iris to the lens (posterior synechias) or to the cornea (anterior synechias), formation of a pupillary membrane that occludes the pupil and obstructs the flow of aqueous humor (Fig. 24-45), opacification of the cornea, formation of cataracts, diminution of aqueous production, chorioretinal degeneration, and optic atrophy. As a consequence of these complications, the eye may become glaucomatous or hypotonic, or it may first become glaucomatous and then later hypotonic when damage to the ciliary body becomes sufficiently severe. In cases of long-standing severe hypotony, one often sees a detachment of the retina and uvea, papilledema, and shrinkage of the globe or atrophia bulbi (Fig. 24-46).

GLAUCOMA

Glaucoma is the name given to a large group of ocular disorders that have in common a rise in intraocular pressure sufficient to damage various tissues, especially optic nerve fibers. Theoretically, such an increase in intraocular pressure could arise from an excessively rapid production of aqueous humor by the ciliary body or from a great increase in episcleral venous pressure with consequent impairment of aqueous flow out of the globe, but for all practical purposes the cause is almost always found to be an obstruction to aqueous flow within the eyeball.

There are three main sites at which the flow of aqueous humor most often is obstructed: at the pupil, in the angle of the anterior chamber, and within the outflow pathways that lie between the anterior chamber angle and the episcleral veins (Fig. 24-6). When the anatomic obstruction is the result of a developmental malformation, the glaucoma is classified as congenital. All other glaucomas are acquired and traditionally are subdivided into secondary and primary forms. The secondary glaucomas are those that develop as a complication of some other primary disease process (e.g., uveitis, trauma, intraocular hemorrhage, neoplasms, etc.) and are usually unilateral. The primary glaucomas are typically bilateral, occurring in eyes that are not obviously affected by some other condition.

Secondary glaucoma

Secondary glaucoma is produced by one or more of four main types of obstruction:

1. Posterior synechias
2. Anterior synechias
3. Accumulation of cells or cellular debris in the anterior chamber angle
4. Damage to the outflow channels in the trabecular meshwork, canal of Schlemm, ciliary body, scleral spur, etc.

Posterior synechias are adhesions between the pupillary margin of the iris and the anterior surface of the lens that usually develop as a result of inflammation of the iris (iritis). These adhesions may bind the iris to the lens completely, a condition called seclusion of the pupil (Fig. 24-45). Accompanying the formation of posterior synechias one often sees the outgrowth of a fibrovascular membrane from the pupillary margin of the iris across the pupil. Obstruction of the pupil by such a membrane is called occlusion of the pupil. Either seclusion of the pupil or occlusion of the pupil will prevent the flow of aqueous humor from the posterior chamber through the pupil into the anterior chamber. This leads to an increase in pressure within the posterior chamber and a forward ballooning of the iris (iris bombé).

Adhesions between the anterior surface of the iris at its periphery and the trabecular

meshwork and cornea are called peripheral anterior synechias. Inflammation of the iris and ciliary body (Fig. 24-34), neovascularization of the iris (called rubeosis iridis—Fig. 24-47), and organization of hemorrhages and exudates in the anterior chamber angle are the most frequent causes for the development of peripheral anterior synechias.

Particulate matter in the aqueous humor often gets caught in the trabecular meshwork as the aqueous humor drains through this structure into the canal of Schlemm and other related outflow channels (Fig. 24-48). Grossly (and clinically), the angle of the anterior chamber may appear to be completely normal, although careful biomicroscopic examination may reveal evidence of the accumulation of cellular debris in the angle. These, then, are cases of secondary open-angle glaucoma in contrast with the angle-closure secondary glaucomas resulting from the formation of peripheral anterior synechias. Many different pathologic processes may lead to the accumulation of cells and debris in the outflow pathways: hemorrhage into the anterior chamber or the vitreous, uveitis, liquefaction and escape of lens protein in hypermature cataracts, tumor cells shed from uveal melanomas or retinoblastomas, pigmented cells from the iris (in pigmentary glaucoma and pseudoexfoliation of the lens capsule), etc.

Finally, the trabecular meshwork and other tissues containing outflow passages may be-

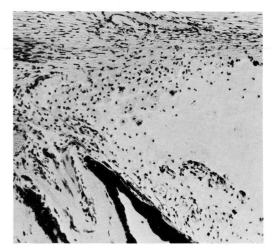

Fig. 24-48 Phacolytic glaucoma. Liquefied lens cortex and macrophages have accumulated in angle of anterior chamber in eye that had hypermature senile cataract. (×150; AFIP 54-25767; from Zimmerman, L. E.: In Maumenee, A. E., and Silverstein, A. M., editors: Immunopathology of uveitis; copyrighted by The Williams & Wilkins Co.)

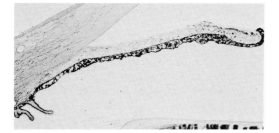

Fig. 24-47 Peripheral anterior synechia resulting in neovascularization of iris in patient with diabetes mellitus (diabetic rubeosis iridis). Thickened and vacuolated pigment epithelium is very characteristic of iris in diabetic patients. (×24; AFIP 55-8505.)

come thickened and their passages narrowed as a result of tissue damage accompanying any of the foregoing conditions that permit cellular debris to become trapped in these tissues. They may become similarly affected after contusions to the eye (Fig. 24-49) or from chemical damage as, for example, in siderosis bulbi resulting from a retained intraocular ferrous foreign body.

Primary glaucoma

Primary glaucoma is of two main types: chronic open-angle (often called chronic simple) glaucoma and acute angle-closure (often called acute congestive) glaucoma.

Chronic open-angle glaucoma appears to be a genetically determined disease that becomes evident with aging. It is characterized by a very insidious onset and slowly progressive rise in intraocular pressure, resulting from an increased resistance to aqueous outflow of undetermined cause and at an undetermined site. Early in the course of the disease, the eyes may seem to be perfectly normal except for the elevated intraocular pressure. Gradually, the increasing rise in intraocular pressure leads to a typically painless loss of vision and eventually to complete blindness.

Acute angle-closure glaucoma is an entirely different form of primary glaucoma occurring most often in individuals who typically have small hyperopic eyes with relatively shallow anterior chambers and very narrow anterior chamber angles. These peculiar anatomic features, which can be readily recognized by ophthalmic examination, predispose the eye to bouts of angle-closure glaucoma, especially as the lens grows larger with aging or with the development of a cataract. Normally in such eyes there is a closer than normal approximation of the iris to the lens so that a relatively small increase in the anteroposterior diameter of the lens may impair the flow of aqueous humor between the lens and the iris at the pupil, even without the formation of synechias (a physiologic block). When this situation develops, the pressure rises in the posterior chamber, the iris becomes bowed forward, and the already very shallow anterior chamber angle becomes obliterated by the apposition of iris to the trabecular meshwork. If this situation is permitted to remain uncorrected by medical or surgical therapy, adhesions between the iris and cornea lead to permanent occlusion of the angle of the anterior chamber. Bouts of angle-closure glaucoma tend to develop very suddenly, and the intraocular pressure rises to very high levels

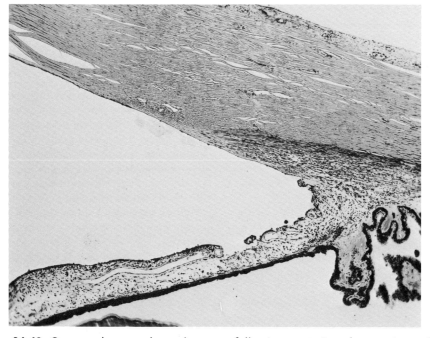

Fig. 24-49 Open-angle secondary glaucoma following contusion damage to outflow pathways. Injury produced tear into face of ciliary body with consequent deepening of angle of chamber. (×50; AFIP 58-5478; from Hogan, M. J., and Zimmerman, L. E.: Ophthalmic pathology, ed. 2, W. B. Saunders Co.)

in a relatively short time. Consequently, the affected eye becomes very red and painful. Often, the patient complains of headache, nausea, and vomiting. The sudden rise in pressure to the very high levels (three to four times normal) produces marked corneal edema and, if unrelieved for more than a few hours, severe damage to the nerve fibers in the optic nerve head. The creation of a new passage for aqueous flow from the posterior chamber into the anterior chamber by peripheral iridectomy or iridotomy overcomes the pupillary block and is therefore a procedure that is used both in the treatment and prevention of attacks of acute angle-closure glaucoma.

Effects

Effects of glaucoma on the eye vary with the type of glaucoma, but common to all is the eventual damage to optic nerve fibers and consequent blindness. When glaucoma develops congenitally or very early in infancy, it typically causes an opacification and enlargement of the cornea (Fig. 24-50) even though the elevation of intraocular pressure may not be very great. Thus, the corneal findings are of great significance in the clinical recognition of congenital and infantile glaucoma.

The optic nerve tolerates marked elevation in intraocular pressure very poorly and, regardless of cause, a sudden rise of pressure into the range of 50 mm to 90 mm Hg, if unrelieved for more than a day or two, may produce such ischemic necrosis of the optic

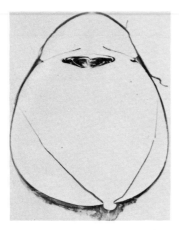

Fig. 24-50 Congenital glaucoma has led to marked enlargement of cornea and deep cupping of optic nerve head. (AFIP 38269; from Friedenwald, J. S., Wilder, H. C., Maumenee, A. E., Sanders, T. E., Keyes, J. E., Hogan, M. J., Owens, W. C., and Owens, E. U.: Ophthalmic pathology, W. B. Saunders Co.)

nerve head that all vision is destroyed. Corneal edema, but without enlargement of the cornea, is a characteristic feature of acute glaucoma, regardless of its specific cause. Marked elevations in intraocular pressure also often produce areas of ischemic necrosis in the iris and foci of opacification in the superficial lens cortex.

On the other hand, the eye often tolerates small or moderate rises of pressure remarkably well, particularly when the elevation in pressure has developed very slowly, as it does in the chronic forms of primary and secondary glaucomas. Eventually, however, chronic glaucoma leads to an atrophy of optic nerve fibers, usually, however, sparing those from the macula until very late, so that the patient who has lost most of his peripheral field of vision may still retain good visual acuity. This fact accounts for the not unusual experience that a patient with chronic glaucoma may suffer optic nerve damage and be unaware of his visual loss as long as his macular function remains reasonably good. This is why a routine check of intraocular pressure and of the peripheral field of vision is recommended as part of the annual physical examination of all adults.

After glaucoma has produced atrophy of the optic nerve fibers, the physiologic cup that is normally observable in the optic nerve head gradually becomes larger and deeper. The elevated intraocular pressure tends to bow the lamina cribrosa backward, accentuating the enlargement of the cup. This is called glaucomatous cupping (Fig. 24-50). It is a late complication of glaucoma.

Other late complications include atrophy of all ocular tissues and chronic corneal edema leading to bullous keratopathy. Atrophy of the ciliary body eventually will lead to a diminution of aqueous formation, compensating somewhat for the impaired outflow of aqueous humor. Although this tends to relieve the elevated intraocular pressure, it is not without sequelae, for the normal production and circulation of aqueous humor are necessary for the nutrition of such avascular tissues as the lens, vitreous, and cornea. Advanced glaucoma, therefore, often is complicated by cataract formation, severe degenerative keratopathy, and alterations in the vitreous body.

CATARACT

Opacification of the lens, regardless of its cause, is termed a cataract. Some cataracts are present at birth. These congenital cataracts may be genetically determined, the result of rubella acquired in utero, or associated with other malformations produced by chromosomal abnormalities (e.g., 13-15 trisomy) or they may be sporadic and idiopathic. Opacification of the lens acquired after birth may be the result of ocular trauma (traumatic cataracts), a complication of some other primary ocular or systemic disease such as uveitis, malignant melanoma of the uvea, or diabetes mellitus (complicating cataracts), a consequence of chemical intoxication as occurred when dinitrophenol was used for weight reduction and MER-29 was employed for the reduction of blood cholesterol levels, or simply a manifestation of aging (senile cataracts).

The lens is one of the most unusual tissues of the body. Derived from the surface ectoderm, it is a mass of modified epithelial cells that become sequestered in the posterior chamber very early in embryologic development. Devoid of stroma and containing no blood supply, the lens depends upon the circulating aqueous humor for its nutrition, oxygenation, and removal of catabolites. It is also a unique epithelial tissue in that it has no way of desquamating its oldest cells. These merely get compressed into the central (nuclear) part of the lens as new lenticular cells (cortical fibers, as they are generally called) are formed at the equator from the epithelial layer. The mystery, therefore, is not why the lens sometimes becomes opaque but rather how it generally remains optically clear for so many years in most individuals.

Microscopically, the changes observed in cataractous lenses are not specifically related to the cause of the cataract. Very minimal variations in the size, shape, and water content of cortical cells may cause opacification readily detectable by the ophthalmologist on slit-lamp examination, yet the pathologist may find it impossible to be certain whether he sees any abnormalities. With more advanced cortical degeneration, the integrity of the cells breaks down. Fragmentation and dissolution of the tissue become very obvious (Fig. 24-51).

With the breakdown of lens protein and because of associated alterations in the lens epithelium, movement of water into the lens may become increased and the lens swells (intumescent cataract), leading to an increase mainly in its anteroposterior diameter. This is one factor that may produce a block of aqueous flow through the pupil and provoke an attack of acute congestive glaucoma.

With more complete breakdown of lens protein, total liquefaction of the cortex may be observed. In such cases, the hard yellowish nucleus may be observed to float about within the milky liquefied cortex. This type of hypermature senile cataract is called a morgagnian cataract (Fig. 24-52). Often, the lens epithelium becomes completely necrotic in these morgagnian cataracts, and as the lens protein

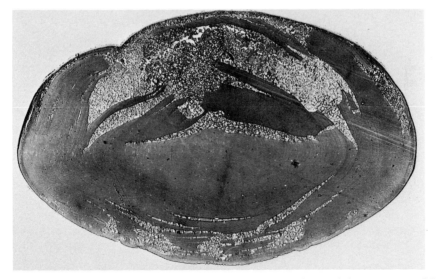

Fig. 24-51 Mature cortical and nuclear cataract. There is advanced degeneration of lens fibers which are markedly fragmented. (×27; AFIP 66872; from DeCoursey, E., and Ash, J. E.: Atlas of ophthalmic pathology, American Academy of Ophthalmology and Otolaryngology.)

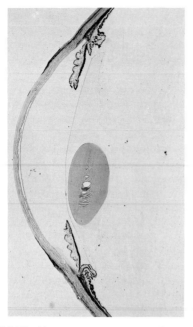

Fig. 24-52 Hypermature cataract (morgagnian type). Lens cortex has become completely liquefied and dense nuclear portion has settled downward (vertical plane of section). (×7; AFIP 54-25766; from Flocks, M., Littwin, C. S., and Zimmerman, L. E.: Arch. Ophthal. [Chicago] **54**:37-45, 1955.)

breaks down into smaller molecules, the latter diffuse out through the lens capsule, carrying water along. This leads to a shrinkage of the lens, and in advanced states only the nucleus remains within the capsule. Only rarely does the entire lens substance become absorbed in this fashion, but it accounts for some of the rare spontaneous cures of blindness due to cataract. Posterior dislocation of a cataractous lens provides another explanation of such "cures."

The passage of liquefied cortex of a hypermature cataract through the lens capsule into the aqueous humor often provokes an outpouring of macrophages which then phagocytize the escaped lens matter. These macrophages, together with the remaining liquefied lens cortex in the aqueous humor, often obstruct the outflow of aqueous humor in the anterior chamber angle (Fig. 24-48). Typically, this produces a rapidly developing form of open-angle acute congestive glaucoma that is called "phacolytic glaucoma" because pathogenetically it is the result of lysis of the lens (phacolysis). Cataract extraction and irrigation of the anterior chamber may control the glaucoma and restore vision if performed soon after the onset of glaucoma.

Because the lens does become sequestered and encapsulated by a remarkably thick basement membrane (called the lens capsule) so early embryologically, the body's immunologic system for recognizing its own unique proteins never gets the opportunity to recognize those of the lens. Thus, later on in life, when as a result of accidental trauma or a surgical procedure the lens capsule is ruptured, lens protein escapes into the aqueous humor, from which it can be absorbed into the bloodstream. The reticuloendothelial system then gets its first opportunity to encounter these proteins. Autosensitization may ensue, but, fortunately, lens proteins seem to be very weakly antigenic, even when injected in a different species, and it is believed that some other factor acting as an adjuvant is necessary to permit significant autosensitization to develop. There is one condition believed to be at least partially dependent on autosensitization to lens protein for its occurrence—*phacoanaphylaxis*. This is almost always a complication of some injury that ruptures the lens capsule. In the days when extracapsular cataract extraction was the standard operation for senile cataracts, phacoanaphylactic endophthalmitis was relatively more important because if the operation performed on the first eye sensitized the patient, then when the operation was subsequently performed on the second eye, the stage was set for a severe immunopathologic reaction when the aqueous became flooded with antigen released from the lens.

The histopathologic picture of phacoanaphylactic endophthalmitis is very characteristic (Fig. 24-53). An intense inflammatory reaction is seen centered about the lens. In those cases that follow a penetrating wound, one sees a massive invasion of the lens by inflammatory cells at the site where the lens capsule is ruptured. A typically granulomatous reaction develops in the lens. Necrotic lens tissue infiltrated by polymorphonuclear leukocytes becomes surrounded by a zone of epithelioid cells and giant cells about which there develops an even broader zone of granulation tissue heavily infiltrated by lymphocytes and plasma cells. The iris becomes firmly adherent to the inflammatory mass that surrounds the lens and it, too, is diffusely infiltrated by lymphocytes and plasma cells. The inflammatory reaction spreads into the vitreous and, as a result, retinal detachment often complicates the situation.

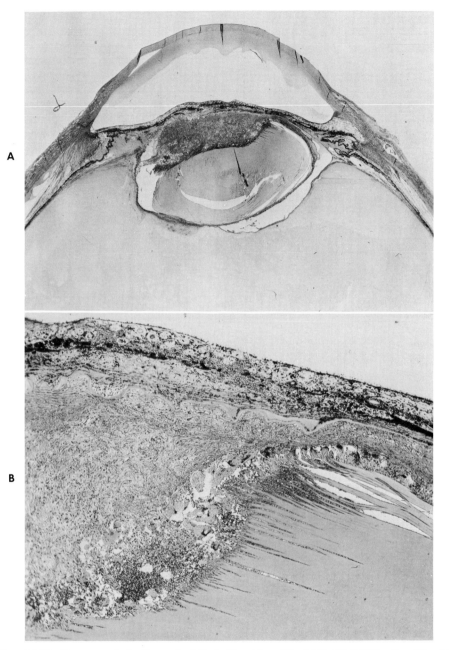

Fig. 24-53 Phacoanaphylactic endophthalmitis. (**A,** ×10; AFIP 55-22260; **B,** ×53; AFIP 55-22261; from Zimmerman, L. E.: In Ackerman, L. V. [in collaboration with Butcher, H. R., Jr.]: Surgical pathology, The C. V. Mosby Co.)

DISLOCATION OF LENS

The lens is held in place by the bundles of collagenous filaments passing from the ciliary epithelium to the lens capsule (the zonular ligament). These zonular fibers may be ruptured as a result of trauma, and the lens may lose all or a part of its support. If only a part of the zonular ligament is ruptured, the lens becomes only partially dis-

located or subluxated to one side. When all of the support has been lost, the lens may become completely dislocated posteriorly or anteriorly. When dislocated into the anterior chamber, there is often obstruction to aqueous outflow and an acute secondary glaucoma develops. Thus, surgical removal is usually undertaken when anterior dislocation is observed. If the lens capsule has not been

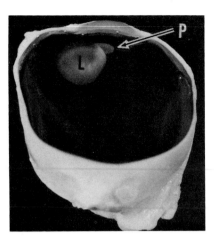

Fig. 24-54 Spontaneous subluxation of lens, **L,** in homocystinuria. Note that lens is dislocated to left of its normal position behind pupil, **P.** (AFIP 64-3737.)

broken, the eye usually tolerates posterior dislocation quite well. If the lens is ruptured, however, phacoanaphylactic endophthalmitis may develop. Dislocated lenses usually become cataractous and also may give rise to a phacolytic glaucoma.

Dislocation or subluxation of the lens also may develop spontaneously as a result of damage to the zonular ligament in certain ocular or systemic diseases. Two notorious examples are Marfan's syndrome and homocystinuria (Fig. 24-54). Patients with late syphilis also are thought to be prone to develop spontaneous dislocation of the lens.

INTRAOCULAR NEOPLASMS

There are only two important primary intraocular malignant neoplasms, malignant melanoma of the uvea and retinoblastoma. All others are so rare that no mention of them need be made here. In addition, there is the problem of metastatic tumors that must be considered.

Malignant melanoma

Malignant melanoma of the uvea is observed almost exclusively in white adults. Because of its selective occurrence in whites, it rarely is encountered in Africa, the Orient, and in those parts of Central and South America where there has been a large degree of intermarriage among Indians, blacks, and whites. In North America and in Europe, it is the most common of all intraocular tumors (primary or secondary, benign or malignant).

Uveal melanomas usually are slow growing and late in metastasizing. They have a much better prognosis than malignant melanoma of the skin (60% ten-year survival after enucleation of the eye). Two main cell types are observed: spindle and epithelioid (Fig. 24-55). Melanomas composed entirely of slender spindle-shaped cells with thin, elongated nuclei and no nucleoli (spindle cell A type) have the most favorable prognosis (85% ten-year survival). Those composed of larger, plumper spindle-shaped cells containing more ovoid nuclei with nucleoli (spindle cell B type) have a slightly less favorable prognosis (80% ten-year survival). Those composed entirely of large, pleomorphic cells with hyperchromatic nuclei and large, prominent nucleoli (epithelioid cells) carry the worst prognosis (35% ten-year survival). When there is a mixture of spindle and epithelioid cells, the tumors are said to be of the "mixed cell type." The ten-year survival for this group is 45%. Regardless of cell type, uveal melanomas show great variations in the production of melanin. Some are totally devoid of pigment, whereas others are jet black, and between these extremes are all shades of gray.

Melanomas arising in the choroid and ciliary body generally attain a fairly large size (10 mm to 20 mm in diameter) before they are detected, whereas those arising in the iris, where they can be seen by the patient and his family, are usually very much smaller. For this reason and because they are more accessible for surgical excision, iris tumors rarely have to be treated by enucleation of the eye, which operation must be done for most melanomas of the choroid and ciliary body. Since most iris tumors are not only small but also are frequently composed of the most favorable cell type (spindle cell A), which grows in a compact cohesive manner, they generally can be removed by iridectomy or iridocyclectomy without tumor cells being disseminated throughout the anterior chamber. Thus, recurrence is usually not a problem, and metastasis is very rare. The overall mortality rate from iris melanomas is less than 5%.

Melanomas of the choroid and ciliary body typically grow inward, toward the vitreous body, producing first an elevation and then a detachment of the retina. This causes visual disturbance for which the patient seeks ophthalmologic examination. Other complications of uveal melanomas include intraocular hemorrhage, inflammation (especially when the tumor develops areas of necrosis), cataract formation, and glaucoma. Thus, the possibility

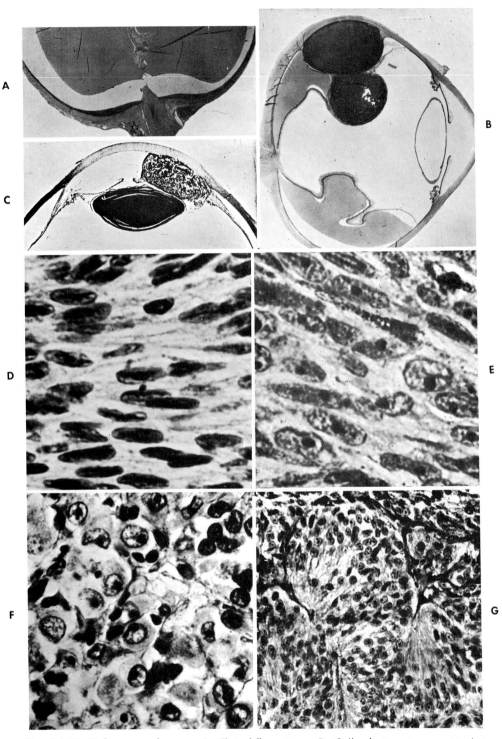

Fig. 24-55 Melanoma of uvea. **A,** Flat diffuse type. **B,** Collar-button type, extension through break in Bruch's membrane. **C,** Tumor in ciliary body and iris. **D** to **F,** Callender cell types. **D,** Spindle cell A. **E,** Spindle cell B. **F,** Epithelioid cell. **G,** Fascicular type. (AFIP; **A, B, D, E,** and **G,** from DeCoursey, E., and Ash, J. E.: Atlas of ophthalmic pathology, American Academy of Ophthalmology and Otolaryngology.)

of an intraocular melanoma often must be considered in the differential diagnosis of many ocular disorders.

Retinoblastoma

Retinoblastoma, in sharp contrast with uveal melanomas, is observed almost exclusively in very young children, and no racial group is spared. For this reason, it is encountered in all parts of the world. Often, if not always, it is present at birth, although it may take two to three years or more before it is discovered. Some cases are genetically determined, and in these patients there is a very high incidence of multicentricity and bilaterality. Survivors of bilateral retinoblastoma are very likely to transmit the disease to about one-half of their progeny. Sporadic unilateral retinoblastomas are believed to be the result of a somatic mutation, in which case the survivor would not be capable of transmitting the disease to his offspring. Unfortunately, however, one can never be certain that a unilateral sporadic retinoblastoma appearing in a family in which there is no known history of retinoblastoma will not turn out to be the result of a genetic mutation that has expressed itself in only one eye.

Retinoblastoma, as the name implies, is a retinal neoplasm composed of anaplastic, poorly differentiated retinal cells (Fig. 24-56). These cells tend to grow in all directions—into the vitreous, beneath the retina, and along the retina. By each of these routes the tumor tends to invade the optic nerve head, through which it spreads back into the optic nerve and meninges. A fatal outcome often is attributable to intracranial spread via the optic nerve and subarachnoid fluid. The tumor also has the capability for vascular invasion and hematogenous dissemination. It also can spread back into the orbit, and in neglected cases the child may present with a large fungating mass that fills the orbit (Fig. 24-57). Before the turn of the century, this was the typical picture of retinoblastoma. Fortunately, today—at least in our more highly civilized countries, where the public as

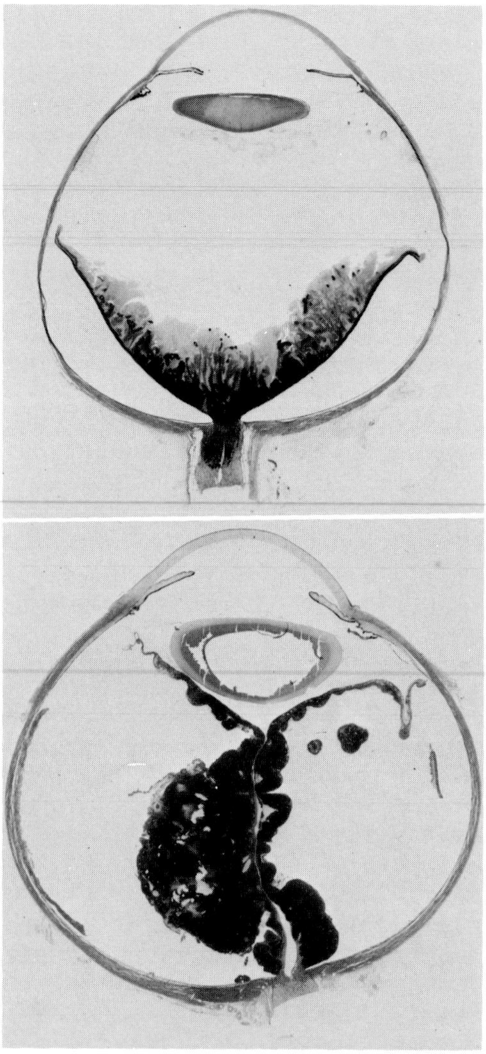

Fig. 24-56 Retinoblastoma. **A,** Endophytic pattern of growth with invasion of optic nerve. **B,** Exophytic growth with total detachment of retina. (**A,** AFIP 211405; **B,** AFIP 183030; from Friedenwald, J. S., Wilder, H. C., Maumenee, A. E., Sanders, T. E., Keyes, J. E., Hogan, M. J., Owens, W. C., and Owens, E. U.: Ophthalmic pathology, W. B. Saunders Co.)

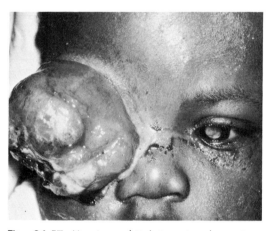

Fig. 24-57 Massive orbital invasion by retinoblastoma of right eye. Left eye also affected, as evident from leukokoria. (Courtesy Dr. V. T. Curtin; from Zimmerman, L. E.: Med. Annual D.C. **38:**366-374, 1969.)

well as physicians are better educated—such advanced stages rarely are seen.

The great majority of cases are detected when a parent first notices something peculiar about the child's eye. Usually, this is a change in the appearance of the normally jet black pupil. The white mass in the retina tends to reflect light rays entering the eye, producing a white, yellow, or grayish discoloration of the pupil (a sign called leukokoria—Fig. 24-57). Other pathologic processes in the retina and/or vitreous body may produce similar pupillary changes and thus lead to enucleation in the mistaken belief that the eye contains a malignant neoplasm. Congenital malformations, endophthalmitis produced by wandering larvae of *Toxocara canis,* exudative retinopathies (e.g., Coats' disease), traumatic or idiopathic retinal detachment, and the retinopathy of prematurity are some of the more important causes for leukokoria, leading to confusion with retinoblastoma. Besides leukokoria, other manifestations of retinoblastoma include strabismus, inflammation, glaucoma, and intraocular hemorrhage.

Metastatic tumors

Metastatic tumors of many different types have been encountered in the eye, but metastasis from two sources are notorious. In women, metastasis from carcinoma of the breast is by far more frequent than from all other sources combined. Usually, metastasis to the eye occurs after mastectomy has been performed, although rarely the ocular tumor may be the initial clinical manifestation. If the ocular metastasis occurs long after mastectomy at a time when the patient appears to be in good general health, the possibility of metastatic carcinoma may not be suspected by either the patient or ophthalmologist. In such cases, enucleation may be performed in the mistaken belief that the eye contains a malignant melanoma.

In men, bronchogenic carcinoma is the most frequent source of metastasis to the eye. This tumor is more likely than breast cancer to remain undetected until after enucleation has been carried out because of a suspected uveal melanoma. Thus, in the differential diagnosis of malignant melanoma of the uvea, one must always be alert to the possibility of metastatic carcinoma, and appropriate studies should be undertaken before enucleation is recommended. Some ophthalmologists still seem to want to rush a patient suspected of having an intraocular melanoma to surgery

for enucleation, afraid that any delay might jeopardize the patient's chances for a cure. Melanomas, however, are slow growing and generally have been present for a very long time before they have been discovered, so that taking the additional time for a thorough clinical, laboratory, and radiologic work-up would be time well spent.

Metastatic tumors in the eye almost always selectively involve the uvea rather than the retina, optic nerve, or any other tissue. The choroid is by far the part of the uvea most frequently involved (Fig. 24-58), and the iris is the least frequently affected. In the iris, however, the metastatic carcinoma very characteristically produces clinical signs and symptoms of a uveitis, whereas the metastatic tumor in the choroid rarely is accompanied by such manifestations. The reason for this difference is unknown.

Benign tumors

Benign tumors include nevi of the uveal tract, melanocytomas of the optic disc, hemangiomas of the choroid, and other hamartomatous lesions of the phakomatoses (Sturge-Weber syndrome, Lindau-von Hippel disease, Recklinghausen's disease, and Bourneville's disease). It should be noted that the various ocular lesions typical of the phakomatoses also may be observed as isolated lesions in individuals who seem to have no systemic manifestations.

In the Sturge-Weber syndrome, there is a

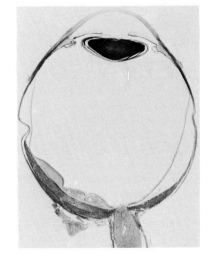

Fig. 24-58 Metastatic carcinoma in choroid from breast cancer. (AFIP 37637; from DeCoursey, E., and Ash, J. E.: Atlas of ophthalmic pathology, American Academy of Ophthalmology and Otolaryngology.)

cavernous hemangioma of the choroid (Fig. 24-59) and often an ipsilateral congenital glaucoma associated with an extensive cavernous hemangioma (nevus flammeus) of the face, involving the eyelids. In Lindau-von Hippel disease, the characteristic ocular lesion is angiomatosis retinae (Fig. 24-60). Huge, tortuous vessels course to a vascular tumor of the retina that microscopically resembles closely a hemangiopericytoma. In Reckling-hausen's neurofibromatosis, the eye may show any one or more of many different lesions,

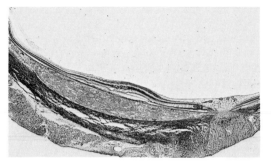

Fig. 24-59 Cavernous hemangioma of choroid. (×8; AFIP 171647-26081; from Friedenwald, J. S., Wilder, H. C., Maumenee, A. E., Sanders, T. E., Keyes, J. E., Hogan, M. J., Owens, W. C., and Owens, E. U.: Ophthalmic pathology, W. B. Saunders Co.)

including discrete nevi and/or neurofibromas, diffuse neurofibromatous thickening of the uvea with or without hyperpigmentation, plexiform neurofibromas of the ciliary nerves, juvenile astrocytoma of the optic nerve, congenital glaucoma, congenital enlargement of the globe, atrophia bulbi, etc. In Bourne-ville's disease, the characteristic lesion is the astrocytic hamartoma that involves the optic nerve head or the retina, or both. These benign astrocytic tumors tend to undergo calcification, giving rise to the giant drusen that are seen most frequently protruding from the nerve head.

RETINAL DISEASES

Retinal diseases are extremely important not only because the retina is the single most important ocular tissue but also because it often is affected by a very broad spectrum of systemic as well as ocular disease processes, far too many to be considered here. Only a few of the most important will be considered.

Retinopathy of prematurity

Retinopathy of prematurity, also called retrolental fibroplasia, is a curious condition that first made its appearance early in the 1940's when modern incubators fed by pure

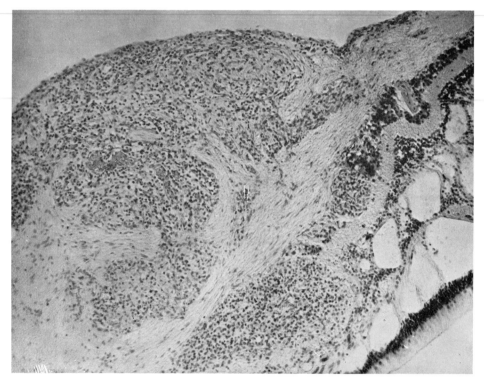

Fig. 24-60 Angiomatosis retinae.

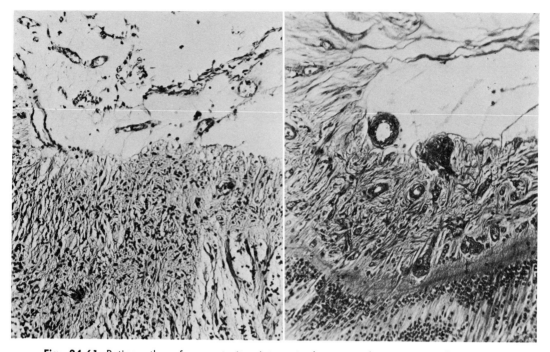

Fig. 24-61 Retinopathy of prematurity. Intraretinal neovascularization can be seen on right and proliferation of vessels in vitreous on left. (From Friedenwald, J. S., Owens, W. C., and Owens, E. U.: Trans. Amer. Ophthal. Soc. **49:**207-234, 1951.)

oxygen became available for the routine treatment of premature babies. Soon the disease became a leading cause of blindness in children. After much intensive research, it was shown that the incompletely vascularized retina of the premature baby is exquisitely sensitive to hyperoxia. The proliferating retinal capillaries under the influence of continuous high-oxygen tension not only cease their normal growth to the retinal periphery but also may become permanently obliterated. After oxygen therapy is discontinued, abnormal vasoproliferative changes occur proximal to the points where the retinal vessels are permanently obliterated. These proliferating new vessels often penetrate the internal limiting membrane of the retina and grow into the vitreous (Fig. 24-61). There they leak fluid and blood which may subsequently lead to organization, produce traction on the retina, and cause retinal detachment and blindness. After the cause of this retinopathy of premature babies was discovered, appropriate control measures were instituted, and the disease virtually disappeared.

Diabetic retinopathy

Diabetic retinopathy is the second leading cause of new adult blindness in the United States, and it is one of the most dreaded of all the vascular complications that await the diabetic patient. It is particularly among those who developed diabetes in childhood and who have had the disease for fifteen to twenty years that retinopathy is most frequently observed and is most disabling, just when the patient is in what should be his most productive years. The duration of diabetes rather than the adequacy of its control seems to be the most significant pathogenetic factor, for diabetic retinopathy was not a significant problem in the preinsulin era when young diabetic patients rarely survived more than a few years.

The selective retinal capillary microangiopathy of diabetes seems to begin with a degeneration of the mural cells or pericytes, but in patchy areas one also observes capillaries that appear to be totally ischemic, showing a loss of endothelial cells as well as pericytes (Fig. 24-62). Immediately adjacent to these ischemic foci are focal saclike aneurysmal dilatations of the capillaries. Most of these microaneurysms are too small to be visible by ordinary ophthalmoscopy, but some of the larger ones do become visible, especially when associated with a diapedesis of erythrocytes, producing the small dot hemorrhages.

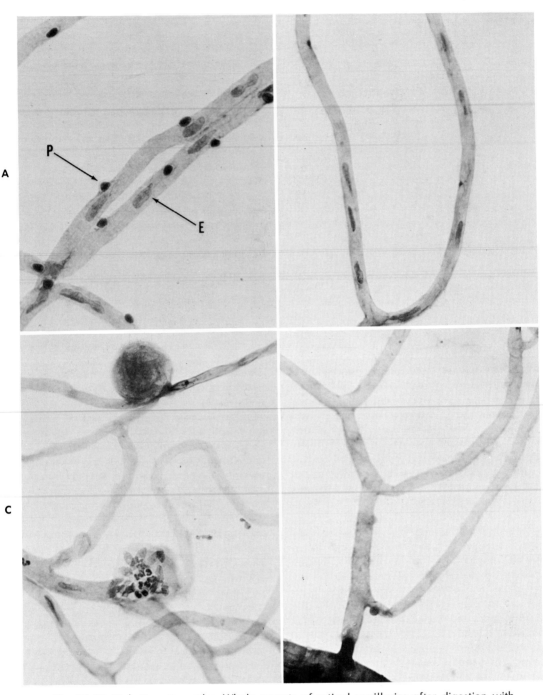

Fig. 24-62 Diabetic retinopathy. Whole mounts of retinal capillaries after digestion with trypsin. **A,** Nuclei of endothelial cells, **E,** and of pericytes or mural cells, **P,** are normally observed in about 1:1 ratio. **B,** Selective loss of mural pericytes, one of earliest changes in diabetes. **C,** Saccular microaneurysms characteristic of diabetic retinopathy. One in upper part of field is hyalinized, whereas one in lower part shows endothelial proliferation and adherent leukocytes. **D,** Many of ischemic vessels showing loss of all nuclei in advanced diabetic retinopathy. (**A,** AFIP 64-7004; **B,** AFIP 64-7010; **C,** AFIP 64-7009; **D,** AFIP 64-7008.)

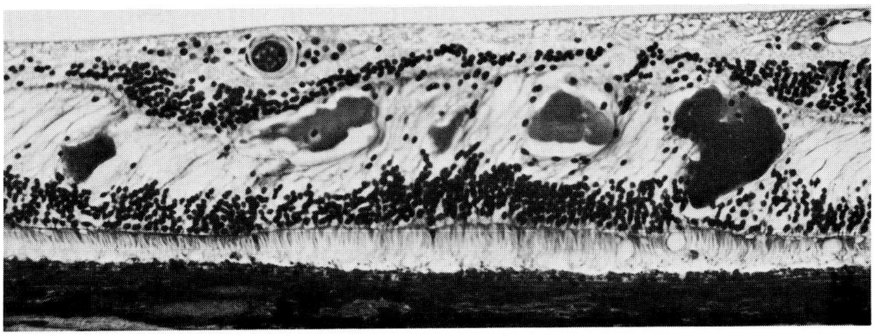

Fig. 24-63 Diabetic retinopathy. Ischemic degeneration of inner layers and exudates in outer plexiform layer. (×205; AFIP 84800; from Friedenwald, J. S., Wilder, H. C., Maumenee, A. E., Sanders, T. E., Keyes, J. E., Hogan, M. J., Owens, W. C., and Owens, E. U.: Ophthalmic pathology, W. B. Saunders Co.)

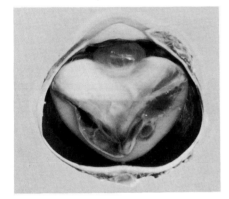

Fig. 24-64 Diabetic retinopathy has led to retinitis proliferans, intravitreal hemorrhage, and retinal detachment. (AFIP 57-5060.)

At about the same time that microaneurysms and dot hemorrhages make their appearance, "soft exudates" in the superficial layers of the retina also are seen. These are believed to be microinfarcts involving the nerve fiber layer, similar to those responsible for the cotton wool spots of hypertensive retinopathy (see below). Venous dilatation and irregularity are typically present. The microangiopathy includes a loss of permeability with the formation of hard exudates in the deeper layers of the retina (Fig. 24-63). These are rich in proteins and lipids and have a yellowish appearance. Histiocytes swollen with ingested lipids often are present in large numbers in these deeply situated exudates.

Midway in the course of diabetic retinopathy, new capillaries proliferate, often at the optic disc or along one of the major veins. These erupt through the internal limiting membrane of the retina into the vitreous. These also leak, and an accumulation of connective tissue develops along the preretinal vessels. Hemorrhage from these intravitreal

vessels and contraction of connective tissue eventually lead to traction on the retina and its detachment (Fig. 24-64).

It is clear, therefore, that visual loss from diabetic retinopathy may be ascribed to a number of pathologic processes—retinal ischemia, formation of hemorrhages and exudation in the retina, presence of microinfarcts, proliferation of new vessels and connective tissue on the retinal surface, hemorrhages into the vitreous, and retinal detachment.

Hypertensive retinopathy

Hypertensive retinopathy is observed most frequently and in its most severe forms in the acutely progressive type of malignant hypertension. There is a generalized narrowing of retinal arterioles leading to retinal ischemia. Microinfarcts are commonly present. Clinically, these appear as soft, fluffy, superficial exudates (called cotton wool spots) protruding forward from the retina. Microscopically, however, these are not exudates but focal areas of ischemic infarction, typically involving only the nerve fiber and ganglion cell layers of the retina (Fig. 24-65). The lesion is associated with edematous swelling and a disappearance of nuclei. Within the swollen nerve fiber layer one sees peculiar cell-like structures (cytoid bodies), which are tremendously swollen necrotic axons (end bulbs of Cajal). In hypertensive retinopathy, flame-shaped superficial hemorrhages and watery exudates in the deeper retinal layers frequently are present. Often, the retina is diffusely edematous, and there may be marked papilledema. The accumulation of protein-rich exudate and lipid-laden macrophages in the outer plexiform layer of the macula leads to the formation of a series of linear hard exudates radiating out from the foveal area

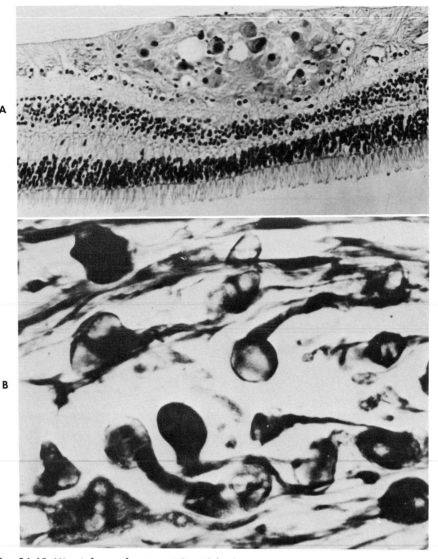

Fig. 24-65 Microinfarct of retina. "Cytoid bodies" are axonal enlargements in infarcted nerve fiber layer. **A,** Paraffin section. **B,** Frozen section stained by Hortega's method. (**A,** ×210; AFIP 69808; from Friedenwald, J. S., Wilder, H. C., Maumenee, A. E., Sanders, T. E., Keyes, J. E., Hogan, M. J., Owens, W. C., and Owens, E. U.: Ophthalmic pathology, W. B. Saunders Co.; **B,** from Wolter, J. R.: Amer. J. Ophthal. **48:**473-485, 1959.)

(macular star figure). Retinal changes similar to those observed in malignant hypertension also may be observed in other conditions such as eclampsia, periarteritis nodosa, lupus erythematosus, etc.

Vascular occlusive disease

Vascular occlusive disease may affect either the arterial or the venous side and may develop suddenly or slowly. Sudden total occlusion of the central retinal artery is usually the result of atherosclerosis leading to hemorrhage and/or thrombosis in the vicinity of a subintimal plaque that has already markedly narrowed the lumen. This vascular accident produces complete ischemic infarction of those retinal layers that are totally dependent on the central retinal artery, and the patient experiences a sudden loss of vision (Fig. 24-66).

The same clinical and histopathologic picture may be observed when an embolus obstructs the central retinal artery. Endocardial vegetations, mural thrombi after myocardial infarction, and the cardiac myxoma are sources of large emboli. Smaller emboli from atherosclerotic plaques in the great vessels of the neck more frequently lodge in branches of

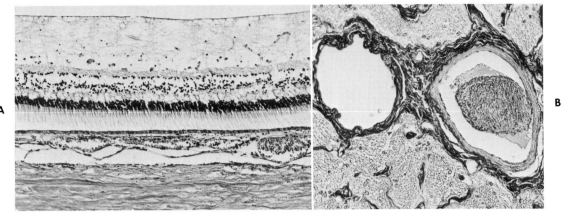

Fig. 24-66 Acute ischemic infarction of retina, **A,** produced by embolus in central retinal artery, **B,** from mural thrombus in left ventricle of patient who had sustained myocardial infarction. (AFIP 951983; **B,** from Zimmerman, L. E.: Arch. Ophthal. [Chicago] **73:**822-826, 1965.)

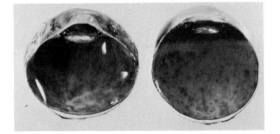

Fig. 24-67 Hemorrhagic infarction of retina. (AFIP 64-2232.)

the central retinal artery, producing smaller areas of retinal infarction. Microscopically, the retinal infarct is characterized by an early edematous thickening of the inner half of the retina and a dissolution of nuclei in the ganglion cell and inner nuclear layers. Clinically, the edematous retina appears gray, and only in the fovea where the inner layers of the retina are normally absent does the choroidal circulation give the fundus its normal pink hue. Later on, as the edema subsides, the retina regains its transparency, and microscopically one sees only a marked thinning of the inner retinal layers from which the nerve fibers, ganglion cells, and almost all of the cells in the inner nuclear layer have disappeared.

Thrombosis of the central retinal vein leads to hemorrhagic infarction of the entire retina (Fig. 24-67). All of the retinal veins and capillaries are engorged. Rupture of the latter leads to bleeding into all retinal layers. Bleeding into the vitreous or beneath the retina may also be observed. An important complication of thrombosis of the central retinal vein is hemorrhagic glaucoma, which typically makes

its appearance after about three months. This is the result of a proliferation of capillaries in the anterior chamber angle from the root of the iris and face of the ciliary body, obstructing the outflow of aqueous humor and leading to hemorrhage into the anterior chamber. Similar anterior segment changes may be observed after occlusion of the central retinal artery, but much less frequently. They also may be seen with other retinopathies, especially diabetic retinopathy, and it is suspected that the cause is a vasostimulatory factor liberated from the hypoxic retina.

Slowly progressive vascular insufficiency most often affects not just the retinal circulation but also the uveal blood supply, because it is observed mainly in those occlusive vascular diseases that affect the aortic arch and/or the great vessels of the head and neck (e.g., atherosclerosis of the carotid arteries, cranial arteritis, pulseless disease, etc.).

Retinal detachment

Retinal detachment is a separation of the sensory retina from its normally tenuous juxtaposition to the retinal pigment epithelium. The tips of the rods and cones normally are interdigitated with villous projections from the retinal pigment epithelium, but they are not attached by any specialized structures such as desmosomes. Thus, these two tissues separate very readily—artifactitiously when a normal eye is opened in the laboratory without prior fixation or in vivo as a result of many pathologic processes. In general, retinal detachment can be expected to occur as a consequence of any of the following three pathogenetic mechanisms: (1) traction on the

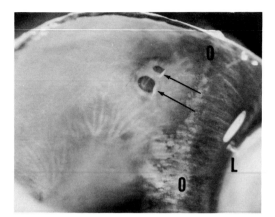

Fig. 24-68 Two holes are present in peripheral retina. Dense white retinal tissue at anterior border of each hole (arrows) is retracted operculum torn away in formation of holes. **O—O**, Ora serrata. **L**, Posterior surface of lens. (AFIP 65-3203-1.)

retina resulting from pathologic processes developing in the vitreous or in the anterior segment of the eye, including abscesses and hemorrhages in the vitreous, complications of intraocular surgery, or accidental trauma, etc., (2) exudation of fluid from the choroid opening up the potential subretinal space, as often occurs when there is an inflammatory process or tumor in the choroid, or (3) passage of liquefied vitreous and/or aqueous humor through a hole or tear in the retina.

It is the latter type that generally is treated by various surgical procedures designed to drain off the subretinal fluid and then to seal off the hole or tear by creating permanent adhesions between the adjacent retina and the pigment epithelium.

Since the outer layers of the retina are dependent upon the choroidal circulation for nutrition and oxygenation, retinal detachment leads to a spatial separation of the retina from the choroid and a consequent ischemic loss of function. The aim of surgical reattachment of the retina is to get the retina back in place before irreparable damage has occurred in the retinal rods and cones.

REFERENCES
General

1 Boniuk, M., editor: Ocular and adnexal tumors; new and controversial aspects, St. Louis, 1964, The C. V. Mosby Co.
2 Hogan, M. J., and Zimmerman, L. E.: Ophthalmic pathology; an atlas and textbook, Philadelphia, 1962, W. B. Saunders Co.
3 New Orleans Academy of Ophthalmology: Industrial and traumatic ophthalmology, St. Louis, 1964, The C. V. Mosby Co.
4 New Orleans Academy of Ophthalmology: Symposium on surgical and medical management of Congenital anomalies of the eye, St. Louis, 1968, The C. V. Mosby Co.
5 Reese, A. B.: Tumors of the eye, ed. 2, New York, 1963, Hoeber Medical Division, Harper & Row, Publishers.
6 Zimmerman, L. E., editor: Int. Ophthal. Clin. 2:237-557, 1962, (tumors of eye and adnexa).

Eyelids

7 Boniuk, M.: In Zimmerman, L. E., editor: Int. Ophthal. Clin. 2:239-317, 1962 (tumors of eyelids).
8 Boniuk, M.: In Boniuk, M., editor: Ocular and adnexal tumors; new and controversial aspects, St. Louis, 1964, The C. V. Mosby Co., pp. 75-100 (differentiation of squamous cell carcinoma from other epithelial tumors of eyelid).
9 Boniuk, M., and Zimmerman, L. E.: Trans. Amer. Acad. Ophthal. Otolaryng. 72:619-642, 1968 (sebaceous carcinomas).

Conjunctiva and cornea

10 Ashton, N., Kirker, J. G., and Lavery, F. S.: Brit. J. Ophthal. 48:405-415, 1964 (ochronosis).
11 Cogan, D. G., and Kuwabara, T.: Arch. Ophthal. (Chicago) 61:553-560, 1959 (arcus senilis).
12 Cogan, D. G., and Kuwabara, T.: Arch. Ophthal. (Chicago) 63:51-57, 1960 (cystinosis).
13 Cogan, D. G., Albright, F., and Bartter, F. C.: Arch. Ophthal. (Chicago) 40:624-638, 1948 (hypercalcemia).
14 Finley, J. K., Berkowitz, D., and Croll, M. N.: Arch. Opthal. (Chicago) 66:211-213, 1961 (arcus senilis).
14a Goldberg, M. F., Maumenee, A. E., and McKusick, V. A.: Arch. Ophthal. (Chicago) 74:516-520, 1965 (mucopolysaccharidoses).
14b McKusick, V. A.: Amer. J. Med. 47:730-747, 1969 (mucopolysaccharidoses).
15 Newell, F. W., and Koistinen, A.: Arch. Ophthal. (Chicago) 53:45-62, 1955 (gargoylism).
16 Reese, A. B.: Amer. J. Ophthal. 61:1272-1277, 1966 (acquired melanosis).
17 Spaeth, G. L., and Frost, P.: Arch. Ophthal. (Chicago) 74:760-769, 1965 (Fabry's disease).
18 Witschel, H., and Mathyl, J.: Klin. Mbl. Augenheilk. 154:599-605, 1969 (Fabry's disease).
19 Zimmerman, L. E.: Arch. Ophthal. (Chicago) 76:307-308, 1966 (acquired melanosis).
20 Zimmerman, L. E.: In Rycroft, P. V., editor: Corneo-plastic surgery, London/New York, 1969, Pergamon Press, Inc., pp. 547-555 (cancerous, precancerous, and pseudocancerous lesions).

Orbit

21 Anderson, D. R.: Amer. J. Ophthal. 68:46-57, 1969 (endocrinopathic exophthalmos).
22 Ashton, N., and Morgan, G.: J. Clin. Path. 18:699-714, 1965 (rhabdomyosarcoma).
23 Dutcher, T. F., and Fahey, J. L.: J. Nat. Cancer Inst. 22:887-917, 1959 (macroglobulinemia).
24 Font, R. L., Yanoff, M., and Zimmerman, L. E.:

Amer. J. Clin. Path. **48**:365-376, 1967 (benign lymphoepithelial lesion of lacrimal gland and Sjögren's syndrome).

25 Forrest, A. W.: In Zimmerman, L. E., editor: Int. Ophthal. Clin. **2**:543-553, 1962 (tumors following radiation about eye).

26 Godwin, J. T.: Cancer **5**:1089-1103, 1952 (benign lymphoepithelial lesion of salivary gland).

27 Hoyt, W. F., and Baghdassarian, S. A.: Brit. J. Ophthal. **53**:793-798, 1969 (natural history of optic gliomas).

28 Jones, I. S., Reese, A. B., and Krout, J.: Trans. Amer. Ophthal. Soc. **63**:223-255, 1965 (rhabdomyosarcoma).

29 Kroll, A. J., and Kuwabara, T.: Arch. Ophthal. (Chicago) **76**:244-247, 1966 (endocrinopathic exophthalmos).

30 Little, J. M.: Trans. Amer. Acad. Ophthal. Otolaryng. **71**:875-879, 1967 (macroglobulinemia).

31 Porterfield, J. F., and Zimmerman, L. E.: Virchow Arch. Path. Anat. **335**:329-344, 1962 (rhabdomyosarcoma).

32 Straatsma, B. R., Zimmerman, L. E., and Gass, J. D. M.: Lab. Invest. **11**:963-985, 1962 (phycomycosis).

33 Werner, S. C.: Amer. J. Ophthal. **68**:646-648, 1969 (endocrinopathic exophthalmos).

34 Zimmerman, L. E., Sanders, T. E., and Ackerman, L. V.: In Zimmerman, L. E., editor: Int. Ophthal. Clin. **2**:337-367, 1962 (epithelial tumors of lacrimal gland).

Inflammations

35 Ashton, N.: In Rycroft, P. V., editor: Corneoplastic surgery, London/New York, 1969, Pergamon Press, Inc., pp. 579-591 (Toxocara canis and the eye).

36 Fine, B. S.: Lab. Invest. **11**:1161-1171, 1962 (intraocular mycotic infections).

37 Gould, H. L., and Kaufman, H. E.: Arch. Ophthal. (Chicago) **65**:453-456, 1961 (sarcoidosis).

38 Wilder, H. C.: Trans. Amer. Acad. Ophthal. Otolaryng. **55**:99-109, 1950 (ocular larva migrans).

39 Wilder, H. C.: Arch. Ophthal. (Chicago) **48**: 127-136, 1952 (Toxoplasma chorioretinitis).

40 Zimmerman, L. E.: Lab. Invest. **11**:1151-1160, 1962 (mycotic keratitis).

41 Zimmerman, L. E.: Amer. J. Ophthal. **60**:1011-1035, 1965 (juvenile xanthogranuloma).

42 Zimmerman, L. E., and Maumenee, A. E.: Amer. Rev. Resp. Dis. **84**(Nov. suppl.):38-44, 1961 (sarcoidosis).

Glaucoma; cataract

43 Flocks, M., Littwin, C. S., and Zimmerman, L. E.: Arch. Ophthal. (Chicago) **54**:37-45, 1955 (phacolytic glaucoma).

44 Kolker, A. E., and Hetherington, J., Jr.: Becker-Shaffer's Diagnosis and therapy of the glaucomas, ed. 3, St. Louis, 1970, The C. V. Mosby Co.

45 Wolff, S. M., and Zimmerman, L. E.: Amer. J. Ophthal. **54**:547-563, 1962 (postcontusion glaucoma).

46 Zimmerman, L. E.: In Maumenee, A. E., and Silverstein, A. M., editors: Immunopathology of uveitis, Baltimore, 1964, The Williams & Wilkins Co., pp. 221-242 (lens-induced inflammation in human eyes).

47 Zimmerman, L. E.: In New Orleans Academy of Ophthalmology: Symposium on glaucoma, St. Louis, 1967, The C. V. Mosby Co., pp. 1-30 (histology and pathology of outflow channels).

48 Zimmerman, L. E.: Amer. J. Ophthal. **65**:837-862, 1968 (congenital rubella syndrome).

49 Zimmerman, L. E., and Font, R. L.: J.A.M.A. **196**:684-692, 1966 (congenital malformations).

Retinal diseases

50 Cant, J. S., editor: The William Mackenzie Centenary Symposium on The ocular circulation in health and disease, St. Louis, 1969, The C. V. Mosby Co.

51 Goldberg, M. F., and Fine, S. L., editors: Symposium on The treatment of diabetic retinopathy, Washington, D. C., 1968, U. S. Government Printing Office, U.S.P.H.S. Publ. no. 1890.

52 McPherson, A., editor: New and controversial aspects of retinal detachment, New York, 1968, Hoeber Medical Division, Harper & Row, Publishers.

53 Schepens, C. L., and Regan, C. D. J., editors: Controversial aspects of the management of retinal detachment, 1965, Boston, Little, Brown and Co.

54 Wolter, J. R.: Amer. J. Ophthal. **48**:473-485, 1959 (pathology of cotton wool spot).

55 Wolter, J. R.: Trans. Amer. Ophthal. Soc. **65**: 106-127, 1967 (cytoid bodies).

56 Wolter, J. R., Philips, R. L., and Butler, R. G.: Arch. Ophthal. (Chicago) **60**:49-59, 1958 (macular star figure and hypertensive retinopathy).

57 Zimmerman, L. E.: Discussion of Wolter, J. R.: Trans. Amer. Ophthal. Soc. **65**:106-127, 1967 (historical review of cytoid bodies as axonal enlargements).

Chapter 25

Upper respiratory tract and ear

J. Daniel Wilkes

■ Upper respiratory tract

The anatomic and histologic structure of the upper respiratory tract influences the clinical course and pathology of lesions developing in this area. The thin walls of the paranasal sinuses allow inflammatory processes and neoplastic lesions to spread easily from one section to another by pressure atrophy or invasion. Therefore, a lesion that is innocuous in another site could result in a fatal outcome if located in the sinuses. A tumor originating in the maxillary sinus may remain clinically silent until it has produced pressure symptoms by completely filling the space, and then it is very difficult to eradicate. A small benign papilloma or an inflammatory polypoid swelling may prove fatal if located on a vocal cord but be innocuous on the palate.

Another anatomic factor is the close relationship of mucosa and skin to underlying cartilage, as in the anterior nasal septum, the nasal alae, the epiglottis, and the larynx. This factor is of particular importance when squamous cell or basal cell carcinoma arises in the overlying epithelium, for invasion of underlying cartilage occurs early.

The presence of special structures in an area is another modifying factor: (1) pilosebaceous elements of the nares, (2) mucous glands, abundant vascular tissue (some erectile in type), and the nerve elements of the nasal cavity, (3) mucous glands, abundant lymphoid tissue, and possible embryonal remnants in the nasopharynx and bones of the face, (4) simple squamous mucosa of the oral pharynx and tonsils, and (5) glands of the epiglottis, larynx, and trachea.

Some lesions also are specific to certain locations in these areas—e.g., epithelial papilloma of the nasal turbinates, neurogenous tumor arising from the olfactory placode, hemangioma of the nasal septum, juvenile hemangiofibroma of the nasopharynx, nasal polyps (inflammatory or allergic), and laryngeal nodules.

Modifying factors also include age and sex. Polypoid epithelial lesions of the turbinates in the younger age groups, especially in females, rarely become malignant. The epithelial papilloma (Ewing) of the turbinates occurs most frequently in men and is more likely to undergo malignant deterioration into squamous cell carcinoma. The evaluation of papillomatous lesions is clearly dependent upon the age of the patient. The juvenile papilloma occurring in the larynx may recede at puberty. It rarely, if ever, becomes malignant, so that its location is its menace.

The type of inflammatory and neoplastic lesions that develop in the upper respiratory tract depends upon the structure of the mucosa in the specific regions. The nares are lined by stratified squamous epithelium and have pilosebaceous elements. The alae nasi are covered by stratified squamous epithelium and contain mucous glands. The stratified squamous epithelium also extends onto the cartilaginous septum. Respiratory-type epithelium (i.e., pseudostratified columnar), mucous glands, and erectile blood vessels are present in the nasal cavity of the choana and line the turbinates and paranasal sinuses. Stratified squamous epithelium overlying lymphoid tissue covers the tonsils, adenoids, and pharyngeal bursa of the nasopharynx, and fewer mucous glands are present. The nasopharynx is lined by respiratory-type epithelium overlying lymphoid tissue. The tonsils are covered by stratified squamous epithelium in close approximation to lymphoid tissue. The tonsillar pillars, oral pharynx, epiglottis, and hypopharynx are lined by simple stratified squamous epithelium with few glands being present. The glottis, false cords, lower larynx, and trachea are covered by respiratory epithelium. However, the true vocal cords are

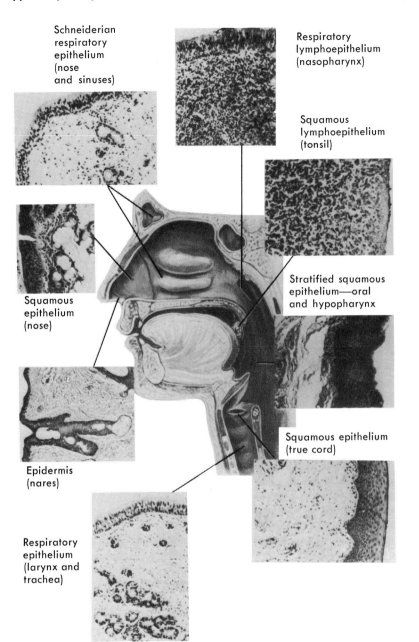

Schneiderian
respiratory
epithelium
(nose
and sinuses)

Respiratory
lymphoepithelium
(nasopharynx)

Squamous
lymphoepithelium
(tonsil)

Squamous
epithelium
(nose)

Stratified squamous
epithelium—oral
and hypopharynx

Epidermis
(nares)

Squamous epithelium
(true cord)

Respiratory
epithelium
(larynx and
trachea)

Fig. 25-1 Hemisection of head showing various types of epithelium that line specific anatomic sites of upper respiratory tract. (From Ash, J. E., Beck, M. R., and Wilkes, J. D.: Tumors of the upper respiratory tract and ear. In Atlas of Tumor pathology, Sect. IV, Fascs. 12 and 13, Washington, D. C., 1964, Armed Forces Institute of Pathology; AFIP 70-1150-3.)

covered by stratified squamous epithelium (Fig. 25-1).

Rare **malformations** occur in the upper respiratory tract, a few examples of which are as follows: **epignathus,** parasitic attachment of a twin embryo to the palate or pharynx; **agnathia,** in which the ears are deformed and usually united below the face due to the mandible being totally absent; **cyclops,** in which both eyes are fused into one and often associated with developmental failure of the frontal nasal process.

NOSE AND PARANASAL SINUSES
Lesions of skin

Lesions of the skin may involve the nose. These include all of the miscellaneous benign conditions as well as some specific inflammatory lesions such as lupus vulgaris and lupus erythematosus. **Rhinophyma** is a sequela of extreme hypertrophy of the sebaceous glands of the alae of the nose. It is characterized by a nodular enlargement of the lower part of the nose that may present as a lobulated mass. The characteristic histologic features are hypertrophy and hyperplasia of the sebaceous glands, dilatation of the ducts, which are filled with keratinaceous material, exaggerated vascularity, a chronic inflammatory infiltrate, and progressive fibrosis.

Inflammation

Acute catarrhal rhinitis. Acute catarrhal rhinitis is characterized by hyperemia of the mucous membrane, edema, and exudation of serous and mucinous fluid. The most common etiologic agents are viruses. The nasal mucous membrane contains abundant mucous glands in the lower and middle turbinates and a network of erectile vascular tissue. In performing the function of cleansing, warming or cooling, and humidifying inspired air, the nasal mucosa is constantly challenged by antigens in the environment. Lymphoid elements readily synthesize immunoglobulins, with a resulting antigen-antibody reaction occurring. Histamine is released along the proteolytic enzymes. With recurrent immunologic responses, allergic rhinitis and sinusitis occur. There is usually a gray mucinous discharge with numerous eosinophils.

Histologically, there is marked edema of the stroma with a cellular infiltrate composed of eosinophils, lymphocytes, and plasma cells. As the condition progresses, squamous metaplasia occurs along with marked fibroblastic formation of the stroma. Eventually, the subepithelial basement membrane shows characteristic thickening and hyalinization.

Atrophic rhinitis (ozena). Atrophic rhinitis affects predominantly the inferior turbinate. It is characterized clinically by marked crusting of the nasal mucosa and a characteristic foul offensive odor. The histologic appearance varies with the stage of the condition. Primarily, there is an abundant lymphocytic and plasma cell exudate with desquamation of epithelium and squamous metaplasia. Atrophy of the mucosal glands and stromal fibrosis occur later. The condition occurs more frequently in young females.

Rhinitis caseosa. A rare disease, rhinitis caseosa is characterized by accumulation in the nose of an extremely offensive cheesy mass accompanied by a seropurulent discharge. It is usually unilateral and may be polypoid but eventually results in marked deformities. The pathologic changes are not specific and merely reflect a chronic inflammatory process, the cause of which is not clear. The disease is comparable to cholesteatoma of the ear.

Sinusitis. Sinusitis usually accompanies acute rhinitis and may be acute or chronic, infectious or allergic. The paranasal sinuses are poorly drained, and the ostia are easily occluded by the resulting edema of an acute infection. The histologic features of sinusitis are identical to those of rhinitis. Due to the peculiar location of the sinuses, otherwise innocuous infections may result in lethal complications. A purulent ethmoiditis may result in orbital cellulitis and intracranial infection. Frontal sinusitis may be complicated by osteomyelitis of the frontal bone because of the peculiarity of the vascular supply. Thrombophlebitis occurs readily, and the infection has access to the surrounding cancellous bone. Retrobulbar neuritis may result from sphenoidal sinusitis.

Syphilis. Primary syphilis rarely occurs at the mucocutaneous border. Chronic coryza and bony destruction with saddlenose deformity are characteristic of congenital syphilis. Tuberculosis and leprosy also may involve the nasal cavity.

Rhinoscleroma. A chronic granulomatous inflammation, rhinoscleroma involves the nose and nasopharynx and may extend into the oral pharynx, larynx, and trachea. Deforming nodular masses eventually result in marked obstruction of the nose, nasal cavity, and nasopharynx. The disease is rare in the United States, although over one hundred cases have been reported. It is seen more frequently in the Mediterranean areas, especially Egypt. A gram-negative diplobacillus, *Klebsiella rhinoscleromatis,* always is found in the lesion, usually in foamy mononuclear cells (Mikulicz's cells). However, the organism also is found in the nasal mucosa and throat of healthy individuals. The disease has never been produced in experimental animals. The etiologic agent is unknown.

The inflammatory process confines itself to soft tissue. Cartilage and bones are not involved. This is an important differential point, because neoplasms will invade all tissues. Rhinoscleroma is characterized by an accumulation of plasma cells and foamy histiocytes and, later, proliferation of fibrous tissue with the formation of dark red nodular masses in the nasal mucosa with subsequent scarring and contraction with resulting deformities. Ulceration is not a constant feature.

Rhinosporidiosis. Rhinosporidiosis is caused by a fungus, *Rhinosporidium seeberi*. It usually presents as a bleeding nasal polyp but may involve the conjunctiva and urethral mucosa. The organism is transmitted chiefly in swimming pools. The polyps have a rough surface in contrast to the smooth appearance of allergic polyps. Among the vascular myxomatous fibrous connective tissue are fungi in all stages of development. The earliest stage is a small round cell, the size of an erythrocyte, containing clear vacuolated protoplasm with a distinct membrane. The spore enlarges to form a mature cyst approximately 200μ in diameter and containing thousands of spores. This entire structure ultimately ruptures, disseminating the spores in and onto the mucosa and into the submucosa (Fig. 25-2).

Phycomycosis. Phycomycosis is a generic term designating a group of infections caused by large nonseptate fungi belonging to the class Phycomycetes. The term mucormycosis also has been used. The Phycomycetes are ubiquitous opportunistic molds that produce airborne spores in tremendous numbers. This class of molds is probably as familiar to the housewife as to the bacteriologist, since the spores find their way into refrigerators and bread boxes as well as into incubators. Because of their saprophytic nature, great cau-

tion must be exercised in evaluating the significance of the recovery of one of these molds from body fluids, biopsies, and exudates.

The syndrome of nasal, paranasal sinus, orbital, and central nervous system disease has been an outstanding feature in one-third of the cases reported since 1943. Almost all of the lethal infections have occurred in severely acidotic patients, most commonly in those with uncontrolled diabetes mellitus. The occurrence of an acute necrotizing inflammatory process in the nasal or orbital area in a debilitated patient demands immediate consideration of phycomycosis. Smears, cultures, and biopsy specimens are necessary for diagnosis.

The histopathologic features are characteristic in that the fungi have a greater affinity for hematoxylin than most other organisms. The large irregular hyphae seem to twist upon their long axis, vary in caliber, and branch dichotomously and laterally in a haphazard fashion. They grow profusely in tissues, invading by direct penetration and extending along tissue planes. There is a remarkable tendency to infiltrate the walls of blood vessels, especially arteries (Fig. 25-3).

Lethal midline granuloma. An aggressive necrotizing inflammatory process, lethal midline granuloma leads to destruction of soft

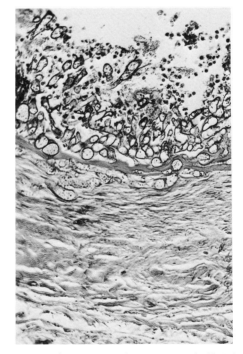

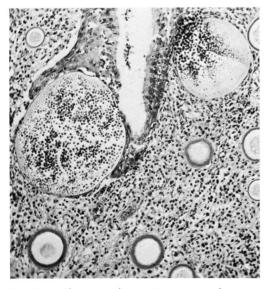

Fig. 25-2 Rhinosporidiosis. Mature cyst has ruptured and small spores are disseminating onto mucosa. (AFIP 70-1150-1.)

Fig. 25-3 Phycomycosis (mucormycosis). Twisting, branching, large nonseptate hyphae have peculiar tendency to invade vessels. (AFIP 58-7380.)

tissues, bones, and cartilage of the nose, paranasal sinuses, soft palate, and pharynx. The inflammatory exudate is pleomorphic, consisting of histiocytes, plasma cells, and giant cells in varying proportions. Vascular lesions are usually secondary.

A prodromal period of months to years is characterized by nasal congestion with obstruction and rhinorrhea. In the active stage, there is progressively spreading inflammation and ulceration beginning at the nose and extending to involve other structures of the midface. The disease slowly progresses, with death resulting from hemorrhage, meningitis, or inanition. Abortive self-limited forms have been reported.

Reticulum cell sarcoma and lymphoblastic lymphoma may present clinically as lethal midline granuloma. Sufficient material must be examined to recognize the malignant cellular characteristic of the tumors in contrast to the pleomorphic infiltrate of lethal midline granuloma.

Wegener's granulomatosis. A syndrome of unknown etiology, Wegener's granulomatosis is characterized by necrotizing granulomatous lesions, generalized arteritis, and glomerular nephritis. The pathologic changes are similar to those present in various hypersensitivity diseases. The disorder generally is believed to be a disease involving the immune mechanisms (see also p. 926).

The patient may present with intractable rhinitis, sinusitis, otitis, or ocular symptoms. Nodular or diffuse infiltration with cavitation is present in both lungs. Necrotizing granulomatous lesions of the upper and lower respiratory tract, necrotizing vasculitis involving arteries and veins, and glomerulitis characterized by necrosis and thrombosis of loops of the capillary tuft are seen. The granulomatous reaction is an immunologic response to an unknown antigen. The disease is more active and fulminant than lethal midline granuloma. Immunosuppressive chemotherapy has produced effective prolonged remissions.[20a]

Relapsing polychondritis. Relapsing polychondritis most frequently involves the cartilages of the ear, but the nasal cartilage, larynx, trachea, joints, and sclera of the eye also are involved. The disease is basically a metabolic disorder of chondromucin in cartilaginous structures and has been associated with immunologic processes, including rheumatoid arthritis, systemic lupus erythematosus, and Hashimoto's thyroiditis.

Polyps

Nasal polyps are most often the result of allergic rhinosinusitis. The allergic polyp is clinically the more common. The inflammatory polyp is associated with trauma, chemical irritation, and local bacterial infection. **Choanal polyp** is a clinical entity. The term is applied to either the inflammatory or al-

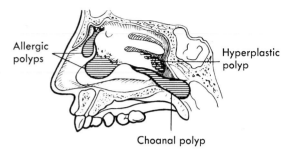

Fig. 25-4 Location of nasal polyps. Allergic polyps occur more commonly in upper area of lateral nasal wall, involving anterior middle turbinate especially. Chonal polyps have long pedicle and present in nasopharynx. Hyperplastic or neoplastic polyps and epithelial papilloma are not so pedunculated and involve posterior aspect of middle turbinate. (AFIP 70-1150-2.)

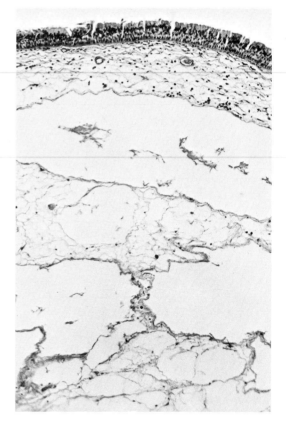

Fig. 25-5 Nasal polyps, allergic type. Stromal edema with pseudocyst formation.

lergic polyp that has extended by an elongated pedicle from the nasal cavity through the carina and presents in the nasopharynx. The pure forms of allergic and inflammatory polyps are distinct (Fig. 25-4).

Polyps, especially those of allergic origin, enlarge chiefly from accumulation of interstitial fluid. The gland content and vascularity vary with the site of origin. Blood vessels may be particularly prominent in polyps of the turbinates, where the mucosa is of an erectile type.

Allergic polyps. The **allergic polyp** is usually bilateral and multiple. It is more common in the upper part of the lateral nasal wall, involving especially the middle turbinate and the ethmoidal sinuses. It also arises commonly in the maxillary sinuses, emerges through the sinus osteum, and hangs free in the nasal cavity. The fact that it does not bleed readily is an important point of clinical differentiation from neoplastic polypoid lesions such as the epithelial papilloma and inverted papilloma. After excision, it recurs consistently unless the allergic background is eliminated.

In the allergic polyp, marked stromal edema with pseudocyst formation is striking (Fig. 25-5). An eosinophilic exudate is prominent, epithelial metaplasia results from chronic irritation, hyaloid thickening of the mucosal basement membrane is striking, and there is an increase in interstitial reticulin fibrils (Fig. 25-6).

Inflammatory polyps. The **inflammatory polyp** developing on a basis of local infection or trauma is usually unilateral and solitary. It does not recur after excision. There is much less polypoid edema with an exudate composed of neutrophilic leukocytes and a few mononuclear cells. Epithelial metaplasia is not so frequent, and thickening of the mucosal basement membrane is not a significant feature.

Hemangioma. Hemangioma of the nasal septum is frequently a polypoid lesion occurring predominantly in the mucosa of the cartilaginous septum within Little's triangle. It rarely occurs before puberty and usually is a reactive vascular proliferation, not a neoplasm. Groups of dilated, thin-walled blood vessels with relatively little stroma constitute characteristic histologic features. The squamous epithelium may show varying degrees of acanthosis, but malignant change has not been reported.

Occasionally, marked vascular proliferation occurs in the early months of pregnancy. When situated on the nasal septum, it may be misinterpreted as a hemangioma. The lesion usually disappears when the pregnancy is terminated.

Pseudotumors

The mucosa of the upper respiratory tract is so exposed to clinical and physical trauma and to the influence of infections and allergies that it is a favorite site for the formation of inflammatory pseudotumors. These may present as an edematous polypoid lesion with cellular fibrosis and exudate or as granulation tissue. Where fibrous tissue predominates, the proliferation may be pleomorphic and confused with fibrous neoplasms.

The inflammatory pseudotumors are most common on lower portions of the nasal septum, on the hypopharynx, and on the sublottic area of the larynx (usually following instrumentation) and appear as small elevated nodules. Features that differentiate the pseudotumor from the true neoplasm are the presence of exudate, vascular sclerosis, maturation of connective tissue elements, rapid growth, and calcification in pseudotumors.

Tumors

The nasal cavity is the site of the greatest variety of tumors in the upper respiratory

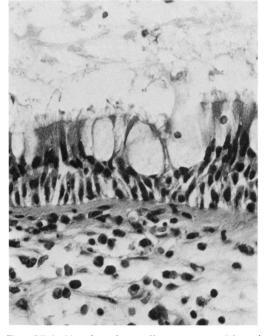

Fig. 25-6 Nasal polyp, allergic type. Ciliated pseudostratified columnar respiratory epithelium shows increased mucin production. Thickened basement membrane is evident. Inflammatory infiltrate is predominantly plasma cell.

tract. Adenoid cystic carcinoma occurs more frequently in the nose than do mixed tumors of the salivary gland type, but the latter do occur. Neurogenous tumors comprise a significant proportion of all of the tumors of the nose. Approximately one-half of the intranasal neoplasms are malignant.

The paranasal sinuses are unique in that one-fourth of all tumors that develop in these sinuses are lesions of bone. However, squamous cell carcinoma is the most frequent neoplasm encountered. Colloid and papillary adenocarcinoma in this region are of low-grade malignancy and locally invasive and rarely metastasize (Fig. 25-7). Adenocarcinoma and adenoid cystic carcinoma are more frequently noted than are mixed tumors of the salivary gland type. Extracranial extensions of meningiomas may involve the sinuses. Most neoplasms of the sinuses originate in the maxillary sinuses. The next most frequently involved sinuses are the ethmoidal, frontal, and sphenoidal in that order. About two-thirds of the neoplasms in the sinuses are malignant.

Epithelial papilloma. Epithelial papilloma occurs most commonly in the adult male and arises usually from the middle turbinate toward the posterior portion of the nasal cavity

but occasionally in a sinus. The tumors may be multiple and have a tendency to recur. Histologically, there are squamous components, papillary in character, and columnar, ciliated, and mucous cells (Fig. 25-8). Although the microscopic appearance is often benign, the tumors constitute a distinct threat to the patient. They are prone to recur even after wide excision. When malignant deterioration occurs, it usually is a squamous cell carcinoma.

The term *inverted papilloma* is used by some as a designation for a separate entity when invagination of the surface epithelium occurs. Since this occurs not only in the epithelial papillomas but also in ordinary nasal polyps and in the squamous cell papillomas, especially those of the larynx, it is only a morphologic variation of several entities—not a distinct single one. The invaginating epithelium may be squamous, glandular, or transitional.

Carcinomas of nasal mucosa. Carcinomas of the nasal mucosa usually occur in adult life and are slightly more common in females. They rarely metastasize. The nasal and sinus cavities are obstructed, and the tumor erodes bones by expansion and invasion. The *nasopharyngeal carcinoma* occurs most commonly in males and metastasizes early to cervical lymph nodes.

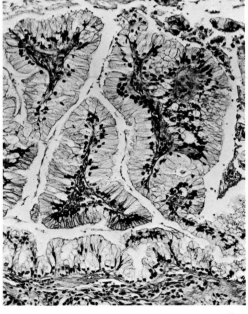

Fig. 25-7 Recurrent nonmetastasizing papillary adenocarcinoma from ethmoidal sinus of 82-year-old woman. Tumor recurred locally over ten-year period but did not metastasize. Epithelium well differentiated, and copious mucin present.

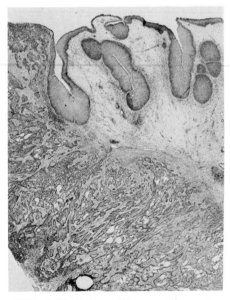

Fig. 25-8 Epithelial papilloma with carcinoma. Metaplastic squamous epithelium covers most of lesion. Malignant epithelial proliferation extensive in underlying portion. (AFIP 56-1576-5.)

NASOPHARYNX AND PHARYNX
Inflammations

Pharyngitis. The vast majority of the inflammatory diseases of the pharynx and nasopharynx are viral in origin. Congestion, edema, and lymphoid hyperplasia are characteristic findings.

The entire pharynx is encircled by aggregations of lymphoid tissue forming Waldeyer's ring, consisting principally of four aggregates:

1 Faucial tonsils, which are located laterally at the orifice of the oropharynx
2 Nasopharyngeal lymphoid tissue, which extends behind the orifices of the eustachian tubes and downward on the lateral walls of the pharynx
3 Adenoids, which are located in the posterior wall of the nasopharynx
4 Lingual tonsils, which are located at the base of the tongue

Bacterial and viral inflammatory processes may originate in any of these areas. Pharyngeal ulcers also may be noted in acute leukemia. Secondary tuberculosis involving the nasopharyngeal mucosa usually is located in the posterior wall of the nasopharynx.

Plummer-Vinson syndrome. The Plummer-Vinson syndrome is associated with chronic inflammatory changes in the mucosa of the pharyngoesophageal junction in women past the age of 40 years. In addition, there are mucosal atrophy, scarring, iron-deficiency anemia, and an increased incidence of hypopharyngeal, postcricord, extrinsic carcinoma.

Tornwaldt's syndrome. Tornwaldt's syndrome results from the obstruction of the orifice of the nasopharyngeal bursa. The obstruction usually results from an acute or chronic inflammatory process. The bursa normally is lined by respiratory-type epithelium, but in chronic inflammation squamous metaplasia usually occurs.

Tumors

Nasopharyngeal carcinoma. Nasopharyngeal carcinoma arises more commonly near the fossae of Rosenmüller, spreading widely beneath the mucosa without ulceration. The malignancy usually metastasizes to lateral retropharyngeal lymph nodes early. It is more common in males than in females and has a particular predilection for Orientals. It is the most common malignant tumor of the Chinese in Hong Kong.

Adenoid cystic carcinoma (cylindroma) is derived from minor salivary glands in the upper respiratory tract. Malignant melanoma and other miscellaneous tumors also occur rarely in the pharynx and nasopharynx. It is a common site for neurilemoma and ganglioneuroma.

Juvenile nasopharyngeal angiofibroma. Juvenile nasopharyngeal angiofibroma is a relatively rare tumor occurring almost exclusively in young males and becoming manifest in early adolescence. Growth of the tumor is accelerated at puberty, and spontaneous regression may occur at approximately 25 years of age. Since this type of hemangiofibroma has such distinctive clinical features, a hormonal relationship is suggested.

The tumor originates from the fibrocartilaginous tissue of the upper cervical vertebrae or from the fascia basalis located in the pharynx at the base of the skull. It most frequently develops in the nasopharyngeal recess but occasionally may arise in the anterior wall of the sphenoid bone.

Although basically hemangiomatous, it is clinically a specialized fibrous lesion. The fibrous component develops secondarily and is responsible for its final sclerotic and regressive course. The vascular and connective tissue elements vary in amount. The blood vessels at the base of the tumor are often large (Figs. 25-

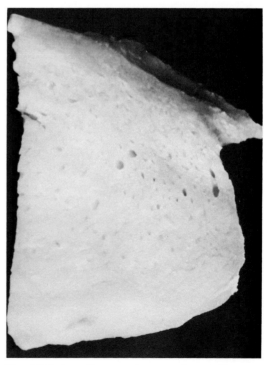

Fig. 25-9 Juvenile nasopharyngeal angiofibroma. Large blood vessels apparent on cut surface of portion of large tumor. (AFIP 56-18303-2.)

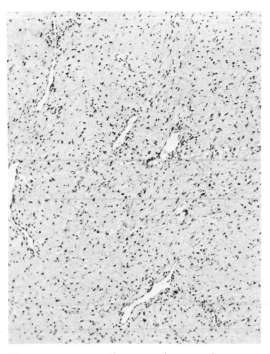

Fig. 25-10 Juvenile nasopharyngeal angiofibroma. Stroma consists of vascular spaces and dense cellular fibrous tissue. (AFIP 56-9683.)

9 and 25-10). Hemorrhage is the chief hazard, especially at surgery. Since malignant deterioration of the tumor is rare, its dangerous potential depends on its location, its marked vascularity, and its tendency to invade contiguous bony structures.

Synovial tumors of hypopharynx. Synovial tumors of the hypopharynx resemble synovial sarcomas of the joints. There are ample normal synovial tissues in the neck to provide a source for the tumor, including the bursae associated with the hyoid bone and the cricoarytenoid joints and those in the upper posterior portion of the neck. The mesothelial portion of the pharyngeal tumor usually is more differentiated than in the joint tumor.

Extramedullary plasmacytoma. Extramedullary plasmacytoma occurs most commonly in the nasal cavity and nasopharynx. Diagnosis usually is based on histologic features which include orientation of plasma cells in broad sheets on a delicate stroma and replacement of other tissue by such plasma cell sheets (Fig. 25-11). Since there is a definite relationship between extramedullary plasmacytoma and multiple myeloma, appropriate diagnostic studies to detect the latter are necessary. These include immunoelectrophoresis, bone x-ray studies, and bone marrow examination.

Neurogenic tumors. A review of neurogenic tumors in the upper respiratory tract indicates that the majority of fibrillar tumors are of

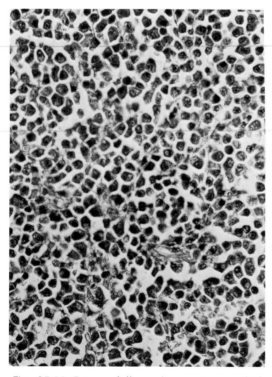

Fig. 25-11 Extramedullary plasmacytoma, which occurs predominantly in nasal cavity. Pleomorphic plasma cells completely replace stroma. (AFIP 870263.)

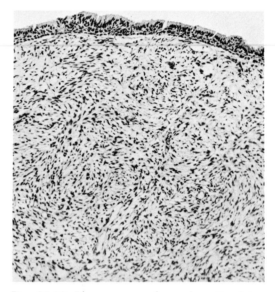

Fig. 25-12 Fibrosarcoma of nasal cavity. Interlacing fascicles of neoplastic fibrous cells evident. (AFIP 831866.)

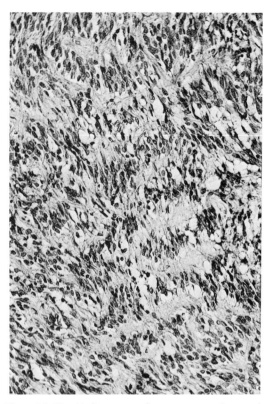

Fig. 25-13 Malignant schwannoma of nasal cavity, which originally was interpreted as fibrosarcoma. Palisading of nuclei became apparent when tumor recurred. Nuclear palisading characteristic of neurogenic tumors but not of fibrosarcomas. (AFIP 304290.)

neural origin and often are confused with fibrous mesenchymal tissue (Fig. 25-12).

The sources of origin of the neurogenous tumors may be divided into three categories:

1 Peripheral neural elements
2 Central neural elements
3 Extrusions of brain tissue through defects in the cribriform plate and glabellar and occipital sutures

Tumors originating from peripheral nerve elements include the neuroma, neurofibroma, neurilemoma (schwannoma), malignant schwannoma (Fig. 25-13), ganglioma, and gangliofibroma. Central neural crest elements that have migrated simultaneously with cranial nerve are the source of origin of the ganglioglioma, neuroblastoma (esthesioneuroepithelioma), and medulloblastoma. Sympathetic neural elements that are derived from central neural elements give rise to the ganglioneuroma, sympathicoblastoma, and paraganglioma. Secondary neurogenous tumors include the meningioma, ependymoma, and retinoblastoma.

The olfactory neuroblastoma is a neoplasm that originates in the olfactory placode. It is presumed that the tumor arises from a stem cell, termed esthesioneuroblast, because the usual location is in the olfactory area of the

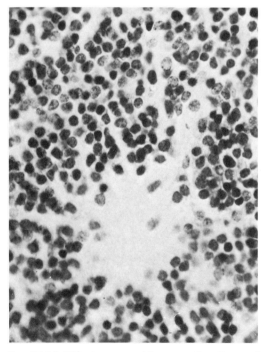

Fig. 25-15 Olfactory neuroblastoma. Small, round or oval, primitive neuroepithelial cells grow in rosette clusters around bundle of fine fibrillar neural stroma. (AFIP 64-8034-2.)

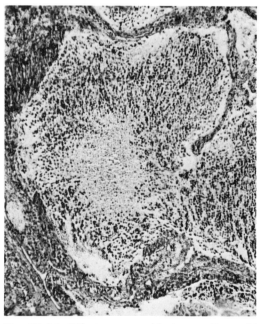

Fig. 25-14 Olfactory neuroblastoma. Organoid masses of neurocytoblasts associated with delicate neural fibrils pathognomonic for this lesion. (AFIP 64-8034-1.)

nasal cavity. The architecture varies, especially the proportion and arrangement of the cellular and fibrillar elements. Small, round or oval, primitive neural epithelial cells which are slightly pointed at one end grow in clusters that are closely associated with bundles of fine neural fibrils (Figs. 25-14 and 25-15). Although rosette formation among the cells occurs, it is not so prominent a feature as in sympathicoblastoma and retinoblastoma. Olfactory neuroblastoma is apparently the most sensitive neurogenous tumor to irradiation therapy.

The **nasal glioma (congenital ganglioglioma)** occurs in the newborn infant, in whom the presence of an intranasal polypoid mass is almost pathognomonic of brain extrusion. Wide separation of the infant's eyes usually is associated with this condition. The lesion results from a congenital herniation of the cerebral vesicle through the skull, most commonly in the occipital and nasal frontal areas.

A nasal glioma may present as a smooth, nonulcerated, subcutaneous mass in the nasofrontal area attached by a fibrous stalk to the brain through the glabellar sutures. Intranasally, the mass may seem to arise from a turbinate, but its attachment to the cribriform plate is usually obvious. When the lesion is an encephalocele that communicates with the cerebral ventricles, it will enlarge when the patient cries or strains. Most nasal gliomas present a monotonous pattern of brainlike adult glial tissue interspersed with fine fibrous septae (Fig. 25-16). Meningitis may occur if an encephalocele is removed intranasally through a communicating ependymal-lined sinus.

Sarcoma botryoides (malignant mesenchymoma). Sarcoma botryoides is a recognized entity of the urogenital tract in children (p. 578). Recently, it has also become recognized as an equally specialized entity in the upper respiratory tract. The lesion occurs in the nasopharynx, palate, and ear. Although usually classified as a form of rhabdomyosarcoma, we have seen some congenital mesenchymal tumors containing no recognizable striated muscle elements. They are composed of neoplastic fibrous tissue, bone, or cartilage.

Since embryonal mesenchyme is the tissue of origin, the histologic appearance is varied because many of the tissues that normally are derived from embryonal mesenchyme are represented in the neoplastic growth. Fibromatous and myomatous elements usually are present in varying proportion. The large strap cell is characteristic of the primitive muscle component (Fig. 25-17). Neoplastic bone and cartilage may be present. Typically, the tumor metastasizes early and death rapidly ensues.

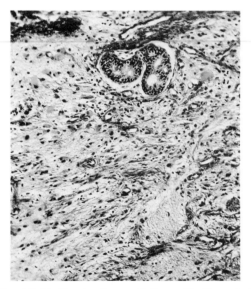

Fig. 25-16 Nasal glioma. Delicate fibrillar glial tissue with plump gemistocytic astrocytes extends to level of sweat gland in skin of glabellar region.

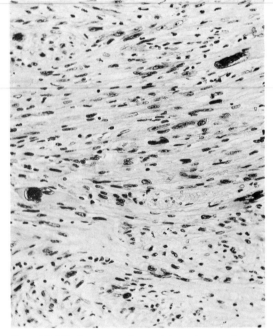

Fig. 25-17 Sarcoma botryoides. Large hyperchromatic nuclei in cells with abundant cytoplasm characteristic of primitive striated muscle components.

LARYNX

Infectious inflammatory lesions. Infectious inflammatory lesions of the larynx are rarely seen. Laryngeal diphtheria has been virtually eliminated in the United States by the use of antibiotics and immunization.

Hyperkeratotic papilloma. The hyperkeratotic papilloma resembles the verrucal type of senile keratosis. In the larynx, it is solitary and does not cause fixation of the cords. Microscopically, it may resemble keratotic acanthosis of the skin, but more commonly it resembles senile keratosis with varying degrees of dyskeratosis. Squamous cell papilloma occurs in the larynx and may show varying degrees of epithelial dysplasia.

Pachyderma laryngis. Pachyderma laryngis is a diffuse epithelial thickening with a surface layer of true keratin that involves the true cords and occurs most commonly in men (Fig. 25-18).

Nodules. The laryngeal nodule originates as a focal fibrosis that is generally of short dura-

tion. Constant irritation of the true cord produces interstitial edema and dilatation of the thin-walled blood vessels. Hyaline material is deposited in the walls of the blood vessels and in the interstitial tissue. The various histologic appearances of the nodules suggest subdivision into four stages; fibrous, polypoid, varicose, and fibrinoid (Fig. 25-19). In general, elimination of the cause, especially correction of voice misuse, and simple excision have proved to be adequate therapy.

Leukoplakia. Although literally meaning white patch, leukoplakia is a term that implies potential malignant change. It is similar to senile or actinic keratosis in the epidermis. Leukoplakia is a more desirable term than *carcinoma in situ* because caution must be exercised in interpreting laryngeal lesions. Obviously, a laryngectomy is a devastating experience for the patient. Laryngectomies have been performed for carcinoma in situ without carcinoma being found in the surgical specimen.

Of the two clinical and pathologic forms of leukoplakia, the more common is the flat relatively smooth lesion. The other form presents

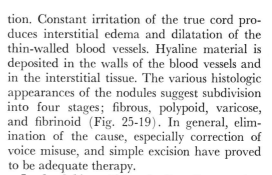

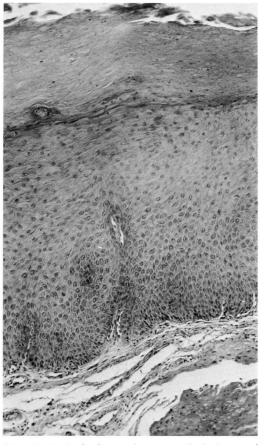

Fig. 25-18 Pachyderma laryngis. Thick layer of keratin not normally present on true vocal cords. Squamous epithelium thickened.

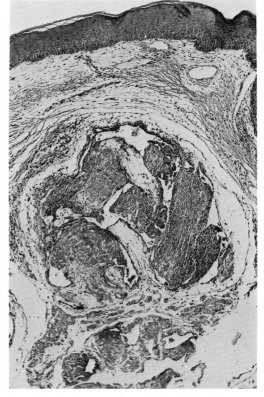

Fig. 25-19 Laryngeal nodule—fibrinoid stage. Darker staining material in edematous stroma characteristic of this stage.

localized changes and verrucous architecture. Dyskeratosis is characterized by cells that are irregular in size and shape with abnormal chromatin pattern. In addition, atypical mitotic figures and premature keratinization as evidenced by cells containing eosinophilic homogeneous droplets of intracellular keratin are evident (Fig. 25-20).

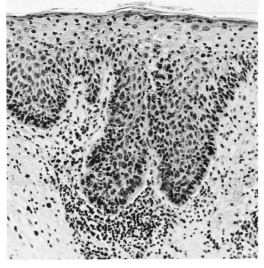

Fig. 25-20 Leukoplakia of larynx. Epithelium shows premature keratinization, mitotic figures, and disorderly maturation sequence. Chronic inflammatory infiltrate can be noted in subjacent stroma. (AFIP 56-11557.)

Carcinoma. The older classification divided carcinoma of the larynx into (1) an extrinsic type originating in the hypopharynx, arytenoid folds, epiglottis, and pyriform fossae and (2) an intrinsic type involving the mucosa lining the larynx. The clinical course of these two categories differs widely, although the pathology may not be strikingly different.

Extrinsic laryngeal carcinoma grows more rapidly than intrinsic. Diffuse extension of extrinsic carcinoma renders it less amenable to treatment. Intrinsic carcinoma of the larynx is overwhelmingly squamous and usually is a well-differentiated tumor. It occurs predominantly in older men. The majority of the tumors arise on the vocal cords. They grow relatively slowly and remain superficial for prolonged periods. When they infiltrate, however, the extension is rapid.

■ Ear

EXTERNAL EAR

Onchocerciasis, as well as leprosy, blastomycosis, and coccidioidomycosis may involve the external ear. Keloids develop on the pinna

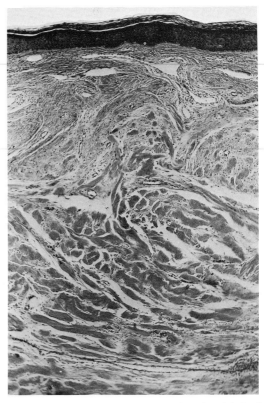

Fig. 25-22 Keloid of ear. Dense bands of keloid collagen in subcutaneous tissue.

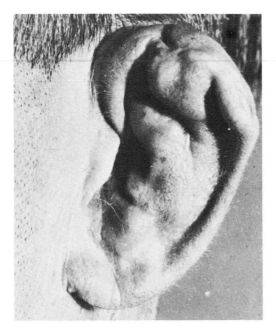

Fig. 25-21 Keloids of ear (cauliflower ear).

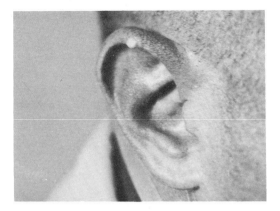

Fig. 25-23 Chondrodermatitis nodularis chronica helicis. Location and clinical appearance characteristic of this painful nodule. (From Shuman, R., and Helwig, E. B.: Amer. J. Clin. Path. **24:**126-144, 1954; AFIP 165134.)

Chondrodermatitis nodularis chronica helicis specifically involves the external ear and presents as a painful tumorlike nodule on the superior edge of the helix (Fig. 25-23). At this site, the skin is in direct contact with cartilage without a protective vascular subcutaneous layer (Fig. 25-24). The pathogenesis is unknown. A compromised blood supply has been suggested. The lesion is benign.

EXTERNAL AUDITORY CANAL; MIDDLE EAR; TEMPORAL BONE
Tumors and tumorlike lesions

Tumors of the external auditory canal are rare. The majority of them arise in the skin that lines the canal. These tumors include the junctional nevus, an occasional malignant

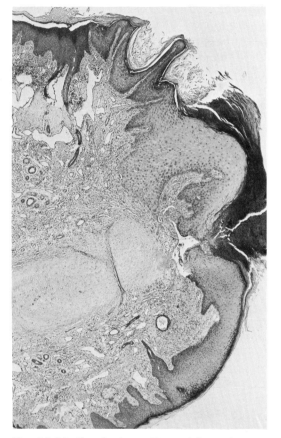

Fig. 25-24 Chondrodermatitis nodularis chronica helicis. Superficial parakeratotic plaque with acanthotic squamous epithelium overlying cartilage showing fibrinoid degeneration.

(cauliflower ear) after repeated trauma (Fig. 25-21) such as experienced by boxers and wrestlers. Subcutaneous hemorrhage occurs originally, and keloid collagen forms subsequently (Fig. 25-22). Squamous cell carcinoma and basal cell carcinoma also occur in this area.

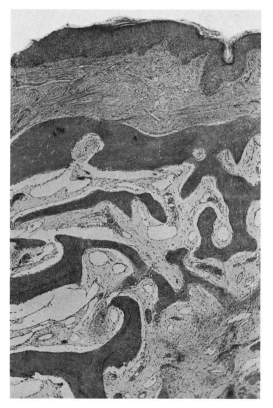

Fig. 25-25 Osteoma of external auditory canal. Spicules of hypertrophic bone apparent.

melanoma, and the squamous cell papilloma that has histologic characteristics similar to those of the lesion arising in the mucosa of the upper respiratory tract. Special entities of this area are osteoma and exostosis, ceruminal adenoma, and otic polyp.

Osteoma. Osteomas appear most often in adolescent boys and young men, arising most commonly at the chondro-osseous junction of the external auditory canal (Fig. 25-25). These lesions of bone occur more frequently in persons who habitually swim in cold water. Experimental support for this observation was furnished when overgrowths of bone were produced in the otic canals of guinea pigs by injecting cold water into the canals at intervals for long periods. The lesions are benign and do not recur after excision.

Ceruminal adenoma. Although ceruminal adenoma occurs in man, it is more common in lower animals, especially dogs and cats (Fig. 25-26). The ceruminal glands are modified sweat glands of the apocrine type, normally situated deep in the dermis near the cartilage of the canal. The tumor is particu-

larly pleomorphic histologically. Squamous metaplasia is not uncommon, although its basic epithelial cell retains similarity to the apocrine type of the parent gland (Fig. 25-27). Although frequently interpreted as an adenocarcinoma, we have no record of an authentic ceruminal gland tumor that has metastasized.

Polyps. Polyps arise in the middle ear as a complication of chronic otitis media and protrude into the external canal through a perforated tympanic membrane. They are composed chiefly of granulation tissue and chronic exudate, but wide variations are also possible in the proportion of their other constituents—epithelium, blood vessels, and fibrous tissue (Fig. 25-28). The lesion most often is covered by squamous epithelium that has resulted from metaplasia of the normally modified respiratory epithelium of the middle ear.

Cholesteatoma. Cholesteatoma is most frequently a postinflammatory pseudotumor and is classified as a primary lesion when it arises from an embryonal inclusion of squamous epithelium in the temporal bone, especially in

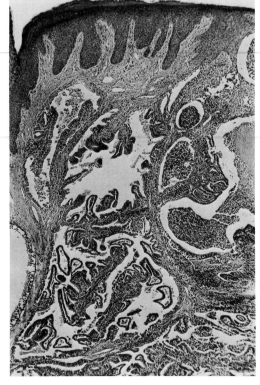

Fig. 25-26 Ceruminal adenoma of external auditory canal in cat. Papillary character seen more frequently in lesions in dogs and cats than in those in human beings.

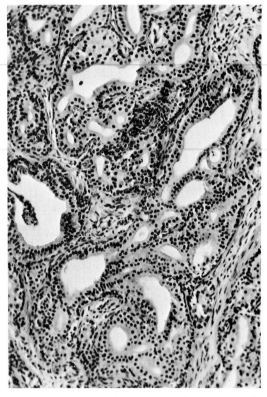

Fig. 25-27 Ceruminal adenoma of external auditory canal. Glandular pattern retained.

the petrous portion. The lesion is almost always a consequence of chronic otitis media in which there is marginal perforation of the external tympanic membrane. Through this opening, squamous epithelium from the external canal gains access to the middle ear and either reepithelializes the denuded surface or burrows under the epithelium normally present and replaces it (Fig. 25-29). From this epithelium, flaky keratin is constantly being shed, the accumulation of which eventually causes pressure erosion of bone. The term *cholesteatoma* is an unsatisfactory one in that the occasional cholesterol deposits are the result of hemorrhage or chemical degradation of the keratin lipid. However, this nomenclature is universally accepted and would be difficult to change.

Nonchromaffin paraganglioma (glomus jugulare tumor). Nonchromaffin paraganglioma arises from structures in the human temporal bone similar to the carotid bodies, the glomus jugularis. In the middle ear, more than 90% of the tumors arise from the glomus jugularis that lies in the jugular canal immediately under the floor of the middle ear (Figs. 25-30 and 25-31). Additional foci of chemoreceptor glomera in the temporal bone region

are located along the tympanic branch of the glossopharyngeal nerve along the auricular branch of the vagus nerve and in the jugular ganglion of the vagus nerve.

For many years, chemoreceptor structures have been classified as nonchromaffin paraganglionic tissue to differentiate them from the catecholamine-containing, chromaffin-reacting paraganglonic tissue such as the adrenal medulla and autonomic nervous system. However, recent observations suggest that the normal paraganglionic structures of the neck and temporal bone, and the tumors of these structures, contain and may secrete physiologically active catecholamines. Until the true frequency of functioning tumors is known, all patients with suspected paragangliomas or chemodectomas arising in the glomus jugularis complex should have routine preoperative determinations of urinary catecholamines and their metabolites. If these are found to be elevated before operation, the management is similar to that of pheochromocytoma.

These tumors may be misdiagnosed as hemangioendotheliomas. However, the structure

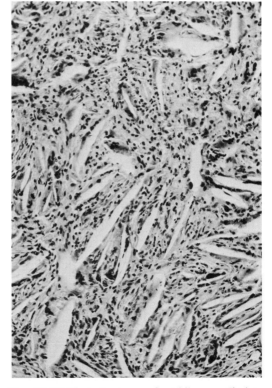

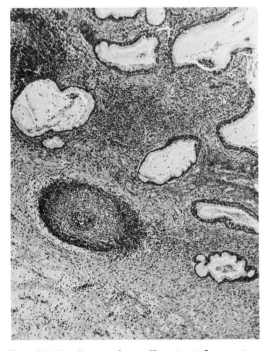

Fig. 25-28 Otic polyp. Chronic inflammation, pseudogland formation, and lymphoid follicle present.

Fig. 25-29 Cholesteatoma of middle ear. Cholesterol-slit spaces, foreign body type giant cells, and chronic inflammatory changes evident. (AFIP 56-2028-2.)

of the glomus is readily recognized in that the lesion tends to retain the characteristic pattern and cell type (Fig. 25-32). The tumor cells are arranged in organoid intercapillary clumps which sometimes assume an acinar pattern around small capillaries (Fig. 25-33).

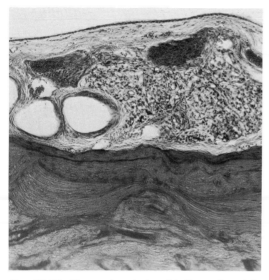

Fig. 25-30 Glomus jugularis with floor of middle ear below.

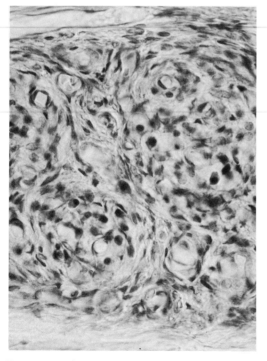

Fig. 25-31 Glomus jugularis, middle ear, showing characteristic histologic details of glomus body (high power).

Since the tumor is difficult to excise, it usually recurs locally. Instances of metastasis have been reported.

Sarcoma botryoides. Sarcoma botryoides occurs most commonly between the ages of 1 and 6 years. It usually presents as a swelling situated either in the temporal bone posterior to the auricle or in the external auditory canal. The histologic characteristics of this tumor are similar to those of sarcoma botryoides in other sites. Occasionally, a large protoplasmic strap cell is noted (see p. 1058).

Only a few cases of primary squamous cell carcinoma and adenocarcinoma of the temporal bone have been reported.

Otosclerosis

Otosclerosis generally is considered a primary, often symmetrical, dystrophic disease involving the labyrinth of the temporal bone adjacent to membranous inner ear structures. There is replacement of the altered bone by localized foci of abnormal weblike bone

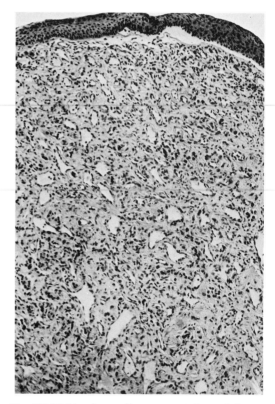

Fig. 25-32 Nonchromaffin paraganglioma (glomus tumor) of middle ear originally diagnosed as hemangioma because of prominent vascular component. However, nests of epithelioid cells with hyperchromatic oval nuclei can be noted protruding into vascular spaces.

exhibiting prominent cement lines, irregularly shaped and distributed osteocytes, and prominent vascular connective tissue marrow spaces (Fig. 25-34). This process can, over many years, replace extensive adjacent areas of temporal bone surrounding inner ear structures, or the disease may become inactive or quiescent in whole or in part at any time, with the formation of a histologically more sclerotic, mosaic type of bone. A definite etiology has not been established. Certain peculiarities have been confirmed such as occurrence only in human beings, a prominent familial predisposition, a predominance in males over females in a ratio of 2:1, and its rarity in blacks and Orientals as compared to whites. A high incidence of otosclerosis has been established in association with osteogenesis imperfecta. The onset of clinical otosclerosis varies from midchildhood to late middle adult life, with the great majority of patients noting hearing loss soon after puberty.

The primary foci of otosclerotic bone most

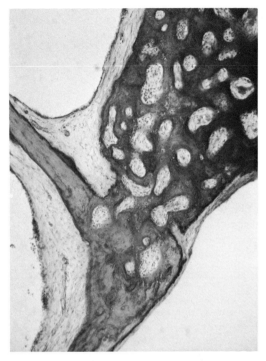

Fig. 25-34 Otosclerosis. Hypertrophic bone.

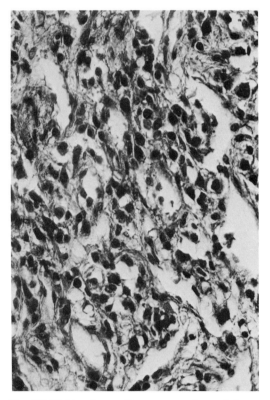

Fig. 25-33 Nonchromaffin paraganglioma (glomus tumor) of middle ear. Organoid nests of epithelioid cells in close proximity to capillary spaces. Note that nests tend to protrude into vascular spaces, retaining characteristic pattern of chemoreceptor organs.

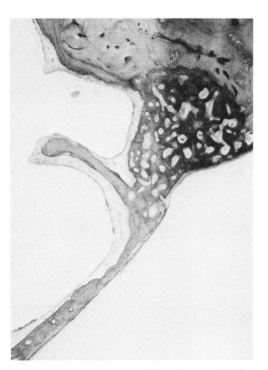

Fig. 25-35 Otosclerosis. Ankylosed stapedial foot plate.

frequently are found in an area of the temporal bone just anterior to the oval window, with other primary sites, listed in order of frequency, being the bone surrounding the round window, the internal auditory canal, and the semicircular canals. Extension of the foci usually is found to involve the bony wall adjacent to the membranous cochlear structures. The auditory ossicles, with the exception of the footplate of the stapes, have not been clearly determined as primary foci of the disease.

Otosclerosis found in the majority of routinely examined temporal bones produces no appreciable clinical symptoms, being referred to in such cases as histologic otosclerosis. When the disease process advances to either impact or ankylose the stapedial footplate (Fig. 25-35), a conduction type of deafness results. It is then that surgical intervention may ensue, with an attempt to mobilize the fixed footplate or complete removal of the stapes with replacement by various types of prostheses. The pathologist should be reminded that the surgeon must submit the stapedial footplate if a histologic diagnosis of otosclerosis is likely to be made, for seldom will the disease be found to involve the crura or head of the stapes. A sensoneural type of deafness has been described in clinical otosclerosis and is believed to be in some way due to involvement by the disease of the bone adjacent to the membranous cochlear structures.

REFERENCES

Miscellaneous

1 Ash, J. E., and Raum, M.: Atlas of otolaryngic pathology, Washington, D. C., 1956, American Academy of Ophthalmology and Otolaryngology, American Registry of Pathology, and Armed Forces Institute of Pathology (general).
2 Holdcraft, J., and Gallagher, J. C.: Ann. Otol. 78:5-20, 1969 (malignant melanomas).
3 Kraus, F. T., and Perez-Mesa, C.: Cancer 19: 26-38, 1966 (verrucous carcinoma).
4 Masson, J. K., and Soule, E. H.: Amer. J. Surg. 110:585-591, 1965 (embryonal rhabdomyosarcoma).
5 Pang, L. Q.: Arch. Otolaryng. (Chicago) 82: 622-628, 1965 (carcinoma of nasopharynx).
6 Prior, J. T., and Stoner, L. R.: Cancer 10:957-963, 1957 (sarcoma botyroides).
6a Al-Saleem, T., Harwick, R., Robbins, R., and Blady, J. V.: Cancer 26:1383-1387, 1970 (malignant lymphomas of pharynx).

Upper respiratory tract
Nasal and paranasal sinuses
Phycomycosis

7 Battock, D. J., Grausz, H., Bobrowsky, M., and Littman, M. L.: Ann. Intern. Med. 68:122-137, 1968.
7a Bergstrom, L., Hemenway, W. G., and Barnhart, R. A.: Ann. Otol. 79:70-81, 1970 (mucormycosis).
8 Berk, M., Fink, G. I., and Uyeda, C. T.: J.A.M.A. 177:511-513, 1961.
9 Hoagland, R. J., Sube, J., Bishop, R. H., Jr., and Holding, B. F., Jr.: Amer. J. Med. Sci. 242:415-422, 1961.
10 McBride, R. A., Corson, J. M., and Dammin, G. J.: Amer. J. Med. 28:832-846, 1960.
11 Straatsma, B. R., Zimmerman, L. E., and Gass, J. M.: Lab. Invest. 11:963-985, 1962.

Lethal midline granuloma; Wegener's granulomatosis

12 Alarcon-Segovia, D., and Brown, A. L. Jr.: Proc. Mayo Clin. 39:205-222, 1964.
13 Berman, D. A., Rydell, R. E., and Eichenholz, A.: Ann. Intern. Med. 59:521-530, 1963.
14 Byrd, L. J., Shearn, M. A., and Tu, W. H.: Arthritis Rheum. 12:247-253, 1969 (Wegener's granulomatosis).
14a Cassan, S. M., Divertie, M. B., Hollenhorst, R. W., and Harrison, E. G., Jr.: Ann. Intern. Med. 72:687-693, 1970 (orbital pseudotumor and Wegener's granulomatosis).
15 Edgerton, M. T., and Desprez, J. D.: Brit. J. Plast. Surg. 9:200-211, 1956.
16 Elsner, B., and Harper, F. B.: Arch. Path. (Chicago) 87:544-547, 1969 (Wegener's granulomatosis).
17 Feldman, F., Fink, H., and Gruezo, Z.: Amer. J. Dis. Child. 112:587-592, 1966 (Wegener's granulomatosis).
18 Fisher, J. H.: Canad. Med. Ass. J. 90:10-14, 1964 (Wegener's granulomatosis).
19 Greenspan, E. M.: J.A.M.A. 193:74-76, 1965 (therapy).
19a Kunkel, G., Hüttemann, U., and Nickling, H. G.: Deutsch. Med. Wschr. 94:959-965, 1969 (Wegener's granulomatosis).
20 McIlvanie, S. K.: J.A.M.A. 197:130-132, 1966 (therapy).
20a Novack, S. N., and Pearson, C. M.: New Eng. J. Med. 284:938-942, 1971 (therapy—Wegener's granulomatosis).

Relapsing polychondritis

21 Dolan, D. L., Lemmon, G. B., Jr., and Teitelbaum, S. L.: Amer. J. Med. 41:285-299, 1966.
22 Kaye, R. L., and Sones, S. A.: Ann. Intern. Med. 60:653-664, 1964.
23 Spritzer, H. W., Weaver, A. L., Diamond, H. S., and Overholdt, E. L.: J.A.M.A. 208:355-357, 1969.

Nasopharynx and pharynx
Juvenile nasopharyngeal angiofibroma

24 Apostol, J. V., and Frazell, E. L.: Cancer 18: 869-878, 1965.
25 Furstenberg, A. C., and Boles, R.: Trans. Amer. Acad. Ophthal. Otolaryng. 67:518-523, 1963.
26 Schiff, M.: Laryngoscope 69:981-1016, 1959.

Synovial tumors of hypopharynx

27 Cadman, N. L., Soule, E. H., and Kelly, P. J.: Cancer 18:613-627, 1965.
28 Harrison, E. G., Jr., Black, B. M., and Devine, K. D.: Arch. Path. (Chicago) 71:137-141, 1961.

29 Jernstrom, P.: Amer. J. Clin. Path. 24:957-961, 1954.
30 McCormack, L. J., and Parker, W.: Cleveland Clin. Quart. 23:260-264, 1956.
31 Mackenzie, D. H.: Cancer 19:169-180, 1966.
32 Martens, V. E.: J.A.M.A. 157:888-890, 1955.

Extramedullary plasmacytoma

33 Rawson, A. J., Eyler, P. W., and Horn, R. C., Jr.: Amer. J. Path. 26:445-461, 1950.
34 Stout, A. P., and Kenney, F. R.: Cancer 2:261-278, 1949.
35 Webb, H. E., Hoover, N. W., Nichols, D. R., and Weed, L. A.: Cancer 15:1142-1155, 1962.

Neurogenic tumors

36 Berger, L., and Coutard, H.: Bull. Ass. Franc. Cancer 15:404-414, 1926.
36aCummings, C. W., Montgomery, W. W., and Balogh, K., Jr.: Ann. Otol. 78:76-95, 1969 (neurogenic tumors of larynx).
37 Fisher, E. R.: Arch. Path. (Chicago) 60:435-439, 1955.
38 Fruhling, L., and Wild, C.: Arch. Otolaryng. (Chicago) 60:37-48, 1954.
39 Lewis, J. S., Hutter, R. V. P., Tollefsen, H. R., and Foote, F. W.: Arch. Otolaryng. (Chicago) 81:169-174, 1965.
40 McCormack, L. J., and Harris, H. E.: J.A.M.A. 157:318-321, 1955.
41 Mendeloff, J.: Cancer 10:944-956, 1957.
42 Oberman, H. A., and Sullenger, G.: Cancer 20:1992-2001, 1967.
43 Schall, L. A., and Lineback, M.: Ann. Otol. 60:221-229, 1951.
44 Seaman, W. B.: Radiology 57:541-546, 1951.
45 Thaler, S. U., and Smith, H. W.: Arch. Otolaryng. (Chicago) 83:233-236, 1966.

Ear

46 Batsakis, J. G., Hardy, G. C., and Hishiyama, R. H.: Arch. Otolaryng. (Chicago) 86:66-69, 1967 (ceruminal gland tumors).
47 Cankar, V., and Crowley, H.: Cancer 17:67-75, 1964 (ceruminal gland tumors).
48 Kingery, A. J.: J.A.M.A. 197:137, 1966 (chondrodermatitis helicis).
49 Levit, S. A., Sheps, S. G., Espinosa, R. E., Remine, W. H., and Harrison, E. G., Jr.: New Eng. J. Med. 281:805, 1969 (glomus tumors).
50 Rosenwasser, H.: Arch. Otolaryng. (Chicago) 88:1-40, 1968 (glomus tumors).
51 Schermer, K. L., Pontius, E. E., Dziabis, M. D., and McQuiston, R. J.: Cancer 19:1273-1280, 1966 (glomus tumors).
52 Shuman, R., and Helwig, E. B.: Amer. J. Clin. Path. 24:126-144, 1954 (chondrodermatitis helicis).
53 Simonton, K. M.: J.A.M.A. 206:1531-1534, 1968 (glomus tumors).

Otosclerosis

54 Altman, F.: Henry Ford Hospital International Symposium on Otosclerosis, Boston, 1960, Little, Brown and Co.
55 Guild, S. R.: Ann. Otol. 53:246-266, 1944.
56 Gussen, R.: Acta Otolaryng. (Stockholm) suppl. 248, pp. 1-38, 1969.
57 Shambaugh, G. E., Jr.: Surgery of the ear, ed. 2, Philadelphia, 1967, W. B. Saunders Co., p. 475.
58 Transactions of the American Otological Society, Inc., vol. LIV, (Ninety-ninth annual meeting, April 18 and 19, 1966), St. Louis, 1966, American Otological Society, Inc. (Z-P Graphic Arts Service, Inc.).

Chapter 26

Face, lips, mouth, teeth, jaws, salivary glands, and neck

Robert J. Gorlin and Robert A. Vickers

DEVELOPMENTAL ANOMALIES
Facial and oral developmental malformations

Facial cleft. A facial cleft, occurring in approximately 1 of every 800 white infants, may exist as an isolated anomaly or in combination with other developmental disturbances (about 15%) such as hydrocephalus, syndactyly, hypertelorism, etc.[1, 9] At times, the combination is so well known as to constitute a syndrome. About the head and neck, these symptom complexes are legion, and only a few may be considered here. For a comprehensive survey, the reader is referred to Gorlin and Pindborg.[2]

Facial clefts arise from the failure of the mesenchyme to cross the junction of fusion of facial processes about the sixth or seventh week in utero. Thus, *cleft upper lip (harelip)*, the most common facial cleft, results from failure of fusion of the lower part of the median nasal (globular) process with the maxillary process. Unilateral cleft is about eight times as common as bilateral involvement. It is more common in males (about 60%) and on the left side (about 2:1), and it is unusual in black infants. The degree of cleavage may vary from a slight notch at the lateral border of the philtrum to a complete separation extending into the nostril.[1, 9]

Commonly (in about 50% of cases), cleft lip (cheiloschisis) is associated with *cleft palate* (palatoschisis). When the cleft extends through the line of fusion between the premaxilla and the maxilla, the area subsequently to be occupied by the developing lateral incisor frequently is disturbed. Supernumerary, impacted, or (most commonly) missing maxillary lateral incisors often are observed.

Cleft palate also may exist to varying degrees, ranging from fissure of the azygos or tip of the uvula (uvula fissa) to complete cleft. Not uncommonly, a submucous palatal cleft may remain undetected. Cleft palate unassociated with cleft lip (about 25%) is seen more commonly in females. Associated with abnormally small mandible (micrognathia) and tongue (microglossia) and posterior displacement of the tongue (glossoptosis), it is known as *Robin's syndrome*. Cleft lip and/or cleft palate may be associated with chromosomal abnormalities—e.g., cleft lip with cleft palate is seen in trisomy 13-15, cleft palate occurs in about 15% of the cases of the XXXXY syndrome, and cleft lip–cleft palate occurs in about 15% of the cases of trisomy 18.

The tongue is cleft into two to four lobes in association with asymmetric cleft palate, pseudocleft of the upper lip, and digital anomalies in the *orofaciodigital syndrome*.[13]

Congenital lip pits. Congenital lip pits, first described by Demarquay in 1845, almost always involve the lower lip. They vary in size from small bilateral dimples on the vermilion border to large snoutlike structures in the midline (Fig. 26-1). The fistulas are lined by stratified squamous epithelium and are connected at the base with the mucous glands of the lip by means of communicating ducts. Not uncommonly, mucus may be observed exuding from the openings.

Familial occurrence is common. The pits may occur alone or in common with cleft palate or cleft lip as part of a syndrome (66%). Most cases (75%) show an autosomal dominant pattern of inheritance due to a single gene of variable expressivity.[7, 26] An un-

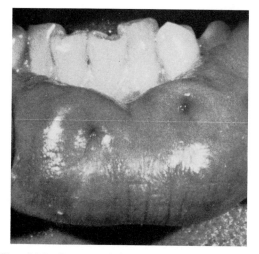

Fig. 26-1 Congenital lip pits (fistulas). Usually bilateral, frequently associated with facial clefts, and symmetrically situated on vermilion border of lower lip, fistulas represent failure of closure of evanescent sulci that appear in 10 mm to 14 mm embryo.

related condition, *commissural lip pits,* is observed on one or both sides in frequencies up to 15% of those examined.

Median rhomboid "glossitis." Median rhomboid "glossitis" is manifest as a roughly diamond-shaped reddish pattern on the dorsum of the tongue, immediately anterior to the circumvallate papillae. Occurring in somewhat less than 1% of individuals, it reportedly represents developmental failure of coverage of the tuberculum impar by the lateral tubercles of the tongue. It may arouse suspicion of malignant neoplasm in the minds of clinicians unaware of the nature of this condition.[1, 3, 18]

Fissured tongue. Fissured tongue occurs in about 5% of the population, the frequency increasing with age. It is noted more commonly in mongolism, being present in about 30% of affected individuals, and is also part of the Melkersson-Rosenthal syndrome (upper facial edema, facial palsy, cheilitis glandularis, etc.).[15, 25]

Fordyce's granules. Fordyce's granules are collections of sebaceous glands symmetrically located on the lateral vermilion part of the upper lip and on the buccal mucosa of about 65% of adults. The lower lip is seldom involved. The most common oral mucosal sites are lateral to the angle of the mouth, about Stensen's papilla, and lateral to the anterior pillar of the fauces.[1, 15]

Klinefelter's and Turner's syndromes. Examination of cytologic smears of buccal mucosa for sex chromatin (Barr bodies) in cases of Klinefelter's, Turner's (gonadal agenesis), and other sex chromosome syndromes has become a widespread technique.[8, 21] Aceto-orcein–fast green stain usually is employed to demonstrate the rounded chromatin masses adjacent to the nuclear membrane. There is one less nuclear membrane mass than the number of X chromosomes. In the normal female, more than 25% of the epithelial cells manifest the sex chromatin. Males do not have these nuclear membrane masses.

Demonstration of the so-called fluorescent Y body is useful in determining the number of Y chromosomes. This can be accomplished on buccal cytologic smears by use of Atabrine or quinacrine mustard.[8]

Developmental anomalies of teeth

Anomalies of number. Rarely is there complete absence of teeth (**anodontia**) or marked suppression in tooth formation (**oligodontia**). More commonly, a mild reduction in number (**hypodontia**) is observed.[1, 28, 29, 32] The third molars, less commonly the maxillary lateral incisors and second premolars, are the teeth most likely to be missing. Radiation to the jaws may injure and/or inhibit developing tooth buds. Supernumerary teeth occasionally are observed—most commonly mesiodens in the midline of the maxilla and extra molars, posterior to the third molars.[33]

Anomalies of size. Rarely are all of the teeth too large or small. More frequently, a single tooth is reduced in size (**microdontia**) or disproportionately enlarged (**macrodontia**).

Anomalies of shape. An anomaly called **dens invaginatus** (dens in dente) is manifest most commonly in the maxillary lateral incisor. A similar anomaly may occur in premolars.[1]

Anomalies of eruption. Rarely (1 in 2,000 white infants; more common among Amerindians) are teeth present at birth (**natal teeth.**) This condition may occur idiopathically or, occasionally, in association with other anomalies (chondroectodermal dysplasia, pachyonychia congenita, oculomandibulodyscephaly) in the neonatal period. Adrenogenital syndrome may be associated with premature eruption. Delay in eruption may be related to physical obstruction (impaction), endocrine disturbances (cretinism), or a multitude of other causes (cleidocranial dysostosis, fibromatosis gingivae, etc.).[1]

Anomalies of pigmentation. The teeth may be discolored as a result of exogenous (usually chromogenic bacteria) or endogenous (usually altered blood pigments) factors—internal hemorrhage due to trauma, congenital porphyria, erythroblastosis fetalis, etc.[1] Tetracyclines administered to the mother during the last trimester of pregnancy or to the infant are also incorporated in developing teeth, producing a yellow to gray color. Their presence may be demonstrated by a marked yellow fluorescence under ultraviolet light.[1]

Premature loss of teeth. Premature loss of a tooth or teeth may be due to trauma, mercury poisoning, hypophosphatasia, cyclic neutropenia, premature periodontoclasia with hyperkeratosis of palms and soles (Papillon-Lefèvre syndrome), or histiocytosis X.[1]

Hereditary enamel defects. These occur in about 1 in 16,000 children, affecting both dentitions. According to Witkop and Rau,[35] there appear to be at least ten distinct types.[33, 35] In the hereditary enamel dysplasias, the teeth are frequently brown and the enamel has a tendency to flake off, but the enamel varies in hardness and thickness according to the specific type. The underlying dentin and the root formation are entirely normal, in contrast to dentinogenesis imperfecta and dentin dysplasia.

Hereditary dentin defects. Two distinct dentin defects are recognized: dentinogenesis imperfecta (hereditary opalescent dentin) and dentin dysplasia. Both are transmitted as autosomal dominant traits.[30, 31, 33]

Dentinogenesis imperfecta usually occurs as an isolated phenomenon (1 in 8,000 individuals). A somewhat similar condition may occur as part of Lobstein's or van der Hoeve's syndrome (osteogenesis imperfecta, blue sclerae, otosclerosis, laxity of ligaments, etc.). Both deciduous and permanent teeth have an opalescent blue to brown color. Due to poor attachment at or near the dentinoenamel junction, the enamel fractures off. The roots are frequently thin and short and the canals obliterated. Microscopically, irregularly arranged dentinal tubules and defective matrix formation are noted.[30]

Dentin dysplasia is characterized by rootless malaligned teeth, generally exhibiting an absence of pulp chambers and canals but normal-appearing crowns.[35] Many teeth exhibit large periapical radiolucencies, and a pathognomonic half-moon–shaped pulp chamber may be seen on roentgenographic examination.

Other enamel disturbances. Nonhereditary enamel disturbances may affect either dentition, and they may be widespread or involve

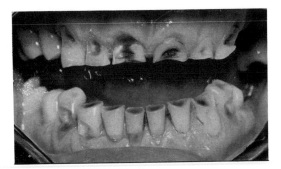

Fig. 26-2 Dental erosion. Characterized by smooth surface dissolution of enamel, especially at cervical portion, condition is of unknown etiology.

but a single tooth. The disturbance may be severe, causing deep pitted grooves, or so mild as to be manifest by only a small chalky spot. Defective enamel may result from injury to the enamel organ at any time from the earliest period of matrix formation to the last stage when calcification is taking place or result from acquired abnormalities such as in dental erosion (Fig. 26-2).

Nutritional deficiencies (calcium, phosphorus, vitamin D), endocrine and related disorders (hypoparathyroidism, pseudohypoparathyroidism, hypophosphatasia, rickets), congenital syphilis, infection of the deciduous precursor *(Turner's tooth)*, ingestion of excessive fluoride (in excess of 1.5 ppm), and a plethora of miscellaneous conditions can injure the developing ameloblast, producing enamel hypoplasia.

Other dentin disturbances. Nonhereditary dentin disturbances may occur in scurvy. The rate of dentin formation is less than normal in scurvy. Irregular deposits of cell-containing dentin (osteodentin) occur in severe experimental vitamin C deficiency states. Histologically, similar defective dentin formation is found in experimental vitamin A deficiency. In rickets, the developing dentin is hypocalcified, with a wide margin of predentin analogous to the wide osteoid seams in forming bone.

Vitamin D–resistant rickets, an X-linked dominant trait, is associated with defective dentin formation and resultant periapical abscess development. Similar changes have been reported in a variety of related metabolic disorders.[35]

ORAL LESIONS
Lesions of dermatologic type

Oral lesions that appear very red and severe, produce blisters, involve the skin, or are otherwise remarkable frequently are dis-

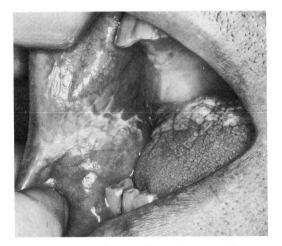

Fig. 26-3 Lichen planus of buccal mucosa. Dorsum of tongue also involved. (Courtesy Dr. J. O. Andreasen.)

cussed under the heading "dermatologic." Although they constitute, in reality, a heterogeneous group that may not have skin abnormalities, they are conveniently discussed together.

Lichen planus. Lichen planus usually appears as an irregular, lacelike whitening of the buccal mucosa (Fig. 26-3), but other oral areas (gingiva, tongue, palate, etc.) also may be involved and the clinical appearance also may be bullous or erosive. Approximately one-third of affected patients have only oral lesions. The other two-thirds have only cutaneous or skin and oral manifestations. Mucosal surfaces of other body sites are much less frequently involved. The diagnosis may be suspected when the lacelike whitening of the surface of the buccal mucosa (Wickham's striae) is seen. Biopsies of nonulcerated whitenings support the diagnosis.[42]

The cause of lichen planus is not known. Patients are most frequently between 40 and 60 years of age. Oral lesions of lichen planus do not itch. Symptoms may not be present, but pain and discomfort have been observed, especially with bullous or atrophic types of the disease. Approximately one-half of the patients observe concurrent "nervous stress" and express unwarranted anxiety or fear of having oral cancer.

Pemphigus. Pemphigus, especially pemphigus vulgaris, characteristically involves the oral mucosa during its course and may be manifested initially in this location. The oral tissues are very red, friable, and pebbly. Vesicle and bulla formation is observed, but the blisters do not remain intact for long periods in the mouth. Smear preparations, biopsies of

oral sites, and immunofluorescence are most useful in establishing a diagnosis.[39]

Benign mucous membrane pemphigus. Benign mucous membrane pemphigus is a vesicular or bullous disease involving the oral mucosa. Conjunctival tissues are frequently affected also, and the associated inflammation and scarring of this site are most serious sequelae.[37, 39] Microscopically, vesicle formation occurs immediately below the epithelium, and biopsy specimens of the short-lived vesicles are helpful in establishing the diagnosis, as are immunofluorescence studies.

Erythema multiforme. Erythema multiforme is characterized by large, erosive, frequently hemorrhagic lesions of the lips, buccal mucosa, and tongue. Oral and facial tissues are involved in approximately 25% of the patients. *Erythema multiforme exudativum* and *Stevens-Johnson syndrome* are terms applied to clinically severe examples of erythema multiforme, especially when the conjunctiva, genitalia, and, often, lungs are involved. Further, many consider these conditions closely related to Reiter's syndrome and Behçet's and Sutton's diseases.[1]

Epidermolysis bullosa. Oral tissues are involved in clinical and genetic types of epidermolysis bullosa. Microstoma, following the scarring of buccal mucosa, and dental abnormalities are complications of the dystrophic forms of this disease.

Chronic desquamative gingivitis and gingivosis. Dental specialists note that there is a disease limited to the maxillary and mandibular gingival tissues called chronic desquamative gingivitis or gingivosis. It is characterized by diffuse erythema, lack of known cause, no vesicles, and chronic course. Although bullous lichen planus, chronic candidal infections, benign mucous membrane pemphigus, and other conditions may present similar symptoms and manifestations, it appears likely that this may represent a specific and uncommon gingival inflammation. The diagnosis should be made following exclusion of other, better understood conditions.

Other lesions of dermatologic type. *Keratosis follicularis* (Darier's disease),[1] *lupus erythematosus,* and *herpes zoster* are additional examples of so-called dermatologic conditions with oral manifestations.

Lipoidproteinosis (Urbach-Wiethe syndrome) causes extreme induration of the oral mucosa, especially that of the lips and the tongue, which becomes atrophic and bound down to the oral floor. In *primary amyloidosis,* infiltration of the tongue may be associated with *macroglossia*. Enlargement of the tongue also may be seen in an unusual form of glycogen-storage disease of muscle. Deposits of secondary amyloid in the gingiva are not clinically manifested. *Scleroderma* and *acrosclerosis* occasionally are (about 7%) associated with a widening of the periodontal ligament of the teeth.

Hairy tongue is associated with proliferation of saprophytic organisms that cause extrinsic staining of elongated filiform papillae. Although the etiology is unknown, hairy tongue may follow therapeutic use of antibiotics or radiation. *Benign migratory glossitis* (geographic tongue), also of unknown etiology, is characterized by irregular superficial areas devoid of filiform papillae. It is more common in females and is seen in about 2% of the population.[1]

Oral and labial *papillomatosis* may be associated with both the juvenile (benign) and adult (malignant) forms of *acanthosis nigricans*.[2] The oral lesions, in contrast to the cutaneous, are not pigmented.

White lesions of mucosa

A change in color of the normally reddish oral mucosa to white constitutes one of the most frequently encountered oral abnormalities. Failure to recognize and identify the cause of this alteration can be a serious omission, since early squamous cell carcinoma may appear white.

The term leukoplakia has been used so differently by so many that it has come to signify only a "white patch" that does not rub away.[45, 47, 49, 54, 56]

Hyperkeratoses. An increased retention and production of keratin by mucosal stratified squamous epithelium is the most frequent cause of white patches of the oral cavity. This is termed hyperkeratosis and may be associated with chronic mechanical irritation and other factors. Biopsies of oral white patches may demonstrate cytologic alterations of a degree to warrant consideration as "premalignant." Specific alterations of dysplastic or "premalignant" character include those of dyskeratosis—abnormal nuclear shapes and size and increased numbers of mitotic figures. Most pathologists alter the terminology in such circumstances to *epithelial dysplasia* or similar designations. Microscopic examination of oral white patches that do not resolve with conservative management within a short time (e.g., one to two weeks) is indicated. *Leukoedema* is a slight whitening of oral mucosa

without dysplasia or abnormalities of keratinization.[43]

"Snuff box granuloma" is a term denoting the white, leathery, oral patches seen in patients using snuff. Patients using snuff have an increased incidence of oral carcinoma. The microscopy is characteristic.[57, 117]

Other white lesions. The *white oral lesions of lichen planus* were discussed previously (p. 1071). Wickham's striae or lacelike patterns in this condition are characteristic. Several hereditary conditions feature whitenings of the oral cavity. *Hereditary benign intraepithelial dyskeratosis, white sponge nevus (leukokeratosis heredita), pachyonychia congenita, Darier's disease,* and *dyskeratosis congenita (Zinsser-Engman-Cole syndrome)* are examples.[44, 58]

Aspirin burns resulting from the unprescribed use of tablets as dental topical anesthetics or troches frequently are seen. Soft, focal, oral whitenings that peel away easily, leaving a raw, bleeding surface, are seen in *candidosis*.

Disturbances of pigmentation

Melanotic pigmentation. Melanin may occur in the oral mucosa and about the lips under both normal and pathologic conditions.[60] Racial pigmentation, especially of the gingiva, is the most common type and appears to be directly related to skin color. It is present not only in nearly all blacks but also in Oriental peoples and those of Mediterranean background. Little melanin is present at birth. It is deposited largely during the first decade.

Chronic adrenocortical insufficiency (Addison's disease), hemochromatosis, and Albright's syndrome (polyostotic fibrous dysplasia, precocious puberty) may be associated with pigmentation of the oral mucosa as well as of the skin. Pigmentation also is seen in chronic steatorrhea and in the Peutz-Jeghers syndrome. The latter is characterized by gastrointestinal polyposis, mucocutaneous pigmentation, and autosomal dominant inheritance.[2] Palatal melanotic pigmentation may be seen after extensive use of various antimalarial drugs, such as Camoquin or chloroquin.[61] It also may be seen in patients with oral lichen planus ("melasmic" staining).

All types of melanotic nevi have been reported in oral surroundings, as has malignant melanoma.

Nonmelanotic pigmentation. Nonmelanotic pigmentation usually is due to heavy metals.[4, 60] Amalgam tattoo results from implantation of particles of filling material under the mucosa at the time of dental procedures. Lead, bismuth, arsenic, and mercury intoxications may be associated with a deposit of the metallic sulfide in the inflamed gingival margin.

MOUTH

Dental caries

Dental caries is a disease of the enamel, dentin, and cementum that produces progressive demineralization of the calcified component and destruction of the organic component, with the formation of a cavity in the tooth.[63] Microorganisms are present at all stages of the disease and, from the results of animal experiments, appear to be essential etiologic factors. Destruction of tooth structure by caries is to be differentiated from erosion and abrasion. In these latter instances, there is no bacterial invasion, and the affected tooth surface is hard and appears polished.

Tooth decay commonly is stated to be the most frequent disease of civilized man.[62] Certainly, it occurs or has occurred in the great majority of individuals living in the United States, Canada, and Europe. Once a carious cavity has formed, the defect is permanent. The designation DMF (decayed, missing, filled) has proved useful in comparative studies of the frequency of dental caries, particularly in children and young adults. After the introduction of fluoride to the drinking water (1 ppm), the DMF rate has generally decreased over a period of years by more than 50%.[62, 70]

Studies in many cities in the United States, Canada, and abroad have given striking evidence of the efficiency of fluoridation of communal water supplies in reducing the rate of tooth decay in children. Partial control of tooth decay by this method constitutes an important public health achievement. Excessive amounts of fluoride cause a condition called "mottling" of the enamel. It occurs in children who have consumed drinking water containing 1.5 ppm fluoride or more during the time when tooth enamel is being deposited in the developing, unerupted teeth. Drinking water had long been suspected as causing the disfigurement. In 1931, excessive amounts of fluoride were demonstrated in such waters.

The mechanism of fluoride in controlling the incidence of dental caries is not fully understood. An optimal amount of fluoride built into the apatite crystal during tooth formation decreases the acid solubility of enamel. Topical applications of fluoride solu-

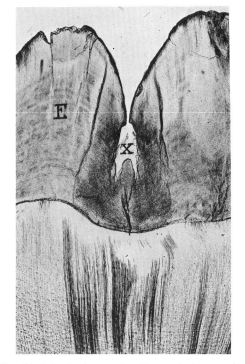

Fig. 26-4 Beginning caries. Fissure lesion resulted in establishment of cavity, **X**, in enamel, **E**. Ground section of molar.

tions to recently erupted tooth surfaces and brushing the teeth with dentifrices containing fluoride appear to be effective in reducing susceptibility to dental caries. Teeth with a relatively high content of fluoride are relatively free from caries.

Caries occurs in areas on tooth surfaces where saliva, food debris, and bacterial plaques accumulate. These areas are chiefly the cervical part of the tooth, interproximal surfaces, and pits and fissures. Surfaces that are self-cleansing by the excursion of food and the action of the tongue and cheeks are usually free of caries. If the cleansing process is interfered with (e.g., by prosthetic appliances), caries may develop rapidly. Dental caries does not occur in germ-free animals or in animals fed an otherwise cariogenic diet by stomach tube.[66, 67] Specific strains of streptococci have been shown to induce dental caries in rats and in hamsters.[66]

The formation of bacterial plaques (Fig. 26-5) in areas of stagnation precedes cavity formation. Acidogenic and aciduric bacteria, together with filamentous forms, are present in such plaques.[63, 64, 69] Once a cavity has been produced in the enamel, with exposure of the underlying dentin, proteolytic microorganisms complete the destruction of the decalcified

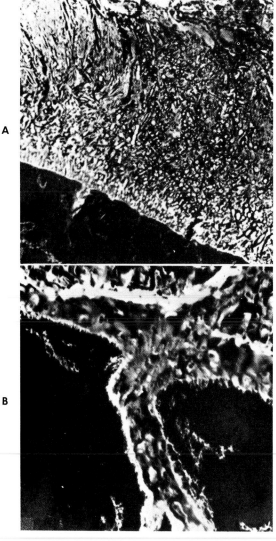

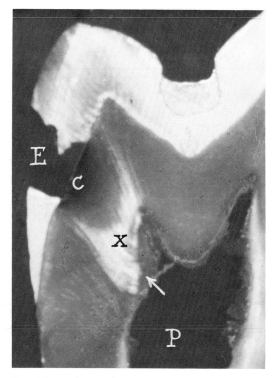

Fig. 26-6 Advanced caries of enamel and dentin in proximal surface of molar. Ground section photographed in reflected light. Lesion shows cavitation in enamel, **E**, softened carious dentin, **C**, sclerotic dentin appearing white in reflected light, **X**, and secondary dentin (arrow). **P**, Space occupied by dental pulp. (Courtesy Dr. V. Kalnins and Dr. L. Masin.)

Fig. 26-5 A, Bacterial plaque isolated by acid flotation from clinically noncarious enamel. **B,** Mass of bacteria at enamel surface extending from plaque into lamella. (**A,** ×2,000; **B,** ×6,000; **A** and **B,** from Scott, D. B., and Albright, J. T.: Oral Surg. Oral Med. Oral Path. **7:**64-78, 1954.)

tooth structure. The process may be slow, with extensive sclerosis of dentin (Fig. 26-6) in advance of the carious process and formation of secondary dentin in the pulp, which may even justify the term "arrested caries." More commonly, caries spreads laterally at the dentino-enamel junction, weakening and undermining the enamel (Fig. 26-7). It also progresses along dentinal tubules, and, especially in the young, may rapidly lead to exposure of the underlying pulp tissue (acute caries).

Another concept has been advanced, according to which an active bacterial penetra-

tion occurs along the relatively organic parts of the enamel (lamellae), with development of subsurface defects (Fig. 26-8) that subsequently cause collapse of the undermined enamel, with the formation of a cavity.[72] Formation of microscopic spaces in the enamel is postulated as the result of removal of the enamel protein. Dilute acid from the oral environment may be important in this initial step and in the dissolution of mineral crystallites embedded in the enamel protein. Pathways thus opened allow penetration by microorganisms, which have been demonstrated by conventional histologic techniques and by electron micrographs. Dissolution of the nonsoluble (keratinous) portion of the enamel by proteolytic (keratinolytic) microorganisms has been postulated. Removal of minerals by chelating agents also has been suggested.

Pulp and periapical periodontal disease

The tooth, projecting into the oral cavity through the mucous membrane and extending deep into the jawbone, affords two major

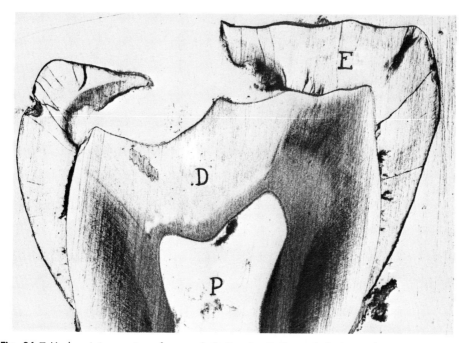

Fig. 26-7 Undermining caries of enamel. **D,** Dentin. **E,** Enamel. **P,** Space formerly occupied by pulp. Ground section of molar. (Courtesy Dr. G. Bergman.)

pathways of infection—one via the pulp and periapical tissue, which is usually a sequel to dental caries, with eventual exposure and infection of the dental pulp, and the other beginning at the gingival margin and leading to periodontal disease (see following discussion).

Inflammatory processes in the tooth pulp may be infected or noninfected. Trauma to the tooth from a blow, which may or may not fracture the tooth, from dental operations, or from excessive thermal changes may induce inflammation. This may be minimal with recovery, particularly in teeth with incompletely formed roots, or it may be severe. Since the rigid walls of the tooth do not permit expansion of the inflamed pulp, the circulation may be cut off and the pulp become an infarct that is later replaced by fibrous connective tissue.

Bacterial infection is the common sequel to

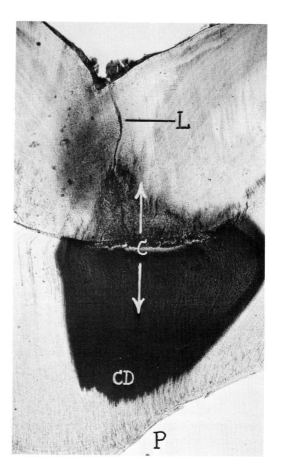

Fig. 26-8 Penetrating caries that started in fissure of molar. Ground section. Through lamella, **L,** carious nidus, **C,** became established at dentino-enamel junction. Arrows show progress of decay from nidus toward surface of enamel and toward pulp. Note close proximity of carious dentin, **CD,** to pulp, **P,** and almost intact surface enamel. **P,** Space formerly occupied by dental pulp. (×35.)

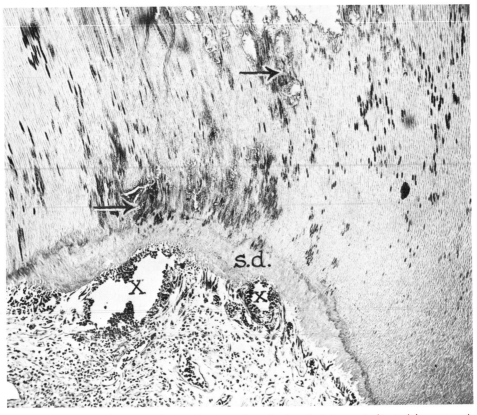

Fig. 26-9 Section of carious dentin showing liquefaction foci (some indicated by arrows) and formation of secondary dentin, **s.d.** Pulp infiltrated by inflammatory cells. Adjacent to secondary dentin, two small abscesses, **X,** are formed. (From Hill, T. J.: A text-book of oral pathology, Lea & Febiger.)

dental caries or to mechanical exposure of the tooth pulp.

Pulpitis may be acute or chronic. In acute pulpitis, pain is usually severe and increased by heat or cold. It often is aggravated by lying down (increased vascular pressure) and may be accompanied by a mild fever and leukocytosis. Histologically, microabscesses may be observed, surrounded by acutely inflamed pulpal tissue (Fig. 26-9). Characteristically, the purulent process spreads to involve the entire pulp, and unless the tooth is opened to establish drainage, the periapical tissues become involved in an acute alveolar abscess. Once the tissues about the root apex become involved, the tooth becomes sensitive to percussion.

In teeth in which the pulp is open to the oral cavity and where microorganisms of low virulence are responsible for the inflammatory reaction, the clinical symptoms may be minimal. Gradual necrosis of the pulp occurs, with drainage into the oral cavity. Since the nerve tissue of the pulp is involved in the necrotic process, pain may be minimal or absent.

Acute alveolar abscess is usually the result of spread of suppurative infection—from the tooth pulp through the root canals to the periodontal ligament about the tooth root ends. The inflammation characteristically follows the blood vessels into the bone marrow spaces. Suppuration follows pathways determined by the location of the tooth roots and the characteristics of adjacent structures. Usually, the periosteum overlying the tooth root end is destroyed, and eventually pus is drained through a fistula (gumboil). In maxillary teeth, drainage may occur into the antrum or the palate. Occasionally, the soft tissues are extensively involved, and, if untreated, drainage to the surface of the skin of the face or neck may occur. Osteomyelitis, cavernous sinus thrombosis, and Ludwig's angina are serious complications.

A much more common sequel to dental pulp infection is the dental granuloma. Clinically, this may be completely symptomless. Radiographic examination frequently discloses an area of bone rarefaction about a tooth root apex, with a chronically infected

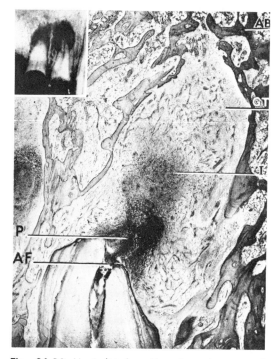

Fig. 26-10 Mesiodistal section through apex of maxillary first premolar with granuloma. Roentgenogram of specimen (inset) shows large areas of bone destruction around root ends of both maxillary premolars. **AF,** Apical foramen. **P,** Breaking down of tissue and formation of pus at foramen. **I,** Dense cellular infiltration next to foramen. **GT,** Granulation tissue. **AB,** Alveolar bone. (From Boyle, P. E., editor: Kronfeld's Histopathology of the teeth and their surrounding structures, Lea & Febiger.)

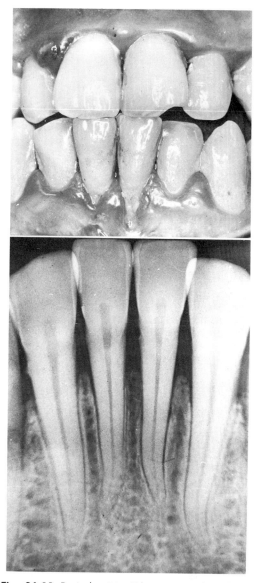

Fig. 26-11 Periodontitis. Edema, periodontal abscess, hemorrhage upon slight pressure, tissue recession with retraction of gingival margin, color change from light pink to deep red, loss of tissue in interdental area, horizontal bone loss, and widening of periodontal space. Compare clinical appearance and radiographs of this case with those shown in Fig. 26-12. (Courtesy Dr. S. R. Suit.)

or partially obliterated root canal. This area is usually spherical and well demarcated. Histologically, the tissue consists of granulation tissue, often heavily infiltrated by lymphocytes and plasma cells, surrounding necrotic tissue at the apex of the root canal foramen or within the pulp canal. Peripherally, loose and dense connective tissue merges into the surrounding bone, which may develop a definite cortical layer (Fig. 26-10).

A granuloma represents a balance between the defense forces of the body and a chronic area of necrotic tissue in the tooth root that is acting as an infected sequestrum. Very rarely, such a dental sequestrum is subject to osteoclastic resorption, as necrotic bone would be. If the tooth is extracted, the granulation tissue usually disappears during the healing process. Occasionally, a granuloma may persist as an area of "residual infection" after the tooth is extracted. Common oral organisms, chiefly streptococci and staphylococci, have been demonstrated in many dental granulomas, although some lesions appear to be sterile.

Remnants of epithelium (rests of Malassez) are found in the periodontal ligament, surrounding the teeth. In granulomas, this epithelium may proliferate. The root end may become surrounded by fluid with epithelium lining the surface, thus forming a radicular cyst. The cyst may enlarge to a considerable size. Although epithelium is present in prac-

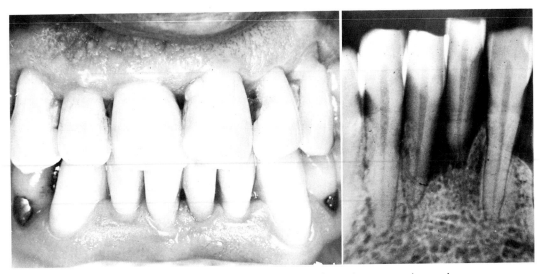

Fig. 26-12 Periodontitis with occlusal traumatism. Pale pink gingiva, hemorrhage upon heavy pressure, moderate recession, some exudate upon firm palpation, extreme mobility of individual teeth, and extensive bone loss in vertical pattern in localized areas. Correct diagnosis cannot be made by visual examination alone. It is necessary to probe, palpate, and use radiographs and other diagnostic methods to determine type and extent of periodontal inflammation. In comparing clinical appearances, although condition shown in Fig. 26-11 appears to be more serious than that illustrated here, prognosis is much better. (Courtesy Dr. S. R. Suit.)

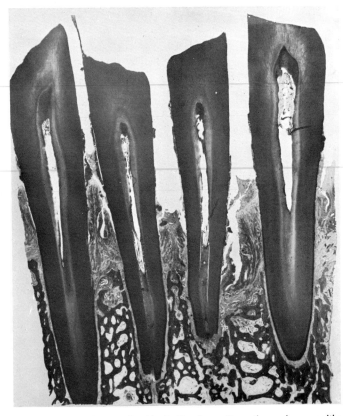

Fig. 26-13 Periodontitis (advanced), Mesiodistal section through mandibular incisors. Chronic inflammation of gingiva followed by proliferation of epithelium of gingival attachment along cementum, excessive osteoclastic resorption of interdental bone, and deep periodontal pocket formation between gingiva and surface of roots.

tically all granulomas and often proliferates to line small cystic cavities, the development of large cysts is relatively uncommon.

Periodontal disease

The inflammatory and degenerative processes that develop at the gingival margin and progress until the tooth-supporting structures are lost have much in common with periapical periodontal disease. In both instances, chronic asymptomatic infection by the common oral pathogens is usual, although episodes of acute suppuration may occur. The reactions in both are a walling-off process, with a marked chronic inflammatory cell infiltration. The proliferation of epithelium is always present in the marginal form of periodontal disease. It represents an attempt to cover the surface of the chronic ulcer that develops about the involved tooth root area. Histologically, the lesion is indistinguishable from the epithelium-lined granuloma unless identifying tooth structure is included in the tissue section.

Two cases of periodontal disease are illustrated in Figs. 26-11 and 26-12. That illustrated in Fig. 26-11 clearly shows evident signs of inflammation, bleeding, and recession of tissue, particularly about the mandibular left incisor. An acute periodontal abscess is apparent between the maxillary right central and lateral incisors. The roentgenogram of the mandibular incisors shows the presence of calculus on tooth root surfaces, slight loss of alveolar bone support, and widened periodontal ligament areas.

The case shown in Fig. 26-12 is one in which alveolar bone loss has progressed over a number of years. Signs and symptoms are minimal except for the development of excessive tooth mobility. The roentgenogram of the mandibular incisors shows an extreme degree of bone loss. The prognosis for restoring these periodontal tissues to health is poor, and extraction of one or more teeth is indicated. A histologic section through a closely similar area is shown in Fig. 26-13.

The disease commonly begins as a gingivitis. Deposits of plaque and calculus upon the tooth surfaces, impaction of food, decayed teeth, overhanging margins of dental restorations, and ill-fitting dental appliances are among the local causes.[77, 79] Once a "pocket" has been established below the gingival margin, calcified deposits form on the tooth root surfaces and act as an infected foreign body, thus prolonging and promoting

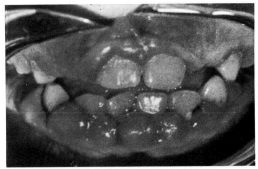

Fig. 26-14 Dilantin hyperplasia of gingiva.

the inflammatory process, with progressive resorption of the fibrous and bony tooth-supporting structures. Proliferation of epithelium to line the pocket occurs concomitantly with the loss of tissue. A purulent discharge from periodontal pockets can be elicited by digital pressure in many adult patients and even may occur in adolescents. Some individuals may show great resistance to the development of periodontal pockets in spite of adverse local factors, just as others have an extraordinary resistance to dental caries. Periodontal disease is more common in older individuals, and after middle age it becomes the chief cause of tooth loss.[75, 78]

Patients with diabetes mellitus are especially susceptible to periodontal disease, and an alert dentist may be led to suspect this condition because of oral signs and symptoms.[78]

Pregnancy with its change in endocrine balance frequently is accompanied by gingivitis and hyperplastic inflammatory responses. Gingivitis may be somewhat more frequent during puberty.[75]

Drug action, too, may cause gingival response. The hyperplasia associated with the use of Dilantin sodium may be so extensive that the teeth are almost completely covered by gingival enlargement[1] (Fig. 26-14).

Inflammatory diseases

Acute herpetic gingivostomatitis. Acute herpetic gingivostomatitis is the most common manifestation of primary infection with the herpes simplex virus. It is frequently misdiagnosed as necrotizing ulcerative gingivitis or Vincent's stomatitis. Occurring in less than 1% of the population, it is rarely, if ever, seen in a child under 1 year of age. It reaches its peak between the ages of 1 and 3 years, although it also is observed in older children and in young adults. The incubation period is four to six days. The gingiva is red and swollen, is exquisitely tender, and bleeds easily. Numerous vesicles and bullae are present on the labial, lingual, and buccal mucosae.[1, 85, 86, 95]

Microscopically, the herpes simplex vesicle shows multinucleated giant cells having two to fifteen nuclei per cell, and eosinophilic "inclusion bodies" are seen within the nuclei. Intraepithelial edema (ballooning degeneration) and intracellular edema are especially marked.

The herpes simplex virus may be identified by determination of neutralizing antibody titer, complement fixation, or specific skin test following the infection. There is a high incidence (70% to 90%) of neutralizing antibody in the adult population.

Hand-foot-and-mouth disease. Generally unrecognized, hand-foot-and-mouth disease is a self-limited, febrile disease caused by group A coxsackieviruses, principally type 16, less often types 5 and 10. It is manifest by many small vesicles or punched-out ulcers of the lips and buccal mucosa. The gingiva characteristically is spared, in contrast to herpetic stomatitis. Those affected are principally children under 10 years of age. Cutaneous involvement is usually limited to the palms, soles, and ventral surfaces and sides of fingers and toes.[1]

Recurrent herpes (cold sore; fever blister). Recurrent herpes occurs most frequently about the face and lips and tends to recur at the same site. The condition is characterized by groups of small clear vesicles on an erythematous base. The recurrent lesions seem to be induced by such agents as sunshine, fever, mechanical trauma, menses, and allergy.[1] Intraoral involvement is rare but may involve the hard palate and gingiva with pinhead-sized, grouped ulcers.

Recurrent aphthae (canker sores). Although resembling the lesions of recurrent herpes, recurrent aphthae are not caused by the herpes simplex virus. Somewhat similar lesions are seen on the oral mucosa in *Reiter's syndrome* (arthritis, conjunctivitis, and urethritis) and Behçet's syndrome (orogenital ulcerations and iridocyclitis).[84, 92]

Infectious mononucleosis. Infectious mononucleosis may present pronounced oral signs. In addition to inflammation of the oral pharynx and lymphadenopathy, about one-third of patients will exhibit a grayish or grayish green membrane resembling that of diphtheria or Vincent's angina over the throat or posterior buccal mucosa. The gingiva bleeds easily and becomes enlarged, resembling that in leukemia or scurvy.[80]

Agranulocytosis. Agranulocytosis often is manifest by ragged necrotic ulcers of the gingiva, palate, tonsils, or oropharynx.[1, 91] Sialorrhea may be marked. Drug sensitivity, especially to the barbiturates, amidopyrine, and the sulfonamides, is the best-known cause. Similar lesions are seen in *cyclic neutropenia,* a heritable disorder in which the neutrophils are decreased every twenty-one days.[88] Various *cytotoxic agents* employed in cancer chemotherapy produce severe oral ulceration.

Lethal granuloma (midline lethal granuloma). Probably a form of malignant reticulosis, lethal granuloma involves the palate, sinuses, and nasopharynx in a severe, progressive, ulcerative, destructive process.[83, 94]

Wegener's granulomatosis. Considered to be a form of hypersensitivity, Wegener's granulomatosis, a possible variant of polyarteritis nodosa, may be heralded by "multiple pyogenic granulomas" of the interdental papillae of the gingiva.[1]

Acute necrotizing gingivitis (Vincent's disease; fusospirochetosis). Acute necrotizing gingivitis is far less common than supposed.[98] Often the term "trench mouth" is used as a catchall to include primary herpetic gingivostomatitis, herpangina, infectious mononucleosis, etc. This is especially true in children, for fusospirochetosis is extremely uncommon in childhood (except in Africa), afflicting instead young and middle-aged adults. The disease is almost exclusively limited to the interdental papillae and the free gingival margin, rarely extending to the faucial area *(Vincent's angina)*. Necrosis and ulceration of one or more interdental gingival papillae, mild fever, fetid breath, malaise, and local discomfort characterize the condition. Predisposing conditions seem to allow penetration of the oral tissues by several symbiotic organisms normally inhabiting the mouth, among these a fusiform bacillus and an oral spirochete, *Borrelia vincenti.*

Noma (cancrum oris; gangrenous stomatitis). Noma may occur as a complication of acute necrotizing gingivitis in children or, rarely, in adults debilitated by infectious disease or possibly malnourishment. It is rare other than in the Far East and Africa. The process usually begins in a gingival ulceration and rapidly spreads to involve the cheeks, lips, and jawbones. The tissues become blackened and necrotic. Pneumonia and toxemia are common sequelae.[97]

Syphilis. In both the prenatal and the acquired forms, syphilis may be manifest about the mouth.[1] In the acquired form, the primary lesion or *chancre* may appear on the lips or tongue, simulating a squamous cell carcinoma. The secondary stage is characterized by the mucous patch (a milky white, focal, superficial ulcer of the oral mucosa), sore throat, and occasionally condyloma at the corner of the mouth (split papule). The hard palate may be perforated in the tertiary stage as a result of gumma formation. The tongue may be involved with a diffuse inflammatory process *(syphilitic glossitis)* that may predispose to the development of squamous cell carcinoma. Prenatal syphilis may be demonstrated by rhagades or radiating scars about the mouth and characteristic alteration in the form of the permanent teeth *(Hutchinson's incisors* and *mulberry molars),* in addition to the changes seen in the secondary and tertiary stages of acquired syphilis.[1]

Yaws. Yaws presents lesions somewhat similar to those of syphilis. The secondary papular lesions are commonly perioral. Tertiary lesions *(gangosa)* result in extensive destruction of the soft palate, hard palate, and nose.

Granuloma inguinale. Oral lesions of granuloma inguinale occur and are the most common extragenital (about 5% to 6%) manifestations of the disease[87] (p. 344).

Actinomycosis. Actinomycosis of the cervicofacial type arises through invasion of oral mucous membranes or a tooth socket, spreading to involve the jawbones, musculature, and salivary glands. Multiple foci of suppuration lead into sinus tracts that drain to the cutaneous surface or oral mucosa, liberating pus containing the typical and diagnostic "sulfur granules" of *Actinomyces israelii* or *Nocardia asteroides*[82] (see p. 411).

Histoplasmosis. Oral lesions of histoplasmosis are common and appear most frequently as nodular or ulcerated areas on the tongue or palate. *Tuberculosis* of the oral tissues is rare and usually is associated with advanced pulmonary disease. The typical lesion is an irregular, slowly enlarging, painful ulcer of the base of the tongue or palate.[81]

Many other fungal and tropical diseases have oral lesions—among them tropical sprue, leishmaniasis, scleroma, leprosy, and South American blastomycosis.

Candidosis (thrush). Candidosis is a fungal disease occurring most often in debilitated persons, infants, or especially individuals who have been taking oral antibiotics. It also may be associated in the form of a syndrome with hypoparathyroidism, keratoconjunctivitis, and Addison's disease. A chronic hyperplastic candidosis often is present. It is characterized by a pseudoepitheliomatous hyperplasia, with fungal invasion and a marked chronic inflammatory reaction. The fungus may invade the oral mucosa, skin, female genitalia, or urinary tract. Since the fungus *Candida albicans* is a normal oral inhabitant, the diagnosis cannot be made by smear alone. The presence of large numbers of oral spores of *Candida albicans* is strongly suggestive, however. The clinical appearance is that of numerous milk-white plaques—occasionally covering the entire oral mucosa—that are easily stripped off, leaving a bleeding surface due to penetration of the mycelia. Overclosure of the jaws in the edentulous patient or in the patient with poorly constructed dentures commonly results in low-grade chronic infection at the corners of the mouth, due at least in part to *Candida* organisms. This is called *perlèche* or *angular cheilitis.* True cheilosis, due to deficiency of one or more of the B complex vitamins, is far less common.[1]

Childhood exanthematous diseases. The childhood exanthematous diseases frequently manifest oral lesions. *Koplik's spots,* one of the prodromal signs of measles, are pinhead-

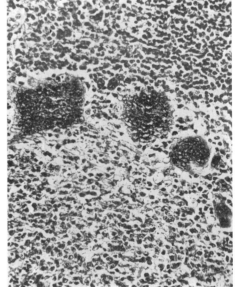

Fig. 26-15 Warthin-Finkeldey giant cells. These huge multinucleated cells appear in lymphoid follicles in prodromal stage of measles. These were found in lingual tonsils at base of tongue.

sized, bluish white spots surrounded by erythematous halos. They appear on the buccal or labial mucosa about eighteen hours prior to the skin rash. *Warthin-Finkeldey* giant cells may be observed in the tonsils or other lymphatic tissues if these structures happen to be biopsied during prodromal measles (Fig. 26-15).

Tumors and tumorlike lesions

Benign tumors and tumorlike lesions of oral soft tissues

Generalized or localized enlargement of the gingiva may arouse clinical suspicion of neoplastic disease. Enlarged gingival papillae, with bleeding upon slight pressure, are found in vitamin C deficiency (scorbutic gingivitis). Clinically similar appearances may indicate the local infiltration of the gingiva with immature leukocytes characteristic of one variety or another of leukemia.

In contrast, the gingiva may show localized or generalized enlargements that are dense and firm and that show little or no tendency to hemorrhage upon pressure. These may be associated with chronic local irritation and represent a formation of scar tissue. Diphenylhydantoin sodium (Dilantin) frequently causes a striking enlargement of the gingiva associated with a dense overgrowth of fibrous tissue.

All gingival enlargements become traumatized during mastication, toothbrushing, etc. Plasma cells, characteristically present in the gingiva in small numbers, may increase under inflammatory stimuli to simulate plasma cell myeloma or solitary plasmacytoma, but the presence of other inflammatory cells suggests the correct diagnosis of plasma cell granuloma.

Fibromatosis gingivae. Fibromatosis gingivae represents a proliferation of the entire gingiva. Inflammation is characteristically absent, the gingiva being of normal color and hard texture. The normal eruption of teeth is prevented. Fibromatosis gingivae may rarely be associated with hypertrichosis, seizures, and mental retardation. An autosomal dominant genetic pattern is common.[125]

Papilloma. Papilloma is an arborescent growth consisting of numerous squamous epithelial fingerlike projections, each of which contains a well-vascularized, fibrous connective tissue core. Although it may be seen throughout the mouth, the tongue and periuvular area are especially common sites.[1]

Fibroma. The most common benign oral mucous membrane "tumor," fibroma occurs as a discrete superficial pedunculated mass. Such lesions appear to be nonneoplastic in nature, arising in response to physical trauma. An example of this type of reaction is the so-called denture injury tumor. Microscopically, fibromas are composed of collagenic fibrous connective tissue covered by keratinized or parakeratinized stratified squamous epithelium. Not uncommonly, myxomatous degeneration, metaplastic bone formation, or fatty infiltration is noted in the connective tissue.[125]

Lipoma and "amputation neuroma." Although uncommon, lipoma and "amputation neuroma" may occur, particularly in the mandibular gingivobuccal sulcus. The former probably is derived from the buccal fat pad. The amputation neuroma is a pseudotumor consisting of congeries of nerve bundles that have proliferated into a knotlike mass, usually subsequent to surgery in the region of the mental foramen.[125]

Neurilemoma and neurofibroma. Neurilemoma and neurofibroma are also observed in oral environs, especially the tongue. Neurofibroma may occur as an isolated lesion or as part of Recklinghausen's *neurofibromatosis*. The lesions of the latter condition may be of at least three types: discrete, diffuse, or plexiform.[125] Both *osteoma* and *chondroma* have been reported in the tongue.

Granular cell tumor or granular cell myoblastoma. First described by Abrikossoff in 1926 and assumed initially to be of striated muscle origin, granular cell tumor has, in recent years, been the subject of considerable controversy. Many investigators now believe it to be of neural origin, whereas others suggest that it represents not a true neoplasm but a special type of muscle degeneration. Recently, histochemical and electron microscopic investigations have added support to the neural theory of origin.[99, 124, 125, 127]

Granular cell myoblastoma is usually benign. Although having its origin in many tissues, especially the skin, about 40% arise in the tongue. There appears to be no age preference except for an interesting variant that occurs at birth on the anterior alveolar ridges and has been called *congenital epulis of the newborn*. It is seen almost exclusively in female infants.

Microscopically, the tumor consists of large polyhedral cells with an acidophilic granular cytoplasm. Ultrastructural studies have demonstrated that the "granules" are lysosome-

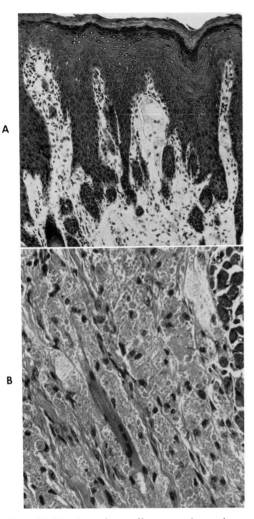

Fig. 26-16 Granular cell tumor (granular cell myoblastoma). Tongue and skin are two most frequent sites. Also occurs in gingiva of female infants as so-called congenital epulis of newborn. **A,** Pseudoepitheliomatous proliferation may be marked, simulating squamous cell carcinoma. **B,** Tumor consists of sheets of large cells with granular eosinophilic cytoplasm and small hyperchromatic nuclei.

like structures.[127] The nucleus is small, somewhat pyknotic, and eccentrically placed. Pseudoepitheliomatous hyperplasia, characteristically absent in the congenital epulis, may be so marked in the tongue lesion that a diagnosis of squamous cell carcinoma may be erroneously made (Fig. 26-16). While the histology of this lesion is specific, its histogenesis is not. Other benign muscle tumors, *leiomyoma* and *rhabdomyoma*, have been reported in the tongue, lip, and uvula but are rare.[125]

Hemangioma. Hemangioma of the oral mucous membranes is essentially similar to that of the skin and may occur in any area of the mouth. Although it is most commonly of the capillary type, cavernous and mixed types also are seen. These often congenital lesions should not be confused with the exuberant overgrowth of granulation tissue designated as *granuloma pyogenicum,* which apparently arises as the result of trauma and nonspecific infection. The granuloma pyogenicum is indistinguishable, microscopically, from the so-called *"pregnancy tumor"* that arises on the gingiva during the second trimester of gestation in at least 10% of gravid females. Consisting of new capillaries, fibroblasts, and polymorphonuclear neutrophils, these lesions frequently last long after termination of pregnancy, eventuating in a fibroma-like lesion.[125]

Hereditary hemorrhagic telangiectasia (Osler-Rendu-Weber disease). Hereditary hemorrhagic telangiectasia is manifest by numerous spiderlike angiomatoses of the lips and tongue. Nasal mucosal involvement results in frequent epistaxis. Usually noted at puberty, the condition is inherited as an autosomal dominant characteristic. Microscopically, the individual lesion is a superficial blood vessel surrounded by abnormal elastic fibers that permit dilatation.[125]

Encephalofacial angiomatosis (Sturge-Weber syndrome). Encephalofacial angiomatosis consists of superficial and deep-seated hemangiomas, usually of the upper two-thirds or half of the face, associated with leptomeningeal angiomas, cerebral calcifications, seizures, glaucoma, and mental retardation. There are many clinical variations.[125]

Lymphangioma. The majority of lymphangiomas are found at birth in the head and neck region and may cause enlargement of the tongue (macroglossia) and the lip (macrocheilia). *Cystic hygroma* is a special type of lymphangioma occurring in the cervical region in the newborn infant.

Solitary plasmacytoma. Solitary plasmacytoma of the mouth occurs as a soft tissue lesion without bone involvement (especially about the tonsillar area and antrum) or as part of a generalized myeloma. About one-third of the cases of solitary plasmacytoma eventuate in multiple myeloma. There is a very definite predilection for males (about 2:1). Rarely are they seen in individuals under 30 years of age. Grossly, they are smooth, soft, and somewhat rubbery tumors. Microscopically, they are indistinguishable from plasma cell myeloma. Differential diagnosis includes *plasma cell granuloma.*[116]

Malignant tumors of oral cavity
Squamous cell carcinoma

Squamous cell carcinoma (epidermoid carcinoma) is the most common oral malignant neoplasm, and approximately 7 per 100,000 deaths in the United States are currently attributed to it annually. Further, investigations in Minnesota indicate that among adults 45 years of age or older, 1 in every 1,000 examined has this lesion of the lip or other oral structure.[126] Tobacco, syphilis, and alcohol have been etiologically implicated for many years, although they are not considered primary causes.[1, 122] Chronic inflammations, such as caused by poorly fitting prostheses, poor oral hygiene, or inadequate dental restorations, probably are not important etiologic factors. Approximately 10% of patients having or having had oral carcinoma have or will have another.[101] Oral white patches are observed in association with squamous cell carcinoma in up to 75% of instances, and it is considered likely that many superficial malignancies evolve in this fashion.[1]

The clinical appearance of small or early examples of the malignancy may vary from white, thickened, or verrucous to soft, red, velvety or ulcerative. Induration is also clinically indicative of oral malignancy.

Squamous cell carcinomas of the lip or oral cavity are, generally, histologically well differentiated and occur in males 40 years of age and older. This may yield an erroneous impression, however, for the oral cavity offers neoplasms with as great a clinicopathologic diversity as any body part. Metastasis most frequently occurs first in ipsilateral, submandibular, or cervical lymph nodes. The presence or absence of lymph node metastasis is an important index of the clinical stage of the disease. A sarcoidal reaction may be seen in regional cervical lymph nodes in perhaps 6% of cases of carcinoma of the tongue, parotid gland, and oral cavity, especially after radiation therapy, probably as a result of the necrotic products of the tumor.[108]

Squamous cell carcinoma of lip. Squamous cell carcinoma of the lip is almost exclusively a male disease, less than 3% of the cases occurring in women. Originating most frequently in the sixth to eighth decades, approximately 90% arise on the vermilion border of the lower lip, usually on one side of the midline. It presents as a painless, characteristically indurated, ulcerated or exophytic lesion. Usually, lip carcinoma is well differentiated (about 60%) and slow to metastasize to the

submental and submandibular nodes. Prognosis is good[100] whether the lesion is treated by radiation or by surgery, five-year cure rates being about equal (80%). Carcinoma of the lip is more common in individuals of light complexion, especially in those who, because of their occupation, receive an unusual amount of actinic radiation, such as farmers, sailors, and policemen. About 6% have multiple lip carcinomas, either simultaneously or at intervals. Over 10% have at least one cancer of the skin, and over 3% have an oral, pharyngeal, laryngeal, or esophageal carcinoma.[100, 115]

Early malignant alterations of lip epithelium appear as localized keratotic plaques that may resolve, only to reappear. Alternately, malignant degeneration is indicated by diffuse, thin whitening of superficial portions of the vermilion border of the lip.

Squamous cell carcinoma of tongue. Squamous cell carcinoma of the tongue is the most frequent intraoral malignant lesion, comprising about one-half of the cases.[106] It is less exclusively a male disease (about 75% in males) than is carcinoma of the lip. Approximately 80% of the cases arise in the sixth to eighth decades. In Scandinavia, however, the disease is not rare in women and commonly is associated with *Plummer-Vinson syndrome* (atrophy of mucous membrane, iron deficiency anemia, and dysphagia). There appears to be a positive correlation between carcinoma of the tongue, especially of the dorsal surface, and syphilitic glossitis, the incidence of carcinoma of the tongue being about four times as common in individuals with syphilis (Fig. 26-17).

The lateral border and ventral surfaces of the tongue are frequent sites of carcinoma (about 65%). Metastases, frequently bilateral (about 20%), are present in about 35% of

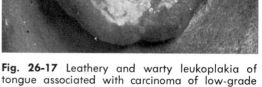

Fig. 26-17 Leathery and warty leukoplakia of tongue associated with carcinoma of low-grade malignancy.

the patients at the time of hospital admission. Contralateral metastasis occurs in less than 3%.

Survival figures indicate that the prognosis for patients with squamous cell carcinoma of the tongue is dependent on several factors. The small, early lesion of low-grade malignancy without evidence of metastasis or marked local invasion may be successfully managed by surgery or radiation therapy. Approximately 60% of such patients live five years or more. This figure is reduced to 30% in instances where the tumor is anaplastic or has metastasized.[1]

Squamous cell carcinoma of floor of mouth. Squamous cell carcinoma of the floor of the mouth (about 15% of oral cases) is typically manifest as an indurated ulcer in the anterior portion about the openings of the sublingual and submandibular glands, with over 80% occurring in males.[104] The carcinoma invades rapidly, spreading to the submandibular lymph nodes (about 50%) and to the submandibular and sublingual salivary glands, tongue, and mandibular gingiva. Treatment, usually radiation, yields a survival rate similar to that for carcinoma of the tongue. While white patches are observed throughout the oral cavity in a variety of clinical circumstances, the white patch on the mouth floor, however subtle, should be thoroughly investigated. Early squamous cell carcinoma of the area frequently will be overlooked if this is not done.

Squamous cell carcinoma of buccal mucosa. Squamous cell carcinoma of the buccal mucosa constitutes from one-fourth to one-third of all oral carcinomas and varies in frequency in different geographic areas.[104] In India and other countries in which betel nut and tobacco chewing are commonplace, buccal carcinomas are the major cancer.[117] Abnormal keratinization is especially common in this group. Oral submucous fibrosis may be another premalignant mucosal alteration.[115a] Progressive infiltrative growth, local recurrence following treatment, and local lymph node metastasis characterize squamous cell carcinoma originating in the cheeks. Five-year survival figures vary, but approximately 50% of affected patients survive this period after diagnosis and adequate surgical or radiation therapy. Patients rarely succumb to the disease from complications associated with distant metastasis. Rather, malnutriiton, asphyxia, pneumonia, etc. complicate local tumor growth and lead to death.

An unusual form of epidermoid carcinoma most frequently involving the buccal mucosa and mandibular gingiva is *verrucous carcinoma*.[107] In the United States, in the midsouth, it is commonly associated with the prolonged use of snuff placed in the gingivobuccal sulcus. It is characteristically associated with leukoplakia, growing into large, fungating, soft, papillary masses. Microscopic diagnosis may be difficult and delayed, for the tumor presents an unusually well-differentiated pattern. Although destruction may be extensive and recurrence frequent (about 75%), metastasis is unusual. Patients are especially prone to develop additional, sometimes less differentiated oral carcinomas.

Squamous cell carcinoma of gingiva. Squamous cell carcinoma of the gingiva constitutes about 10% of oral malignancy and is more common in men than women (about 4:1). It has been more frequent on the mandibular gingiva, and its early, clinical resemblance to more common inflammatory conditions in this location may lead to delayed diagnosis. Tobacco and syphilis are less clearly related etiologically to gingival carcinoma than to carcinomas of the tongue or cheek. Early involvement of contiguous structures, such as bone and lymph nodes, characterizes the tumor.[1, 102]

Squamous cell carcinoma of palate. Squamous cell carcinoma of the palate may be ulcerative and/or tumorous. The tumors are more often of high grade malignancy and occur about four times more frequently in men than in women. Although the lesions often are symptomless, patients may complain of a dental prosthesis that has become ill-fitting. Pain may be a late clinical feature. Early involvement of underlying bone is a common feature. The soft palate is the more frequent site.[1, 120]

Pseudosarcoma (carcinosarcoma)

Pseudosarcoma (carcinosarcoma) occasionally is associated with an intramucosal or in situ squamous cell carcinoma of the mouth or oral pharynx. Bizarre, sarcoma-like proliferation of neoplastic cells results in bulky polypoid masses that may only faintly resemble carcinoma.[110, 111]

Carcinoma in situ

An occasional oral carcinoma, regardless of location, may demonstrate all cytologic criteria of malignant neoplasia yet fail to show any histologic evidence of invasion. The term *carcinoma in situ* is used in this case.[119] Considerable variability in the clinical appearance of carcinoma in situ has been experienced. The terms bowenoid (see Bowen's disease of skin, p. 1649), erythroplastic (see erythroplasia of Queyrat, p. 855), and leukoplakia-like are used to describe the variable clinical appearance.

Lymphoepithelial carcinoma

Lymphoepithelial carcinoma may be found in the faucial area and base of the tongue, as well as in the nasopharynx and nasal cavity. Since the primary lesion is frequently small and undiscovered, the first clinical sign is often regional adenopathy and dysphagia. The "lymphoepithelioma" consists of syncytial masses of large polyhedral cells with eosinophilic cytoplasm, a large nucleus, large eosinophilic nucleoli, and a stroma infiltrated by numerous small lymphocytes (Regaud type). The cells of the "transitional cell carcinoma" are large, poorly differentiated, and anaplastic (Schmincke type). Radiation therapy is employed for both neoplasms, the survival rate approaching 30%.[1]

Other tumors

Kaposi's sarcoma, liposarcoma, rhabdomyosarcoma, embryonal rhabdomyosarcoma, alveolar soft part sarcoma, etc. have been reported but are uncommon. Leukemic infiltration of the gingiva is seen with regularity in affected patients.[113, 125]

Primary malignant melanoma

Primary malignant melanoma of the oral cavity is relatively rare. About twice as common in males as in females, the peak incidence is in the sixth decade. Seldom has a case been reported in anyone under 20 years of age. Approximately 80% arise in the hard palate, alveolar ridge, or soft palate. Metastatic spread is exceedingly common. The five-year survival rate appears to be about 5%.[121]

JAWS
Developmental lesions

Exostoses (tori). Exostoses or bony protuberances are not uncommon about the mouth. The most frequent is *torus palatinus,* which occurs in the midline of the hard palate in about 20% of the white population. *Torus mandibularis* is less frequent (about 7% of the white population), generally bilateral (80%), and is found on the lingual surface of the mandible, usually opposite the premolars. It

is inherited as an autosomal dominant trait.[1, 128, 140] *Multiple exostoses* are still less common and occur as small nodular outgrowths on the buccal surface of the maxilla and mandible, opposite the premolars and molars.

Osteomatosis. Osteomatosis may be associated with polyposis and adenocarcinoma of the colon and multiple cutaneous and mesenteric fibromas and lipomas. Epidermoid inclusion cysts are scattered over the body. The syndrome (Gardner's) is transmitted as an autosomal dominant trait.[2, 147, 153]

Microscopically, the bony growths consist of dense, irregular bone with well-marked haversian systems and fibrous medullary portions. Cartilage is never observed. Blood calcium, phosphorus, and alkaline phosphatase levels are within normal limits.

Pigmented neuroectodermal tumor of infancy (retinal anlage tumor; melanoameloblastoma; melanotic progonoma). A tumor of the jaws, the pigmented neuroectodermal tumor is a rare benign lesion of neural crest origin, largely restricted to the maxilla of infants.[109, 125, 142] At time of discovery of the tumor, the infant is nearly always under 6 months of age. A few similar tumors have been reported in the shoulder, epididymis, man-

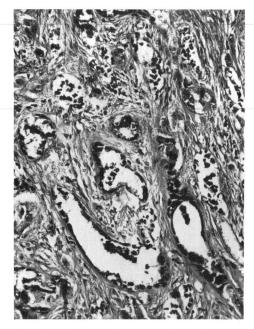

Fig. 26-18 Pigmented neuroectodermal tumor of infancy. This hamartomatous lesion is composed of numerous tubules in fibrous connective tissue stroma. Tubules lined by large cuboidal cells containing melanin. Within lumina are cells resembling neuroblasts.

dible, calvaria, and brain. There is little evidence of odontogenic origin and insufficient evidence to imply origin in the retinal anlage. Borello and Gorlin[131] have demonstrated that the tumor elaborates vanilmandelic acid, and neural crest origin appears likely. Ultrastructural evidence supports this view.[109]

Grossly, the tumor is pigmented and well circumscribed, although no well-defined capsule is present. Microscopically, the tumor consists of a fibrous connective tissue stroma in which tubules or spaces are present in large numbers (Fig. 26-18). The spaces are lined by a single layer of large cuboidal cells with abundant cytoplasm in which are found numerous melanin granules. The spaces frequently are filled with many deeply staining cells that are smaller than the duct cells and contain much less cytoplasm.

Inflammatory and metabolic lesions

Acute suppurative osteomyelitis. Acute suppurative osteomyelitis of the jaws has become a relatively rare disease with the advent of antibiotics.[1] Usually due to infection of the marrow cavity with *Staphylococcus aureus* subsequent to jaw fracture or severe periapical disease, the process spreads, especially in the lower jaw, causing severe pain and facial cellulitis. When the resistance of the host is high or the virulence of the organism low, a chronic focal sclerosing osteomyelitis or condensing osteitis is seen.

Osteomyelitis of jaw of newborn infant. A distinct clinical entity, osteomyelitis of the jaw of the newborn infant almost exclusively involves the upper jaw.[145]

Garré's chronic sclerosing osteomyelitis with proliferative periosteitis. Garré's chronic sclerosing osteomyelitis with proliferative periosteitis is a nonsuppurating type seen most often in the lower jaw in children and young adults.[1]

Infantile cortical hyperostosis (Caffey's disease). Infantile cortical hyperostosis appears in infants, usually within the first three months of life, as a bilateral cortical thickening of the mandible, being inherited as an autosomal dominant trait.[144]

Osteoradionecrosis of the jaws. Osteoradionecrosis of the jaws, principally affecting the mandible, follows extensive therapeutic radiation in about 5% of patients. The severity seems to be proportional to the radiation dose, the presence of peridental sepsis, and the degree of trauma to the tissue by ill-fitting dentures, etc.[143]

Osteitis deformans (Paget's disease of bone). Osteitis deformans may involve the jaws, especially the maxilla, with progressive enlargement and displacement of teeth. This becomes especially apparent if the patient wears dentures.[135]

Histiocytosis X (Letterer-Siwe disease; Hand-Schüller-Christian disease; eosinophilic granuloma). In histiocytosis X, the jaws are sites of deposits of foamy histiocytes. It has been reported that 93% of patients had sore, swollen necrotic gingivae and 78% had loose, sore teeth that rapidly exfoliated. The premolar-molar region of the mandible more frequently than the maxilla is the most common area of involvement. Loss of trabeculae, pseudocyst formation, and dental root resorption are typical roentgenographic findings.[141, 148]

Giant cell granuloma. Giant cell "reparative" granuloma is a nonneoplastic lesion of unknown etiology that appears to be limited to the jaws.[1] Treatment consists of simple excision and curettage. Although resembling true giant cell tumor of bone, it has certain properties and microscopic characteristics that separate it as a distinct entity. It constitutes about 3% of benign jaw tumors. It is found either centrally or peripherally (epulis), being about equally distributed. It is somewhat more common in the mandible and in females. The roentgenographic appearance is not pathognomonic, being solitary, radiolucent, and sharply delineated. The lamina dura may be displaced. Grossly, the tissue is usually reddish brown or black, depending upon the amount of hemorrhage. Not uncommonly, the surface is eroded or ulcerated.

Microscopically, the giant cell granuloma consists of an admixture of multinucleated giant cells scattered in a very cellular stroma from which the giant cells probably are derived (Fig. 26-19). The stromal cell has a round or oval nucleus, small nucleolus, prominent nuclear membrane, and poorly delineated cytoplasmic boundaries. Nuclear pleomorphism, hyperchromatism, and marked mitotic activity are characteristically absent. Hemosiderin pigment, evidence of old hemorrhage, often is seen lying free or ingested by mononuclear phagocytes. Collagen production is quite common, whereas osteoid is present less often, and both are nearly always absent from the true giant cell tumor.

Microscopic differentiation should include true giant cell tumor (extremely rare in the

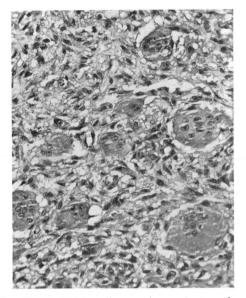

Fig. 26-19 Giant cell granuloma. Lesion characterized by numerous multinucleated giant cells in fibrous cellular stroma from which giant cells are derived. Collagen, osteoid, or bone frequently formed.

jaws), cherubism, fibrous dysplasia, aneurysmal bone cyst, benign chondroblastoma, chondromyxoid fibroma, and nonosteogenic fibroma. The lesions of *hyperparathyroidism* cannot be differentiated on a microscopic basis from central giant cell granuloma, and in the case of recurrence or multiple or satellite lesions, blood and urinary calcium levels always should be determined. Also suggestive of hyperparathyroidism is disappearance of the lamina dura about the teeth, but this is less common than is generally believed.

Tumors and tumorlike lesions

Fibrous dysplasia. The jaws are frequently involved in fibrous dysplasia of the monostotic or polyostotic types.[1, 146, 152] The monostotic form is the more common and seems to be more frequent in children and young adults. Clinically, it is manifest by a painless swelling of the bone. Displacement of teeth may be present. Polyostotic fibrous dysplasia, in addition to manifestation in several or many bones, may be accompanied by melanotic pigmentation of the skin and oral mucosa and endocrine disturbances, including precocious puberty in females *(Albright syndrome)*.

Cherubism. Cherubism is an autosomal dominantly inherited disease essentially limited to the jawbones. It has been imprecisely referred to as familial fibrous dysplasia.[1, 151] This condition is characterized by enlarge-

ment of the jaws during the second or third year of life, especially in the mandibular molar area. Bony expansion increases for a few years and then tapers off, finally regressing by puberty. Associated with the jaw anomaly are upturning of the eyes, revealing a rim of sclera, and nonspecific submandibular lymphadenopathy.

Microscopically, the bony lesion consists of vascular and usually collagenic fibrous connective tissue, having an abundant admixture of perivascular osteoclastic giant cells. Not uncommonly, fibrin is deposited around small capillaries.

Malignant tumors metastatic to jaws. Malignant tumors metastatic to the jaws are relatively uncommon, spread probably taking place through the vertebral system of veins. In an extensive survey, there was an indication of the following order of frequency: carcinoma of breast, lung, large intestine, prostate and kidney, thyroid gland, and testis.[134]

The tooth-bearing area of the body and the molar regions of the mandible are the most frequent sites, possibly because of greater arterial blood supply in these regions. In about one-half of the cases, the oral metastasis is the first sign of the generalized cancer. Swelling, pain, and anesthesia are the most common symptoms.

Osteosarcoma (osteogenic sarcoma). Approximately 10% of osteosarcomas occur in the jaws. Accessibility, a feature leading to early treatment, and greater histopathologic differentiation likely contribute to the relatively more favorable prognosis appreciated by this malignant tumor when observed in oral sites.[130]

Chondrosarcoma. Less frequently encountered in the jaws than osteosarcoma, chondrosarcoma has been less successfully managed and may be more biologically malignant than chondrosarcoma of long bones. Microscopically, chondrosarcoma and osteosarcoma may appear benign early in their development. While both these nosologic entities may contain bone and cartilage, only the neoplastic cells of the latter, osteosarcoma, produce osteoid.[133]

Fibrosarcoma. Fibrosarcomas of jaws also have been observed. They may originate in periosteal or central locations. Histopathologic interpretation and diagnosis are complicated by the numerous other fibrous or spindle cell neoplasms observed in the jawbones.

Multiple myeloma and Ewing's sarcoma. Multiple myeloma and Ewing's sarcoma may be initially manifest as a lesion of the jaws, but this is uncommon. Usually, jaw involvement is merely a part of the generalized disease.[138]

Malignant lymphoma. In contrast to most other primary malignancies of the jawbones, malignant lymphomas of the jaws occur more frequently in the maxilla.[149]

Burkitt's lymphoma. An undifferentiated lymphosarcoma, Burkitt's lymphoma, has been described in the jaws and abdominal viscera of equatorial African children from 3 to 8 years of age, constituting about 50% of all malignant tumors in this age group. Arising most often in the maxillary alveolar process, it is destructive, effecting loss of deciduous molars. The process extends to involve the parotid gland, antrum, nasopharynx, and orbit. Usually, there is no associated lymphadenopathy.[132, 154]

Recent evidence suggests that the Epstein-Barr virus is immunologically associated with Burkitt's tumor and infectious mononucleosis[1] (see also p. 1354).

Cysts

Cysts of the jaws and mouth usually are classified according to their odontogenic or nonodontogenic origin. However, a number of oral lesions called "cysts" on clinical or roentgenographic evidence alone do not fall within the definition of a pathologic, epithelium-lined cavity containing fluid or debris. The salivary gland retention "cyst" (mucocele), ameloblastoma, traumatic bone "cyst," static bone cyst, and the lesions of hyperparathyroidism all fall within this category.[1]

Odontogenic cysts

Periodontal cyst. The most common odontogenic cyst is the periodontal cyst. Most often it is observed at the apex of an erupted tooth *(radicular type)*. The origin of this cyst appears to be in the cystic degeneration of epithelialized granulomas that have resulted most frequently as sequelae to dental caries and pulpitis. The origin of the stratified squamous epithelium lining these cysts is the epithelial rests of Malassez, which lie in the periodontal ligament. They are derived from Hertwig's root sheath. The walls of smaller cysts usually are infiltrated with chronic inflammatory cells.

Gingival cyst. The gingival cyst, multiple as a rule, occurs in the anterior jaws of infants and children.[137] This type becomes uncommon with increasing age. Those situated on the lat-

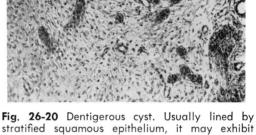

Fig. 26-20 Dentigerous cyst. Usually lined by stratified squamous epithelium, it may exhibit epithelial rests of Malassez within connective tissue wall.

eral surface of the root of erupted teeth have been called *lateral periodontal cysts.*

Dentigerous cyst. If the crown of the permanent tooth has been formed, fluid accumulation between the crown of the tooth and the reduced enamel epithelium results in the dentigerous cyst (Fig. 26-20).[1, 3, 4] The mandibular third molars and maxillary cuspids are most often involved. This cyst has significance because of the occasional massive resorption of involved jawbone that results from its unhampered expansion. Whereas the incidence of ameloblastomatous transformation within dentigerous cysts has not been precisely determined, the fact that such transformation does occur, the fact that ameloblastomas may appear cystic, and, finally, that histopathologic examination is required for these determinations render pathologic examination of such material mandatory.[172a]

Eruption cyst. A special type, occasionally bilateral, that does not involve bone, the eruption cyst, is seen rarely in the gingiva overlying erupting deciduous cuspids or molars.

Multiple cysts (odontogenic keratocysts). Multiple cysts of the jaws are associated in a syndrome with multiple nevoid basal cell carcinomas and skeletal anomalies, especially bifid rib and kyphoscoliosis.[136] The syndrome is inherited as an autosomal dominant trait. Lamellar calcification of the dura is common. Medulloblastoma also may be part of the syndrome.

Calcifying odontogenic cyst. The calcifying odontogenic cyst (Fig. 26-21) is characterized by masses of "ghost" or aberrantly keratinized

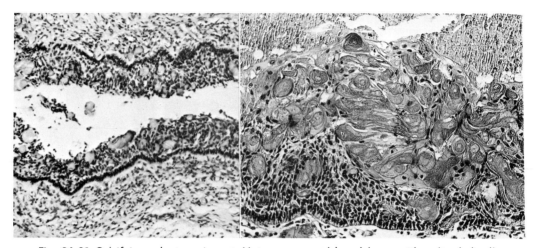

Fig. 26-21 Calcifying odontogenic cyst. Note pronounced basal layer with palisaded cells and large masses of partially keratinized "ghost" cells.

epithelium intermixed with the cells lining the cystic cavity. About one-third of these cysts occur extraosseously.

Nonodontogenic cysts

As the name implies, nonodontogenic cysts are not derived from the tissues of the developing tooth. Many have been classified as *fissural* or *inclusion cysts,* since they are believed to have their origin in epithelial rests in bone resulting from fusion of two or more embryologic processes.

Median anterior maxillary cyst (nasopalatine duct cyst; incisive canal cyst; cyst of palatine papilla). The most common nonodontogenic cyst is the median maxillary cyst, which arises from the epithelial remnants of the nasopalatine duct. It often is discovered in routine dental roentgenograms. It lies above and midway between the roots of the maxillary central incisors.

Globulomaxillary cyst. The globulomaxillary cyst is intraosseous and is located between the maxillary lateral incisor and cuspid at the embryologic junction of the globular process with the palatine process of the maxilla.

Nasoalveolar (nasolabial) and dermoid cysts. In contrast to the intraosseous cysts just mentioned, the nasoalveolar cyst and dermoid cyst are formed within soft tissue. The nasoalveolar cyst is formed at the junction of the globular, lateral nasal, and maxillary processes, being located at the ala of the nose and frequently extending into the nostril. The dermoid cyst is especially common in the head and neck, the floor of the mouth being the principal site. Dermoid cysts probably are derived from enclavement of epithelial debris in the midline during closure of mandibular and branchial arches.

■ ■ ■

From the practical standpoint, few cysts of the jaws can be differentiated from each other on microscopic basis alone. Generally, roentgenographic evidence and further information such as history, clinical appearance, and evidence derived from tooth vitality tests are necessary to establish a definite diagnosis. However, the following hints may help. Gingival, periodontal, dentigerous, primordial, and fissural (globulomaxillary, median anterior maxillary, nasoalveolar, etc.) cysts usually are lined by nonkeratinizing, stratified squamous epithelium overlying dense fibrous connective tissue. The dermoid cyst, on the other hand, is lined by a keratinized stratified squamous epithelium plus skin appendages. The radicular, periodontal, and fissural cysts commonly show secondary chronic inflammatory infiltrate especially rich in plasma cells. Far less frequently is this seen in dentigerous or gingival cysts. Fissural cysts of the maxilla not uncommonly are lined by ciliated columnar epithelium, at least in their superior part. The odontogenic keratocyst is lined by a thin layer of keratinized epithelium. Mucous glands and congeries of blood vessels and nerves frequently are noted in the connective tissue wall of the median anterior maxillary cyst. The mandibular dentigerous cyst occasionally may be lined in part by goblet cells or have lymphoid follicles or epithelial cell rests beneath the lining in the cyst wall. These proliferated rests of Malassez are responsible occasionally for an incorrect diagnosis of ameloblastoma.

Traumatic bone "cyst" (solitary or unicameral bone cyst). The traumatic bone "cyst" is not a true cyst. It is not lined by epithelium but by a thin membrane of connective tissue. Usually, no content is found other than a small amount of blood, serum, or granulation tissue laden with hemosiderin, macrophages, and a few foreign body giant cells.

Static or latent bone cyst (Stafne's cyst). The static or latent bone cyst is not a cyst but is a developmental defect usually containing salivary gland tissue. It is located on the inferior surface of the mandible just in front of the angle.

Gastric or intestinal epithelium–lined cyst. The gastric or intestinal epithelium–lined cyst

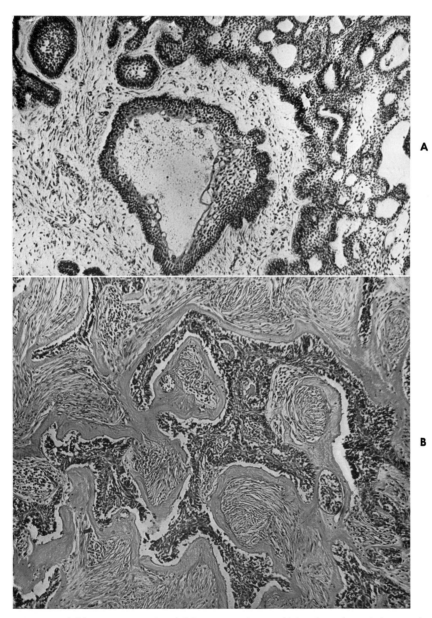

Fig. 26-22 Ameloblastoma. **A,** Ameloblastoma of mandible showing solid strands of enamel organs with formation of cystic spaces. Fibrous stoma. **B,** Atypical solid ameloblastoma of mandible. Cords of irregularly shaped epithelial cells surrounded by hyaline zone of very dense fibrous stroma.

is rare. It has been observed almost exclusively in males. The most common location is in the anterior portion of the oral floor or body of the tongue. It corresponds to developmental abnormalities ("duplications") seen elsewhere in the gastrointestinal tract.

Odontogenic tumors

Odontogenic tumors of the jaws arising from tooth-forming tissues are uncommon. There has been an interest in them, however, and classifications have been relatively numerous dating from that of Broca in 1867. Goldman and Thoma classified odontogenic tumors according to their tissue origin as epithelial, mesodermal, and mixed. Pindborg and Clausen, in 1958,[167] presented a classification that stressed the phenomenon or phenomena of induction in addition to histogenesis. Subsequent authors have expanded on this slightly.

While suffering, as it were, from a certain necessary complexity, the World Health Organization recently adopted a classification that allows for evaluation of the numerous transition forms. The interested reader is referred to this work and that of Gorlin[1] for a comprehensive discussion of the subject.

The classification that follows presents odontogenic tumors in a fashion that attempts simplification without sacrifice of histogenetic considerations. Moreover, it emphasizes clinical behavior in the traditional manner.

Benign
1 Ameloblastoma
2 Adenomatoid odontogenic tumor
3 Calcifying epithelial odontogenic tumor
4 Ameloblastic fibroma
5 Odontomas
6 Cementomas
7 Myxoma/myxofibroma

Malignant
1 Ameloblastic carcinoma (malignant ameloblastoma)
2 Ameloblastic fibrosarcoma

Ameloblastoma. Ameloblastoma is the most common of epithelial odontogenic tumors. It is comparatively uncommon, reportedly comprising about 1% of tumors and cysts arising in the jaws. It may arise from the epithelial lining of a dentigerous cyst, the remnants of dental lamina and enamel organ, or from the basal layer of the oral mucosa.

Analysis of over 1,000 cases reveals that ameloblastoma appears most commonly in the third to fifth decades.[168] No sex or racial preference is noted. Over 80% occur in the man-

dible, and 70% of these arise in the molar-ramus area. Rarely, an extraosseous example is discovered.[158, 159]

Because of its invasive property and tendency to recur, the ameloblastoma has been usually considered "locally malignant" but is benign. Distant metastases, especially to the lungs, have been reported in rare instances, but factors such as aspiration and transplantation are considered significant in these examples.[1, 160] Frankly carcinomatous neoplasms resembling dental organ epithelium are best considered *ameloblastic carcinoma*. Traditionally, ameloblastoma has been divided into solid and cystic types, but nearly all ameloblastomas demonstrate some cystic degeneration. Microscopically, many subtypes or patterns have been suggested: follicular, plexiform, acanthomatous, granular cell (Figs. 26-22 and 26-23), and vascular varieties. However, two or more types may occur within the same tumor, and there is no evidence that any subtype is more aggressive than any other.

The majority of ameloblastomas demonstrate one of the two predominant patterns, follicular and plexiform, the former being the more common. In the follicular type there is an attempt to mimic the dental organ epithe-

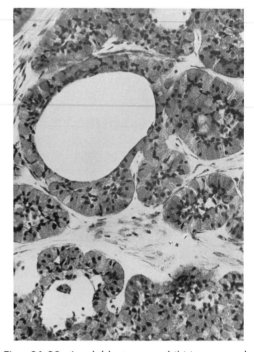

Fig. 26-23 Ameloblastoma exhibiting granular cell pattern. Occasionally, whole tumor may be composed of large granular cells with eosinophilic granular cytoplasm.

lium. The outermost cells resemble those of the inner dental epithelium of the developing tooth follicle—i.e., the ameloblastic layer. The cells are tall columnar, with marked polarization of the nuclei away from the basement membrane.[172a] The central portion of the epithelial island is composed of a loose network of cells resembling stellate reticulum. Squamous metaplasia within the stellate reticulum gives rise to the acanthomatous type. The epithelial islands demonstrate no inductive influence upon the collagenized connective tissue stroma. Enamel and dentin are never formed by the ameloblastoma. The plexiform pattern demonstrates irregular masses and interdigitating cords of epithelial cells with a minimum of stroma.

Adenomatoid odontogenic tumor (ameloblastic adenomatoid tumor). A benign lesion, the adenomatoid odontogenic tumor probably arises from the preameloblast or inner enamel epithelium.[1, 164] It appears to be more common in females, arises somwhat more often in the anterior region of the upper jaw, and occurs most frequently in the second decade of life. Frequently it is associated with an unerupted cuspid. Although the tumor expands, it is not invasive and does not recur even after extremely conservative surgical therapy.

Microscopically, the lesion consists of con- geries of ductlike structures, lined by medium to tall columnar epithelium, in an extremely scant fibrous connective tissue stroma (Fig. 26-24). Small calcified deposits are often seen scattered throughout the epithelial tissue.

Calcifying epithelial odontogenic tumor. The calcifying epithelial odontogenic tumor is a rather rare lesion. The tumor has been invasive and may be locally recurrent. It seems to occur more commonly in the fourth and fifth decades. There is no sex predilection. Several of the reported cases have arisen in the mandibular premolar-molar area in association with an embedded tooth.[1, 157]

Microscopically, the tumor is composed of polyhedral epithelial cells with scanty stroma. The closely packed cells frequently demonstrate nuclear pleomorphism. Intracellular degeneration results in numerous spherical spaces filled with eosinophilic homogeneous material that in time becomes calcified. This has been shown to be amyloid by Vickers et al.[172] (Fig. 26-25).

Ameloblastic fibroma. The ameloblastic fibroma (soft mixed odontoma) is characterized by proliferation of both epithelial and mesenchymal elements in the absence of hard tooth structure, i.e., enamel and/or dentin. In contrast to ameloblastoma, the tumor for which it is most commonly mistaken, the

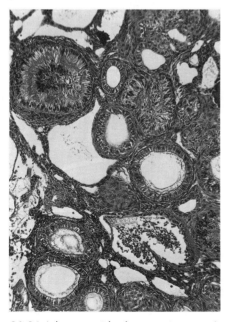

Fig. 26-24 Adenomatoid odontogenic tumor (ameloblastic adenomatoid tumor). Consists of congeries of tubules. Possibly arises from preameloblast.

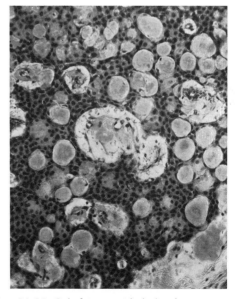

Fig. 26-25 Calcifying epithelial odontogenic tumor. Very rare, somewhat aggressive tumor arising from reduced enamel epithelium. Droplets of calcified amyloid material frequently exhibit Liesegang rings.

ameloblastic fibroma usually occurs in a young age group, rarely being seen in individuals over 21 years of age. Clinical behavior is entirely benign.[1, 156]

Microscopically, the ameloblastic fibroma is composed of strands and buds of epithelial cells in a very cellular connective tissue stroma (Fig. 26-26). The presence of this reactive stroma clearly differentiates this lesion from ameloblastoma. For the most part, the cells composing the strands of epithelial cells are cuboidal and are one cell layer thick. Only occasionally a stellate reticulum is present. In contrast to ameloblastoma, simple curettement of the ameloblastic fibroma is adequate treatment.

Odontomas. Three subtypes or varieties of odontogenic tumors featuring production of calcified parts of teeth are usually considered: *complex odontoma,* in which enamel, dentin, cementum, etc., have not differentiated to the point where an actual tooth can be recognized; *compound odontoma,* in which a tooth or teeth, regardless of size or fine form, can be discerned; and *ameloblastic odontoma,* in which an additional component resembling dental organ epithelium (ameloblastomatous) is observed in addition to enamel, dentin, etc.[1]

Complex odontoma has been most frequently encountered in molar areas of the mandible and more often observed in female patients. Differentiation is poor, and a variety of calcified patterns is observed. The enamel, dentin, and cementum may be virtually unidentifiable. While the tumors occasionally achieve considerable proportions, they are entirely benign. Growth and symptomatology are slight. They are frequently diagnosed following routine radiographic examinations.

Compound odontoma presents a higher degree of differentiation than complex odontoma, and the individual lesion characteristically consists of masses of small, misshapen teeth. Some may have as few as three teeth, whereas the exception has been reported containing 2,000 denticles. These odontomas behave in an entirely benign fashion. They are more commonly encountered in anterior regions of the jaws and in the maxilla more often than in the mandible.

Ameloblastic odontoma is much less frequent than either complex or compound odontoma. While dental hard tissues such as enamel and dentin in the odontomas under discussion necessarily form through action of ameloblasts and odontoblasts, certain odontomas are encountered that possess a striking epithelial component. In these instances, the

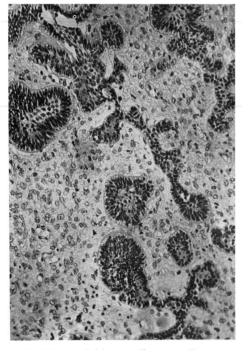

Fig. 26-26 Ameloblastic fibroma. Consists of numerous islands of odontogenic epithelium in cellular mesenchymal matrix. This tumor is nonaggressive and must be differentiated from ameloblastomas, which lack mesenchymal matrix.

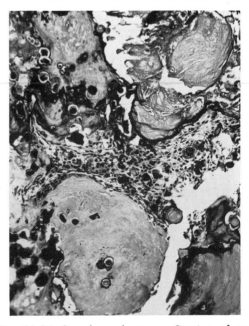

Fig. 26-27 Complex odontoma. Consists of unorganized mass of dentin, enamel, cementum, and pulpal tissue and occasional areas of enamel epithelium.

term *ameloblastic odontoma* has been employed. They are considered benign but may, on occasion, behave more aggressively and recur locally following conservative surgical removal.[1, 161]

Cementomas. Three, possibly four, apparently unrelated lesions of the jaws can be identified within this group characterized by benign neoplastic formation of cementum or cementum-like hard tissue within a cellular fibrous connective tissue.[1, 173]

Cementoma or periapical fibrous dysplasia (periapical cemental dysplasia) has been the most frequently encountered, and estimates place the prevalence at 2 to 3 per 1,000 individuals. Females are principally affected. Multiple mandibular teeth are usually involved by asymptomatic, small radiolucencies or, later, radiopacities that may be confused with dental inflammations. Treatment is not required.

Familial multiple cementomas, much less frequently encountered, have been reported with varying terminology in middle-aged black females. There are swelling and deformity, and multiple areas of both jaws appear to be affected.[31]

Diagnosis of the several fibrous, ossifying, and/or "cementifying" jaw lesions, such as the so-called true cementomas, cementoblastomas, cementifying fibromas, fibrous dysplasias, etc., represents a most consuming exercise of pathology. In each instance, the clinical history, radiographic examination, histopathology, and, occasionally, blood chemistry are required.

Myxoma and/or myxofibroma; odontogenic fibroma. Myxoma of bone does not occur outside of the jaws.[155] Most investigators believe that this lesion is of tooth germ origin (dental papilla) and have called it **odontogenic myxoma.** Some examples are associated with the proliferation of large numbers of small epithelial rests of Malassez. The **odontogenic fibroma** differs microscopically from the myxoma only by the presence of collagenic fibrous connective tissue and greater numbers of odontogenic epithelial rests.

About 60% of odontogenic myxomas and fibromas occur during the second and third decades. The maxilla and mandible are equally affected. The tumors are slow growing. Bony expansion may be great, however, producing marked facial deformity. Microscopically, the myxoma consists of loose stellate cells with long, anastomosing cytoplasmic processes (Fig. 26-28). Occasionally, an inactive strand of odontogenic epithelium is noted around the edge of the tumor.

Malignant ameloblastoma (ameloblastic carcinoma). We have encountered four neoplasms, three maxillary and one mandibular, that besides possessing histologic criteria of ameloblastoma manifest malignant cytologic features such as numerous mitotic figures and marked clinical aggressiveness. While one is struck by the relative rarity of malignant odontogenic neoplasms, this possibility may not at the present time be excluded.

Ameloblastic fibrosarcoma. Ameloblastic fibrosarcomas have also been rarely observed. Initially, these pathologic "curiosities" presented histopathologic features of ameloblastic fibroma. Recurrences were marked by an increasingly malignant-appearing connective tissue portion, diminution or absence of the epithelial component, and malignant behavior. Pain has preceded the nine instances available for analysis, a feature differing from other odontogenic tumors. In no case yet studied has metastasis occurred. Death follows extensive local recurrence and extension.

SALIVARY GLANDS
Development

Both the major and the minor salivary glands develop as buds of oral ectoderm, arising in much the same manner as teeth. The epithelial bud proliferates into the adjacent

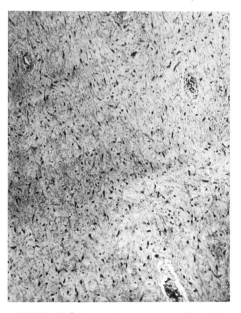

Fig. 26-28 Odontogenic myxoma. Consists of loose, embryonal connective tissue. Occasionally, strands of odontogenic epithelium are present.

mesenchyme, enlarging at its most distal end to form alveoli, the epithelial cords becoming hollow to form ducts. The parotid and submandibular gland anlagen first become apparent by the sixth fetal week (13 mm to 15 mm embryo), although acini are not developed until the fifth month in utero. During the eighth week (19 mm to 25 mm embryo), the buds of the sublingual gland become apparent. The minor salivary glands are initiated by the tenth week.

Labial glands arise as epithelial buds of the vestibular epithelial plate prior to the opening of the alveolabial sulcus. Buccal and molar glands arise at the same time, associated with the terminal portion of Stensen's duct. Retromolar glands develop in the fifth fetal month.

The major salivary glands are subject to many developmental anomalies. One or more lobes (rarely, whole glands) may be congenitally absent or aplastic. Total absence of all major glands also has been reported. Accessory glands and glands ectopically placed within the body of the mandible have been noted. Major salivary ducts may be congenitally atretic or, rarely, imperforate.

Structure and types

The salivary glands, both major and minor, are tubuloalveolar structures. Both the parotid and submandibular glands are well encapsulated, although the sublingual is not. The adult parotid gland is serous in type, whereas the submandibular and sublingual glands are mixed, the former being predominantly serous and the latter mucous. Minor salivary glands are widespread, being scattered over the lips, buccal mucosa, palate, and tongue. Pure serous glands are seen about the circumvallate papillae (glands of von Ebner); pure mucous glands, in the palate and base of the tongue (Weber's glands). All others are of the mixed type.

Function

Saliva, the product largely of the major salivary glands, varies in quantity from 150 ml to 1,300 ml per day (mean, 345 ml). The amount and the degree of viscosity depend upon many factors (mechanical, chemical, and psychologic) but ultimately upon the type of nerve stimulus received by the glands.

The secretory nerve fibers to the salivary glands are under both parasympathetic and sympathetic control. Sympathetic stimulation of the submaxillary gland via the superior cervical ganglion, for example, evokes a secretion of thick viscous mucus, while parasympathetic stimulation via the chorda tympani elicits a copious, thin watery flow.

The saliva performs several known functions, the most important being lubrication for deglutition and speech. Both mucin, a glycoprotein elaborated by mucous glands, and the voluminous watery secretion of the parotid glands aid in this process. In cases of diminished flow (xerostomia), poor oral hygiene and increased dental decay are observed. Taste is altered markedly. Saliva has antibacterial properties and a high buffering capacity. It probably contributes little toward digestion, although it contains a salivary amylase (ptyalin) capable of transforming starch to maltose and of splitting glycogen.

Disturbances of salivary flow

Increased salivary flow, sialorrhea (ptyalism),[223] can result from many causes. It most commonly is associated with acute inflammation of the oral cavity, such as herpetic or aphthous stomatitis, and with "teething." It often is seen in mentally retarded individuals, in deteriorated schizophrenics, and in patients with neurologic disturbances with lenticular involvement. Mercury poisoning, acrodynia, pemphigus, pregnancy, rabies, epilepsy, nausea, and ill-fitting dentures all may be accompanied by an increased degree of salivation. Also, increased gastric secretion is accompanied by increased salivary flow. These may be marked sialorrhea in familial autonomic dysfunction and in one of the periodic diseases, periodic sialorrhea.

Recurrent sialadenitis and periodic sialorrhea. Recurrent sialadenitis and periodic sialorrhea are similar to other periodic diseases in their regular recurrence at short intervals, chronic course, resistance to therapy, and generally benign behavior.[223]

Single pairs or all glands, most commonly the parotid, enlarge at regular intervals of weeks or months. Periodic sialorrhea is more common in women and may be an autosomal dominant trait. It not uncommonly accompanies other recurrent periodic diseases such as periodic abdominalgia or periodic neutropenia.

Familial autonomic dysfunction (Riley-Day syndrome). Familial autonomic dysfunction is characterized by excessive perspiration, sialorrhea, erythematous blotching of the skin, defective lacrimation, wide blood pressure fluctuation, emotional instability, cold hands and feet, and hyporeflexia. It is first manifest in infancy by impaired sucking and swallowing and an absence of tears. Growth is retarded, and the ability to sit, walk, and speak is delayed. It occurs almost exclusively in Jews of Ashkenazi extraction. The sialorrhea is especially marked during excitement.[219, 235] The disorder is inherited as an autosomal recessive trait.

Xerostomia. Decreased salivary flow, xerostomia, is also associated with many conditions. Rarely, there is congenital absence[247] of one or more major glands or ducts.[230] Epidemic parotitis (mumps) and sarcoidosis (uveoparotitis) are associated with reduced flow. Sjögren's syndrome[184, 185, 189] (keratoconjunctivitis sicca, rhinitis sicca, polyarthritis) and the other so-called "autoimmunization" syndromes and diseases (Mikulicz's, Felty's, Waldenström's, lupus erythematosus, etc.) also exhibit xerostomia. Therapeutic radiation to the lateral cervical area commonly produces fibrotic changes following acinar destruction of the parotid glands. Megaloblastic anemias (pernicious anemia, anemia of pregnancy) are not uncommonly associated with decreased salivary output. The majority of cases of xerostomia appear to be idiopathic. Many of these are associated with a smooth atrophic tongue.

Enlargements

Enlargement of one or more salivary glands may be associated with sialorrhea, xerostomia, or normal salivary secretion. A single glandular enlargement may denote localized inflammation, cyst, or neoplasm. Bilateral enlargement may signify an inflammatory process, such as mumps or sarcoid, or a diffuse neoplastic infiltrate (leukemia or lymphoma), or it may be due to unknown factors related to malnutrition, alcoholic cirrhosis, or hormonal disturbance.

Cysts

Cysts of salivary gland origin fall under three categories: true cysts, ranula, and mucocele or superficial retention cyst.

True cyst. The true cyst is usually small, 1 cm or less in diameter, and located within the body of the parotid or submandibular gland. It is lined by stratified squamous epithelium.[208]

Ranula. Ranula is a term used rather

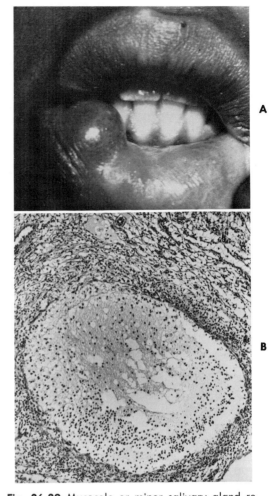

Fig. 26-29 Mucocele or minor salivary gland retention "cyst." **A,** Most commonly observed on lower lip, mucoceles are observed throughout oral cavity. They arise from spillage of mucus into surrounding connective tissue. **B,** Low-power photomicrograph illustrating extraductal mucus surrounded by inflammation. Note absence of epithelium.

loosely to indicate a thin-walled, cystic lesion located on the floor of the mouth, and it includes sublingual gland mucoceles and a deep burrowing lesion that frequently extends through the mylohyoid muscle.[186]

Mucocele (retention "cyst"). The mucocele is a cavity lined by granulation tissue containing an eosinophilic hyaline material (mucus) composed of a variable number of mucus-laden macrophages (Fig. 26-29). Trauma, chiefly mechanical, appears to be responsible for damage to the ducts of minor salivary glands, resulting in the spillage of mucus into the lamina propria and submucous tissue.[226] This mucous pool may be localized and surrounded by a wall of granulation tissue.

Mucocele of the glands near the tip of the tongue is called cyst of Blandin-Nuhn.

Enlargements related to malnutrition

The relationship of parotid gland enlargement to malnutrition has been pointed out by many investigators. Hypertrophy also has been noted in cases of alcoholism and cirrhosis. Enlargement of the submandibular glands also has been noted occasionally in these cases. It is well known that both restricted dietary intake and alcohol contribute toward hepatic cirrhosis. The enlargement may be associated with excessive salivation. Experimentally, parotid enlargement can be produced in rats on a protein-free diet or by feeding proteolytic enzymes.[229]

Parotid enlargement has also been reported in mental patients and in American Indian hospital patients who were assumed to be receiving adequate diets. Past dietary history was not known, however. Cases also have been cited in association with diabetes mellitus, pregnancy and lactation, thyroid disease, cardiospasm, and menopause. In association with diabetes, the parotid swelling may precede the elevation in blood sugar by many months.

Microscopic changes consist of acinar hypertrophy, swelling of cells, and fatty infiltration. No inflammatory changes are observed. The pathogenesis is unknown, although reference is often made to morphologic and functional similarities between the parotid gland and the pancreas.[191]

Inflammatory diseases

Acute parotitis (secondary suppurative type). Acute parotitis is due to ascent of microorganisms, usually *Staphylococcus aureus,* up Stensen's duct when salivary flow is reduced by inadequate fluid balance due to fever, diuretics, starvation, etc. This may become recurrent, leading to scarring and chronic parotitis. Experimental production of secondary parotitis has confirmed clinical evidence. Experimental obstruction alone does not produce the classic microscopic change.

Microscopically, there are widespread destruction of acini and replacement with fibrous connective tissue. Plasma cell and lymphocytic infiltration usually is marked. Ducts and acini frequently are dilated.

Chronic submandibular adenitis. Chronic submandibular adenitis is almost always due to blockage by stricture and/or calculi (sialoliths). This, in turn, renders the gland susceptible to retrograde bacterial invasion.

Sjögren's syndrome. Sjögren, in 1933, first described a syndrome consisting of conjunctivitis sicca, pharyngolaryngitis sicca, rhinitis sicca, polyarthritis, parotid (occasionally submandibular) enlargement, and xerostomia.[191, 198] This syndrome subsequently was shown to have a relationship to other disorders such as Felty's syndrome, polyarteritis, lupus erythematosus, purpura and hypergammaglobulinemia of Waldenström, scleroderma, and Hashimoto's thyroiditis. Patients with Sjögren's syndrome reportedly have a higher incidence of lymphomas[240] (see also p. 504).

The patient, usually a postmenopausal female, clinically presents red, burning eyes, photophobia, and lack of tears. Dysphagia and dysphonia may be marked, and the oral mucosa, especially that of the tongue, is atrophic and shiny. Dental caries is usually widespread.

Sjögren's syndrome has been designated by many authors as an autoimmune disorder.[214] It has been suggested that an antigen released from damaged acini coming in contact with lymphatic tissue (normally present with parotid gland) would result in the production of antibodies that, in turn, would damage more acinar epithelium, continuing the cycle. Arguing for the autoimmune nature of the disease are the following:

1 The associated rheumatoid arthritic changes in over 50%
2 The hypergammaglobulinemia
3 The rheumatoid factor found in over 75%
4 The antithyroglobulin antibodies (about 35%) and antinuclear factors (about 65%)
5 The autoantibody reaction with salivary duct cytoplasm noted in over 50%

It has been suggested that there is impaired IgG autoantibody production. A model for the syndrome has been described in NZB mice.

Microscopically, the changes were long recognized under the name of either *Mikulicz's disease* or *benign lymphoepithelial lesion.* Initially, there is a periductal mononuclear cell infiltrate consisting predominantly of small lymphocytes. Later, large lymphocytes and reticular cells appear. The acinar tissue is eventually totally replaced (Fig. 26-30). Epimyoepithelial islands arising from ductal proliferation are scattered throughout the tissue. Similar changes have been described in the lacrimal glands and the minor salivary glands of the lip and palate.[175, 189, 198]

Sialolithiasis. Sialolithiasis, the occurrence

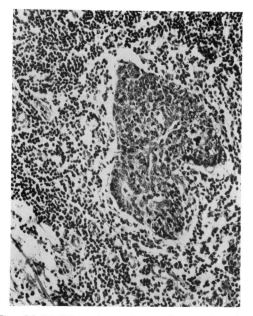

Fig. 26-30 Sjögren's syndrome (benign lympho-epithelial lesion). Acini replaced by marked lymphocytic infiltrate. Differentiation from lymphosarcoma made with difficulty.

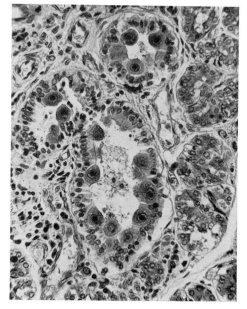

Fig. 26-31 Cytomegalic inclusion disease illustrating numerous, large, doubly contoured inclusion bodies within cytoplasm of duct cells of parotid gland. (Courtesy Dr. R. Marcial-Rojas.)

of salivary stone or calculus, is found most commonly in the submandibular gland or especially its duct. Involvement of the parotid gland is relatively unusual (estimates ranging from 4% to 21%). Calculus in the sublingual and minor salivary glands, although not unknown, is rare.[1]

Although the etiology is unknown, theories have been advanced that salivary retention, with resultant precipitation of calcium salts, is the significant factor. Whether the retention is preceded by inflammation of the duct due to foreign body, bacteria, or other factor is debatable.

Because of the intermittent obstruction of the duct system, inflammation of the proximal portion of the gland occurs. Contrast media may be employed to demonstrate tortuous dilatation of the principal ducts and the presence of strictures. There is atrophy of the acinar cells, with replacement by scar tissue and fat cells if the obstructive process continues.

Cytomegalic inclusion disease. Cytomegalic inclusion disease is a widespread viral disease that becomes clinically manifest in only a small percentage of the population. It appears to be largely harmless outside infancy but remains a risk to the fetus if first contracted by the mother during pregnancy (see p. 402).

Described in 1932 by Farber and Wolbach as coincidental findings in intact salivary and lacrimal gland epithelium in more than 10% of all infant autopsies, the disease was proved to have viral etiology in 1956.[1]

Although initially thought to be limited to salivary and lacrimal glands, it was subsequently shown to be generalized, producing a clinical picture resembling erythroblastosis or hepatitis in neonates and characterized by a train of events: mild jaundice, hepatosplenomegaly, bruising, and, finally, purpura. Interstitial pneumonitis, Addison's disease, or interstitial nephritis with hematuria also may eventuate. A high proportion of fatal cases have exhibited a peculiar laminar necrosis immediately beneath the ependyma of the brain. These areas become calcified and simulate congenital toxoplasmosis.

Microscopically, the inclusions may be seen in the salivary glands, lacrimal glands, liver, kidney, lung, etc. In the salivary gland, the inclusions are seen as round, highly refractile, homogeneous, eosinophilic bodies within the cytoplasm and/or nucleus of ductal cells (Fig. 26-31). These cells also may be seen with standard Wright's stain in gastric washings, subdural fluid, or sediment from freshly voided urine.

Epidemic parotitis (mumps). Epidemic parotitis is an acute, highly contagious viral disease. In spite of the name, it is systemic, affecting many organs other than the parotid gland. It is probable that some degree of

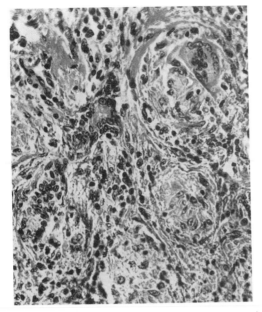

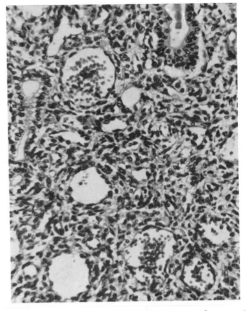

Fig. 26-32 Heerfordt's syndrome (uveoparotid fever) or sarcoidosis. Acini replaced by multiple, usually discrete, sarcoidal granulomas. Lacrimal glands, as well as major salivary glands, enlarged and associated with facial nerve paralysis.

Fig. 26-33 Hemangioendothelioma of parotid gland—most common tumor of parotid gland in children under 1 year of age. Usually of capillary type, with few well-defined lumina.

pancreatitis (and orchitis in male adults) occurs in nearly every case, but severe complication is rather uncommon. Oophoritis also may occur but is quite rare[1] (see p. 399).

There is diffuse tender enlargement of one or both parotid glands, accompanied by mild fever. Less commonly, the submandibular and sublingual glands are involved and, very rarely, the lacrimal glands. Examination of the buccal mucosa during the active state usually will reveal an erythematous halo about the opening of Stensen's duct.

In adolescents and adult males, clinical orchitis (usually unilateral) is present in about 25%. Only rarely is sterility produced, however. Pancreatitis, manifested by epigastric pain and nausea, although not very common as a severe complication, is probably a constant factor, causing elevated serum amylase and lipase levels.

Microscopically, in the parotid glands there are degenerative changes of the ductal epithelium, with infiltration of lymphocytes and macrophages about the ducts. The acini may undergo pressure atrophy.

Uveoparotid fever (Heerfordt's syndrome). Uveoparotid fever is a form of sarcoidosis originally described by Heerfordt in 1909. The syndrome consists of a triad of signs: parotid enlargement, uveitis, and facial paralysis. It usually is seen in the second and

third decades and is decidedly more common in black females. It represents about 10% of the cases of sarcoidosis.

The parotid swelling, which is bilateral in over half of the cases, often is preceded by mild fever, lassitude, and anorexia. The swelling, in contrast to mumps, is not painful and is firm and nodular. The lacrimal glands occasionally are involved (Fig. 26-32). Ocular involvement, usually bilateral, may be severe and prolonged. Uveitis, iridocyclitis, and optic neuritis are not uncommon complications. Paralysis of the facial nerve is common in about 25% of the patients in uveoparotid fever.[2]

Tumors

Benign hemangioendothelioma. The benign hemangioendothelioma is the most common tumor of the parotid gland during the first year of life, usually appearing within the first three months (Fig. 26-33). It occasionally is noted at birth. It also may arise in the submandibular gland. Skin hemangiomas may overlie the salivary gland hemangioendothelioma.

Histologically, the benign hemangioendothelioma is composed of capillary vessels lined by two or more layers of endothelial cells. The vessel lumina often are obscured as a result of the marked cellularity. It is never

Table 26-1. Tumors of major and minor salivary glands

Tumor type	Major	Minor
Benign		
Pleomorphic adenoma (mixed tumor)	55-65%	45-55%
Papillary cystadenoma lymphomatosum	5-6%	—
Oxyphil granular cell adenoma (oncocytoma)	Rare	Rare
Papillary cystadenoma	Rare	2-3%
Benign hemangioendothelioma	Rare, except in infants	—
Miscellaneous (adenoma, lipoma, neurilemoma, neurofibroma, sebaceous adenoma, etc.)	Rare	Rare
Malignant		
Carcinoma in pleomorphic adenoma[217]	3-5%	2-3%
Adenocarcinoma (includes "classic," trabecular, etc.)	4-5%	10-18%
Cylindroma (adenocystic carcinoma)	4-5%	16-20%
Mucoepidermoid carcinoma	12-15%	10-12%
Acinic cell adenocarcinoma	2-3%	Rare
Squamous cell carcinoma	3-4%	?
Undifferentiated carcinoma	Rare	Rare
Miscellaneous (unclassified, oxyphil adenocarcinoma, melanoma, lymphoma, etc.)	Rare	1-2%

encapsulated, infiltrating the gland, replacing the acini, and leaving only the ductal elements.[244]

Pleomorphic adenoma or mixed tumor. The benign pleomorphic adenoma is the most common tumor of the major (about 60%) and minor (about 50%) salivary glands.[179, 180, 183, 187, 190] It occurs most frequently in the parotid gland and less commonly in the submandibular gland—in the ratio of about 9:1. Only rarely does it occur in the sublingual gland.

It arises most frequently in the fourth to sixth decades and is found somewhat more commonly in women. It is extremely rare in children. The primary growth occurs as a single nodule or mass in contrast to the recurrence, which is usually multilobulated. Although usually single, multiple mixed tumors[211] have been reported, arising either in two independent sites within the same gland, bilaterally, or within the homolateral parotid and submandibular glands.

Numerous theories of origin have been postulated: mesenchymal, branchiogenic, embryonal gland anlagen, and adult epithelial and/or myoepithelial tissue.[245] Only the last has received rather general support. Of special interest are the histochemical studies,[177, 200] which support a theory of histogenesis from intercalated ducts. Two types of mucus have been demonstrated: an epithelial type elaborated by glandular structures and a "mesenchymal" type found in myxomatous areas, apparently the product of myoepithelial cells.[207]

Grossly, the pleomorphic adenoma is not truly encapsulated, a condition that was responsible for its high rate of recurrence in the past. Most tumors are from 2 cm to 5 cm in size, although some have attained gigantic proportions. The cut surface is grayish white and translucent. Areas containing cartilage appear bluish. Secondary cyst formation or hemorrhage is rare.

Microscopically, a wide variety of patterns may be found, both within the same tumor and in different tumors (Fig. 26-34). Myxoid areas occur in possibly 90%, whereas over one-third exhibit such an area as a dominant feature. One-half will contain pseudocartilage. Squamous epithelial masses are seen in about 25%, and a pseudoadenoid arrangement of epithelial cells resembling cylindroma (adenoid cystic basaloid carcinoma) is manifest in about 10% of the cases.

A histologic feature in many pleomorphic adenomas is the presence of well-differentiated ductlike structures. Some tumors are composed entirely of these structures, having well-defined lumina with no admixture of mucoid material. These have been called *adenoma*. Other pleomorphic adenomas are composed almost entirely of mucoid pools, with only scant evidence of epithelial elements.

The epithelial cells vary in appearance from single-layered or double-layered high columnar to low cuboidal. Material found in the ductlike lumina in some cases resembles colloid and in others, mucin. The former has been called epithelial mucin, whereas the lat-

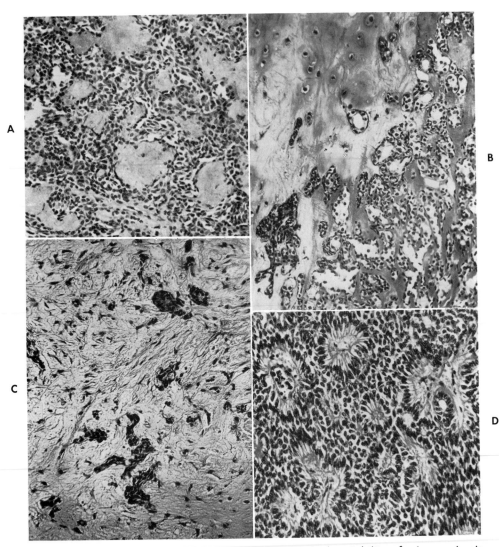

Fig. 26-34 Pleomorphic adenoma or mixed tumor. Marked variability of microscopic picture. **A,** Some tumors are exceedingly cellular, consisting of masses or sheets of small oval or rounded cells exhibiting little tendency to form ducts. **B,** Some tumors exhibit large masses of cartilage-like tissue. True cartilage occasionally produced by metaplasia of fibrous connective tissue stroma. Numerous ductlike structures manifest in this tumor. **C,** Certain tumors contain only few islands of epithelial cells in sea of loose mucoid matrix. **D,** Unusual variant of pleomorphic adenoma, so-called "adenomyoepithelioma."

ter has been characterized as being of mesenchymal origin. This mesenchymal product may simulate cartilage. True cartilage and even bone are observed in a small percentage of these tumors. In some, islands of acidophilic granular cells (oncocytes) are noted. Cylindromatous areas may cause considerable difficulty in diagnosis, especially if the biopsy specimen is small. Fortunately, cylindroma rarely, if ever, arises in mixed tumor.

Although several investigators have attempted to classify the mixed tumor into numerous subtypes on the basis of histologic pattern, clinical behavior is in no way correlated with microscopic variation. The local recurrence rate is low. Various investigators have estimated this to be in the range of 0% to 5%. Because there is seldom any change in histologic pattern with recurrence, poor encapsulation or pseudoencapsulation has been suggested by many as the responsible factor.

Papillary cystadenoma lymphomatosum. (Warthin's tumor; adenolymphoma). Papillary cystadenoma lymphomatosum is a benign

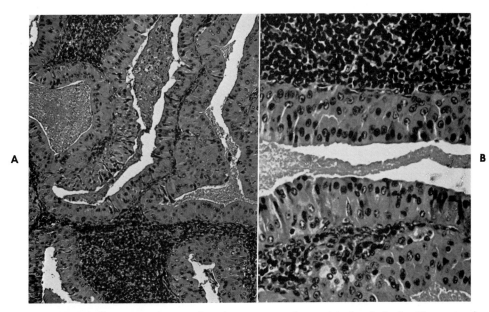

Fig. 26-35 Papillary cystadenoma lymphomatosum of parotid gland. **A,** Papillae extending into cavity contain lymphoid core covered by columnar epithelium. **B,** High magnification of area of **A** showing layer of columnar epithelium and lymphoid tissue.

tumor of the parotid gland, arising most commonly in the lower portion of the gland overlying the angle of the mandible. It comprises from 2% to 6% of all parotid neoplasms. It chiefly affects males (5:1) from 40 to 70 years of age.[181] About 7% of the tumors occur bilaterally. The tumor may be superficial or deep to parotid fascia, within the substance of the gland or occasionally posterior to it. Rarely, an extraparotid lesion is encountered. A malignant variant has been described.[182, 227]

There have been numerous theories of the histogenesis of papillary cystadenoma lymphomatosum.[243] The most plausible theory is that proposed by Albrecht and Arzt in 1910 and supported by numerous investigators. According to this concept, the tumor represents neoplastic proliferation of heterotopic salivary gland rests entrapped during growth and development in lymph nodes adjacent to or within the parotid gland.[232, 243, 246]

Grossly, this well-encapsulated tumor is round or oval or often flattened. Its surface is usually smooth, occasionally lobulated, and commonly pinkish gray in color. The cut surface is studded with whitish nodules that correspond to the germinal centers. Irregular cystic spaces filled with serous or milky fluid and containing papillary projections are observed.

Microscopically, the essential components

of the neoplasm are epithelial parenchyma and lymphoid stroma. The parenchymatous tissue is composed of tubules and dilated cystic spaces into the lumina of which project slender, fingerlike, papillary processes, giving the neoplasm its characteristic appearance (Fig. 26-35). The lining epithelium is composed of two rows of cells, the inner row of tall nonciliated columnar cells with oxyphilic granular cytoplasm and the outer layer of cuboidal, polygonal, or rounded cells. The cell nuclei of the inner layer tend to be deeply stained and are evenly arranged toward the luminal end. The nuclei of the basal layer are round or vesicular, with a distinct nuclear membrane and one or two nucleoli. Occasionally a mucous or goblet cell is observed. Within the tubular and cystic spaces, a pink, granular or, more often, homogeneous substance is seen, probably a product of the lining epithelial cells. A thin basement membrane separates the epithelium from the lymphoid stroma. When present in abundant quantities, the lymphoid stroma contains numerous germinal centers.

Electron microscopic studies have demonstrated that the epithelial cells are oncocytic (i.e., essentially bags of mitochondria).[246] The mitochondria are of two types, the usual form and the giant form, which is two to three times the size of the former. The cristae of the giant form are in the shape of closely

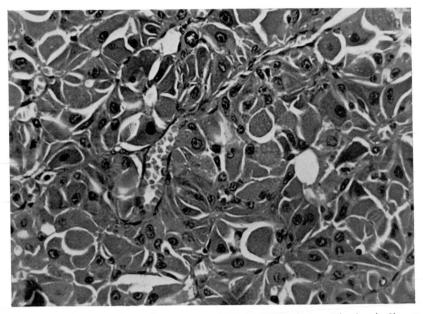

Fig. 26-36 Oxyphil granular cell adenoma (oncocytoma) of parotid gland. Sheets and glandular formations of tall columnar cells with eosinophilic granular cytoplasm.

packed lamellae. Preoperative diagnosis has been aided by scanning with technetium.

Oxyphil granular cell adenoma (oncocytoma). A rare, benign neoplasm of glandular origin, oxyphil granular cell adenoma is composed of large epithelial cells containing oxyphil granular cytoplasm. Although cases have been reported in other major and minor salivary glands, it occurs almost exclusively in the parotid gland. Similar tumors may occur in the thyroid gland (Hürthle cell adenoma), parathyroid glands, kidney, adrenal glands, and pancreas. The tumor apparently arises from oxyphil granular cells (oncocytes), which have been reported to be present in a large number of organs (thyroid gland, parathyroid glands, pituitary gland, testicles, pancreas, liver, etc.) as well as in normal salivary glands. Hamperl[201, 202] has suggested that the oncocyte is derived by a special degenerative metaplasia that does not prevent the cell from dividing.

Clinically, the tumor is indistinguishable from pleomorphic adenoma. It is usually firm, well demarcated, and freely movable. The facial nerve is almost never involved. Grossly, the tumor is round or oval, solid, and well encapsulated. The cut surface is usually grayish red and is divided into lobules by thin strands of fibrous connective tissue.

Microscopically, the oxyphil granular cell adenoma is composed of large cells of different sizes and shapes, sharply delineated from one another, somewhat resembling hepatic or adrenal cortical cells (Fig. 26-36). The abundant eosinophilic cytoplasm contains numerous small, uniform granules. The nuclei are usually single and small, with one or more prominent nucleoli. The cells are commonly arranged in columns or cords, occasionally in tubular or acinar fashion. Rarely, an occasional focus of cartilage is found. Rarely also, diffuse collections of oncocytes or even focal oncocytomas are seen in typical pleomorphic adenomas.

Electron microscopic studies have shown a mitochondria-rich cytoplasm.[178, 213] This is borne out by the histochemical demonstration of an abundance of oxidative enzymes and adenosine triphosphatase. A marked metachromasia is noted with thionine or cresyl violet.[178]

Oxyphil granular cell carcinoma (malignant oncocytoma). The oxyphil granular cell carcinoma has been described in the salivary, thyroid, and adrenal glands[71, 82, 201, 202]

Sebaceous lymphadenoma. Sebaceous lymphadenoma is a rare benign lesion of the parotid gland. Microscopically, it is composed of a well-demarcated mass of lymphoid tissue in which there are numbers of islands of ductlike structures exhibiting sebaceous cell differentiation.[176, 188]

Mucoepidermoid carcinoma. Of ductal origin, mucoepidermoid carcinoma exhibits cells of various ranges of activity, from the mucus-secreting cell to those that are quite squamous in character.[204]

Although originally considered to be of two types, benign and malignant, further observation has indicated that occasionally the most benign-appearing ones have metastasized. All are now classified as carcinoma, and the degree of malignancy is estimated as low or high. It should be realized that this is purely an arbitrary microscopic classification and not a hard-and-fast clinical evaluation.

Clinically, mucoepidermoid carcinoma of low-grade malignancy usually resembles the pleomorphic adenoma. It presents itself as a painless swelling, usually of the parotid gland. The appearance depends upon the stage of differentiation, the mature tumor being smaller, less firm, more movable, and more prone to mucous cyst formation than is the more malignant type. Encapsulation, although not uncommon in the better-differentiated tumor, is quite rare in the more anaplastic type. The low-grade tumor is more commonly found in females in the fourth to fifth decades. Involvement of the facial nerve in patients not operated upon is exceedingly rare.

In contrast, the high-grade (more malignant) mucoepidermoid tumor not uncommonly manifests pain and/or facial nerve paralysis as an initial symptom. Sex predilection is not observed. Metastases to lung, brain, and bone frequently occur early in the course. The five-year survival rate is about 25%.

The tumor also may occur within the body of the jaws, principally the mandible, in the retromolar area, where it makes its presence known early.[233] The prognosis of the tumor in this location is good.

Microscopically, the appearance is quite variable and depends upon the degree of differentiation of the tumor, those of low-grade malignancy having an abundance of mucous cells, whereas the more anaplastic have few to no mucous cells and may be mistaken for squamous cell carcinomas (Fig. 26-37). A mucin stain such as Meyer's mucicarmine or Schiff stain should be employed in all doubtful cases. There are three cell types evident: those that are frankly mucoid, others that are evidently epidermoid, and an intermediate type that is neither but has the capacity of maturing in either direction. Not uncommonly, the squamous epithelial cell nests of low-grade malignant tumors become hydropic. The presence of small cysts is very common in these well-differentiated tumors. The cysts become filled with mucus and com-

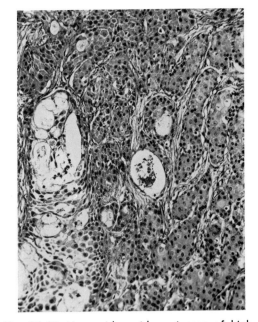

Fig. 26-37 Mucoepidermoid carcinoma of high-grade malignancy, strongly resembling squamous cell carcinoma. Careful search usually will reveal few cells that are producing mucus. Periodic acid–Schiff stain may aid in diagnosis.

monly rupture. Cystic arrangement is uncommonly seen in the more malignant variety. Here, the pattern is more nestlike or sheetlike, mucous cells being uncommon in the primary tumor. However, metastases from these tumors not rarely manifest mucous cells.[1, 204, 231, 237]

Cylindroma (adenocystic carcinoma; cylindromatous adenocarcinoma). Cylindroma constitutes about 5% to 10% of parotid gland tumors, 18% submandibular gland tumors, 25% malignant oral salivary gland tumors, and over 50% of the glandular tumors of the tongue. Its origin appears to be the intercalated duct.[218, 236] The same tumor occurs in the nasopharynx, paranasal sinuses, and lower respiratory system. It is most commonly observed in the sixth decade. The tumor is slow growing and of a moderate to low-grade malignancy but is widely infiltrative. It is poorly encapsulated. Facial nerve involvement is common, invasion of perineural lymphatics usually being readily demonstrated in section. The tumor is usually small (2 cm to 4 cm), firm, homogeneous, and grayish white in cross section. Multiple recurrence is common, with regional and finally generalized metastasis. The five-year survival rate is about 35%. Prognosis for the palatal cylindroma is far better than that for cylindromas in the major salivary glands.

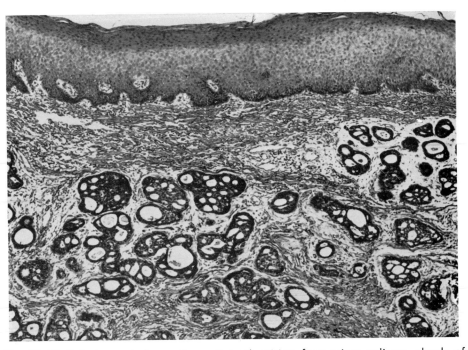

Fig. 26-38 Cylindroma (adenocystic carcinoma) arising from minor salivary glands of palate.

Microscopically, the tumor demonstrates a striking pattern of anastomosing cords of small, darkly staining cells with scant cytoplasm (Fig. 26-38). These cords are separated by acellular areas containing hyalin or mucicarmine-positive material. The cells have regular, rounded, rather vesicular nuclei. Chromatin clumping, mitotic figures, and prominent nucleoli are characteristically absent. There are two principal patterns: cribriform and solid. There appears to be a better prognosis if the pattern is cribriform rather than solid. Frequently, centripetal perineural extension can be demonstrated.[197, 215]

Although the tumor is moderately radiosensitive, recurrence after radiation therapy is rather common in spite of an initially favorable response.

Acinic cell adenocarcinoma (clear cell carcinoma; serous cell adenocarcinoma). Acinic cell adenocarcinoma appears to arise from the intercalated duct cells of normal glands, chiefly the parotid gland. It is uncommon, constituting about 2.3% of major salivary gland tumors.[174] It occurs about twice as frequently in women as in men.

The tumor is usually rounded and is well encapsulated in about one-half of the cases. It is slow growing but has a tendency to recur, especially when poorly encapsulated. The recurrent lesion is usually multiple. Character-istically, metastasis occurs to the lungs, bones, and brain. Regional spread is rather uncommon. The tumor occurs most commonly in the third and fourth decades. On cut section, it is gray to reddish tan, soft, friable, and, occasionally, somewhat cystic.

Histologically, acinic cell adenocarcinoma occurs in two distinct forms—the granular cell, which is the more common, and the clear cell. Some tumors are admixtures of the two types. The granular cell type is composed of large polyhedral or rounded cells with small, dark, eccentrically placed nuclei. The cytoplasm is abundant, granular, and somewhat basophilic. PAS-positive material may be present, especially in microcystic areas. Occasionally, a lymphoid stroma is present. In over 10% of the tumors, the principal cell is clear, at times exhibiting a pseudoglandular papillary or cystic arrangement, markedly resembling adenocarcinoma (hypernephroma) of the kidney (Fig. 26-40). Ultrastructural studies have demonstrated that the granular cell variety is composed of cells that resemble the serous acinar cells of normal glands—i.e., they contain secretory granules and histochemically are identical with serous cells.[194, 199, 203]

The clear cell variety, as the name implies, does not stain with hematoxylin and eosin and does not react with stains for glycogen or mucin. Electron microscopic studies have

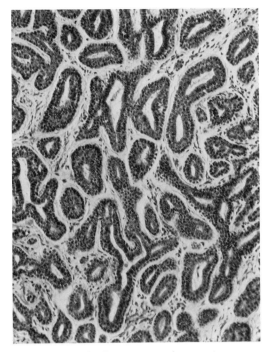

Fig. 26-39 Cylindromatous adenocarcinoma or cylindroma (adenocystic carcinoma). Tumor consists of cylinders or tubules of small polymorphic cells with hyperchromatic nuclei. Cells frequently surrounded by hyaline stroma.

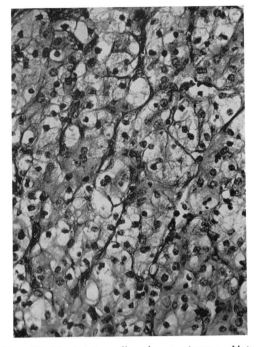

Fig. 26-40 Acinic cell adenocarcinoma. Note hypernephroid appearance.

demonstrated a large number of free ribosomes and few mitochondria and other organelles. The clear appearance is due to the clumping and margination of the free ribosomes after formalin fixation. Presumably, the clear cell variety arises from the striated ducts.[194, 203]

Carcinoma in pleomorphic adenoma. Confusion exists regarding the "malignant mixed tumor," and two separate views regarding it are available. One ascribes the term to those salivary gland neoplasms that are histologically similar to pleomorphic adenoma but, because of cellular activity (mitotic index), nuclear pleomorphism, and growth characteristics, are felt more likely to recur and/or metastasize. On the other hand, if serial sections are made on examples of all proved salivary gland malignancies, a focus of "typical" mixed tumor may be found, allowing the diagnosis. Obviously, divergent clinicopathologic data ensue from these two tumor groups.[217]

Squamous cell carcinoma. Squamous cell carcinoma comprises about 4% of major salivary gland tumors, arising predominantly in males in the sixth or seventh decade. The high degree of malignancy indicated by its histologic appearance is confirmed by its ag-

gressive clinical behavior. Completely replacing salivary gland acini, the tumor infiltrates the skin and involves the facial nerve early in its clinical course. Pain may be marked. Metastatic spread is common. Care must be exercised to differentiate the squamous cell carcinoma from the poorly differentiated malignant mucoepidermoid carcinoma.

Papillary cystadenoma and cystadenocarcinoma. Papillary cystadenoma and cystadenocarcinoma occur most frequently in the parotid gland, less commonly in the submandibular and minor salivary glands. The majority of the adenocarcinomas are slow growing, somewhat invasive, and slow to metastasize. Microscopically, the tumor consists of glandlike spaces lined with tall columnar epithelium having eosinophilic cytoplasm. Mucin is commonly produced and may fill the glandlike spaces. Metastasis usually occurs to the regional lymph nodes and vertebrae.[222]

Undifferentiated carcinoma. Undifferentiated carcinoma consists of sheets or cords of anaplastic epithelial cells surrounded by varying amounts of fibrous stroma. Pleomorphism usually is marked, and mitotic figures are abundant. At times, some degree of differentiation into glandlike structures is noted, but this does not seem to have any effect upon prognosis. Invasion of adjacent structures such

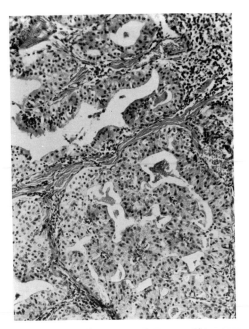

Fig. 26-41 Papillary cystadenoma. This tumor arises from neoplastic proliferation of ducts, being essentially a Warthin tumor without lymphoid stroma.

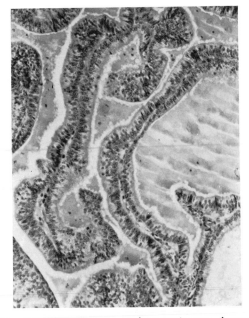

Fig. 26-42 Papillary cystadenocarcinoma. A most uncommon tumor, it occurs in both major and minor salivary glands.

as auditory canal, paranasal sinuses, and mandible is common, as well as local and widespread metastasis. Prognosis is poor—only radical surgery being of any value, for the tumor is characteristically radioresistant. It appears to run a more malignant course in children than in adults.[241]

Other tumors of salivary glands. Several other tumors having their origin in the stromal tissues of salivary glands have been described: lipoma, rhabdomyosarcoma, leiomyoma, neurofibroma, neurilemoma, leiomyosarcoma, xanthoma, lymphangioma, malignant hemangioendothelioma, and fibromatosis.[221]

Tumors of minor salivary glands. Tumors of the minor salivary glands include all those that occur in the major glands (parotid, submandibular, sublingual), with the exception of sebaceous cell adenoma and hemangioendothelioma.[187]

Pleomorphic adenoma appears to be the most common tumor arising from the intraoral minor salivary glands. Next in order of frequency are cylindromatous adenocarcinoma, mucoepidermoid tumor, and adenocarcinoma. Benign tumors occur most frequently in the fourth and fifth decades. The malignant tumors are most common in the sixth decade. The palate is the site of greatest predilection, followed by the upper lip, buccal mucosa, tongue, oral floor, and retro-

molar region. Cylindroma occurs about twice as frequently in women and in a slightly older age group. Minor salivary gland tumors rarely may occur entirely within the mandible.[180, 183, 212]

NECK
Tumors

Carotid body tumor. Carotid body tumor (nonchromaffin paraganglioma; chemodectoma) arises in the carotid bodies, small ovoid nodules situated on the medial aspect of the bifurcation of the common carotid arteries. Histologically identical tumors are found in the aortic bodies, the glomus jugulare (paraganglion tympanicum), and the ganglion nodosum of the vagus nerve. All of these structures are apparently derived from neuroepithelial elements of the cranial nerves. They subsequently migrate to areas of mesodermal concentration about the vessels of the embryonic branchial arches.[125, 252, 258, 259]

The tumor may become manifest at any age but rarely before puberty. There is a slight female predilection. About 5% are bilateral.

Microscopically, the tumor is lobulated and thinly encapsulated or embedded in loose connective tissue. It consists of nests of rather large polyhedral cells grouped together in an alveolar or organoid pattern (Fig. 26-43).

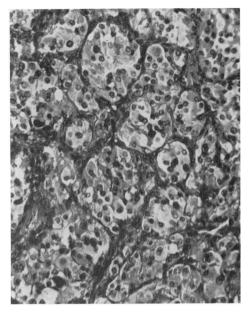

Fig. 26-43 Carotid body tumor.

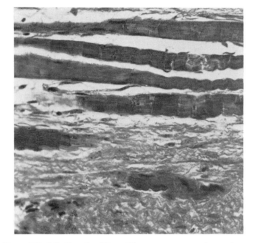

Fig. 26-44 Torticollis. Fibrous connective tissue replaces striated muscle fibers.

The cell nests are separated by loose connective tissue and a vascular stroma. The individual epithelial cells present rounded vesicular nuclei with pronounced nucleoli. Their cytoplasm is pale, eosinophilic, and frequently vacuolated, with indistinct cell boundaries. Rarely, bizarre, hyperchromatic cells, active mitoses and capsular invasion may be observed. Spread to regional nodes or even distant dissemination has been noted but does not seem to adversely affect the patient.[261]

Fibromatosis colli

Fibromatosis colli (torticollis; wryneck) occurs both as a primary and as a secondary disease.[255] Primary or congenital torticollis is manifest by a firm, fusiform swelling of the sternocleidomastoid muscle either at birth or within the first few weeks of life. The swelling usually increases for several weeks and then regresses, occasionally disappearing between the sixth and eighth month.

Grossly, the muscle is shortened, contracted, and fibrous. Clinically, the chin becomes tilted upward and toward the unaffected side. If untreated, facial asymmetry results, with adaptive scoliosis of the lower cervical and upper thoracic spine, foreshortening of the skull, and flattening of the facial bones on the involved side. Etiology is unknown, but theories have implicated birth trauma or, especially, uterine malposition. Often (35% to 50%) it is associated with breech delivery. Microscopically, the muscle fibers are widely separated by dense, scarlike fibrous connective tissue (Fig. 26-44). Secondary torticollis is usually due to a myositis that is attributed to a "chill." Occasionally it follows poliomyelitis or a tumor of the cervical cord, or it may be a hysterical manifestation.

Cysts

Thyroglossal duct cysts. The thyroid gland arises as an anlage in the region of the foramen cecum of the tongue and descends into the anterior neck. If it persists in its embryonal position, it is spoken of as lingual thyroid.[253, 254] Rarely, a strand of epithelium persists and connects the base of the tongue with the normally positioned thyroid gland. The thyroglossal duct cyst results from cystic degeneration of this tract. It is situated in the midline of the neck in the region of the hyoid bone, through which the tract usually passes. The cyst is lined by respiratory and/or stratified squamous epithelium. The cyst may become infected and drain, becoming a thyroglossal duct fistula[250] (see also p. 1431).

Lymphoepithelial cyst. The lateral cervical cyst (branchial cyst) is located anterior to the sternocleidomastoid muscle near the angle of the mandible.[249, 262] The alleged association of these cysts or sinuses with squamous carcinoma appears unwarranted. Microscopically, the cyst is lined by either stratified squamous or pseudostratified ciliated columnar epithelium. Beneath the epithelium is abundant lymphoid tissue with germinal centers. The cysts are thought to arise from cystic degeneration of epithelium enclaved in cervical lymph nodes.[249] The cyst usually becomes apparent during the third decade. Similar lesions may occur in the parotid gland or on the oral floor.[262]

Parathyroid cyst. Microscopic cysts of the parathyroid glands are seen in at least 50% of normal specimens. Nevertheless, cysts large enough to produce clinical symptoms are rare.[256, 263]

The parathyroid cyst is solitary and slow growing and may cause dysphagia and displacement of the trachea to the contralateral side, producing hoarseness by pressure on the recurrent laryngeal nerve. In several instances, this symptom has led to a preoperative diagnosis of thyroid carcinoma. It is found anywhere in the lateral neck from the angle of the mandible deep to the sternocleidomastoid muscle to the mediastinum. Most of the patients have been over 30 years of age, and a 2:1 female and left-sided predilection is evident.

The cyst is usually very thin and filled with a clear, watery fluid. Microscopically, it is lined by a somewhat flattened cuboidal to low columnar epithelium. Within the collagenic connective tissue wall, one usually notes several types of parathyroid cells: water-clear cells, chief cells, and, occasionally, oxyphil cells. Not all three types are always present.

Cervical thymic cyst. Occasionally, remnants of thymus primordium are left in the neck, where they may remain undisturbed or, rarely, may undergo cystic alteration and subsequent enlargement. The cysts probably arise from degeneration of Hassall's corpuscles.[248] They present clinically most often at about the age of 3 to 6 years, and there appears to be a 2:1 male sex predilection. The cysts

are usually elongated and may assume quite large proportions. They usually are located in the lateral neck at the angle of the mandible just anterior to the sternocleidomastoid muscle.

Microscopically, the cysts are lined by stratified squamous epithelium and often contain a thick reddish-brown fluid. Rarely, cuboidal epithelium is found. In the walls, thymic structures (i.e., Hassall's corpuscles) may be identified. The cyst is well encapsulated and often exhibits cholesterol crystals among the connective tissue fibers (p. 1399).

Cystic hygroma colli. The cystic hygroma or diffuse lymphangioma is manifest as a rather poorly defined soft tissue mass in the neck. It is present at birth. Usually located behind the sternocleidomastoid muscle, it may extend to involve the shoulder or mediastinum.[251]

Microscopically, it consists of large endothelium-lined lymphatic spaces in a loose connective tissue stroma (Fig. 26-45).

Inflammatory disease

Ludwig's angina. Ludwig's angina is a severe, boardlike cellulitis of the neck involving all of the submandibular spaces. Prior to the advent of antibiotics, this was a rare complication of periapical infection of the mandibular molars or extension from an acute osteomyelitis following compound fracture of the mandible. Drainage of a mixed infection through the lingual plate of the mandible into one or more spaces and subsequent extension with marked edema of the glottis commonly resulted in death through severe toxemia and asphyxiation.[257]

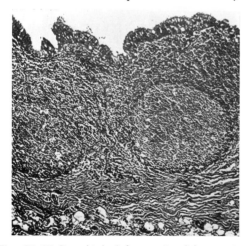

Fig. 26-45 Branchial cleft cyst lined by respiratory epithelium with lymphoid tissue in connective tissue wall.

REFERENCES
General

1 Gorlin, R. J., and Goldman, H.: Thoma's Oral pathology, ed. 6, St. Louis, 1970, The C. V. Mosby Co.
2 Gorlin, R. J., and Pindborg, J. J.: Syndromes of the head and neck, New York, 1964, McGraw-Hill Book Co.
3 Pindborg, J. J.: Pathology of the dental hard tissues, Philadelphia, 1970, W. B. Saunders Co.
4 Shafer, W. G., Hine, M. K., and Levy, B. M.: Oral pathology, ed. 2, Philadelphia, 1963, W. B. Saunders Co.

Developmental anomalies
  Facial and oral developmental malformations

5 Ardran, G. M., Beckett, J. M., and Kemp, F. H.: Arch. Dis. Child. **39**:389-392, 1964 (aglossia).
6 Beckwith, B.: Birth Defects: Original Article

Series V(2):188-196, 1969, The National Foundation, New York (macroglossia-omphalocele syndrome).

7 Cervenka, J., Gorlin, R. J., and Anderson, V. E.: Amer. J. Hum. Genet. **19:**416-432, 1967 (congenital lip fistulas).

8 Cervenka, J., Jacobson, D. E., and Gorlin, R. J.: New Eng. J. Med. **284:**856-857, 1971 (Y chromosome staining).

9 Drillien, C. M., Ingram, T. T. S., and Wilkinson, E. M.: The causes and natural history of cleft lip and palate, Edinburgh, 1966, E. & S. Livingstone, Ltd. (cleft lip and palate).

10 Fernandez, A. O., and Ronis, M. L.: Arch. Otolaryng. (Chicago) **80:**505-520, 1964.

11 Fogh-Andersen, P.: Acta Chir. Scand. **129:**275-281, 1965 (macrostomia).

12 Glass, D.: Brit. J. Oral Surg. **1:**194-199, 1964 (hemifacial atrophy).

13 Gorlin, R. J.: Cutis **4:**1345-1349, 1968 (orofaciodigital syndrome).

14 Gorlin, R. J., and Meskin, L. H.: J. Pediat. **61:**870-879, 1962 (hemifacial hypertrophy).

15 Halperin, V., Kolas, S., Jefferis, K. R., Huddleston, S. O., and Robinson, H. B. G.: Oral Surg. Oral Med. Oral Path. **6:**1072-1077, 1953 (developmental oral anomalies).

16 Hubinger, H. L.: J. Oral Surg. **10:**64-66, 1952 (bifid tongue).

17 MacMahon, B., and McKeown, T.: Amer. J. Hum. Genet. **5:**176-183, 1953 (cleft lip and palate—associated malformations).

18 Martin, H. E., and Howe, M. E.: Ann. Surg. **107:**39-49, 1938 (median rhomboid glossitis).

19 Miles, A. E. W.: Advances Biol. Skin **4:**46-77, 1963 (Fordyce granules).

20 Monroe, C. W.: Plast. Reconstr. Surg. **38:**312-319, 1966 (median cleft of mandible).

21 Moore, K. L.: The sex chromatin, Philadelphia, 1966, W. B. Saunders Co. (sex chromatin).

22 Randall, P., Krogman, W. M., and Jahins, S.: Cleft Palate J. **2:**237-246, 1965 (Robin's syndrome).

23 Rogers, B. O.: Brit. J. Plast. Surg. **17:**109-137, 1964 (mandibulofacial dysostosis).

24 Schaumann, B. F., Peagler, F. J., and Gorlin, R. J.: Oral Surg. Oral Med. Oral Path. **29:** 566-575, 725-734, 1970 (minor craniofacial anomalies).

25 Tobias, N.: Arch. Derm. Syph. (Chicago) **52:** 266, 1945 (fissured tongue—heredity).

26 Watanabe, Y., Igaku-Hakushi, M. O., and Tomida, K.: Oral Surg. Oral Med. Oral Path. **4:**709-722, 1951 (congenital lip fistulas).

Developmental anomalies of teeth

27 Chaudhry, A. P., Johnson, O. N., Mitchell, D. F., Gorlin, R. J., and Bartholdi, W. L.: J. Pediat. **54:**776-785, 1959 (amelogenesis imperfecta).

28 Gorlin, R. J., Old, T., and Anderson, V. E.: Z. Kinderheilk. **108:**1-11, 1970 (hypohidrotic ectodermal dysplasia—genetic heterogeneity).

29 Grahnen, H.: Odont. Rev. (Malmo) **7**(suppl. 3):1-100, 1956 (hypodontia).

30 Johnson, O. N., Chaudhry, A. P., Gorlin, R. J., Mitchell, D. F., and Bartholdi, W. L.: J.

31 Rushton, M. A.: Ann. Roy. Coll. Surg. Eng. **16:**94-117, 1954 (dentin anomalies).

32 Sackett, L. M., Marans, A. E., and Hursey, R. J., Jr.: Oral Surg. Oral Med. Oral Path. **9:**659-665, 1956 (congenital ectodermal dysplasia.).

33 Schulze, C.: In Gorlin, R. J., and Goldman, H. M., editors: Thoma's Oral pathology, ed. 6, St. Louis, 1970, The C. V. Mosby Co. (teeth—developmental abnormalities).

34 Witkop, C. J., Jr.: Oral Surg. Oral Med. Oral Path. **23:**174-182, 1967 (amelogenesis imperfecta—X-linked).

35 Witkop, C. J., Jr., and Rau, S.: Birth Defects: Original Article Series, The National Foundation, New York (in press) (hereditary defects in enamel and dentin).

Oral lesions
Lesions of dermatologic type

36 Clement, D. H., and Godman, G. C.: J. Pediat. **36:**11-30, 1950 (glycogen-storage disease—macroglossia).

37 Cook, B. E. D.: Brit. Dent. J. **109:**83-96, 131-138, 1960 (oral bullous lesions).

38 Green, D.: Oral Surg. Oral Med. Oral Path. **15:**1312-1324, 1962 (scleroderma—oral changes).

39 Lever, W. F.: Pemphigus and pemphigoid, Springfield, Ill., 1965, Charles C Thomas, Publisher (pemphigus and pemphigoid).

40 Simpson, H. E.: J. Oral Surg. **24:**463-466, 1966 (familial white folded hypertrophy).

41 Soderquist, N. A., and Reed, W. B.: Arch. Derm. (Chicago) **97:**31-33, 1968 (pachyonychia congenita).

White lesions of mucosa

42 Andreasen, J. O.: Oral Surg. Oral Med. Oral Path. **25:**31-42, 158-166, 1968 (lichen planus).

43 Archard, H. O., Carlson, K. P., and Stanley, H. R.: Oral Surg. Oral Med. Oral Path. **25:**717-728, 1968 (leukoedema).

44 Browne, W. G., Izatt, M. M., and Renwick, J. H.: Ann. Hum. Genet. **32:**271-281, 1969 (white sponge nevus).

44a Clausen, F. P., Mogeltoft, M., Roed-Petersen, B., and Pindborg, J. J.: Scand. J. Dent. Res. **78:**287-294, 1970 (focal epithelial hyperplasia).

45 Einhorn, J., and Wersäll, J.: Cancer **20:**2189-2193, 1967 (oral cancer and oral leukoplakia).

46 Forman, G.: Brit. Dent. J. **119:**83-84, 1965 (occupational oral keratosis).

47 Hansen, L. S.: J. Oral Surg. **17:**60-66, 1959 (white lesions—histology).

48 Jepsen, A., and Winther, J. E.: Acta Odont. Scand. **23:**239-256, 1965 ("speckled leukoplakia").

49 MacComb, W. S.: Postgrad. Med. **27:**349-355, 1960 (oral leukoplakias).

50 Phillips, H., and Williams, A.: Oral Surg. Oral Med. Oral Path. **26:**619-622, 1968 (focal epithelial hyperplasia).

51 Pindborg, J. J., and Sirsat, S. M.: Oral Surg. Oral Med. Oral Path. **22:**764-779, 1966 (oral submucous fibrosis).

52 Pindborg, J. J., Renstrup, G., Silverman, S.,

Jr., and Poulsen, H. E.: Acta Odont. Scand. **21**:407-414, 1963 (clinical and histologic signs of malignancy—leukoplakias).

53 Renstrup, G., Pindborg, J. J., and Joist, O.: Ugeskr. Laeg. **129**:1539-1545, 1967 (oral leukoplakias).

54 Shafer, W. G., and Waldron, C. A.: Surg. Gynec. Obstet. **112**:411-420, 1961 (oral leukoplakia).

55 Shedd, D. P., Hukill, P. B., Kligerman, M. M., and Gowen, G. F.: Amer. J. Surg. **106**:791-796, 1963 (oral carcinoma in situ).

56 Sprague, W. G.: Oral Surg. Oral Med. Oral Path. **16**:1067-1074, 1963 (terminology of "leukoplakia").

57 Van Wyk, C. W.: Med. Proc. (Johannesb.) **11**:531-537, 1965 (oral lesion caused by snuff).

58 Young, W. G.: Brit. J. Oral Surg. **5**:93-98, 1967 (white sponge nevus).

Disturbances of pigmentation

59 Bowerman, J. E.: Brit. J. Oral Surg. **6**:188-191, 1969 (oral pigmentation—Albright's syndrome).

60 Dummett, C. O., and Barens, G.: J. Periodont. **38**:369-378, 1967 (oral pigmentation—review).

61 Zachariae, H.: Acta Dermatovener. (Stockholm) **43**:149-153, 1963 (palatal pigmentation—antimalarial drugs).

Mouth
Dental caries

62 Ast, D. B., Kantwell, K. T., Wachs, B., and Smith, D. J.: J. Amer. Dent. Ass. **53**:314-325, 1956 (Newburgh-Kingston caries-fluorine study).

63 Darling, A. I.: In Gorlin, R. J., and Goldman, H. M., editors: Thoma's Oral pathology, ed. 6, St. Louis, 1970, The C. V. Mosby Co. (dental caries).

64 Gustafsson, B. E., Quensel, C.-E., Lanke, L. S., Lundqvist, C., Grahnen, H., Bonow, B. E., and Krasse, B. O.: Acta Odont. Scand. **11**:232-364, 1954 (carbohydrates and caries).

65 Holloway, P. J.: Brit. Dent. J. **126**:161-165, 1969 (diet and caries).

66 Keyes, P. H.: Arch. Oral Biol. **1**:304-320, 1960 (caries-infectious nature).

67 Keyes, P. H.: J. Amer. Dent. Ass. **76**:1357-1373, 1968 (research in dental caries).

68 Mandel, I. D.: J. Amer. Dent. Ass. **51**:432-441, 1955 (caries—histology, histochemistry).

69 Marthaler, T. M.: Caries Res. **1**:222-238, 1967 (carbohydrate and caries).

70 Murray, J.: Brit. Dent. J. **126**:352-354, 1969 (fluoride and caries).

71 Naylor, M. N.: Proc. Roy. Soc. Med. **62**:839-844, 1969 (caries research).

72 Schatz, A., and Martin, J. J.: J. Amer. Dent. Ass. **65**:368-375, 1962 (proteolysis—chelation theory of caries).

73 Scott, D. B., and Albright, J. T.: Oral Surg. Oral Med. Oral Path. **7**:64-78, 1954 (electron microscopy of caries).

Periodontal disease

74 Barros, L., and Witkop, C. J., Jr.: Arch. Oral Biol. **8**:195-206, 1963 (periodontal disease—nutritional factors).

75 Boyle, P. E.: Milit. Med. **128**:493-498, 1963 (periodontal disease—review).

76 Goldman, H. M., and Cohen, D. W.: Periodontal therapy, ed. 4, St. Louis, 1968, The C. V. Mosby Co. (experimental periodontal disease).

77 Hodge, H. C., and Leung, S. W.: J. Periodont. **21**:211-221, 1959 (calculus formation).

78 Ruben, M. P., Goldman, H. M., and Schulman, S. M.: In Gorlin, R. J., and Goldman, H. M., editors: Thoma's Oral pathology, ed. 6, St. Louis, 1970, The C. V. Mosby Co. (periodontal disease).

79 Waerhaug, J.: J. Periodont. **26**:107-118, 1955 (periodontal disease—occlusal factors).

Inflammatory diseases

80 Banks, P.: Brit. J. Oral Surg. **4**:227-234, 1967 (infectious mononucleosis—oral lesions).

81 Bennett, D. E.: Arch. Intern. Med. (Chicago) **120**:417-427, 1967 (histoplasmosis).

82 Bronner, M., and Bronner, M., editors: Actinomycosis, London, 1969, John Wright & Sons, Ltd.

83 Burston, H. H.: Laryngoscope **69**:1-43, 1959 (lethal granuloma—oral changes).

84 Cook, B. E. D.: Brit. Dent. J. **109**:83-96, 1960 (recurrent aphthae).

85 Crouse, H. V., Coriell, L. L., Blank, H., and Scott, T. F. M.: J. Immun. **65**:119-128, 1950 (herpes—cytochemical studies).

86 Dudgeon, J. A.: J. Clin. Path. **3**:239-247, 1950 (herpes simplex—complement fixation).

87 Ferro, E. R., and Richter, J. W.: J. Oral Surg. **4**:121-126, 1946 (granuloma venereum—oral lesions).

88 Gorlin, R. J., and Chaudhry, A. P.: Arch. Derm. (Chicago) **82**:344-348, 1960 (cyclic neutropenia—oral manifestations).

89 Huebner, R. J., Beeman, E. A., Cole, R. M., Beigelman, P. M., and Bell, J. A.: New Eng. J. Med. **247**:249-256, 285-289, 1952 (herpangina).

90 Komet, H., Schaefer, R. F., and Mahoney, P. L.: Arch. Otolaryng. (Chicago) **82**:649-651, 1965 (tuberculosis—oral manifestations).

91 Krill, C. E., Jr., and Mauer, A. M.: J. Pediat. **68**:361-366, 1966 (agranulocytosis).

92 Lehner, T., and Sagebiel, R. W.: Brit. Dent. J. **121**:454-456, 1966 (aphthae-electronmicroscopic changes).

93 Pindborg, J. J., Gorlin, R. J., and Asboe-Hansen, G.: Oral Surg. Oral Med. Oral Path. **16**:551-560, 1963 (Reiter's syndrome—oral lesion).

94 Snijman, P. C.: Brit. J. Oral Surg. **4**:106-110, 1967 (gangrenous stomatitis).

95 Southam, J. C., Colley, I. T., and Clarke, N. G.: Brit. J. Derm. **80**:248-256, 1968 (herpetic gingivostomatitis).

96 Taylor, R., Shklar, G., Budson, R., and Hackett, R.: Arch. Derm. (Chicago) **89**:419-425, 1964 (mucormycosis).

97 Tempest, M. N.: Brit. J. Surg. **53**:949-969, 1966 (noma).

98 Uohara, G. I., and Knapp, M. J.: Oral Surg. Oral Med. Oral Path. **24**:113-123, 1967 (oral fusospirochetosis).

Tumors and tumorlike lesions

99 Aparacio, S. R., and Lumsden, C. E.: J. Path. 97:339-355, 1969 (granular cell tumor—ultrastructure).

100 Ashley, F. L., McConnell, D. V., Machida, R., Sterling, H. E., Galloway, D., and Grazer, F.: Amer. J. Surg. 110:549-551, 1965 (carcinoma of lip).

101 Barron, S. L., Roddick, J. W., Jr., Greenlaw, R. H., Rush, B., and Tweeddale, D. N.: Cancer 21:672-681, 1968 (multiple primary cancers).

102 Cady, B., and Catlin, D.: Cancer 23:551-569, 1969 (gingival carcinoma).

103 Colberg, J. E.: Int. Abstr. Surg. 115:205-213, 1962 (granular cell tumor—review).

104 Feind, C. R., and Cole, R. M.: Amer. J. Surg. 116:482-486, 1968 (carcinoma of oral cavity and floor of mouth).

105 Fisher, E. R., and Wechsler, H.: Cancer 15: 936-954, 1962 (granular cell tumor).

106 Frazell, E. L., and Lucas, J. C., Jr.: Cancer 15:1085-1099, 1962 (cancer of tongue).

107 Goethals, P. L., Harrison, E. G., Jr., and Devine, K. D.: Amer. J. Surg. 106:845-851, 1963 (verrucous oral carcinoma).

108 Gorton, G., and Linell, F.: Acta Radiol. (Stockholm) 47:381-392, 1957 (malignant tumors—sarcoidal reaction in lymph nodes).

109 Hayward, A. F.: Brit. J. Cancer 23:702-708, 1969 (pigmented tumor of infancy—ultrastructure).

110 Himalstein, M. R., and Humphrey, T. R.: Arch. Otolaryng. (Chicago) 87:389-395, 1968 (pseudosarcoma).

111 Lane, N.: Cancer 10:19-41, 1957 (pseudosarcoma with squamous cell carcinoma).

112 Masson, J. K., and Soule, E. H.: Amer. J. Surg. 110:585-591, 1965 (rhabdomyosarcoma).

113 O'Day, R. A., Soule, E. H., and Gores, R. J.: Oral Surg. Oral Med. Oral Path. 20:85-93, 1965 (oral embryonal rhabdomyosarcoma).

114 Pearse, A. G. E.: J. Path. Bact. 62:351-362, 1950 (granular cell tumor).

115 Plaza, F. L., and Avello, A.: Brit. J. Oral Surg. 4:26-28, 1966 (carcinoma of lip).

115a Pindborg, J. J., and Sirsat, S. M.: Oral Surg. Oral Med. Oral Path. 22:764-774, 1966 (oral submucous fibrosis).

116 Poole, A. G., and Marchetta, F. C.: Cancer 22:14-21, 1968 (plasmacytoma).

117 Rosenfeld, L., and Callaway, J.: Amer. J. Surg. 106:840-844, 1963 (snuff dipper's cancer).

118 Sharp, G. S., Bullock, W. K., and Helsper, J. T.: Cancer 14:512-516, 1961 (multiple oral carcinoma).

119 Shedd, D. P., Hukill, P. B., Kligerman, M. M., and Gowen, G. F.: Amer. J. Surg. 106:791-796, 1963 (oral carcinoma in situ).

120 Shirokov, E. P.: Amer. J. Surg. 100:530-532, 1960 (carcinoma of palate).

121 Simons, J. N.: Amer. J. Surg. 116:494-498, 1968 (oral malignant melanoma).

122 Trieger, N., Ship, I. I., Taylor, G. W., and Weisbarger, D.: Cancer 11:357-362, 1958 (cirrhosis and oral cancer).

123 Tsukada, Y., and Pickren, J. W.: Oral Surg. Oral Med. Oral Path. 20:640-644, 1965 (oral rhabdomyoma).

124 Vance, S. F., III, and Hudson, R. P., Jr.: Amer. J. Clin. Path. 52:208-211, 1969 (granular cell tumor).

125 Vickers, R. A.: In Gorlin, R. J., and Goldman, H. M., editors: Thoma's Oral pathology, ed. 6, St. Louis, 1970, The C. V. Mosby Co. (oral soft tissue neoplasms).

126 Vickers, R. A., Gorlin, R. J., and Lovestedt, S. A.: Northwest Dent. 44:339-342, 1965 (oral cancer—mass screening).

127 Whitten, J. B.: Oral Surg. Oral Med. Oral Path. 26:202-213, 1968 (granular cell tumor—ultrastructure).

Jaws

128 Austin, J. E., Redford, G. H., and Banks, S. O., Jr.: New York Dent. J. 31:187-191, 1965 (torus palatinus and torus mandibularis—Negroes).

129 Bender, I. B.: Oral Surg. Oral Med. Oral Path. 12:546-561, 1959 (Gaucher's disease—oral findings).

130 Bennett, J. E., Tignor, S. P., and Shafer, W. G.: Amer. J. Surg. 116:538-541, 1968 (osteosarcoma of jaw).

131 Borello, E., and Gorlin, R. J.: Cancer 19:196-206, 1966 (pigmented neuroectodermal tumor of infancy).

132 Burkitt, D.: Cancer 20:756-759, 1967 (Burkitt's lymphoma—review).

133 Chaudhry, A. P., Robinovitch, M. R., Mitchell, D. F., and Vickers, R. A.: Amer. J. Surg. 102:403-411, 1961 (chondrosarcoma—jaws).

134 Clausen, F., and Poulsen, H.: Acta Path. Microbiol. Scand. 57:361-374, 1963 (carcinoma—metastatic to jaws).

135 Gardner, A. F., Drescher, J. T., and Goodreau, G. J.: J. Calif. Dent. Ass. 39:105-116, 1963 (Paget's disease—oral aspects).

136 Gorlin, R. J., Vickers, R. A., Kelln, E., and Williamson, J. J.: Cancer 18:89-104, 1965 (nevoid basal cell carcinoma syndrome).

137 Harless, C. F., Jr.: Oral Surg. Oral Med. Oral Path. 20:684-689, 1965 (gingival cysts).

138 Henderson, D., and Rowe, N. L.: Brit. J. Oral Surg. 6:161-172, 1969 (multiple myeloma—jaw).

139 Jones, E. L., and Cornell, W. P.: Arch. Surg. (Chicago) 92:287-300, 1966 (osteomatosis-polyposis or Gardner's syndrome).

140 Kolas, S., Halperin, V., Jefferis, K., Huddleston, S., and Robinson, H. B. G.: Oral Surg. Oral Med. Oral Path. 6:1134-1141, 1953 (torus palatinus and torus mandibularis).

141 Lichtenstein, L.: J. Bone Joint Surg. 46A:76-90, 1964 (histiocytosis X—critical review).

142 Lurie, H. I.: Cancer 14:1090-1108, 1961 (pigmented anlage tumor).

143 MacDougall, J. A., Evans, A. M., and Lindsay, R. K.: Amer. J. Surg. 106:816-818, 1963 (osteoradionecrosis of jaw).

144 Macleod, W., Douglas, D. M., and Mahaffy, R. G.: Clin. Radiol. 16:269-273, 1965 (infantile cortical hyperostosis).

145 Norgaard, B., and Pindborg, J. J.: Acta Ophthal. (Kobenhavn) 37:52-58, 1959 (osteomyelitis of jaw—infants).

146 Ramsey, H. E., Strong, E. W., and Frazell,

E. L.: Amer. J. Surg. **116**:542-547, 1968 (fibrous lesions—jaws).

147 Rayne, J.: Brit. J. Oral Surg. **6**:11-17, 1968 (osteomatosis-polyposis or Gardner's syndrome).

148 Sedano, H. O., Cernea, P., Hosxe, G., and Gorlin, R. J.: Oral Surg. Oral Med. Oral Path. **27**:760-771, 1969 (histiocytosis X—oral changes).

149 Steg, R. F., Dahlin, D. C., and Gores, R. J.: Oral Surg. Oral Med. Oral Path. **12**:128-141, 1959 (malignant lymphoma).

150 Thoma, K. H.: Oral Surg. Oral Med. Oral Path. **7**:1091-1107, 1954 (tumors of temporomandibular joint).

151 Topazian, R. G., and Costich, E. R.: J. Oral Surg. **23**:559-568, 1965 (cherubism).

152 Waldron, C. A.: J. Oral Surg. **28**:58-64, 1970 (fibrous lesions of jaws).

153 Weary, P. E., Linthicum, A., Cawley, E. P., Coleman, C. C., Jr., and Graham, G. F.: Arch. Derm. (Chicago) **90**:20-30, 1964 (osteomatosis-polyposis or Gardner's syndrome).

154 Wright, D. H.: Brit. J. Surg. **51**:245-251, 1964 (Burkitt's lymphoma—jaws).

Odontogenic tumors

155 Barros, R. E., Dominguez, F. V., and Cabrini, R. L.: Oral Surg. Oral Med. Oral Path. **27**: 225-236, 1969 (odontogenic myxoma).

156 Cina, M. T., Dahlin, D. C., and Gores, R. J.: Mayo Clin. Proc. **36**:664-678, 1961 (ameloblastic fibroma).

157 Gardner, D. G., Michaels, L., and Liepa, E.: Oral Surg. Oral Med. Oral Path. **26**:812-823, 1968 (calcifying odontogenic tumor).

158 Gorlin, R. J., and Meskin, L. H.: Ann. N. Y. Acad. Sci. **108**:722-771, 1963 (odontogenic tumors—review).

159 Gorlin, R. J., Chaudhry, A. P., and Pindborg, J. J.: Cancer **14**:73-101, 1961 (odontogenic tumors—review).

160 Hoke, H. F., and Harrelson, A. B.: Cancer **20**: 991-999, 1967 (ameloblastoma—metastatic).

161 Jacobsohn, P. H., and Quinn, J. H.: Oral Surg. Oral Med. Oral Path. **26**:829-836, 1968 (ameloblastic odontoma).

162 Kramer, I. R. H.: Brit. J. Oral Surg. **1**:13-28, 1963 (ameloblastoma).

163 O'iver, R. T., McKenna, W. F., and Shafer, W. G.: J. Oral Surg. **19**:245-248, 1961 (ameloblastoma—vascular variety).

164 Philipsen, H. P., and Birn, H.: Acta Path. Microbiol. Scand. **75**:375-398, 1969 (adenomatoid odontogenic tumor).

165 Pincock, L. D., and Bruce, K. W.: Oral Surg. Oral Med. Oral Path. **7**:307-311, 1954 (odontogenic fibroma).

166 Pindborg, J. J.: Acta Path. Microbiol. Scand. suppl. 105, pp. 135-144, 1955 (dentinoma).

167 Pindborg, J. J., and Clausen, F.: Acta Odont. Scand. **16**:293-301, 1958 (odontogenic tumors—classification).

168 Small, I. A., and Waldron, C. A.: Oral Surg. Oral Med. Oral Path. **8**:281-297, 1955 (ameloblastoma).

169 Smith, J. F., Blankenship, J., Drake, J., and Robbins, M.: Oral Surg. Oral Med. Oral Path.

17:618-627, 1964 (ameloblastoma—granular cell variety).

170 Spouge, J. D.: Oral Surg. Oral Med. Oral Path. **24**:392-403, 1967 (odontogenic tumors).

171 Spouge, J. D., and Spruyt, C. L.: Oral Surg. Oral Med. Oral Path. **25**:447-457, 1968 (odontogenic tumors).

172 Vickers, R. A., Dahlin, D. C., and Gorlin, R. J.: Oral Surg. Oral Med. Oral Path. **20**: 476-480, 1965 (calcifying odontogenic tumor—amyloid).

172a Vickers, R. A., and Gorlin, R. J.: Cancer **26**: 699-710, 1970 (ameloblastoma—histopathologic criteria).

173 Zegarelli, E. V., Kutscher, A. H., Napoli, N., Iurono, F., and Hoffman, P.: Oral Surg. Oral Med. Oral Path. **17**:219-224, 1964 (cementoma; periapical fibrous dysplasia).

Salivary glands

174 Abrams, A. M., Cornyn, J., Scofield, H. H., and Hansen, L. S.: Cancer **18**:1145-1162, 1965 (acinic cell carcinoma).

175 Abramson, A. L., Goodman, M., and Kolodny, H.: Arch. Otolaryng. (Chicago) **88**:91-94, 1968 (Sjögren's syndrome—palatal salivary glands).

176 Assor, D.: Amer. J. Clin. Path. **53**:100-103, 1970 (sebaceous lymphadenoma).

177 Azzopardi, J. G., and Smith, O. D.: J. Path. Bact. **77**:131-140, 1959 (salivary gland tumors—histochemistry of mucins).

178 Balogh, K., and Roth, S. I.: Lab. Invest. **14**: 310-320, 1965 (oncocytoma—electron microscopy).

179 Bardwil, J. M.: Amer. J. Surg. **114**:498-502, 1967 (parotid tumors).

180 Bardwil, J. M., Reynolds, C. T., Ibanez, M. L., and Luna, M. A.: Amer. J. Surg. **112**:493-497, 1966 (minor salivary gland tumors).

181 Baum, R. K., and Perzik, S. L.: Amer. Surg. **30**:420-422, 1964 (papillary cystadenoma lymphomatosum—review).

182 Bazaz-Malik, G., and Gupta, D. N.: Z. Krebsforsch. **70**:193-197, 1968 (malignant oncocytoma).

183 Bergman, F.: Cancer **23**:538-543, 1969 (minor salivary gland tumors).

184 Bloch, K. J., Buchanan, W. W., Wohl, M. J., and Bunim, J. J.: Medicine (Balt.) **44**:187-231, 1965 (Sjögren's syndrome—review).

185 Bunim, J. J., Buchanan, W. W., Wertlake, P. T., Sokoloff, L., Bloch, K. J., Beck, J. S., and Alepa, F. P.: Ann. Intern. Med. **61**:509-530, 1964 (Sjögren's syndrome—review).

186 Catone, G. A., Merrill, R. G., and Henny, F. A.: J. Oral Surg. **27**:774-786, 1969 (ranula).

187 Chaudhry, A. P., Vickers, R. A., and Gorlin, R. J.: Oral Surg. Oral Med. Oral Path. **14**: 1194-1226, 1961 (minor salivary gland tumors—review).

188 Cheek, R., and Pitcock, J. A.: Arch. Path. (Chicago) **82**:147-150, 1966 (sebaceous lymphadenoma).

189 Chisholm, D. M., and Mason, D. K.: J. Clin. Path. **21**:656-660, 1968 (Sjögren's syndrome—labial salivary glands).

190 David, H., and Korth, I.: Zbl. Allg. Path. **106**: 78-85, 1964 (mixed tumors).

191 Davidson, D., Leibel, B. S., and Berrie, B.: Ann. Intern. Med. 70:31-38, 1969 (Sjögren's syndrome).

192 Deppisch, L. M., and Toker, C.: Cancer 24:174-184, 1969 (mixed tumor—ultrastructure).

193 Deysine, M., and Mann, B. F., Jr.: Ann. Surg. 169:437-443, 1969 (sebaceous lymphadenoma).

194 Echevarria, R. A.: Cancer 20:563-571, 1967 (acinic cell carcinoma, clear cell carcinoma—ultrastructure).

195 Eneroth, C. M., Blanck, C., and Jakobsson, P. A.: Acta Otolaryng. (Stockholm) 66:477-492, 1968 (malignant mixed tumor).

196 Eneroth, C. M., Hjertman, L., and Moberger, G.: Acta Otolaryng. (Stockholm) 64:514-536, 1967 (submandibular gland tumors).

197 Eneroth, C. M., Hjertman, L., and Moberger, G.: Acta Otolaryng. (Stockholm) 66:248-260, 1968 (cylindroma).

198 Font, R. L., Yanoff, M., and Zimmerman, L. E.: Amer. J. Clin. Path. 48:365-376, 1967 (Sjögren's syndrome—lacrimal glands).

199 Fox, N. M., ReMine, W. H., and Woolner, L. B.: Amer. J. Surg. 106:860-867, 1963 (acinic cell carcinoma).

200 Grishman, E.: Cancer 5:700-707, 1952 (histochemistry of mixed tumors).

201 Hamperl, H.: Cancer 15:1019-1027, 1962 (oncocytoma—benign and malignant).

202 Hamperl, H.: Virchow Arch. Path. Anat. 335:452-483, 1962 (oncocytoma).

203 Hübner, G., Klein, J., and Kleinsasser, O.: Virchow Arch. Path. Anat. 345:1-14, 1968 (acinic cell carcinoma—ultrastructure).

204 Jakobsson, P. A., Blanck, C., and Eneroth, C. M.: Cancer 22:111-124, 1968 (mucoepidermoid carcinoma).

205 Kauffman, S., and Stout, A. P.: Cancer 16:1317-1331, 1963 (salivary gland tumors—children).

206 Kessler, H. S.: Amer. J. Path. 52:671-685, 1968 (Sjögren's syndrome—animal model).

207 Kierszenbaum, A. L.: Lab. Invest. 18:391-396, 1968 (mixed tumor—ultrastructure).

208 Kini, M. G.: Brit. Med. J. 2:415, 1940 (parotid cyst).

209 Kleinsasser, O., and Klein, H. J.: Arch. Klin. Exp. Ohr. Nas. Kehlkopfheilk. 190:272-285, 1968 (malignant mixed tumor).

210 Kleinsasser, O., Klein, H. J., and Hübner, G.: Arch. Klin. Exp. Ohr. Nas. Kehlkopfheilk. 192:100-105, 1968 (salivary duct carcinoma).

211 Lenson, N., and Strong, M. S.: New Eng. J. Med. 254:1231-1233, 1956 (multiple mixed tumors—review).

212 Luna, M. A., Stimson, P. G., and Bardwil, J. M.: Oral Surg. Oral Med. Oral Path. 25:71-86, 1968 (minor salivary gland tumors).

213 McGavran, M. H. P.: Virchow Arch. Path. Anat. 338:195-202, 1965 (papillary cystadenoma lymphomatosum—electron microscopy).

214 Macsween, R. N., Goudie, R. B., Anderson, J. R., Armstrong, E., Murray, M. A., Mason, D. K., Jasani, M. K., Boyle, J. A., Buchanan, W. W., and Williamson, J.: Ann. Rheum. Dis. 26:402-411, 1967 (Sjögren's syndrome—autoimmune studies).

215 Market, J.: Arch. Klin. Exp. Ohr. Nas.

Kehlkopfheilk. 184:496-500, 1965 (cylindroma—ultrastructure).

216 Marsden, A. T. H.: Brit. J. Cancer 5:375-381, 1951 (salivary gland tumors in Malaya).

217 Moberger, J. G., and Eneroth, C. M.: Cancer 21:1198-1211, 1968 (malignant mixed tumor).

218 Moran, J. J., Becker, S. M., Brady, L. W., and Rambo, V. B.: Cancer 14:1235-1250, 1961 (cylindroma).

219 Moses, S. W., Rotem, Y., Jagoda, N., Talmor, N., Eichhorn, F., and Levin, S.: Israel J. Med. Sci. 3:358-371, 1967 (familial dysautonomia).

220 Myerson, M., Crelin, E. S., and Smith, H. W.: Arch. Otolaryng. (Chicago) 83:488-490, 1966 (salivary gland duct duplication).

221 Postoloff, A. V., and Kaiser, F. F., Jr.: Cancer 9:1116-1119, 1956 (rhabdomyosarcoma—salivary gland).

222 Rawson, A. J., Howard, J. M., Royster, H. P., and Horn, R. C., Jr.: Cancer 3:445-458, 1950 (papillary cystadenoma and cystadenocarcinoma).

223 Reimann, H. A., and Lindquist, J. N.: J.A.M.A. 149:1465-1467, 1952 (periodic sialorrhea).

224 Reynolds, C. T., McAuley, R. L., and Rogers, W. P., Jr.: Amer. J. Surg. 111:168-174, 1966 (minor salivary gland tumors).

225 Richard, E. L., and Ziskind, J.: Oral Surg. Oral Med. Oral Path. 10:1086-1090, 1957 (ectopic salivary glands).

226 Robinson, L., and Hjørting-Hansen, E.: Oral Surg. Oral Med. Oral Path. 18:191-205, 1964 (mucocele).

227 Ruebner, B., and Bramhall, J. L.: Arch. Path. (Chicago) 69:110-117, 1960 (malignant papillary cystadenoma lymphomatosum).

228 Sachs, R. L.: Metastatic carcinoma of jaw bones, M.S. Thesis, New York University, 1962 (metastatic carcinoma to jaws).

229 Sandstead, H. R., Koehn, C. J. and Sessions, S. M.: Amer. J. Clin. Nutr. 3:198-214, 1955 (parotid enlargement—malnutrition).

230 Scher, I., and Scher, L. B.: Brit. Dent. J. 98:324-325, 1955 (imperforate salivary ducts).

231 Schwartz, I. S., and Feldman, M.: Cancer 23:636-640, 1969 (mucoepidermoid tumors).

232 Shklar, G., and Chauncey, H. H.: J. Oral Surg. 23:222-230, 1965 (papillary cystadenoma lymphomatosum—histochemistry).

233 Silverglade, L. B., Alvares, O. F., and Olech, E.: Cancer 22:650-653, 1968 (jaws—central mucoepidermoid tumors).

234 Singleton, A. O.: Surg. Gynec. Obstet. 74:569-572, 1942 (salivary gland tumors).

235 Smith, A. A., Taylor, T., and Wortis, S. B.: New Eng. J. Med. 268:705-707, 1963 (familial dysautonomia—metabolic defect).

236 Smith, L. C., Lane, N., and Rankow, R. M.: Amer. J. Surg. 110:519-526, 1965 (cylindroma).

237 Smith, R. L., Dahlin, D. C., and Waite, D. E.: J. Oral Surg. 26:387-393, 1968 (mucoepidermoid tumors).

238 Stebner, F. C., Eyler, W. R., DuSault, L. A., and Block, M. A.: Amer. J. Surg. 116:513-517, 1968 (papillary cystadenoma lymphomatosum—technetium).

239 Swinton, N. W., and Warren, S.: Surg. Gynec.

Obstet. **67:**424-435, 1938 (salivary gland tumors).

240 Talal, N., Sokoloff, L., and Barth, W. F.: Amer. J. Med. **43:**50-65, 1967 (Sjögren's syndrome—lymphoma).

241 Tefft, M., Vawter, G., and Neuhauser, E. B.: Amer. J. Roentgen. **95:**32-40, 1965 (parotid adenocarcinoma).

242 Thomas, W. H., and Coppola, E. D.: Amer. J. Surg. **109:**724-730, 1965 (malignant mixed tumor).

243 Thompson, A. S., and Bryant, H. C., Jr.: Amer. J. Path. **26:**807-849, 1950 (papillary cystadenoma lymphomatosum—histogenesis).

244 Walsh, T. S., Jr., and Tompkins, V. N.: Cancer **9:**869-904, 1956 (hemangioma).

245 Welsh, R. A., and Meyer, A. T.: Arch. Path. (Chicago) **85:**433-447, 1968 (mixed tumors—histogenesis).

246 Yarington, C. T., Jr., and Zagibe, F. T.: J. Laryng. **83:**361-365, 1969 (papillary cystadenoma lymphomatosum—ultrastructure).

247 Zaus, E., and Tuescher, G. W.: J. Dent. Res. **19:**326, 1940 (absence of salivary glands).

Neck

248 Barrick, B., and O'Kell, R. T.: J. Pediat. Surg. **4:**355-358, 1969 (thymic cysts).

249 Bhaskar, S. N., and Bernier, J. L.: Amer. J. Path. **35:**407-423, 1959 (lymphoepithelial cyst).

250 Brintnall, E. S., Davies, J., Huffman, W. C., and Lierle, D. M.: Arch. Otolaryng. (Chicago) **59:**282-289, 1954 (thyroglossal duct cysts).

251 Broomhead, I. W.: Brit. J. Plast. Surg. **17:**225-244, 1964 (cystic hygroma).

252 Chambers, R. G., and Mahoney, W. D.: Amer. J. Surg. **116:**554-558, 1968 (carotid body tumors).

253 Dodds, W. J., and Powell, M. R.: Amer. J. Roentgen. **100:**786-791, 1967 (lingual thyroid scanning with technetium).

254 Downton, D., and O'Riordan, B. C.: Brit. J. Oral Surg. **1:**29-32, 1963 (lingual thyroid).

255 Gruhn, J., and Hurwitt, E. S.: Pediatrics **8:**522-526, 1951 (fibroblastic sternomastoid tumor of infancy).

256 Haid, S. P.: Arch. Surg. (Chicago) **94:**421-426, 1967 (parathyroid cysts).

257 Herd, R. M., and Hall, J. F.: Oral Surg. Oral Med. Oral Path. **4:**1523-1527, 1951 (Ludwig's angina).

258 LeCompte, P. M.: In Atlas of tumor pathology, Sect. IV, Fasc. 16, Washington, D. C., 1951, Armed Forces Institute of Pathology (tumors of carotid body; chemoreceptor system).

259 Marshall, R. B., and Horn, R. C., Jr.: Cancer **14:**779-787, 1961 (nonchromaffin paraganglioma).

260 Masson, J. K., and Soule, E. H.: Amer. J. Surg. **112:**615-622, 1966 (head and neck desmoid tumors).

261 Reese, H. E., Lucas, R. N., and Bergman, P. A.: Ann. Surg. **157:**232-243, 1963 (malignant carotid body tumors).

262 Vickers, R. A., Gorlin, R. J., and Smart, E. A.: Oral Surg. Oral Med. Oral Path. **16:**1214-1222, 1963 (lymphoepithelial cyst—oral).

263 Wood, J. W.: Arch. Surg. (Chicago) **92:**785-790, 1966 (parathyroid cysts).

Chapter 27

Alimentary tract

Robert C. Horn, Jr.

CONGENITAL ANOMALIES
Atresia

The most common anomaly of the esophagus is atresia. It results from failure of pharyngeal and gastric outpouchings to meet and form a continuous lumen. Since there is frequently associated faulty development of the septum between the trachea and esophagus, tracheoesophageal fistula is a common accompaniment. The atresia may take one of several forms. Both the pharyngeal and gastric pouches may be blind, or either or both may communicate with the trachea or a bronchus near the bifurcation via a fistulous tract. In its commonest form, the pharyngeal diverticulum is a blind sac, and the distal segment communicates with the trachea. Infants with this anomaly will not survive unless surgical correction is carried out promptly.

Atresias also may affect the intestinal tract. Although any part of the gut may be involved, the anomaly occurs most frequently in the ileum and least so in the colon. Usually, it takes the form of complete interruption of the continuity of the intestine, the blind ends being connected by a thin fibrous cord. However, there are variations. Such a cord may be absent, or the atresia may be in the form of a diaphragm or web (Fig. 27-1)—a focal remnant of the solid core of the epithelium that fills the intestinal "lumen" at one stage of embryologic development. The diaphragm may be incomplete, resulting in stenosis.

At times, intestinal atresia is associated with *meconium ileus* (see discussion of cystic fibrosis, pp. 1145 and 1279). It has been argued that in this situation the atresia is an acquired defect—acquired in fetal life—the result of scarring secondary to volvulus and gangrene, or perforation and meconium peritonitis, both common complications of meconium ileus.

Still another manifestation of intestinal atresia is *imperforate rectum* or *anus*. Faulty development of the hindgut may result in a rectum terminating in a blind pouch at or below the rectosigmoid junction. Because of the intimate relationship of the descent of the hindgut with the development of the cloacal septum, which ultimately separates the terminal portions of the genitourinary and gastrointestinal systems, this malformation frequently is associated with fistulous communication between the rectum and the bladder or urethra in the male or between the rectum and uterus or vagina in the female. Occasionally, there is a fistulous opening on the perineum. Failure of the proctodeum to invaginate or of the anal plate to be absorbed results in imperforate anus.

All these gastrointestinal atresias are manifested clinically very early in the infant's life

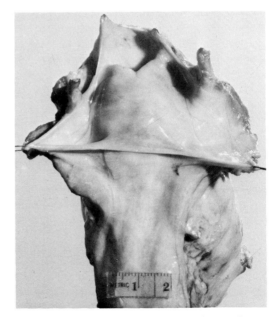

Fig. 27-1 Congenital esophageal web. Esophagus has been opened posteriorly.

and must be treated promptly by surgical means if the infant is to survive.

Heterotopia

Patches of *heterotopic gastric mucous membrane* occur not uncommonly in the esophagus, most frequently in the cervical region. Rarely do they occur elsewhere in the gut. This anomaly frequently is associated with other malformations, such as Meckel's diverticulum.

Heterotopic pancreatic tissue occurs in the form of discrete nodules, usually submucosal, in the stomach or duodenum within 5 cm of the pylorus or, less frequently, in the jejunum or in Meckel's diverticulum. Although commonly an incidental finding, it may give rise to symptoms of "indigestion." It usually is composed of ducts and acinar tissue, but islets of Langerhans are occasionally present as well. At times, the continuity of one or more ducts with invagination of the mucous membrane may give rise to a "dimple" or "diverticulum" that may be observed on roentgen examination. A possibly related lesion is the so-called *adenomyoma*—an intramural nodule composed of ducts mingled with hypertrophied, irregularly oriented bundles of smooth muscle, most frequently encountered in the stomach or gallbladder.

Duplications and cysts

Duplications are segments of gastrointestinal tube situated in apposition to any portion of the alimentary canal. The gut epithelium at one stage in the embryo proliferates rapidly, more or less filling the lumen. This solid core is canalized by the progressive development of vacuoles that coalesce. The persistence of more than one group of vacuoles, and ultimately lumen, at any level results in a duplication. They usually are situated between the leaves of the mesentery. (Failure of this epithelial proliferation at one or more levels is another mechanism accounting for congenital stenosis.) Duplications may be completely independent of the adjacent normal intestine, or they may share mesentery (or mesentery and one or more muscle coats) with it; the lumina may or may not communicate. Duplications may give rise to symptoms of obstruction or, if they contain gastric mucous membrane, peptic ulceration and hemorrhage, or even perforation.

Some of the enteric or enterogenous cysts (often labeled duplications) probably arise in the same way. Others develop through the persistence, growth, and sequestration of minute diverticular buds of the intestinal epithelium that represents a normal developmental stage in the embryo. Enteric cysts are very similar to duplications but are more or less spherical and regularly lacking communication with the gut lumen.

Although both occur in relation to any portion of the alimentary tract, duplications are commonest in the region of the terminal ileum, and cysts occur most often in relation to the esophagus, where they are often intramural. Regardless of location, both duplications and cysts are lined by mucous membrane of any of the types normally occurring in the gastrointestinal tract—e.g., a duplication or cyst adjacent to the ileum may be lined by small intestinal or gastric mucous membrane or both. Many esophageal (as well as enteric) cysts are lined partially or wholly by bronchial mucosa, and the wall may contain cartilage. At least some of the intrathoracic cysts probably arise as pinched-off accessory buds from the primitive foregut.

Meckel's diverticulum

The only commonly occurring congenital diverticulum of the gastrointestinal tract is Meckel's diverticulum, which represents persistence of the proximal (intestinal) part of the omphalomesenteric duct. Any portion of the duct may persist as such or as a fibrous cord, accounting for a variety of anomalies—e.g., in addition to simple Meckel's diverticulum, Meckel's diverticulum attached to the umbilicus by a fibrous cord (which can give rise to volvulus), a cyst suspended between ileum and umbilicus, fistula between ileum and umbilicus, etc.

The diverticulum itself is on the antimesenteric aspect of the terminal ileum one inch to six feet[14] proximal to the ileocecal valve. It varies greatly in length and usually has an opening only slightly smaller than the lumen of the ileum (Fig. 27-2). Typically, its lining resembles that of the adjacent small intestine, but in roughly 25% of cases the mucous membrane of other parts of the gastrointestinal tract, especially the stomach, is represented; pancreatic tissue is also not uncommon. Thus, peptic ulceration may occur and call attention to the diverticulum by hemorrhage or perforation. The most frequent complications are hemorrhage, intestinal obstruction, diverticulitis, inversion with intussusception, and tumor formation.

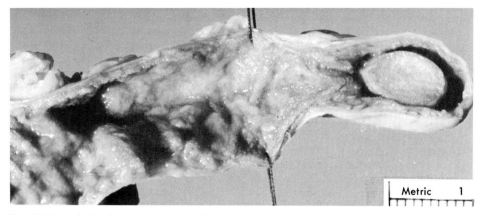

Fig. 27-2 Meckel's diverticulum. Note fruit pit in tip of diverticulum.

Aganglionic megacolon (Hirschsprung's disease)

Congenital aganglionic megacolon is characterized by symptoms of partial or complete intestinal obstruction usually from birth or very early in life, with great dilatation and hypertrophy of the colon. It must be differentiated from megacolon of functional origin or the result of mechanical obstruction.

The underlying anatomic defect is a lack of ganglion cells in Auerbach's (myenteric) plexus and Meissner's (submucous) plexus in a narrowed, nonhypertrophied segment of intestine distal to the extremely distended colon, which is innervated normally and shows marked muscle hypertrophy (Plate 3, *A*). The aganglionic area usually does not extend higher than the sigmoid colon, but instances of involvement of the entire colon and even the small intestine occur. The lack of coordinated propulsive movement in this segment is combined with spasm, the result of unopposed sympathetic nervous activity. The diagnosis can be made on the failure to find ganglion cells on adequate rectal biopsy. Surgical resection of the aganglionic segment relieves the condition. The disease may be complicated by pseudomembranous enterocolitis (p. 1135), the usual situation in fatal cases.

Pyloric stenosis

It has been suggested, but not demonstrated, that a mechanism similar to that in aganglionic megacolon may be operative in the pathogenesis of *congenital pyloric stenosis*. The latter, a condition almost exclusively of male infants (Hirschsprung's disease also predominates in males), is manifested at about the age of 3 weeks by vomiting, with attendant dehydration and malnutrition. The hypertrophied pyloric muscle frequently forms a palpable tumor. Prompt surgical incision of the pyloric ring muscle usually results in cure. The untreated patient does not usually survive long enough to develop generalized gastric muscular hypertrophy.

A similar condition is occasionally encountered in adults, and the condition can be simulated by a redundant fold of antral mucous membrane, producing intermittent obstruction by prolapsing through the pylorus.

Achalasia of esophagus

Achalasia of the esophagus predominates in women, usually becomes manifest in adult life, and is associated with a marked degree of dilatation and hypertrophy of the entire esophagus, except the distal spastic segment.

Although ganglia are not regularly absent in the spastic segment of the esophagus, at times they are. Frequently they are degenerate and/or deficient in number. There is evidence to implicate degenerative disease of the vagus nerve.[18]

Miscellaneous

A variety of anomalies of position may involve the gastrointestinal tract—presence of portions of the tract in internal or external or diaphragmatic hernial sacs, malrotation or failure of descent of the intestine, transposition associated with transposition of other viscera, and variations in development and/or attachment of the mesentery. Any or all of these anomalies may be responsible for volvulus and intestinal obstruction.

Abnormal peritoneal bands also may produce obstruction. A *congenitally short esophagus* may be associated with herniation of a portion of the gastric cardia into the thoracic cavity—so-called *hiatus hernia* (p. 1124).

ACQUIRED MALFORMATIONS
Diverticula

Acquired diverticula of the gastrointestinal tract are, for the most part, "false" diverticula —i.e., they represent herniations of the mucous membrane and muscularis mucosae through weakened areas or defects in the muscularis propria. Thus, the walls of such diverticula do not have all the layers of the segment of alimentary tract from which they arise but are composed simply of mucous membrane, muscularis mucosae, and areolar tissue (Fig. 27-3). One example is the *pulsion diverticulum* (Zenker's diverticulum), which occurs posteriorly at the junction of the esophagus and hypopharynx where the cricopharyngeal muscle is attached. It is a lesion of adults, occurring more frequently in men than in women.

The *traction diverticula* that occur in the esophagus and duodenum are exceptions to the statement that the acquired lesions are false diverticula. Diverticula occur anteriorly in the esophagus at the level of the bifurcation of the trachea secondary to inflammatory disease of hilar or mediastinal lymph nodes and in the first portion of the duodenum just distal to the pylorus in association with the scarring of duodenal or pyloric ulcers.

Diverticula occur infrequently in the duodenum and small intestine and rarely are the cause of clinical disease. In the duodenum, they usually occur in the second portion and tend to be large, with large openings. They are usually single but may be multiple. In the small intestine, on the other hand, they are generally multiple, occurring along the mesenteric attachment and herniating through the gaps by which the blood vessels and nerves penetrate the muscle coat.

Diverticula of colon. The most frequently occurring diverticula of the gastrointestinal tract, and by far the most important in causing clinical disease, are those of the colon. They are found throughout the colon but most commonly in the descending and sigmoid colon, where they are said to occur in 5% or more of all patients over 50 years of age. Diverticulum of the cecum is usually single. When acutely inflamed, it is readily misdiagnosed as acute appendicitis. When the inflammation is chronic and an inflammatory mass is formed, it is readily mistaken clinically, and even at operation, for carcinoma.

Diverticula of the left colon are almost invariably multiple. They develop more frequently in men than in women, presumably on the basis of loss of muscle tone and elasticity of the intestine. Morson[22] has emphasized abnormality, essentially thickening, of the muscle as an important factor in the development of colonic diverticula. They occur on the convexity of the intestine opposite the mesenteric attachment and between the longitudinal muscle bands (taeniae). They frequently are seen in two parallel rows along these bands (Fig. 27-4). Their average diameter is about 1 cm, and their opening into the intestinal lumen is usually small (Fig. 27-3). These herniations of mucosa and submucosa often take place into epiploic appendages and are surrounded and obscured by fat, making their recognition on external inspection difficult. Similarly, muscle contraction may serve to hide their openings from casual inspection of the mucosal aspect of the involved intestinal segment. Colonic diverticula are important because they are prone to the complication of inflammation (10% to 15% of patients). At times, in the absence of overt inflammatory change, they may be associated with sufficient spasm to produce a degree of intestinal narrowing, with appropriate roentgenologic findings suggesting the diagnostic possibility of obstructing carcinoma.

Fecal matter readily accumulates in these colonic diverticula, becoming inspissated to

---

Plate 3

A, Congenital aganglionic megacolon (Hirschsprung's disease).
B, Multifocal epidermoid carcinoma of esophagus. Photograph of gross specimen superimposed upon radiographic film, demonstrating lesion with aid of contrast medium.
C, Familial multiple polyposis of colon.
D, Multiple chronic gastric (peptic) ulcers. Pylorus is just to left of ulcer on left.
E, Carcinomatous ulcer of stomach. Lesion presumed to have been malignant from its inception.
F, Carcinoma of stomach, linitis plastica type. Surgically resected specimen.
G, Multiple carcinoid tumors of ileum. Patient had lymph node and liver metastases and demonstrated carcinoid syndrome.

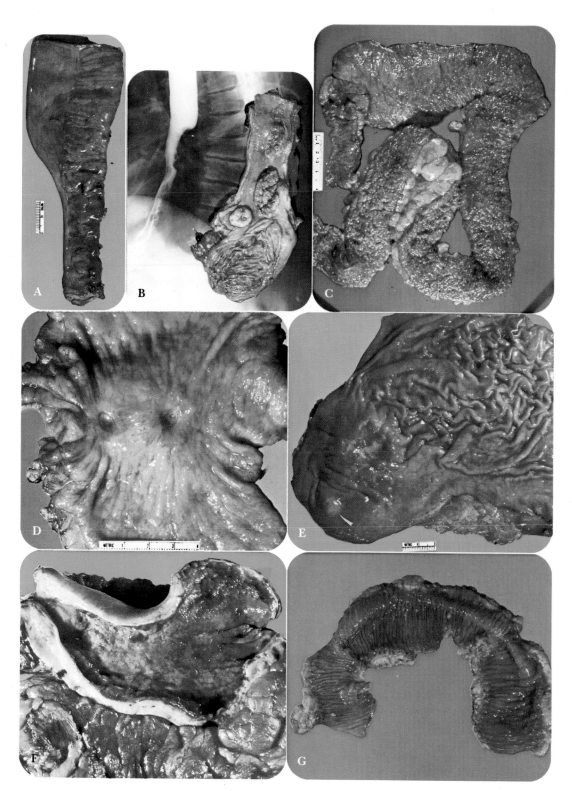

Plate 3

For legend see opposite page.

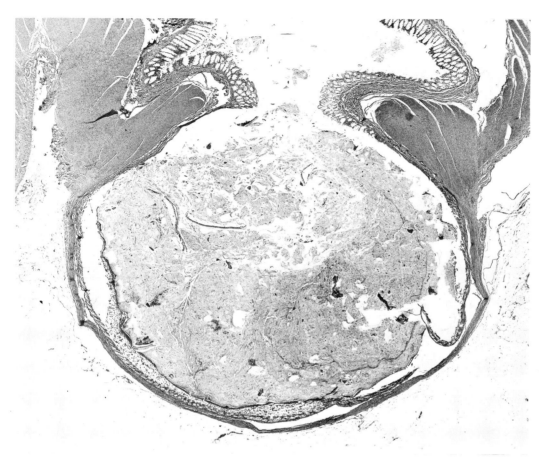

Fig. 27-3 Diverticulum of sigmoid colon, demonstrating hernia-like nature. Note fecal content. (×17.)

form fecaliths, obstructing their orifices and predisposing to inflammation. (Conversely, in the small intestine, where the intestinal content is fluid, inflammation of diverticula is unusual.) Perforation is a not infrequent sequel of diverticulitis. Commonly, such perforation is localized in its effects rather than freely extending through the peritoneal cavity. Focal abscesses are produced, or peridiverticular or periocolonic inflammation occurs, which frequently becomes chronic. In this fashion, inflammatory masses may develop that can produce intestinal obstruction and mimic carcinoma.

Pneumatosis intestinalis

In pneumatosis intestinalis, gas-filled cysts are found in the submucosa and/or subserosa of the small intestine and, less frequently, of the colon (Fig. 27-5). More than half of the reported cases have been associated with gastric or duodenal ulcers, and a high degree of association with respiratory disease, notably asthma, has been observed.

Although there have been much discussion and speculation about pathogenesis, it now appears that the development of pneumatosis can be explained on a mechanical basis in association with:

1 Obstruction with ulceration
2 Trauma from biopsy, sigmoidoscopic examination, etc., or
3 Respiratory disease with severe cough

In the latter case, it is postulated that pneumomediastinum follows pulmonary alveolar rupture, the air then dissecting retroperitoneally and reaching the intestine along the path of the mesenteric blood vessels. Some of the gas cysts, which range in diameter from a few millimeters to a centimeter or more, are lined by flattened, endothelium-like cells and resemble lymphatic vessels, but others are lined by, or contain multinucleated giant cells, and still others appear to have no cellular lining. There may be some associated inflammation and fibrosis. The cysts do not communicate with the intestinal lumen or with each other. In association with other lesions (ulcer,

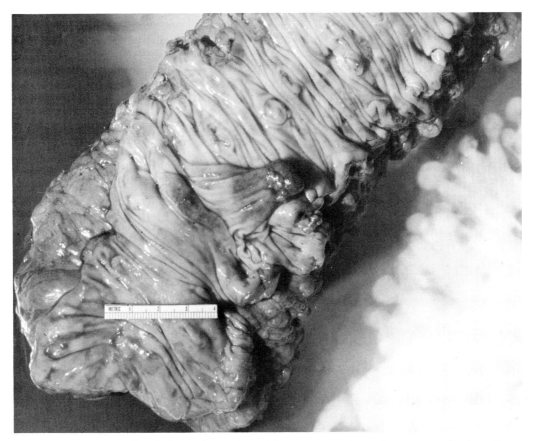

Fig. 27-4 Diverticula of descending colon. Adenomatous polyps also present. Portion of radiograph taken following barium enema on right.

etc.) of the gastrointestinal tract, subserosal cysts are usual. In the absence of such an association, cysts are more often seen in the submucosa. The symptoms of pneumatosis are generally nonspecific. Apparently the gas cysts can resolve.

Melanosis of colon

In some individuals the mucous membrane of the colon may acquire brown pigmentation of varying depth—the result of the presence in the lamina propria of numerous pigment-bearing phagocytes. Although the pigment is referred to as melanin, its exact nature is unknown. The condition is not of clinical significance; it has been suggested that it is related to colonic stasis and the habitual use of anthracene laxatives.

Endometriosis

Foci of endometrial glands with characteristic endometrial stroma may involve the colon, usually the sigmoid or rectum, or the appendix, generally as part of more widespread disease of the pelvic organs (Fig. 27-6).

Endometriosis may be responsible for obstructive symptoms, colic and diarrhea, or even rectal bleeding. Obstruction is the result of fibrosis or muscle spasm, and cancer can be simulated closely, both radiographically and at operation.

Miscellaneous

Many of the malformations more commonly seen as congenital lesions also may be acquired. For example, **esophagotracheobronchial fistulas** may result from infections or trauma, and **acquired megacolon** in the adult may result from a destructive lesion of the myenteric plexus.

MECHANICAL DISTURBANCES
Obstruction

Achalasia of the esophagus and congenital pyloric stenosis have already been briefly discussed. Both the esophagus and stomach are subject to obstruction by some of the causes

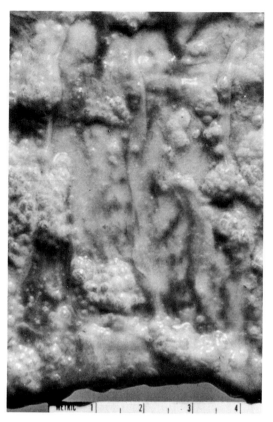

Fig. 27-5 Pneumatosis cystoides intestinalis.

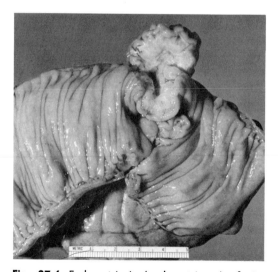

Fig. 27-6 Endometriosis (endometrioma) of sigmoid colon.

of intestinal obstruction mentioned in the following discussion. In addition, it should be noted that peptic ulcers located in the distal part of the stomach or proximal part of the duodenum may produce pyloric obstruction as the result of scarring and muscle spasm.

The end result of esophageal obstruction is starvation. In pyloric obstruction, dehydration and alkalosis from loss of chlorides by vomiting are additional factors.

Although in the experience of any single individual or group (because of the varying composition of patient populations studied), the relative incidence of the various causes of *intestinal obstruction* varies, hernias, adhesions, and neoplasms are always among the more common. Other causes are volvulus, foreign objects, inflammatory disease, stricture, and external compression by tumors, cysts, enlarged viscera, etc., as well as such congenital lesions as annular pancreas, meconium ileus (p. 1279), and the atresias, bands, etc., previously noted.

Hernia

Hernia is the protrusion of tissue or of an organ or part of an organ through an abnormal opening in the wall of the body cavity in which it is normally confined. The great majority of hernias are abdominal and consist of the extension of a peritoneal pouch (the hernial sac) through a defect or a weakened area in the abdominal wall. Of first importance is the indirect inguinal hernia—herniation of abdominal contents through the internal inguinal ring and along the inguinal canal into the scrotum—as a result of persistence, actual or potential, of the vaginal process of peritoneum that normally accompanies the testis on its descent into the scrotum, to become obliterated subsequently.

Herniation may take place through the external inguinal ring of the male (direct inguinal hernia) or through the femoral ring beneath the inguinal ligament, usually of the female (femoral hernia). Umbilical hernias may be congenital, in which case they are often huge, or they may be acquired. Ventral hernias are related to traumatic abdominal wall defects, usually resulting from improper healing following a surgical procedure. All types of hernias involve an increase of intra-abdominal pressure (as produced by lifting or straining) and a defect or a weakened area in the abdominal wall.

Abdominal hernial sacs may contain any of the mobile viscera, most commonly the omentum and/or portions of the intestinal tract. When they contain intestine, it is usually the small intestine. Hernias are not of serious import so long as they remain uncomplicated and reducible (i.e., subject to return of their visceral content to the abdominal cavity).

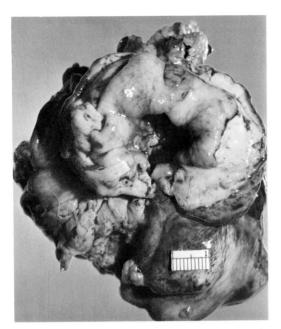

Fig. 27-7 Peptic ulceration in portion of stomach herniated through esophageal hiatus (hiatus hernia).

However, they may become irreducible or incarcerated, usually as the result of adhesions. Obstruction to the passage of the intestinal contents may then occur, and strangulation may follow. In the latter situation, obstruction to venous blood flow in the mesentery produces congestion and edema, setting up a vicious circle culminating in arterial obstruction and hemorrhagic infarction.

Less common are internal hernias, wherein loops of intestine penetrate normally small peritoneal recesses, such as the fossa at the junction of duodenum and jejunum.

Diaphragmatic hernias will be considered briefly; they are not a significant cause of intestinal obstruction. Herniation of abdominal viscera occasionally occurs through congenital defects in the diaphragm, but the so-called *hiatus hernia* is the only one that is encountered with any degree of frequency. It is the protrusion, often intermittent ("sliding" hernia), of a portion of the stomach and abdominal esophagus through the esophageal hiatus of the diaphragm into the thoracic cavity. Symptoms are related to the reflux of gastric secretions into the esophagus, with resultant so-called peptic esophagitis and ulceration (Fig. 27-7). The esophagus is commonly shorter than normal, either congenitally or as a result of inflammation with scarring. Symptomatic hiatus hernia is usually a disease of obese, middle-aged individuals (see Mal-

lory-Weiss syndrome, p. 1126). Herniation of the gastric cardia through the esophageal hiatus also may occur alongside the esophagus—paraesophageal hernia.

Adhesions

It has been noted that congenital peritoneal bands may produce intestinal obstruction. Similarly, peritoneal adhesions between loops of intestine or between the intestine and other viscera or the abdominal parietes, acquired as the result of previous inflammation and usually after laparotomy, may cause kinking or compression of intestinal loops or be the focal point of a volvulus and thus be responsible for intestinal obstruction. Again, the occluding band also may compress the blood vessels, causing infarction. It is usually the small intestine that is obstructed by adhesions.

Neoplastic obstruction

Neoplastic intestinal obstruction usually occurs in the large intestine because it is one of the more common sites of cancer in man, whereas cancer is much less common in the small intestine.

The most common obstructing tumors are the encircling carcinomas that occur in the left half of the colon, where the intestinal content is semisolid. The intestine proximal to the tumor is commonly dilated and hypertrophied. Metastatic tumors and tumors involving the peritoneal surfaces also can cause obstruction by external compression and by producing adhesions.

Intussusception

Intussusception is the invagination of a segment of the intestinal tract (the intussusceptum) into the immediately adjacent (almost always distal) intestine (the intussuscipiens). It is primarily a disease of infants and young children, but it does occur in adults, in whom it may be initiated by a pedunculated or mucosal tumor projecting into the intestinal lumen. The tumor, usually benign, but sometimes carcinoma or metastatic malignant melanoma, is propelled along the intestine by peristalsis, pulling its attachment and the proximal intestine along with it.

In children, intussusception is most common in the region of the ileocecal valve, the ileum telescoping into the colon and the ileocecal valve retaining its normal position (Fig. 27-8). Ileoileal intussusception is less common, and colocolonic even more so. At times, abnormally large masses of lymphoid tissue ap-

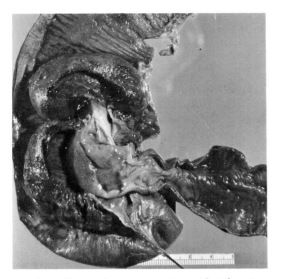

Fig. 27-8 Ileocecal intussusception with infarction.

parently form the advancing head of the intussusception. At other times, the ileocecal valve itself may do so. No such specific cause can be incriminated in many childhood cases, and the disease is attributed to uncoordinated muscle contractions. Males are more frequently affected than females.

Intussusception tends to be progressive, and as the intussusceptum pulls its mesentery with it, a point is reached where the blood supply is compromised. Hemorrhagic infarction and acute inflammation follow. The clinical manifestations are those of intestinal obstruction, with violent pain and bloody stools. A sausage-shaped abdominal mass may be palpable. In some cases, recurrent episodes of intussusception may follow reduction, either spontaneous or induced by enema. Generally, however, the condition constitutes a surgical emergency, and, if operation is prompt, reduction generally can be effected. If not, or if the lesion has progressed to gangrene, resection, with an attendant high mortality rate, is required.

Multiple foci of intussusception, unassociated with any reaction, are seen occasionally at autopsy. They are believed to be agonal.

Volvulus

Volvulus is the twisting of a loop (or loops) of intestine upon itself through 180° or more that produces obstruction of both the intestine and the blood supply of the affected loop. Predisposing factors are unusually long mesenteric attachment, redundant intestine, abnormal bands, congenital or acquired, or abnormal attachments of the intestine.

The lesion is most common in the sigmoid

colon and predominates in males. Because strangulation occurs almost simultaneously with obstruction, operative treatment must be prompt to avoid a prohibitive mortality rate.

Obturation obstruction

A wide variety of ingested foreign bodies or objects of endogenous origin not natural to the intestinal tract may be responsible for intestinal obstruction—obturation obstruction. If large, a foreign body may produce obstruction on that basis alone, but a smaller object may also produce obstruction by irritation and secondary spasm, or if the object becomes lodged in an area where narrowing due to other causes is already present—e.g., impaction of a fruit pit in a radiation-induced stricture.

Gallstones, entering the intestine via a cholecystogastric or cholecystoduodenal fistula (the late result of cholecystitis with perforation) and becoming impacted, are the most common examples of obstruction by an endogenous foreign object (often referred to as "gallstone ileus"). Enteroliths and fecaliths are others. Gallstones usually cause obstruction of the small intestine and enteroliths of the large intestine. Fecaliths frequently are implicated in appendiceal disease.

In addition to the fruit pits cited, almost any conceivable sort of foreign body may be ingested—usually by the very young, the mentally deficient, or the insane. At times, the object does not pass the esophagus. Bezoars—masses of ingested hair (trichobezoars) or of vegetable residues (phytobezoars), most notably of persimmons—are worthy of special mention. They usually are found in the stomach. Masses of parasites, particularly *Ascaris lumbricoides,* are another potential cause of intestinal obstruction.

Stricture

The most commonly occurring stricture of the alimentary canal is that of the esophagus following chemical injury, usually due to accidental ingestion of lye by small children. The cicatricial scarring produces stenosis at the points of natural narrowing (i.e., the levels of the cricopharyngeal muscle, the bifurcation of the trachea, and the cardia), but narrowing may extend over a considerable distance. Stenosis also may be associated with peptic ulceration of the lower esophagus or esophageal involvement in scleroderma.

Years after x-ray irradiation, usually in the treatment of cancer of the pelvic organs of the female, radiation ulcers of the small intestine, less often of the colon, may develop. If they heal without perforating, the final result may be one or more strictures. Rarely, scarring at the site of anastomosis following resection of a segment of intestine or healing of an infarct (p. 1127) produces a stricture.

Effects of intestinal obstruction

Obstruction of the small intestine is usually acute and complete. The higher in the tract it occurs, the more profound are the systemic effects and the more immediate is the threat to life. The large amount of fluid normally secreted into the gastrointestinal tract is augmented under the stimulus of intestinal distention, and its absorption in the lower portion of the ileum is decreased or entirely abolished, depending upon the site of the obstructing lesion. There is also transudation of edema fluid and blood into the intestinal wall and lumen. Gas, consisting largely of swallowed air, but including some gases from the blood and some from bacterial action on the intestinal content, also accumulates.

The significant electrolyte content of the intestinal fluid is lost to the organism. Vomiting tends to minimize distention when obstruction is high in the intestine but accentuates the fluid and electrolyte loss. If the obstruction is at the pylorus, the predominant loss of chloride leads to alkalosis. If obstruction is lower and significant amounts of bile and pancreatic and intestinal secretions also are lost, the noncompensable sodium deficit leads to acidosis. Dehydration occurs, and with it, hemoconcentration. Decrease in intracellular fluid follows, and finally renal suppression and nitrogen retention result. The loss of potassium is also an important factor in the morbidity of intestinal obstruction.

Obstruction low in the small intestine does not produce the dramatic systemic effects described. Vomiting cannot completely empty the intestine proximal to the block, and as a result the distention of the intestine with fluid, blood, and gas, instead of electrolyte alteration, dominates the picture. As intraluminal pressure rises, the viability of the intestinal wall is compromised, and it becomes permeable to bacteria. Thus, peritonitis can develop, even without actual gangrene and/or perforation. Depending upon the cause of the obstruction, it may be associated with infarction, the result of obstruction to the blood supply of the involved intestine, its venous drainage, or both.

Obstruction in the colon is usually incom-
plete and chronic, carcinoma being by far the most frequently encountered underlying lesion. It does not produce the striking clinical picture just described. However, if complete and unrelieved, it is incompatible with life. So-called "closed loop" obstruction occurs in the presence of a competent ileocecal valve. Since colonic obstruction is usually incomplete and chronic, the intestine proximal to the obstructing lesion is hypertrophied as well as dilated. It is when the hypertrophy fails to compensate for the obstruction that clinical disease becomes manifest.

Adynamic (paralytic) ileus

The clinical picture of acute intestinal obstruction may occur in the absence of mechanical or organic obstruction as the result of paralysis of the musculature of a portion or all of the intestinal tract. Abdominal distention and accumulation of gas and fluid in the intestine may be extreme. Such paralytic ileus frequently occurs following laparotomy, usually in a mild form. Otherwise, it may be associated with intra-abdominal infection, trauma, or other disease (e.g., ureteral stone) or systemic infection (e.g., pneumonia in children).

Peritonitis secondary to acute appendicitis with perforation, perforated peptic ulcer, etc. is probably the most important single underlying cause. Paralytic ileus may be superimposed upon partial organic intestinal obstruction, producing effective complete obstruction. A related condition is *acute dilatation of the stomach,* which occasionally complicates surgery, usually abdominal.

Mallory-Weiss syndrome

Any action that increases intra-abdominal pressure, but particularly bouts of repeated and forceful vomiting, may produce one or more lacerations of the gastric cardia that may be the source of gastrointestinal hemorrhage, sometimes massive. This syndrome, known eponymically by the names of those who first described it, frequently occurs in alcoholics or is associated with atrophic gastritis. Dagradi et al.[48] consider the Mallory-Weiss lesion a complication of a sliding hiatus hernia. The tears occur in the long axis of the stomach and esophagus, occasionally crossing the esophagogastric junction.

VASCULAR DISTURBANCES
Esophageal varices

Elevated pressure in the portal venous system, most often the result of cirrhosis of the liver but, at times, due to such other lesions as portal vein thrombosis, commonly results in esophageal varices. The esophageal venous plexus receives blood from the gastric vein and the coronary vein of the stomach, forming part of one of the routes by which portal venous blood may bypass the liver to reach the right atrium. As a result, the submucosal veins of the lower part of the esophagus, and sometimes of the upper part of the stomach as well, become greatly dilated, tortuous, and engorged. They are covered by a thinned mucous membrane. The increased venous pressure, with or without inflammation and/or ulceration, often results in massive and frequently fatal hemorrhage.

Infarction of intestine

Excluding instances of strangulation as discussed previously, the most common cause of intestinal infarction is sclerosis of the mesenteric arteries, with or without associated thrombosis. Embolism and venous thrombosis are less frequently encountered causes, and still rarer are such vascular diseases as arteriolar sclerosis, thromboangiitis obliterans, periarteritis nodosa, etc. Emboli may be from vegetations in the diseased left side of the heart or from atheromatous material dislodged from aortic plaques, but more often they are related to intracardiac mural thrombi, usually in hearts damaged by rheumatic disease. In some instances, complete vascular occlusion may not be demonstrated. Lowering of the systemic blood pressure, as in shock, may be sufficient to cause an infarct in an intestine whose blood supply is compromised by nonoccluding atheromatous plaques. The superior mesenteric vessels and consequently the jejunum and proximal part of the ileum are involved most frequently, although any part or all of the gastrointestinal tract may be affected.

In a majority of instances of arterial occlusion, the infarct is initially anemic. With time, it becomes hemorrhagic. Infarction caused by strangulation, where venous occlusion usually precedes arterial blockage, is hemorrhagic from the beginning. Hemorrhage takes place into both the intestinal wall and the lumen. The affected intestine is a dusky, purplish red. Necrosis without inflammatory exudation progresses to gangrene, with ultimate perforation and peritonitis. Inasmuch as the musculature becomes paralyzed soon after interference with the blood supply takes place, effective intestinal obstruction, with its attendant physiologic alterations and clinical manifestations, compli-

cates the disease solely because of the interruption of the blood supply.

Ischemic enteritis

Infarction of limited extent or of less than the full thickness of the intestinal wall or reduction in blood flow due to arteriosclerosis or arteriolar sclerosis may be responsible for a variety of lesions, all nonspecific in character. They are ulceration, nonspecific inflammation, cicatrization with stricture formation and incomplete intestinal obstruction, and "intestinal angina." The distinction between such lesions and those believed to be related to potassium ingestion (p. 197) is not always clear.

Hemorrhoids

Hemorrhoids are varicosites of the hemorrhoidal veins—"internal" and covered by mucous membrane if of the superior hemorrhoidal plexus and "external" and covered by skin if of the inferior hemorrhoidal plexus. The former are the more important and the more troublesome. Any mechanism that increases the pressure in these veins may be the proximate cause—e.g., portal hypertension or cardiac failure. However, increased pressure from some local cause, such as carcinoma of the rectum, myomatous or pregnant uterus, or, above all, chronic constipation, is far more important.

The coincidence of hemorrhoids and rectal carcinoma is sufficiently great to make search for the latter mandatory in every patient with hemorrhoids.

The principal complication of hemorrhoids is thrombosis, with associated inflammation and scarring and resultant pain. Hemorrhage (bright red blood passed by rectum) is a common clinical manifestation.

Gastrointestinal hemorrhage

A wide variety of diseases or lesions that involve the gastrointestinal tract give rise to bleeding. A number have already been considered. In many cases, blood loss is not great, and the bleeding is merely an evidence of the presence of disease, although, if continued over a long period of time, anemia may develop (e.g., in hiatus hernia or carcinoma of the right side of the colon). In others, the bleeding is massive and significant in itself, even of life-threatening proportions. If the blood is vomited or passed by rectum soon after escaping from the vascular system, it is, of course, bright red. If, on the other hand, the shed blood remains in the alimentary canal for a period of time or has to traverse a considerable length of the gut before emerging, it is partially digested and its color altered to brown or black (coffee-ground vomitus and tarry stools or melena).

The most important sources of massive hematemesis (vomiting of blood), the majority of which are proximal to the ligament of Treitz, are esophageal varices, gastric or duodenal (peptic) ulcer, and leiomyoma. Other tumors (benign or malignant), hiatus hernia, gastritis, etc. usually produce bleeding of lesser degree. Massive bleeding from the rectum and/or anus is less common than massive hematemesis. Hemorrhoids, diverticular disease, or the polyps of Peutz-Jeghers syndrome may cause it. However, these lesions also may be associated with bleeding of small amount, as is commonly found in carcinoma of the large intestine and, less often, with other tumors, regional enteritis, ulcerative colitis, and anal fissure. The lesions causing hematemesis are also associated with blood in the stool, which may be occult (i.e., detectable only by chemical means). Other conditions that should be considered as potential causes of any type of gastrointestinal bleeding include hereditary telangiectasis (Rendu-Osler-Weber disease), other vascular malformations, any of the blood dyscrasias, and anticoagulant therapy.

INFLAMMATIONS
Esophagitis

Reference already has been made to the peptic esophagitis that may occur in the distal part of the esophagus as the result of reflux of acid gastric secretion in such conditions as hiatus hernia and scleroderma. It may progress to peptic ulceration, with scarring and stricture formation. The cicatricial stricture due to ingestion of corrosive substances (usually lye) follows an acute ulcerative inflammatory process, although the immediate effect of ingestion is fixation in situ of the tissue with which the lye, or other corrosive, comes in contact.

In rare instances, the virus of *herpes simplex* is responsible for ulcers in the esophagus, usually occurring in older patients with malignant disease. Eosinophilic intranuclear inclusions are present in the preserved epithelium adjacent to the ulcers.

Gastritis and gastroenteritis

The gastritis and gastroenteritis that are such common clinical complaints rarely come to the attention of the pathologist. There is described, however, a *phlegmonous gastritis,* or cellulitis of the stomach, of streptococcal origin. Nonspecific inflammatory changes occur in association with other gastric lesions, especially ulcer.

The pathologic changes in the occasionally fatal *diarrhea of newborn and older infants* are nonspecific and frequently unimpressive. The disease probably has multiple bacterial and viral etiologic agents.

Eosinophilic granuloma and eosinophilic gastroenteritis

Two different but possibly related conditions in which eosinophilic leukocytes make up a prominent part of the histopathologic picture occur in various parts of the gastrointestinal tract. One lesion is a localized, fibrotic, granulomatous, polypoid tumorlike mass including many eosinophils ("inflammatory fibroid polyp"[60]). The other is a diffuse infiltration of eosinophilic leukocytes throughout all coats of the gut wall. The pyloric region is affected more commonly than the small or large intestine. This is particularly true of the diffuse infiltration, which readily produces pyloric obstruction. Some of the patients, more often those with a diffuse infiltration, have had histories of allergic disease, and at times there is a striking peripheral blood eosinophilia.

Nonspecific ulceration

In recent years, nonspecific ulcerations of the small intestine have been encountered with sufficient frequency to command attention. Some cases have been complicated by perforation and some by scarring and partial intestinal obstruction. A large percentage of the patients presenting with such lesions were

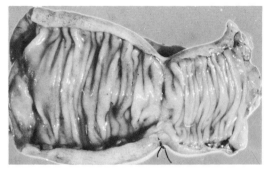

Fig. 27-9 Ulceration of small intestine with scarring and stenosis, possibly secondary to potassium chloride administration or ischemia.

receiving enteric-coated potassium chloride therapeutically, and potassium, a known tissue irritant, has been implicated as the etiologic agent. The relationship has not been established, however, and there is evidence in the form of vascular changes to suggest that vascular disease may be a more important factor (Fig. 27-9).

Ulcers of stomach and duodenum

Ulcers, usually small and superficial and frequently multiple, occur in the stomach as a terminal event in a variety of disease states. Many of them might be better termed erosions. Acute ulcers of the stomach or duodenum, *Curling's ulcers,* are an important complication of extensive cutaneous burns (Fig. 27-10). They have been reported as occurring in as many as one-third of autopsied cases.[64] They may be fatal as the result of uncontrolled hemorrhage or spontaneous perforation and peritonitis. Similar ulcers may be associated with Cushing's disease, therapeutic administration of adrenocorticosteroids, lesions of the hypothalamus, or with such causes of stress as trauma. They are considered to be mediated through central hypothalamic stimulation, together with anterior pituitary stimulation of the adrenal cortex and/or excessive vagal activity.

Peptic ulcer

Incidence and etiology. Chronic ulcers that have certain similarities occur in both the stomach and the duodenum. However, they also manifest distinct differences, and it is not certain that they represent the same fundamental disease process. *Duodenal ulcers* are

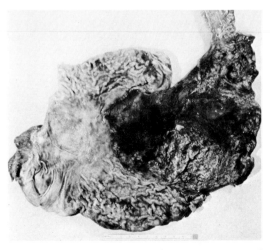

Fig. 27-10 Curling's ulcer of proximal part of stomach.

much more common and occur most often in young adult and middle-aged males, whereas gastric ulcers occur more frequently in females and at older ages. It is the duodenal ulcer particularly that is thought of as a "disease of civilization." We have drawn a picture of the patient with duodenal ulcer as a successful, hard-driving young man unable to relax and continually confronted with the necessity of making important decisions—or, more generally, an individual in a life situation of continuous or oft-repeated severe stress. However, this is by no means always the case, and there is no agreement on the importance of stress in the pathogenesis of chronic peptic ulcer.

It is certain that peptic ulcers occur only in the environment of acid gastric secretion: the stomach, duodenum, lower esophagus, jejunum just distal to the site of surgical gastroenteric anastomosis, and malformations containing gastric mucosa. In each instance, ulceration does not occur in the acid-secreting mucous membrane but adjacent to it in mucous membrane not naturally accustomed to an acid-pepsin environment. Thus, gastric ulcers occur in the antrum, infrequently in the cardia, whereas acid secretion usually is limited to the fundus.

Dragstedt[66] contends that peptic ulcers are caused by hypersecretion of gastric juice and, furthermore, that there is no solid evidence for the existence of a localized area of decreased resistance in the involved mucosa. The gastroduodenal mucous membrane is protected against digestion by normal gastric secretions not only by its mucous coating, but also by prompt dilution and neutralization by swallowed food, saliva, mucus from the antrum, and regurgitated duodenal fluids. Pure gastric juice as it is secreted is capable of digesting any living tissue. In the case of duodenal ulcer, Dragstedt[66] states that patients secrete three to twenty times as much hydrochloric acid into the fasting stomach at night as do normal persons. This hypersecretion is the result of vagal stimulation and can be abolished by section of the vagus nerves. Gastric ulcer, on the other hand, occurs in an atonic stomach in which the stasis of ingested food is responsible for a humoral (gastrin) stimulus to hypersecretion. Dragstedt[66] cites experimental work and clinical observations of his own and others to support his theory, adding that his findings do not support the postulate that stress plays a part in the pathogenesis of peptic ulcer.

On the other hand, Wolf[69] has produced considerable evidence that emotional factors do affect gastric function. There remains much support for the thesis that the hypothalamus–anterior pituitary–adrenal cortex stress mechanism is of importance in the genesis of ulcer, perhaps mediated through vagal stimulation. Ulcers similar to those under discussion develop not infrequently in patients on prolonged *steroid therapy* for such diseases as rheumatoid arthritis and systemic lupus erythematosus. These steroid ulcers are usually gastric and more acute and shallower than the typical chronic peptic ulcer. They may be asymptomatic until some dramatic event, such as hemorrhage, calls attention to their presence. Steroid administration also may activate an existing ulcer and be responsible for perforation or hemorrhage. Occasionally, *single acute ulcers* differing from typical peptic ulcers only in their lack of evidence of chronicity are encountered.

Morbid anatomy and histology. Gastric ulcers most commonly occur on or near the lesser curvature of the stomach, usually within about 5 cm of the pylorus. They are more numerous on the posterior than the anterior wall. A few occur in the cardia, and a few seemingly straddle the pylorus, making it difficult to assign them definitely to either stomach or duodenum. Duodenal ulcers usually occur in the first centimeter or two distal to the pylorus on the anterior or posterior wall rather than laterally.

Although some gastric ulcers are large and irregular, the typical peptic ulcer is small (± 1 cm in the duodenum, 1 cm to 2.5 cm in the stomach). It is characteristically "punched out," with sharply defined margins, sometimes sloping distally. The ulcer penetrates deeply. Its edges are neither raised nor overhanging (Plate 3, *D*). The mucosal folds converging upon the ulcer are distinct to the edge of the lesion. In the case of *gastric ulcer,* it is important, although often difficult and sometimes impossible, to differentiate the lesion from a *malignant ulcer.* The latter is usually a bowl-shaped lesion, and the entire ulcer tends to be raised above the surface of the rest of the stomach (Plate 3, *E*). Penetration is not usually deep, and the progress of the mucosal folds toward the crater is interrupted by nodular mucosal or submucosal thickening.

Microscopically, the bed of the ulcer is seen to be covered by fibrinous exudate containing fragmented leukocytes. Separating this from the scar tissue base is fibrotic granulation tissue with a plasma cell and lymphocytic infiltrate. Occasionally, eosinophils are prominent. The scar tissue is dense and avascular and occupies a full-thickness defect in the muscularis. Hypertrophic nerve bundles may be conspicuous, and at times a large artery, often thrombosed or sclerotic, may be seen. In some bleeding ulcers, such a vessel may be recognized on gross examination.

Many ulcers heal, and epithelium grows over the defect in a single layer. In time, glandlike structures may develop, but a completely normal mucous membrane is not regenerated. Because of the dense scar, the muscle does not regenerate, and evidence of the ulcer will remain indefinitely.

Complications. The principal complications of peptic ulcer are hemorrhage, perforation, and obstruction. Which, if any, occurs is dependent in part on the location of the ulcer. Both gastric and duodenal ulcers are subject to massive hemorrhage. Duodenal ulcers are especially prone to perforation. Any ulcer, but especially those located posteriorly, may bleed in smaller amounts, producing melena or evidence of occult blood in the stool.

Anterior duodenal ulcers may perforate into the free peritoneal cavity, with resultant generalized peritonitis. Perforating posterior ulcers more often penetrate into the pancreas, producing intractable pain. Posterior perforation also may occur into the lesser peritoneal sac, leading to localized peritonitis. The omentum or adhesions to adjacent organs also may serve to localize peritoneal inflammation. The peritonitis due to perforated peptic ulcer is initially a chemical inflammation, but bacterial contamination soon follows.

Pyloric obstruction may be a complication of an ulcer, gastric or duodenal, situated near the pylorus. It usually results from a combination of cicatricial narrowing and spasm. The stomach becomes greatly dilated and hypertrophied.

The development of carcinoma has been referred to as one of the complications of peptic ulcer. It seems probable that carcinoma can develop in a preexisting ulcer, but it is equally probable that it is a rare event. It is extremely difficult to establish the fact of such a sequence of events in any particular case.

A complication of surgical treatment of ulcer is the development of a *marginal (stomal) ulcer*—peptic ulceration of the jejunum just distal to the site of anastomosis with the stomach following gastroenterostomy or gastric resection with gastrojejunostomy. Such ulcers may perforate. If perforation into the transverse colon takes place, gastrojejunocolic fistula is the result.

Regional enteritis

Regional enteritis (Crohn's disease) is a chronic inflammatory disease of unknown etiology affecting a portion of the intestinal tract, occurring in young adults, and frequently producing partial intestinal obstruction. The disease most commonly involves the terminal ileum, often with extension into the cecum and sometimes into the ascending colon as well. It is usually in the terminal ileum that narrowing produces partial obstruction. In more than half the cases, multiple areas of both small and large intestine are involved in segmental fashion—i.e., lengths of normal intestine separate areas of disease (so-called skip areas). Occasionally, changes are limited to the colon, and such involvement may be extensive.

The inflammatory changes are nonspecific and more or less granulomatous. The mucosal surface has a reddened, nodular, cobblestone-like appearance, with multiple, linear ulcerations. All coats of the diseased intestine are thickened—the mucosa by inflammatory infiltrate, chiefly of lymphocytes and plasma cells, the submucosa and subserosa by fibrosis, and the muscularis by hypertrophy (Fig. 27-11). The fibrosis and infiltrate extend into the mesentery.

Histologically, irregular ulceration with a neutrophilic leukocytic reaction is seen. In the preserved mucous membrane, the glands are dilated, goblet cells are absent or decreased in number, and Paneth cells are more prominent than usual. Peculiar glands resembling Brunner's glands of the duodenum or pyloric glands frequently are seen. The muscularis mucosae is hypertrophied, and nerves in the involved segment are increased in number, size, and prominence. Lymphoid nodules are conspicuous in the submucosa, and often in the subserosa as well. Tubercles composed of epithelioid cells, with occasional multinucleated giant cells but without necrosis, are conspicuous in some cases. They have given rise to the speculation of etiologic identity with Boeck's sarcoid, an idea that has been abandoned. Deep ulcers may give rise to sinus tracts and perforations, which usually are walled off by omentum or adhesions. Fistulas may complicate long-standing cases. The fistulas may be internal, involving other organs or other segments of intestine, or external, opening on the skin of the abdomen, following surgical procedures. The regional lymph nodes are enlarged. They usually show nonspecific inflammatory changes but may contain granulomas like those in the intestine.

Lymphatic obstruction is believed to play a primary role in the pathogenesis of regional enteritis, giving rise to submucosal edema. This, in turn, is followed by fibrosis, lymphoreticular hyperplasia, and, ultimately, secondary mucosal ulceration, inflammation, and the other changes described. Ammann and Bockus[70] suggest that ulceration results from shortening and distortion of Kerkring's folds, in turn the result of shortening of the muscularis mucosae early in the development of the disease.

Appendicitis

Acute appendicitis is the most common intra-abdominal condition that constitutes a surgical emergency. The appendix has been considered functionless and vestigial, but it may make a contribution to the development of the body's immune defense mechanism. It varies greatly in size and position—from a tiny stump or mere cord without a lumen to a completely patent structure as long as 9 cm or 10 cm (or rarely more) with a wall 2 mm to 4 mm thick. It extends medially from the cecum, lying behind it or hanging down into the pelvis.

An important feature of the appendix is the presence in the mucosa of abundant lymphoid tissue in the form of large follicles

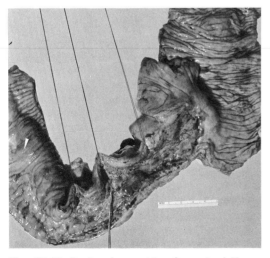

Fig. 27-11 Regional enteritis of terminal ileum. Note abrupt cessation of pathologic change at ileocecal valve.

with conspicuous "germinal centers." These are most striking in the young, reaching maximum development in adolescence and undergoing atrophy with age. Eosinophilic leukocytes and plasma cells are regularly present in the mucosa of the uninflamed appendix.

Acute appendicitis is a disease of the western world and has been related to a high protein and/or high fat content of the diet. It is uncommon at the extremes of age and is most frequently seen in older children and young adults. The most important factor in the pathogenesis of appendicitis is obstruction of the lumen, and the most frequent cause of obstruction is a fecalith—a molded mass of inspissated fecal material that may develop rock-hard consistency. Fecaliths are found in at least three-fourths of acutely inflamed appendices and in virtually all that are gangrenous. In youth, the lymphoid tissue of the mucous membrane may become sufficiently hyperplastic, at times in association with systemic infection, to produce obstruction leading to appendicitis or to cause symptoms and signs indistinguishable from those of mild acute appendiceal inflammation. Other causes of obstruction are scars that represent the residua of previous attacks of appendicitis, tumors, external bands, and adhesions, and, rarely, masses of parasites (especially pinworms), foreign bodies, and possibly spasm of the muscle at the base of the appendix. The immediate cause of acute appendicitis is bacterial infection. Although infection via the bloodstream in systemic disease is possible, the usual source of bacteria is from the intestinal lumen. Many species of bacteria can be identified—all those common to the intestinal tract. Multiple organisms usually can be isolated from an individual case.

In instances of inflammation of limited extent, grossly visible evidences of disease may be only mild hyperemia, and microscopic examination may show mainly small amounts of purulent exudate in the lumen, although careful study reveals one or more foci of inflammation, with ulceration, in the mucosa. Many examples of *focal appendicitis* are not merely an early phase of diffuse inflammation but a milder form of the disease, perhaps dependent upon temporary or incomplete obstruction by such mechanisms as lymphoid hyperplasia or muscle spasm. Although, at times, the inflammation appears limited to the muscle coat and/or subserosa, examination of sufficient microscopic sections usually shows mucosal involvement.

The trauma of a surgical procedure, particularly if appendectomy is performed incidentally following a more complex operation, may be responsible for hyperemia and margination of leukocytes in the peripheral blood vessels of the appendix, or even for infiltration of some polymorphonuclear leukocytes into the subserosal tissues. More intense inflammatory change in the serosa and subserosa may be associated with disease primary outside the appendix (e.g., salpingitis). Also, at times a few neutrophilic leukocytes may be found in the lumen of an incidentally removed appendix without there being any evidence of inflammation of the appendiceal wall.

Diffuse acute appendicitis almost always occurs in an obstructed appendix, usually one with an obstructing fecalith. With obstruction, secretions accumulate and distention occurs. The appendiceal wall is thinned, and the arterial blood supply to that portion of the organ distal to the obstruction is compromised and ultimately cut off completely. The pressure of an impacted fecalith may well contribute directly to this process. Thus, bacterial infection and infarction proceed together. There is relatively free communication between the submucosal and subserosal coats of the appendix, and the inflammation soon involves the full thickness of the wall and ultimately the whole organ. The exact anatomic picture will depend upon the time when the surgeon removes the appendix, interrupting the progression. The inflammatory process is one of infiltration of polymorphonuclear leukocytes, with progressive, usually hemorrhagic, necrosis. The mucous membrane is patchily ulcerated or completely destroyed, and fibrinous or fibrinopurulent exudate is present on the serosal surface. Peritonitis precedes perforation of the wall of the appendix, which is a common event. The final stage may be gangrene of the appendix.

Grossly, the diffusely inflamed appendix is distended, at least distal to obstruction, its blood vessels are engorged, and its surface is dulled by a delicate or shaggy layer of fibrin. Purulent exudate, which also may be hemorrhagic, is present in the lumen. The mucous membrane may be visibly ulcerated. With progression to gangrene, the colors change to grayish green, reddish black, or almost black, the wall becomes friable, and one or more perforations may be apparent, usually on the antimesenteric border at the site of, or just distal to, a fecalith. The appendix, or part of it, may slough. If a perforation is walled off by the cecum, omentum, or other organs, an *appendiceal abscess* develops. If no such walling off takes place, *generalized suppurative peritonitis* is the result. An infrequently encountered complication of acute suppurative appendicitis is pylephlebitis, wherein the appendiceal veins are involved and the infection is carried to the liver by way of the portal venous system. Pyogenic liver abscesses result.

Not every instance of inflammation of the appendix follows this course. At times, appendicitis may subside. If tissue destruction is minimal, resolution follows. However, if significant tissue destruction has occurred, healing will be by cicatrization. Depending upon the time relationships of the onset of appendicitis and appendectomy, evidences of subsiding acute inflammation or of scarring may be observed. There may be recurrent attacks of acute appendicitis, with resolution or healing and scar formation following each episode. Occasionally, true chronic inflammation of the appendix occurs, usually associated with fistula formation or a foreign body (intestinal content) after acute appendicitis with perforation. Otherwise, true chronic appendicitis as a distinct disease entity does not exist.

In as many as one-fourth of all appendices, all or a part of the lumen is *obliterated* by fibrous tissue that replaces the mucous membrane and within which there may be scattered lymphocytes, lymph follicles, or nerve bundles. When such obliteration is only partial, it is the tip that is involved. The obliterated appendix is usually small and appears atrophic. Although frequently referred to by such terms as "obliterative appendicitis," there is no evidence that this state is the result of inflammatory disease.

The appendix may be involved in diseases primarily affecting other portions of the gastrointestinal tract, such as regional enteritis, typhoid fever, and amebiasis, and in certain systemic diseases (e.g., measles). In the prodromal stage of measles, characteristic giant cells are seen in the lymphoid tissue of the appendix, as well as in the lymphoid tissues of the rest of the body.

Many parasites may be found in the appendix. *Enterobius vermicularis* (pinworm) is the parasite most often encountered. It may be seen on gross inspection as well as in histologic sections (Fig. 27-12). Ordinarily, these worms merely inhabit the appendix and have no relationship to appendiceal disease. On occasion, however, they may penetrate the wall and become the center of a granulomatous

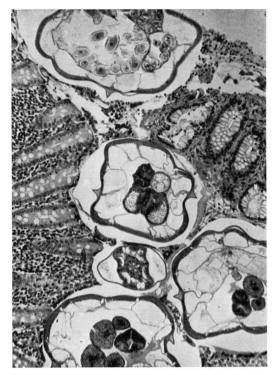

Fig. 27-12 Cross sections of pinworms *(Enterobius vermicularis)* in appendix. (From Anderson, W. A. D.: Synopsis of pathology, The C. V. Mosby Co.)

inflammatory reaction. Their eggs have been observed in similar peritoneal lesions.

Chronic ulcerative colitis

Chronic (idiopathic) ulcerative colitis is usually a disease of young adults, although its onset may be at any age. It runs a very protracted course. It frequently has been suggested that ulcerative colitis and regional enteritis might represent expression in different sites of an identical or related fundamental disease process. However, there are many differences, and although some features are common to both conditions, each generally forms a distinctive total pathologic picture. Although there are instances difficult to assign to one or the other category, it is now generally accepted that the distinction usually can be made between Crohn's disease involving the colon (granulomatous colitis) and chronic ulcerative colitis.

In many respects, ulcerative colitis appears to be a systemic disease rather than a condition affecting only the colon. It is generally believed that psychogenic factors are frequently of etiologic importance. Evidence has been accumulating recently to implicate hypersensitivity as a factor in causation, very likely secondary, since an immune basis for the disease has not been demonstrated. In patients with ulcerative colitis, the occurrence of drug and transfusion reactions, erythema nodosum, iritis, arthritis, hemolytic anemia, and elevated serum gamma globulin support this concept. In 1960, Priest et al.[91] demonstrated, in "skin windows" in patients with ulcerative colitis, the exudation of an unusually large number of basophilic leukocytes in response to a nonspecific injury. This was followed by the demonstration of increased numbers of mast cells in the exudate in the lesions of at least some cases of ulcerative colitis.

It frequently is stated that ulcerative colitis begins in the rectum or sigmoid and progresses proximally to involve the left side of the colon or the whole colon. This is not universally accepted, and it is possible that the theory is based upon the relative ease of establishing the diagnosis by proctoscopic examination. When the whole colon is examined, all or almost all of it is affected in the majority of cases. When a limited segment is involved, it is usually in the left half. It is probable that some of the instances of segmental distribution really represent regional enteritis (or enterocolitis). The terminal ileum is involved in approximately one-fourth of cases, almost always in direct continuity with colonic disease.

The pathologic appearance of the colon varies greatly in different stages of the disease. Invariably, there is hyperemia, and the mucosa is dark red or purplish red and velvety (Fig. 27-13). At first, tiny erosions appear,

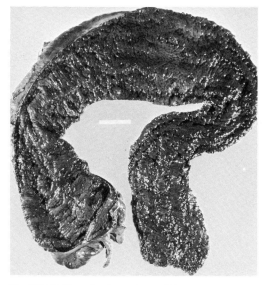

Fig. 27-13 Chronic ulcerative colitis.

later becoming deeper and coalescing to form linear ulcers, which have the appearance of longitudinal furrows distributed in the long axis of the colon. The ulcers are often undermining, partially freeing ragged remnants of mucous membrane. In occasional acutely progressing cases, the entire colon may be extremely friable and bleed freely. The muscle is thickened, apparently by contraction, and rigid, having lost, in whole or in part, its distensibility. This produces shortening as well as narrowing, and as the disease progresses, the colon comes more and more to resemble the garden hose to which it has been compared. Inasmuch as chronic ulcerative colitis is a disease of remissions and exacerbations, periods of relative quiescence and healing alternate with periods of activity.

The earliest histologic lesion in most cases is a crypt abscess—the accumulation of polymorphonuclear leukocytes in the crypts of Lieberkühn, with breakdown of the crypt wall. The crypt abscesses tend to coalesce to form enlarging, shallow ulcers. Along with the neutrophilic exudate are noted the other usual changes of inflammation—i.e., hyperemia, edema, hemorrhage, and, more deeply, accumulation of lymphocytes and plasma cells. Frequently, eosinophils as well as basophils are present in impressive numbers. The former are readily seen in routine histologic preparations, but special techniques are necessary to demonstrate basophils. Some authors have emphasized vasculitis as an early feature, but this is striking only in occasional cases. Ulcerative colitis is primarily a mucosal disease, with infrequent and usually limited involvement of the other layers, whereas regional enteritis is a disease of the submucosa and deeper tissues. Also, the inflammation of ulcerative colitis is not characteristically productive of abundant fibrous scar tissue. Granulomas with giant cells, like those of regional enteritis, are only an occasional finding in ulcerative colitis. When the ulcers heal, they are covered by a single layer of epithelium. Although there is an attempt to reform crypts, regeneration is not complete, and structural abnormalities persist. In quiescent chronic disease, the mucosa remains red and granular.

Pseudopolyps are a frequent and striking finding in ulcerative colitis. They consist of polypoid masses of granulation tissue that include distorted, inflamed crypts, often with hyperplastic epithelium. In contrast to adenomatous polyps, they vary greatly in size and shape, may be long and pendulous, and show no clear distinction between stalk and main body of the polyp. True adenomatous polyps do occur, however, in association with these inflammatory pseudopolyps.

There is a distinctly increased incidence of carcinoma of the colon in patients with ulcerative colitis of very long standing, particularly when the onset has been in childhood or adolescence. There may be multiple carcinomas. Whether or not this complication represents progression from pseudopolyp to adenomatous polyp to carcinoma is debated. Another important complication is acute dilatation of the colon in fulminant disease— so-called toxic megacolon. It constitutes an emergency and may progress to perforation.

Pseudomembranous enterocolitis

Pseudomembranous (staphylococcal) enterocolitis is an occasional complication of a major surgical procedure (usually on the intestinal tract) and is highly lethal. It almost invariably occurs in patients who have had antibiotic therapy, and it results from disturbance of the normal balance of the intestinal flora and infection by *Micrococcus pyogenes (Staphylococcus aureus),* which elaborates a potent enterotoxin. The condition occurs more rarely as a terminal phenomenon in diverse other diseases, among them treated leukemia and lymphoma.

Pseudomembranous enterocolitis may involve any portion of the gastrointestinal tract from the lower esophagus to the rectum, most often the ileum. The lesion is an acute in-

flammation with necrosis, initially patchy, of the mucous membrane, producing focal erosions leading to diffuse ulceration. There are intense hyperemia, edema, and neutrophilic infiltration, often with perivascular hemorrhages. Characteristically, the ulcerated surface is covered by a pseudomembrane consisting of a fibrin mesh and mucus with entrapped inflammatory and blood cells and bacteria (Fig. 27-14). Large amounts of fluid distend the intestine. The disease usually develops between the third and seventh postoperative days and is attended by profuse watery diarrhea, dehydration, and profound shock.

Bacillary dysentery

Bacillary dysentery is an acute inflammatory disease of the colon, occasionally involving the ileum as well, caused by microorganisms of the genus *Shigella.* Infection is the result of contamination of food or water supplies with the feces of individuals who either have the disease or, less often, are symptomatic carriers of the organism.

The anatomic changes are not characteristic. They are those of an acute, pyogenic inflammation that may progress from edema and leukocytic infiltration of the mucous membrane to necrosis and ulceration, usually superficial. In contrast to amebic colitis, the ulcers are not undermined. Healing is with granulation tissue formation, but in the usual case there is little scarring. It is postulated that the lesion is caused by the action of a bacterial endotoxin upon the deeper cells lining the intestinal crypts.

Diarrhea, abdominal pain, and fever are the outstanding clinical manifestations of the disease, which is usually self-limited and resolves completely. However, on occasion the acute infection may evolve into chronic recurrent disease with episodes of diarrhea or dysentery or, rarely, into the asymptomatic carrier state.

The epidemiology of bacillary dysentery and the severity of the individual case vary greatly with the species of *Shigella* involved, as well as with the character of the population at risk. Thus, the disease is particularly severe in infants and young children, as well as in the case of *Shigella dysenteriae (shiga)* infections in the tropics.

Typhoid fever

Typhoid fever is the prototype and the best known of the infections with organisms of the

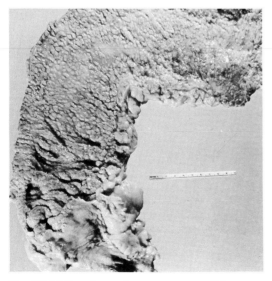

Fig. 27-14 Pseudomembranous enterocolitis.

genus *Salmonella*. Typhoid fever differs from bacillary dysentery in being essentially systemic rather than limited to the gastrointestinal tract. Its main consideration will be found on p. 305. In typhoid fever, there are striking local manifestations in the gastrointestinal tract. Inasmuch as the principal lesions are those of lymphoid tissue, the ileum is most affected, although the jejunum, appendix, and colon also may be involved.

The early changes are degeneration and proliferation in the intestinal epithelium, inflammatory cell infiltrate of the lamina propria, and hyperplasia of the lymphoreticular tissue of Peyer's patches and of the solitary lymphoid follicles of the intestine. Large mononuclear cells, actively phagocytic macrophages, are found in large numbers, constituting the most conspicuous histologic feature of the disease. In approximately the second week of the disease, necrosis of the lymphoid tissue takes place, and as it progresses to sloughing, ulceration occurs. The ulcerations have the configuration of the lymphoid aggregates, elongated with the long axis in line with that of the intestine in the terminal ileum and more or less rounded elsewhere. Peripheral remnants of preserved hyperplastic lymphoid tissue usually elevate their margins. The ulcers extend down to the submucosa or muscularis, their bases covered with greenish yellow exudate. They may be confluent. A striking feature of typhoid lesions is the virtual absence of polymorphonuclear leukocytes. The characteristic large macrophages contain phagocytized erythrocytes, lymphocytes, and necrotic cellular debris. They may occur in sufficiently large numbers to occlude capillaries, contributing to the process of tissue necrosis. These large cells are also conspicuous in the spleen and liver. In the latter situation, they are usually in focal collections and associated with foci of necrosis. In the typhoid fever case that resolves, ulceration is followed by granulation tissue formation, and ultimately epithelial regeneration takes place. Scarring is not usually a feature.

The toxemia of typhoid fever is often extreme, especially early in the disease. The two life-threatening complications are hemorrhage and perforation. If they occur, the hemorrhage usually takes place during the second week of the disease and perforation in the third week. Hemorrhage is often massive. Perforation and the resultant peritonitis are associated with secondary infection by a variety of bacteria.

Asiatic cholera

Cholera is an acute diarrheal disease caused by *Vibrio cholerae*. Like *Shigella* and *Salmonella* infections, it is dependent upon contamination with human excrement, usually of water supplies. Like the former but in contrast to typhoid fever, the disease is one manifested principally in the intestinal tract but coupled with the production of a potent endotoxin. It is seen almost exclusively in tropical countries, not infrequently in epidemic proportions, as well as endemically.

Cholera varies greatly in severity, probably as the result of both variations in individual susceptibility and the presence or absence of predisposing factors such as fatigue and/or nonspecific gastrointestinal derangements, etc. The incubation period varies from one to five days. It is shortest in the most severe, fulminant cases, which may be rapidly fatal. Initially, the disease is characterized by profuse diarrhea, with so-called rice water stools (stools composed of tremendous amounts of fluid containing mucus and bacteria) and vomiting. In the severe cases, this is rapidly followed by extreme dehydration, circulatory collapse, and anuria. Except for the nonspecific changes associated with dehydration, acidosis, etc., the pathologic findings are limited to the intestines.

The entire intestinal tract is involved, usually the small intestine being most severely affected. For many years, it has been considered that the intestinal mucosa was denuded by desquamation of the superficial epithelium, but biopsy studies indicate that this desquamation is an agonal event or the result of postmortem autolysis. There are, of course, vascular engorgement and inflammatory cell infiltration of the mucous membrane, but the outstanding finding is the accumulation of tremendous amounts of proteinaceous edema fluid in the interstices of the lamina propria, to such a degree that the fluid serves to obscure widening of the epithelial basement membrane. A great deal of this fluid passes into the intestinal lumen to be excreted in the rice water stools.

Tuberculosis

Primary intestinal tuberculosis, ordinarily the result of ingestion of foods (especially dairy products) infected with the bovine tubercle bacillus, has become rare in the United States. Tuberculosis of the gastrointestinal tract is almost invariably associated with advanced, open pulmonary disease with discharge from the lung lesions, and subsequent swallowing, of large numbers of bacilli. In fatal pulmonary tuberculosis, gastrointestinal involvement is quite common, and in disseminated disease, gastrointestinal lesions may be widespread.

The usual isolated gastrointestinal lesion of tuberculosis involves the ileocecal region. It is the same as that of tuberculosis elsewhere—a granulomatous inflammation with the formation of tubercles featuring epithelioid cells, giant cells of the Langhans type, caseation necrosis, and fibrous tissue production. The caseation necrosis progresses to sloughing, and ulceration is a regular feature. The ulcers are said to lie with their long axes perpendicular to the long axis of the intestine. Contracting scar tissue may produce a degree of stricture formation, usually with partial rather than complete intestinal obstruction. A characteristic macroscopic feature of intestinal tuberculosis is the presence of small white or yellowish white tubercles arranged longitudinally on the serosa overlying the lesion. The mesenteric lymph nodes are commonly involved. An occasional complication is tuberculous fistula in ano, a lesion that does not occur in the absence of intestinal disease.

Fungal infections

Intestinal histoplasmosis may mimic the picture described previously for tuberculosis, just as it may mimic, even in histopathologic detail, the pulmonary lesion due to the tubercle bacillus. Differentiation of histoplasmosis and tuberculosis is made with assurance only by the demonstration of the causative organisms, either in microscopic sections by appropriate staining techniques or in cultures.

Although most common in the ileocecal region, gastrointestinal lesions also may be widespread as a part of a generalized histoplasmosis. When *actinomycosis* involves the gastrointestinal tract, it too shows predilection for the ileocecal region or the appendix (p. 411).

Lymphopathia venereum

Lymphopathia (lymphogranuloma) venereum is a venereal disease caused by a filtrable virus, involving primarily the external genitalia and secondarily the lymphatics and lymph nodes draining them (p. 346). In the male, primary lymphatic drainage of the genitalia is by way of the inguinal lymph nodes, whereas in the female the pelvic and perirectal lymphatic structures are involved.

Hence, lymphopathia venereum involving the anorectal region is a disease of females or male homosexuals.

Initially, the perirectal fat is involved by chronic inflammatory change and fibrosis, rendering it very firm. The lymphatic lesions commonly suppurate, and the inflammation spreads to involve the rectal wall proper. Characteristically, stricture formation follows.

Other forms of enteritis and colitis

Several other forms of enteritis and/or colitis should be considered briefly. Reference already has been made to the stricture, single or multiple, that may be produced by *ionizing radiation,* usually given for treatment of cancer of the female generative organs. Inflammation in one or more focal areas of the small intestine or colon is more common than stricture formation, the latter occurring only as the result of healing of a penetrating ulcer of significant size (Fig. 27-15). The inflammatory changes in themselves are not specific, although vascular changes (fibrous intimal

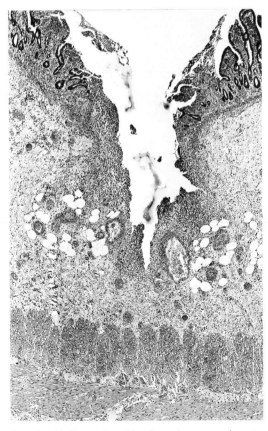

Fig. 27-15 Enteritis with ulceration secondary to therapeutic irradiation for carcinoma of uterine cervix. (×55.)

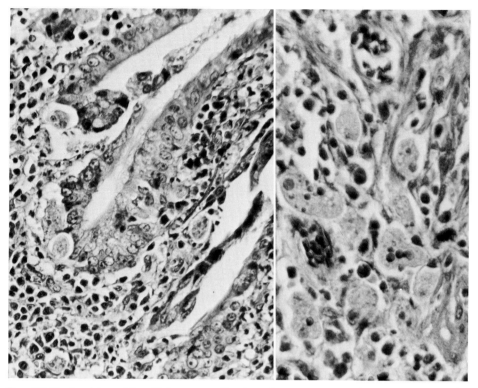

Fig. 27-16 Amebic colitis. Higher magnification demonstrates erythrocyte ingestion by trophozoites.

thickening of medium-sized and small arteries and hyalinization of arterioles) are often conspicuous. Radiation ulcers in the rectum may be associated with marked scarring.

In *mercurial poisoning,* the colon and the kidney are the two organs that show the principal anatomic changes, since they are the organs chiefly responsible for excretion of the poison. Colonic involvement is especially conspicuous in the more acute cases, the changes varying from those of minimal nonspecific inflammation to widespread necrosis of the mucous membrane, with sloughing of appreciable portions of it.

The gastrointestinal tract also reflects *arsenical poisoning.* Both the small intestine and the colon are involved, and in the case of ingestion of certain inorganic arsenical compounds such as Paris green, the stomach also may show changes. The inflammation, like that due to poisoning with mercury, is essentially nonspecific, but ulceration is less apparent and less extensive.

Nonspecific inflammation of the gastrointestinal tract, especially the colon, occurs in patients dying with *uremia.* Changes range from minimal to those of an extensive necrotizing colitis. It seems likely that some, perhaps all,

of the extensive lesions really represent pseudomembranous enterocolitis, or even some other specific infection.

Parasitic infestations
Amebiasis

Amebiasis, infestation with *Entamoeba histolytica,* is the most important of the parasite-caused gastrointestinal diseases, at least in the United States. The lesions of amebic colitis are located most frequently in the cecum or rectum, but extensive segments of the large intestine may be involved.

In the earliest lesions, the trophozoites (vegetative forms) penetrate the epithelium at the base of the colonic crypts, reaching the lamina propria and producing coagulation necrosis with little or no associated inflammatory reaction. This produces grossly visible, tiny, yellowish, nodular elevations of the mucosa, which slough, producing minute ulcers. Typically, the ulcers are flask shaped. Their edges are undermined, and they frequently coalesce. Mononuclear and eosinophilic leukocytes predominate in the inflammatory infiltrate at this stage.

The fully developed ulcers are ragged and

covered with whitish exudate. Organisms may be present in the tissues in large numbers, or they may be difficult to find and identify with certainty, especially after secondary bacterial invasion has elicited a polymorphonuclear leukocytic response (Fig. 27-16). In the advanced case, the mucosa may have a shaggy appearance, with shreds of fibrin and tags of undermined mucous membrane attached to the margins of the ulcers. The colon may be greatly thickened, and there may be many adhesions to adjacent loops of intestine or to the mesentery. Amebic granulomas (amebomas) may develop (p. 437).

Schistosomiasis

In areas in which infection with *Schistosoma* is common, ova may be found in the submucosa and mucosa of the colon and, less often, adult worms may be found in the submucosal veins. The eggs excite a tubercle-like foreign body reaction and commonly are associated with polyps showing inflammatory changes and what is described as adenomatoid hyperplasia. The latter is not regarded as truly neoplastic (p. 451).

Various other parasites that inhabit the intestinal tract are considered in Chapter 13.

Anorectal lesions

Stercoraceous (**stercoral**) ulcers are irregular ulcers of the mucous membrane of the rectum and, less often, of the colon, resulting from trauma caused by impacted, inspissated fecal masses. They may be associated with perforation and peritonitis or with hemorrhage.

Although **colitis cystica profunda** may be diffuse and involve extensive areas of the large intestine, it usually is confined to the rectum. It is characterized by mucous cysts and glands lined by goblet cells in the submucosa. There are often associated chronic inflammatory change and extraglandular accumulation of mucin. The condition may result from extension of surface epithelium along granulation tissue tracts following deep ulceration.

The crypts of Morgagni have traditionally been implicated in the causation of most anorectal inflammatory disease, specifically perirectal **abscesses** and **anorectal fistulas.** Corresponding to the columns and sinuses of Morgagni is a circular band 0.3 cm to 1.1 cm wide of "transitional" or "cloacogenic" epithelium interposed between rectal and anal mucous membrane. This transitional epithelium,

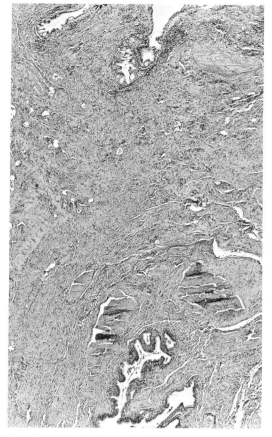

Fig. 27-17 Anal ducts. Small portion of epithelial lining of anal canal visible above, and anal ducts present both superficially and deep within muscle. (×55.)

often including mucus-secreting cells, lines the sinuses of Morgagni and the anal ducts or glands that communicate with them. These anal ducts can be demonstrated in a majority of anatomic specimens if searched for. Their development and distribution vary greatly. They commonly extend caudally, penetrating the musculature of the internal anal sphincter. Less frequently, they extend cephalad beneath the rectal mucosa. They may branch in very complex fashion. On occasion, such glands have no connection with the lumen (Fig. 27-17). It is infection in the crypts of Morgagni and of these anal ducts that is responsible for the very troublesome perianal and ischiorectal abscesses. Such abscesses, in turn, and again dependent upon the anal duct system, are responsible for the equally troublesome anal fistulas. These are infected sinus tracts opening internally in the region of the anorectal junction and externally on the perianal skin. Histologically, they frequently show, in addition to nonspecific inflammation, a foreign body reaction, no doubt because of contamination with fecal matter.

Anal fissures are acute or chronic ulcers situated posteriorly in the anal canal just distal to the anorectal junction. These various anal, perianal, and anorectal lesions are insignificant in themselves, but they may be the source of great discomfort and disability.

PERITONEUM, OMENTUM, RETROPERITONEUM, AND MESENTERY
Peritonitis

The most frequently occurring and important disease condition involving the peritoneum is acute inflammation. Peritonitis usually is associated with acute inflammatory disease of one of the abdominal hollow viscera, often with rupture or perforation, although rare instances of so-called "primary" peritonitis are encountered, and some degree of peritonitis follows all surgical procedures in which the peritoneal cavity is opened. The typical example of primary peritonitis is that occurring in children suffering from nephrosis and usually caused by pneumococci or streptococci. The incidence has been reduced by current methods of management of nephrosis, especially with steroid hormones, and its seriousness has been lessened by use of anti-infective drugs.

Peritoneal inflammation accompanies all surgical transgressions of the peritoneal membrane, but in the absence of visceral inflammation and in the presence of maximum effort on the part of the surgeon to avoid trauma, it is minimal and is followed by complete restoration to normal. If the gastrointestinal tract is entered at the time of operation, bacterial contamination is inevitable and the inflammatory reaction is more marked. Even in this circumstance, resolution follows in the usual case, and it is only with grosser contamination or, more especially, visceral inflammation and usually perforation that severe peritonitis with the late formation of adhesions is the sequel. Hemorrhage into the peritoneal cavity, the result of trauma, ruptured tubal pregnancy, rupture of a graafian follicle or corpus luteum, tumor, etc., may be responsible for clinical manifestations simulating those of peritonitis. There may be actual inflammatory change as the result of this irritation, especially reactive proliferation of serosal cells.

Peritonitis is also commonly associated with inflammation of abdominal organs in the absence of perforation. Acute cholecystitis and intestinal infarction are two examples. In acute appendicitis, involvement of the serosal coat occurs early in the disease process, microorganisms penetrating the partially devitalized wall before actual perforation takes place. It is in the case of perforation or rupture of viscera that are the seat of inflammatory disease that violent, severe, acute peritonitis is encountered. The commonest visceral perforations occur in association with appendicitis and peptic ulcer, although many other gastrointestinal lesions (e.g., diverticulum, tumor, etc.) may perforate. As previously noted, the peritonitis secondary to perforated peptic ulcer is initially chemical because the hydrochloric acid of the gastric juice maintains sterility, but without treatment, bacterial invasion soon ensues.

The organisms that can cause peritonitis are of many varieties, including the normal flora of the gastrointestinal tract. *Escherichia coli, Proteus,* and the enterococci are the most frequent, but bacteroides and clostridia are also important. The process may be localized or diffuse, but in general there is a distinct tendency for the omentum and mobile viscera to become so arranged, and held in apposition by plastic exudate, that more or less complete "walling off" of the inflammation occurs. The initial hyperemia, edema, and extravasation of blood cells, with the concomitant loss of the serous membrane's normal glistening sheen, is followed by exudation of leukocytes and fibrin. The character of the exudate varies in the individual case according to the relative proportions of serum, fibrin, leukocytes, and red blood cells. Thus, it may be serous, fibrinous, purulent, hemorrhagic, or any combination of these. To a limited extent, the character of the peritoneal exudate may depend upon a particular dominant organism. Athough it may be thin, watery, and only slightly turbid, it usually is frankly purulent or fibrinopurulent.

The process progresses to a stage at which the plastic exudate causes involved viscera (especially loops of intestine, omentum, and abdominal parietes) to become stuck together, forming abscesses in localized areas, rather than permitting general spread of the process. There are certain specific anatomic sites where such abscesses are prone to develop—the lumbar gutters, the subphrenic space (between the liver and diaphragm), the subhepatic area, and the pelvic cul-de-sac especially. After widespread peritonitis subsides, such focal accumulations of exudate may persist and necessitate surgical drainage.

A common complication of acute peritonitis is adynamic or paralytic ileus (p. 1126). Another important complication is the development of *fibrous peritoneal adhesions,* the late result of organization of exudate that is not absorbed. It is probable that most of the exudate is usually absorbed and that it is only in the more severe and extensive cases that adhesions form. Peritoneal adhesions, however, are a significant cause of intestinal obstruction.

The adhesions associated with inflammatory disease of the female pelvic organs, most importantly the fallopian tubes, are especially noteworthy. The causative infections are usually primarily of gonococcal etiology, but secondary superinfection is common. This pelvic inflammatory disease is usually marked by recurring episodes of acute but low-grade inflammation, and the resulting adhesions may become very dense and complicated, although generally limited to the pelvis.

Tuberculous peritonitis may occur as a manifestation of disseminated tuberculosis, miliary or otherwise, or in association with intestinal involvement. It also may be secondary to disease of the female generative organs. The disease process is the same as that in other parts of the body. It may be productive of widespread, dense adhesions.

Bile peritonitis is produced by leakage of bile into the peritoneal cavity as the result of perforative disease of the gallbladder, bile ducts, or duodenum or as an untoward complication of operative procedures involving these structures. Bile peritonitis itself may produce a profound initial systemic reaction in the host, but the nature of the resulting pathologic process is dependent upon the source of the contaminating bile and the type and number of associated bacteria.

The peritoneum gives rise to certain *foreign body granulomas.* The best known were reactions to *Lycopodium* spores and to talc (magnesium silicate) crystals. Both of these have been used in the past as dusting powders for surgical rubber gloves. The resultant lesions are characteristic foreign body granulomas, often productive of adhesions, in which the foreign material may be identified on microscopic examination. Today, it is customary to use an absorbable substance as a dusting powder for surgical gloves. However, this has not proved to be completely innocuous, and instances of peritonitis and foreign body granuloma have been reported, presumably developing on the basis of hypersensitivity.

The prognosis is said to be good. Infrequently, oily materials used in salpingography, parasites or their ova, barium sulfate administered for diagnostic radiologic study and escaping into the peritoneum as the result of perforation, and sclerosing agents used in the treatment of hernia may be incitants of a peritoneal foreign body reaction.

Ascites

Ascites is the condition of transudation of clear, low–specific gravity fluid into the peritoneal cavity. The protein content is less than 3%. It is most commonly seen with portal cirrhosis of the liver but may result from other causes of hypertension in the portal venous system, such as thrombosis or cardiac decompensation, or from hypoalbuminemia. *Chylous ascites,* in which the fluid appears milky and has a high fat content, usually is related to neoplastic obstruction of the thoracic duct.

Retroperitoneal lesions

The retroperitoneum is an ill-defined area that may share in the complications of diseases of the many organs that lie within it or impinge upon it. Hemorrhage, infections, and extensions of neoplasms are the important complications and may be related to the urinary tract, adrenal glands, pancreas, gastrointestinal tract, retroperitoneal lymph nodes, blood vessels, including the aorta and vena cava, etc.

A number of possibly related conditions involve the mesenteric and retroperitoneal adipose tissue. At one end of the spectrum is a self-limited, chronic, productive inflammation of the mesentery, usually of the small intestine. This has been variously termed "mesenteric panniculitis," "lipogranuloma," and "isolated lipodystrophy" and likened to Weber-Christian disease. It may produce a significant mass and may or may not be symptomatic. Retractile mesenteritis is a similar condition, distinguished by fibrosis and hyaline scarring and retraction of the mesentery, with distortion of intestinal loops productive of episodes of pain, constipation, and obstruction.

Idiopathic retroperitoneal fibrosis is a lesion characterized by dense fibrosis and a limited, nonspecific inflammatory reaction that frequently presents with ureteral obstruction.[128] The disease also occurs in the mediastinum. A similar lesion has been observed in association with methysergide therapy. It usually regresses after withdrawal of the drug.

Torsion
of omentum

Omental torsion, secondary to adhesions, tumors, etc. or, at times, of unknown cause, may result in infarction and give rise to signs and symptoms simulating those of acute appendicitis but usually without vomiting. Similarly, epiploic appendages may become infarcted. Fat necrosis of an appendage, presumably a late result, is not uncommon.

FUNCTIONAL STATES
Gastric atrophy
(atrophic gastritis)

So-called atrophic gastritis is not properly classified as an inflammatory condition. The term is used by some as a synonym for gastric atrophy. Others consider the two as different stages of the same pathologic process.

In atrophic gastritis, the mucous membrane is greatly thinned, and the gastric

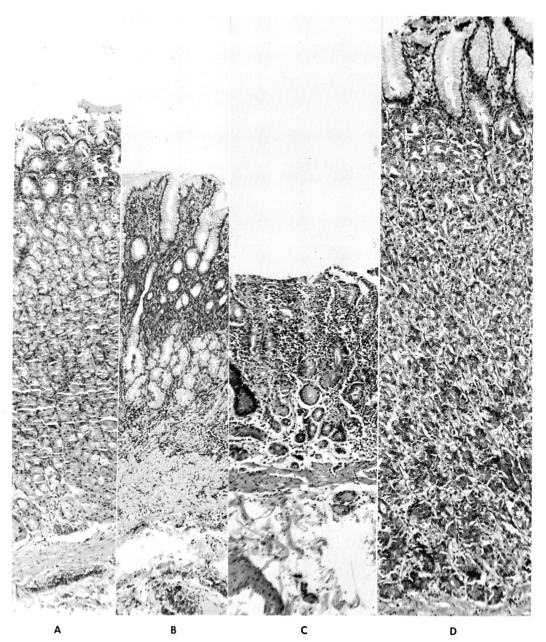

A B C D

Fig. 27-18 A and **B,** Normal stomach. **A,** Fundus. **B,** Antrum. **C,** Atrophic gastritis. **D,** Gastric rugal hypertrophy. (**A** to **D,** ×90.)

glands are correspondingly shortened and also widely separated. On naked-eye inspection, the mucosa in advanced atrophy is smooth, is patently thinned, and has a waxy cast. The striking cellular changes in the gastric glands are two: (1) a decrease in number or, in the fully developed case, complete absence of parietal cells and (2) the occurrence, usually in the deeper part of the mucosa, of glands identical with those of the small intestine (Fig. 27-18, *C*). All cell types normally found in the glands of the small intestine may be represented. This change has been regarded as "intestinal metaplasia" by some and as heterotopia by others. The decrease or absence of parietal cells, which has been demonstrated to be associated with an autoantibody in a high percentage of patients with atrophic gastritis, accounts for deficient hydrochloric acid secretion or complete achlorhydria. Large numbers of lymphocytes and plasma cells are present in the lamina propria, but the increase may be more apparent than real. The changes described occur focally in many stomachs without overt disease. They are seen more often and in more widespread and advanced degree with increased age.

Atrophic gastritis commonly is associated with gastric carcinoma, but a postulated predisposing role has not been demonstrated. Advanced atrophy regularly accompanies polypoid carcinoma and adenomatous polyp. Indeed, the appearance of many of the latter and of some polypoid carcinomas strongly suggests origin from glands typical of the small intestine. Gastric atrophy also regularly accompanies pernicious anemia, a disease associated with achlorhydria and a high incidence of gastric carcinoma. However, in general, it has been difficult to correlate the pathologic findings of atrophic gastritis with clinical disease or with radiologic or gastroscopic findings.

Gastric rugal hypertrophy

Gastric rugal hypertrophy (called hypertrophic gastritis by some) is characterized by enlargement of the gastric mucosal folds in both length and breadth, producing thickening and convolution of the mucous membrane reminiscent of the appearance of the cerebral convolutions (Fig. 27-19). Histologically, it appears to be a true thickening, and there is an apparent striking increase in the depth of the glands and in the number of parietal cells. At times, glands penetrate the muscularis mucosae (Fig. 27-18, *D*). The changes may be diffuse and marked or localized and of limited degree. It seems likely that pathologists have failed to recognize localized instances or

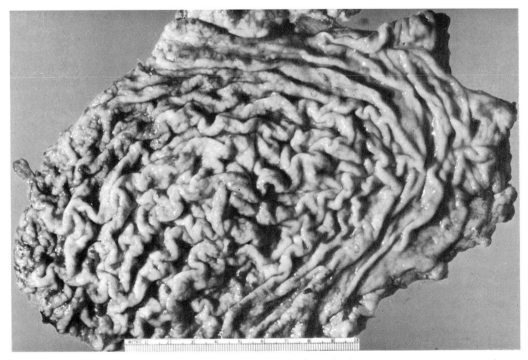

Fig. 27-19 Gastric rugal hypertrophy. Patient had marked gastric hypersecretion and duodenal ulcer.

minor degrees of the condition, accounting, perhaps, for the difficulty they have had in supporting clinical and/or radiologic diagnoses of "hypertrophic gastritis."

Gastric rugal hypertrophy has been associated with hyperchlorhydria (in some instances with extreme gastric hypersecretion), hypoproteinemia, and *tumors or hyperplasias of multiple endocrine glands.* It is postulated that gastric rugal hypertrophy is one manifestation of a syndrome consisting additionally of islet cell tumor, primary chief cell hyperplasia of the parathyroid glands, and, at times, abnormalities of other endocrine glands, especially the adrenal cortex and pituitary, and having several different modes of clinical expression. The principal ones are as follows:

1 The *Zollinger-Ellison syndrome,* with intractable peptic ulcer, often in an unusual location

2 The *Verner-Morrison syndrome,* with intractable watery diarrhea, the result of incomplete neutralization in the intestine of the very large amounts of highly acid gastric juice

3 Hyperparathyroidism

These syndromes are familial in some instances. In the Zollinger-Ellison syndrome, the islet cell tumor is often malignant, often in the duodenum instead of the pancreas, and characteristically composed of alpha cells that secrete gastrin, which, in turn, stimulates gastric secretion. However, insulin-secreting beta cell tumors also occur.

Malabsorption syndrome

The malabsorption syndrome is characterized by impaired intestinal absorption, especially of fats, and is manifested by diarrhea with bulky, foul stools, abdominal distention, and malnutrition with attendant vitamin deficiencies, all in varying degree. The clinical picture may be associated with a wide variety of underlying diseases, and the cases may be conveniently subdivided into primary and secondary groups. Among the numerous causes of secondary malabsorption are the following: cystic fibrosis of the pancreas, chronic incomplete intestinal obstruction, surgical resection of significant segments of the gastrointestinal tract, infections (especially enteric), antibiotics, biliary tract disease, scleroderma, Whipple's disease, parasitic infestations, regional enteritis, diabetes, neoplasms (notably lymphoma), possibly allergy, etc.

Celiac disease and sprue. The names given to primary malabsorption or steatorrhea are *celiac disease* in infants and children, *nontropical sprue* in the adult, and *tropical sprue.*

In the first two conditions there seems to be an identical, genetically controlled, enzymatic or metabolic defect that is converted to overt clinical disease by a number of possible triggering mechanisms, the most important and most frequently occurring of which is sensitivity to, or intolerance of, gluten. In this case, the elimination of gluten from the diet usually relieves the symptoms and permits normal development, although it does not cure

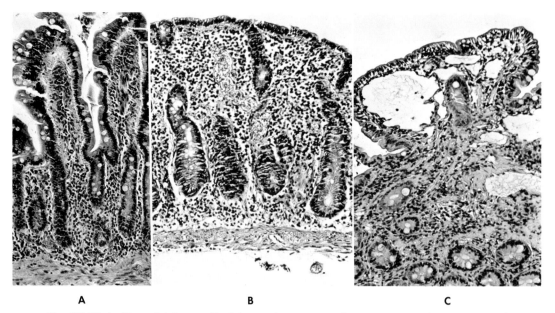

A   B   C

Fig. 27-20 A, Normal jejunum. **B,** Jejunum in nontropical sprue. **C,** Lymphangiectases of jejunum in protein-losing enteropathy. (**A** to **C,** ×150.)

the underlying defect. The small intestine in this state has a flat surface, partially or completely lacking villi. The mucosal crypts appear elongated, dilated, and more widely spaced than normal. The surface epithelial cells are cuboidal or low columnar with irregular nuclei (Fig. 27-20, *B*). When a gluten-free diet produces clinical remission, the anatomic lesion can be reversed to some degree, although usually not completely. The change is most marked in the upper part of the jejunum, becoming less so in the ileum and duodenum. This pathologic picture is not specific for nontropical sprue or celiac disease, but when full-blown is very nearly so.

Tropical sprue is very similar to nontropical sprue in its clinical and morphologic expressions. The pathologic changes usually are not so marked and are reversible with folic acid therapy, but they are unaffected by elimination of gluten from the diet. Macrocytic anemia is usually a feature.

Protein-losing enteropathy (exudative enteropathy)

In protein-losing enteropathy, which also may be associated with steatorrhea, large amounts of serum protein are lost in the intestine, and serum levels (of both globulin and albumin) are abnormally low. Like the malabsorption state, it may be secondary to some specific gastroenteric disease state or congestive heart failure, or it may be idiopathic.

Some of the gastrointestinal diseases that may be associated with marked protein loss are gastric rugal hypertrophy, sprue, regional enteritis, and ulcerative colitis. Constrictive pericarditis is the most important underlying cardiac lesion. In some patients with "idiopathic" protein-losing enteropathy, dilatation of lymphatic channels (lymphangiectasia) in the intestinal mucosa and mesentery has been demonstrated (Fig. 27-20, *C*). Some of these latter patients have had systemic lymphatic abnormalities, but in others no cause of lymphatic obstruction is found.

GASTROINTESTINAL MANIFESTATIONS OF SYSTEMIC DISEASE
Cystic fibrosis

Cystic fibrosis of the pancreas *(mucoviscidosis)* is an hereditary, generalized disturbance of exocrine glands, manifest in pancreatic insufficiency, chronic respiratory disease, increased sweat electrolytes, and sometimes cirrhosis of the liver. In its more severe forms, it is seen in infants and young children. The most important gastrointestinal manifestation

is malabsorption with steatorrhea and azotorrhea, secondary to pancreatic achylia and deficient secretion of the intestinal glands themselves. Approximately 10% of patients have intestinal obstruction in the newborn period as the result of *meconium ileus*. The lumen of the small intestine, usually the terminal ileum, is plugged with inspissated, rubbery, tenacious meconium. Proximally, abnormal meconium accumulates in distended loops of intestine, which in one-third of the cases rotate upon themselves, producing a volvulus with strangulation. Another complication is intestinal perforation in utero with the development of sterile peritonitis—so-called *meconium peritonitis*. The escaping epithelial cells, mucus, and cellular debris usually stimulate a foreign body reaction. Calcification, visible roentgenographically, frequently takes place (see also p. 1277).

Progressive systemic sclerosis (scleroderma)

It has long been known that there was disease of the esophagus in an appreciable proportion of cases of progressive systemic sclerosis. The most consistent findings are hyaline sclerosis of the submucosa with lymphocytic infiltrate and atrophy of the muscularis with fibrosis. The mucous membrane is thinned. Ulceration, frank inflammation, and stricture may occur distally and are secondary to regurgitation of acid gastric juice, consequent to the rigidity of the sclerotic esophagus. More recently, it has become apparent that the remainder of the alimentary canal, from the stomach to the rectum and including the appendix, also may be involved. There are varying degrees of replacement of the submucosa, muscularis, and subserosal tissues with dense, hyalinized fibrous connective tissue and similarly varying infiltrates of lymphocytes and plasma cells.

Whipple's disease (intestinal lipodystrophy)

Originally considered to be a disorder of intestinal function involving lipid metabolism, Whipple's disease has been generally recognized more recently as a systemic disease. Aggregates of large pale macrophages bearing intracytoplasmic inclusions in the intestinal mucous membrane and mesenteric lymph nodes dominates the anatomic picture, but similar deposits have now been described in virtually every organ of the body. Involvement of tissues outside the intestine and mesenteric nodes regularly occurs. Lipid deposits are also striking in lymph nodes, espe-

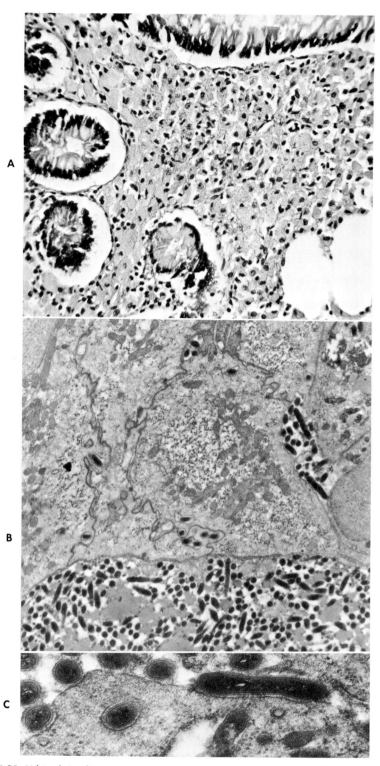

Fig. 27-21 Whipple's disease involving mucous membrane of small intestine. **A,** Pale macrophages in mucosa. **B,** Bacilliform bodies are extracellular. **C,** Encapsulated bodies are seen both intracellularly and extracellularly. (**A,** ×300; **B,** ×8,100; **C,** ×45,000.)

cially those of the mesentery. The sickle-shaped inclusions just referred to react strongly with the periodic acid–Schiff staining procedure.

Clinically, Whipple's disease is characterized by diarrhea, gradual wasting, and migratory polyarthritis. It is generally a condition of adult males and may be familial. It is another of the potential causes of the malabsorption syndrome. Whipple's disease is no longer regarded as a disorder of lipid metabolism, and a strong body of opinion has developed favoring an infectious etiology. This is based largely on the belief, generated from electron microscopic studies, that the "inclusions" are in fact bacilliform microorganisms (Fig. 27-21). Thus far, it has not been possible to identify or culture organisms from material from patients with Whipple's disease. Previously considered a progressive and usually fatal disease, it has been found to respond favorably to antibiotic therapy.

Many other systemic diseases have gastrointestinal manifestations. *Amyloid* disease and *hemochromatosis* are two examples, in both of which gastric or intestinal biopsy by intraluminal tube has been used to establish the diagnosis.

NEOPLASMS
Adenomatous polyps, papillary adenomas, and miscellaneous polyps

The term adenomatous polyp, although widely used, is a poor designation, since a wide variety of lesions (neoplastic, inflammatory, and others) may present as polyps. At the same time, the common use of the term has inevitably led to the incorrect use of the single word "polyp" as a synonym. Nevertheless, "adenomatous polyp" has assumed precedence over "polypoid adenoma" in the language of most physicians.

These polypoid, benign glandular neoplasms occur throughout the gastrointestinal tract, from the stomach to the rectum, occurring in greatest numbers in the colon and rectum. Because of the high incidence of the neoplasms in the latter situation, these will be described and discussed first. Estimates of their incidence range as high as 25% to 50% in an autopsy population of the older age groups (60 to 80 years). Their incidence increases after 30 years with advancing age. In one-fourth or more of cases, they are multiple, frequently but not regularly limited to one part of the intestine. Approximately 75% of adenomatous polyps occur in the

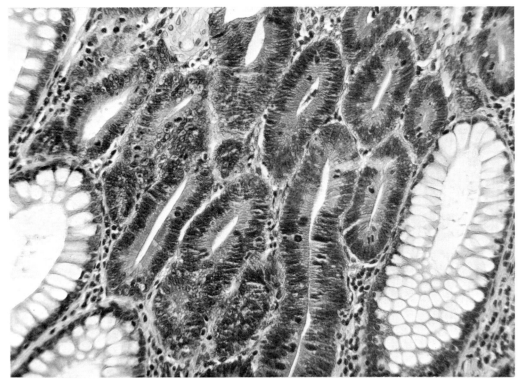

Fig. 27-22 Adenomatous (neoplastic) change in glands of colon in contrast to normal glands at left and in right lower corner. (×300.)

rectum and sigmoid colon, although their exact incidence in various segments of the large intestine varies from one reported series to another, in part because of varying criteria for recognition and in part because of variations in the manner of designating intestinal segments.

The earliest adenomatous change that can be recognized is the replacement of some of the lining cells of the crypts, beginning at the base, by cells that are generally taller, more slender, and more deeply stained than the normal. They have hyperchromatic nuclei and lack vacuoles indicative of mucin secretion (Fig. 27-22). Mitotic figures may be numerous. Proliferation progresses to the formation of a focal nodule. At this point, the adenoma (or "polyp") is presenting grossly as a nodular pinkish or whitish elevation of the mucous membrane. As the lesion enlarges, it projects into the lumen and becomes subject to the drag of peristalsis, becoming ultimately pedunculated. At this stage, the polyp is represented by a pink or red, lobulated berrylike nodule usually less than 2 cm in diameter, composed of neoplastic glands (the adenoma proper) attached to the intestinal wall by a pedicle composed of normal mucous membrane (Fig. 27-23).

There are a number of polypoid epithelial lesions of the colon that bear a general resemblance to the adenomatous polyp and are commonly confused with it. At times, *ab-normal folds* or minute elevations of the mucous membrane are mistaken for adenomas on proctoscopic or sigmoidoscopic examination. Rather frequently occurring polyps, best termed *hyperplastic* or *metaplastic*, are lesions composed of enlarged, regular glands with a scalloped luminal border showing excessive mucin secretion but lacking the neoplastic change of the adenomatous polyp described previously (Fig. 27-24). Another lesion in this group that must be distinguished from the neoplasms and does not have any relationship to cancer is the *juvenile polyp*. Also referred to as a retention polyp, it is usually single—a smooth, rounded nodule 1 cm to 3 cm in diameter, composed of large hyperplastic or cystic glands with a very abundant, well-vascularized fibrous stroma infiltrated by inflammatory cells (Fig. 27-25). It is supported on a stalk of normal mucous membrane. The most frequent clinical manifestation is bleeding. As the name indicates, it is a lesion of children, although similar polyps occasionally occur in adults. Polypoid inflammatory or nonspecific granuloma-like nodules—*inflammatory polyps*—are occasionally seen as solitary le-

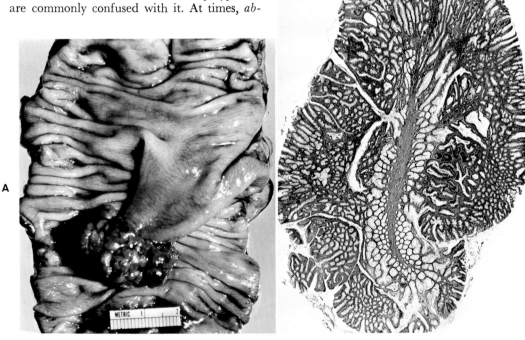

Fig. 27-23 A, Adenomatous polyp of colon. **B,** Adenomatous polyp of colon, with stalk of normal mucous membrane visible at bottom center. (**B,** ×20.)

sions, but the typical inflammatory polyp or pseudopolyp is that seen in long-standing chronic ulcerative colitis.

The *papillary adenoma* (which is known by many other names, including chiefly *villous adenoma* or *villous papilloma*) is a neoplasm related to, but much less common than, the adenomatous polyp. It is encountered more often in the rectum than in other parts of the large intestine. It is characterized by neoplastic proliferation from the mucosal surface into the lumen and develops a gross papillary configuration (Fig. 27-26), as opposed to the lobulated, berrylike nodule of the polyp. It frequently retains evidence of mucin secretion. Characteristic examples are large (several centimeters in diameter) and sessile (Fig. 27-26, *B*). Large papillary adenomas have been recognized as the occasional cause of severe fluid and electrolyte loss, especially of potassium. Electrolyte imbalance may develop suddenly and even threaten life.

Papillary adenomas and adenomatous polyps may coexist, and many lesions have morphologic characteristics of both. The distinction is particularly difficult in small lesions and especially when study is limited to small fragments of biopsy material. Both papillary adenomas and adenomatous polyps occur rarely in the small intestine.

In *familial multiple polyposis,* the entire colon is studded with polyps, usually tiny and sessile (Plate 3, *C*). The disease is transmitted

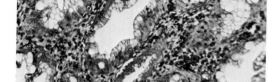

Fig. 27-24 Hyperplastic polyp of colon. (×175.)

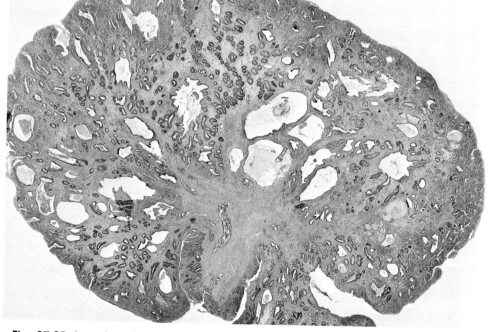

Fig. 27-25 Juvenile polyp of rectum. Cystic dilatation of glands and abundant stroma. (×13.)

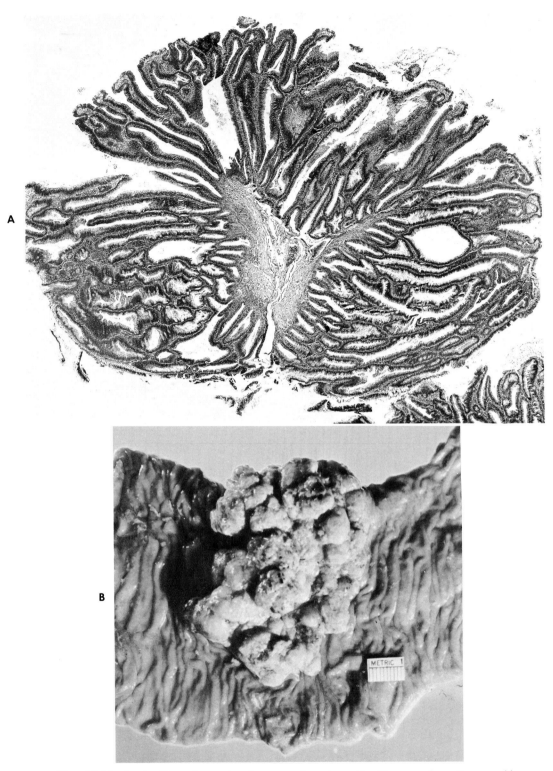

Fig. 27-26 A, Papillary (villous) adenoma of rectum. Papillary configuration readily apparent. **B,** Papillary adenoma of colon. (**A,** ×25.)

as an autosomal dominant trait and usually makes its existence known in childhood or adolescence. The incidence of carcinoma in this disease is so high and the cancers occur so often in young adults (or even adolescents) that total colectomy is generally regarded as the treatment of choice once the diagnosis has been established. Some patients, however, survive to develop intestinal cancer at the more usual age for that disease, and it is not uncommon for patients with familial multiple polyposis to give a history of relatives' having succumbed to various clinically diagnosed enteric conditions, without definite knowledge of the presence or absence of polyposis or carcinoma.

The *Peutz-Jeghers* syndrome is characterized by polyps, almost invariably pedunculated, throughout the stomach and small and large intestines associated with a peculiarly distributed melanin pigmentation of the face, lips, oral mucous membranes and digits. The disease is transmitted as a simple mendelian dominant trait (roughly half the children of a sufferer are affected) and makes its clinical appearance in childhood. The polyps, at least those of the stomach and small intestine, differ from those already described in that they are hamartomatous (i.e., they are composed of normal-looking but irregularly arranged glands of any of the types normally occurring in the mucous membrane of origin and may include bands of smooth muscle; Fig. 27-27). Thus, parietal cells may be present in gastric polyps, Brunner's glands in duodenal lesions, etc. The polyps of the large intestine are not always readily distinguishable from adenomatous polyps. The principal clinical manifestations of the Peutz-Jeghers syndrome are hemorrhage and intussusception.

Instances of the development of gastrointestinal carcinoma in patients with this syndrome have been documented, but progression of the Peutz-Jeghers polyps to genuine cancer must be rare. Although cytologic atypia is frequent, it is apparently not of significance, nor is the pseudoinvasive appearance suggested by the smooth muscle within the polyps. Rarely encountered are isolated polyps resembling the Peutz-Jeghers polyp, but without the other features of the syndrome. A number of other syndromes including gastrointestinal polyposis have been described. Some are familial, but all are rare.

Relationship of adenomatous polyps and papillary adenomas to carcinoma of colon

It has been usual to regard the benign epithelial proliferations of the large intestine as precursors of cancer, but in recent years this point of view has been seriously challenged. There is now a large body of opinion to the effect that a small or even insignificant number of carcinomas have their origin in preexisting "polyps." The belief in a direct sequential relationship between the benign polyps and carcinomas was based chiefly on the following observations:

1 The similarity between the relative incidence of carcinoma in the various parts of the colon to that of adenomatous polyps

2 The frequency of adenomas in segments of colon surgically resected for carcinoma

3 The finding of so-called carcinoma in situ in adenomatous polyps

In opposition to this "precancerous" point of view is the lack of general agreement about the relative distribution of carcinomas and adenomas in the various segments of the colon. As noted previously, differing views about distribution may depend, at least in

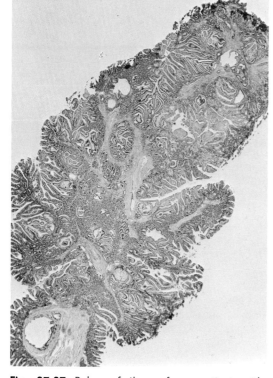

Fig. 27-27 Polyp of ileum from patient with Peutz-Jeghers syndrome. Note irregularities and variegated appearance. (×16; from Horn, R. C., Jr., Payne, W. A., and Fine, G.: Arch. Path. [Chicago] **76:**29-37, 1963.)

part, upon differences in defining the various segments of the large intestine, as well as upon differences in criteria for recognition of a benign or malignant neoplasm. A second countering argument to the traditional view is the documented frequency of carcinoma in colons without polyps. Also, there is no unanimity of opinion as to the criteria necessary for the diagnosis of carcinoma in situ. Cytologic evidences of cancer such as cellular pleomorphism, nuclear hyperchromatism, mitotic activity, variations in nuclear polarity, etc. receive varying interpretation in lesions without evidence of invasive growth. The histopathologic diagnosis of carcinoma in situ is being made with increasing frequency in cases of both adenomatous polyps and papillary adenomas, and atypical cellular features are observed even more often. There is growing recognition, however, that these changes, in the absence of the invasive growth characteristic of malignancy, are by no means necessarily associated with the biologic evolution we expect of malignant tumors. It has been emphasized by several observers that small polyps (diameter of 12 mm or less) almost never contain foci of cancer and also that metastases are extremely rare from microscopic foci of cancer in predominantly benign-appearing polyps. Finally, study of small (diameter of 2 cm or less) carcinomas of the colon and rectum has not revealed consistent, or even frequent, association with benign neoplastic histologic change to support the concept of origin in a preexisting benign tumor.

In summary, it appears that carcinomas of the large intestine can, and do, take origin in adenomatous polyps. However, in all probability, carcinomas arising on this basis are infrequent, and most colonic carcinomas are malignant neoplasms from their inception. This statement may not be true for the papillary adenoma, concerning which the consensus continues to be that the danger of cancer is great. This is based upon the frequent finding, by study of numerous blocks and sections, of associated foci of invasive growth and of lymph node metastasis, as well as upon the frequency of locally recurrent growth following excision, and upon recurrence as frank invasive cancer. There is little evidence of progression from adenoma to carcinoma.

Gastric polyps

The belief that adenomatous polyps of the stomach offer the threat of transformation into cancer is held by many, although the seriousness of the threat is not a matter of general agreement. It is incorrect to infer, because a gastric carcinoma has a polypoid configuration, that it had its origin in a benign "polyp." Among the reasons given for relating gastric polyps to carcinoma are the relatively frequent occurrence of both lesions in the same stomach and the fact that both lesions are regularly associated with atrophic gastritis and achlorhydria, or at least significant hypochlorhydria.

Just as "intestinal metaplasia" is a striking feature of atrophic gastritis, so also are many of the gastric polyps composed of glands resembling those of the small intestine. This is also true of many gastric carcinomas, especially those with a gross polypoid growth pattern. In fact, the frequent or usual resemblance of the glands of gastric polyps to those of the small intestine, along with cystic dilatation and inflammatory cell infiltrate, suggest a similarity between such polyps and the inflammatory or retention polyps of the large intestine rather than similarity to the adenomatous polyps.

In the stomach, polyps are commonly associated with carcinomas, and when polyps are multiple, as is the case in one-third to one-half of instances, there is almost always an associated carcinoma. In addition, atypical cytologic changes, consistent with interpretation as carcinoma in situ, are not uncommonly present in parts of gastric polyps. Nevertheless, despite the fact that some gastric cancers may arise in preexisting polyps, not all polyps will become invasive cancers, and relatively few cancers can be traced to polyps as precursors. Gastric polyps have an incidence less than 10% of that of gastric cancer.

Carcinoma of colon and rectum

Incidence. The colon and rectum constitute the body site that accounts for the highest incidence of cancer. This area ranks with the lung and breast as one of the most frequent sites of fatal malignant disease. Carcinoma of the colon and rectum has become the most frequently encountered of the numerous cancers of the gastrointestinal tract, its incidence now exceeding that of gastric cancer. Roughly three-fourths of carcinomas of the large intestine occur in the rectum and sigmoid colon. Of the remainder, a majority arise in the cecum and ascending and descending colon, the flexures and transverse colon being least often affected.

Histology and morbid anatomy. The great

majority of carcinomas of the large intestine show a fair to excellent degree of glandular differentiation, reproducing the appearance of normal colonic glands more or less faithfully (Fig. 27-28). There are cellular pleomorphism, nuclear hyperchromatism, loss of nuclear polarity, usually increased mitotic activity, etc. The secretion of some mucin by tumor cells is quite common. Occasionally one encounters tumors capable of secreting very large amounts of mucin. A majority of these present a histologic picture of pools of mucin separated from one another by thin stromal septa, in which float groups of tumor cells, sometimes in glandular orientation. Signet-ring cells (cells in which a large vacuole of mucin pushes the nucleus off to one side) may be conspicuous in some of these tumors (Fig. 27-29). In others, signet-ring cells may dominate the picture and produce a tumor quite like the linitis plastica type of gastric carcinoma (described later), without any readily apparent mucosal lesion.

There are usually distinct differences between the growth patterns of carcinomas of the right half of the colon and those of the left half, with a gradual transition from one to the other. In the right half of the colon, where the fecal stream is normally fluid, carcinomas are usually bulky and, as such, commonly outgrow their blood supply and undergo extensive necrosis (Fig. 27-30, A). Occult bleeding is common, and the presenting symptoms may be generalized weakness and anemia. With progress distally in the colon, the fecal content becomes progressively more solid, and, with the "napkin-ring" configuration of the cancer typical of the descending and sigmoid colon, the clinical manifestations of left-sided colonic cancer are those of low intestinal obstruction. The typical left-sided colonic cancers are small, grow to extend around the intestine circumferentially, and are accompanied by considerable fibrous tissue stroma, with subsequent contraction and, of course, luminal narrowing (Fig. 27-30, B). The colon proximal to such a lesion becomes dilated and hypertrophied, but ultimately this compensatory mechanism becomes inadequate, and clinical evidences of obstruction ensue. With carcinomatous obstruction of the left side of the colon and a competent ileocecal valve, closed loop obstruction and even perforation of the cecum may occur.

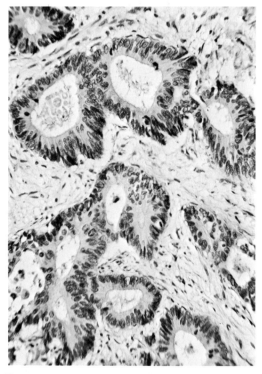

Fig. 27-28 Typical well-differentiated adenocarcinoma of colon. (×300.)

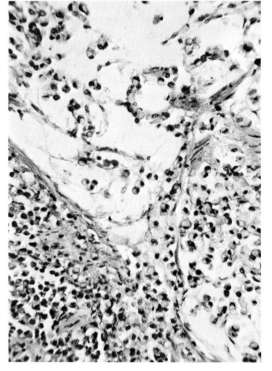

Fig. 27-29 Colloid (mucinous) carcinoma of cecum. Both patterns of pools of mucin and of sheets of individual signet-ring cells are seen. (×300.)

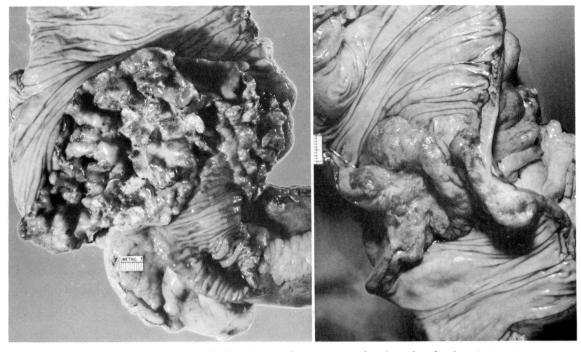

Fig. 27-30 A, Characteristic bulky, ulcerated carcinoma of right side of colon. Lesion in cecum. **B,** Characteristic constricting, "napkin-ring" carcinoma of left side of colon. Lesion in sigmoid. Tumor does not quite involve full circumference. Hypertrophied proximal bowel above.

Carcinomas primary in the rectum do not have a characteristic gross anatomic pattern but vary a great deal. Bleeding is a common symptom. Many are discovered on routine proctoscopic or digital examination. The diffusely infiltrating linitis plastica–like lesion composed of mucin-secreting signet-ring cells and often having an abundant fibrous stroma has already been referred to. More common are bulky "colloid" carcinomas presenting a varicolored mucosal aspect with extensive ulceration. The smaller, more or less flat carcinomas that occur in the rectum and sigmoid colon commonly undermine the peripheral normal mucous membrane as they grow centrifugally. Thus, it is readily possible, on proctoscopic or sigmoidoscopic biopsy, to obtain a specimen containing only overlying normal mucosa if the forceps bite is not deep enough.

Spread. The initial spread of most colonic carcinomas is directly through the intestinal wall by locally invasive growth. Penetration of the muscular wall and involvement of the serosa and subserosa have usually occurred by the time the lesion is observed. Of greater significance to the patient's longevity is spread by way of the lymphatics. Extension generally is to anatomically predictable lymph node groups by embolization rather than by permeation. Ordinarily, lymphatic spread takes place in a proximal direction (i.e., proximal in regard to the direction of flow of intestinal content). Knowledge of the anatomy of the lymphatic circulation and associated lymph nodes is the basis for properly planned surgical treatment of carcinoma in general, as well as specifically of carcinoma of the colon and rectum. Spread to collateral lymph nodes or to nodes farther along the chain of progression (by collateral channels) occurs when metastatic deposits are so extensive as to block the main routes. Metastatic spread bypasses uninvolved nodes infrequently. Study of surgically resected specimens utilizing special "clearing" techniques reveals more regional lymph nodes and more lymph node metastases than is possible with conventional methods. Penetration of lymph node capsules takes place only when disease is advanced.

Blood vascular spread of colonic cancer is also highly significant. Cancer cells have been found circulating in the bloodstream with greater frequency than previously realized, but the significance of this finding remains incompletely understood. The finding of cancer cells in the circulating blood and the establishment of metastatic foci are not synonymous.

In general, when venous invasion and blood-borne metastases are present, local growth and lymphatic spread are also extensive. However, striking examples are encountered of extensive venous dissemination of otherwise localized carcinomas and of locally far-advanced, highly invasive tumors without significant lymphatic or venous spread.

The colloid or mucoid carcinomas—of the type characterized grossly by bulky tumor masses and histologically by large pools of mucin and relatively few cells—are prone to spread widely over the peritoneal surface. Similar peritoneal seeding occurs less frequently with the more usual carcinomas of the large intestine. At times, peritoneal spread may result in formation of a metastatic tumor mass palpable on rectal examination in the rectovesical or rectouterine space—so-called rectal (Blumer's) shelf. It is also possible for implantation of cancer cells at the suture line of intestinal anastomosis, or in the peritoneum, to follow intestinal resection for carcinoma.

A number of classifications of colonic and rectal carcinoma, the most important of which are based on degree of differentiation and on the extent of spread both directly through the intestinal wall and by way of the lymphatics following a proposal by Dukes,[175] correlate reasonably well with the end results of surgical treatment. The five-year survival rates following intestinal resection vary from 15% to 20% to better than 60% depending upon the part of the intestine involved and the extent of the disease at the time of diagnosis and treatment. The foregoing figures take into account only those tumors not so far advanced as to be considered inoperable.

Carcinoma of stomach

Incidence. Although the relative incidence of gastric cancer has been decreasing, it still occurs with sufficient frequency to maintain its position as a very important form of cancer. Its incidence varies greatly in various parts of the world and among various peoples. For example, it is known to be particularly frequent in Japan, very rare among the Malay population of Java, but by no means rare among the Chinese inhabitants of Java. Iceland is one of the countries in which it is a common disease, and there it accounts for 35% to 45% of all fatal cancers in males. Dungal and Sigurjonsson[184] have produced evidence linking this high incidence to the consumption of considerable amounts of smoked fish and meat, particularly the former.

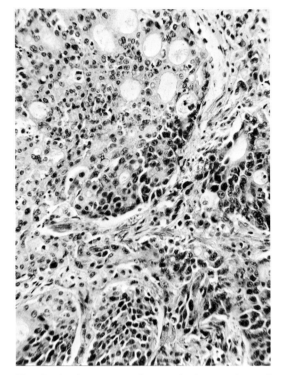

Fig. 27-31 Carcinoma of stomach showing limited degree of glandular differentiation. (×300.)

These points suggest that geographic variations in the incidence of gastric carcinoma may depend, at least in part, upon dietary customs and resultant exposure to carcinogens. The incidence in women is about half of that in men.

Classification. Most carcinomas of the stomach arise from the mucus-secreting cells. Their differentiation is variable as to extent and regularity of gland formation, mucus secretion, cytologic features, etc., but in general they tend to be less well differentiated and less characteristic than the carcinomas of the colon and rectum (Fig. 27-31). All parts of the stomach may be involved, but most gastric carcinomas occur in the antrum and on or near the greater curvature. Ulcerative cancers in particular have a predilection for location in proximity to the greater curvature and/or the pylorus.

Of the many classifications of gastric carcinoma that have been devised, a large proportion lack the merit of clinical significance. An exception is that of Borrman,[182] which has been widely accepted. It is based upon the extensiveness of the lesion as judged by gross examination, showing a gradual gradation between the less malignant tumors that grow mainly within the lumen of the stomach and those prognostically less favorable, which are deeply invasive and penetrate the gastric wall. Stout's classification is somewhat similar, being based upon direction of growth and the resultant gross configuration of the tumor. He recognized (1) a fungating or polypoid type, (2) an ulcerating type (ulcer-cancer), (3) a superficial spreading type, and (4) a diffusely spreading type (linitis plastica).[190]

Polypoid or fungating gastric carcinomas have a particularly favorable prognosis. Fungating carcinomas that arise in the region of the cardioesophageal junction are exceptions, for they may become very extensive, both locally and in terms of lymph node spread, before giving rise to symptoms. Superficial spreading carcinoma is also a relatively favorable type. These two forms of gastric carcinoma having a reasonably good prognosis are relatively infrequent varieties. The linitis plastica type, equally or more rare, is hopeless in its outlook.

These various classifications and their clinical correlations all support the concept that the tumor that grows by frank infiltration offers a greater and more immediate threat to the life of the host than does the gastric cancer that grows expansively, essentially "pushing" aside the host tissues. An important defect in Stout's classification is the fact that some two-thirds of gastric carcinomas cannot be assigned to any one of these categories—either because they are too far advanced to yield a clue to their initial gross configuration or because they show features of tumors of two or more growth types.

Morbid anatomy. *Polypoid gastric carcinomas* resemble adenomatous polyps except that they are usually larger and have a less delicate and often less distinct pedicle because of carcinomatous invasion. Benign polyps are commonly seen, and atrophic gastritis is always present in stomachs that are the site of polypoid carcinomas. Pernicious anemia may be associated. Carcinomas of this gross type usually show good glandular differentiation, and the neoplastic glands very often resemble those of the small intestine.

The macroscopic differences between ulcer-cancers and peptic ulcers have been described in the discussion of peptic ulcer (Plate 3, *D* and *E*). The old controversy over how many gastric cancers have their origins in peptic ulcers (if any) seems to have been largely resolved. Current prevailing opinion is that a small number of gastric carcinomas may arise in preexisting ulcers. Conviction of such

an occurrence in any given case must rest upon demonstration of a characteristic peptic ulcer with cancer limited to one portion of its base or margin. Caution must be exercised not to misinterpret cytologically atypical, proliferative epithelial changes in the mucous membrane at the edge of the ulcer as malignant. It has been said that fusion of the fibers of the muscularis propria with those of the muscularis mucosae at the periphery of an ulcer is an indication of its originally benign nature, but this is probably not invariably true. A majority of the ulcer-cancers are malignant lesions from their inception, either because of primarily deeply penetrating growth or because of early peptic ulceration of a small cancer. Ulcerative cancer has no specific histologic features.

Superficial spreading type. Infrequently, carcinomas arise and spread superficially in the mucosa or submucosa of the stomach to form a serpiginous lesion that may cover a large portion of the mucosal surface. Even without extensive deeper penetration, lymph node metastasis may take place. This type of tumor may be multicentric.

In the *linitis plastica* or *diffusely spreading* type of carcinoma, the wall of the entire stomach is thickened more or less uniformly to as much as 1 cm or 1.5 cm by neoplastic infiltration and new fibrous tissue production. The shrunken stomach with its relatively rigid wall earned the old descriptive term "leather-bottle stomach" (Plate 3, *F*). Characteristically, the mucosa displays no focal lesion, although it may show thickening and irregularities, with flattening and distortion of its folds. Tumor infiltration involves all layers, but the submucosa and subserosa are chiefly affected. In addition to showing infiltration, the muscularis often is hypertrophied. Lymphatic permeation is usual within the gastric wall proper, as well as into the adjacent omentum. Extension into the duodenum is generally sharply limited, although the subserosa may be involved to some extent.

Histologically, carcinomas of linitis plastica type tend to be undifferentiated, and at times distinction from malignant lymphoma is difficult or impossible. If a tumor secretes mucin, this may be a helpful diagnostic feature. At times, mucin secretion may be abundant, and signet-ring cells may be the predominant cells. Desmoplasia often is marked, and in some cancers dense fibrous stroma may so dominate the histologic picture that recognition of cancer cells is difficult. Because of the extent of the disease by the time it is recognized in the usual case, the prognosis is essentially hopeless. Occasionally, focal fibrotic thickening of the antrum, apparently of inflammatory nature, may simulate cancer clinically and on naked-eye inspection of the specimen.

The majority of gastric carcinomas, which do not meet the criteria of any one of these groups, are extremely variable in gross appearance and histologic pattern. Again, because they are usually far advanced before an opportunity for treatment is offered, the outlook is poor.

Spread. Direct spread and spread by way of the lymphatics are of foremost importance in dictating principles of surgical treatment and in assessing the individual patient's prognosis. Metastasis to lymph nodes along both the greater and lesser curvature, depending upon both the location and the size of the primary lesion, is frequent. Extension into the next zone, the para-aortic nodes and those about the celiac axis, is often seen.

Metastasis to the left supraclavicular lymph nodes by way of the thoracic duct may be a presenting sign of gastric carcinoma—the so-called *Virchow's (Ewald's) node*. With lesions high in the stomach, spread into the esophagus, especially submucosal, and to mediastinal lymph nodes is a feature. In occasional cases, there may be permeation of pulmonary lymphatics and the bone marrow (with clinically unexplained anemia) as early manifestations of the disease.

Liver metastases, common even in cases believed to be "early," result from invasion of tributaries of the portal venous system. Peritoneal spread and carcinomatosis occur, and gastric cancer is an important diagnostic consideration when a rectal shelf is demonstrated clinically. Carcinoma of the stomach, as well as of other parts of the gastrointestinal tract, may metastasize early to the ovaries so that the ovarian tumors dominate the clinical picture—so-called *Krukenberg tumors*. The typical Krukenberg tumor is characterized by signet-ring cancer cells with abundant fibrous tissue stroma.

Carcinoma of esophagus

Among gastrointestinal cancers, **epidermoid carcinoma of the esophagus** ranks behind only carcinoma of the colon and rectum and carcinoma of the stomach in frequency. It is a disease of older age groups, affecting men more often than women. Roughly half of the esophageal cancers arise in the mid-third of the organ, the remainder being approximately equally distributed between the upper and lower thirds. The typical epidermoid carcinoma of the esophagus is ovoid, with its long axis parallel to the long axis of the esophagus, and elevated to form a plaquelike lesion, with central ulceration and undermining of the peripheral mucous membrane (Plate 3, *B*). Growth to involve the full circumference of the esophagus occurs. The usual presenting problem is dysphagia. Extension through the full thickness of the esophageal wall is the rule, and since the esophagus has no serous coat, spread in the mediastinum is facilitated. Lymphatic spread is as readily accomplished. As a result, carcinoma of the esophagus is generally well established when recognized, and the results of treatment, as measured in terms of five-year survivals, are, as might be expected, quite poor.

Although primary glandular carcinomas occur rarely in the esophagus, most adenocarcinomas seen in the esophagus are primary tumors of the gastric cardia that have grown upward into the esophagus.

Carcinoma of small intestine

Carcinoma of the small intestine is rare. Primary carcinoma of the duodenum invading the pancreas may be very difficult to distinguish with certainty from pancreatic carcinoma secondarily invading the duodenum. In the region of the ampulla of Vater, carcinomas of the common bile duct or of the ampulla proper must be included in the differential diagnosis.

With the exception of some of the periampullary carcinomas, many of which resemble the biliary duct system tumors morphologically, carcinomas of the small intestine are similar in appearance and behavior to those of the large intestine, although their clinical diagnosis may be more difficult and their evolutionary stage more advanced when they are diagnosed. An occasional carcinoma of the small intestine may take origin in a papillary adenoma.

Carcinoma of appendix

Carcinoid is the most frequently encountered tumor of the appendix, but carcinomas essentially indistinguishable from those of the colon occur rarely. Cancer of the appendix appears to be particularly malignant, presumably because the anatomic structure of the appendix permits the growth ready access to the serosal layer as well as to the lymphatics.

Carcinoma of anal region

A number of different epithelial tumors take origin in the vicinity of the anus and anorectal junction. Among **epidermoid carcinomas of the anus** are "ordinary" epidermoid carcinomas arising from the squamous epithelium of the anal mucous membrane. They appear and behave like epidermoid carcinomas of other squamous epithelial mucous membranes. These malignant tumors spread freely by way of the rich perianal lymphatic plexuses to the lymph nodes of the groin.

Another group of anal tumors are so-called **basaloid tumors** that have epidermoid features only in the centers of the clusters of basaloid cells. The name "basaloid" points up their histologic resemblance to the common basal cell epitheliomas of the skin, from which they must be distinguished. Presumably these tumors arise from the mucosa of the transitional or cloacogenic zone separating the rectal and anal mucous membranes and are believed to have a more favorable prognosis than the anal epidermoid carcinomas.

Occasional epidermoid tumors in this area include some glandular elements or individual cells with the demonstrable ability to secrete mucin—**mucoepidermoid carcinomas.**

Anal duct carcinoma is an infrequent tumor, usually glandular and mucin-secreting, that occurs in the anorectal area without apparent involvement of anal skin or anal or rectal mucous membrane. These tumors arise from anal glands or ducts and usually are not recognized as being malignant until some time has elapsed, often while treatment has been directed toward such conditions as fistula in ano. Similar tumors (of mucinous or mucoepidermoid type) have apparently arisen in long-standing anal fistulas.

Rarely, **epidermoid carcinomas** arise in the rectum, with or without squamous metaplasia, where anatomic continuity with the anus can be excluded with certainty. They also occur, but even more rarely, in the stomach, as do mixed glandular and epidermoid tumors—adenoacanthomas. Apparently, epidermoid carcinoma can develop, under particular circumstances, from epithelium of any type.

Malignant melanoma

Malignant melanomas have been encountered in many parts of the gastrointestinal tract. Most such lesions are metastatic. Metastases may lodge superficially in the mucous membrane, and the resultant tumor masses trigger intussusceptions.

Primary malignant melanomas arise from the anus, and examples believed to be primary have been reported in the esophagus. Their appearance and behavior do not differ from those of the corresponding skin lesions. Anal malignant melanomas may present primarily as rectal lesions because anal sphincteric action may cause them to grow in a cephalad direction initially.

Establishment of the primary nature of gastrointestinal malignant melanomas rests upon demonstration of junctional change—the recognition of neoplastic proliferation in the area of the junction of epithelium and subepithelial stroma.

Carcinoid tumor

Carcinoid (argentaffin) tumors are relatively uncommon neoplasms that have excited a degree of interest out of proportion to their frequency. This is partly because of vagaries in their clinical behavior, but more especially because of the recognition of their endocrine secretion and its effects upon the body. They are found throughout the gastrointestinal tract from the stomach to the rectum, as well as in the gallbladder and in teratoid ovarian tumors. Morphologically and functionally identical tumors arise from the bronchial and tracheal mucous membrane. The cell of origin has been thought to be the Kulchitsky cell, one of the cell types occurring in the crypts of Lieberkühn, characterized morphologically by the presence of cytoplasmic granules capable of reducing ammoniacal silver nitrate (argentaffin granules). Recently, it has been suggested that more than one cell type may be involved, argentaffin granules being found only in midgut and bronchial carcinoids. Those of the stomach may contain so-called argyrophil granules, which stain with metallic silver after the addition of an exogenous reducing substance. Those of the hindgut also contain granules, but they are neither argentaffin nor argyrophil. The argentaffin cells secrete serotonin (5-hydroxytryptamine), a hormone carried in the circulation by the blood platelets and concerned with blood coagulation, probably through a vasoconstrictive action. Serotonin also has been shown to have a normal central nervous system function, and these facts, together with its pathologic role in the development of cardiovascular lesions and the "carcinoid syndrome," account for the widespread interest it has generated.

Some carcinoid tumors are indistinguishable

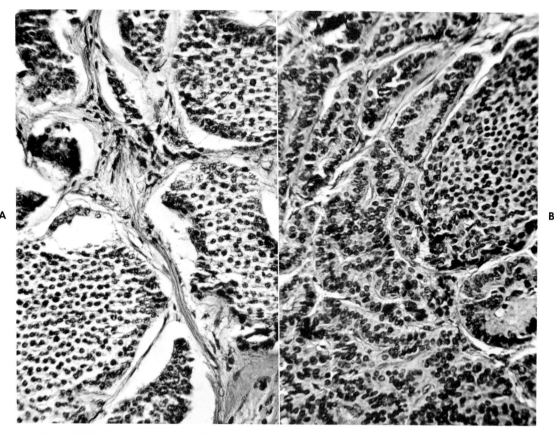

Fig. 27-32 Carcinoid (argentaffin) tumor. **A,** "Classic" pattern. **B,** Trabecular pattern. (**A** and **B,** ×300.)

grossly from carcinomas, but the characteristic lesions are small submucosal nodules or merely focal areas of submucosal thickening. Their yellow color has been emphasized, but many are actually gray or grayish white. Muscle hypertrophy often is marked in the involved area, and this, together with the characteristic fibrosis and perhaps peritoneal adhesions, may produce kinking and partial obstruction (Plate 3, *G*).

Histologically, carcinoid tumors are of two types. The "classic" variety is composed of solid nests of uniform small cells with nuclei that are round or ovoid and usually regular. There is a tendency for the argentaffin granules to be concentrated in the peripheral border of the cells at the periphery of the nests. The second and less common variety is composed of similar cells, but there is a distinctive trabecular pattern of interanastomosing bands or ribbons. Rosettelike formations may occur with either type, and both patterns are seen in some tumors (Fig. 27-32). Occasional tumors of intermixed carcinoid and mucus-secreting type are encountered. Characteristically, a carcinoid tumor grows

invasively. It has the potential for metastasizing by way of both the lymphatics and the bloodstream. However, carcinoid tumors grow slowly, and it is not uncommon for a patient with disseminated disease to live an essentially asymptomatic life for many years.

Carcinoid tumors occur more frequently in the appendix than elsewhere. They are usually incidental findings at autopsy or in appendices removed surgically for acute inflammation or other reason. As such, they are rarely observed to metastasize. Much the same is true with respect to the rectum, another common site, where most of the tumors are asymptomatic and are found incidentally on proctoscopic examination carried out as a routine procedure. However, roughly 10% to 15% of rectal carcinoid tumors, usually those more than 2 cm in diameter and found to be invading the muscularis propria, behave like rectal carcinomas, although perhaps progressing more slowly. Occasionally, very small tumors may be associated with distant, even widespread, metastases. Carcinoid tumors that metastasize and prove fatal, as well as those associated with the "carcinoid syndrome," most often are encountered in the ileum and commonly are multiple.

The principal components of the "carcinoid syndrome" are diarrhea, a peculiar cyanotic flushing of the skin, and right-sided heart failure, the latter based on organic disease of the tricuspid and/or pulmonic valves. Almost invariably, extensive liver metastases are present in patients with the syndrome, which is believed to occur only when a large bulk of tumor tissue can account for the secretion of a large quantity of serotonin. In the usual functioning carcinoid tumor, 5-hydroxy-indole acetic acid (5-HIAA), a degradation product of 5-hydroxytryptamine (5HT), can be demonstrated in the urine. The cardiac lesion consists of dense, fibrous endocardial thickening, the fibrous tissue apparently being deposited upon the surface of the endocardium. The pulmonic valve usually shows the greatest change, but the tricuspid valve and the endocardium of the right auricle and even the other chambers of the heart, the great vessels, and the coronary sinus may be involved. The usual functional valvular lesions are pulmonic stenosis and tricuspid insufficiency. Normally, serotonin is destroyed in the lung by monoamine oxidase, accounting for the preponderance of right-sided cardiac disease.

It has been suggested that serotonin releases histamine and mucopolysaccharides from mast cells and that this causes local edema in the loose connective tissues generally, but especially in those of the subendocardium. Fibrinolysis of the fibrin deposited on the damaged endocardium may be prevented by oxidized serotonin, and organization and fibrosis follow. Similarly, local edema may be the direct precipitating factor of the striking fibrosis so commonly seen in the immediate vicinity of primary carcinoid tumors.

Williams and Sandler[208] have subdivided carcinoid tumors into three groups:

1 Those of the bronchus and stomach, arising from the foregut
2 Those of the jejunum, ileum, and cecum, arising from the midgut
3 Those of the rectum, developing from the hindgut

They point out that those from the foregut are often of trabecular pattern and sometimes secrete 5-hydroxytryptophan, a precursor of serotonin, and store the latter poorly; those of midgut origin are the classic lesions, both morphologically and tinctorially (positive argentaffin reaction) and in the ability to store large amounts of serotonin; those of the hindgut are usually of trabecular pattern and lack secretory function. The syndrome, as well as 5-HIAA excretion, is frequent with both foregut and midgut tumors.

Neoplasms of smooth muscle

With the exception of the uterus, the muscle of the gastrointestinal tract gives rise to more tumors of smooth muscle than any other organ or organ-system of the body. As is true

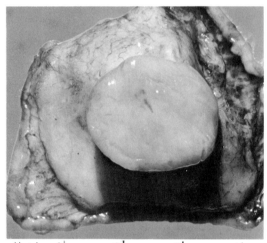

Metric 1 2 3 4

Fig. 27-33 Leiomyoma of stomach. Growth essentially endogastric.

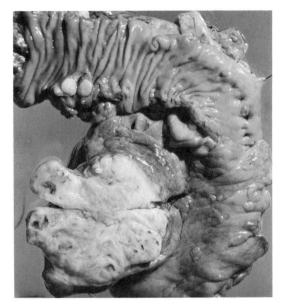

Fig. 27-34 Leiomyosarcoma of descending colon. Lesion almost wholly exoenteric. Note openings of diverticula at right.

also of the uterus, **leiomyomas** far outnumber **leiomyosarcomas.** They arise in any portion of the alimentary tract, from the esophagus to the rectum (and including the retroperitoneum, mesentery, etc.) but are more common in the stomach than elsewhere. The small intestine is next most frequently involved. Myomas may grow primarily into the gut lumen (Fig. 27-33), and in that part of the intestine supported on a mesentery they may become pedunculated and form the head of an intussusception. They also may project primarily from the serosa and grow to a large size without producing gastrointestinal symptoms (Fig. 27-34). Some tumors are dumbbell-shaped lesions, projecting in both directions. It is common for gastrointestinal smooth muscle tumors to ulcerate and undergo extensive central necrosis. For this reason, the presenting symptom is often hematemesis (or melena), and a small leiomyoma of the small intestine may be the cryptic source of massive, even exsanguinating, hemorrhage.

The smooth muscle neoplasms are composed of interlacing bundles of fusiform cells, with long processes and nuclei with blunted ends, often bearing a very striking resemblance to normal smooth muscle. Although

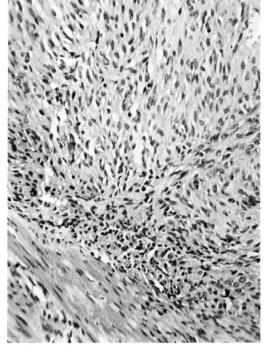

Fig. 27-35 Leiomyoma of small intestine. Portion of normal musculature present at lower left. (×300.)

they appear well delineated grossly, under the microscope no capsule is seen, and tumor muscle fibers usually can be seen to interdigitate with those of the muscularis propria or, occasionally, the muscularis mucosae (Fig. 27-35). The histologic distinction between leiomyoma and leiomyosarcoma may be very difficult. Occasional sarcomas appear very orderly and well differentiated, giving no hint of malignancy until metastases occur. More often, however, completely benign tumors show great cellularity and nuclear pleomorphism, even to the presence of bizarre giant cells. The presence of mitotic figures in appreciable numbers is generally a reliable indication of malignancy.

Like sarcomas in general, distant metastases of leiomyosarcomas are usually blood-borne, but some display a tendency to spread over the peritoneal surface and some are only locally invasive. A capacity for local invasion only is particularly true of those arising in the retroperitoneum, most of which are classified as sarcomas, largely because of the impossibility of removing them completely and thus effecting cure, although they metastasize infrequently.

Lymphoma

A benign lesion, often referred to as *lymphoma of the rectum,* but also known as *lymphoid polyp* or rectal tonsil, is occasionally encountered on proctoscopic examination and removed as a "polyp." It is usually only a few millimeters in diameter but may reach a dimension as great as 1.5 cm. It can be recognized microscopically as benign by its excellent organization with "germinal centers" and its usual limitation to the mucosa and submucosa without invasion of the muscle coat. It is of significance only in differential diagnosis.

With this exception, the lymphomas of the gastrointestinal tract are malignant. Such *malignant lymphomas* may arise as primary or apparently primary gastrointestinal tumors or may be but one manifestation of generalized disease. The latter situation is more common, and all varieties of malignant lymphoma encountered in the lymphoid tissues of the body generally may involve the alimentary tract. The same varieties also occur as "primary" lesions, but some (e.g., Hodgkin's disease and plasmacytoma) are very rare, whereas lymphosarcoma and reticulum cell sarcoma are relatively more frequent. Gastrointestinal lesions in generalized malignant

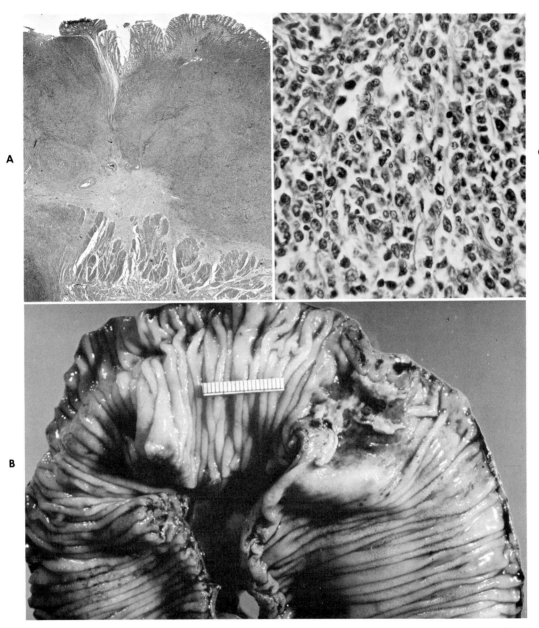

Fig. 27-36 A, Malignant lymphoma of stomach. Characteristic plateaulike elevation of mucosa and marked thickening of submucosa well demonstrated. At left, muscle has been freely invaded. **B,** Malignant lymphoma of small intestine, with multiple sites of involvement. Note similarity to gross appearance of carcinoid tumor illustrated in Plate 3, G. **C,** Malignant lymphoma of stomach showing considerable pleomorphism. (**A,** ×13; **C,** ×625.)

lymphoma (including the leukemias) are of importance in and of themselves, and they may demand treatment when they are responsible for problems relative to gastrointestinal hemorrhage or obstruction. Malignant lymphomas readily perforate, occasionally at multiple sites, especially following radiation therapy.

"Primary" malignant lymphoma of the gastrointestinal tract is most often seen in the stomach, less commonly in the rectum, cecum, and ascending colon, and infrequently elsewhere. Gastric malignant lymphomas usually simulate carcinoma in their clinical manifestations, and they may do so as far as their gross pathologic appearance is concerned as well.

However, many have a characteristic gross morphology. They appear as flat, disklike, or plateaulike elevations with rather sharply defined borders (Fig. 27-36, *A*). They are raised only a few millimeters or a centimeter or so above the surrounding mucous membrane, and if they involve the antrum, their pyloric margin is abrupt. Frequently involvement is multifocal, and ulceration is usual, producing shallow saucerlike lesions. In the intestine, involvement of submucosa, as opposed to mucosa, is a prominent feature, and, again, multicentric origin is frequent. As with carcinoid tumors, kinking and incomplete obstruction may bring the disease to the patient's attention (Fig. 27-36, *B*).

Many lymphomas are distinguishable from carcinoma only on microscopic examination, and at times even histologic differentiation may be difficult. Gastrointestinal lymphomas are subject to the same classifications that are applied to neoplasms arising from the lymphoreticular tissues of the rest of the body, although there is a tendency to classify them more simply as of large (reticulum) cell or of small (lymphocytic) cell type or as Hodgkin's disease. Many of the gastric lymphomas show marked pleomorphism, making precise classification according to the usual criteria difficult (Fig. 27-36, *C*). Some of the gastric lymphoid neoplasms can be distinguished from inflammatory hyperplasias only with great difficulty. At times, the distinction requires observation of the clinical course over a period of years.

It is noteworthy that malignant lymphomas of the gastrointestinal tract, although they have their greatest incidence in the same age range as carcinoma, have an appreciably greater incidence during early ages, including childhood. Primary malignant lymphoma of the stomach, the most common malignant gastric tumor next to carcinoma, offers a distinctly better prognosis than carcinoma in terms of five-year survival after surgical treatment. On the other hand, so-called primary malignant lymphomas of the colon and rectum in a majority of instances prove to be manifestations of systemic disease, although the extraintestinal involvement may not be apparent at the time of recognition of the colonic or rectal lesion.

Occasional cases of multiple, polypoid, relatively well-differentiated and organized lymphoid lesions of the gastrointestinal tract (so-called gastrointestinal pseudoleukemia) are encountered. Many of these eventuate as disseminated malignant lymphoma.

Miscellaneous rare tumors

Although **mucocele of the appendix** is not a true neoplasm, it will be considered here. It is a cystic dilatation of the appendix distal to a complete obstruction, usually the result of cicatricial stricture following inflammation. The mucocele is distended with thick, glairy mucus, its wall is thinned, and the normal mucous membrane is replaced by glands resembling those of the colon or by a single layer of mucus-secreting cells. In a number of cases, there are associated pseudomucinous ovarian cysts. Rupture of a mucocele (or of a pseudomucinous cyst) results in the lesion known as **pseudomyxoma peritonei**—spread of mucus-secreting cells over the peritoneal surfaces, with accumulation of mucoid material in the peritoneal cavity. A difference of opinion exists as to whether pseudomyxoma represents actual neoplastic epithelial proliferation or a nonneoplastic proliferation of serosal cells under the stimulus of irritation. It seems likely that either or both mechanisms may be operative in individual cases.

Lipomas occasionally are encountered in various parts of the gastrointestinal tract, most often in the colon and rectum and particularly in the vicinity of the ileocecal valve, where appreciable submucosal adipose tissue is usually present. They are submucosal, often

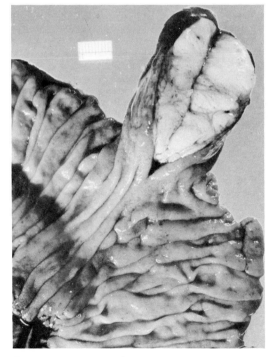

Fig. 27-37 Lipoma of jejunum.

superficially ulcerated, and may lead to an intussusception (Fig. 27-37). In instances of incipient intussusception, there may be puckering of the overlying serosa, and this, coupled with induration as the result of inflammation, may account for their being mistaken for carcinoma at operation.

Vascular tumors, especially cavernous **hemangiomas,** have been reported as occurring in various parts of the gastrointestinal tract. **Lymphangiomas** occur less frequently. Characteristic **glomus tumors** may form polypoid, sometimes painful, gastric tumors. Rarely, gastrointestinal lesions occur in **Kaposi's sarcoma.**

The gastrointestinal tract may be involved in **Recklinghausen's disease (neurofibromatosis).** Many of the reported isolated schwannian tumors of the gut are very likely leiomyomas. **Adenomas** or papillary cystadenomas arise from the apocrine sweat glands in the region of the anus.

Carcinosarcoma is a rare but spectacular tumor of the esophagus, incorporating both epithelial growth (usually epidermoid) and a sarcomatous or sarcoma-like stroma, which

may dominate the picture. Many such tumors are polypoid. There is no agreement as to the nature of the stromal change—whether it is genuinely malignant or pseudosarcomatous. The carcinosarcomas are distinctly less malignant than the much more common epidermoid carcinomas. Metastases, which are relatively infrequent, may be carcinomatous, sarcomatous, or mixed.

Mesothelial cysts are encountered rarely in the mesentery or retroperitoneum. Of greater importance and slightly greater frequency are tumors arising from the serosal lining cells—**mesotheliomas.** They may be solitary and fibrous, in which case they may be amenable to surgical removal, but more often the peritoneal mesotheliomas, in contrast to most of those of the pleura, are diffuse and result in widespread adhesions. They have a tubular pattern, forming multiple small spaces lined by mesothelium, and may secrete mucin (Fig. 27-38). The histologic picture may simulate carcinoma very faithfully. Rare peritoneal mesotheliomas may present as multiple small papillary growths.

Metastatic tumors

Metastatic tumors, especially carcinomas, are very common in the peritoneal cavity. Spread over the serosal surfaces to involve multiple organs and produce widespread adhesions is a frequent autopsy finding in disseminated cancer. The primary tumor may not be readily apparent without complete autopsy study. Therefore, the assured diagnosis of primary diffuse tubular mesothelioma of the peritoneum may be impossible during life.

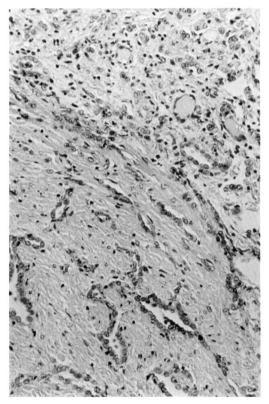

Fig. 27-38 Tubular mesothelioma of peritoneum. (×240.)

REFERENCES
Congenital anomalies
General

1 Estrada, R. L.: Anomalies of intestinal rotation and fixation, Springfield, Ill., 1958, Charles C Thomas, Publisher.
2 Gross, R. E.: The surgery of infancy and childhood, Philadelphia, 1953, W. B. Saunders Co.

Atresias

3 DeLorimier, A. A., Fonkalsrud, E. W., and Hays, D. M.: Surgery 65:819-827, 1969.
4 Dykstra, G., Sieber, W. K. and Kiesewetter, W. B.: Arch. Surg. (Chicago) 97:175-182, 1968.

Imperforate anus

5 Kiesewetter, W. B., Turner, C. R., and Sieber, W. K.: Amer. J. Surg. 107:412-421, 1964.

Heterotopia
Heterotopic gastric mucous membrane

6 Bosher, L. H., Jr., and Taylor, F. H.: J. Thorac. Surg. **21**:306-312, 1951.
7 Rector, L. E., and Connerley, M. L.: Arch. Path. (Chicago) **31**:285-294, 1941.

Heterotopic pancreatic tissue

8 Martinez, N. S., Morlock, C. G., Dockerty, M. B., Waugh, J. M., and Weber, H. M.: Ann. Surg. **147**:1-12, 1958.
9 Tonkin, R. D., Field, T. E., and Wykes, P. R.: Gut **3**:135-139, 1962.

Duplications and cysts

10 Bremer, J. L.: Arch. Path. (Chicago) **38**:132-140, 1944.
11 Desforges, G., and Strieder, J. W.: New Eng. J. Med. **262**:60-64, 1960.

Meckel's diverticulum

12 Johns, T. N. P., Wheeler, J. R., and Johns, F. S.: Ann. Surg. **150**:241-256, 1959.
13 Seagram, C. G. F., Louch, R. E., Stephens, C. A. and Wentworth, P.: Canad. J. Surg. **11**:369-373, 1968 (achalasia of esophagus).
14 Weinstein, E. C., Cain, J. C., and ReMine, W. H.: J.A.M.A. **182**:251-253, 1962.

Aganglionic megacolon (Hirschsprung's disease)

15 Gherardi, G. J.: Arch. Path. (Chicago) **69**:520-523, 1960.
16 Swenson, O.: Arch. Dis. Child. **30**:1-7, 1955.

Pyloric stenosis

17 Benson, C. D., and Lloyd, J. R.: Amer. J. Surg. **107**:429-433, 1964.
18 Cassella, R. R., Brown, A. L., Jr., Sayre, G. P., and Ellis, F. H., Jr.: Ann. Surg. **160**:474-487, 1964.

Acquired malformations
Diverticula

19 Borow, M., Smith, M., Jr., and Soto, D., Jr.: Amer. Surg. **33**:373-377, 1967 (duodenum).
20 Edwards, H. C.: Ann. Surg. **103**:230-254, 1936 (jejunum).
21 King, B. T.: Surg. Gynec. Obstet. **85**:93-97, 1947 (esophagus).
22 Morson, B. C.: Brit. J. Radiol. **36**:385-392, 1963 (colon).
23 Reichmann, H. R., and Watkins, J. B.: J.A.M.A. **182**:1023-1028, 1962 (colon).

Pneumatosis intestinalis

24 Culver, G. J.: J.A.M.A. **186**:160-162, 1963.
25 Doub, H. P., and Shea, J. J.: J.A.M.A. **172**:1238-1242, 1960.
26 Keyting, W. S., McCarver, R. R., Kovarik, J. L., and Daywitt, A. L.: Radiology **76**:733-741, 1961.
27 Skendzel, L. P.: Arch. Path. (Chicago) **67**:333-338, 1959.
28 Smith, B. H., and Welter, E. H.: Amer. J. Clin. Path. **48**:455-465, 1967.

Melanosis of colon

29 Ecker, J. A., and Dickson, D. R.: Amer. J. Gastroent. **39**:362-370, 1963.

Endometriosis

30 Tagart, R. E. B.: Brit. J. Surg. **47**:27-34, 1959.

Esophagotracheobronchial fistula

31 Wychulis, A. R., Ellis, F. H. Jr., and Andersen, H. A.: J.A.M.A. **196**:117-122, 1966.

Mechanical disturbances
Obstruction
Hernia
Inguinal hernia

32 Mayo, C. W., Stalker, L. K., and Miller, J. M.: Ann. Surg. **114**:875-885, 1941.

Hiatus hernia

33 Barrett, N. R.: Brit. J. Surg. **42**:231-243, 1954.
34 Grimes, O. F., and Stephens, B. H.: Ann. Surg. **152**:743-766, 1960.
35 Marchand, P.: J. Thorac. Surg. **37**:81-92, 1959.

Intussusception

36 Benson, C. D., Lloyd, J. R., and Fischer, H.: Arch. Surg. (Chicago) **86**:745-751, 1963.
37 Ladd, W. E., and Gross, R. E.: Arch. Surg. (Chicago) **29**:365-384, 1934.

Obturation obstruction

38 Norberg, P. B.: Amer. J. Surg. **104**:444-447, 1962.

Stricture

39 Fabrikant, J. I., Anlyan, W. G., and Creadick, R. N.: Southern Med. J. **52**:1136-1191, 1959 (irradiation).
40 Norton, J. H., Jr., Rev-Kury, H., and White, H. J.: Gastroenterology **46**:471-473, 1964.
41 Perkins, D. E., and Spjut, H. J.: Amer. J. Roentgen. **88**:953-966, 1962 (irradiation).
42 Sauer, W. G.: J. Iowa Med. Soc. **50**:1-7, 1960 (irradiation).

Effects of intestinal obstruction

43 Storck, A., Rothschild, J. E., and Ochsner, A.: Ann. Surg. **109**:844-861, 1939.
44 Tumen, H. J.: In Bockus, H. L.: Gastroenterology, ed. 2, Philadelphia, 1964, W. B. Saunders Co.
45 Wangensteen, O. H.: Intestinal obstructions, ed. 3, Springfield, Ill., 1955, Charles C Thomas, Publisher.

Adynamic (paralytic) ileus

46 Ochsner, A., and Gage, I. M.: Amer. J. Surg. **20**:378-404, 1933.

Mallory-Weiss syndrome

47 Baue, A. E.: J.A.M.A. **184**:325-328, 1963.
48 Dagradi, A. E., Broderick, J. T., Juler, G., Wolinsky, S., and Stempien, S. J.: Amer. J. Dig. Dis. **11**:710-721, 1966.
49 Dobbins, W. O., III: Gastroenterology **44**:689-695, 1963.

Vascular disturbances
Esophageal varices

50 Baker, L. A., Smith, C., and Lieberman, G.: Amer. J. Med. **26**:228-237, 1959.
51 Liebowitz, H. R.: J.A.M.A. **175**:874-879, 1961.

Infarction of intestine

52 Glotzer, D. J., and Shaw, R. S.: New Eng. J. Med. **260:**162-167, 1959.

53 Marston, A.: Lancet **2:**365-370, 1962.

Ischemic enteritis

54 Frengley, J. D., and Reid, J. D.: New Zeal. Med. J. **63:**212-218, 1964.

Gastrointestinal hemorrhage

55 Brief, D. K., and Botsford, T. W.: J.A.M.A. **184:**18-22, 1963.

56 Ecker, J. A., Doane, W. A., Dickson, D. R., and Gebhardt, W. F.: Amer. J. Gastroent. **33:** 411-421, 1960.

57 Thompson, H. L., and McGuffin, D. W.: J.A.M.A. **141:**1208-1213, 1949.

Inflammations
Esophagitis

58 Moses, H. L., and Cheatham, W. J.: Lab. Invest. **12:**663-669, 1963 (herpetic).

Gastritis
Phlegmonous gastritis

59 Cutler, E. C., and Harrison, J. H.: Surg. Gynec. Obstet. **70:**234-240, 1940.

Eosinophilic granuloma and eosinophilic gastroenteritis

60 Helwig, E. B., and Ranier, A.: Surg. Gynec. Obstet. **96:**355-367, 1953.

61 Ureles, A. L., Alschibaja, T., Lodico, D., and Stabins, S. J.: Amer. J. Med. **30:**899-909, 1961.

Nonspecific ulceration

62 Boley, S. J., Allen, A. C., Schultz, L., and Schwartz, S.: J.A.M.A. **193:**997-1000, 1965.

63 Wayte, D. M., and Helwig, E. B.: Amer. J. Clin. Path. **49:**26-40, 1968.

Ulceration of stomach and duodenum
Stress ulcers

64 Goldman, H., and Rosoff, C. B.: Amer. J. Path. **52:**227-244, 1968.

65 Pruitt, B. A., Jr., Foley, F. D., and Moncrief, J. A.: Ann. Surg. **172:**523-539, 1970 (Curling's ulcer).

Peptic ulcer

66 Dragstedt, L. R.: J.A.M.A. **169:**203-209, 1959.

67 Illingworth, C. F. W.: Peptic ulcer, Edinburgh, 1953, E. & S. Livingstone, Ltd.

68 Kirsner, J. B., Kassriel, R. S., and Palmer, W. L.: Advances Intern. Med. **8:**41-124, 1956.

69 Wolf, S.: Ann. Intern. Med. **31:**637-649, 1949.

Regional enteritis*

70 Ammann, R. W., and Bockus, H. L.: Arch. Intern. Med. (Chicago) **107:**504-513, 1961.

71 Lockhart-Mummery, H. E., and Morson, B. C.: Gut **1:**87-105, 1960 (and ulcerative colitis).

72 Meadows, T. R., and Batsakis, J. G.: Arch. Surg. (Chicago) **87:**976-982, 1963.

73 Saltzstein, S. L., and Rosenberg, B. F.: Amer. J. Clin. Path. **40:**610-623, 1963 (and ulcerative colitis).

Appendicitis

74 Altemeier, W. A.: Ann. Surg. **107:**517-528, 1938 (bacteriology).

75 Bowers, W. F.: Arch. Surg. (Chicago) **39:**362-422, 1939.

76 Collins, D. C.: Surg. Gynec. Obstet. **101:**437-455, 1955.

77 Davidsohn, I., and Mora, J. M.: Arch. Path. (Chicago) **14:**757-765, 1932 (measles).

78 Fitz, R. H.: Amer. J. Med. Sci. **92:**321-346, 1886.

79 Gray, S. H., and Heifetz, C. J.: Arch. Surg. (Chicago) **35:**887-900, 1937.

80 Schenken, J. R., and Moss, E. S.: Amer. J. Clin. Path. **12:**509-517, 1942 (parasites).

81 Schenken, J. R., Anderson, T. R., and Coleman, F. C.: Amer. J. Clin. Path. **26:**352-359, 1956.

82 Tashiro, S., and Zinninger, M. M.: Arch. Surg. (Chicago) **53:**545-563, 1946.

83 Therkelsen, F.: Acta Chir. Scand. **94** (suppl. 108)**:**1-48, 1946.

84 Wangensteen, O. H., and Dennis, C.: Ann. Surg. **110:**629-647, 1939.

85 Wilkie, D. P. D.: Brit. Med. J. **2:**959-962, 1914.

Chronic ulcerative colitis*

86 Hawk, W. A., Turnbull, R. B. Jr., and Farmer, R. G.: J.A.M.A. **201:**738-746, 1967.

87 Kent, T. H., Ammon, R. K., and DenBesten, L.: Arch. Path. (Chicago) **89:**20-29, 1970 (ulcerative colitis and regional enteritis).

88 Kirsner, J. B.: J.A.M.A. **191:**809-814, 1965.

89 Lewin, K., and Swales, J. D.: Gastroenterology, **50:**211-223, 1966.

90 Lumb, G.: Gastroenterology **40:**290-298, 1961.

91 Priest, R. J., Rebuck, J. W., and Havey, G. P.: Gastroenterology **38:**715-720, 1960.

92 Warren, S., and Sommers, S. C.: Amer. J. Path. **25:**657-679, 1949.

Pseudomembranous enterocolitis

93 Altemeier, W. A., Hummel, R. P., and Hill, E. O.: Ann. Surg. **157:**847-858, 1963.

94 Prohaska, J. V., Mock, F., Baker, W., and Collins, R.: Int. Abstr. Surg. **112:**103-115, 1961.

Bacillary dysentery

95 Morgan, H. R.: In Dubos, R. J., and Hirsch, J. G., editors: Bacterial and mycotic infections of man, ed. 5, Philadelphia, 1965, J. B. Lippincott Co.

96 Mosley, W. H., Adams, B., and Lyman, E. D.: J.A.M.A. **182:**1307-1311, 1962.

Typhoid fever

97 Goodpasture, E. W.: Amer. J. Path. **13:**175-186, 1937.

98 Sprinz, H., Gangarosa, E. J., Williams, M., Hornick, R. B., and Woodward, T. E.: Amer. J. Dig. Dis. **11:**615-624, 1966.

*See also reference 86.

*See also references 71 and 73.

99 Stuart, B. M., and Pullen, R. L.: Arch. Intern. Med. (Chicago) **78**:629-661, 1946.
100 Szanton, V. L.: Pediatrics **20**:794-808, 1957.

Asiatic cholera

101 Fresh, J. W., Versage, P. M., and Reyes, V.: Arch. Path. (Chicago) **77**:529-537, 1964.
102 Sheehy, T. W., Sprinz, H., Augerson, W. S., and Formal, S. B.: J.A.M.A. **197**:321-326, 1966.
103 Sprinz, H.: Fed. Proc. **21**:57-64, 1962.

Tuberculosis

104 Abrams, J. S., and Holden, W. D.: Arch. Surg. (Chicago) **89**:282-293, 1964.
105 Cullen, J. H.: Quart. Bull. Sea View Hosp. **5**:143-160, 1940.

Fungal infections

106 Putnam, H. C., Jr., Dockerty, M. B., and Waugh, J. M.: Surgery **28**:781-800, 1950.
107 Rubin, H., Furcolow, M. L., Yates, J. L., and Brasher, C. A.: Amer. J. Med. **27**:278-288, 1959 (histoplasmosis).

Lymphopathia venereum

108 Grace, A. W.: J.A.M.A. **122**:74-78, 1943.

Other forms of enteritis and colitis*

109 Abrahamson, R. H.: Arch. Surg. (Chicago) **81**: 553-557, 1960 (radiation).
110 Gonzales, T. A., Vance, M., Helpern, M., and Umberger, C. J.: Legal medicine, pathology and toxicology, ed. 2, New York, 1954, Appleton-Century-Crofts (chemicals).

Colitis—general

111 McGovern, V. J.: In Pathology annual, vol. 4, (S. C. Sommers, editor), New York, 1969, Appleton-Century-Crofts, pp. 127-158.

Parasitic infestations†

112 Arean, V. M., and Koppisch, E.: Amer. J. Path. **32**:1089-1115, 1956 (balantidiasis).
113 Dimmette, R. M., Elwi, A. M., and Sproat, H. F.: Amer. J. Clin. Path. **26**:266-276, 1956 (schistosomiasis).
114 Frye, W. W.: J.A.M.A. **183**:368-370, 1963 (small intestine).
115 Juniper, K., Jr.: Amer. J. Med. **33**:377-386, 1962 (amebiasis).
116 Kean, B. H., Gilmore, H. R., Jr., and Van Stone, W. W.: Ann. Intern. Med. **44**:831-843, 1956 (amebiasis).
117 Koppisch, E.: J.A.M.A. **121**:936-942, 1943 (schistosomiasis).
118 Prathap, K., and Gilman, R.: Amer. J. Path. **60**:229-245, 1970 (amebiasis).

Anorectal lesions

119 Grinvalsky, H. T., and Bowerman, C. I.: J.A.M.A. **171**:1941-1946, 1959 (stercoraceous ulcers).
120 Grinvalsky, H. T., and Helwig, E. B.: Cancer **9**:480-488, 1956.

121 Parks, A. G.: Brit. Med. J. **1**:463-469, 1961.
122 Wayte, D. M., and Helwig, E. B.: Amer. J. Clin. Path. **48**:159-169, 1967.

Peritoneum, omentum, retroperitoneum, and mesentery

123 Altemeier, W. A., and Holzer, C. E.: Surgery **20**:810-819, 1946 (torsion of omentum).
124 Eiseman, B., Seelig, M. G., and Womack, N. A.: Ann. Surg. **126**:820-832, 1947 (talc).
125 Horsley, J. S.: Arch. Surg. (Chicago) **36**:190-224, 1938 (peritonitis).
126 Means, R. L.: Amer. Surg. **30**:583-588, 1964 (bile peritonitis).
127 Mitchison, M. J.: J. Clin. Path. **23**:681-689, 1970 (idiopathic retroperitoneal fibrosis).
128 Ormond, J. K.: Henry Ford Hosp. Bull. **10**: 13-20, 1962 (idiopathic retroperitoneal fibrosis).
129 Pflaum, C. C.: Amer. J. Clin. Path. **5**:131-150, 1935 (peritonitis).
130 Rogers, C. E., Demetrakopoulos, M. S., and Hyamns, V.: Ann. Surg. **153**:277-282, 1961 (mesenteric lipodystrophy).
131 Schwartz, F. D., Dunea, G., and Kark, R. M.: Amer. Heart J. **72**:843-844, 1966 (methysergide and retroperitoneal fibrosis).
132 Sobel, H. J., Schiffman, R. J., Schwarz, R., and Albert, W. S.: Arch. Path. (Chicago) **91**: 559-568, 1971 (starch granulomas).
133 Tedeschi, C. G., and Botta, G. C.: New Eng. J. Med. **266**:1035-1040, 1962 (retractile mesenteritis).

Functional states
Gastric atrophy (atrophic gastritis)

134 Bernhardt, H., Burkett, L. L., Fields, M. L., and Killian, J.: Ann. Intern. Med. **63**:635-641, 1965.
135 Cox, A. J.: Amer. J. Path. **19**:491-501, 1943.
136 Magnus, H. A.: J. Clin. Path. **11**:289-295, 1958.

Gastric rugal hypertrophy

137 Moldawer, M.: Metabolism **11**:153-156, 1962.
138 Morrison, A. B., Rawson, A. J., and Fitts, W. T., Jr.: Amer. J. Med. **32**:119-127, 1962.
139 Murphy, R. T., Goodsitt, E., Morales, H., and Bilton, J. L.: Amer. J. Surg. **100**:764-778, 1960.

Malabsorption syndrome

140 di Sant'Agnese, P. A., and Jones, W. O.: J.A.M.A. **180**:308-316, 1962.
141 Rubin, C. E., Brandborg, L. L., Phelps, P. C., and Taylor, H. C., Jr.: Gastroenterology **38**: 28-49, 1960.
142 Shiner, M.: J.A.M.A. **188**:45-48, 1964.
143 Shiner, M., and Doniach, I.: Gastroenterology **38**:419-440, 1960.

Protein-losing enteropathy (exudative enteropathy)

144 Davidson, J. D., Waldmann, T. A., Goodman, D. S., and Gordon, R. S., Jr.: Lancet **1**:899-902, 1961.
145 Pomerantz, M., and Waldmann, T. A.: Gastroenterology **45**:703-711, 1963.
146 Waldmann, T. A., Steinfeld, J. L., Dutcher,

---

*See also references 39, 41, 42.

†See also reference 80.

T. F., Davidson, J. D., and Gordon, R. S., Jr.: Gastroenterology **41**:197-207, 1961.

Gastrointestinal manifestations of systemic disease
Cystic fibrosis

147 Bernstein, J., Vawter, G., Harris, G. B., Young, V., and Hillman, L. S.: Amer. J. Dis. Child. **99**:804-818, 1960.
148 di Sant'Agnese, P. A., and Lepore, M. J.: Gastroenterology **40**:64-74, 1961.
149 Donnison, A. B., Schwachman, H., and Gross, R. E.: Pediatrics **37**:833-850, 1966.

Progressive systemic sclerosis (scleroderma)

150 Goldgraber, M. B., and Kirsner, J. B.: Arch. Path. (Chicago) **64**:255-265, 1957.
151 Hoskins, L. C., Norris, H. T., Gottlieb, L. S., and Zamcheck, N.: Amer. J. Med. **33**:459-470, 1962.

Whipple's disease (intestinal lipodystrophy)

152 Maizel, H., Ruffin, J. M., and Dobbins, W. O., III: Medicine (Balt.) **49**:175-205, 1970.
153 Ruffin, J. M., Kurtz, S. M., and Roufail, W. M.: J.A.M.A. **195**:476-478, 1966.
154 Sieracki, J. C., and Fine, G.: Arch. Path. (Chicago) **67**:81-93, 1959.
155 Watson, J. H. L., and Haubrich, W. S.: Lab. Invest. **21**:347-357, 1969.

Neoplasms
Adenomatous polyps, papillary adenoma, and miscellaneous polyps

156 Dukes, C. E.: Proc. Roy. Soc. Med. **40**:829-830, 1947 (difference between adenomatous polyp and papillary adenoma).
157 Dukes, C. E.: Canad. Med. Ass. J. **90**:630-635, 1964 (familial polyposis).
158 Helwig, E. B.: Dis. Colon Rectum **2**:5-17, 1959.
159 Horn, R. C., Jr., Payne, W. A., and Fine, G.: Arch. Path. (Chicago) **76**:29-37, 1963 (Peutz-Jeghers syndrome).
160 Klepinger, C. A., and Pontius, E. E.: Amer. J. Clin. Path. **42**:371-380, 1964 (inflammatory polyp).
161 Lane, N., and Lev, R.: Cancer **16**:751-764, 1963.
162 McKusick, V. A.: J.A.M.A. **182**:271-277, 1962 (genetic factors).
163 Roth, S. I., and Helwig, E. B.: Cancer **16**:468-479, 1963 (juvenile).
164 Sunderland, D. A., and Binkley, G. E.: Cancer **1**:184-207, 1948.
165 Wells, C. L., Moran, T. J., and Cooper, W. M.: Amer. J. Clin. Path. **37**:507-514, 1962 (electrolyte imbalance).
166 Wheat, M. W., Jr., Ackerman, L. V.: Ann. Surg. **147**:476-487, 1958.

Relationship of adenomatous polyps and papillary adenomas to carcinoma of colon

167 Enterline, H. T., Evans, G. W., Mercudo-Lugo, R., Miller, L., and Fitts, W. T., Jr.: J.A.M.A. **179**:322-330, 1962.
168 Horn, R. C., Jr.: Cancer **28**:146-152, 1971 (malignant potential of polypoid lesions).

169 Spratt, J. S., Jr., Ackerman, L. V., and Moyer, C. A.: Ann. Surg. **148**:682-698, 1958.

Gastric polyps

170 Eklof, O.: Acta Radiol. (Stockholm) **57**:177-198, 1962 (also duodenum).
171 Ming, S. C., and Goldman, H.: Cancer **18**:721-726, 1965.
172 Monaco, A. P., Roth, S. I., Castleman, B., and Welch, C. E.: Cancer **15**:456-467, 1962.
173 Tomasulo, J:. Cancer **27**:1346-1355, 1971.

Carcinoma of colon and rectum

174 Cooper, W. L.: Kentucky Med. J. **46**:423-427, 1948.
175 Dukes, C. E.: J. Path. Bact. **35**:323-332, 1932.
176 Dukes, C. E.: J. Path. Bact. **50**:527-539, 1940.
177 Gilchrist, R. K.: Dis. Colon Rectum **2**:69-76, 1959.
178 Grinnell, R. S.: Cancer **3**:641-652, 1950.
179 Laufman, H., and Saphir, O.: Arch. Surg. (Chicago) **62**:79-91, 1951.
180 Moore, G. E., and Sako, K.: Dis. Colon Rectum **2**:92-97, 1959.
181 Southwick, H. W., Harridge, W. H., and Cole, W. H.: Amer. J. Surg. **103**:86-89, 1962.

Carcinoma of stomach

182 Borrman, R.: In Henke, F., and Lubarsch, O., editors: Handbuch der speziellen pathologischen Anatomie und Histologie, Berlin, 1926, Julius Springer.
183 Boswell, J. T., and Helwig, E. B.: Cancer **18**:181-192, 1965 (squamous cell carcinoma and adenoacanthoma).
184 Dungal, N., and Sigurjonsson, J.: Brit. J. Cancer **21**:270-276, 1967.
185 Friesen, G., Dockerty, M. B., and ReMine, W. H.: Surgery **51**:300-312, 1962.
186 Golden, R., and Stout, A. P.: Amer. J. Roentgen. **59**:157-167, 1948.
187 Horn, R. C., Jr.: Gastroenterology **29**:515-525, 1955.
188 Monafo, W. W., Jr., Krause, G. L., Jr., and Medina, J. G.: Arch. Surg. (Chicago) **85**:754-763, 1962.
189 Saphir, O., and Parker, M. L.: Surg. Gynec. Obstet. **76**:206-213, 1943.
190 Stout, A. P.: Arch. Surg. (Chicago) **46**:807-822, 1943.

Carcinoma of esophagus

191 Block, G. E., and Lancaster, J. R.: Arch. Surg. (Chicago) **88**:852-859, 1964 (cardioesophageal adenocarcinoma).
192 Burgess, H. M., Baggenstoss, A. H., Moersch, H. J., and Clagett, O. T.: Surg. Clin. N. Amer. **31**:965-976, 1951.
193 Kay, S.: Surg. Gynec. Obstet. **117**:167-171, 1963.

Carcinoma of small intestine

194 Benson, R. E.: Ann. Surg. **157**:204-211, 1963.
195 Darling, R. C., and Welch, C. E.: New Eng. J. Med. **260**:397-408, 1959 (tumors of small intestine).
196 Wiancko, K. B., and MacKenzie, W. C.: Canad. Med. Ass. J. **88**:1225-1230, 1963.

Carcinoma of appendix

197 Sieracki, J. C., and Tesluk, H.: Cancer **9**:997-1011, 1956.

Carcinoma of anal region*

198 Helwig, E. B., and Graham, J. H.: Cancer **16**:387-403, 1963.
199 Kline, R. J., Spencer, R. J., and Harrison, E. G., Jr.: Arch. Surg. (Chicago) **89**:989-994, 1964.
200 Lone, F., Berg, J. W., and Stearns, M. W., Jr.: Cancer **13**:907-913, 1960.
201 Zimberg, Y. H., and Kay, S.: Ann. Surg. **145**:344-354, 1957.

Malignant melanoma

202 Quan, S. H. Q., White, J. E., and Deddish, M. R.: Dis. Colon Rectum **2**:275-283, 1959.

Carcinoid tumor

203 Bates, H. R., Jr., and Clark, R. F.: Amer. J. Clin. Path. **39**:46-53, 1963.
204 Black, W. C., III: Lab. Invest. **19**:473-486, 1968.
205 Hernandez, F. J., and Reid, J. D.: Arch. Path. (Chicago) **88**:489-496, 1969.
206 Horn, R. C., Jr.: Cancer **2**:819-837, 1949.
207 Moertel, C. G., Sauer, W. G., Dockerty, M. B., and Baggenstoss, A. H.: Cancer **14**:901-912, 1961.
208 Williams, E. D., and Sandler, M.: Lancet **1**:238-239, 1963.

Neoplasms of smooth muscle

209 Berg, J., and McNeer, G.: Cancer **13**:25-33, 1960.
210 Bogedain, W., Carpathios, J., and Najib, A.: Dis. Chest **44**:391-399, 1963.
211 Camishion, R. C., Gibbon, J. H., Jr., and Templeton, J. Y., III: Ann. Surg. **153**:951-956, 1961.
212 Skandalakis, J. E., Gray, S. W., and Shepard, D.: Int. Abst. Surg. **110**:209-226, 1960.
213 Starr, G. F., and Dockerty, M. B.: Cancer **8**:101-111, 1955.
214 Wald, M.: Aust. New Zeal. J. Surg. **33**:147-154, 1963.

Lymphoma

215 Azzopardi, J. G., and Menzies, T.: Brit. J. Surg. **47**:358-366, 1960.
216 Cornes, J. S.: Cancer **14**:249-257, 1961.
217 Cornes, J. S., Wallace, M. H., and Morson, B. C.: J. Path. Bact. **82**:371-382, 1961 (benign lymphoma of rectum).
218 Dawson, I. M. P., Cornes, J. S., and Morson, B. C.: Brit. J. Surg. **49**:80-89, 1961.
219 Jacobs, D. S.: Amer. J. Clin. Path. **40**:379-394, 1963 (malignant lymphoma and pseudolymphoma).
220 Joseph, J. I., and Lattes, R.: Amer. J. Clin. Path. **45**:653-669, 1966.
221 Welborn, J. K., Rebuck, J. W., and Ponka, J. L.: Arch. Surg. (Chicago) **94**:717-723, 1967.

Miscellaneous rare tumors

222 Ackerman, L. V.: In Atlas of tumor pathology, Sect. VI, Fascs. 23 and 24, Washington, D. C., 1954, Armed Forces Institute of Pathology, (tumors of the retroperitoneum, mesentery, and peritoneum).
223 Grodinsky, M., and Rubnitz, A. S.: Surg. Gynec. Obstet. **73**:345-354, 1941 (mucocele and pseudomyxoma).
224 Hughes, J.: Ann. Surg. **165**:73-76, 1967 (mucocele and pseudomyxoma).
225 Hyun, B. H., Palumbo, V. N., and Null, R. H.: J.A.M.A. **208**:1903-1905, 1969 (hemangioma).
226 Kay, S., Callahan, W. P., Jr., Murray, M. R., Randall, H. T., and Stout, A. P.: Cancer **4**:726-736, 1951 (glomus tumor).
227 Lane, N.: Cancer **10**:19-41, 1957 (carcinosarcoma).
228 Perea, V. D., and Gregory, L. J., Jr.: J.A.M.A. **182**:259-263, 1962 (neurofibromatosis).
229 Sahai, D. B., Palmer, J. D., and Hampson, L. G.: Canad. J. Surg. **11**:23-26, 1968 (lipoma).
230 Stout, A. P.: Cancer **3**:820-825, 1950 (mesothelioma).
231 Stout, A. P.: J. Tenn. Med. Ass. **44**:409-411, 1951 (mesothelioma).
232 Stout, A. P., Hendry, J., and Purdie, F. J.: Cancer **16**:231-243, 1963 (omentum).
233 Talbert, J. L., and Cantrell, J. R.: J. Thorac. Cardiovasc. Surg. **45**:1-12, 1963 (carcinosarcoma).
234 Wesser, D. R., and Edelman, S.: Ann. Surg. **153**:272-276, 1961 (mucocele).
235 Winslow, D. J., and Taylor, H. B.: Cancer **13**:127-136, 1960 (mesothelioma).
236 Wychulis, A. R., Jackman, R. J., and Mayo, C. W.: Surg. Gynec. Obstet. **118**:337-340, 1964 (lipoma).
237 Yannopoulos, K., and Stout, A. P.: Cancer **16**:914-927, 1963 (mesentery).

*See also reference 120.

Chapter 28

Liver

**Hugh A. Edmondson and
Robert L. Peters**

Liver disease has steadily gained recognition as a major health problem principally because of the worldwide distribution of epidemic hepatitis and the ubiquity of cirrhosis of the liver. The symptoms of liver disease, such as jaundice, fever, abdominal enlargement, and encephalopathy, are striking phenomena that bring the patient to the physician. The interpretation of the increasing number of laboratory and radiologic tests plus needle biopsy of the liver now makes it imperative that the physician have a sound knowledge of the pathology of this most interesting organ and its multitudinous functions.

STRUCTURE AND CIRCULATION
Structure and embryology

The liver arises from the primitive duodenum in the fourteen-somite embryo as an epithelial-lined outpouching. This grows into the coelomic mesoderm and septum transversum, where the entodermal cells proliferate rapidly, while at the same time rapid growth of the mesoderm produces angioblasts and sinusoids. In the third month, the liver begins to store glycogen and iron, and at the same time it becomes the chief blood-forming organ of the embryo. The site of hematopoiesis is the extravascular component of the lobule.[15, 16] This function is gradually transferred to the bone marrow as the latter develops, so that by time of birth, only an occasional focus of hematopoiesis remains. In premature infants, areas of hematopoiesis are abundant. At birth, the liver weighs about 300 gm and projects well below the costal margin. The left lobe is relatively large in the newborn infant. During fetal life, this lobe receives well-oxygenated blood from the umbilical vein. The latter structure atrophies and becomes the round ligament. The omphalomesenteric veins drain into the larger right lobe

of the liver, and from these develops the portal vein.

The liver grows at a relatively slower rate than the rest of the body, so that in an adult it weighs approximately 1,350 gm. At maturity, the liver is located most commonly at or above the costal margin. However, it is not unusual for the lower edge to be 1 cm to 3 cm below the costal margin.[11] The right lobe has become much larger than the left, and the organ is held firmly in the right hypochondrium and epigastrium by the falciform and triangular ligaments. Anatomically, the dividing line between the right and left lobe is 1 cm to 1.5 cm to the right of the falciform ligament, approximating the gallbladder-caval line.

A firm, smooth layer of connective tissue (Glisson's capsule) encloses the liver and is continuous with the connective tissue of the porta hepatis, the latter forming a sheath around the portal vein, hepatic artery, and bile ducts that enter the hilum of the liver. This connective tissue surrounds all subdivisions of the blood vessels and ducts to the finest radicles, where it joins the inner aspect of Glisson's capsule. The portal vein, hepatic artery, and common hepatic duct divide in the porta hepatis into right and left branches that supply the two lobes of the liver. In their subsequent ramification through the liver, the branches of the artery, vein, and hepatic duct are always together in the portal canals. Injection and corrosion methods have shown that, among the structures of the portal triad, the portal vein is the largest. The hepatic artery, being much smaller, tends to twine about it like a vine over the trunk of a tree.[5] The size of the branches of the hepatic duct is about the same as that of the hepatic artery. The latter is subject to many gross anatomic variations.[9]

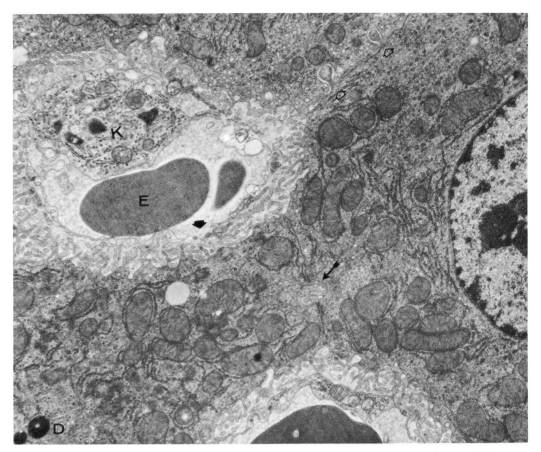

Fig. 28-1 Interlocking of liver cells is furnished by studlike projections of intercellular membrane (open arrowheads). Erythrocyte, **E,** in sinusoid. Kupffer cell, **K.** Dense body, **D.** Bile canaliculus indicated by arrow.

The hepatic parenchyma, as may be seen with the naked eye, or more clearly with the microscope, is composed of innumerable small lobules, each with a diameter of 0.5 mm to 2 mm and the shape of an irregular and somewhat pyramidal hexahedron. At the center of each lobule is the intralobular or central efferent vein, while around the periphery are four or five portal spaces arranged at regular intervals. This is the classic lobule of the liver.[6] Rappaport et al.[12] have described the functioning lobule or liver acinus that has at its center a portal triad and around its periphery portions of several classic lobules. The liver acinus probably represents the true functioning unit of the liver, but because it is difficult to recognize, grossly and microscopically, pathologists in their gross and microscopic descriptions use the term *lobule* in its classic sense.

The lobules are composed of hepatocytes so arranged between sinusoids that at least two cells at their poles opposite the sinusoids may form bile canaliculi.[6] Depending on the angle at which the cells are sectioned for histologic preparations, one may see cell groups of variable thickness. It is important from the functional standpoint that a hepatocyte-sinusoidal system does exist, so that every hepatic cell abuts upon a sinusoid through which blood passes from the portal vessels to the central veins and that the cell has access to the bile canalicular system. These canaliculi are formed by liver cell membranes that form the lining of the canaliculi and are seen to be arranged as microvilli when viewed with the electron microscope.[13] The canaliculi form an interlacing network that impinges upon at least one side of every hepatic cell. These lead into larger channels that finally join the bile ductules at the margin of the lobule. At the junction, biliary duct epithelium and liver cells join in an uneven manner over a short distance.[13] Just before the passage is surrounded by a rosette of biliary epithelium, it has been termed *duct of Hering* or *bile preductule*.[13] The sinusoids form a radial network that allows the blood to come into contact with every parenchymal cell as it flows to the central veins. The lining cells of the sinusoidal system are best known as Kupffer cells. They apparently are held in place by interdigitations of their microvilli with the microvilli of the parenchymal cells. The Kupffer cells form an incomplete lining of the sinusoidal system, so that blood plasma may circulate freely in the space between the Kupffer cells and the parenchyma (Fig. 28-1). This space is known as Disse's space. It is not large enough to accommodate erythrocytes or leukocytes but averages around $1/3 \mu$ or 3,000 Å to 4,000 Å in width. The cytoplasm of the Kupffer cells usually contains many lysosomes and vacuoles. The rough endoplasmic reticulum and mitochondria are abundant.[10] Isolated Kupffer cells are similar in many respects to circulating monocytes. Actually, it has been proposed that Kupffer cells are derived from monocytes. Kupffer cells are actively phagocytic, taking up many kinds of particulate matter.

The liver cells have a polyhedral shape, a round nucleus, and a fairly prominent nucleolus. The fine structure of liver cells has been extensively investigated in recent years.[7] The surface of the liver cell is in contact with (1) its neighbors, from whom it is separated by narrow intercellular spaces, (2) Disse's space, and (3) the bile canaliculus (Fig. 28-1). Along the intercellular space, the outer leaflet of the plasma membranes of adjacent liver cells often fuse to form tight junctions. Near the canaliculus, desmosomes are often found, and it is probable that very little, if any, fluid can flow through this area under normal conditions. The bile canaliculi are lined by rather short microvilli of adjoining liver cells. A large portion of the surface of the parenchymal cell is exposed to Disse's space. This approximates about 40% in the mouse.[7] Triangular extensions of Disse's space may extend fairly deep into the space between the cells, thus increasing the surface of the liver cell that is exposed to the blood plasma. Electron microscopic studies disclose further that the liver cell has abundant mitochondria as well as rough and smooth endoplasmic reticulum. The latter usually is located near the nucleus. A Golgi apparatus is present between the nucleus and the bile canaliculus. Normally, glycogen is abundant throughout the cytoplasm. Lysosomes are numerous and, in the functioning liver, vesicles and vacuoles of variable size are present near Disse's space. Vesicular invaginations of the plasma membrane are noted to occur between the bases of the microvilli that project into Disse's space. Bile canaliculi form a polygonal network throughout the lobule, so that a small portion of every liver cell contributes to the canalicular system.[4] The central veins course through the centers of the lobules in a longitudinal fashion and empty into sublobular veins. The sublobular veins have specialized connective tissue walls and are distinguished from branches of the portal vein by the fact that they are not associated with arteries and bile ducts. The sublobular veins unite to form the hepatic veins. The latter combine to form two large trunks and several smaller ones that open into the inferior vena cava where it passes through a groove on the posterior surface of the liver. Large trunks of the hepatic vein form a simple branching system that is not nearly so angulated and tortuous as are the large branches of the portal vein.

Circulation

The liver receives into its sinusoidal system about 1,500 ml of blood per minute. It is estimated that about 600 ml comes from the hepatic artery and 900 ml from the portal vein. Some 50% to 60% of the oxygen is supplied by the portal vein.[14] The latter system differs from the systemic venous system in that the blood is under a pressure of 8 mm to 10 mm Hg and has a relatively high oxygen content, usually about 80% saturated. The mixture of blood from a high-pressure arterial system (90 mm Hg) and a low-pressure venous system (8 mm to 10 mm Hg) is accomplished by a drop in arterial pressure consequent to the fine subdivisions of the hepatic arterioles before the blood enters the peripheral sinusoids at a pressure of 5 mm Hg.

Some degree of control of blood flow through the liver is no doubt exercised by the tonus of the hepatic arteriolar system and also by the regulation of blood flow into the gastrointestinal tract and spleen. Studies of the microcirculation of the liver in experimental animals has shown that reticuloendothelial cells in the peripheral sinusoids and also at the outlet bordering the central veins act as sphincters to control the flow of blood through the lobules.[8] The sphincters at the periphery may allow arterial blood, portal blood, or a mixture of the two to flow through the sinusoids. Small twigs from the hepatic artery flow directly into the peripheral sinusoids.

FUNCTION AND LABORATORY DIAGNOSIS

Most chemical constituents and even some of the formed elements of the blood are maintained at physiologic levels by some specific activity of the liver. In order to accomplish these physiologic objectives, the liver cells contain hundreds of enzymes whose function has to do with the following:

1 The intermediary metabolism of protein, lipids, and carbohydrates
2 The storage of certain foodstuffs and minerals
3 The production of bile that is secreted externally[18]
4 The purification or cleansing of the blood of useless and toxic substances

The mechanisms concerned with these functions have been and still are being elucidated by research techniques that include the study of the fine structure of the hepatocytes and of the various cell fractions for enzyme function. In liver disease, one or more vital functions may be disturbed. When possible, this malfunction is measured by some chemical analytical procedure performed on the blood. A single abnormal biochemical finding rarely is the basis for diagnosis. Other hepatic tests, as well as the radiologic findings, and even biopsy of the liver, may have to be considered. A needle biopsy, studied by means of light microscopy and, on occasion, by electron microscopy, may help establish a morphologic basis for malfunction. It is important in the evaluation of each laboratory test that the physician have an understanding of the normal physiologic mechanisms involved as well as the various diseases that cause the abnormal findings. The laboratory evaluation of an organ system with such diverse functions as the liver requires considerable experience and skill.

Among the laboratory tests used in the evaluation of liver disease are those:

1 That measure the capacity of the liver to remove and secrete certain substances, such as sulfobromophthalein and bilirubin, from the bloodstream. These substances pass through the liver cell plasma membrane and then are conjugated and excreted into the bile.
2 That measure the capacity to synthesize certain proteins, such as albumin, prothrombin, and fibrinogen, that are then secreted into the blood. The production of protein is a function of the rough endoplasmic reticulum.
3 That quantitate the serum level of certain soluble enzymes that are normally present in high concentration in the cytoplasm of the liver cell but enter the blood when the cells are injured by any one of many injurious agents.
4 That measure a nonspecific reticuloendothelial response of chronic inflammation by the serum globulin level.
5 That measure abnormal substances, proteins or otherwise, elaborated by the liver cell.

Hepatic tests

The most commonly used tests are determinations of serum bilirubin, sulfobromophthalein (BSP) retention after injection, serum albumin and globulin, prothrombin time, serum alkaline phosphatase, serum glutamic–oxaloacetic transaminase (SGOT), and serum glutamic pyruvic transaminase (SGPT).

Serum bilirubin and BSP. One of the most common findings in liver disease is the accumulation of bilirubin in serum and tissue fluids. Approximately 300 mg per day of bilirubin are formed in the reticuloendothelial system from the catabolism of heme, 80% to 90% of which is a component of hemoglobin released from senescent erythrocytes. The remainder arises from certain hepatic enzymes such as cytochromes and catalases or from precursors of hemoglobin in the marrow.[18, 32, 33] This early labeled bilirubin is derived from two sources, one related to erythropoiesis and the other is nonerythropoietic. The latter is apparently synthesized mostly in the liver, from "free" heme and heme proteins.[38] The erythrocyte component probably comes from the bone marrow, but its source is yet to be determined.[43] Arriving in Disse's space as an albumin-linked, lipid-soluble nonpolar substance, bilirubin is freed of albumin and enters the liver cell, where it is accepted by two specific binding proteins, Y and Z.[37] These same proteins also bind BSP. In the endoplasmic reticulum, the bilirubin is converted to an excretable, water-soluble form by conjugation to 2 molecules of glucuronide per bilirubin molecule. In this process, glucuronide is transferred from uridine pyrophosphate glucuronate by means of the enzyme glucuronyl transferase. Conjugated bilirubin leaves the liver cell by what must be an active transport mechanism to enter the canaliculus. From the canaliculi, it passes into the small bile ducts and finally enters the gut by way of the biliary duct system. Bilirubin levels will rise in the serum and tissues, producing jaundice:

1 If a markedly increased load of bilirubin must be removed from the blood for conjugation and excretion

2 If abnormal liver cell function either prevents removal of "unconjugated" bilirubin from serum or inhibits the conjugation of the bilirubin with glucuronide in the liver cell, or both

3 If the excretion of bile via the duct system is impeded

The adult liver has sufficient reserve to handle much more than the normal quantity of bilirubin formed by the breakdown of erythrocytes, but the liver of the newborn infant or of the patient with parenchymal cell disease is often unable to cope with an increased pigment load that results from hemolysis. Hyperbilirubinemia is a common early sign of liver disease, but its detection and fractionation is usually of little help in the differential diagnosis. The "direct-reacting" bilirubin, which is a rough quantitation of the polarized water-soluble or conjugated bilirubin, will rise in about equal proportions to the indirect-reacting bilirubin in most jaundice disorders except those that are associated with an increase in pigment load (hemolysis) or in the hereditary hyperbilirubinemias (specific enzymic deficiency disorders). Unconjugated bilirubin, due to its lipid solubility, may pass in small amounts through the intestinal mucosa into the gut.[36, 46, 47] Conjugated bilirubin is water soluble and is excreted by the kidney. It is probable that serum levels become elevated because conjugated bilirubin becomes loosely associated with albumin. In biliary tract obstruction, bilirubin levels generally do not rise above 25 mg/100 ml because of the excretion of bilirubin through the kidney. However, in the presence of kidney disease, the hyperbilirubinemia may exceed this level.

Among the dyes excreted by the liver, the one most commonly used for diagnostic purposes is sulfobromophthalein (BSP). It quickly binds to plasma proteins after intravenous injection. From 70% to 80% is removed by the liver and the remainder by muscle, kidney, and other organs.[35] BSP is conjugated by the liver cell to glucuronide and excreted by way of the biliary passages in a fashion similar to that in which bilirubin is secreted. The disappearance rate is measured as an indication of the removal and excretory ability of the liver cell. The laboratory determination of the dye level is much more precise than the methods of establishing the amount to be given. Although the test is sensitive to minimal liver disease of almost any type, interpretative errors may occur. First, the amount of intravenously injected dye is calculated on the basis of patient weight, in order to give a certain initial plasma concentration of dye, but variations in plasma volume for any given body weight can cause erroneous amounts of dye to be injected. Second, the removal depends upon hepatic blood flow that is altered in some conditions that are unrelated to liver disease, such as heart failure and shock. It is probable that much of the BSP retention observed in cirrhotic patients is the result of inadequate exposure of liver cells to sinusoidal blood. Furthermore, some blood may not enter the sinusoids because of intrahepatic shunts. Obviously, either liver cell damage or biliary tract obstruction will produce BSP retention in serum. In biliary obstruction, much of the serum BSP is conjugated to BSP-glucuronide.[25] The BSP test is valuable in the diagnosis of mass lesions as well as of infiltrative diseases but is of little value in most jaundice disorders, since dye will obviously be retained. An exception is seen in some of the familial indirect hyperbilirubinemias.

Serum proteins. The major fractions of serum proteins, the albumin and the globulins, usually are measured simultaneously. The albumin level is a measure of liver cell function, but globulins are derived from many sources. Hypoalbuminemia is most often caused by one of the following:

1 Building blocks are inadequate. Hypoalbuminemia may be seen in starvation or in conditions in which the amino acid components are used preferentially in production of other proteins.

2 The liver cell in advanced chronic disease or in severe acute damage is incapable of sustaining normal levels of albumin. The serum albumin level often is closely monitored in order to judge the course of disease.

3 Excessive loss of albumin from the gastrointestinal system or the kidneys produces a low serum level.

The albumin is synthesized by the ribosomes of the rough endoplasmic reticulum but, after detachment of the ribosomes, the albumin remains attached to the smooth membrane.[39] The albumin is apparently then transported to the plasma membrane for release into the bloodstream.

The serum globulin level may become elevated in the course of any chronic inflammatory disease. Usually, it is the gamma fraction that increases. In the United States, where the incidence of parasitic and mycotic disease is small, chronic liver disease is one of the more common causes of prolonged hyperglobulinemia. Several studies indicate that a selective increase of specific immunoglobulin occurs in certain liver diseases,[20, 34, 48] but such specificity is denied in other studies.[29, 42]

The numerous flocculation and turbidity tests used in the past were based on a poorly understood insolubility of gamma globulin in certain reagents when the quantity of albumin was reduced or its quality was altered. There seems to be little use for such tests in a modern laboratory.

Prothrombin. Of the known coagulation factors, prothrombin (factor II), labile factor (factor VII), fibrinogen (factor I), and PTC (factor IX), as well as PTA (factor XI) and Stuart factor (factor X), are produced by rough endoplasmic reticulum in hepatocytes.[27] All of these components may be partially depleted in advanced chronic or severe acute liver disease, and their quantitation may be used in prognosis. The coagulation test used most commonly in assessment of liver disease is the prothrombin time. Because of its shorter half-life,[21] however, factor VII is theoretically superior, for the serum level reflects the parenchymal cell status more closely.

It has been shown that prothrombin synthesis by hepatocytes is cyclic. Usually only 10% to 30% of the cells are active at any one moment. The rate depends upon the level of prothrombin in the blood,[19] and the synthesis of prothrombin factors V and VII is dependent upon the availability of vitamin K. This vitamin is stored in the liver. The warfarin (Coumadin) anticoagulants all act by blocking vitamin K utilization. It is uncommon for dietary deficiency of vitamin K to occur, but impaired absorption of lipids from the gut will include inadequate assimilation of vitamin K. Those conditions that inhibit the absorption of lipid-soluble vitamin K from the gastrointestinal system include the spruelike diseases, pancreatic insufficiency, impaired bile flow, and chronic use of mineral oil. Sterilization of the gut by antibiotics will reduce available vitamin K made by bacteria.

A normal flow of bile into the intestine allows emulsification of lipids, including vitamin K. This emulsification is necessary for esterification and absorption. Thus, either chronic biliary obstructive disease or liver cell disease may be associated with a low prothrombin time. If vitamin K is administered parenterally, the reduction of prothrombin activity associated with chronic obstructive biliary tract disease is quickly reversed, whereas that related to parenchymal cell disease is not.

Alkaline phosphatase activity. The phosphomonoesterases with optimal activity in the alkaline pH range are grouped together and called *serum alkaline phosphatase.* Alkaline phosphatases are present in endothelium, surface epithelia of many mucosal surfaces, neutrophils, placenta, bone, renal tubules, and, to some extent, in liver canaliculi.[26] In spite of its uncertain source and largely undetermined function, serum alkaline phosphatase activity is a valuable and sensitive liver test. For practical purposes, only liver diseases, bone abnormalities, bone growth, and late pregnancy produce elevations in activity. Although the serum alkaline phosphatase activity may rise in the presence of any liver disease, the greatest elevations occur in biliary tract obstruction. This increase, plus BSP retention, may be the only laboratory alterations detected in a patient with a space-occupying mass in the liver.

Although there has been much investigation on the sources, the mechanisms of action, and isoenzymes of alkaline phosphatase, the basic character of the enzyme group is still largely unexplained.

Transaminases. SGOT and SGPT are the two parenchymal cell enzymes that are most frequently quantitated in the evaluation of liver cell necrosis. Hepatocellular damage brings about the release of many cytoplasmic components. Some are unstable, and others that may also originate in extrahepatic tissues are unsuitable for diagnosis. GPT is fairly restricted to liver tissue. It is unbound to ultrastructures and is quite soluble,[44] and it apparently leaks through damaged but viable cell membranes. GOT is present in other tissues but in smaller quantities than in the liver.[41] In hepatocytes, the GOT is found in the soluble fraction (GOT I) and in mitochondria (GOT II) in a ratio of 1:4.[22] The different electrophoretic activities, pH optima, and substrate affinities[23, 24, 31] have prompted some investigators to attempt to separate the

Table 28-1 Laboratory findings in acute and chronic liver disease*

Normal values	Transaminases SGPT, 5-35 units; SGOT, 8-40 units	Bilirubin (1.2 mg. % or less)	Urine urobilinogen (positive in 1:4 dilution)	Alkaline phosphatase (depends on methods†)	Prothrombin— % of normal level (100%)	Response to vitamin K	Serum proteins Albumin, 3.5-4.5 gm; Globulin, 3.0-4.0 gm
Acute liver disease							
1 Necrosis							
A Viral hepatis	Marked elevation (500-4,000) early; SGPT usually > SGOT	Mild to marked elevation (2-40)	Increased early and late but may be absent during phase of deepest jaundice	Normal or mild increase	Moderate to marked decrease (10%-80%)	Poor	Normal except in a prolonged course or in elderly patients
B Mononucleosis	Moderate elevation (100-500)	Normal or mild increase (2-5)	Mild or moderate increase	Normal or mild increase	Normal or mild decrease	Poor	Normal
C Chemical (CCl₄, monamine oxidase inhibitors)	Marked elevation (500-5,000); SGPT usually > SGOT	Mild to marked increase (2-40)	Usually increased but may be decreased during period of deepest jaundice	Normal or mild increase	Moderate to marked decrease (5%-80%)	Poor	Normal
D Acute alcoholic liver disease	SGOT, 75-300; SGPT, 50	Usually moderately elevated	Mild to moderate increase	Slight elevation	Normal to marked decrease	Poor	Albumin acutely decreased; globulin normal in early stage
2 Cholestasis							
A Drug-induced	Mild to moderate elevation (usually < 300); SGOT and SGPT approximately equal	Mild to moderate increase (3-15)	Variable—mild decrease to mild increase	Moderate or marked increase	Normal or mild decrease (50%-100%)	Good	Normal
B Extraheptic obstruction **a** Stone	Mild to moderate increase (100-300); SGOT and SGPT equal	Mild to moderate increase; fluctuations 2-15)	Variable—may be absent but occasionally increased	Moderate to marked increase	Normal or moderate decrease (40%-100%)	Good	Normal

b Cancer	Same as for stone	Moderate elevation without fluctuation (10-20)	Absent	Moderate to marked increase	Variable decrease, mild to marked (20%-80%)	Good	Normal except for possible decrease in albumin due to malnutrition
Chronic liver disease						
1 Biliary cirrhosis A Secondary	Mild to moderate increase (100-300); SGOT often > SGPT	Mild to moderate increase (3-15)	Variable—decreased to increased	Moderate to marked increase	Mild to moderate decrease	Variable, poor to good	Albumin decreased; globulin increased
B Primary	Same as for secondary	Same as for secondary	Same as for secondary	Marked increase	Mild to moderate decrease	Variable, poor to good	Albumin decreased; globulin increased
2 Portal cirrhosis	Same as for biliary cirrhosis	Anicteric to episodes of jaundice (2-40)	Usually increased	Normal or mild increase	Moderate to marked decrease	Poor	Albumin decreased; globulin increased
3 "Lupoid" cirrhosis or chronic active hepatitis	Marked increase during jaundice episodes (500-1,500); SGOT often > SGPT	Mild to moderate increase (2-20)	Usually increased	Variable—normal to marked increase	Moderate to marked decrease	Poor	Albumin decreased; globulin increased (often markedly)
Other lesions						
1 Abscess	Mild increase (< 200)	Normal or slightly elevated	Normal	Normal to moderate increase	Normal		Albumin may be decreased if chronic
2 Cancer, primary or metastatic	Mild increase (< 200)	Normal unless major bile ducts involved	Normal	Usually a moderate to marked increase	Normal		Usually normal, but albumin may be decreased
3 Granulomas	Mild increase (< 200)	Normal	Normal	Same as for cancer	Normal		Normal

*Many tests are necessarily omitted—e.g., the BSP retention test is valuable but it is used only for anicteric patients.

†May be measured in King-Armstrong units, Bodansky units, or Bessey-Lowry units.

types or extent of cell necrosis by differential analysis of transaminase isoenzymes, but the technique awaits thorough clinical trials. The GOT not only is tissue-bound and less soluble than GPT, but also is cleared more rapidly from blood. GOT II is cleared more rapidly than GOT I.[30] Thus, SGPT is a more satisfactory indicator of liver cell damage.

Needle biopsy

A needle biopsy of the liver is now frequently obtained for study by means of both light and electron microscopy. These studies have added immeasurably to the knowledge of liver disease. Morphologic details unobtainable in autopsy material are seen and are useful in the diagnosis, prognosis, and treatment of hepatic disease.[28, 45]

The clinician is careful not to perform a biopsy on a patient with common bile duct obstruction because of the danger of bile leakage. A prothrombin value below 40% of normal also is a contraindication because of the possibility of hemorrhage. Portions of the biopsy often are used for bacterial cultures, for analysis of iron or copper, and for other analyses heretofore impossible. Study with the electron microscope is most valuable in research, but this instrument is not yet used in the routine surgical pathology laboratory.

Angiography and scintiscans

Hepatic angiography and scintiscans have become important aids in the diagnosis of liver disease. Angiograms of a liver that contains a space-occupying lesion discloses its size and location and often is helpful in differentiating neoplasms from other diseases.[17] Scintiscans likewise may show the location and size of similar lesions.[40]

CLASSIFICATION OF LIVER DISEASES

The discussion of liver disease in this chapter will generally follow the clinicopathologic concept shown in Table 28-1. Acute disorders of the liver may be subdivided into those in which there is primarily necrosis and those in which there is predominantly cholestasis. Chronic liver disease includes the many stages of precirrhosis and cirrhosis as well as other disorders. There may be episodes of jaundice or other indications of acute liver disease. The onset of chronic liver disease is often insidious. Sooner or later, however, the clinical and laboratory evidence of cirrhosis becomes manifest in most patients. A heterogeneous group includes those acute and chronic liver diseases in which the principal finding is hepatomegaly. Although the latter may be due to some relatively acute disease like amebic abscess, most often it is of long standing and the patient has few or no symptoms.

NECROSIS

Liver cells may be injured sufficiently to undergo necrosis by any one of many agents of infectious, chemical, metabolic, or nutritional origin, as well as by ischemia. The microscopic recognition of liver cell necrosis is dependent upon irreversible pathobiologic changes of several hours' duration. The point of irreversibility is not distinguishable by present histotechniques. From a diagnostic standpoint, the limited forms that the necrotic liver cell may assume are expanded by differences in distribution and extent of necrosis and by the variable inflammatory responses that occur in diseases of diversified etiology. The different patterns of necrosis that are observed must reflect distinct pathways of molecular pathology, but there is little understanding of the pathogenesis of necrosis at the ultrastructural level.

Necrosis of liver cells is most frequently of a *lytic* type, as though early lysosomal release had caused self-destruction. Experimentally,[59] other changes occur before lysosomal destruction. Lytic necrosis usually involves only parenchymal cells, sparing the stroma. After lysis, the necrotic cell or cells are not visualized—only the area of dropout or hepatocytolysis.

Coagulative necrosis, on the contrary, is a mummified change of cells in which an eosinophilic granular cytoplasm develops, the nucleus disappears, and the shadow of the cell persists. Such cells are only slowly removed. Coagulative necrosis is a characteristic feature of anoxia and suggests that aerobic conditions are necessary for lytic necrosis. *Caseous and gummatous necrosis,* as well as *liquefactive necrosis,* may be observed in the liver.

Acidophilic necrosis is a singular type of unicellular death in which the cell becomes globular and small, and it loses its pyknotic nucleus by extrusion. On ultrastructural examination, the cytoplasm seems to have become dehydrated and the organelles compressed (Fig. 28-2). The acidophilic body is expelled into the sinusoid, where it may be ingested by a Kupffer cell.

Hyaline necrosis is another type of single

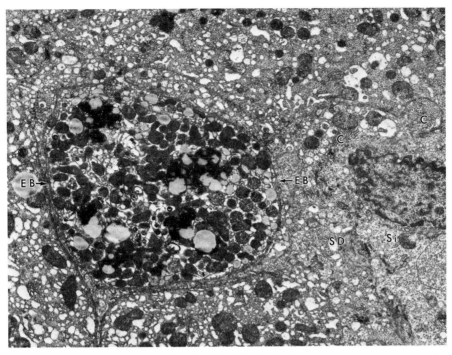

Fig. 28-2 Electron photomicrograph of acidophilic body just prior to extrusion into sinusoid. Note collagen in Disse's space not generally detectable on light microscopy. **EB**, Eosinophilic (acidophilic) body. **SD**, Disse's space. **Si**, Sinusoid. **C**, Collagen.

cell necrosis that seems to follow hydropic degeneration of the liver cell. A deeply eosinophilic coagulum of cytoplasmic components, believed by some to be clumped mitochondria[56] but by other investigators to be a coagulum that incorporates the endoplasmic reticulum,[50] forms in a perinuclear location. This relatively insoluble, poorly digestible coagulum is seen most frequently in alcoholic liver disease and thus is called either the "alcoholic hyaline body" or "Mallory body" after the investigator who originally described it. Hyaline necrosis also is observed in Wilson's disease, in infantile cirrhosis in India, and, rarely, in primary biliary cirrhosis.

Liver cell necrosis, depending upon its distribution, has been divided into *focal, zonal,* and *diffuse* types. Further definition is achieved by grading the severity as focal, submassive, and massive necrosis. There is a lack of uniformity, however, among pathologists as to the use of these descriptive terms. Nevertheless, *the distribution* of cell necrosis and the particular kind of necrosis are important features in microscopic diagnosis.

Focal necrosis

Focal necrosis has no zonal pattern. Generally, single cells or small clusters of cells undergo lytic necrosis and are immediately replaced by swollen macrophages, Kupffer cells, and lymphocytes. Often, rapidly dividing adjacent liver cells will quickly heal the defect. Focal necrosis usually is related to an infective agent; viral hepatitis is the prototype. Rare foci of unicellular necrosis may be found in the liver of patients who have extrahepatic infections. In tuberculosis, sarcoidosis, and other granulomatous disorders, both hepatocellular focal necrosis and granulomas may occur. Focal necrosis is seen in typhoid fever, tularemia, and certain cases of rapidly progressive Hodgkin's disease. Biliary obstruction also may lead to focal necrosis and "bile lake" formation.

Zonal necrosis

Zonal necrosis is the usual reaction to toxins. Apparently, liver cells in corresponding lobular areas have a similar sensitivity. Depending upon the noxious agent, necrosis may be centrilobular, midzonal, or peripheral (periportal).

Centrilobular necrosis is the commonest type of zonal necrosis. It most often is due to ischemia and may be seen in patients with congestive failure or shock due to any cause. Most necrotizing hepatotoxins have a centrilobular effect. The best known of these because it is used so frequently in experimental pathology is carbon tetrachloride (Fig. 6-42). Compounds such as chloroform and trinitrotoluene have a similar effect. Centrilobular necrosis in the fatty liver of alcoholic patients is discussed on p. 1201.

Midzonal necrosis is characteristic of yellow fever but may be seen in other infective conditions. The midzonal lesions are sharply delineated (Fig. 11-23) and are characterized by a round hyaline cytoplasmic mass (Councilman body) and intranuclear inclusions. The sequence of nuclear and cytoplasmic changes has been studied in yellow fever–injected rhesus monkeys.[49] The Councilman bodies are not specific for yellow fever, for they also are seen in other liver diseases.

Peripheral necrosis has been described in phosphorus poisoning and in eclampsia. Yellow phosphorus in sufficient doses leads to peripheral fatty change and necrosis of liver cells.[51] In addition, centrilobular necrosis has been described after phosphorus poisoning.[55]

Diffuse necrosis

Viral hepatitis is by far the most common cause of the diffuse, submassive, or massive necrosis of the liver that has commonly been called *acute yellow atrophy*. Furthermore, massive or submassive hepatic necrosis may be seen after therapy with monamine oxidase inhibitors,[52] zoxazolamine, iproniazid, ethionamide, diphenylhydantoin,[53] and others.[57]

Although the mechanisms of liver cell damage undoubtedly differ for many agents, certain features of pathogenesis are common. The initial molecular pathophysiologic change is generally unknown but is often specific for the liver cell, since many of the toxic agents enter other cells without ill-effect. Carbon tetrachloride, for example, is thought to be split by microsomal enzymes to produce free radicals.[54] The latter attack methylene bonds of the unsaturated fatty acids of microsome membranes, producing lipoperoxidases that cause severe membrane alterations. The single layer membranes of the rough endoplasmic reticulum are more vulnerable to peroxidase action than are the double layered ones of mitochondria. The lipid solvent action of carbon tetrachloride could have some direct action on membranes, but isolated endoplasmic reticulum membranes show no ultrastructural effect of treatment by carbon tetrachloride and only a little decrease of protein formation.[58]

VIRAL HEPATITIS

Viral hepatitis is a necrotizing inflammatory disease of liver parenchymal cells. Its etiology is presumed, but not yet proved, to be viral. It is the most common acute liver disease of children and young adults and has assumed epidemic proportions in many parts of the world. Most of the population is presumed to have had the disease by the age of 30 years. Classically, an orally acquired variety of viral hepatitis with an incubation period of fifteen to forty-five days has been referred to in the United States as infectious hepatitis (IH) or viral hepatitis type A (infective hepatitis in the United Kingdom, Botkin's disease in Russia, epidemic jaundice and catarrhal jaundice in older literature), whereas a parenterally transmitted disease with an incubation period of fifty to 180 days has been called serum hepatitis (SH) or viral hepatitis type B.

Detailed epidemiologic and inoculation studies indicate that at least two viruses or strains of viruses cause epidemics in pediatric institutions.[107] One strain, called MS-1, was initially obtained from the pooled serum of hepatitis patients and was highly contagious by the oral route. A short incubation type of hepatitis (thirty to thirty-eight days) resulted. The MS-1 agent appeared in the stool, from which extracts were also infective parenterally. It maintained its relatively short incubation period on serial passage. A second agent was demonstrated, known as MS-2, whose infectivity was highest when administered parenterally, but also showed a low infectivity by the oral route. The incubation period for this agent is between forty-one and 108 days. It generally is believed that the MS-1 hepatitis agent is similar to, if not the same as, infectious hepatitis and that the MS-2 agent bears a similar relationship to serum hepatitis.

History

In the United States, hepatitis became known during the Civil War when 10,929 Northern troops developed the disease in the first year of the war.[118, 121] Similar epidemics occurred in subsequent wars.[94, 118]

Serum hepatitis has been recognized in more contemporary times, but an epidemic retrospectively interpreted as serum hepatitis occurred in 1885, when inoculation of 1,289 workmen against smallpox by human lymph resulted in 199 cases of hepatitis.[113] The increasing incidence of arsphenamine jaundice in 1920 led some investigators to suggest that some infective rather than toxic basis might exist.[132] Observations of liver necrosis after insulin therapy in 1931 were ignored.[131] Reports in 1937 and 1938 dealing with hepatitis following yellow fever vaccination[92, 130] and two reports in 1938 of a highly fatal jaundice disorder after injection of human measles convalescent serum were largely overlooked.[115, 121] However, recognition of serum hepatitis was forced on medical science in 1942, when 24,664 United States troops contracted hepatitis after receiving injections from nine of the lots of yellow fever vaccine made with pooled human sera, an incidence of 56.64 cases per 1,000 doses.[125]

Etiology and immunology

None of the viruses that has been isolated or propagated from tissues and fluids of patients with hepatitis has proved to be the etiologic agent of either infectious or serum hepatitis. Although attempts to reproduce the disease or propagate the infective agent in animals generally have been disappointing,[102] recent observations of outbreaks of hepatitis in animal handlers,[103] confirming a 1927 report,[139] have spawned extensive experimental work. Apparently, human material can produce a disease in chimpanzees that is similar to human hepatitis.[66, 129]

In 1965, a major breakthrough occurred when an immunologically distinct serum factor was discovered[70] that was later found to occur in sera of 65% to 95% of patients in early stages of serum hepatitis (hepatitis B).[128] Administration of blood containing the antigen produced some manifestation of viral hepatitis in 75% of recipients.[64, 96] By mid-1969, reports from many parts of the world confirmed the immunologic identity of the agent, which was ultimately named *hepatitis-associated antigen* (HAA) (previously called Australia antigen, hepatitis antigen, and SH antigen). The incidence of antigen positivity is 30% to 65% in the acute stage of adult hepatitis in patients who give no history of contact of any type with potentially infected material. However, 100% of institutionalized children who were inoculated with MS-2 hepatitis agent had HAA in their sera after developing hepatitis, but none of the patients administered MS-1 hepatitis agent developed HAA with their disease.[95] Epidemic outbreaks of viral hepatitis (hepatitis A) have all been HAA negative.[76]

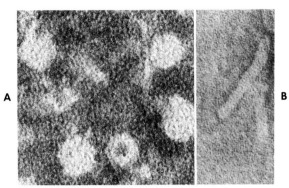

Fig. 28-3 Electron photomicrographic appearance of particles in serum of patient with hepatitis antigen. Particles are 200 Å in diameter. **A,** Note that one particle is hollow. **B,** Some forms are tubular.

Studies with the electron microscope disclose that HAA is a 200 Å globose unit that occasionally has branching and filamentous forms (Fig. 28-3). Concentration and biochemical analysis of this particle have yielded too low a nucleoprotein content to satisfy the requirements for a replicating virus. A somewhat larger 450 Å particle much more sparsely distributed in serum may be the virus.[81, 84, 101, 136] During 1970 and 1971, antigenic subtypes became demonstrable with selectively absorbed antisera.[104, 110] The significance of antigenic subgroups is not yet established.

The antibody and the cellular and immune responses to HAA vary qualitatively and quantitatively from one patient to another. Complexes of antigen and antibody may be detected in sera of certain patients, and a variety of hepatic and extrahepatic disorders have been ascribed to the formation of immune complexes of HAA and its antibody,[63, 98] but evidence is far from conclusive.[120] Immunization against HAA or MS-2 hepatitis agent by a boiled preparation of antigen is being initiated and offers promise of protective effect.[108] An indirect demonstration of hepatitis B on tissue culture has been described.[75]

Only 25% to 30% of instances of post-transfusion hepatitis are derived from HAA-positive donor blood.[64, 97] There have been a report of immunologic identification of a fecal agent[83] and other reports of demonstration of a short incubation agent.[89] These may both represent hepatitis A, but further work is necessary.

Long incubation hepatitis (serum hepatitis, HAA-positive hepatitis, or hepatitis B) can be transmitted by means that are not obviously percutaneous. In addition, short incubation hepatitis (or infectious hepatitis, hepatitis A) can be passed in serum. Since the incubation periods overlap, it has been recommended that the terminology and definitions be based on presence or absence of HAA. Reversion to the terminology *hepatitis A and B* is also recommended*:

Hepatitis A—The serum is HAA negative during all stages of the disease. The agent is highly infectious orally, usually being responsible for epidemics. It is shed in feces and urine but may be transmitted in serum. Most patients with hepatitis A have an incubation period between twenty and fifty days.

Hepatitis B—The serum is HAA positive during some stage of the disease. The agent is most infective parenterally, perhaps only by this route. The majority of cases of adult viral hepatitis in the United States are of this type. Most patients have an incubation period between forty and 180 days, but occasional short incubation cases occur.

We refer to the disease of the patients whose sera were not tested for HAA and who have no epidemiologic background as viral hepatitis, NOS (not otherwise specified).

Clinical features

The agent for hepatitis A apparently is shed in the stool of the infected individual and is transmitted by ingestion of fecally contaminated material.[109] Consequently, the disease is most common where there is poor sanitation or overcrowding. Recently, certain mollusks harvested from polluted sea water have been shown to concentrate the virus, and ingestion of raw or partially cooked mollusks has been associated with epidemics.[90] Although the usual route of entry of the agent for hepatitis A is oral, it can be transmitted parenterally if inoculated. In children, the disease is probably common but passes as a mild flulike illness. Even in adults, it is estimated that only 33% of patients with viral hepatitis are ill enough for the condition to be diagnosed.[123]

During the incubation period of fifteen to forty-five days, the site of proliferation of the infective agent is unknown. Volunteer studies have shown that the serum does contain the infective agent two to three weeks before onset of jaundice.[95, 109] The initial symptoms, known as the prodrome, are nonspecific but include vague gastrointestinal discomfort,

*Abstract in Hepatitis Scientific Memoranda of June, 1971, on the Conference of the National Institute of Arthritis and Infectious Diseases of April 30, 1970.

muscle or joint pains, skin rash, and fatigue. Toward the end of the prodrome, fatigue becomes more marked, nausea, vomiting, and anorexia are frequent and the patient often complains of a distaste for cigarettes. Fever usually is prominent. The liver may be slightly firm and tender, reflecting the liver cell damage, and the spleen and posterior cervical lymph nodes may be palpable. Bile appears in the urine, followed in most instances by jaundice or at least hyperbilirubinemia. The highest bilirubin level usually is reached one to two weeks after the onset of jaundice, at which time the patient usually feels better. Most patients steadily improve and are free of signs and symptoms by six weeks after onset of jaundice. Aplastic anemia may follow recovery from viral hepatitis in rare instances and may be responsible for death.[88, 126] Although there is one report of sixteen cases seen in a two-year period,[126] this particular sequela is rarely seen at the Los Angeles County–University of Southern California Medical Center in spite of more than 800 patient admissions for viral hepatitis per year.

Hepatitis B generally is transmitted by inoculation of human blood products or material contaminated with blood. One study indicates that it may be acquired by the oral route.[107] Hepatitis B has increased at alarming rates in large cities, where the practice of needle sharing by parenteral drug users is common. The sale of blood by this segment of the population to commercial blood banks has resulted in increased infectivity of those who receive blood products. In some cities, the incidence of clinically apparent hepatitis acquired from a blood transfusion is as high as 20 per 1,000 units of blood, although two-thirds of the patients contracting hepatitis have subclinical disease.[64, 99, 134] Pooling of blood products obviously increases the risk of transmitting the agent. For years, it was believed that storage of plasma for six months at room temperature was effective in inactivating the agent,[61] but such treated plasma recently has been shown to transmit hepatitis.[124] Blood fibrinogen carries a particularly high risk of transmitting hepatitis B.[72] Only the heat-treated serum albumin and Cohn-fractionated gamma globulin are free of the agent.[117]

Hepatitis B usually is associated with fewer system symptoms than is hepatitis A. Gastrointestinal symptoms and fever are uncommon, but severe weakness may be a feature.

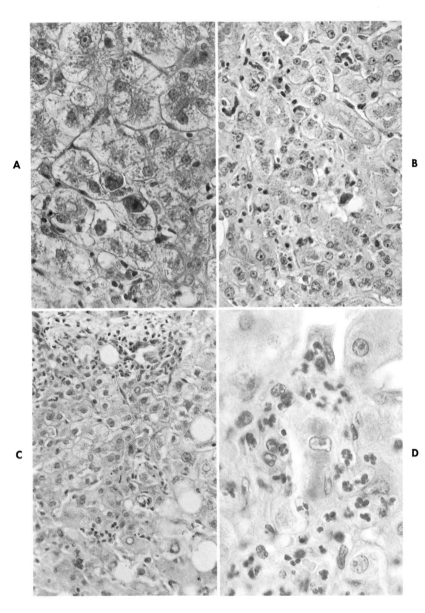

Plate 4
A, Needle biopsy in epidemic hepatitis. Two acidophilic bodies present near bottom. Cytoplasm swollen and granular and cell membranes indistinct.
B, Centrilobular bile stasis in patient taking oral contraceptive.
C, Acute pericholangitis and cholestasis in needle biopsy. Later at surgery, stone removed from common bile duct.
D, Hyaline necrosis in alcoholic. Many neutrophils in sinusoids.

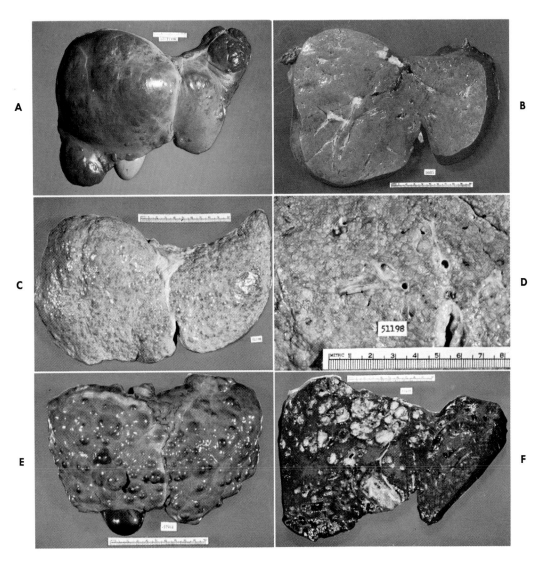

Plate 5

A, Submassive hepatic necrosis from viral hepatitis, with bulging areas of residual liver and much shrinkage and collapse of left lobe. Patient lived twenty-four days after onset of clinical symptoms.

B, Large, deep, yellow fatty liver, etiology unknown.

C, Granular to nodular liver of advanced Laennec's cirrhosis (65-year-old man with history of chronic alcoholism).

D, Nodules of variable size surrounded by dense connective tissue septa. Same liver as that shown in **C.**

E, Small liver with bulging nodules (20-year-old woman with postnecrotic cirrhosis).

F, Suppurative cholangitis with multiple abscesses secondary to carcinomatous obstruction of common duct.

Pathologic changes

Hepatitis A and B produce morphologic lesions indistinguishable from one another. Histologic changes vary, depending upon the temporal stage of the disease, severity of the process, and individualized cellular and reparative response.

Pathologic changes prior to onset of clinical symptoms. In a liver biopsy taken prior to the onset of symptoms, and before there is biochemical evidence of cell necrosis, the liver parenchymal cells have slightly enlarged nuclei and sharp nuclear membranes. The size and number of Kupffer cells, as well as the number of lymphocytes in the sinusoids, are increased. Sparse areas of cell dropout may be seen, but generalized liver cell damage develops just prior to the onset of symptoms and concurrently with serum biochemical abnormalities.

Pathologic changes with onset of symptoms. Three nearly concurrent morphologic changes occur at the height of clinical disease that characterize viral hepatitis: liver cell *damage*, liver cell *regeneration*, and lymphoid and reticuloendothelial *reaction*. The liver cell *damage* is generalized. All parenchymal cells become swollen and hydropic with a watery-appearing cytoplasm, a change that is most severe in the centrilobular regions. The liver cell cytoplasm assumes a ground-glass appearance in many damaged cells. In others, the watery vacuolization at the sinusoidal margin contrasts sharply with the perinuclear condensation of cytoplasm. Even in the early stage, the liver cell cord arrangement becomes disrupted because of the cytoplasmic swelling and early onset of cell regeneration (Fig. 28-4). The nuclei are enlarged with a finely granular or vesicular nucleoplasm and a sharp nuclear membrane. Liver cell dropout is focal throughout the lobule, but it is more striking in the centrilobular regions, where the intercellular membranes between adjacent parenchymal cells often become indistinct. Breakdown of intercellular membrane results in syncytial giant cells. In fairly severe hepatitis, centrilobular cell destruction may be sufficiently extensive to leave only the spongy network of the stroma. The destruction and absorption of dying cells must be rapid, since dead liver cells as such usually are not identifiable on biopsy. An exception is the type of cell death that results in the acidophilic body (see discussion of necrosis, Fig. 28-2, and Plate 4, *A*).

Concurrently with acute cell damage and

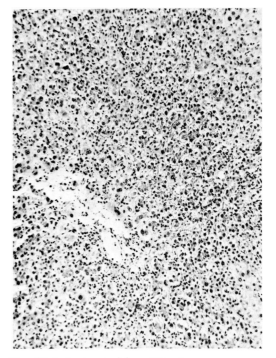

Fig. 28-4 Acute viral hepatitis. Appearance generally seen on needle biopsy. Note swollen liver cells, lack of cord pattern, and focal necrosis.

necrosis, *regeneration* without nodularity occurs, and mitoses often are abundant. Regeneration is manifest by massing of cells, so that the usual sinusoid cell–canaliculus cell–sinusoid order is replaced by more solid pavement of parenchymal cells. Canalicular cholestasis is variable. Some patients have extensive bile stasis in canaliculi without apparent differences of clinical pattern of viral hepatitis.[80] If jaundice is prolonged, the Kupffer cells also contain bile pigment, but usually there is little bile staining of the cytoplasm of the swollen liver parenchymal cells.

The *lymphoid and reticuloendothelial response* is often the most obvious histologic change. Kupffer cell activity is markedly increased, and small unicellular foci of cell dropout usually are replaced by macrophages and Kupffer cells that have ingested lipochrome pigment. These foci are further marked by numerous lymphocytes and a few plasma cells. In the portal areas, proliferative cholangiolar epithelium and poorly formed duct structures are found, and lymphoid tissue traverses the limiting plate.

Late histologic changes. Histologic changes in the liver persist even after the patient is well and the transaminase levels are normal. Pigmented Kupffer cells remain in the scattered foci of previous cell necrosis, and the liver parenchymal cells maintain a pavement configuration with a slow reestablishment of the sinusoidal and cord pattern without the marked hydropic swelling, cytoplasmic condensation, and centrilobular accentuation of cell damage seen earlier. Often, the portal lymphoid hyperplasia remains prominent.

Electron microscopic changes. Electron microscopic changes have been described by many investigators. These changes include intracellular structures resembling viral agents in human hepatitis. Some have described 200 Å particles in intracytoplasmic saccules[67] and others intranuclear inclusions from invaginated nuclear membranes with 200 Å bodies in the inclusions,[140] whereas earlier reports described 400 Å to 600 Å bodies arising from endoplasmic reticulum.[100] Since the characterization of HAA in serum, similar particles have been demonstrated in both liver cell cytoplasm and nuclei, but principally in patients with impaired immunity.[62]

Other ultrastructural changes observed in liver cells and Kupffer cells have been nonspecific.[135] In the early stages, the endoplasmic reticulum becomes irregularly dilated and vesicular and often is separated or destroyed by ballooning of the cytoplasm. The nuclei enlarge and nucleoli are prominent. Free ribosomes increase in the cytoplasm, and glycogen deposition is irregular. The intercellular membranes, instead of being destroyed as one would anticipate from light microscopy, actually develop microvilli, and the space between adjacent cells is widened. Fine strands of collagen often are found in Disse's space and in the intercellular space (Fig. 28-2).

The acidophilic, or Councilmanlike, body is observed most often in viral hepatitis, although it may be seen in many other diseases in man and animals. Councilman described acidophilic bodies in yellow fever.[82] There is some doubt as to whether or not the bodies are the same as those seen in viral hepatitis.[116] The acidophilic body is composed of condensed cytoplasm from which ribosomes have largely disappeared but in which the shadowy, electron-dense remains of many cell organelles are still visible.[69, 77, 106]

In addition to the clinical and hepatic morphologic features of acute viral hepatitis just described, several variants may occur. The current evidence suggests that these are based not on different viral strains nor antigenic subgroups but on host response. The principal host responses in viral hepatitis include im-munologic reaction and parenchymal reparative properties. Obviously, many external environmental factors may affect both.

Fatal viral hepatitis
Fulminant viral hepatitis

Fulminant viral hepatitis is the clinical designation for massive or submassive hepatic necrosis. Fewer than 1% of patients admitted to the hospital with viral hepatitis develop such abrupt and complete liver cell necrosis that hepatic insufficiency ensues. Death in hepatic coma occurs from twenty-four hours to a few days from the onset of such symptoms. The liver morphology depends upon the extent of necrosis, amount of regeneration, and duration of survival of the patient. In *acute massive necrosis* that is most severe and rapidly progressive, the liver weighs from 1,000 gm to 1,200 gm, only slightly less than normal. Its capsule is smooth, but the liver is limp. On sectioning, the centrilobular areas are red and retracted and may closely resemble severe acute passive congestion, a pattern once referred to as *acute red atrophy*.

Histologically, the hepatocytes are destroyed, the Kupffer cells are large and numerous, and there is a variable amount of lymphocytic infiltrate and hyperplasia (Fig. 28-5). The liver stroma is intact, and little collapse is noted. The bile ducts may show some hyperplasia. After a week of survival, the stroma is collapsed, the liver is shrunken to about

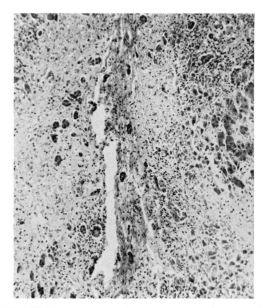

Fig. 28-5 Liver in acute hepatic necrosis from viral hepatitis.

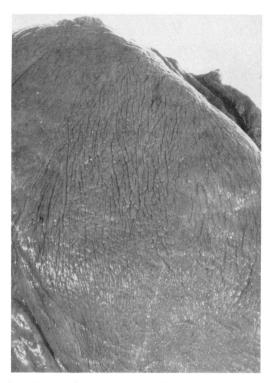

Fig. 28-6 Fulminating serum hepatitis following blood transfusions given 140 days before onset of jaundice. Note typical wrinkling of capsule of liver when flexed.

600 gm to 900 gm, and it is wrinkled and deeply icteric (Fig. 28-6).

A patient with *submassive necrosis* of the liver may die in less than one week or may live for two or three weeks when there is sufficient surviving liver parenchyma. The deeply icteric swollen parenchymal cells impart the golden yellow color that caused Rokitansky to use the term *acute yellow atrophy* to describe the liver of the patients who survived only a few days. By the time the patient has survived two to three weeks, the red collapsed areas contrast sharply with the bulging yellowish residual liver (Plate 5, *A,* and Fig. 28-7). Some pathologists have called this stage *subacute hepatic necrosis* or *subacute yellow atrophy.* However, the necrosis is acute, even though the patient may have a prolonged survival when there is enough residual liver. If the patient lives for several weeks following submassive hepatic necrosis, the blood channels in the collapsed stroma of the liver may sclerose—thus areas of collapse become pale.

At autopsy following death from massive or submassive necrosis, there may be damage in organs other than the liver. Extrahepatic changes include minimal ascites and sometimes pleural effusion and peripheral edema. The regional lymph nodes and spleen are en-

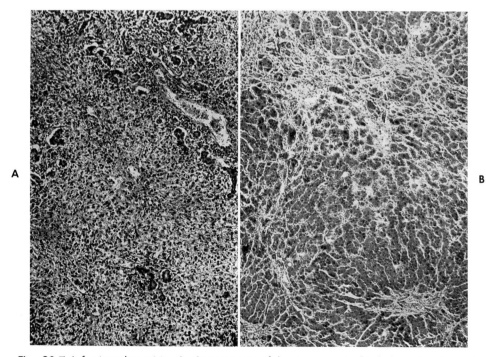

Fig. 28-7 Infectious hepatitis. **A,** Appearance of liver on ninety-third day, showing collapsed areas. **B,** Residual liver. (From Lucké, B.: Amer. J. Path. **20:**595-619, 1944.)

larged. Hemorrhagic phenomena may be seen in various tissues due to disturbances of prothrombin deficiency as a result of hepatic destruction. Gross hemorrhages are often present in the intestine and mesentery. Gastrointestinal bleeding may contribute to death. Acute pancreatitis occasionally is noted at autopsy.

At the Los Angeles County–University of Southern California hospitals from 1919 to 1969, over 90% of the fatal cases of viral hepatitis occurring in patients under 20 years of age were those with massive hepatic necrosis. About one-half of the patients over 30 years of age had massive hepatic necrosis, and one-half had submassive necrosis of the liver. Probably younger patients have sufficient regenerative capacity, so that if they do not expire in the initial fulminant phase, complete recovery is the rule. Some of the older patients may have enough residual liver to allow survival for a short period, but regeneration is apparently inadequate to permit recovery.[74]

Mortality rates. Estimates of the survival rates that follow clinically diagnosed fulmi-

nant viral hepatitis have ranged between 10% and 35%.[86] The more favorable survival figures noted during the past five years probably reflect the striking increase of drug-associated serum hepatitis in younger individuals (Fig. 28-8) with a consequently larger proportion of fulminant hepatitis in the younger group (Fig. 28-9). Most of the survivors of fulminant hepatitis since 1965 have been under 30 years of age. Survival statistics for patients in hepatic coma will differ, depending in part on whether they were taken from areas in the United States where there is a heavy illicit drug traffic or from regions with a minimal drug problem, since the average age of the patients with fulminant hepatic necrosis will differ in the two environments.

At the Los Angeles County–University of Southern California Medical Center, none of the survivors of fulminant hepatitis has developed cirrhosis nor any other hepatic sequela.

Viral hepatitis, protracted course

In contrast to patients with massive or submassive hepatic necrosis who generally have an acute clinical course, some patients have a slower onset and a prolonged course. We call this *protracted viral hepatitis*. The mean age of patients who develop protracted viral hepatitis is greater than that of patients with ordinary viral hepatitis. This form of hepatitis may be ultimately fatal in some older individuals but rarely in those patients under 30 years of age. The onset is similar to that in

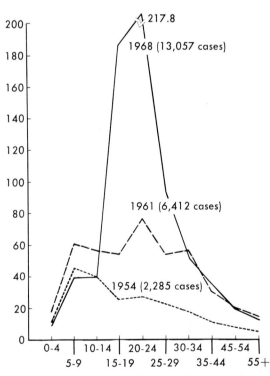

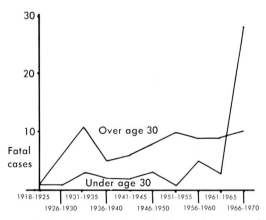

Fig. 28-8 Comparison of reported age incidence of viral hepatitis (rates are per 100,000 population) in California in 1954, 1961, and 1968. (Courtesy Department of Health, State of California.)

Fig. 28-9 Demonstration of abrupt increase of fatal viral hepatitis in patients under 30 years of age, coinciding with increased incidence of disease in younger individuals. (Courtesy Los Angeles County–University of Southern California Hospitals; John Wesley Hospital.)

the usual mild case of viral hepatitis. The etiologic agents are believed to be the same. In fatal cases, the prothrombin activity drops to about 10%, serum albumin levels slowly drop without an increase in globulin levels, and somnolence is followed by coma and death. Younger patients generally recover over a period of several months. In our experience, such patients may or may not have hepatitis-associated antigen (HAA) in their sera, they do not have positive-reacting lupus erythematosus preparations (LE preps), nor do they have smooth muscle antibodies (SMA) in their sera.

Ultimate recovery from hepatitis depends upon the amount of necrosis, the duration of necrosis, and the rapidity of repair. Protracted viral hepatitis is apparently characterized as much or more by impaired regeneration than by continuing necrosis or severity of initial necrosis.

Because of the risk of hemorrhage due to a low prothrombin time, biopsies that have been studied from the liver of patients with protracted viral hepatitis are not usually representative of the later stages or the more severe varieties of the disease. Most often the changes are indistinguishable from those of ordinary acute viral hepatitis. However, it has been demonstrated that the protracted clinical course may be predicted if there is evidence of areas of more confluent or extensive liver cell necrosis to the extent that bridging bands of collapsed stroma infiltrated by lymphocytes connect adjacent portal areas or central regions. When such bridging is apparent, the lesion has been referred to as *subacute hepatic necrosis* (SHN)[73] and has been shown to be associated with a high frequency of progression to chronic liver disease or death. There is difficulty distinguishing the lesion of SHN from that of *chronic active viral hepatitis,* which even more uniformly is associated with a poor prognosis. Indeed, the diseases may have common features or be different stages of the same process. However, protracted viral hepatitis is characterized by impaired regeneration of liver cells, whereas chronic active viral hepatitis features striking hepatocellular regenerative activity. Patients who have recovered from fulminant hepatitis may have bridging between adjacent central areas resembling the SHN lesion, but patients who recover from the acute necrosis associated with fulminant hepatitis have an excellent long-term prognosis and recover rapidly.

The liver of older patients who succumb after a protracted course of viral hepatitis is shrunken and slightly toughened but limp. Since the patient's regenerative capacity is impaired, the surface is bumpy or irregular with few regenerative areas. On microscopic examination, liver cells are shrunken and there is little exudative reaction, but hyperplastic response of the lymphoid and reticuloendothelial system is similar to that in ordinary viral hepatitis. There is considerable collapse within each lobule, and thin fingers of collapsed stroma and collagen extend from both the portal and the central areas. Regenerative areas are poorly developed.

Nonfatal variants
Relapse of viral hepatitis

Most patients have no further symptoms nor complaints following the initial bout of hepatitis, but about 2% have a relapse of viral hepatitis occurring within a three month period. The symptomatology at the time of the relapse often is indistinguishable from the initial episode, although it is usually somewhat milder. Occasionally, the relapse may be more severe but rarely fatal. Histologic changes in the liver are similar to those of the initial bout of hepatitis.

Unresolved viral hepatitis (transaminitis; asymptomatic carrier state; chronic persistent hepatitis)

Between 10% and 12% of patients who contract viral hepatitis maintain smoldering or episodic elevations of SGPT activity indefinitely, even though they are usually asymptomatic after recovery from the initial disease. This condition is called unresolved viral hepatitis. Twenty-five percent of patients with unresolved hepatitis have HAA in their sera.[65]

On liver biopsy, the hepatocytes are hydropic and are of uniform size throughout the lobule. The cord pattern usually is replaced by a cobblestone-like configuration. There are occasional small foci of hepatocytolysis surrounded by rosettes of lymphocytes (Fig. 28-10). The Kupffer cells may be slightly hypoplastic, and there is a variable amount of portal lymphoid hyperplasia. No patient in the ten-year follow-up studies of patients with unresolved hepatitis from the Los Angeles County–University of Southern California Medical Center has developed fibrosis or cirrhosis, but, conversely, none has recovered.

In addition to the 10% to 12% incidence of

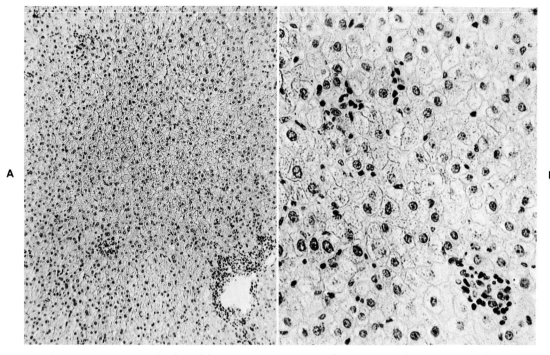

Fig. 28-10 A, Unresolved viral hepatitis in same case shown in Fig. 28-3 two years later. Note cobblestone pattern of liver cells and scattered areas of focal necrosis. **B,** Higher magnification, emphasizing focal necrosis.

unresolved viral hepatitis following the acute disease in otherwise ordinary individuals, patients with immune deficiencies have a much higher frequency of unresolved hepatitis following contact with the hepatitis agent. Often, the initial acute disease has minimal symptoms. Thus, patients with lymphomas,[71] those on chronic renal dialysis programs,[112] mongoloids,[133] lepromatous leprosy patients,[71] and individuals receiving immunosuppressant therapy develop unresolved hepatitis readily. In addition, asymptomatic HAA positivity develops at about 2 months of age in children of mothers who have HAA-positive viral hepatitis at the time of delivery. Such infants continue to have HAA-positive sera thereafter.[127]

Unresolved viral hepatitis patients probably represent the endemic pool for the disease. Persons in close contact with patients who have unresolved hepatitis, particularly spouses of such patients, are at high risk to developing acute viral hepatitis, although the transmission mode from those who are HAA positive is unknown.

The incidence of unresolved hepatitis in the general population differs in various parts of the world from less than 0.1%[105] in some parts of the United States to 15% in Tai-

wan.[137] In the larger cities of the United States, such as Los Angeles, where intravenous drug usage is a problem, the incidence of unresolved viral hepatits in the "normal" population is about 0.4%.

A low-grade type of "hepatitis" has been studied in Korea[78] and Taiwan[80] that has clinical and histologic findings similar to those described in the United States. Some of the cases studied in the Orient have been described as progressing to cirrhosis, but the follow-up data is incomplete.

Prior to the establishment of the relationship between HAA and hepatitis B, the term *chronic persistent hepatitis* was applied to a a histologic pattern in which there was portal lymphoid "infiltration" and little other hepatic histologic alteration.[87] Many of the patients had slight elevation of SGPT activity to about 100 units. Those who coined the term did not suggest nor deny that chronic persistent hepatitis was related to viral hepatitis but were attempting to delineate the lesion from *chronic active hepatitis,* then generally considered to be an autoimmune disorder. But ultimately many investigators adopted the term of that designation for the asymptomatic carrier state of viral hepatitis just described as *unresolved viral hepatitis.* The histologic pattern that has been described in chronic persistent hepatitis is, in fact, a nonspecific lymphoid and Kupffer cell hyperplasia that may develop in any of several conditions that stimulate the reticuloendothelial system, including the late stage of viral hepatitis as well as many remote infections. The confusion is increased by the fact that most intravenous drug users, by virtue of repeated injections of infectious and pyrogenic materials, have striking lymphoid and reticuloendothelial proliferation. In addition, many have HAA-positive unresolved viral hepatitis or are recovering from a bout of hepatitis. One of the characteristic features of unresolved hepatitis that is not a part of the nonspecific pattern of the liver in chronic persistent hepatitis[68] is the continuing low-grade hepatocyte regeneration that prevents the establishment of a regular sinusoidal cord pattern and imparts a cobblestone appearance to liver sections. Another feature is the diminution of Kupffer cell activity in unresolved hepatitis in contrast to the hyperplasia usually seen in chronic persistent hepatitis.

Hepatitis in intravenous drug users

An increased frequency of serum hepatitis among drug addicts has been recognized for many years.[111, 119] The development of the "hippie" culture with its philosophy of greater sharing of earthly goods, including needles and a wide variety of intravenous mixtures, has expanded the hepatitis problem enormously. In Los Angeles County, the frequency of hepatitis associated with common needle use has jumped from 19% of all reported cases of hepatitis in 1964 to 56% in 1968. Among patients with serum hepatitis, 78% to 88% are associated with common needle use. At a large drug rehabilitation center in Los Angeles, 21.6% of patients gave a history of jaundice during the time they were using drugs.[123] Since prospective transfusion studies indicate that for every patient with icteric serum hepatitis there are three who have anicteric disease, it would appear that nearly all intravenous drug users develop hepatitis on one or more occasions.

The problem is further compounded by the fact that 27% of drug users admit having sold blood. The anticipated development of icteric serum hepatitis in a recipient who receives blood obtained from an addict is seventy times greater than the incidence of hepatitis in recipients of blood from highly selected donors.[79]

Most singularly, the addict may develop icteric serum hepatitis on more than one occasion. We have observed patients with as many as eight separate episodes. Multiple bouts of icteric viral hepatitis in other patients, including those who receive hundreds of units of blood or blood products, is rare. Immunoglobulin levels of addicts who develop multiple bouts of hepatitis are not depressed.[42]

On biopsy, the liver of the patient who contracts hepatitis associated with needle sharing often will have much more lymphoid proliferation in the portal areas, even to the degree that lymph follicles may be present. Similarly, the patients often have lymph node hyperplasia that may be related to the multiple foreign components repeatedly inoculated. After multiple bouts of hepatitis, the portal areas may become widened, but nodular regeneration does not develop. The liver parenchymal cells often fail to become hydropic, and a cord arrangement is maintained more often than in ordinary viral hepatitis. In the Los Angeles area, heroin and other opiates often are adulterated or "cut" with talcum before being sold to drug addicts. The long-continued intravenous injection of these talcum-containing drugs results in a recognizable lesion in the liver in which the talc crystals are present in the triads and in Kupffer cells. They do not form true granulomas but may result in a mild increase of connective tissue. The crystals are best seen with a polarizing microscope and may be found in the liver of 20% of patients with hepatitis at the Los Angeles County–University of Southern California Medical Center and the John Wesley Hospital. The *laboratory* findings in addicts with viral hepatitis are indistinguishable from those of nonaddicts who have viral hepatitis.

Laboratory diagnosis

Tests that indicate cell necrosis or damage, such as SGPT, SGOT, isocitric dehydrogenase (ICD), lactic acid dehydrogenase (LDH), and LDH isoenzymes, are the most helpful in the diagnosis of viral hepatitis (Table 28-1). The transaminases are more stable than the others under laboratory conditions. Glutamic pyruvic transaminase is more selectively a liver parenchymal cell enzyme than is GOT. Serum GPT and SGOT activities rise above normal about one week prior to symptoms and continue to rise to levels usually above 1,000 units, occasionally to 3,000 units and rarely to 5,000 units. The SGPT is higher than the SGOT in 85% of patients with viral hepatitis.

Serum bilirubin levels do not indicate the severity of disease, although anicteric viral hepatitis is usually a milder disease and never fatal. The direct and indirect fractions are about equally divided. In younger patients, the serum albumin remains within normal range, but in older patients or severely ill younger patients, it may decrease. The change in albumin level is probably a reflection of functioning capacity of liver cells. The prothrombin activity is of little help in making the diagnosis of viral hepatitis, but it is of considerable prognostic value. A fall in prothrombin activity is of serious consequence, although death rarely occurs when the prothrombin activity (by Owren-Ware technique) remains above 5%.[86] The hepatitis-associated antigen (HAA) in sera is strong evidence for hepatitis B. Serum alkaline phosphatase activity usually is slightly elevated (5 to 10 Bessey Lowry units). Although patients who have considerable cholestasis on liver biopsy are often histologically classified as having cholestatic viral hepatitis,[91] such patients usually have only a slight elevation of alkaline phosphatase activity. Conversely, the occasional patient with a fivefold to sevenfold increase in alkaline phosphatase activity rarely has cholestasis on liver biopsy.

In hepatic coma, the clinical and laboratory data are of little help in determining the amount of liver destruction in contrast to that which is viable but temporarily nonfunctional. Furthermore, regenerative capacity cannot be measured. The best prognostic sign is a rise in prothrombin activity or of factor VII levels.

Encephalopathy

The chief manifestation of hepatic failure is encephalopathy. This occurs in both acute and chronic liver disease. In fulminant hepatitis, the onset is sudden and the mortality high.[86] In chronic liver disease, the symptoms of hepatic encephalopathy are more likely to be mild and the onset gradual. The symptoms are of a neuropsychiatric nature, varying from minor disturbances of consciousness and behavior to drowsiness, confusion, and coma. Often, a flapping tremor of the extremities is evident. In spite of the severe neurologic features that may develop, histopathologic changes are minimal, apparently limited to enlargement and increased numbers of proto-plasmic astrocytes.[60] One of the surprising aspects of hepatic coma is the rapid and complete recovery that may occur if hepatic failure is ameliorated.

The etiology of hepatic encephalopathy is probably related to ammonia metabolism.[93, 138] Ammonia, formed by the kidney and by urea-splitting organisms in the gut, is removed from portal blood by the intact liver to form urea. Patients on diuretic therapy or who have potassium depletion have a greater renal production of ammonia. The relative amounts of NH_3 and NH_4 in blood are critical, since only NH_3 passes through the cell membrane. The ratio follows the Henderson-Hasselbach equation of pH = 9.15 + $\log \dfrac{[NH_3]}{[NH_4+]}$. Thus, alkalosis will increase the amount of diffusible NH_3. In the central nervous system, NH_3 is believed to produce its deleterious effects by diverting α-keto-glutarate from the tricarboxylic cycle with consequent loss of high-energy phosphate bond formation and reduction of aerobic metabolism.

It is likely that in hepatic coma toxic substances other than ammonia affect cerebral metabolism. The consequences of other metabolic disturbances in liver failure[85] are yet to be elucidated.

Encephalopathy often increases as a result of vascular bypass of the liver,[114, 122] either as a spontaneous result of portal hypertension or following surgical portacaval anastomosis for bleeding esophageal varices.

OTHER ACUTE INFECTIONS

There are other acute diseases of the liver of infectious origin that occur less frequently than viral hepatitis. Among these are yellow fever (p. 399), typhoid fever, Weil's disease, and infectious mononucleosis. Although rarely accompanied by jaundice, a classic example of focal necrosis of the liver is that produced by typhoid fever. Jaundice, high fever, and sore muscles always should bring to mind Weil's disease (p. 359). Infectious mononucleosis may cause hepatomegaly, extensive infiltration of the liver by mononuclears, and focal necrosis sufficient to produce jaundice. In the past, focal necrosis of the liver due to some of the pyogenic organisms was known to complicate the course of septicemia, but the jaundice that was occasionally seen was possibly secondary to hemolysis caused by the organisms. In fatal chickenpox, irregular areas of necrosis often involve both the triads and portions of the lobules. The blood vessels of the triads usually are included in the necrotizing process.

CHEMICAL AND DRUG INJURY

The role of the liver in the metabolism of chemicals and drugs has been elucidated by many biochemical and electron microscopic studies in recent years.[155] Most therapeutic or noxious substances are detoxified by the activity of membranes located in the endoplasmic reticulum, the microsomal fraction of the liver cell. This process is one of oxidation and is dependent upon nicotinamide adenine dinucleotide (NADPH) as well as cytochrome P450. It is of interest that the microsomal drug–metabolizing mechanism is inducible. For example, repeated doses of phenobarbital and ethanol are powerful stimulants for increased production of smooth endoplasmic reticulum. Once the enzyme activity is increased, apparently one pathway exists so that other drugs or chemicals can be detoxified at an increased rate. This has led to problems in the therapy of alcoholics. While under the influence of alcohol, they are sensitive to barbiturates because the detoxicating mechanisms are occupied with the metabolism of alcohol. But in the sober state, they are resistant to the same drug for obvious reasons. Work on human volunteers has shown that ethanol would double hepatic pentobarbital hydroxylase.[156] The role of the liver in the induction of the microsomal enzymes by phenobarbital and its beneficial effect on the conjugation of bilirubin of the newborn infant is discussed on p. 1221.

Exposure to or ingestion of any one of numerous drugs and chemicals may cause injury to the liver that becomes manifest by jaundice.[146] A number of substances, of both synthetic and natural origin, have a direct toxic action on the liver of man and experimental animals that is dose-related and is fairly prompt. The morphologic expression, known as *toxic hepatitis,* is usually uniform and predictable. Among these hepatotoxins are carbon tetrachloride, chloroform, chlorinated naphthalenes, phosphorus, and the toxin of *Amanita phalloides.* They usually produce a zonal type of necrosis accompanied by fatty change. Other body organs may be affected and, if death does not occur, recovery is complete. The laboratory findings are similar to those in other types of necrosis. In *mushroom poisoning,* there is damage to both

nuclei and cytoplasm at the ultrastructural level, particularly in the periportal zones. The cytoplasmic changes include fat droplets, focal cytoplasmic degradation, and inclusions within mitochondria.[148] The ultrastructural changes in carbon tetrachloride injury include the dislocation of ribosomes and dilatation of cisternae[141, 158] (see also Chapter 6).

A group of therapeutic agents, known as indirect hepatotoxins, cause either necrosis or cholestasis in a high percentage of patients who receive them.[161] These include urethan, 6-mercaptopurine, and many anabolic steroids, especially the 17-alkyl group.

In contradistinction to the hepatotoxins, a drug may affect only an occasional individual. Reactions are not related to the amount of the drug taken nor to any specific time interval but do recur in susceptible patients upon repeated exposure.[145, 161] A patient who has jaundice or biochemical evidence of liver disease following the use of any therapeutic agent is diagnosed as having *drug-induced jaundice or drug-induced liver disease.* The problem of drug-induced liver disease has assumed such proportions that it is now essential to question every jaundiced patient about drug usage. This is especially true when the jaundice is of the obstructive type—i.e., with a high alkaline phosphatase level and normal or slightly elevated transaminase levels. Otherwise, the condition may be misdiagnosed and the patient subjected to unnecessary surgery. The mechanisms by which drugs injure the liver have not been fully explained. Since only a small percentage of patients are affected, it appears that idiosyncrasy is the key.

A useful clinicopathologic classification of drug-induced liver disease is given in Table 28-2. The list of drugs given that are capable of causing liver injury is by no means complete. In the first group, there is usually simple cholestasis without cell necrosis or inflammation, although the effect of drugs or of any single drug can vary considerably, and an occasional necrotic liver cell as well as minimal inflammation is sometimes seen. Rarely, severe necrosis may ensue. As a group, these cholestatic drugs produce reversible injury to the secretory mechanism that prevents bilirubin glucuronide from entering the canaliculi normally. The bilirubin that does enter the canaliculi tends to accumulate and form bile plugs that are obvious on microscopic examination, especially in the centrilobular zone (Plate 4, *B*). There is usually

Table 28-2 Drug-induced liver disease*

Action of drug	Incidence	Pathology—liver and other	Symptoms	Serum bilirubin	Transaminases	Alkaline phosphatase	Prothrombin time	BUN
I Cholestatic								
A Anabolic steroids with a 17-alkyl group† Methyl testosterone	High	Centrilobular cholestasis	Uncomplicated jaundice	Elevated, usually < 15 mg	Normal	Elevated often above 20 BL units	Normal	Normal
B Oral contraceptives	1/10,000	Centrilobular cholestasis	Itching and jaundice	Mild elevation	Mild increase	Elevation mild to moderate		
II Cholestatic, plus variable degree of necrosis Phenothiazine drugs Sulfonamides Thiouracil Tolbutamide‡ TAO Mercaptopurine	<1% 0.6% < 5%	Centrilobular bile stasis and focal necrosis; inflammation of triads in many instances	In addition to jaundice, may be fever, rash, and eosinophilia	Elevated, usually < 15	Mild rise, < 500; occasionally 1,000 or more	Elevated	Normal	Normal
III Necrosis, zonal or massive Halothane Iproniazid Isoniazid Ethionamide PAS Phenurone Phenylbutazone Urethane	1-10,000 1/100-1/2000 Very rare Low High 2% Rare	Liver cell injury, usually zonal or massive necrosis	Severe jaundice usually; may proceed to hepatic coma and death	Moderate to high	> 500 to 1,000	Elevation normal to mild	Decreased	May rise
IV Other Tetracycline, especially in pregnancy	Unknown	Fine, foamy fatty change; cholestasis; pancreas, brain, and kidney also involved	Jaundice; coma	Elevated	< 500	Elevated	Moderate decrease	High, often renal failure
Novobiocin	Unknown		Newborn infants more susceptive	Elevated unconjugated bilirubin	Normal	Normal	Normal	Normal
Oxyphenisatin	Uncommon	Acute cell injury or chronic active hepatitis	Malaise	Mild elevation	> 500	Normal or elevated	Decrease	Normal

*Data, in part from Zimmerman, H. J.: Amer. J. Gastroent. **49:**39-56, 1968.

†Rarely, cases of liver necrosis have been reported.

‡Data from Pannekoek, J. H.: In Meyler, L., and Herxheimer, A., editors: Side effects of drugs, vol. 6, Baltimore, 1968, The Williams & Wilkins Co.

some swelling or hydropic change of the hepatocytes. The electron microscope discloses blunting and disappearance of the microvilli lining the canaliculi. After discontinuing the drug, the liver returns to normal.

It is of interest that women who have had benign jaundice of pregnancy presumably due to excess production of sex hormones, will often have a recurrence of jaundice when they take one of the oral contraceptives.[146] The estrogens appear to be responsible for the rare instances of jaundice that follows the use of oral contraceptives. The 17-alpha-alkyl-19-norsteroids cause the most difficulty with bile secretion.[157] Thrombosis of the hepatic veins, Budd-Chiari syndrome, is a rare complication of oral contraceptive use.[154] We have seen two cases in the Los Angeles area (see also p. 187).

In the second and largest group of patients, there is liver cell injury as well as cholestasis, so that the laboratory findings occasionally include a rise in the serum transaminases. The number of drugs that cause this type of injury seems endless. The phenothiazine drugs, probably because of the amount consumed, are the most common offenders. On microscopic examination, the findings are variable, but cell ballooning, focal necrosis of hepatocytes, cholestasis, and inflammation along the portal tracts usually are present. The triads contain an unusual number of eosinophils in some biopsies. Granulomas with eosinophilic infiltrate may result from sensitivity to one of the sulfonamide drugs. Most patients in this second group recover when the offending drug is discontinued. A few have a long illness with the laboratory findings of biliary cirrhosis,[160] but most of these patients eventually get well.

In the third group of patients, liver cell necrosis with little to moderate inflammatory response occurs. The laboratory findings are principally hyperbilirubinemia and high serum transaminase activity. Although mild centrilobular necrosis that heals rapidly occasionally is seen following the use of isoniazid or para-aminosalicylic acid,[144] both of these drugs, as well as others, such as iproniazid, may cause massive necrosis and death. Halothane and similar compounds—methoxyflurane (Penthrane)—occasionally are associated with liver necrosis.[150] These agents are chemically related to carbon tetrachloride, but their damaging action on the liver cells is delayed, in contrast to the immediate effect of carbon

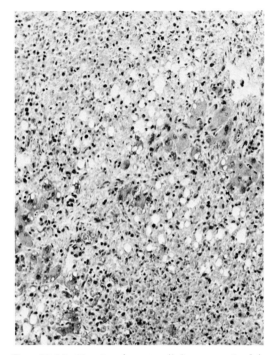

Fig. 28-11 Massive hepatocellular necrosis following halothane anesthesia. (From Peters, R. L., Edmondson, H. A., Reynolds, T. B., Meister, J. C., and Curphey, T. J.: Amer. J. Med. **47**:748-764, 1969.)

tetrachloride. Since halothane and its derivatives are metabolized by the liver,[151, 159] perhaps a metabolic by-product is responsible for necrosis. Clinically, the patient with liver cell necrosis following exposure to halothane initially has hyperpyrexia. The laboratory values resemble those of hepatitis.

In fatal massive necrosis following halothane anesthesia, three stages can be recognized: necrotic, absorptive, and regenerative. In the *necrotic* stage, dead liver cells are still recognizable and occur in the first five days after onset of jaundice (Fig. 28-11). In the *absorptive* stage, the liver cells have disappeared, leaving areas of collapse. This is the period in which most of the patients die, usually one to two weeks after the onset of jaundice. In the *regenerative* stage, submassive necrosis has occurred, and in this stage the patients live from two weeks to a month. These subjects are older and have insufficient regenerative capacity to restore the liver parenchyma. Individuals under 30 years of age who survive for three weeks after the onset of jaundice may be expected to recover.

In a small miscellaneous group (IV in Table 28-2), the abnormalities produced are distinctive for each drug.[143, 149] There are no

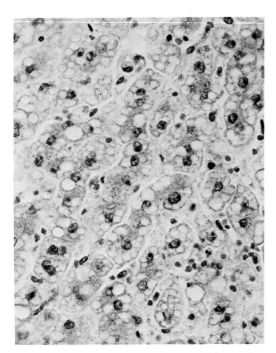

Fig. 28-12 Fine foamy vacuolization of liver after large amounts of intravenously administered tetracycline. (From Peters, R. L., Edmondson, H. A., Mikkelsen, W. P., and Tatter, D.: Amer. J. Surg. **113:**622-632, 1967.)

common findings in the liver. A characteristic foamy type of fatty change occurs in the liver following the use of large amounts of intravenous tetracycline (Fig. 28-12).[142] The intravenous use of this drug in the treatment of pyelonephritis in pregnancy will probably be discontinued. To date, nearly all reported cases have been in women, usually during late pregnancy, although men on estrogen therapy may be affected. The tetracycline interferes with the production of protein by RNA. Thus, formation of lipoprotein necessary for the transfer of fat from the liver is blocked. Novobiocin inhibits the action of glucuronyl transferase, in this way producing an unconjugated hyperbilirubinemia.

Recently, both an acute liver cell damage resembling mild acute viral hepatitis and a disorder indistinguishable from chronic active hepatitis have been described following the chronic use of laxatives that contain the agent oxyphenisatin (acetphenolisatin).[152, 153]

RADIATION INJURY

Heavy irradiation of the liver, 3,000 to 5,900 rads, produces centrilobular necrosis, intense hyperemia, and damage to the small hepatic veins that resembles veno-occlusive disease.[163] The microscopic changes in a needle biopsy specimen taken in the acute stage of irradiation damage are most difficult to disinguish from Budd-Chiari syndrome. In patients who survive more than four months, there is a return toward normal of all structures. Experimentally, irradiation produces a characteristic fine structural change in the rough endoplasmic reticulum, forming dense membranes.[162]

CHRONIC ACTIVE HEPATITIS

Chronic active hepatitis (active chronic hepatitis; chronic aggressive hepatitis) is characterized by recurrent episodes that simulate mild viral hepatitis, yet most patients eventually develop coarsely nodular cirrhosis. Previously under dispute as to whether it represented nonhealing viral hepatitis,[176, 177] an autoimmune disease,[173] or an autoimmune reaction precipitated by a viral infection,[174] it is now generally believed that multiple etiologies may produce the same morphologic lesion and similar clinical patterns.

Most patients have a chronic recurrent disease, with the development of symptoms of portal hypertension, including esophageal varices and ascites. Some have borderline encephalopathy for years. Eventually, chronic liver disease leads to death. Only a few patients survive for ten years or more. Although rare, a patient may die a few weeks after the diagnosis is made.

Since at least one drug can produce all of the features of chronic active lupoid hepatitis, including the positive LE preparation and histologic pattern, it is necessary to consider exogenous agents in the etiology of a disease that has been considered autoimmune in type.

Biopsies taken at the onset of symptoms usually disclose both acute and chronic liver disease. Cirrhosis may be present, but the liver parenchyma also has changes that resemble those of viral hepatitis, with unicellular cytolytic foci surrounded by lymphocytes or plasma cells. Kupffer cell hyperplasia is prominent. The residual parenchymal cells are hydropic with large nuclei that are often vesicular. The normal cord pattern is absent. In contrast to acute viral hepatitis, there is no predilection for greater cytoplasmic changes in the centrilobular areas, nor are the lobules uniformly affected (Fig. 28-13).

During periods of clinical quiescence, the acute changes disappear but regenerative activity continues and progresses toward a coarsely nodular cirrhosis (Plate 5, *E*). The

It is convenient to separate chronic active hepatitis into four groups based on presumed differences in etiology and a few subtle differences in clinical pattern.[152, 166, 169] The names used are chronic active lupoid hepatitis, chronic active viral hepatitis, chronic active toxic hepatitis, and cryptogenic chronic active hepatitis.

Chronic active lupoid hepatitis

Cirrhosis is usually present when the patients are first studied, and the disease generally progresses over a period of years to death by hepatic failure, bleeding esophageal varices, or other complication of chronic liver disease. Early reports[164, 172] indicated a preponderance of women, with findings of recurrent fever, menstrual irregularities, arthralgia, and hyperglobulinemia. Some patients with the same symptom complexes were found to have positive lupus erythematosus (LE) cell tests,[164, 165, 170, 171] and the term *lupoid hepatitis* was used. Although chronic active lupoid hepatitis was originally described in young women,[164] it may affect anyone from childhood to senility[175] but remains preponderantly a disease of women.

Biologic false positive reactions to serologic tests for syphilis occur in 25% or less of patients with chronic active lupoid hepatitis.[174, 175]; 50% have a positive latex fixative reaction for rheumatoid arthritis, 75% have antinuclear antibodies,[174] and 90% or more have a positive reaction for smooth muscle antibodies.[177] The latter seems to be the most reliable, if poorly understood, test. The antibody reaction is to a component of smooth muscle taken from any mammalian species.

Chronic active viral hepatitis

Since discovery of HAA, it has been recognized that a large percentage of patients with chronic active hepatitis who have negative LE cell preparations, and who lack smooth muscle antibodies, do have circulating HAA in their sera.[168, 178] About 0.1% of patients with viral hepatitis who are ill enough for hospitalization will develop a progressive pattern of chronic active viral hepatitis that leads to cirrhosis. About four to five times as many patients will develop the disease without a clinically apparent acute attack. In contrast to chronic active lupoid hepatitis, there is no sex predilection, and systemic symptoms such as amenorrhea, skin rashes, and joint pains, or psychiatric problems, are much fewer. The serologic changes of autoimmune

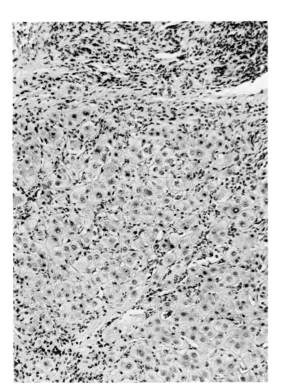

Fig. 28-13 Diffuse inflammation and liver cell necrosis in regenerative nodule from liver in chronic active hepatitis.

regenerative nodules may become large, and the cells may reassume a cord arrangement. The intervening regions of collapse may contain small islands of liver cells. They are heavily infiltrated by lymphocytes and plasma cells. The collagen in the areas of collapse is loose and permits the ready growth of large nodules. Recrudescence of necrosis may not affect all nodules to the same extent or severity.

Although serum albumin is moderately depressed, the striking aberration is in the globulin level. During active stages of the disease, the serum globulin levels become markedly elevated, usually over 6 gm per 100 ml, occasionally over 8 gm per 100 ml. Most patients have elevations of IgG and IgM, and some have elevation of IgA.[29] Serum transaminase activities are elevated, often in the range of 1,000 units. In contrast to those in patients with viral hepatitis, the SGOT level is usually elevated to a greater degree than the SGPT. During the periods when the patient becomes anicteric and asymptomatic, the serum globulin levels may drop to normal or near normal ranges, and the transaminase activities either remain in the range of 100 to 200 units or reach normal levels.[175]

disease are absent, but the microscopic and gross findings in the liver are indistinguishable from those of chronic active lupoid hepatitis.

The pathogenesis of chronic active viral hepatitis remains unknown. Because of the complexing of HAA in serum with the patient's own antibody, there has been speculation that the disease is based on a hyperimmune reaction or an immune complex disease; however, this is a disputed point.[167] We have observed no patients with unresolved viral hepatitis who developed chronic active viral hepatitis, nor have we found patients with chronic active viral hepatitis who lost their HAA.

As with chronic active lupoid hepatitis, the course of the disease is characterized by remissions and exacerbations. It is possible that patients with chronic active viral hepatitis may have an increased propensity to develop liver cell carcinoma.[137]

The differential diagnosis of chronic active viral hepatitis from a combination of viral hepatitis superimposed upon preexisting cirrhosis due to other causes may be difficult or impossible. Alcoholic cirrhosis with superimposed viral hepatitis may be recognizable on biopsy unless the patient has discontinued alcohol for two or three months. Such patients will generally have a greater elevation of SGOT than SGPT activity. The serum globulin level may approach that observed in chronic active hepatitis.

Chronic active toxic hepatitis

At least one drug, oxyphenisatin, when used habitually, may produce chronic active hepatitis. Some patients have even developed positive LE cell preparations and smooth muscle antibodies, all of which disappear with discontinuance of the laxative and reappear with challenge.[152] The fact that a drug may precipitate a disease previously believed to be autoimmune makes it mandatory that other types of exogenous sensitization be excluded in all cases of chronic active lupoid hepatitis.

Cryptogenic chronic active hepatitis

Many patients have the clinical, laboratory, and hepatic morphologic pattern described for chronic active hepatitis but have no evidence of exogenous sensitization. They do not have the LE factor, antinuclear antibody, smooth muscle antibody, or HAA. This form of cryptogenic chronic active hepatitis could have the same etiology as one of the types previously described, the patient lacking

demonstrable quantities of the serum factors that would allow classification as either lupoid or viral types of disease. Alternatively, a toxic agent not yet recognized may be at fault, or hepatitis A may occasionally give rise to chronic active hepatitis.

ACUTE BILIARY OBSTRUCTION

Another group of active acute liver diseases includes the disorders that cause obstruction to the outflow of bile. These may be intrahepatic and of chemical or therapeutic origin, as already discussed. A poorly understood chronic disease of the liver, primary biliary cirrhosis, may begin in much the same way as drug-induced jaundice. In fact, a few cases have been known to follow drug therapy. A most important subgroup is that due to extrahepatic biliary obstruction, sometimes called surgical jaundice.

The most common causes of obstruction of the extrahepatic ducts are stones, carcinoma, or stricture. When secondary to calculous obstruction, there is often a history of gallbladder disease, and jaundice is accompanied by pain. Carcinoma of the ducts or of the head of the pancreas is more likely to produce jaundice with no pain or with a different pain pattern. Postoperative or congenital strictures of the common duct are much less frequent.

The microscopic changes that commonly follow obstruction of the extrahepatic bile ducts are rather characteristic. In biopsy material, the earliest change is mild dilatation of the ducts, with a few periductal neutrophils situated just beneath the basement membrane of the ductal epithelium, and centrilobular cholestasis (Plate 4, *C*). Later, in unrelieved obstruction, the ducts enlarge further and may proliferate. Periductal neutrophils are more numerous and penetrate the lumen of the ducts. This combination of changes is known as acute cholangitis. Clinically, the term signifies that the patient has jaundice, fever, and often chills. The bile canaliculi become more distended with yellow to yellow-green bile plugs. The etiology of acute cholangitis is presumed to be of bacterial origin. Organisms often are found in stagnant bile when obstruction is due to stone or stricture but are not present in surgical specimens when the obstruction is caused by tumor.[182] Electron microscopic studies show flattening of the canalicular microvilli and condensation of the pericanalicular ectoplasm.[179] The liver cells often contain intracytoplasmic bile, and Kupffer cells are enlarged by easily discernible masses of bile pigment. Foci of necrosis may appear within the lobules, accompanied by bile lakes. Often, a feathery type of degeneration of liver cells is noted.[180] Increased connective tissue around the bile ducts may assume a lamellar arrangement, and small prolongations enter the periphery of the lobules. Chronic biliary obstruction is discussed on p. 1210.

Effects. Complete obstruction of the common duct by carcinoma causes a prompt rise in the serum bilirubin level and a slower but fairly constant rise in the serum alkaline phosphatase level (Table 28-1). The blood prothrombin decreases but responds to parenterally administered vitamin K. Bile appears in the urine, and there is an absence of stercobilin in the stool. A calculus usually does not produce complete obstruction of the common duct. The serum bilirubin level does not go so high and tends to fluctuate. The alkaline phosphatase level likewise does not show the constant rise usually seen in cancerous obstruction. An increase in bile acids in the serum is held responsible for the pruritus that is so common in patients with biliary obstruction.[181]

CIRRHOSIS

Cirrhosis results from a series of alterations that lead to a quantitative increase of dense fibrous connective tissue that subdivides the liver into nodules (pseudolobules) of variable size. Most often the fibrous complex includes both the portal tissue and the outflow tract, but one or the other may be almost exclusively involved. Episodes of necrosis and regeneration of the liver parenchyma may occur throughout the course of the disease. Any concept of cirrhosis should include both the morphologic and functional aspects. Although cirrhosis usually is considered to be irreversible, it is now known that the removal of the causative agent may, in some instances, result in a remarkable degree of reversibility. This has been noted in alcoholic cirrhosis, biliary cirrhosis of infants, galactosemia, and hemochromatosis. In cirrhosis, the abnormal architecture is easily recognized on gross examination.

In a broader sense, the term cirrhosis often is applied to any widespread fibrosis or scarring of the liver in which loss of hepatic cells is associated with actual or relative increase of connective tissue. Localized limited inflammatory processes and scarring usually are excluded. Although the term "cirrhosis" (derived from the Greek word *kirrhos,* meaning

tawny or orange-colored) was applied originally because of color changes, it is fibrosis and nodular regeneration of liver cells, with distortion of vascular and achitectural relationships, rather than any distinctive color, that constitute the fundamental features of the condition.

Many injurious agents that affect the liver may, over a period of time, lead to cirrhosis. This is a long-continued process, the early stages of which by definition cannot be called cirrhosis. Because the liver may react to injury by producing both scar tissue and hyperplastic nodules that eventually lead to vascular obstruction, decreased vital function, and often jaundice, the final results—from the standpoint both of symptoms and of pathologic findings—may be similar regardless of the etiologic agent. There are, however, certain distinctive changes in cirrhosis that point to one etiologic factor or another, and when these are correlated with the clinical history, a useful classification of cirrhosis emerges:

1 Laennec's or alcoholic cirrhosis—most often follows the chronic use of ethanol but may be of undetermined etiology

2 Coarsely nodular cirrhosis—a type that follows long-continued necrosis and fibrosis, the nature of which is poorly understood

3 Pigmentary cirrhosis—consequent to excess storage of iron within the liver

4 Wilson's disease (hepatolenticular degeneration)—a nodular type of cirrhosis associated with excess storage of copper

5 Biliary cirrhosis—of chologenic origin and associated with obstruction of bile ducts, either within the liver or extrahepatically

6 Syphilitic cirrhosis—extensive scarring or a diffuse fibrosis that results from syphilitic infection

7 Parasitic cirrhosis—due to infection by schistosomes or the liver fluke, *Clonorchis sinensis*

8 Congestive or cardiac cirrhosis—usually the result of prolonged congestive cardiac failure

9 Miscellaneous types—including cases of cirrhosis of unknown cause that often complicate other diseases

Laennec's or alcoholic cirrhosis

On a worldwide basis, the most common type of cirrhosis that has been described has had a multitude of names. Among these are alcoholic cirrhosis, portal cirrhosis, diffuse cirrhosis, nutritional cirrhosis, septal cirrhosis, and hobnail cirrhosis, but the one that has had the most usage is Laennec's cirrhosis. It is impossible for any author to know exactly how the latter term is used in various geographic regions. It is probable that there is considerable variation, depending upon the morphologic criteria used by individual pathologists in various countries. Since the most common type of cirrhosis seen in the United States occurs in the alcoholic, we have come to use the term *alcoholic cirrhosis* to indicate this background. This is not to imply that alcohol is the sole etiologic agent in the production of the cirrhosis in the alcoholic.

Incidence

Laennec's cirrhosis is a common disease in most parts of the world, forming a large proportion of all types of cirrhosis.[270] The reported autopsy incidence of cirrhosis varies between 1% and 10% throughout most of the world. In various centers in the United States, it has varied from 1.6% to 9%. It may occur at any age, but the peak incidence is in late middle life (50 to 55 years), with most patients between 40 and 65 years of age. It appears to occur more frequently in males than in females, and in women the peak age incidence is about a decade earlier than in men. In the Los Angeles County–University of Southern California Medical Center in 1970, the frequency of cirrhosis at autopsy was 11%. The highest frequency was among Mexican-American and Caucasian men over 20 years of age, with an incidence of 25% and 18%, respectively.

Etiology

In the United States, cirrhosis most commonly follows the long-continued use of ethanol. The epidemiologic evidence indicates that the mortality rate from cirrhosis is directly related to the per capita consumption of ethanol from wine and spirits.[310] In India, Africa, and other parts of the world in which cirrhosis is common, malnutrition and hepatitis appear to be more important factors. The relationship between alcoholism and cirrhosis is unquestioned, but the exact mechanism of its injurious effect is not known. It would appear that the development of cirrhosis in the alcoholic depends upon three factors:

1 The susceptibility to hepatic injury, which varies among alcoholics, the often-quoted figure of 8% of all alcoholics developing cirrhosis being probably too low[233, 242]

2 The amount of ethanol consumed daily and the duration of excessive consumption

3 The degree and duration of malnutrition, particularly of protein containing the essential amino acids

It is difficult to define chronic alcoholism other than to say that the individual drinks to such excess that he is incapable of leading a normal existence, primarily from the social and economic standpoints. The basis for this is the individual's loss of control for ethanol consumption. Among patients with portal cirrhosis, a history of excessive use of alcohol has been found in 30% to 92% in various series. At the Los Angeles County–University of Southern California Medical Center, more than 900 new patients with cirrhosis are seen annually. About 90% of these have a history of five to fifteen years of heavy consumption of alcohol. Many consume as much as a quart of whiskey or a gallon of wine per day. In addition to steady drinking, most patients will periodically drink excessively for one or two weeks, during which time they eat little or no food. These bouts often terminate in an attack of jaundice, pneumonia, pancreatitis, or delirium tremens.

Metabolism of alcohol

Ethanol in small quantities is metabolized chiefly in the liver cell by a series of reactions that begin with its oxidation to acetaldehyde by alcoholic dehydrogenase (ADH), which is present in the cell sap or cytosol. Beyond this point, the various reactions are still in question, although the conversion of acetaldehyde to acetate and acetyl coenzyme A seems fairly certain.[248] A distinction must be drawn between the metabolism of small quantities of alcohol as might be ingested in medications and the use of larger quantities as is so customary in our contemporary society. In experimental animals, it has been shown that another mechanism exists for the oxidation of ethanol when given in quantity. The ethanol stimulates hyperplasia of the smooth endoplasmic reticulum, and the microsomal fraction from the liver has a greatly increased capacity to form acetaldehyde from ethanol. This process has been called the microsomal ethanol oxidizing system (MEOS).[249] Furthermore, the oxidation in vitro is maximal at physiologic pH in the presence of O_2 and a cofactor NADPH (reduced nicotinamide adenine dinucleotide phosphate). The ratio of the metabolism of ethanol in vivo as

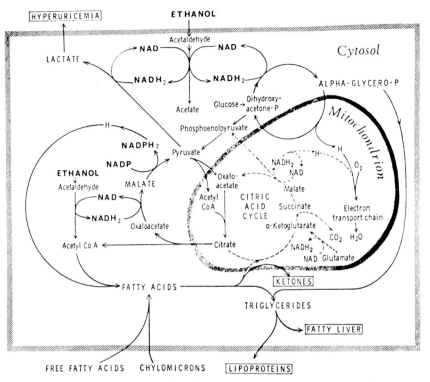

Fig. 28-14 Effects of oxidation of ethanol on intermediary metabolism in liver. Pathways inhibited by ethanol represented by broken lines. Coupling of oxidation of ethanol with reduction of oxaloacetate is hypothetical. (From Lieber, C. S.: Advances Intern. Med. **14:** 151-199, 1968; copyrighted by Year Book Medical Publishers, Inc.; used by permission.)

between the ADH and MEOS system is not known (see also p. 202).

The metabolism of ethanol and its effect on the intermediate metabolism of the liver cell is a most complex problem. A detailed discussion of this has been published, including the outline reproduced in Fig. 28-14.[248] In the oxidation of ethanol to acetaldehyde, the adenine dinucleotide (NAD) to form NADH₂. hydrogen ions are transferred to nicotinamide More NADH₂ results from the formation of acetate or acetyl coenzyme A from acetaldehyde. The net result is an increase of the NADH₂/NAD ratio. This has a marked effect on lipid and glucose metabolism. As shown in Fig. 28-14, excess lactate is formed. This may lead to hyperuricemia and hyperlactacidemia. Intramitochondrial effects of excess NADH₂ include a decrease in the activity of the citric acid cycle and lipid oxidation. These, in turn, could contribute to increased hepatic ketone production and a fatty liver. Hypoglycemia occasionally is seen in alcoholics, especially those who are drinking heavily and taking little or no food. Many mechanisms may contribute to a decrease in

gluconeogenesis.[244, 248] In the presence of decreased carbohydrate stores, glycerol, lactate, and amino acids are precursors for glucose formation. Most of the pathways for the conversion of these substances to glucose are blocked either in the cytoplasm or in the mitochondria by excess NADH₂. The decrease in pyruvate and inability to use lactate have been emphasized.

The increased lipogenesis that leads to a fatty liver arises from multiple defects in intermediary metabolism (Fig. 28-14), with the increased NADH₂/NAD ratio playing a major role. Although many mechanisms have been considered responsible for increased fat in the liver,[2] only two will be considered. In addition to the increased synthesis of fatty acids via many routes (Fig. 28-14), there is also a marked decrease in hepatic lipid oxidation as well as a reduction in the oxidation of chylomicrons.[248] The fatty acids lead to formation of triglycerides that are stored as fat vacuoles. The exact reason for the accumulation of the triglycerides is not known, for phospholipid formation is not decreased. It has been shown that medium-chain fatty acids are oxidized to a greater extent than are the long-chain fatty acids. Another mechanism proposed for the production of the fatty liver after ethanol ingestion deals with the formation of lipoperoxides, hydroperoxides, or other toxic radicals. These, in turn, lead to the storage of fat, an event that can be prevented in rats by the administration of antioxidants.[319]

The deficiency of lipotropic substances, especially choline, has been shown to produce fatty livers that progress to cirrhosis in experimental animals.[308] The fat first occupies a centrilobular position and is present as large vacuoles. Later, the formation of fatty cysts is associated with connective tissue proliferation. The mechanism by which choline prevents or cures the fatty lesion is not yet known. When alcohol is fed to rats that are given a choline-deficient diet, liver changes are produced that are similar to those of alcoholic cirrhosis. Animals given dietary protection did not have any hepatotoxic effect after as long as seven months[273] on appreciable daily quantities of ethanol. A single intoxicating dose of ethanol given rats with fatty liver following choline deficiency results in cell necrosis and a rise in the SGOT levels. Alcohol yields about 7 calories per gram. Thus a chronic alcoholic may consume 2,000 to 2,500 calories per day, with consequent lack of appetite and poor intake of lipotropic substances. Thus, it is possible that in man both a choline-deficient diet and the acute effect of ethanol contribute to increased fat in the liver. The lack of dietary protein and the possible damage to the endoplasmic reticulum by alcohol, especially after the cirrhotic process has begun, may lead to decreased formation of the protein necessary for the synthesis of lipoprotein. It is of interest that in hospitalized patients with a fatty cirrhotic liver who continue on their usual daily intake of ethanol but have a good protein diet, the fat will almost completely disappear.[280] In man, the exact relationship of the fatty change, if any, to the necrosis, fibrosis, and regeneration seen is not clear.

There seems to be very little experimental work that is applicable to the vitally important problem of the marked increase of fibrous connective tissue in alcoholic cirrhosis.

Lesions

The chronic use of ethanol may produce morphologic changes in the liver that are characteristic and allow a presumptive diagnosis to be made on these grounds alone. The study of a large number of biopsies, many of them taken serially, in conjunction with the study of autopsy material has disclosed a number of microscopic features of liver disease in the alcoholic that are helpful in explaining the clinical findings as well as the histogenesis of cirrhosis. In recent years, the term *alcoholic liver disease* has been used for all of the changes that occur, beginning with the earliest seen on needle biopsy and continuing to the end stage of cirrhosis.

Although, broadly speaking, three stages may be recognized—presymptomatic, acute liver disease or "alcoholic hepatitis," and chronic liver disease, which is usually cirrhosis—these may merge one into the other. Furthermore, acute changes sometimes are superimposed upon chronic liver disease. Biopsies and autopsies disclose that the disease often progresses through each of the first two stages before cirrhosis occurs. However, some alcoholics are symptomless until the advanced stage of cirrhosis is reached. In this latter group, the various steps leading to cirrhosis are unknown.

Presymptomatic stage. In the presymptomatic stage before liver disease is manifest, the first discernible alterations may appear after a few years of heavy drinking. The patient may be seen by the physician or be hospitalized for any one of several conditions often seen in the alcoholic. These include delirium tremens, nausea and vomiting, trauma, acute infection, and alcoholic pancreatitis. The liver in presymptomatic disease often is enlarged but not to an unusual degree. The only hepatic tests that may be abnormal are a mild rise in SGOT levels and BSP retention. In a biopsy study of this group,[211] it was noted that fatty vacuolization and hydropic change are the most common abnormalities, having been noted in 95% of biopsies. In addition, a mild but definite increase of connective tissue often thickens the walls of the central veins and centrilobular sinusoids. In an occasional patient, minute foci of hyaline necrosis and sinusoidal sclerosis occur. Most patients entered the hospital because of delirium tremens or nausea and vomiting. They had been drinking excessively for many years, and many had eaten poorly or not at all for short periods before entry.

The time interval between the onset of heavy drinking and microscopic abnormalities in the liver is not known. Alcohol given to young nonalcoholic volunteers produced fatty vacuolation in two days.[285] However, the fat was uniformly distributed throughout the lobule, and droplets were relatively small (usually from 5μ to 15μ) and different from the fat deposition of symptomatic stages of alcoholic liver disease.

Acute alcoholic liver disease. It is difficult to predict when the disease in an alcoholic whose biopsy shows the early changes just described will progress to the point at which symptoms of acute liver disease develop. These symptoms differ somewhat, depending upon the morphologic abnormalities in the liver. Most commonly, however, the patient has a more or less sudden onset of jaundice that often is accompanied by fever. In the literature, these patients have been described as having "alcoholic hepatitis." A liver biopsy usually discloses one of three structural changes, each of which may be rather complex: (1) fatty liver with cholestasis, (2) fatty liver that undergoes a lytic type of necrosis, and (3) liver that undergoes sclerosing hyaline necrosis. There may be some overlap between the three types.

The simplest microscopic change is a fatty liver with cholestasis. A mild thickening of sinusoidal and central vein walls is common, but little or no increase of portal connective tissue is seen. Upon hospitalization, the patients usually recover in a period of a few weeks. It is remarkable how rapidly a large fatty liver shrinks when the patient partakes of an adequate diet and abstains from alcohol. In addition to hyperbilirubinemia, the hepatic tests usually show a moderate rise in alkaline phosphatase levels.

The second microscopic change in acute alcoholic liver disease is a fatty liver that undergoes a lytic type of necrosis. The lytic foci are usually centrilobular and devoid of inflammatory exudate. Cholestasis, bile staining of cytoplasm, and bile in Kupffer cells are uniformly present. Some of the patients become critically ill and may die in hepatic coma. At autopsy, the liver is fatty and deeply icteric and few microscopic details can be seen. Upon the patient's admission to the hospital, the laboratory findings are similar to those in the patients with fatty liver with cholestasis except that the SGOT level may reach 300 units and the SGPT remains normal. The prothrombin activity may be decreased to the range of 20%.

For the third type of microscopic change in acute alcoholic liver disease, we use the term *sclerosing hyaline necrosis*.[212, 278] In sclerosing

hyaline necrosis, the centrilobular cells undergo hydropic and hyaline change that leads to necrosis. This striking change is most often observed in a liver with few fat vacuoles, although fatty livers are not spared. The hyalin first appears as clumps in the cytoplasm and then as large masses that often have an eccentric location in the cell (Plate 4, *D*). Often, there are many neutrophils in the sinusoids around the necrotic cells. They may even penetrate the cytoplasm of the cell and probably assist in its liquefaction. The latter appears to be a slow process. Various stages in the progression of hyaline necrosis are seen in the liver at any one time. A remarkable increase of collagen occurs in the centrilobular areas (Fig. 28-15). This is associated with increased numbers of cells that appear to be derived from Kupffer cells and function as fibroblasts. The increased connective tissue leads to obliteration of many of the central sinusoids and veins. The changes in sclerosing hyaline necrosis may be so severe that death ensues, but many patients recover. The necrotic cells finally disappear, the connective tissue condenses, and, although the regenerative response is poor, the remaining cells in

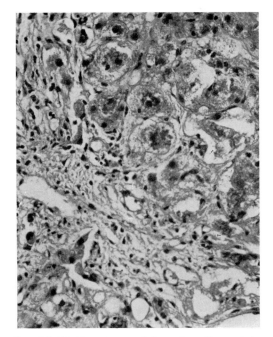

Fig. 28-15 Cytoplasm of hepatic cells contains eosinophilic granular material, so-called alcoholic hyalin. Cells appear swollen, and cell borders are indistinguishable. Sclerosis of vascular walls has begun. Needle biopsy of liver of 42-year-old Indian, chronic alcoholic who had been on long drinking spree before entering hospital.

the altered lobules resume their functions. In the acute phase, the patients often have jaundice, ascites, abdominal pain, and an exceptional neutrophilic leukocytosis.[212]

Cirrhosis. As the *early changes* evolve into cirrhosis, several types are recognizable. In the first type, the fatty liver may retain its lobular pattern, with little or no centrilobular injury, while in the portal tracts an increase of connective tissue and bile duct proliferation is observed. The connective tissue has an irregular distribution as it curves around the periphery of the lobules, and irregular prolongations may extend directly into the lobule along the sinusoids (Fig. 28-16). As the fibrous tissue completely delineates the lobules, it is truly a portal cirrhosis, even though there is little or no necrosis at autopsy, nor are there necessarily any regenerative nodules. The gross appearance of the liver in early cirrhosis is similar to that of fatty change alone. The liver is always enlarged, some-

times weighing as much as 2,000 to 5,000 gm. The capsule is smooth and tense, and the liver is yellow with fat or yellowish green with retention of bile. If early cirrhosis is present, there is slightly increased resistance upon cutting. The parenchyma feels greasy, and thin sections of the liver float in water. The lobules are enlarged, and the central veins may be indistinct.

In the second type, centrilobular fibrosis is the major hepatic change. Portal fibrosis is minor. We call the lesion *chronic sclerosing hyaline disease*. This disorder usually repre-

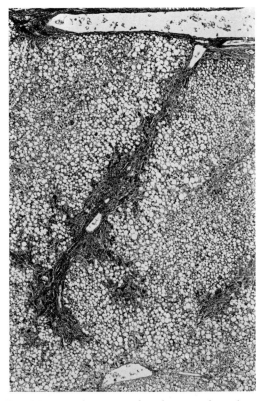

Fig. 28-16 Early stage of cirrhosis in fatty liver of alcoholic. Fibrosis and bile duct proliferation can be seen along terminal branch of portal tree. Irregular manner in which connective tissue invades periphery of lobules clearly shown. Little change around sublobular and central vein at bottom.

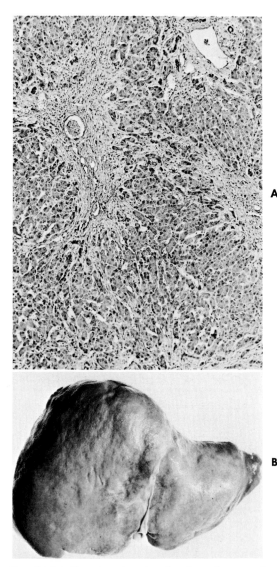

A

B

Fig. 28-17 Chronic sclerosing hyaline disease of liver without nodules. **A,** Fibrous destruction of centrilobular areas and slight widening of portal areas. **B,** Surface has sandstone appearance.

sents a sequela of acute sclerosing hyaline necrosis in which the necrosis and inflammatory reaction has subsided, but the fibrous tissue obstructing the venous outflow tract at the level of the central veins and sublobular veins becomes condensed (Fig. 28-17, *A*). Patients with the chronic sclerosing disease have an indolent clinical course characterized by muscle wasting and resistant ascites and frequently by functional renal failure. Wedged hepatic vein pressure is nearly always elevated.[282] At autopsy, the liver is of normal size or small but has a smooth or fine sandstonelike surface (Fig. 28-17, *B*).

In a third type, which occurs in most patients with early cirrhosis, there is both a a centrilobular and a portal component, and both fatty change and centrilobular sclerosis are observed. The lobular pattern is altered, small regenerative nodules are seen, and communicating septa may connect centrilobular and portal areas.

Although there are all degrees of severity in the cirrhotic process, the next step in progression may be termed *moderate cirrhosis*. The liver is enlarged from slightly above normal to 3,000 or 4,000 gm. A characteristic gross feature of chronic alcoholic liver disease

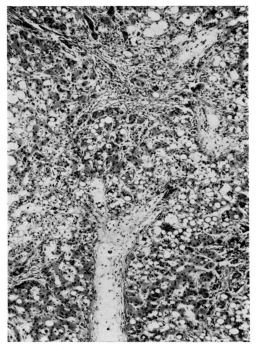

Fig. 28-18 Moderate cirrhosis. Fatty change and early obliteration of central and subhepatic veins. Granular fatty liver of 25-year-old male Mexican with history of chronic alcoholism.

is the firm rubbery quality of the liver. It is more resistant to cutting, and the fibrous septa delineate nodules 1 mm to 3 mm in diameter. Occasional areas of scarring and lobular atrophy may be seen. These scars are irregular in configuration, usually being about 1.5 cm in greatest dimension. Beginning at the margin of the atrophic areas, the pseudolobules become smaller until near the center they disappear completely. Nearly every liver shows severe obliterative change along the outflow tract. The central veins have disappeared or are in the process of obliteration (Fig. 28-18). The small hepatic veins are severely damaged, and even larger veins are sclerosed in some areas, particularly where there is gross scarring. The vascular sclerosis probably follows attacks of hyaline necrosis, although a milder degree of connective tissue proliferation does occur in fatty livers in which there is no hyaline necrosis. There are no lobules with a normal pattern. Instead, connective tissue septa now surround pseudolobules of variable size. Probably as a result of necrosis, regeneration occurs in some portions of the liver, and this further distorts the normal architecture so that the hepatic and portal veins may come to occupy positions near one another in the septa. Infiltration with round cells and, occasionally, neutrophils may occur in the septa. Fatty change is present in the majority, and hyaline necrosis and cholestasis are also frequent.

It is probable that in the histogenesis of moderate cirrhosis, both portal sclerosis and centrilobular sclerosis have played a part, and, when bridging septa connect the two, all normal lobules disappear. Attacks of cellular necrosis also may aid in the disruption of the normal pattern and lead to the formation of larger nodules of regenerative type. The patients in this stage of cirrhosis usually die in hepatic coma, or with bleeding or intercurrent infection, especially pneumonia.

In the advanced stage of Laennec's cirrhosis, the liver is smaller and more nodular, the weight usually being between 1,000 and 1,600 gm. The nodules are most often between 1 mm and 4 mm in diameter but occasionally may be as large as 1 cm or 1.5 cm. The surface is roughened by the projecting nodules (Plate 5, *C*). The liver offers marked resistance to cutting, and, after sectioning, the characteristic yellowish brown nodules are sharply outlined and appear as though they have been embedded in the pale gray bands

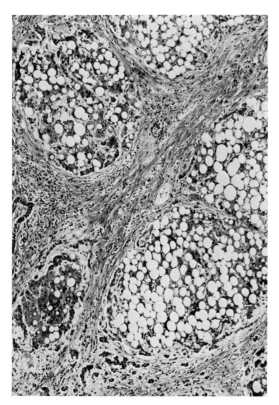

Fig. 28-19 Advanced stage of cirrhosis in 49-year-old white woman, known alcoholic for many years. Increase of connective tissue forms septa that subdivide liver into many small pseudolobules. Patient died in hepatic coma. Portacaval shunt done one year before death, but patient continued to drink excessively.

of connective tissue (Plate 5, *D*). In some irregular areas, there may be complete absence of lobular structure. On microscopic examination, the liver is composed entirely of pseudolobules and wide bands of connective tissue (Fig. 28-19). Much of the outflow tract is obliterated, especially its smaller radicles. The large and thick-walled hepatic veins that remain may be near some of the larger portal triads, the two being separated only by the connective tissue bands.

In the late stage, there is usually diminution or absence of fat. The collagenous connective tissue is dense, but there may be small foci of hyaline necrosis, usually without inflammatory exudate or sclerosis of sinusoids. Focal areas of cholestasis secondary to loss of communication between the regenerative nodules and functioning bile ducts may be observed. Often, the liver cells in the hyperplastic nodules have abnormally large hyperchromic nuclei or even two nuclei. The cells in areas of recent regeneration are distin-

guished by their lack of lipochromic pigment. The problem of increased hepatic iron storage in the alcoholic is discussed on p. 1207.

Following surgery for a portacaval anastomosis, many patients will abstain from further use of ethanol, and a biopsy taken at the time of surgery may be compared with autopsy material many years later. There is usually considerable improvement: the connective tissue septa are thinner and less cellular, the portal lymphatics are less prominent, and the liver cells in the pseudolobules often are normal in appearance.

In some alcoholics, the first symptoms are those of advanced cirrhosis. There is nothing in the history to indicate that the patient ever had a large fatty liver with an attack of jaundice that would indicate necrosis of liver cells. It would seem that in some alcoholics the cirrhotic process may progress through various stages of severity to the atrophic or "hobnail" liver with little or no fat demonstrable on biopsy. The quantitative aspects of alcohol consumption and malnutrition may well determine whether or not fibrosis and pseudolobules occur with or without fatty change. Certainly in the presence of severe fatty change, the sequence of necrosis of hepatic cells, jaundice, and coma is more likely to develop. Also, such patients seem to be more susceptible to fatal infections, pancreatitis, and delirium tremens.

It has been shown by injection-corrosion casts of normal and cirrhotic livers that in cirrhosis there is an enlargement of the hepatic arteries and arterial bed, with an increased number of communications between the hepatic arteries and portal veins.[5] The portal and hepatic venous systems are reduced in size, the change being much more severe on the hepatic vein side. The reduction of venous systems often is associated with fibrosis. Anastomotic channels occasionally are seen between portal and hepatic veins. It is interesting that no significant differences were observed in the vascular pattern of Laennec's and postnecrotic cirrhosis.

In advanced cirrhosis, portal hypertension with variceal bleeding is the most common complication and cause of death. An increased frequency of peptic ulcer also is seen in these patients, and bleeding from this source must always be considered. In some patients, ascites may become chronic and resistant to treatment, while in others the ascites is easily controlled or spontaneously disappears. Hepatic encephalopathy is easily precipitated by hemorrhage, infection, or further insults to the liver.

Coarsely nodular cirrhosis

Coarsely nodular cirrhosis is a morphologic term for a variety of conditions in which the nodules are large, round, and discrete, ranging between 0.5 cm and 1.5 cm in diameter. We include in this category the types of nodular cirrhosis that have been called postnecrotic (Plate 5, *E*), posthepatitic, idiopathic, cryptogenic, and nonalcoholic cirrhosis. We have left as a separate group miscellaneous types of cirrhosis associated with other diseases included in the classification on p. 1197. The connective tissue is softer and more spongy than in most examples of alcoholic cirrhosis. Probbly the resiliency is a prerequisite for the development of larger nodules. Although a large number of cases are of undetermined etiology, subdivisions based upon concepts of pathogenesis and etiology may be formed: (1) chronic active hepatitis and (2) cryptogenic cirrhosis.

Chronic active hepatitis (p. 1194) is a cirrhotic condition in which a hepatitis-like pattern of necrosis and exudate is superimposed. It is characterized by autoimmune features and clinical exacerbations and remissions.

The etiologic factors concerned with the single but changing histologic pattern known as chronic active hepatitis are as follows:

1 Autoimmune (chronic active lupoid hepatitis)—LE cell preparations, antinuclear antibodies, and smooth muscle present

2 Hepatitis B (chronic active viral hepatitis)—HAA is detectable in low titers

3 Drug induced (chronic active toxic hepatitis)

4 Unknown (cryptogenic chronic active hepatitis)

In the category of *cryptogenic (postnecrotic; posthepatitic) cirrhosis* are diseases that vary in etiology, pathogenesis, and morphology. Some may represent the terminal inactive stage of chronic active hepatitis. A small percentage of patients in this group will have hepatitis-associated antigen in their sera, and others have autoimmune factors in their sera. It seems, therefore, that cryptogenic cirrhosis may follow viral hepatitis or chronic active hepatitis. In those patients who have no positive serologic reaction for either the hepatitis-associated antigen or the autoimmune factors and have a negative history of oxyphenisatin use, the condition may represent the inactive

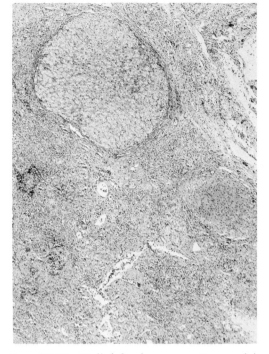

Fig. 28-20 Well-defined regenerative nodule amidst collapsed inflamed stroma in coarsely nodular cryptogenic cirrhosis.

stage of one of the two diseases or is truly cryptogenic in origin. The fact that there have been no symptoms of acute necrosis may attest to the subclinical character of the disease in some individuals until advanced cirrhosis, portal hypertension, and hepatic failure terminate life.

The liver usually weighs about 700 gm to 1,000 gm. The nodules are round, bulging, and discrete and are separated by broad areas of loose, collapsed tissue that usually is heavily infiltrated by lymphocytes. Some patients in whom a diagnosis of cryptogenic cirrhosis is made actually have had alcoholic cirrhosis but have stopped drinking for a prolonged time and deny alcoholism. In such patients, the liver shows revascularization of the dense collagen that classically characterizes alcoholic cirrhosis. The regenerative nodules have continued to grow, losing the poorly defined pattern usually observed in the alcoholic. The newly formed nodules do not have the intrasinusoidal collagen seen in the early stages of alcoholic cirrhosis (Fig. 28-20).

Other patients with coarsely nodular liver may have no symptoms. They actually appear to have only nodular hyperplasia without significant collagen deposition. Many patients with so-called "posthepatitic cirrhosis" fall into this group. Other diverse types of chronic liver disease that may, on rare occasion, terminate with coarse nodules and be no longer identifiable without prior biopsies include Banti's disease, rare cases of primary biliary cirrhosis, a peculiar cirrhosis associated with diabetes mellitus, and cirrhosis occasionally associated with rheumatoid arthritis.

Pigmentary cirrhosis

The liver is a major participant in the metabolism of iron. Normally, the body contains 4 gm to 5 gm of iron, most of which is present in hemoglobin. The amount of iron absorbed in the diet is regulated by the need to replace that lost by hemorrhage or in pregnancy. Iron absorbed from the intestine is transported by transferrin, an iron-binding protein synthesized by hepatocytes. The latter also store unneeded iron as ferritin. The liver cells have only a limited capacity to store iron as ferritin. When this capacity is exceeded, the iron is stored in lysosomes in the form of large aggregates of hemosiderin. The iron leaves the liver cells when needed for hemoglobin synthesis, again attached to transferrin. Iron also may leave the liver by another avenue, for it has been shown that it can be excreted in the bile.[199] In addition to the role of the hepatocyte in iron metabolism, the sinusoidal lining cells, being part of the reticuloendothelial system, break down senescent erythrocytes, thus preserving the iron for reuse by the bone marrow.

There are many conditions in which excess iron may be present in the liver. In one category are those diseases in which there is either hemolysis or inability on the part of the bone marrow to incorporate iron into erythrocytes. In both of these conditions, blood transfusions may add to the body store of iron. Under these circumstances, the liver stores the unused iron. This may be temporary as in folic acid deficiency, where the hemoglobin may be as low as 4 gm per 100 ml and the hepatocytes on biopsy contain a large amount of hemosiderin. When the patient receives remedial therapy, the hemosiderin is again used for hemoglobin synthesis and a biopsy of the liver shows no stainable iron. In any one of many hemolytic disorders or after blood transfusions, the reticuloendothelial system in the liver participates in the breakdown of red blood cells, and, therefore, a large amount of hemosiderin is present in the Kupffer cells. Usually, there is some movement of this iron into the parenchymal cells. In some of the chronic anemias, there is an increased absorption of iron from the intestine so that storage in the hepatocytes is increased. In these anemias, where only a mild to moderate increase of storage iron may involve both Kupffer cells and hepatocytes, there is no damage to the liver and the disorder is usually termed *hemosiderosis* or *siderosis*. However, the interpretation of a needle biopsy of the liver in which there is only a mild to moderate increase of iron in the hepatocytes is difficult for the pathologist, because the excess iron may represent a more serious disease and all the clinical and laboratory data must be taken into account by the clinician.

In contrast to the more simple disorders of iron storage are those diseases in which a great excess of iron is stored, with resultant damage that may progress to cirrhosis. Under these circumstances, the body may contain 20 gm or more of iron and other organs will store the metal. These include the pancreas, myocardium, stomach, skin, and endocrine glands. Once the iron damages any organ, most notably the liver or the myocardium, so that morphologic or functional abnormalities are present, the term *hemochromatosis* is applied. The development of structural change in the liver bears some relation to the amount of iron stored and the duration of storage.

The disorders in which large amounts of iron accumulates include (1) idiopathic hemochromatosis, a familial inheritable disorder, (2) alcoholic liver disease, (3) portacaval shunt siderosis, (4) aregenerative anemias, and (5) excess dietary intake. The latter is seen principally in South Africa, where the Bantus often ingest large quantities of iron in food or drink prepared in iron utensils. This condition has been known as *Bantu siderosis*. It may lead to increased iron absorption and storage within the reticuloendothelial system and liver.[198] When the iron content of the liver is over 2% of the dry weight, full-blown hemochromatosis may develop. Advanced osteoporosis and collapse of vertebrae have been reported in patients with severe siderosis.[232] It is possible that the osteoporosis is consequent to difficulty in phosphate absorption because of large amounts of iron in the diet. In *refractory anemias*, especially those characterized by accelerated erythropoiesis and defects in maturation and in which the patient may receive blood transfusions, secondary hemochromatosis and cirrhosis eventually may develop.[238, 239] In patients with aplastic anemia who have had more than a hundred transfusions, the liver changes at autopsy may simulate hemochromatosis.[266]

The most common form of excess iron storage associated with liver disease occurs in alcoholism. This may be seen in any stage of alcoholic liver disease, from the fatty liver to advanced cirrhosis. It has been stated that ethanol increases the absorption of iron once cirrhosis is present.[228] The reasons for increased iron absorption in alcoholism are not entirely clear. The daily intake of iron, 15 mg or more, in those who drink cheap wine may be of such magnitude that increased absorption results.[254] Both a low-protein diet and chronic anemia favor iron absorption. The effects of the alcoholic beverage itself, pancreatic dysfunction, and portal hypertension are unsettled. We have observed excess iron in those who presumably drank only distilled liquor. In our biopsies from patients with alcoholic liver disease, about 5% have some degree of siderosis. Ordinarily, the iron in alcoholic liver disease is minimal or moderate when compared with the degree of cirrhosis. Fatty change and sclerosis of the outflow veins when present point toward the correct diagnosis. However, there are rare instances in which the amount of iron in a cirrhotic liver is such that it is difficult on biopsy to distinguish alcoholic liver disease with excess iron storage from idiopathic hemochromatosis.

A number of cases of fairly rapid storage of iron in the liver have been observed following portacaval shunts in patients with cirrhosis of the liver.[221] A similar increase has been demonstrated in experimental animals after shunt surgery.[207]

Idiopathic hemochromatosis is an inheritable disorder in which there is increased iron absorption. It affects men far more often than women, in a ratio of about 17:1. Studies of families with the disease have not as yet shown the exact mode of inheritance. It appears that both mendelian dominant and recessive mechanisms may be involved.[186] Women usually are protected until after the menopause because they lose iron during menstruation. Recent studies indicate that there is a marked decrease of iron-binding ability of gastric juice in patients with hemochromatosis as compared with normal subjects. This might allow increased absorption of dietary iron.[253]

In one study of the relatives of patients with idiopathic hemochromatosis, it was found that many of them had excess hepatic iron, whereas the families of those with alcoholic cirrhosis did not have such findings.[274]

Ionic iron does not appear in the serum. Instead, 2 molecules of ferric iron are bound to 1 molecule of a carrier protein, transferrin. Normally, excess transferrin is present. Only one-third is combined with iron. The remainder is unbound. In hemochromatosis, the transferrin levels may be unchanged, but the degree of saturation or binding is usually nearly 100%. Other laboratory results are relatively nonspecific. However, patients with chronic anemia also may have increased iron absorption and saturated iron-binding capacity.

Early in idiopathic hemochromatosis the external surface of the liver may be smooth, but as cirrhosis develops it becomes granular, less often nodular. The weight varies from 1,000 gm to 3,000 gm. On sectioning, the liver has a dark rusty brown appearance. At necropsy, it is rewarding to use the Prussian blue test on all livers that are excessively brown. On analysis, the liver in hemochromatosis contains between 1,000 mg and 10,000 mg of iron per 100 gm of liver, dry weight. This is compared with a normal figure of 188 mg or less.[202] A quantitative determination of iron may be done on a biopsy specimen of the liver. This test uniformly discloses far more iron than is found in alcoholic cirrhosis. In addition to iron, excess quantities of lead, molybdenum, and copper are present.[201]

Microscopically, early in the disease there may be a uniform distribution of hemosiderin (iron-containing pigment) within the liver cells and Kupffer cells without fibrosis. Ordinarily, however, there is a variable degree of proliferation of fibrous tracts, leading to well-defined cirrhosis (Fig. 28-21). Although there is some correlation between the amount of iron present and the severity of cirrhosis, it is not invariable, as some livers with advanced cirrhosis will not have as much stainable iron as will those with poorly developed fibrous septa. The hemosiderin appears to have some predilection for the peripheral portion of the lobules. As the iron increases, the aggregates become larger and cellular detail may be obscured. Masses of hemosiderin are also seen within Kupffer cells, although this does not usually parallel the amount of hemosiderin within the hepatic cells. Focal areas of necrosis may occur, and

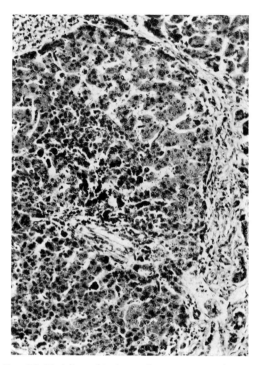

Fig. 28-21 Idiopathic hemochromatosis with pigmentary cirrhosis (54-year-old white man who died of primary carcinoma of liver). Liver cells and Kupffer cells contain fine granules of hemosiderin. In area of recent necrosis near center, histiocytes are filled with hemosiderin.

after healing, such areas are marked by closely packed macrophages whose cytoplasm contains dense accumulations of hemosiderin. Following necrosis, regenerative nodules develop that have little or no stainable iron within their cells. Fibrous tissue septa connecting the portal spaces are similar to those in alcoholic cirrhosis except for iron-filled macrophages and, occasionally, iron-encrusted connective tissue fibers. An iron-free pigment, hemofuscin, may accumulate within both the fibrous tracts and the hepatic cells. Fatty change is seen in a small proportion of patients with pigmentary cirrhosis. It appears to be most prevalent in those who have diabetes mellitus. The latter, when present, is usually mild. The presence of increased iron and/or melanin in the skin may give the patient a blue-gray or bronzed appearance—hence the name *bronze diabetes* for this complication of hemochromatosis. In many patients with pigmentary cirrhosis, there is a long course (ten years or more) that exceeds the duration in most other types of cirrhosis. Portal hypertension and ascites are not common complications, but primary carcinoma of the liver occurs more often than in any other type of cirrhosis.[198, 202]

The mechanism by which iron may damage the liver and pancreas, producing necrosis and fibrosis, is not known. Studies with the electron microscope show that iron is deposited within the lysosomes of the liver cell and, to a lesser extent, in some of the mitochondria. The latter may then degenerate. It is likely that a point is reached where some of the liver cells populating the lobules are unable to survive with so much of their cytoplasm occupied by iron.[314]

Wilson's disease (hepatolenticular degeneration)

Wilson's disease (hepatolenticular degeneration) is an inheritable disorder characterized by the abnormal metabolism of copper.[318] It apparently is inherited in an autosomal recessive manner. Both homozygotes and heterozygotes occur in the same families.[192] Wilson's disease should always be suspected in a child or young person with symptoms of liver disease. The symptoms include abdominal pain, jaundice, ascites, and anemia, especially hemolytic anemia. The presence of brown pigmentation of Descemet's membrane at the limbus of the cornea, the Kayser-Fleischer ring (Plate 6, *C,* and Fig. 24-11) is pathognomonic of Wilson's disease. The hemolytic anemia has been attributed to a flux of copper, for large amounts have been noted in the urine.[255] A similar hemolytic disorder has been studied in sheep grazing on pastures where there is a large content of copper in the forage. It is important that the diagnosis of Wilson's disease be made in its early stages because treatment with penicillamine may restore the patient to health. When the disease is recognized in a family, all of its members should be examined for evidence of presymptomatic disease.

Studies with radioactive copper have shown that 30% to 70% is absorbed in the normal person, most of which is quickly stored in the liver attached to hepatic proteins, but some circulates for a short time loosely bound to serum albumin. A small amount is probably bound to amino acids and can pass through a semipermeable membrane. This portion is probably responsible for the normal excretion of copper in the urine. In patients with biliary fistulas, it has been shown that about 10% of the radioactive copper will be secreted in the bile. The radioactive copper soon disappears from the blood and a secondary rise

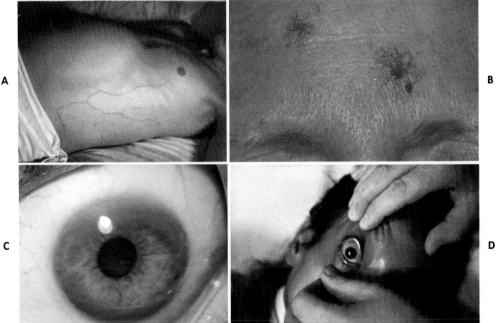

Plate 6

A, Hepatic cirrhosis. Ascites, congested veins, pigmented male nipple, axillary alopecia, and absence of striae.

B, Arteriovenous fistulas (vascular spiders) in diabetic cirrhosis. Arterial blood supply in center of lesion.

C, Kayser-Fleischer ring in Wilson's disease.

D, Jaundice and biliary cirrhosis following ligation of common bile duct.

(**A** and **D,** From Wiener, K.: Skin manifestations of internal disorders, The C. V. Mosby Co.)

in the plasma follows its incorporation into ceruloplasmin (blue protein) by the hepatocytes and secretion of this alpha globulin into the blood. The copper atom is essential for life because it enters into the final reduction of O_2 to H_2O by cytochrome C oxidase.

In Wilson's disease it has been shown that radioactive copper is absorbed in a normal fashion but continues to circulate for the half-life of the metal loosely bound to albumin. Furthermore, larger than normal amounts of copper pass into the urine. No secondary rise in plasma copper bound to ceruloplasmin is noted. This failure is probably the best diagnostic test for Wilson's disease. The physiologic role of ceruloplasmin is unknown. Its plasma level is usually but not always low in Wilson's disease. A less than normal percentage of radioactive copper is found in the stool, and an unanswered question in Wilson's disease is whether or not there is increased intestinal absorption or decreased secretion in the bile.

The failure to excrete absorbed copper leads to its accumulation in the liver. After this organ is saturated, the copper content of the brain, particularly in the basal nuclei, rises to abnormal levels. The kidney also stores the metal. The liver has the capacity to store copper far in excess of that needed in the normal person or in the heterozygote. It has been termed the "copper pot."[309] In the presymptomatic homozygote, the "pot" is not full. Only after it is full does the copper spill over into the blood and other tissues and into the urine in large quantities. In Wilson's disease, the increase in the liver appears to occur first in the cytoplasm,[220] where the copper ion is capable of causing episodes of necrosis. These may produce attacks of jaundice and a rise in serum transaminase levels. The type of hepatocellular necrosis that occurs in the early stages of Wilson's disease has not been well documented. Strangely enough, hyaline necrosis (Fig. 28-22) has been reported,[246] a phenomenon we have also observed. Other changes include fatty vacuolization, increase of lipochrome pigment, and glycogen-filled nuclei. Electron microscopic studies have disclosed marked abnormalities of the mitochondria that may be related to the fatty change.[304] All the stages in liver damage that lead to cirrhosis are not documented, but fibrosis, septal formation, and regenerative nodules may develop over a period of years.

In the advanced stage, the septa are usually

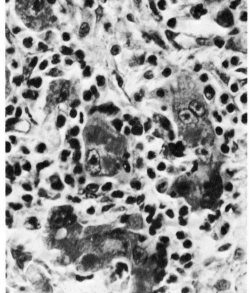

Fig. 28-22 Hyaline necrosis of hepatocytes in Wilson's disease. Abundant neutrophilic and round cell infiltrate in sinusoids.

rather thin, the regenerative nodules are large, and areas of collapse may be present. Abnormalities such as vacuolated nuclei and fatty change may or may not be seen in the advanced stage. Electron microscopic studies have shown that copper is present in lysosomes and presumably not so likely to cause necrosis of hepatocytes.[220]

The laboratory findings in Wilson's disease usually include a low serum copper, low serum ceruloplasmin, and increased copper in the urine. A marked increase in urine copper follows the administration or penicillamine. A needle biopsy of the liver, when analyzed for copper with the emission spectrograph, shows a marked increase of the metal. An amount above 25 mg per 100 gm dry weight of liver is pathognomonic.

Biliary cirrhosis

Obstruction of the biliary tract (either extra-hepatic or intrahepatic) may, if prolonged, lead to cirrhosis of the liver.[270] The causes of biliary obstruction have already been discussed (p. 1196). The appearance of the liver in extrahepatic obstruction depends upon the degree of blockage and the time factor. Neoplastic obstruction is usually complete, and the patient dies before a true cirrhosis develops. The biliary tree proximal to the neoplasm is greatly dilated. The liver is green to greenish brown and finely granular.

An increase of connective tissue along the large bile ducts near the hilum of the liver usually is noted. The organ is usually increased in size and palpable before death, although there is little increase in weight. Occasionally, a carcinoma obstructing the ducts grows very slowly and the increase in connective tissue is such that the liver cuts with increased resistance, and the diagnosis of early biliary cirrhosis is justified. Obstruction of the common duct due to a calculus or a benign stricture is usually incomplete. Therefore, the distention of the ducts and bile stasis in the liver are not so extreme as with cancerous obstruction. On occasion, a stone or a stricture may obstruct the common duct for years and lead to true biliary cirrhosis. The liver has a granular appearance or may even be nodular. It cuts with increased resistance, and fibrosis is as marked as it is in Laennec's cirrhosis. In neglected patients, biliary cirrhosis of this type may cause portal hypertension, splenomegaly, and hemorrhage from esophageal varices. A portacaval shunt may become necessary.[183]

In the early stage of extrahepatic obstruction, microscopic examination reveals that dilatation of the large ducts near the hilum is constant, whereas the size of the smaller ducts is variable. Some increase of fibroblastic activity with the formation of spurs is seen within thirty to fifty days.[297] Bile stasis is predominantly centrilobular. In the intermediate stage, between sixty and 100 days, connective tissue is more abundant and often has a concentric configuration around the bile ducts. Both at this stage and in the later cirrhotic phase, the arrangement of the connective tissue may give a "pipestem" effect (Fig. 28-23). Bile duct proliferation is present in only a small percentage of the total. The mononuclear type of exudate may be increased. Focal necrosis of hepatic cells, of either the lytic or the eosinophilic type, is frequent. Consequent to necrosis, particularly of cells in the peripheries of the lobules, bile lakes may form. The central veins are present and a normal lobular architecture can be seen throughout most of the liver. A few abnormal hyperplastic nodules may make their appearance at this stage. Later, especially in patients with calculus obstruction or stricture, a well-developed cirrhosis is noted, with connective tissue septa outlining pseudolobules. Intralobular bile stasis is irregular but is now both central and peripheral. There is usually no bile stasis within the interlobular ducts,

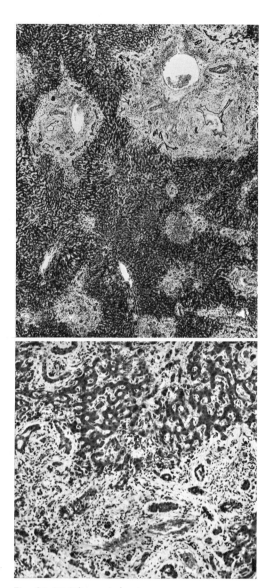

Fig. 28-23 Biliary cirrhosis.

probably because it is absorbed within the lobule. Occasionally, a liver may exhibit wide connective tissue septa, with abundant bile duct proliferation. Fatty change, extensive necrosis of parenchyma, and even abscesses may complicate the disease.

Primary biliary cirrhosis

Primary biliary cirrhosis is a chronic disease of unknown etiology that occurs most frequently in middle-aged women. It primarily affects the intrahepatic bile ducts, although the clinical features are similar to those of prolonged partial obstruction of the extrahepatic bile ducts. The name is somewhat of a misnomer since cirrhosis is a late

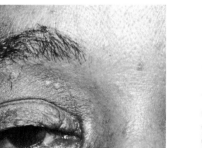

Fig. 28-24 Xanthomas of eyelid in primary biliary cirrhosis.

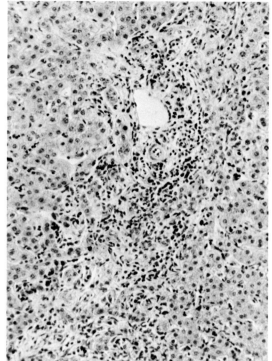

Fig. 28-25 Destruction of bile ducts and limiting plate in primary biliary cirrhosis.

development. However, since the disease progresses to cirrhosis and death, the term primary biliary cirrhosis[184] is widely used.

Primary biliary cirrhosis apparently was described in 1846, 1857, and 1874 but was not recognized until Hanot wrote his thesis on "Hypertrophic cirrhosis with jaundice" in 1876.[284] In the late 1800's, many investigators referred to it as Hanot's disease and believed it to be a variety of "common" cirrhosis related to chronic alcoholism. Others believed it was a rare type of liver disease associated with chronic jaundice and splenomegaly and classified it under the term *hypertrophic biliary cirrhosis* or *Hanot's disease*. Hanot described the initial lesion as a catarrhal inflammation of the small bile ducts that he believed originated from a toxic or possibly an infective process. Early in the twentieth century, some cases were described that seemed to represent an intermediate form between Banti's disease and primary biliary cirrhosis. To this day, occasional patients are seen who have most of the clinical features of Banti's disease but autopsy findings that resemble primary biliary cirrhosis.

Primary biliary cirrhosis is a disease that affects women in the ratio of about 9:1 over men. The onset is generally insidious, beginning with pruritus that may be present for several months to a year before the onset of dark urine or icterus. After jaundice has been present for months, the patient notices foul fatty stools, and slowly the skin manifestations of hyperlipemia become noticeable as xanthomas or fine yellowish deposits in the creases of the palms of the hands, antecubital spaces, and elsewhere (Fig. 28-24).

From the onset, there is hepatomegaly, and about one-half of the patients have splenomegaly. The impaired flow of bile into the intestine causes a deficiency of the absorption of vitamin D and calcium. As a result, the patient develops osteomalacia, often with bone pain and even compression fractures of the vertebrae. Weight loss occurs as greater amounts of the ingested fat are excreted in the stool. The course is slowly downhill, with the duration of life after the diagnosis is established being from five to fifteen years.

By the time a liver biopsy is taken early in the disease, the cholangioles and the limiting plate are destroyed[28, 187] (Fig. 28-25). Lymphocytes, sometimes accompanied by plasma cells, infiltrate and widen the portal areas and often completely surround the larger bile ducts. The arterioles usually are thickened. The liver cords are regular, but the cells generally are shrunken. The Kupffer cells are hyperplastic, and occasional foci of lymphocytes or plasma cells are seen. Bile stasis is more frequently periportal than central. Primary biliary cirrhosis is the only disease in which periportal cholestasis predominates. Bile lakes, an occasional autopsy finding in the liver of patients with extrahepatic biliary tract obstruction, is not a feature of primary biliary cirrhosis.[187] Some studies have shown epithelioid granulomas in the portal areas in as many as one-third of the patients. Granulomas have been encountered much less frequently in our material.

As the disease progresses, the portal areas widen and may unite. Pseudoductules proliferate considerably throughout the later stages of the disease and may be mistaken for ductules. Pseudoductules consist of paired columns of cells rather than round ductular structures with lumina. Regenerative nodules may occur late in the disease, but at autopsy true regenerative nodules are not present. Instead, portal areas have united to produce a finely granular liver. Signs of portal hypertension are a late occurrence. Only an occasional patient will have esophageal varices.

Among the diseases associated with primary biliary cirrhosis is ulcerative colitis. Usually when the bile ducts are affected in ulcerative colitis, the larger ducts are involved and not the ductules. However, in rare instances, classic primary biliary cirrhosis does follow ulcerative colitis.[260]

The laboratory findings in primary biliary cirrhosis resemble those of prolonged obstruction of the extrahepatic bile duct. Total bilirubin levels are usually in the range of 2 mg to 15 mg per 100 ml. The serum alkaline phosphatase activity is elevated, usually to twenty-five times the normal range, levels far greater than those seen in most other obstructive diseases of the biliary tract. The serum cholesterol, triglycerides, and particularly phospholipid levels all are markedly elevated. The serum is not lactescent, apparently because of the high levels of phospholipid. If the serum is frozen, the lipids are deemulsified and form a creamy layer at the meniscus. However, prolonged extrahepatic biliary obstruction or, rarely, prolonged cholestatic reactions to drugs[247] may produce similarly elevated serum lipid levels. Serum albumin levels may drop when the disease progresses. Serum globulin elevations are due to increases in low density β-lipoproteins and in gamma globulin. There is frequently an elevation of serum IgG and IgM levels.[29] Serum transaminase activities generally are elevated in the 200 to 400 unit range. This elevation has led many clinicians to misdiagnose the disease as chronic active hepatitis.

In the past few years, investigators have noted an elevated antiliver antibody level in the sera of patients with primary biliary cirrhosis.[215, 317] This subsequently has proved to be an antibody to the membranes of mitochondria from any cell of any one of several mammalian species. The antimitochondrial antibody test has proved to be most helpful in the diagnosis of primary biliary cirrhosis.[195, 236]

The etiology of primary biliary cirrhosis is unknown. A similar destruction of ductules is found in animals experimentally treated with naphthyl-iso-thiocyanate[252] and in some patients treated with the experimental antineoplastic agent, *methyl methane sulfonate.*[190] Neither immunologic nor toxic damage can be established in any causal relationship, however. Recent reports disclose that in primary biliary cirrhosis the liver copper levels were increased to twenty-five fold.[320] There was no abnormality in the serum ceruloplasmin, but familial studies for liver copper content are not completed.

Recently, an association has been noticed between Osler-Weber-Rendu syndrome (hereditary hemorrhagic telangiectasia) and primary biliary cirrhosis.[283] This is of interest, since the Osler-Weber-Rendu syndrome is a familial disorder, and no familial distribution of primary biliary cirrhosis has been established in the past. In most of our patients who have the combination of these diseases, the major disease was primary biliary cirrhosis. The Osler-Weber-Rendu syndrome was recognized because other members of the family had multiple hemangiomas. The mitochondrial antibodies have not been detected in members of the families of patients with primary biliary cirrhosis in spite of the fact that this factor has been almost uniformly present in the sera of the patients with primary biliary cirrhosis.

In occasional patients with multiple epithelioid granulomas similar to those in sarcoidosis, there is also destruction of the ductules and markedly elevated alkaline phosphatase activity. Most of these patients have had other features of sarcoidosis, such as granulomatous involvement of lymph nodes. Primary biliary cirrhosis has been reported with primary cutaneous amyloidosis.[321]

Syphilitic cirrhosis

In congenital syphilis of the liver, now a rare entity, there is an overgrowth of mesenchymal tissue along the sinusoids that causes wide separation of the hepatic cells. Small gummas or even large soft ones occasionally are seen. Usually, spirochetes are easily demonstrable. Syphilitic cirrhosis rarely eventuates. In the tertiary stage of acquired

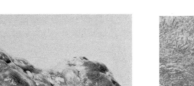

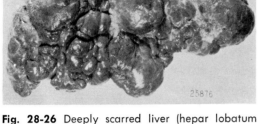

Fig. 28-26 Deeply scarred liver (hepar lobatum syphiliticum) which weighed only 710 gm (79-year-old white woman, known syphilitic, who had received some antisyphilitic therapy three years before death). Several large hyperplastic nodules present. Stringy adhesions bridge some deep transverse fissures.

syphilis, it is stated that about one-sixth of all patients will develop gummas of the liver.[307] Gummas may be solitary or multiple and confluent, sometimes forming a large mass. On sectioning, they have a dull gray-yellow area of central necrosis, an irregular outline, and a marginal zone of gray-white, glassy-appearing granulation tissue. They often are widespread and, in healing, the scar tissue replacing them contracts to form deep scars that may incompletely divide the liver into masses of irregular size—hepar lobatum syphiliticum. In other instances, the crevices are not so deep, but stringy adhesions may bridge the indentations (Fig. 28-26). More rarely, the liver is deformed by linear depressions. This occurs alone or in combination with the deeply scarred organ. Beneath these linear deformities are bands of connective tissue that do not have the appearance of healed gummas. In hepar lobatum syphiliticum, there may be little more than the normal amount of connective tissue, or, on the contrary, the connective tissue may be diffusely increased.

Microscopically, in the gummatous stage there are isolated areas of necrosis surrounded by granulation tissue relatively poor in fibroblasts and usually sparse in epithelioid cells (Fig. 28-27). The granulation tissue impinges upon the liver parenchyma, and necrosis of the latter appears to occur at this junction. Lymphocytes and plasma cells are common, both around the areas of gummatous necrosis and along the portal tracts. Later, wide bands of scar tissue are irregularly distributed throughout the liver, sometimes in combina-

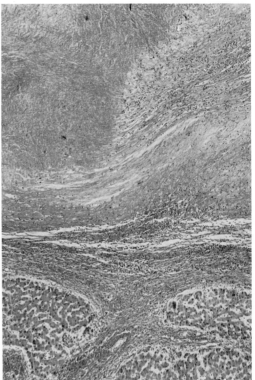

Fig. 28-27 Margin of gumma showing irregular outline, sparsity of epithelioid cells, and zone of granulation tissue (41-year-old woman who died of massive gastrointestinal hemorrhage; syphilis not diagnosed antemortem).

tion with unhealed gummas. In some areas, it appears that connective tissue septa may form without an intervening gummatous stage. The plasma cell infiltrate is helpful in distinguishing gummas from tuberculosis of the liver. Occasionally, a patient with advanced syphilis of the liver is a chronic alcoholic, and in this case the liver will be fatty.

Parasitic cirrhosis

Fibrosis in the liver may result from infection with the liver fluke, *Clonorchis sinensis,* or with schistosomes.

Clonorchis sinensis, prevalent in the Far East and in India, lodges in the biliary system, where it may, at times, cause sufficient obstruction to result in a cholangitic biliary cirrhosis (p. 448).

Schistosomiasis results in hepatic fibrosis due to the lodgment of ova in the liver. Cirrhosis occurs particularly with *Schistosoma mansoni* and less frequently with *Schistosoma japonicum* and *Schistosoma haematobium*. The liver is nodular and firm and shows pale gray fibrotic areas on the cut surface. The fibrosis is particularly evident about portal areas, where ova or their remnants may be seen. Broad bands of fibrous tissue may be formed, with considerable architectural distortion. In later stages, clinical manifestations may be similar to those of portal cirrhosis, with ascites, splenomegaly, anemia, and esophageal varices (p. 451 and Fig. 13-20).

Congestive or cardiac cirrhosis

The condition known as congestive or cardiac cirrhosis is a fibrosis and alteration of architecture of the liver associated with severe and prolonged passive hyperemia of the type that occurs in patients with constrictive pericarditis and rheumatic heart disease.[295] This lesion is seen less commonly with hypertension or other forms of cardiac disease. Repeated bouts of decompensation appear to favor development of fibrosis. Because it is the end result of prolonged passive congestion, it is discussed with this disorder on pp. 108 and 1233.

Miscellaneous types of cirrhosis

Cirrhosis may complicate the course of any one of many serious diseases that are systemic or that primarily involve other organs in the body. The most common lesions of the liver associated with ulcerative colitis are pericholangitis, active chronic hepatitis, fatty liver, cirrhosis, nonspecific hepatitis, bile duct carcinoma, primary biliary cirrhosis, viral hepatitis, and primary sclerosing cholangitis.[260] Pericholangitis and fibrosis may lead to protracted jaundice and finally a biliary type of cirrhosis. Young women with ulcerative colitis may have "lupoid hepatitis" or "chronic active hepatitis" that eventuates in cirrhosis.

In diabetes mellitus, fatty changes and even cirrhosis may occur, especially in patients whose disease is poorly controlled. Cirrhosis in nonalcoholic diabetic patients is rare. It has been observed that patients with alcoholic cirrhosis may secondarily become diabetic.[218] Rheumatoid arthritis,[235] regional enteritis,[205] scleroderma,[189] rheumatic fever, hyperthyroidism,[262] and various bacterial infections[243] occasionally may be complicated by cirrhosis. A mild degree of cirrhosis is not infrequently noted in the liver of elderly persons. This seems to be a slow progressive disease that occurs in patients in whom there are no etiologically demonstrable factors except possibly poor eating habits. In Boeck's sarcoidosis, the lesions in the liver may

progress to cirrhosis.[265] In sickle cell anemia, a postnecrotic type of cirrhosis may be seen. Presumably, this is caused by anoxic necrosis due to stagnation of the sickled red blood cells in the sinusoids.[302] There is also the possibility that patients who receive many transfusions may develop serum hepatitis followed by cirrhosis.

PATHOPHYSIOLOGY OF CHRONIC LIVER DISEASE

Many pathophysiologic phenomena are associated with chronic liver disease. Although some of these are the direct result of hepatic disease, others are unexplained. The concept that hepatic failure or insufficiency may occur to a variable degree is important. The most severe form of hepatic failure that results in coma is discussed on p. 1190. Only occasionally does the cirrhotic patient die in deep coma without some complication. The patient with cirrhosis, however, may from time to time have episodes of encephalopathy that are reversible. Some of these mild forms of encephalopathy are indicated by an inability to perform simple mental tests. More severe forms include flapping tremor, agitation, and disorientation.

Among the most common complications of chronic liver disease that progresses to cirrhosis are portal hypertension, esophageal varices, and ascites.

Portal hypertension

Resistance to the flow of blood within the liver in chronic liver disease is the most common cause of portal hypertension. This is the intrahepatic type, in contrast to the posthepatic type caused by lesions of the hepatic veins and the prehepatic type in which the obstruction is due to disease of the portal vein.

Any form of cirrhosis may be associated with *intrahepatic portal hypertension*. The mechanism of obstruction has been attributed to compression by regenerative nodules.[237] However, at least in the alcoholic patient, significant portal hypertension develops in response to centrilobular intrasinusoidal collagen deposition before the development of regenerative nodules.[282] The normal pressure in the portal vein is 6 mm to 10 mm Hg.[279] In cirrhosis, it may rise to 20 mm or 30 mm Hg. The rise in pressure is directly related to the resistance to blood flow within the liver.

In about 15% of patients in whom portacaval shunt has been performed, the pressure on the hepatic side of a clamp placed on the vein is higher than it is on the splanchnic side, indicating that there is a reversal of portal vein blood flow in these patients.[258] The pressure within the portal system also may be measured with a fair degree of accuracy by introducing a catheter, via an antecubital vein, superior vena cava, and inferior vena cava, into a small branch of the hepatic venous system. The catheter, when wedged into the vein, gives a pressure reading similar to the pressure within the portal vein system.[281] The so-called wedged hepatic vein pressure is quite helpful in determining whether the point of obstruction is within the liver or is extrahepatic. In the latter, normal wedged pressures are observed.

The portal vein averages 7 cm in length and is formed by the confluence of the superior mesenteric and splenic veins. The inferior mesenteric vein joins the latter about 3 cm from its junction point. Thus, the portal blood is received from the gastrointestinal tract, mesentery, spleen, gallbladder, and pancreas. Obstruction to the flow of blood through the portal trunk results in hypertension throughout the system. In cirrhosis, this develops slowly but finally results in chronic passive hyperemia of the tissues drained by the portal vein. The intestines and peritoneum appear congested and edematous. The spleen is enlarged, firm, and dark red, and it may weigh between 300 gm and 1,000 gm. There is poor correlation between the size of the spleen and increased pressure in the portal system.

Posthepatic portal hypertension is rare. It results from impaired entry of hepatic vein blood into the vena cava. Neoplastic obstruction, thrombosis of the hepatic veins or of the inferior vena cava, and prolonged congestive heart failure may transmit elevated pressure through the hepatic vascular bed to the portal vein.

Prehepatic portal hypertension is an uncommon condition in which the liver is presumed not to be involved. Banti's disease (idiopathic portal hypertension) is the principal example (p. 1234). Extrahepatic portal vein thrombosis has been considered a cause of portal hypertension.[291, 294] However, neoplastic occlusion of the extrahepatic portal vein produces neither portal hypertension nor splenomegaly. In thrombosis of the portal vein associated with portal hypertension, it is likely that sludged blood already under increased pressure caused the thrombus to form.[259]

Rarely, myelofibrosis will produce portal hypertension. The elevated pressure probably results from the fibrous involvement of all of the intrahepatic portal structures rather than increased blood flow through the enlarged spleen.

Esophageal varices

As a result of the increase in pressure within the portal system, the blood tends to bypass the liver and return to the heart by various collaterals (Fig. 28-28). These develop more prominently cephalad than caudad. Although hemorrhoids are common, they do not cause serious complications. More important are the large varices susceptible to erosion and fatal bleeding that arise in the mucosa at the lower end of the esophagus (Fig. 28-29). The blood entering these veins is short-circuited from the portal system via the coronary veins of the stomach and also the left gastroepiploic and vasa brevia. In the lower third of the esophagus, the submucosal veins are poorly supported and are subjected to trauma by the passage of food and also may be eroded by regurgitation of gastric juice. In patients with cirrhosis, both esophagoscopy and roentgenograms are used to demonstrate the presence of these varices. The exsanguination that follows rupture of the esophageal varices is a precipitating cause of death in 15% of cirrhotic patients. An additional 35% die of liver failure following esophageal hemorrhage.[268] *Other anastomoses* between the portal circulation and systemic veins may develop between the hilum of the liver and the umbilicus along the paraumbilical plexus of veins. These may cause enlargement of the umbilicus (caput medusae). When greatly enlarged paraumbilical veins are present, the term "Cruveilhier-Baumgarten syndrome" sometimes is applied, especially when a murmur is heard. The cutaneous vessels over the upper abdomen may be enlarged. Other communications may be established through the veins of Retzius in the posterior mesentery and directly through the diaphragm via the veins of Sappey. It has been demonstrated that blood may even find its way through the periesophageal veins directly to the pulmonary veins and the left atrium.[203]

In patients who have esophageal varices demonstrable by esophagoscopy or by roentgenograms and who may or may not have

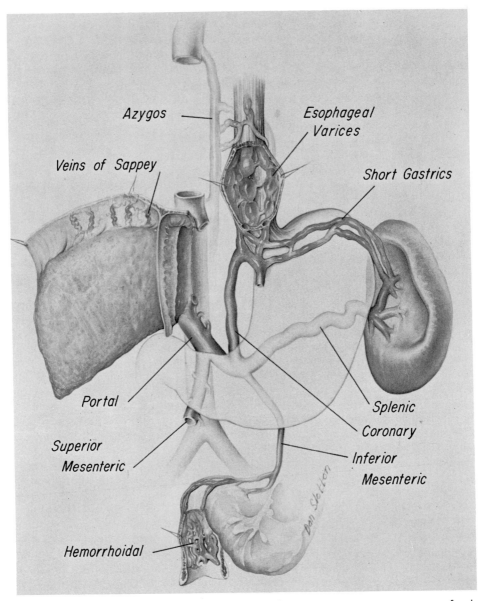

Fig. 28-28 Portal vein and its major tributaries showing most important routes of collateral circulation between portal and caval systems.

had an episode of hemorrhage, an anastomosis of the portal vein to the inferior vena cava often is performed in order to decompress the portal system. If an end-to-side anastomosis is used, it prevents any possible retrograde flow in the portal vein via anastomoses with branches of the hepatic artery within the liver. It has been proposed that a side-to-side anastomosis may help the nutrition of the liver by allowing more hepatic artery blood to circulate through the parenchyma and then out through the portal vein (reversed flow). Following either procedure, the varices tend

to decrease in size, as does the spleen in about one-half of the patients. Further variceal hemorrhage is rare. The status of the fibrotic process in the liver is unaffected by surgery. Proper diet and abstinence from ethanol are of most value in allaying the progress of the disease. In extrahepatic obstruction, a portacaval shunt is usually impossible and a splenorenal shunt may be done.

Ascites

Ascites often accompanies portal hypertension, especially in the advanced stages of cir-

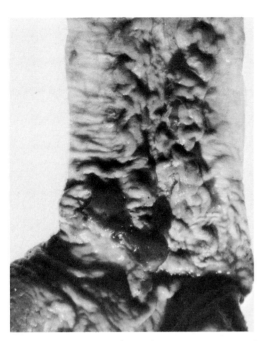

Fig. 28-29 Large esophageal varices on mucosal surface of opened esophagus.

rhosis (Plate 6, *A*). The fluid within the abdomen is in the nature of a transudate, having a specific gravity of around 1.010. The mechanism of formation is complex and many factors are involved.

1 Portal hypertension and increased capillary filtration pressure
2 Postsinusoidal block
3 Hypoalbuminemia
4 Impaired renal function
5 Inferior vena cava hypertension
6 Hyperaldosteronism

The simple *elevation of portal pressure and increased capillary filtration pressure* may produce a soft tissue transudate from the entire splanchnic bed and liver surface. *Postsinusoidal block* is thought to be the fundamental mechanism of ascites formation. Not only does increased lymph form, but the liver surface tends to "weep considerable amounts of fluid." *Hypoalbuminemia* may contribute to ascites by reduction of osmotic pressure in plasma, but its importance is believed to be minimal.

Impaired renal function in cirrhosis may be caused by pooling of splanchnic blood that results in a diminution of *effective* blood volume, reduced glomerular filtration rate, and sodium retention. There is also evidence that renal dysfunction is more directly related to hepatic disease. It has been suggested that in some unexplained fashion the liver may have a direct effect on the kidney's ability to excrete sodium. The failure to excrete sodium would be responsible for increased blood volume and partially responsible for ascites.[250]

Inferior vena cava hypertension has been proposed as a contributing feature in the formation of ascites.[263] Frequently in cirrhosis, an enlarged caudate lobe will compress the inferior vena cava into an elliptical shape that may cause a pressure differential between the abdominal and thoracic inferior vena cavae. It has been suggested that such narrowing may impair both hepatic venous and renal venous return, thus accentuating hepatic postsinusoidal portal hypertension and renal sodium clearance.

Aldosterone has strong sodium retaining properties and is frequently found in increased amounts in the plasma and urine of cirrhotic patients, particularly those with ascites.[251, 267] Whether the elevated levels are a primary or secondary feature in relation to ascites is unknown. Certainly *hyperaldosteronism* is not a prerequisite for ascites.

Other changes

Arteriovenous fistulas of skin. Arteriovenous fistulas of the skin, also called vascular spiders, are often observed in chronic liver disease (Plate 6, *B*). Recently, similar lesions in the lung have been described and recognized as a possible cause of finger clubbing and cyanosis that is common in patients with alcoholic cirrhosis.[196] Other findings in the cirrhotic patient may include palmar erythema,[191] pallor of the fingernails, enlargement of the salivary glands, and Dupuytren's contractures of the palmar fascia. In women with cirrhosis, a decrease in menstruation or amenorrhea is frequent.

Testicular atrophy. Testicular atrophy is a common accompaniment of cirrhosis.[194] Alteration or inactivation of circulating estrogens appears to be a normal function of the liver[231] that is disturbed when the liver is extensively damaged in cirrhosis. The testis is susceptible to excess of circulating estrogens. Hormonal changes, however, are not always accompanied by the physical findings of estrogen excess.[208, 288]

Functional renal failure. Functional renal failure is a common cause of death in cirrhotic patients. Those who develop ascites tend to develop elevated creatinine levels, followed by a less striking rise of serum urea. Although it is well established that functional renal failure follows reduced renal plasma flow and an even more pronounced decrease in glomerular filtration rate, the pathogenesis is unknown. The total plasma volume actually is increased, although it is possible that splanchnic pooling of blood secondary to portal hypertension may reduce *effective* plasma volume.[213, 269] Recent research indicates that the liver disease is linked somehow with the impaired renal capacity to excrete sodium and with consequent fluid retention.[250] Functional renal failure is not associated with any recognized pathologic changes in the kidneys.

Cirrhotic glomerulosclerosis. Cirrhotic glomerulosclerosis, a diffuse thickening of the glomerular basement membrane, occurs in up to 28% of cirrhotic patients.[234] There is disagreement as to functional importance of the lesion. In our experience, it is not associated with impaired renal function. It may represent an agonal edematous thickening of the basement membrane.

Proximal convoluted tubular epithelial proliferation. In patients who die of hepatic failure, the parietal layer of Bowman's capsule may be involved by a peculiar proliferation of swollen eosinophilic cuboidal epithelium like that in the proximal convoluted tubules. Only scattered glomeruli may be involved. The cause of hepatic failure seems unimportant.

Burr cell hemolytic anemia and cirrhosis. Patients with cirrhosis and those with other liver diseases associated with absence of the spleen may develop a hemolytic process with large numbers of circulating erythrocytes that have spurlike projections from their surface producing marked distortion. The syndrome is associated with anemia and hyperbilirubinemia, predominantly in the indirect fraction. Conflicting experimental results have been reported regarding whether or not the defect is in the erythrocytic cell membrane[298] or in a plasma fraction.[222] The prognosis is poor. Occasionally, *hypersplenism* is associated with portal hypertension. The pancytopenia may be a major concern in Banti's disease.

Folate deficiency. Folate deficiency is relatively common in alcoholic liver disease, producing anemia, although rarely to the extent that megaloblastosis is prominent. Usually, folate deficiency is blamed on inadequate dietary intake,[227] but it is possible that the damaged liver may be incapable of adequate storage.

Hemorrhagic phenomena. Hemorrhagic phenomena are common in patients with hepatic disease. A number of defects in the clotting mechanism have been studied.[277] Fibrinogen, prothrombin, and factors VII, IX, X, and V all are produced by the liver parenchymal cell, and the platelet count may be reduced by hypersplenism.

DIFFERENTIAL DIAGNOSIS OF JAUNDICE

A rise in either the indirect-reacting or direct-reacting bilirubin fraction in the blood results in yellow pigmentation of the skin, or jaundice. More than 97.5% of normal patients have serum bilirubin levels between 0.1 mg per 100 ml and 1.0 mg per 100 ml. Although a serum bilirubin above 1.2 mg per 100 ml is abnormal, jaundice does not become manifest until a level of 2 mg per 100 ml or more is reached. Since jaundice is dependent upon bilirubin in tissue fluids, there may be a lag between the rise of the serum bilirubin level and evident jaundice. Minimal jaundice is best detected by examination of the sclerae. Bilirubin has an affinity for elastic connective tissue, so that these structures are more deeply pigmented (Plate 6, *D*). However, in severe jaundice, the skin, interstitial fluids, and most of the body tissue (with the exception of the central nervous system) become bile stained. In chronic jaundice, the skin may appear a deep green-yellow and, in a few instances, an increase in melanin may result in a dark brown to black skin.

Pigments other than bilirubin may cause a yellow skin. Patients who ingest large quantities of carrots or carrot juice may have carotenemia. This pigment is best seen in the palms of the hands but not in the sclerae. Atabrine, an antimalarial drug, also is capable of causing a yellow skin, as is dinitrophenol.

When confronted with a jaundiced patient, the physician has the responsibility for making an etiologic diagnosis as quickly as possible. The use of the terms "medical" and "surgical" jaundice emphasizes the importance of etiology. The most common causes of jaundice are viral hepatitis, cirrhosis, extrahepatic biliary obstruction, and drug-induced liver disease. In patients under 40 years of age, jaundice frequently is caused by viral hepatitis and drug sensitivity. In those over the age of 40 years, extrahepatic biliary obstruction is more common. Cirrhosis is a common cause of jaundice both before and after 40 years of age.

A careful history and physical examination followed by the performance of essential hepatic tests and, on occasion, by a needle biopsy of the liver usually will lead to a correct diagnosis. The patient should be questioned about exposure to other jaundiced individuals, transfusions, and needle sharing, all related to viral hepatitis. Further questioning about ingestion of hepatotoxic drugs or exposure to hepatotoxic chemicals is necessary. A family history of jaundice may suggest an inheritable disease or a common infective, toxic, or dietary disorder. Questions regarding alcohol intake are important but often are ignored in the private hospital. Travel outside the United States may point to infectious hepatitis. If pain is present, its location, type, severity, and radiation are important. The patient should be questioned about pruritus and a change in stool color. The presence or absence of previous attacks of jaundice should be ascertained. Neoplasms usually cause an unremitting jaundice, while calculus obstruction, cirrhosis, and chronic active hepatitis are usually intermittent.

On physical examination, the size and consistency of the liver and the presence or absence of tenderness, nodules, or masses should be determined. A normal liver may extend below the costal margin but is too soft to palpate. The cirrhotic liver has a firm palpable edge. Even in advanced cirrhosis, when the liver is contracted, the lower margin may be felt on deep inspiration. In early to moderate cirrhosis, the liver is enlarged as a rule and the edge may be as low as the umbilicus. A small liver rarely is associated with biliary tract obstruction but often develops after liver cell necrosis. Careful palpation for an enlarged gallbladder, splenomegaly, and minimal ascites is likewise helpful in diagnosis. Splenomegaly, ascites, and many vascular spiders suggest chronic liver disease in the jaundiced patient. Primary carcinoma of the gallbladder may produce a hard palpable organ that is associated with jaundice as the initial symptom. A tense distended gallbladder favors neoplastic obstruction rather than choledocholithiasis. In cholelithiasis, the gallbladder usually becomes too fibrotic to undergo distention when the common bile duct is obstructed by a stone. Usually no single laboratory test is relied upon to diagnose the cause of jaundice, but certain combinations of abnormal tests (Table 28-1) help to delineate various subgroups that narrow the possibilities to be considered by

the clinician. The total serum bilirubin, as well as the direct-reacting and indirect-reacting fractions, always is determined. The test is usually performed at frequent intervals, for it gives valuable information as to the course of the disease.

Jaundice may be associated with an elevation of the indirect-reacting fraction of the serum bilirubin or, as is far more common, an elevation of both the direct-reacting and indirect-reacting fractions. The van den Bergh reaction shows that only a few diseases cause an excess of indirect-reacting bilirubin in the adult. Among these is the excess production of bilirubin that follows severe hemolysis. Congenital hemolytic anemia, mismatched blood transfusions, and severe hemorrhage into tissues or body cavities are examples. A different etiology is noted in Gilbert's disease, in which there is a failure to remove a normal quantity of unconjugated bilirubin from the blood. Jaundice due to a lack of UDP-glucuronyl transferase in the infant, Crigler-Najjar disease, is discussed on p. 1231. A similar disease in the adult has been reported. The drug novobiocin may inhibit glucuronyl transferase and thus cause an unconjugated hyperbilirubinemia. Occasionally, patients with alcoholic cirrhosis may have a predominance of indirect-reacting bilirubin that is often associated with spur cell anemia or hypersplenism. The unconjugated bilirubin does not filter through the glomerulus, so there is no bilirubinuria, as is seen in jaundice due to conjugated hyperbilirubinemia.

In most cases of jaundice (i.e., those caused by viral hepatitis, cirrhosis, biliary tract obstruction, and drugs), there is an increase of both direct-reacting and indirect-reacting bilirubin. Accompanying the rise in direct-reacting bilirubin there is also an increase in indirect-reacting bilirubin, often to as much as 50% in some disorders. The level of the total bilirubin may bear some relationship to the severity of disease in patients with liver cell necrosis and obstruction of the bile ducts but is more useful in following the course of the disorder. Declining levels of the serum bilirubin reflect the healing phase of hepatitis, drug jaundice, and other disorders. The height of the serum bilirubin is regulated not only by degree of hepatic dysfunction and red cell destruction, but also by rate of excretion of the water-soluble conjugated fraction in the urine. This fraction binds to albumin and is not freely excreted. The direct-reacting bilirubin may rise to higher levels in parenchymal cell disease than in obstructive disease for unknown reasons. Although biliuria is prominent early in viral hepatitis, biliuria decreases as jaundice deepens even though the direct-reacting bilirubin in serum rises.

Patients with hyperbilirubinemia who have markedly elevated serum transaminase levels and little or no rise in the alkaline phosphatase are considered to have liver cell necrosis or hepatocellular jaundice. Viral hepatitis, chemicals, poisons, and certain drugs must be considered in differential diagnosis. In some instances, a rise in alkaline phosphatase occurs in viral hepatitis and may, in older patients, be difficult to differentiate from obstructive biliary tract disease, particularly if the patient is at the stage where serum transaminase levels have dropped to a range of 500 units or less. Patients in shock or severe heart failure may have anoxic centrilobular necrosis associated with high serum transaminases and jaundice, but usually the bilirubin levels are in the range of 5 mg or less.

An increase in serum bilirubin levels accompanied by a high alkaline phosphatase usually is associated with intrahepatic or extrahepatic biliary obstruction. Although extrahepatic biliary obstruction due to stone, cancer, or stricture is a well-known cause of jaundice with a high alkaline phosphatase, the possibility of drug-induced liver disease must always be ruled out. On occasion, obstructive disease may be accompanied by a moderate rise in serum transaminase (Table 28-1). The prothrombin activity may be reduced in either hepatocellular or prolonged obstructive disease. Administration of parenteral vitamin K will correct prothrombin deficiency induced by biliary tract obstruction but will have little effect on the impairment caused by liver cell necrosis.

Primary biliary cirrhosis in its early stage is often impossible to differentiate from extrahepatic obstruction on the basis of history and the physical and laboratory examinations. A needle biopsy is sometimes performed, but this may be hazardous if the jaundice is really due to common bile duct obstruction, for bile leakage or hemorrhage may ensue. As a consequence, the diagnosis of obstructive biliary tract disease usually is made by clinical and laboratory means. Patients with choledocholithiasis tend to have a painful disorder that is often associated with cholangitis that produces bed-shaking chills, fever, and a high incidence of gram-negative bacteremia. Similar episodes of cholangitis may develop in the patient with a bile duct stricture. Cholangitis is uncommon in a patient with a malignant obstruction.

Unless the patient is quite ill from duct obstruction, with signs and symptoms of cholangitis not responding to antibiotics, or has diabetes, conservative treatment is the rule for a period of time in the hope that improvement will follow. A drop in bilirubin level or alkaline phosphatase is evidence against a malignant obstruction, except for carcinoma of the papilla of Vater, parts of which may slough periodically. A return of the bilirubin level to normal indicates a benign lesion and a cholecystogram often is performed. In the absence of gallstones, normal concentration by the gallbladder suggests that drug cholestasis is the cause of jaundice.

If jaundice does not abate, and doubt remains as to whether the disease is medical or surgical, a percutaneous cholangiogram may be attempted. A needle is inserted into the liver and, by gentle aspiration, an intrahepatic duct is sought while slowly withdrawing the needle. Contrast material injected into a duct should outline the obstructive site. The failure to enter a duct in this procedure in experienced hands suggests nonobstructive disease, and a needle biopsy may be taken.

In patients suspected of having primary biliary cirrhosis, surgery is sometimes the final resort in order to be certain that a curable lesion does not exist, since a needle biopsy may not be definitive. Further experience with the serum mitochondrial antibody may enable a positive diagnosis of primary biliary cirrhosis to be made without resorting to surgery. Other causes of jaundice and increased alkaline phosphatase include primary and secondary carcinomas and, on occasion, pyogenic and amebic liver abscesses as well as granulomas.

The presence of underlying chronic liver disease in the jaundiced patient usually is manifested by a low serum albumin and a high serum globulin. An enlarged, firm liver, splenomegaly, vascular spiders, and ascites are nearly conclusive evidence of chronicity. The first symptom of chronic active hepatitis and alcoholic liver disease may be jaundice, even though chronic liver disease already is present. The jaundice that occurs in the patient with chronic liver disease is usually of limited duration, but more than one episode is not uncommon.

The diagnosis, care, and management of

the jaundiced patient remain a challenge to the clinical acuity of the physician. This has been true for over one hundred years, since the pioneers in the study of liver disease first published their observations.

DISEASE IN INFANTS AND CHILDREN

Neonates, infants, and children all are subject to liver disease. In the neonate, acute liver disease predominates. In infants and children, both acute and chronic disease occur. Normally an acholuric, nonhemolytic type of jaundice (so-called physiologic jaundice) is noted in most infants from the second to the fourth day of life. This is apparently due to a lack of a normal amount of glucuronyl transferase necessary to form bilirubin glucuronide. This enzyme increases quickly in the full-term newborn infant, and jaundice subsides rapidly. In the premature infant, however, the jaundice may be more severe and prolonged, leading to higher levels of unconjugated bilirubin in the plasma. When the serum bilirubin rises above 20 mg per 100 ml, irreversible damage to the central nervous system, called kernicterus, may be caused by unconjugated bilirubin entering nerve cells, particularly those in the basal ganglia. Inasmuch as unconjugated bilirubin circulates bound to albumin, a low serum albumin or drug therapy that replaces the bilirubin bound to albumin will allow central nervous system damage at levels lower than 20 mg per 100 ml.

The hyperbilirubinemias of the neonate have been classified as unconjugated and conjugated. However, regardless of etiology, this separation does not become too evident before the liver has enough glucuronyl transferase to conjugate bilirubin. This occurs by the fifth to the seventh day of life. The etiology of mild hyperbilirubinemia in the neonate often is not established. In the Los Angeles County–University of Southern California Medical Center, this includes approximately 50% of all neonates with hyperbilirubinemia.

In the premature infant with hyaline membrane disease, jaundice may occur on the third day, and eventually the bilirubin rises to levels that produce kernicterus.

In *hemolytic disease of the newborn*, jaundice is apparent within the first twenty-four hours. When due to ABO incompatibility, the disease is usually mild, although kernicterus can occur if the serum bilirubin level rises

excessively. A far more serious disorder occurs when the Rh factor is involved. In the past, this disease was known as *erythroblastosis fetalis* or *icterus gravis neonatorum*. Usually, the liver is unable to secrete the large amount of unconjugated bilirubin that results from the hemolysis of erythrocytes. In fatal instances, there is an even distribution of bile in canaliculi and also in the hepatic cells. Liver cell necrosis of variable degree may occur and probably accounts for an increase in conjugated bilirubin that is sometimes seen in hemolytic disease of the newborn infant. Extramedullary erythropoiesis is common and may be extensive not only in the liver, but also in other organs. Because of the danger of kernicterus, severe hyperbilirubinemia often is treated by exchange transfusions. More recently, other methods of treating hyperbilirubinemia have been attempted. The mother may be treated with phenobarbital in the last weeks of pregnancy, and the drug is also given to the newborn infant. Phenobarbital is capable of increasing the smooth endoplasmic reticulum of hepatocytes, which is associated with the formation of glucuronyl transferase necessary for the conjugation of bilirubin and glucuronide.[209, 275] It also has been shown that exposure of the newborn infant to blue light will cause a breakdown of the unconjugated bilirubin in the blood.[245]

Other causes of unconjugated hyperbilirubinemia in the neonate include septicemia, especially that due to gram-negative organisms, hematomas, and maternal diabetes mellitus. In the latter, the infant is usually large and hypotonic and has hypoglycemia. Congenital syphilis still occurs and may be manifested by hepatosplenomegaly and unconjugated hyperbilirubinemia. Fibrosis, cellular injury, and cholestasis are the usual microscopic findings. It has been noted that serologic tests on the neonate who has congenital syphilis of the liver may be negative, whereas the tests on the mother will be positive.[290] A newly recognized disease, *fatal neonatal hepatic steatosis*, occurring in siblings, has been reported.[289]

Although any one of several diseases may cause an increase in conjugated bilirubin, it may not become manifest until after the first week of life, for the liver is incapable of conjugating a large amount of bilirubin. The diseases most often responsible are either *infections* or *biliary atresia*.[322] It has been estimated that as many as 90% of infants with an obstructive type of jaundice have either neonatal hepatitis or biliary atresia.[313] It is important to differentiate between these, because surgical exploration is necessary in biliary atresia. There are many morphologic variations in atresia of the extrahepatic bile ducts.[300] When only a segment of the more distal portion of the extrahepatic bile duct system is affected, surgical correction is often possible. When the proximal portion or all of the system is atretic, an anastomosis is impossible. In these patients, liver transplantation has been attempted.[303] On microscopic examination of the liver, there is cholestasis that is predominantly centrilobular (but sometimes also peripheral and within the bile ducts), bile duct proliferation, and periductular fibrosis that is often lamellar (Fig. 28-30). In some instances, foci of necrosis may surround pools of bile in the periphery of the lobules—the so-called bile lakes. Fibrosis along the biliary tracts usually leads to biliary cirrhosis, so that at autopsy one-third or more of the liver is composed of fibrous tissue. However, there is considerable variation in severity not related to the duration of the obstruction. Furthermore, when the obstruction is relieved by surgery, the biliary cirrhosis may regress.[312] Children with unrelieved atresia who survive several years may develop portal hypertension and die of bleeding esophageal varices.

In *neonatal or giant cell hepatitis,* icterus commonly develops in the first or second week of life. Microscopically, the lesion is characterized by bile stasis and the formation of giant multinucleated hepatic cells (Fig. 28-31) that may have from eight to forty nuclei. They usually contain bile pigment in their cytoplasm and appear swollen with excess fluid. With progression of the disease, the giant multinucleated cells become more numerous, bile stasis is more prominent, and often intralobular tubules filled with bile are noted. Rather characteristic is the diffuse formation of intralobular connective tissue that tends to surround rather sharply the circumscribed giant cells. Excess hepatic hematopoiesis is nearly always present. A majority of patients have an increased amount of iron in the liver cells and usually excess iron in the spleen.[286] There is ordinarily some increase of connective tissue in the periportal spaces, but the bile ducts are usually not so prominent as they are in biliary

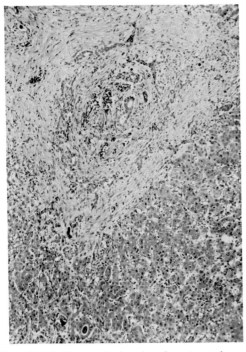

Fig. 28-30 Concentric bands of periportal connective tissue and bile stasis characteristic of biliary cirrhosis (5-month-old infant with atresia of common bile duct).

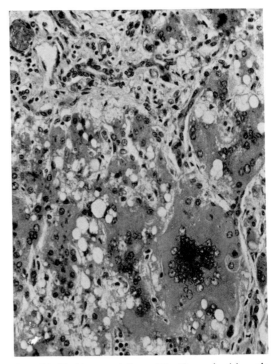

Fig. 28-31 Neonatal hepatitis (3-week-old male infant). Multinucleated giant cells compose most of parenchyma. Increased connective tissue can be seen along sinusoids and in periportal space. Intracanicular bile stasis at upper right and lower left.

atresia. Sometimes they are small and hypoplastic. A cellular exudate composed of mononuclear leukocytes and even eosinophils is often present about the portal triads.

When neonatal hepatitis with giant cell transformation is noted on needle biopsy or at autopsy, every effort should be made to establish its etiology. The rubella syndrome, cytomegalic inclusion disease, galactosemia, and biliary atresia may cause similar microscopic findings. However, there remains a sizable group of patients in whom no etiologic factor is recognized. The majority of these patients recover with no sequelae. Some die in the acute stage, and in a few the liver involvement progresses to cirrhosis. In some instances, giant cell transformation is severe in biliary atresia, before the typical fibrosis around the bile ducts appears, and in a needle biopsy specimen it is impossible to distinguish it from neonatal hepatitis. When the giant cell change is extreme and reaches the limiting plate around the triads, the diagnosis of neonatal hepatitis can be made with a high degree of certainty.

A number of specific infections character-

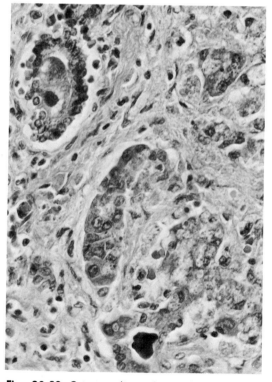

Fig. 28-32 Cytomegalic inclusion body in bile duct epithelial cell at upper left. Cholestasis and liver cell necrosis evident. Patient had jaundice since birth and died at 2½ months of age.

ized by liver cell injury are rare causes of neonatal jaundice. In *cytomegalic inclusion disease,* bile stasis is prominent. Some multinucleated giant cells may be seen, but necrosis of liver cells is variable. When present, the giant intranuclear inclusions are diagnostic (Fig. 28-32). As a rule, they are more easily found in the kidney. Cytomegalovirus hepatitis may produce jaundice in the adult.[315] In *herpes simplex,* the transmission of the disease is probably through the placenta, and the death rate is high.[219] There is a large tender liver and a rise in SGOT but no jaundice as a rule.[193, 256] An extensive coagulation necrosis is seen in the liver. The individual virus particles and the method of their exodus from the nucleus have been studied by electron microscopy.[271] In *Coxsackie viremia,* there may be extensive necrosis of the liver and jaundice.[241] Severe hepatitis with cholestasis and giant cell change has been observed in the rubella syndrome.[214] Coagulative necrosis also has been reported.[306] Many infants with trisomy of number 18 chromosome (E trisomy) have neonatal hepatitis and also may have biliary atresia.[185]

In the first two to three weeks of life, if an infant with *galactosemia* is given cow's milk, the liver may enlarge and jaundice supervene. The diagnosis of this condition is highly important, because the removal of galactose from the diet relieves the symptoms.[206] The newborn infant with galactosemia may present with severe infection and septicemia.

A group of infants, predominantly males (5:1), with neonatal cirrhosis has been described. The course of the disease is relatively short, and its differentiation from neonatal hepatitis is emphasized. The etiology is unknown.[311] Occasional instances of extensive necrosis of the liver in the newborn infant associated with excessive iron have been observed.

During the period of infancy (up to 2 years of age), *infantile cirrhosis* may follow some of the conditions just described, such as atresia of the common bile duct and galactosemia, or it may occur occasionally as a complication of congenital syphilis. In instances of neonatal hepatitis in which the infant survives for a year or more, fibrosis may be of such severity that the liver could be classified as *cirrhotic.*

Galactosemia[224] ordinarily becomes manifest in the first few months of life. In this disease, the toxic effects of galactose accumu-

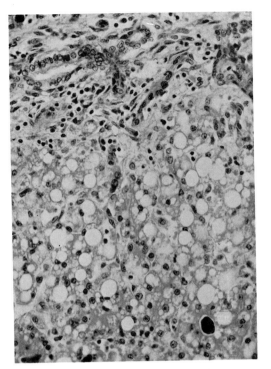

Fig. 28-33 Fatty change, intralobular bile stasis, and some increase of periportal connective tissue characteristic of galactosemia (3-week-old white male infant).

lation is noted in the liver, in the eye where lenticular opacities develop quickly, and in the brain where degeneration and mental retardation may result.[210, 316] The pathology and inheritance of the disease have been studied extensively.[197, 299]

The liver is enlarged and fatty and may become cirrhotic. Microscopically, the lobules are large, a moderate to severe degree of fatty change is present, and bile stasis is the rule. The bile plugs are contained within large acini. Often, numerous bile ducts entering the periphery of the lobules are likewise filled with bile (Fig. 28-33). An irregular increase of connective tissue widens and lengthens the periportal spaces, sometimes connecting adjacent ones, so that cirrhosis can be diagnosed. The combination of large liver lobules, fatty change, and bile stasis seems to be characteristic of galactosemia. More rarely in galactosemia, the liver contains an excess of glycogen, the cytoplasm of the cells being almost water clear, and rather delicate septa connect the periportal spaces, resulting in a different type of cirrhosis. In both of the foregoing types, the central veins are visible and regenerative change seems to be minimal. It is of interest that in children with proved

cirrhosis and ascites, proper treatment results in an apparent cessation of the disease process.

Other rare inheritable disorders of infancy include *tyrosinosis,* in which the liver may become cirrhotic and death is due to liver failure. Apparently the disease is caused by a lack of the enzyme *p*-hydroxyphenylpyruvic acid oxidase. On microscopic examination, regeneration, fatty change, and fibrosis are noted. Liver cell carcinoma may arise late in the disease.[223] In a child with features of tyrosinosis, recovery after dietary treatment has been reported.[225] Tyrosinosis is one of the many causes of the deToni-Debré-Fanconi syndrome, in which there are multiple renal tubular defects that cause the patient to have vitamin D–resistant rickets.[217] In *fructose intolerance,* hepatomegaly and jaundice are noted. This disorder is due to deficiency of the enzyme fructose-phosphate-1-aldolase. In the liver, there is fatty change, fibrosis, and cirrhosis.[272] Cirrhosis in children with *alpha-1-antitrypsin deficiency,* a genetic disorder, has recently been reported.[293]

In *Reye's syndrome,* the infant or child has an upper respiratory infection, apparently recovers, and then has an episode of vomiting, delirium, and coma, followed by death or recovery in one to two days. The liver is enlarged and transaminase levels are elevated, but there is no jaundice. At necropsy, the liver contains fatty vacuoles of the fine foamy type. The etiology of the disorder is unknown.[276]

Niemann-Pick disease usually runs its course during infancy. Cirrhosis occasionally is noted as a complication.[216] Ony a few cases of cirrhosis following proved attacks of *viral hepatitis* before the age of 2 years have been seen. Both grossly and microscopically, the liver is similar to that of coarsely nodular cirrhosis in the adult. In the West Indies, both children and adults who have ingested "bush tea" made from boiling the leaves of *Crotolaria fulva* and *Senecio discolor* may develop occlusive disease of the central and sublobular veins, with resultant hepatomegaly, ascites, and often jaundice[200, 292, 305] (Fig. 28-34). The venous lesion is first characterized by edema and later by collagenization. The large hepatic veins usually are unaffected. The sinusoids are remarkably congested, and the centrilobular hepatic cells atrophy. Later, in chronic cases, a nonportal type of cirrhosis may develop. A similar disease apparently follows the use of flour contaminated with

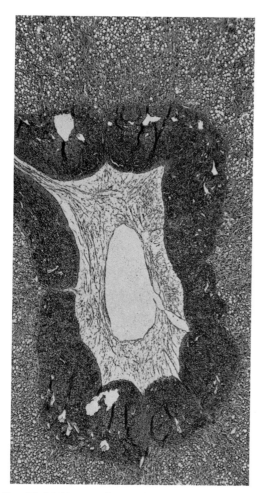

Fig. 28-34 Veno-occlusive disease of liver. (Slide courtesy Dr. G. Bras.)

Senecio in Africa.[292] Egyptian children also suffer from a disease involving the hepatic veins.[226]

In some sections of India, many cases of infantile or childhood cirrhosis are seen. A hereditary factor has been considered likely.[261] Needle biopsies have disclosed a portal type of cirrhosis.[188] In the limited material available, we have noted sclerosing hyaline necrosis similar to that seen in alcoholics.

The term *juvenile cirrhosis* is used for cirrhosis in patients between the ages of 2 and 16 years. In this age group, cirrhosis may follow biliary atresia, be secondary to one of the inborn errors of metabolism, or be of unknown origin. Biliary cirrhosis due to unrelieved atresia may be seen up to 6 or 8 years of age, although most of the patients will die before the age of 2 years.

Several of the inborn errors of metabolism may be responsible for cirrhosis in the ju-

venile patient. In *glycogen-storage disease type III,* liver failure has been observed.[230] In type IV, cirrhosis may be the cause of death.[229] In type II, Pompe's disease, glycogen is stored in excess quantity in abnormal lysosomes called "lysosomal bags." In this disorder, there is an absence of α-1,4-glucosidase.[301] Fibrosis associated with *Gaucher's cells* may lead to scarring and finally a nodular liver. In Hurler's syndrome (gargoylism), the liver may be greatly enlarged, but cirrhosis rarely develops.[257] In this disorder, there is excess accumulation of acid mucopolysaccharide, chondroitin sulfuric acid–B (β-heparin), and heparin monosulfuric acid (heparitin).[204] The hepatocytes are highly vacuolated. When studied with the electron microscope, these vacuoles appear to be a combination of lysosomes and engulfed mucopolysaccharides.

In children with *cystic fibrosis of the pancreas,* the liver may contain focal areas of fibrosis associated with dilated bile ducts containing eosinophilic casts. In more advanced states of liver disease, a true cirrhosis may develop, with formation of nodules of variable size[216, 296] (see also p. 1280).

Congenital hepatic fibrosis is a variant of polycystic disease, for microcysts are present in the dense fibrous tissue that surrounds the lobules, and a medullary sponge kidney may be present.[264] Portal hypertension is the predominating symptom. The disease was first described in children.[240] *Juvenile cirrhosis,* usually termed *posthepatitic* or *Laennec's,* has been reported.[287] This is of unproved etiology, and it is likely that as better diagnostic tests become available, fewer cases will fall into this category. In our experience, the presence of Wilson's disease has been missed most frequently in children with chronic liver disease.

DISEASE IN PREGNANCY

The most common disorder of the liver during pregnancy is obstetric cholestasis or recurrent jaundice of pregnancy, a familial disorder that has its onset in the third trimester. It is accompanied by pruritus and tends to recur with succeeding pregnancies. Pruritus of pregnancy without jaundice is a variant. It is likely that the disorder is due to an increased level of hormones in susceptible patients, especially since it has been shown that after pregnancy the same symptoms follow the use of physiologic doses of estrogens or oral contraceptives. A biopsy discloses centrilobular cholestasis without necrosis. Laboratory findings include a serum bilirubin level of less than 10 mg per 100 ml, a marked elevation of serum alkaline phosphatase, and only a mild rise in SGOT levels. An associated rise in plasma bile acids is probably responsible for the pruritus.

Viral hepatitis occurring during pregnancy seems to be no different than that seen in nonpregnant women. In our series of cases of fulminant hepatitis from 1918 to 1970, none of the patients were pregnant.

Idiopathic *fatty liver of pregnancy,* initially described in 1940,[326] is a rare, highly fatal disorder that occurs in the third trimester. During the early 1960's, many cases of fatty liver of pregnancy were reported, but most of them followed the intravenous administration of tetracycline given for the treatment of pyelonephritis. It became apparent that tetracycline hepatotoxicity in pregnancy produced a fatty liver indistinguishable from the idiopathic type. Both are characterized by epigastric pain, vomiting, jaundice, and symptoms of hepatic and renal failure. The laboratory findings usually consist of hyperbilirubinemia, lactic acidosis, azotemia, hyperamylasemia, and depressed prothrombin activity. The transaminase levels are usually under 500 units. At autopsy, the liver is only moderately decreased in size. It is yellow and has a soft consistency. Fatty change of a foamy type is present, the fat being most prominent on the sinusoidal border of the liver cell with the displacement of the eosinophilic portion of the cytoplasm around the bile canaliculus. Cholestasis is not prominent. Necrosis may vary from a mild unicellular type that follows the use of tetracycline to fairly severe centrilobular necrosis of the idiopathic variety. Pathologic changes also are seen in the renal tubules, pancreas, and brain. It is probable that tetracycline inhibits the synthesis of the proteins essential to the formation of lipoproteins, the principal form by which fat leaves the liver, thus leading to fatty liver.[324]

Eclampsia may produce hepatic symptoms or clinical liver disease. Only one instance of hepatic failure associated with the liver lesion of eclampsia was found at the Los Angeles County–University of Southern California Medical complexes from 1918 to 1970. However, patients who die from eclampsia generally have a mottled discoloration of the liver with hemorrhagic areas alternating with zones of pale ischemic necrosis and intact liver (Fig. 28-35). The periportal

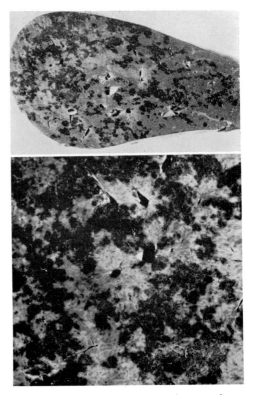

Fig. 28-35 Liver in eclampsia showing hemorrhagic appearance.

regions often have fibrin in the sinusoids and are often necrotic. The small branches of the portal vein may be thrombosed. Zones of infarction may cover several lobules. Occasionally, patients develop such hepatic alterations without the convulsions of eclampsia.[323, 325] Occasionally, diffuse hepatic necrosis occurs as a terminal event. This type of necrosis is coagulative rather than lytic, as it is in viral hepatitis. Spontaneous rupture of the liver in pregnancy is rare but does occur, usually in the third trimester of a multipara who has toxemia with or without eclampsia. The rupture nearly always occurs in the right lobe as a complication of subcapsular hematoma.[327] It is of interest that rupture of the liver may occur in women taking contraceptive drugs.

Most chronic diseases of liver preclude pregnancy, although rarely a cirrhotic patient may become pregnant. Liver disease is often difficult to evaluate because of alterations of laboratory values that are associated with pregnancy. The serum albumin level is ordinarily depressed to 2.8 gm to 3.7 gm per 100 ml (normal is 3.5 gm to 4.8 gm per 100 ml), and the alkaline phosphatase activity often is elevated as much as twice the upper limits of normal.

In the differential diagnosis of liver disease in pregnancy, in addition to the liver diseases occurring almost exclusively in pregnancy, consideration also must be given to more common illnesses, such as stones, toxins, and viral hepatitis, which may occur in a pregnant woman.

DISEASES OF INTRAHEPATIC BILE DUCTS

The most common disease of the intrahepatic bile ducts (i.e., acute cholangitis) is discussed on p. 1196. However, the ducts are subject to other disease, both primary and secondary. Among conditions unique to the ducts alone are sclerosing cholangitis, aneurysmal dilatation of the ducts, intrahepatic calculi, and pneumobilia.

Sclerosing cholangitis is a disease of the common bile duct that often extends into the liver, causing severe deformity of the intrahepatic ducts with characteristic "beading."[328] The cause of the disease is unknown, but the possibility of its being an autoimmune reaction has been considered. A similar cholangitis is sometimes associated with one of the following: ulcerative colitis, retroperitoneal fibrosis, retro-ocular fibrosis, or fibrous mediastinitis. The association of sclerosing cholangitis with ulcerative colitis is not unusual. The patient may be jaundiced for a variable period but often becomes asymptomatic. A few cases will go on to biliary cirrhosis or be complicated by a carcinoma of the ducts.[332, 333]

Aneurysmal dilation of the intrahepatic ducts is a rare disorder that is sometimes associated with polycystic disease of the liver.[329] *Intrahepatic calculi* most often occur as a complication of a chronic obstruction of the extrahepatic biliary tract but may, on occasion, be primary in the liver. An unusual disease seen in Chinese immigrants as well as in East Asia has been called *cholangiohepatitis* (Hong Kong disease). The patients may have calculi in the bile ducts, much sludge, and often remnants of *Clonorchis sinensis*.[331] Air in the intrahepatic biliary tract, or *pneumobilia,* is most often due to a cholecystoduodenal fistula.[330] The diagnosis is usually made on roentgenograms.

REGENERATION

The liver has a marked capacity for regeneration following resection, injury, or destruction of its cells. The organ regenerates rapidly when a large portion is resected. Humoral mechanisms, overloading of excretory function, and changes in hemodynamics have been evoked as possible regulators of regenerative growth. In the adult rat, following amputation of 70% of the liver, there is intense nucleic acid synthesis and mitotic activity for a period of forty-eight hours but is limited thereafter. Finally, the liver is restored to normal size.[339] Much evidence indicates that the control of regeneration is due to a humoral agent that is almost instantaneously responsive to change in liver mass.[341] The cellular changes consist of hypertrophy (DNA synthesis) followed by mitotic activity and hyperplasia.[335] The molecular events that lead to DNA synthesis include the conversion of cytidine to deoxycytidine.[338] Angiographic studies show that during regeneration the arteries probably hypertrophy and appear stretched, but no new vessels are observed.[334]

A major portion of the liver may be extirpated in the treatment of severe traumatic injury and neoplastic disease. Following this, the patient may have hypoglycemia, hypoalbuminemia, and a bleeding diathesis. The latter is caused by decreased levels of prothrombin and fibrinogen but usually is not severe. All of these complications are of short duration.[336]

TRANSPLANTATION

Only a small number of orthotopic liver transplants have been attempted, usually in patients who have a primary carcinoma of the liver or congenital biliary atresia.[303] Some patients have lived for more than a year. At autopsy, in patients who did not die of infection, the microscopic changes in the liver consist of:

1 A mononuclear cell infiltrate around portal and central veins, mostly lymphocytes but including a few eosinophils, macrophages, and plasma cells
2 Arterial intimal thickening
3 Hepatic fibrosis and occasionally cirrhosis
4 Bile thrombi
5 Enlargement of Kupffer cells
6 Necrosis and atrophy of centrilobular hepatocytes

In experimental animals, fulminant necrosis associated with infiltration of the lobular sinusoids by mononuclear cells, either lymphocytes or monocytes, has been observed.[340] A cytotoxic action has been proposed for these cells.

The results of liver transplantation in thirteen patients in England have been published.[337, 342] The histologic changes in the liver are similar to those described in the United States.

DEGENERATIONS

Degenerative changes that affect the liver, such as cloudy swelling and glycogen infiltration, are adequately discussed elsewhere in the text (p. 76).

Amyloidosis. Hepatic involvement is seen with almost equal frequency in primary and secondary amyloidosis.[348] The most common symptom is hepatomegaly, but ascites and jaundice occur in a small percentage of patients. The course is quite variable, and the diagnosis often is established by needle biopsy. The liver is enlarged and firm and has a tense capsule, rounded edges, and pale color. The cut surface is abnormally translucent in the areas of amyloid accumulation. The amyloid appears as a hyaline material between the lining cells of the sinusoids and the liver cells. Its continued accumulation causes compression, atrophy, and disappearance of the liver cells. Amyloidosis of vessel walls exclusively is more likely to be present in the primary form of the disease.

Calcification. When differential diagnosis becomes of clinical importance, calcifications in the liver may be observed on roentgenograms.[347] The most common cause is metastatic mucinous adenocarcinoma from the colon and stomach. Calcifications in other metastatic lesions, such as osteogenic sarcoma, carcinoid, neuroblastoma, and lymphoma, are more rarely seen. Several primary tumors of the liver, including liver cell carcinoma (especially in infants), hemangioendothelioma, and hemangioma, as well as the granulomatous lesions (tuberculosis and histoplasmosis), may cause calcifications. Simple cysts, hydatid cysts, actinomycosis, and pyogenic abscesses are other rare causes.[350]

Fatty change. Fatty change in the liver is common, perhaps more frequent than in any other organ, and it may be of severe degree. Because of the rapid transport of free fatty acids from the peripheral adipose tissue to the liver and the formation of triglyceride, phospholipid, and cholesterol esters that must be secreted into the blood as lipoprotein, anything that interferes with the intracellular metabolism of the lipids can quickly result in recognizable fatty change. Excess mobilization of fat also may result in the accumulation in the liver. The fat usually accumulates in the center of the lobules, where, when abundant, it forms large globules that distend the hepatic cells. Nearer the peripheries of the lobules, the globules tend to be smaller and only partially fill the hepatic cells. In chronic ulcerative pulmonary tuberculosis, a peripheral type of fatty change predominates. In prolonged passive congestion, the fatty change may be most marked at the centers of the lobules. With marked fatty accumulation, the liver is increased in size and has a tense capsule and rounded margins. The cut surface bulges slightly and is pale yellow to yellow (Plate 5, *B*). The lobular markings are obscured.

By far the most common cause of severe fatty change is chronic alcoholism (p. 1198). Fatty livers also are found in association with obesity, malnutrition and wasting diseases (e.g., tuberculosis and malignant tumors) and in some cases of diabetes mellitus. Certain poisons, such as phlorhizin, carbon tetrachloride, chloroform, and ether, may cause fatty change. In kwashiorkor, a common disease in the tropical regions that is associated with protein malnutrition, the fatty change may be extreme.[353] The fat first accumulates in the periportal areas (p. 1201) but later involves the entire lobule. The problem of the relationship of kwashiorkor to cirrhosis is not yet solved.[352]

In experimental animals, a marked centrilobular fatty change may be produced by deficiency of choline, and peripheral fatty changes are produced by certain amino acid deficiencies that must be accompanied by a sufficient intake of carbohydrate.[351]

Fatty change resulting from ethionine administration is apparently due to a lack of adenosine triphosphate (ATP) in the liver cells.[345]

In some cases of sudden death in young adults, marked fatty change in the liver has been the only finding.[346] A peculiar fatty change seen in late pregnancy is described on p. 1226.

Severe fatty change has been noted in obese patients who have had a jejunoileal or jejunocolic bypass for the treatment of obesity. Death has been reported in such cases.[343, 344, 349]

CONGENITAL AND ACQUIRED ABNORMALITIES OF FORM AND POSITION

Congenital abnormalities of the liver are not common. Reidel's lobe is a downward projection of the right lobe, which may be mistaken for a tumor or thought to be a displaced kidney. The liver may be displaced in position in association with a congenital diaphragmatic hernia. Severe abnormalities that require surgery are seen rarely.[354] Atrophy of the left lobe of the liver may be caused by some interference with the left branch of the portal vein.

Acquired abnormalities of position are mainly downward or upward displacement by some extrahepatic cause, such as a subdiaphragmatic abscess or an abdominal tumor. Abnormalities of form may be the result of contraction of scar tissue (e.g., hepar lobatum) or nodularity from irregular regenerative hyperplasia or neoplastic growth, Transverse, oblique, or sagittal grooves on the upper or anterior surface of the liver are common. They have been attributed to pressure of the ribs, folds of the diaphragm, and tight clothing. They often are associated with chronic cough, emphysema, and bronchitis due to pressure from hypertrophied diaphragmatic muscle bundles. The capsule is thickened at the depths of the folds, and adjacent hepatic parenchyma may show slight atrophic changes. Such grooving does not appear to be of any functional significance.

TRAUMATIC INJURY

The liver, because of its size, weight, and soft consistency, is susceptible to blunt injury, especially in vehicular accidents at high speed. Collision with the steering wheel is particularly harmful. Blunt injuries most often affect the right lobe, producing lacerations of variable configuration and severity that may be classified as peripheral, intermediate, or hilar.[336] In the latter, the hepatic veins may be lacerated or torn from the inferior vena cava. Severe injury to the hepatic parenchyma without laceration of the capsule may cause tearing of blood vessels and continued bleeding that results in a subcapsular hematoma. Delayed rupture of such a hematoma into the abdominal cavity twenty-four hours or more after the accident must be treated by surgery. In some instances, an intrahepatic hematoma ruptures into the biliary tract with resultant hemobilia,[356] in which the patient has gastrointestinal bleeding, often with hematemesis. Surgical control of the hemorrhage may necessitate ligature of the common hepatic artery.[358]

Stabbings and gunshot wounds are common causes of injury to the liver.[336] Gunshot wounds may destroy much of the liver (Fig.

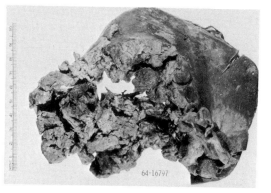

Fig. 28-36 Shattered right lobe of liver following bullet wound. Specimen surgically resected.

28-36). In traumatized liver removed at surgery, there is a variable amount of hemorrhage and necrosis of the injured parenchyma, often with a neutrophilic exudate. On rare occasions, an arteriovenous fistula has been known to follow liver injury.[357] These are often present for many years before they are diagnosed and lead to portal hypertension and ascites. They are curable by surgery.

Subcapsular hematomas, of small or large size, occur occasionally in newborn infants, especially those born prematurely, and require surgery, or prove fatal.[355] These hematomas may be caused by trauma during birth or may accompany blood dyscrasias, such as erythroblastosis fetalis.

PIGMENTATION

Anthrocotic pigment may be carried to the liver by the bloodstream following rupture into the pulmonary veins of a thoracic lymph node containing carbon pigment. The carbon particles are phagocytized by the Kupffer cells and tend to be carried to portal spaces, where they accumulate.

Silver pigment may be found under the sinusoidal endothelial cells of the liver in argyria. After the injection of Thorotrast, macrophages in the periportal areas and Kupffer cells may store thorium for decades.

Hemosiderin accumulation in the liver is common. In hemolytic anemias, the hemosiderin tends to be distributed diffusely. The pigment is found in both the hepatic cells and the phagocytic Kupffer cells of the sinusoids. In hemochromatosis, the pigment is largely hemosiderin, but hemofuscin is present as well.

In malaria, hematin pigment may accumulate in large amount, mainly in the Kupffer cells of the sinusoids. It may be sufficient to

Table 28-3 Hereditary hyperbilirubinemias

Syndrome	Age at onset of jaundice	Symptoms and course	Serum bilirubin			BSP excretion	Cholecystogram	Gallstones	Pathology
			Range	Conjugated	Unconjugated				
Crigler-Najjar	Neonate	Jaundice at birth with or without kernicterus; death in first year of life	>20 mg%		Increased	Normal	Visualization		Few bile thrombi
Gilbert's constitutional hyperbilirubinemia	Birth to 53 yr (av. 18 yr)	Jaundice may be precipitated by fatigue, intermittent infections, alcohol, and stress; nausea, anorexia, and vague abdominal distress may occur	< 5 mg%	Normal	Increased	Normal	Visualization	Increased frequency	None
Dubin-Johnson 1 Classic	Most often 15-25 yr	Pain over liver and hepatomegaly, especially during attacks of jaundice; dyspepsia; problem exists throughout life with fluctuations of jaundice	N to 6 mg%	Increased	Increased	Retention with late rise after 90 min	No visualization	Occur in approximately 10%	Pigment in liver, probably melanins
2 Variants in family	Mild elevation of serum bilirubin after 10 yr	None	> 1 mg in 20% of family	Normal or increased	Normal or increased	Normal	Normal		Pigment in many but not related to increased serum bilirubin
Rotor	Early in life, usually before 20 yr	Jaundice fluctuates	N to 6 mg%	Increased	Increased	Retention with no late rise	Visualization		None

give the liver a dark grayish brown color. A similar pigment may be found in the liver in schistosomiasis.

Bile pigmentation of the liver is seen in any variety of jaundice. When seen fresh, the liver is yellowish but soon changes to green as a result of oxidation of the bilirubin to biliverdin. Masses of pigment may be seen distending the bile capillaries and small ducts and also within the hepatic cells.

The differential diagnosis of increased lipochrome in the liver as seen on biopsies is discussed on p. 1247.

HEREDITARY HYPERBILIRUBINEMIA

Several syndromes that are caused by inborn errors in the metabolism of bilirubin have been described.[367] The essential features of these disorders are given in Table 28-3.

In the *Crigler-Najjar syndrome*, there is an unconjugated hyperbilirubinemia due to hepatic glucuronyl transferase deficiency. The disease occurs in two forms. In one group of patients, there is severe hyperbilirubinemia. The bile is almost completely colorless and contains only traces of unconjugated bilirubin. In the second group of patients, the hyperbilirubinemia is less severe and the bile contains some bilirubin glucuronide. The conjugation defect in the first group is transmitted as an autosomal recessive character and in the second group as an autosomal dominant character.[366] The jaundice appears in the neonate and persists with high concentrations of unconjugated bilirubin in the blood serum. Patients in group 1 often die in infancy, whereas those in group 2 may survive until adult life. A similar disease is seen in the Gunn rat, in which there is a failure to conjugate bilirubin.[362] When given conjugated bilirubin, this animal will secrete a large fraction of unconjugated pigment.[361]

In the *Gilbert syndrome*, the patient usually has intermittent attacks of jaundice, lassitude, and abdominal pain. The jaundice is due to an increase in the unconjugated serum bilirubin. A marked reduction of hepatic bilirubin transferase has been shown in this group.[359]

In the *Dubin-Johnson-Sprinz-Nelson* type, there is chronic or intermittent jaundice, dark urine, and an increase in both conjugated and unconjugated bilirubin. The glucuronyl transferase is presumed to be normal, but the liver cells have difficulty in secreting conjugated bilirubin. Similarly, the secretion of

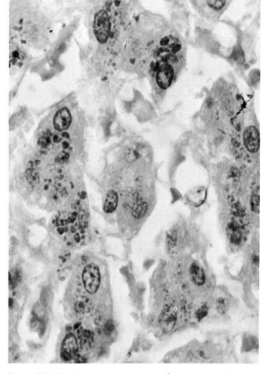

Fig. 28-37 Large masses of intracytoplasmic brown pigment in Dubin-Johnson syndrome.

sulfobromophthalein and iopanoic acid are affected, so that abnormal tests result. The parenchymal cells, especially in the centrilobular zones, contain large granules of lipochrome pigment (Fig. 28-37), often in such amounts that the liver is black. The pigment is apparently a melanin[363] and is located within lysosomes.[365] A similar disease is seen in a Corriedale sheep mutant.[364] The disease in the human being is inherited as an autosomal dominant trait with a variable expression. The study of a large family with the Dubin-Johnson trait disclosed considerable variation in the relation of pigment in the liver to hyperbilirubinemia.[360]

In the *Rotor syndrome*, there is likewise an increase in both conjugated and unconjugated serum bilirubin but no pigmentation of the liver cells. There is sulfobromophthalein retention but normal visualization of the gallbladder. It has been suggested that Rotor's is a variant of the Dubin-Johnson syndrome.

CIRCULATORY DISTURBANCES
Shock

Acute hepatic changes, even centrilobular necrosis, often occur in patients who are in shock. These changes may be observed in a liver that was previously normal or be superimposed upon chronic passive congestion or cirrhosis. Trauma, hemorrhage, myocardial infarction, and endotoxin shock due to septicemia are the more common causes. Shock of more than twenty-four hours' duration usually is associated with liver cell necrosis.[384] Jaundice is rare but does occur in endotoxin shock[386] and in cardiac conditions. Many of the physiologic changes observed in shock are affected by the liver. The key to these changes is the block at the pyruvate acetyl coenzyme A step in intracellular metabolism. This affects the metabolism of glucose, fats, and amino acids, so that they are returned to the bloodstream and the energy produced in the Krebs cycle is reduced.[382] The disappearance of glycogen from liver cells is well known in experimental pathology.

The pathologic changes in the liver that have been described are those seen at autopsy or in experimental animals. A reversible change, fatty vacuolization, has been noted[375] in patients in shock who survived more than eighteen hours. A more severe lesion is anoxic centrilobular necrosis that occurs most often in patients with cirrhosis who die of bleeding esophageal varices. Other causes include shock due to myocardial infarction and exsanguinating hemorrhage from peptic ulcers. Anoxic necrosis also occurs in patients with severe heart failure who have no recognizable episode of shock. On gross examination, centrilobular necrosis may or may not be recognized, but often central zones have a characteristic dull yellow to yellow-brown appearance. The necrosis is of the coagulation type, the cells are intensely acidophilic, and the nuclei stain poorly or have disappeared. Neutrophils may be abundant, especially around the periphery of the necrotic zones. The necrotic cells slowly disappear, and in biopsy material taken in the healing stage, only dilated sinusoids and pigmented macrophages are seen, a histologic picture difficult to distinguish from other types of healing centrilobular zonal necrosis. The cirrhotic liver is particularly prone to anoxic necrosis when there is bleeding from varices. The large pseudolobules of cirrhosis are probably poorly oxygenated as a result of an abnormal outflow pattern. Furthermore, much of the portal vein blood may be shunted around the liver, so that a fall in hepatic artery pressure during shock would lead rapidly to anoxic necrosis. The areas of necrosis are often large and pale

yellow-white and may be surrounded by a thin zone of hemorrhage (Fig. 28-38). It is likely that some of the depressed scars seen in the liver of patients who have bled from varices in the past may be of anoxic origin.

Biopsy material rarely is obtained on patients in shock. In one such case, severe centrilobular necrosis was observed (Fig. 28-39). The recognition of hemorrhage within the necrotic zone is difficult, since the margins of the widened blood-filled sinusoids are difficult to distinguish.

Endotoxin shock in animals produces ex-

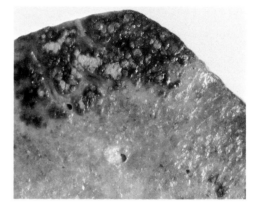

Fig. 28-38 Anoxic necrosis of liver. Alcoholic cirrhosis with fatal hemorrhage from duodenal ulcer.

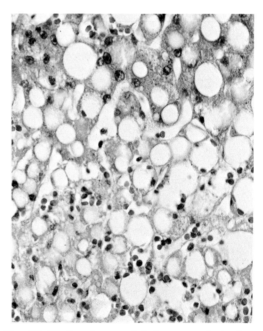

Fig. 28-39 Anoxic centrilobular necrosis in fatty liver of alcoholic who was in shock following variceal bleeding.

tensive damage to the endothelium lining the sinusoids, loss of microvilli in Disse's space, and the production of large intracytoplasmic vacuoles, some of which apparently contain fibrinogen and fibrin.[368] Aggregations of platelets, fibrin, erythrocytes, and leukocytes tend to accumulate in the sinusoids. Erythrocytes enter Disse's space and sometimes are seen between the hepatocytes.

Passive hyperemia and cardiac cirrhosis

Passive hyperemia of the liver is most often the result of cardiac disease with congestive failure but also may result from compression and obstruction of the inferior vena cava or obstructions of the pulmonary circulation leading to right-sided cardiac failure. Increased pressure in the venous system affects the liver severely because of the short distance between the point of entry of hepatic veins into the vena cava and the entry of the latter into the right auricle. Because the liver cells are particularly sensitive to hypoxia, the decreased oxygen content of the hepatic blood[383] and the diminished flow in congestive failure[378] are probably responsible for much of the histologic change that is observed.

In the early stages of passive congestion, only dilatation of central veins and sinusoids are seen. Later, atrophy and disappearance of liver cells lead to larger pools of blood in the dilated channels. Fragments of former sinusoidal walls remain, but the normal archi-

tectural arrangement around the central vein tends to disappear. There is often a lack of correlation between the clinical course and severity of atrophy. When the central one-third to one-half of the lobules has undergone atrophy, fatty change of the remaining liver cells near the margin is often present and is responsible for the gross "nutmeg" appearance (Fig. 28-40). However, in many instances, the pale peripheral lobular zones do not contain fat vacuoles. The reason for their pallor is not apparent. Coincident with the centrilobular atrophy an increase of fibrous tissue may ensue.[381] Occasionally, especially in patients with tricuspid valvular disease, fibrosis links the centrilobular areas together and a diagnosis of cardiac cirrhosis may be made (Fig. 28-41). Portal fibrosis with communicating septa to the central fibrous areas is rare but does occur. Hyperplasia of the peripheral portions of the lobules is occasionally seen. This may or may not be in conjunction with cardiac cirrhosis.

Grossly, the liver is of normal or slightly reduced size, firm in consistency, and dark red-brown or purple-red in color. The surface is only slightly nodular, and the capsule is thickened. The cut surface shows a mottling

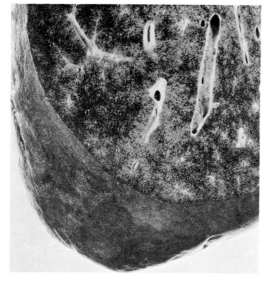

Fig. 28-40 "Nutmeg liver" in chronic passive congestion of liver.

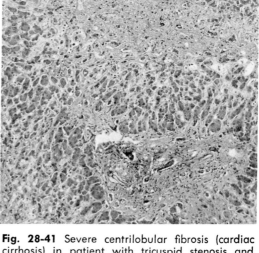

Fig. 28-41 Severe centrilobular fibrosis (cardiac cirrhosis) in patient with tricuspid stenosis and chronic heart failure.

of gray or yellow-gray areas separated by brown-red zones of variable size and shape. The hepatic veins are uniformly dilated, sometimes markedly so, and their walls are thickened. Ill-defined nodules may be present in proximity to the portal tracts. It may be questioned whether or not true cirrhosis of congestive origin exists. A small percentage of patients with long-standing congestive failure do have esophageal varices, but these rarely bleed.[374] In our experience, the wedged hepatic vein pressure is not elevated in patients with congestive failure.

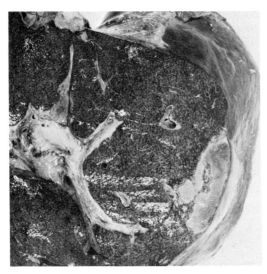

Fig. 28-42 Subcapsular infarct due to periarteritis nodosa.

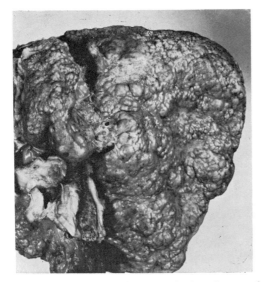

Fig. 28-43 Portal cirrhosis and thrombosis of portal vein. (Courtesy Dr. G. L. Duff.)

Vascular obstruction—infarction

Infarction of the liver is rare, but in most instances it has been due to *obstruction of the hepatic artery* or some of its branches. Bland or septic emboli may reach the hepatic artery from the heart and result in infarction. The presence of congestive failure accentuates the process. The hepatic artery is subject to accidental ligation at surgery. Ligature proximal to the right gastric artery is well tolerated because of retrograde flow of blood through the right gastric artery from its anastomoses. Periarteritis nodosa is a rare cause of multiple infarcts (Fig. 28-42).

Occlusion of the portal vein or of one or more of its branches is usually secondary to another disease (Fig. 28-43). These include cirrhosis of the liver, intravenous invasion by primary carcinoma of the liver that complicates cirrhosis, carcinoma of the pancreas that grows into the intrahepatic portal veins, and pylephlebitis that follows abdominal suppuration or umbilical infection of the newborn infant. Intrahepatic obstruction of the portal vein or one of the major branches usually causes only the atrophic red infarct of Zahn (Fig. 28-44), a discolored zone that does not show any necrosis on microscopic examination. Thrombosis or neoplastic invasion of the trunk of the portal vein occasionally causes areas of necrosis in the liver.

The syndrome first described by Banti in the 1880's and 1890's[371] has recently been

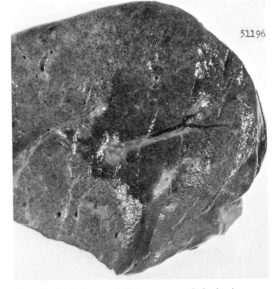

Fig. 28-44 Infarct of Zahn, area of dusky hyperemia due to thrombosis of branch of portal vein.

termed *hepatoportal sclerosis*[377] and *idiopathic portal hypertension*[369] to indicate portal hypertension with esophageal varices but without cirrhosis. It is associated with symptoms of hypersplenism. The etiology and pathogenesis are unknown. Although the entity is rare in the United States, it is more common in India[369] and Japan.[372]

The prominent initial features of Banti's original cases were anemia and splenomegaly, but in the United States most patients first seek medical care for bleeding esophageal varices. At this time, an enlarged spleen and mild pancytopenia are noted. Hepatic function, although initially normal, slowly deteriorates.

On gross examination, the liver surface is smooth, but the edges are blunted and the parenchyma slightly firmer than normal. Microscopically,[28, 377] variations from normal are minor. Usually, the relationship between central veins and portal areas is inconstant. Often, two to four central veins are found in a lobule. The portal area is widened within an intact limiting plate, and there are increased numbers of dilated, thin-walled angiomatous structures (Fig. 28-45). As the disease progresses, collagen becomes more dense in portal areas and may extend beyond the confines of the limiting plate to other portal

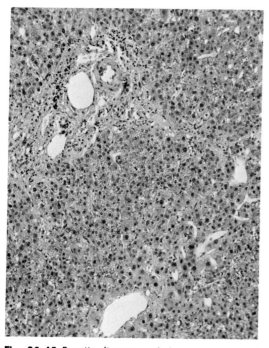

Fig. 28-45 Banti's disease with large vessels and increase of connective tissue in portal areas. Central veins enlarged and prominent.

areas. The portal vein radicles may become thickened. The end stage of idiopathic portal hypertension results in a fibrotic, shrunken liver without regenerative nodules.

A number of patients with the foregoing findings will have thrombotic or sclerotic occlusion of the extrahepatic portal vein. This occlusion is considered by many investigators to be the cause of *extrahepatic portal hypertension,* whereas others[377] have suggested that the portal vein occlusion follows idiopathic portal hypertension, just as it occasionally follows portal hypertension associated with cirrhosis.

Banti and many subsequent investigators[370, 379, 380, 385] believed that primary splenic enlargement resulted in increased portal blood flow and consequent portal hypertension. However, the possibility of the development of abnormal arteriovenous communications either within the liver or in the peripheral splanchnic bed has not been excluded. It has been demonstrated that portal hypertension following acquired extrahepatic arterioportal venous fistulas produces intrahepatic change similar to that in Banti's disease. After such intrahepatic changes have developed, the portal hypertension may not be reversible by surgical correction of the fistula.[370] Investigators in Japan have suggested that the syndrome follows viral hepatitis, a finding not supportable by data from the United States.

The *hepatic veins* are much less frequently involved by thrombosis or other disease than is the portal vein.[373] Small segments may be closed by thrombi or even by tumor thrombi and produce small areas of infarction, but these are almost uniformly symptomless. Primary carcinomas of the liver often grow into the hepatic veins but rarely fill the entire system. However, in rare instances, a large portion of the hepatic vein system is more or less completely obstructed by thromboses or a combination of sclerosis and thrombosis that does produce symptoms of an acute or chronic nature. This condition is known as the *Budd-Chiari* syndrome. A fibrous diaphragm in the inferior vena cava is also capable of blocking the mouth of the hepatic veins. Polycythemia, paroxysmal nocturnal hemoglobinuria, and the use of oral contraceptives also have been associated with the disease.

In the acute type, there is an enlarged, tender, and sometimes painful liver associated with severe ascites. Esophageal varices may develop quickly. Collateral veins appear on the lower abdomen if the vena cava is obstructed. There is usually no jaundice. In the chronic type, essentially the same symptoms develop slowly. In most instances, the hepatic veins are both sclerosed and thrombosed. The remarkable fibrous tissue proliferation in the veins, plus the extreme congestion of the lobules that leads to atrophy of the central one-third to one-half of the lobule, is diagnostic of the Budd-Chiari syndrome. Biopsies taken in the more acute stages of the disease often disclose centrilobular zones of coagulative necrosis or even larger areas of necrosis resembling infarcts.

In *congenital capillary telangiectasia* (Osler-Rendu-Weber syndrome), the lesions in the liver may produce a bruit due to portacaval shunting. Fibrosis and even cirrhosis also may develop.[376]

CHRONIC INFECTIONS AND LIVER ABSCESSES
Chronic infections

Many of the granulomatous diseases, fungal infections, and parasitic infestations are capable of causing liver disease. The term *granulomatous hepatitis* often is used for this group. After the most complete laboratory and clinical study, the etiology of many of the noncaseating granulomas remains obscure.[392] The patient is often febrile, and a needle biopsy of the liver frequently is performed for diagnostic purposes. As a rule, most of the granulomas that involve the liver will cause a rise in the serum alkaline phosphate level and at least a mild retention of BSP. Jaundice is unusual and, when present, is of short duration. The granulomas that are observed on needle biopsy or at autopsy include lesions of tuberculosis, sarcoidosis, larval granulomatosis, Q fever, brucellosis, leprosy, histoplasmosis, secondary syphilis, and tularemia.

Tuberculous and sarcoid granulomas are the most frequently seen, and their differentiation is of practical importance. The lesion of sarcoidosis is composed of epithelioid cells with no particular arrangement. Caseation necrosis is not seen, and a few lymphocytes usually surround the granulomas (Fig. 28-46). Larger lesions are composed of multiple units, often with an occasional multinucleated giant cell. In some instances, the noncaseating lesions of sarcoidosis are observed in the walls of the central and sublobular veins. In healing, sarcoid granulomas usually become sur-

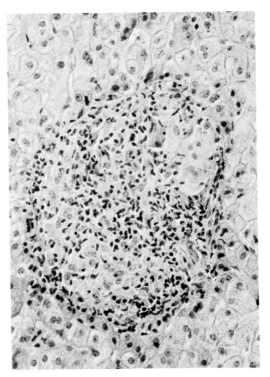

Fig. 28-46 Irregular arrangement of epithelioid cells and scanty lymphoid infiltrate in sarcoid granuloma of liver.

rounded by concentric layers of connective tissue. Tubercles often have a caseous center, the epithelioid cells are arranged in a radial fashion at the periphery, and the exudate contains both lymphocytes and other mononuclear cells. Fibrin is often present, which helps to distinguish tuberculosis from sarcoidosis. In the small early lesions of tuberculosis, there may be no caseation, and the differentiation from sarcoidosis and leprosy is most difficult. An acid-fast stain should always be done on any granulomatous lesion that resembles tuberculosis. Occasionally, the tubercles are concentrated along the portal tracts, and the bile ducts may be destroyed. In a patient so affected, jaundice may occur. More rarely, solitary or multiple tuberculomas have been observed. Tubercle bacilli may reach the liver from either an active pulmonary or abdominal focus.

Lepromatous leprosy may spread to the liver, producing small granulomas that arise in the sinusoids. Studies with the electron microscope have shown that the lysosomes in Kupffer cells fuse with vacuoles containing lepra bacilli and apparently destroy the organisms.[394]

In *visceral larva migrans*, the presence of

the larvae of *Toxocara canis, Toxocara cati,* or other parasites in the liver causes rather distinctive granulomas that may reach a diameter of several millimeters and are composed of a necrotic center surrounded by epithelioid cells having a radial arrangement, many eosinophils, and giant cells (Fig. 13-32). The larvae may be identified on serial sectioning. The disease is seen in children, usually from $1\frac{1}{2}$ to 6 years of age, who eat dirt (pica) and are closely associated with dogs or cats. The syndrome is featured by fever, hepatomegaly, eosinophilia, and hyperglobulinemia.[395] A reliable intradermal test using *Toxocara* antigen has been found useful.[399]

Q fever may cause hepatic enlargement and jaundice. The ringlike necrosis of sinusoidal walls, with the formation of tiny rod-shaped fragments, is characteristic. Large necrotic granulomatous lesions with giant cells and epithelioid cells are also present.[387] Brucellosis occasionally produces caseation necrosis and even abscesses[398] (p. 309). Secondary syphilis is a rare cause of jaundice but can result in small granulomas that are of short duration. Tularemia and leprosy are discussed on pp. 311 and 332. Among the fungal infections, actinomycosis frequently produces hepatic abscesses. Blastomycosis and coccidioidomycosis occasionally may produce small hepatic lesions. Histoplasmosis often involves the liver, the encapsulated organisms being found in large numbers in the Kupffer cells. *Toxoplasma gondii* occasionally causes a granuloma-like lesion of the liver.[389]

Several helminths commonly or characteristically produce lesions in the liver. The larval form of the dog tapeworm, *Taenia echinococcus,* often lodges in the liver, producing there a hydatid cyst (pp. 458 and 1239). Schistosomal infection produces hepatic lesions due to ova that are carried to the liver in the portal blood and produce irritation (p. 451). The liver fluke, *Clonorchis sinensis,* and *Fasciola hepatica* lodge in the bile ducts, which they tend to obstruct (p. 448).

Abscess

Abscesses of the liver are usually of pyogenic, amebic or actinomycotic origin.

Pyogenic liver abscesses occur with equal frequency among men and women, usually past 50 years of age, producing fever and pain in the right upper quadrant.[396] Tenderness over the liver in a jaundiced toxic patient is characteristic. Leukocytosis, an elevated serum alkaline phosphatase level, and a positive blood culture are features expected on laboratory examination. Pyogenic abscesses may result from the following:

1 Extension of organisms to the liver by way of the bile ducts (suppurative cholangitis), secondary to obstruction of the common duct
2 Spread of organisms to the liver by way of the portal vein (pylephlebitis) from the appendix, rectum, or other parts of the intestine
3 Spread to the liver from contiguous infected tissue (e.g., a subphrenic abscess)
4 Infection carried to the liver by hepatic arteries in septicemia
5 Penetrating traumatic injuries

Solitary abscesses have been reported in diabetic patients.[393] On rare occasions, the cysts in polycystic disease of the liver become infected and multiple abscesses result.[390] Aerobic and anaerobic organisms have been cultured from pyogenic abscesses.[388] Most pyogenic abscesses in the adult are a consequence of obstruction of the common bile duct. There is dilatation of the intrahepatic ducts, and the stagnant bile becomes infected with pyogenic organisms (acute cholangitis), an event often accompanied by chills and fever. The cholangitis may or may not proceed to suppuration. When it does, abscesses of variable size involve the entire liver (Plate 5, *F*). Pyogenic abscesses occurring in infants and children usually do so before the age of 5 years and often in patients with acute blastic leukemia.[391] In the neonate liver, abscesses may complicate umbilical infections.

In the past, *pylephlebitis* was seen as an extension from acute suppurative appendicitis or from any suppurative disease in areas drained by the portal vein. Emboli carried by portal venous channels to the liver produce small abscesses at their site of lodgment. The areas of necrosis vary from microscopic size to a diameter of several centimeters and, by coalescence, can form large cavities. Necrosis, cellular disintegration, and leukocyte accumulation are found in the areas of abscess. Occasionally, there is the complication of rupture or spread of the infection to adjacent tissues.

Pyogenic hepatic abscesses due to spread of organisms to the liver by hepatic arteries are usually but part of a general septicemia, with abscesses present in other organs as well.

Amebic abscess of the liver is due to spread of *Entamoeba histolytica* from intestinal lesions by way of the portal vein. It is almost

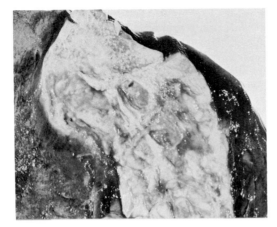

Fig. 28-47 Amebic liver abscess with rough, irregular lining of necrotic tissue.

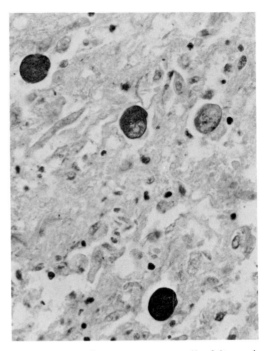

Fig. 28-48 Amebae in necrotic wall of liver abscess. (PAS stain.)

exclusively a disease of men, occurs before the age of 50 years, and is one of the serious diseases noted among travelers exposed to the organism. A history of diarrhea weeks or months before onset of symptoms is given in approximately 50% of patients. However, trophozoites are not always demonstrable in the stools. Fever, leukocytosis, pain in the right upper quadrant, and tender enlarged liver are common findings. Many patients will have a visible bulge of the rib margin and even edema over the right lower anterior portion of the chest. Roentgenograms and a liver scan usually will disclose the location of the abscess. Needle aspiration is usually successful, and as much as a pint or more of purulent material having the appearance of anchovy sauce may be evacuated. Antiamebic therapy usually leads to rapid recovery. Scintiscans show that healing takes two to four months in most patients[397] (see also p. 434).

The abscesses may vary greatly in size but are usually solitary and located in the superoposterior portion of the right lobe (Fig. 28-47). A biopsy taken at surgery discloses the abscess wall with its irregular lining composed of exudate and necrotic liver tissue. Amebae are most easily found in the marginal liver tissue, often in colonies with a clear zone about each ameba. A PAS stain accentuates the contrast between ameba and body cells (Fig. 28-48).

Actinomycotic abscesses of the liver usually have a pathogenesis similar to the pyogenic pylephlebitic abscesses. Spread to the liver from intestinal lesions is by the portal venous channels. Multiple, small, ragged abscess cavities are produced, in which the actinomycotic colonies can be found. A honeycomb type of calcification sometimes is seen on roentgenograms (see also p. 411 and Fig. 12-2).

POSTMORTEM CHANGES

Postmortem autolytic changes develop rapidly in the liver, producing a soft, even mushy, organ. Microscopically, all cell detail may be lost. Portions of the liver adjacent to the transverse colon often develop a bluish black discoloration. The most striking postmortem change is the so-called "foamy" liver, which is due to postmortem growth in the liver of anaerobic gas-producing organisms from the intestinal tract. The liver becomes soft and spongy, the bubbles of gas produced honeycombing the hepatic tissue. Numerous bacilli may be evident, particularly in blood vessels.

CYSTS

Cysts in the liver are commonly of three types: congenital, solitary, and hydatid (*Echinococcus*).

Congenital cysts are not common,[400] but sometimes are found associated with congenital cystic disease of the kidneys or other organs. They are usually small and cause no disturbance, but cysts of large size have been reported. They may be prominent just under the capsule, contain clear fluid, and are lined by flattened or cylindrical epithelium (Fig. 28-49). In some instances, small gray-white

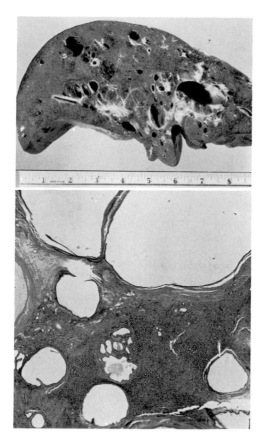

Fig. 28-49 Congenital cysts of liver.

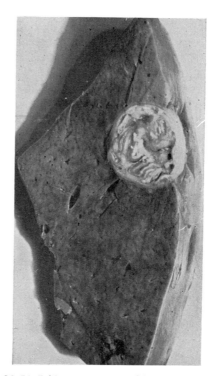

Fig. 28-50 *Echinococcus* cyst of liver. Note convoluted membranous content.

areas are seen throughout the liver, and the cysts are barely visible or are of microscopic size. In this microcystic form of polycystic disease, the tubules are surrounded by dense connective tissue and may contain bile pigment. Rarely, the amount of connective tissue and number of ducts is so great that entire lobules are surrounded, a condition that has been called *congenital hepatic fibrosis.* Under these circumstances, a presinusoidal type of hypertension may develop, and variceal bleeding ensues that necessitates shunt surgery.[240]

Solitary or *nonparasitic cysts* may reach several centimeters in diameter and become clinically manifest. They occur more often in women and are best treated conservatively.[401] The cysts have a cuboidal to columnar epithelial lining and a circumscribed connective tissue wall.

Hydatid cysts are due to the lodgment in the liver of the larval form of the dog tapeworm, *Taenia echinococcus.* The liver is a commonly involved organ. The cyst wall is composed of concentric hyaline laminae lined by germinal cells from which grow "daughter"

cysts. Scolices and hooklets of the worm may be identified in cyst wall or its contents by microscopic examination (Fig. 28-50).

Old cysts, in which the parasites are dead, contain a yellowish gray puttylike material.

TUMORS

The liver provides a most suitable environment for the growth of neoplastic cells, being the favorite site for metastatic cancer. In addition, the lymphomas, leukemias, and primary carcinoma all grow readily within this organ. Its size, anatomic location, and dual blood supply and the ready availability of nutritional material are factors that influence the deposition and growth of neoplasms. Between 40% and 50% of all primary cancers in the body will be noted at death to have metastases within the liver. Primary neoplasms and tumorlike lesions occur much less frequently but nevertheless are important, inasmuch as they may enter into the differential diagnosis of an enlarged liver noted clinically or observed at laparotomy. Hepatomegaly, often symptomless, is a common finding in neoplastic liver disease. Malignant tumors usually are associated with weight loss. Fever and jaundice are less common. Laboratory findings often include an elevation of the serum al-

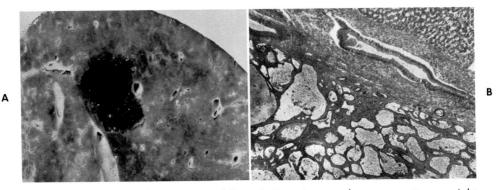

Fig. 28-51 A, Cavernous hemangioma of liver. **B,** Hepatic parenchyma seen at upper right.

kaline phosphatase level and sulfobromo-phthalein retention. Angiograms made by the injection of an iodine compound into the hepatic artery are most helpful in the diagnosis of neoplasms.[17] Scintiscans of the liver following the injection of colloidal gold are also useful as a diagnostic tool.

Primary growths may arise from hepatic cells, bile duct epithelium, or mesodermal structures. Benign tumors are uncommon but include cavernous hemangiomas, hemangio-endotheliomas, bile duct adenomas and cyst-adenomas, and, most rarely, liver cell adenomas.

Benign tumors

Cavernous hemangiomas. Cavernous he-mangiomas usually are noted incidentally at necropsy, but a few become manifest clinically,[407, 430] especially in multiparous women, possibly as a result of an increase of circulating estrogenic hormones during pregnancy. Calcified hemangiomas of the liver have been reported in older women in association with hypertension.[434] Angiomatous lesions of the gingiva and skin may likewise appear. Rarely, a hemangioma may rupture into the peritoneal cavity, necessitating emergency surgery.

Hemangiomas appear as circumscribed, dark red-purple areas that vary from a few millimeters to several centimeters in diameter. They may bulge beneath Glisson's capsule or may be located deep within the liver (Fig. 28-51, *A*). The presence of cavernous spaces gives them a spongy appearance. Microscopically, the large, blood-filled spaces are lined by a single layer of endothelium and are separated by connective tissue that often has a myxomatous appearance (Fig. 28-51, *B*). Hemangiomas apparently grow for a limited length of time and some eventually undergo fibrosis that obliterates the cavernous spaces.

Rarely, the liver may be diffusely involved by small hemangiomas.

Hemangioendotheliomas. The *hemangio-endothelioma of infancy* is an unusual tumor that arises within the first few months of life and tends to undergo involution. However, in a large percentage of patients, an arterio-venous shunt occurs that causes hypertrophy and dilatation of the heart, with resulting congestive failure and death. In about one-third of the patients there are similar growths at extrahepatic sites, especially in the skin. Recent reports indicate that the skin lesions and even the hepatic lesion may involute rapidly under corticosteroid therapy. The reason for this favorable response is not known.[413, 416]

Microscopically, hemangioendotheliomas are characterized by anastomosing vascular channels that are lined with one or more layers of hyperchromatic endothelial cells. The tumor grows along the sinusoids of the lobules, often replacing liver tissue.

Adenomas and cystadenomas. *Bile duct adenomas* are firm, gray-white areas, rarely over a centimeter in diameter, and usually are located beneath Glisson's capsule. They are composed of a multitude of tiny acinar structures that are lined with bile duct type epithelium. The connective tissue stroma is sparse.

Bile duct cystadenomas are extremely rare.[407] They may reach a diameter of several centimeters. The cysts are lined with mucin-secreting columnar epithelium, and the connective tissue stroma is quite cellular. The stroma may contain areas of smooth muscle. Malignant change in a cystadenoma has been reported.[427]

Adenomas derived from *hepatic cells* are actually rare. Many cases so diagnosed have eventually proved to be low-grade carcinomas. Occasionally, large hyperplastic nodules in a cirrhotic liver qualify as adenomas. A true adenoma is one in which there are discrete, sharply delineated areas of uniform-appearing hepatic cells that are usually somewhat larger than the surrounding normal cells. Some of the cells may have an acinar arrangement. There are no bile ducts or other evidence of portal triads. To date, we have seen several liver cell tumors that have not metastasized. They have a uniform acinar arrangement, and the individual cells often contain an unusually large amount of lipochrome pigment. All the neoplasms have been in women, and many have been resected surgically. Tentatively, these tumors have been diagnosed as aggressive adenomas. Malignant change in adenomas has not been proved.

· · ·

Aberrant adrenal tissue is sometimes seen beneath the capsule of the right lobe, and at least one functioning adrenal cortical tumor of the liver has been reported.[405]

Several tumorlike lesions are seen in the liver, many of which are of importance because they may be palpable and lead to surgery. Among these are focal nodular hyperplasia, nodular hyperplasia of cirrhosis, mesenchymal hamartoma, and peliosis hepatis.

Focal nodular hyperplasia. In focal nodular hyperplasia, there is a firm, circumscribed, gray-brown tumor that usually measures from 1 cm to 8 cm in diameter. It is always lighter in color than the surrounding liver. Although sharply circumscribed, the tumors do not have a true capsule. They may be single or multiple. Most often, they are seen beneath the capsule, but they can arise deep within the liver.

Rarely are the tumors pedunculated. Ordinarily, there is a stellate-shaped mass of connective tissue in the center of the lesion with radiation of the connective tissue toward the periphery. The nodules are composed of fairly normal-appearing liver cells arranged in small pseudolobules. Often, the liver cells are arranged in individual units that surround small ducts and vessels. So far, there have been no proved instances of malignant change.[406]

Nodular hyperplasia of cirrhosis. In postnecrotic cirrhosis and, more rarely, in Laennec's cirrhosis, areas of nodular hyperplasia or regeneration may assume tumorlike proportions and become palpable. Sometimes this has led to unnecessary surgery. Localized areas of nodular hyperplasia differ little from smaller nodules in cirrhosis.

Microscopically, there are large areas of regeneration of liver cells, usually with minor subdivisions by connective tissue septa.

Mesenchymal hamartomas. Mesenchymal hamartomas are gray-white to red-purple cystlike lesions that most often arise at the lower margin of the right lobe of the liver in the first two years of life. They tend to grow rapidly because of accumulation of fluid in the cystlike areas.

Microscopically, they are composed of relatively acellular collagenous connective tissue, remnants of bile ducts, and fluid-filled spaces. It is probable that they represent an abnormal development of mesenchymal tissue in the infant.[406, 418, 444]

Peliosis hepatis. Peliosis hepatis is a rare, diffuse angiomatoid change of the liver.[450] Minute angiomatoid spaces of hemorrhagic appearance are distributed throughout the liver. The pathogenesis is uncertain, but it possibly follows miliary necrosis. The disease has been produced experimentally with the 9H virus[404] and has been reported after the use of norethandrolone.[414]

Primary carcinoma

Primary carcinoma of the liver occupies a unique position among neoplasms because of its propensity for arising in an organ that is already severely damaged by another disease—cirrhosis. More rarely, cancer may arise in a noncirrhotic liver. Carcinomas most often are derived from the hepatic cells, but a small percentage (15% to 25%) are of bile duct origin.

Clinically, carcinoma of the liver complicating cirrhosis is difficult to distinguish from cirrhosis alone. An enlarging abdominal mass, pain in the right upper quadrant (often severe), weight loss, rapidly accumulating ascites, and blood-stained ascitic fluid on paracentesis point toward a diagnosis of carcinoma of the liver. Elevation of the right hemidiaphragm and other findings on radiographs are helpful in the diagnosis of primary carcinoma of the liver.[438]

Among patients with primary liver cell carcinoma, an amazing number of abnormal laboratory findings have been noted, including cystathioninuria,[448] dysfibrinogenemia,[447] erythrocytosis,[431] presence of a fetoprotein in the blood,[403] hypercalcemia,[421] hypercholesterolemia,[424] and hypoglycemia.[425] Two types of neoplasms causing hypoglycemia have been studied. In one of these, there is acquired glycogenosis.[425] In patients with erythrocytosis, it has been shown that the blood plasma, urine, and tumor tissue all contain erythropoietin.

Natural history

There is a striking difference in the frequency of carcinoma of the liver in various parts of the world.[409] In Europe and the United States, this varies from 0.1% to 0.7% of all autopsies, whereas in some parts of Africa the frequency is between 10% and 20% of all autopsies. In portions of Southeast Asia, there is also a high frequency of carcinoma of the liver.[445] It is well known that carcinoma of the liver most often arises within a cirrhotic liver, yet there are great differences in the frequency of this complication. Where the incidence of carcinoma of the liver is low, usually between 4% and 6% and, rarely, 10% of patients with cirrhosis eventually develop a carcinoma of the liver. In some geographic areas, particularly Africa, where the frequency of carcinoma of the liver is great, as many as 60% of men with cirrhosis develop carcinoma.

Exactly how cirrhosis predisposes to carcinoma of the liver is not known. Carcinoma most often arises in advanced cirrhosis, especially when large regenerative nodules are present. Precancerous changes, in the form of large atypical cells that contain hyperchromatic nuclei and even binucleate forms, are common in these nodules. It seems that cirrhosis in the native African has a more progressive and intense course, occurs in younger people, and proceeds more often to carcinoma.[412]

In hemochromatosis, cirrhosis evolves slowly and the disease is of long duration. As might be expected, the frequency of carcinoma in this group is high.[449] At the Los Angeles County–University of Southern California Medical Center, the frequency of carcinoma in pigmentary cirrhosis is at least twice as great as carcinoma complicating Laennec's cirrhosis.

The recognition of a high frequency of HAA in sera of patients with liver cell carcinoma has suggested a relationship of carcinoma to hepatitis.[137, 446] It appears that in geographic areas with a high prevalence of asymptomatic antigenemia (chronic active viral hepatitis and unresolved hepatitis), there is an increased frequency of liver cell carcinoma. Thus, in Taiwan, where 80% of patients with liver cell cancer have HAA and where 15% of the population have HAA, liver cell cancer is very frequent. In Uganda, where 3% of the population is HAA positive and 40% of the patients with liver cell carcinoma have antigenemia, there is also a high incidence of liver cancer. In the United States, liver cell carcinoma is not a common tumor. Yet, among those patients whose cirrhosis is nonalcoholic, 60% are HAA positive.

It is possible that the relationship may only be by virtue of the production of cirrhosis, with carcinoma as part of the end stage of cirrhosis. However, we have seen at least one patient with HAA positivity and liver cancer in a noncirrhotic liver. If hepatitis B virus is oncogenic, some additional factor or factors, such as those mentioned below that are common to the tropics, may be a necessary additional factor.

The possibility that *aflatoxins,* the metabolic product of the fungus *Aspergillus flavus,* might be involved in the etiology of liver cell carcinoma has received considerable attention. This fungus has widespread distribution. It has been studied particularly because of its growth on groundnuts in Africa. Aflatoxin B_1 is the most toxic of the aflatoxins. It is highly carcinogenic for some species, including the rat. As little as 15 μg per kilogram daily will produce cancer. To date, there is no direct evidence that aflatoxin is carcinogenic for man.[402, 423]

There is also the possibility that pyrrolizidine alkaloids may be carcinogenic for man. These alkaloids are derived from plants that have a wide distribution in Africa, Asia, and South and Central America. Among these are *Senecio jacobaea, Crotalaria, Cynoglossum, Heliotropium,* and *Trichodesma.* Some of these alkaloids, when given in small quantities, cause immediate effects that are negligible, but cancer of the liver develops in experimental animals weeks or months later. The young are particularly susceptible. The doses given to a pregnant animal may do no damage to the liver of the mother, but the offspring develops cancer.[440] The mechanism of carcinogenesis is not yet understood. Nucleolar segregation and inhibition of RNA synthesis has been shown to occur following acute toxic doses of lasiocarpine.[436]

Among other etiologic factors that may be of significance are infestations due to *Clonorchis sinensis* or *Opisthorchis felineus.* These lead to epithelial hyperplasia of the bile ducts, and either bile duct or liver cell carcinoma

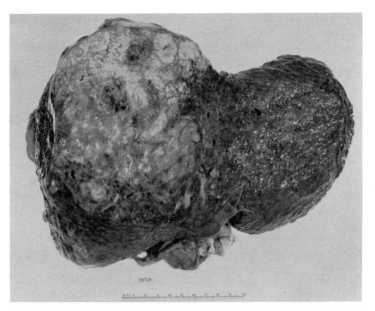

Fig. 28-52 Large nodular liver cell carcinoma of right lobe arising in cirrhotic liver of 57-year-old black man.

may arise. Schistosomiasis, particularly prevalent in Portuguese East Africa, appears to be associated with a high frequency of carcinoma complicating cirrhosis, both in man and in cattle.[412] Intrahepatic calculi, ionizing radiation, and some pharmaceutical preparations also have been mentioned as having etiologic significance.[442] A large number of agents have been used in production of experimental tumors of the liver.[422, 428]

Carcinoma of the liver may occur in infancy and childhood, especially in male infants before the age of 2 years.[441] Among adults, the disease is seen most often in men between the ages of 40 and 60 years in Europe and the United States, whereas in Africa the average is nearer 30 years of age. Carcinoma rarely arises in the absence of cirrhosis, but when it does, females are affected as often as males and they usually live fewer than six months.

Pathologic anatomy

Primary carcinomas may be massive, nodular, or diffuse. They usually arise in a liver that is the seat of advanced cirrhosis.[408] The liver usually weighs between 2,000 gm and 3,000 gm, but some may be of normal size and weight. The right lobe is the more frequently involved in both the massive and the nodular forms. The cancer nodules often bulge beneath Glisson's capsule and are much softer to palpation than are areas of nodular regeneration. The nodules are rarely umbili-

cated. In the massive form of carcinoma, the right lobe particularly may be largely replaced by a well-circumscribed, soft yellow-brown tumor. This type is the more common in noncirrhotic livers. Small secondary nodules are sometimes present in other parts of the liver.

In the nodular type, there is usually one mass that is larger, appears older, and is more circumscribed than any other lesion. Such a tumor may be regarded as the primary lesion (Fig. 28-52). Ordinarily, nodules of smaller size are present throughout the remainder of the liver. Invasion of branches of the portal vein is usually demonstrable and is probably responsible for the rapid spread to all parts of the liver. Hemorrhage, necrosis, and bile-staining may produce a wide variety of color changes within the nodules. It would appear that the nodular type may arise in multicentric foci. This has been emphasized by the African investigators.[412]

The growth of carcinoma in the branches of the portal vein may lead to a tumor thrombus of the portal trunk. Less often, the hepatic veins are invaded, and a tumor thrombus extends into the inferior vena cava. By this route, the cancer may spread to the lungs and more distant structures.

Fully 75% of primary carcinomas are derived from the hepatic cell. These have variously been termed liver cell carcinoma, hepatocellular carcinoma, and hepatoma. They simulate normal liver cells, being char-

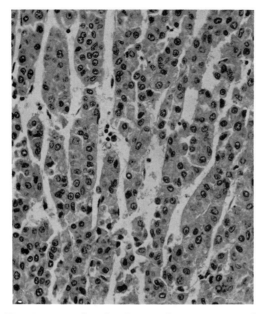

Fig. 28-53 Trabecular liver cell carcinoma with characteristic capillary pattern.

acterized by large, round, hyperchromatic nuclei, prominent nucleoli, abundant granular eosinophilic cytoplasm, and a tendency toward arrangement in trabeculae that are usually two to eight cells in width (Fig. 28-53). They retain another feature indicative of their origin—i.e., the trabeculae are covered (as are liver cords) by a thin basement membrane envelope having, external to this, endothelial cells. This arrangement is particularly well noted when the cancer grows into blood vessels. In the massive carcinomas, the trabecular pattern is not so obvious. But regardless of variations in pattern, most liver cell carcinomas are composed only of malignant cells and a capillary stroma. The excess connective tissue that characterizes most adenocarcinomas is usually absent. Some carcinomas will form acini that may or may not contain bile. Many of the functions of normal liver cells are retained in carcinomas, such as the ability to secrete bile and to store fat and glycogen. It has been suggested that the large amount of glycogen stored in a liver cell carcinoma is not available to form glucose, and this may result in hypoglycemia. Cytoplasmic hyaline inclusions, either globular or small Mallory bodies, are present in some carcinomas.[432] A few carcinomas of liver cell origin are highly undifferentiated, forming spindle and giant cell types. In some carcinomas complicating cirrhosis, there is a combination of liver cell and bile duct carcinoma, with the former predominating as a rule.

Liver cell carcinomas in infants and children are large, multinodular lesions that, with rare exception, arise in noncirrhotic livers. Congenital defects have been noted in an abnormally high percentage of these patients.[411] The cell type is smaller than that seen in adults, and bile plugs are frequent. Some of the tumors contain mesenchymal sarcoma and osteoid tissue. The name *mixed hepatoblastoma* has been suggested for this type.[417] The electron microscopic studies of the epithelial component of these hepatoblastomas disclose immature cells that contain poorly developed organelles. In contrast, the pure hepatomas are composed of more differentiated cells.[419] Surgical treatment of malignant tumors in infants affords the only chance for cure.[426]

Carcinomas may arise from bile ducts within the liver, most often from the large perihilar ducts or ducts of intermediate size. These are usually mucin-producing, well-differentiated sclerosing adenocarcinomas that, on histologic examination, are difficult to distinguish from metastatic adenocarcinomas. Some of these arise in cirrhotic livers. A cholangiolar type of carcinoma has been described.[443] Bile duct carcinoma is known to arise in patients who have had Thorotrast injection,[433] *Clonorchis sinensis* infestation, hemochromatosis, or polycystic disease[415] and occasionally in patients with chronic ulcerative colitis.[435] Bile duct cancer is not so likely to grow within branches of the portal and hepatic veins, although it metastasizes just as widely to the lungs and other organs.

The surgical treatment for carcinoma of the liver has resulted in only a few five-year survivals.[429]

Mesodermal tumors

Malignant tumors of mesodermal origin are rare. *Hemangioendothelial sarcomas* form rather bulky hemorrhagic masses and may metastasize to the lungs, portal lymph nodes, and spleen. Microscopically, they are vasoformative tumors characterized by malignant endothelial lining cells. They may occur following ionizing radiation due to Thorotrast.[433] They also have been seen following exposure to arsenic, both in vineyard workers and following the ingestion of arsenic used for therapeutic purposes.[437]

Embryonal rhabdomyosarcoma, malignant mesenchymoma, and *hepatic mixed tumors* occasionally are seen, especially in infancy

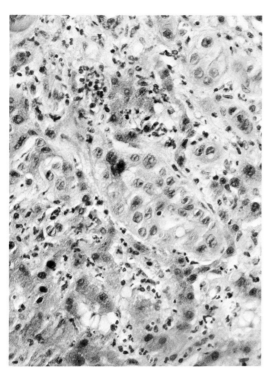

Fig. 28-54 Intrasinusoidal growth of metastatic carcinoma of liver.

and childhood.[407] Although Kupffer cell sarcomas have been reported, this term may be restricted to vasoformative tumors in which the malignant cells are actively phagocytic. Some highly vascular sarcomas of the liver contain large stromal cells in variable quantity that appear to be myosarcomatous.

Metastatic tumors

In *metastatic cancer,* both lobes of the liver usually are involved, producing an enlarged nodular organ that is easily palpable in life. The cancer cells may reach the liver via the portal vein, hepatic artery, or the hilar lymphatics or, occasionally, by direct extension. Once implanted, the cells may, with growth, form small or large nodules or grow diffusely throughout the liver. Metastatic carcinoma often grows within sinusoids. The sinusoidal lining cells may be seen on biopsy around tiny metastatic growths (Fig. 28-54). In about 10% of cases, metastatic nodules are solitary. Characteristically, nodules of irregular size bulge beneath Glisson's capsule and are consistently depressed in their central portions (umbilicated) because of necrosis and/or fibrosis with contraction. Umbilication is practically never seen in liver cell carcinoma.

The pattern of growth of metastatic cancer appears to depend somewhat upon the source —e.g., carcinoma of the colon or stomach often produces large mucin-containing nodules that have a pebbled appearance (Fig. 28-55). Breast cancer often forms smaller, discrete lesions, often oval in outline, as seen beneath Glisson's capsule.

Metastatic carcinoma is usually gray to grayish white, but necrosis, hemorrhage, and mucus may add a variety of colors. Extensive hemorrhagic lesions are characteristic of choriocarcinoma, pancreatic carcinoma, and metastatic carcinoid. Malignant melanoma is black or brown but sometimes only faintly so.

Occasionally, metastatic carcinoma may grow from the hilum outward along the portal tracts, causing them to be unusually prominent. Cancer from the gallbladder may grow directly into the liver, forming a solid mass, along with smaller satellite deposits that decrease in size with increase in distance from their origin.

A needle biopsy of the liver in patients with metastatic carcinoma has proved to be positive in some 60%. If possible, a biopsy should be taken from a palpable nodule.

Metastatic carcinoma usually grows rapidly in the liver, patients rarely living more than a year after the diagnosis is made.[420] There are two notable exceptions: metastatic malignant carcinoid is not incompatible with survival of five to twenty-five years, and metastatic neuroblastoma of the adrenal gland in infancy may apparently be cured with roentgen therapy. Satterlee[439] has given tables indicating the frequency of metastatic tumors in the liver and the probabilities regarding the original site. According to his figures, metastasis to the liver occurs in 36% of all cancers, in 50% of cancers of the portal areas, in 48% of breast cancers, and in 44% of gastric cancers.

INTERPRETATION OF NEEDLE BIOPSIES

The interpretation of needle biopsies of the liver is of such practical importance in the diagnosis and treatment of liver disease that the pathologist should always follow an orderly method of microscopic examination. The following comments are based upon some 13,000 needle biopsies studied by us over the past twelve years.

First, each anatomic subunit is carefully scrutinized for normality. The structures in the triads must be recognized and studied.

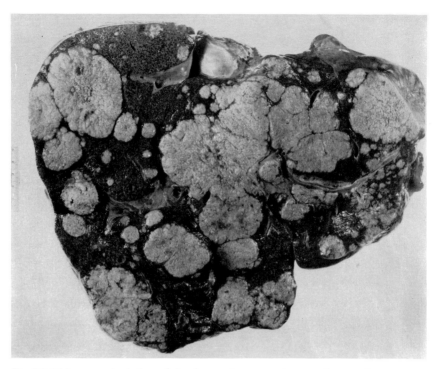

Fig. 28-55 Large metastatic nodules from primary carcinoma of stomach.

The size of the hepatic artery approaches that of the bile duct, whereas the portal vein branch is much larger. The connective tissue within the portal triad is scanty in infants, develops with maturity, and often increases moderately in old age. The borderline between a normal and an abnormal amount of portal lymphoid tissue is difficult to establish. The triads may be considered somewhat analogous to the submucosa of the gut, where the lymphoid tissue has the capacity to become hyperplastic under conditions that cause lymphoid hyperplasia elsewhere. Such hyperplasia may widen the triads, but the limiting plate is intact. Although lymphoid and reticular elements may proliferate, follicles rarely appear. In the absence of intralobular disease, this hyperplasia should not be considered an infiltrate or exudate, and the term "triaditis" is misapplied to this nonspecific lymphoid response.

The lobules are examined for size, cord pattern, sinusoidal appearance, and the presence of central veins. Individual attention must be given to the hepatocytes, bile canaliculi, and Kupffer cells.

Normally, hepatocytes do not differ greatly from one biopsy to another. In old age, atrophy of the cells, as well as decrease in individual size, may decrease lobular diam-

eter. Liver cells may lose glycogen and appear shrunken in starvation, in conditions causing negative nitrogen balance, and in biliary tract obstruction. The hydropic change in any one of many acute liver diseases already has been mentioned. A similar hydropic change occurs in patients with a high fever, in a liver undergoing regeneration, and in diabetic patients treated for hyperglycemia where there is a marked glycogen influx. There may be considerable variation in hepatocytic nuclear size both in specific diseases such as viral hepatitis and in nonspecific reactions. Often, centrilobular liver cells have numerous polyploid nuclei that may be related to an abortive attempt at regeneration in those who are extremely ill, elderly, or undergoing chemotherapy. Vacuolated glycogen-filled nuclei are observed in a variety of metabolic disorders, especially in diabetic patients.

Kupffer cells, as part of the reticuloendothelial system, proliferate in any chronic inflammatory reaction. Inflammatory conditions within the liver, extrahepatic infections, and fever of unknown origin may be responsible for Kupffer cell hyperplasia.

The differential diagnosis of cholestasis often arises in the various forms of acute liver disease. Rarely is viral hepatitis difficult to diagnose, but the differentiation between drug-induced jaundice, extrahepatic biliary obstruction, and simple cholestasis is often difficult or impossible. In extrahepatic bile duct obstruction, the prominence of the small interlobular bile ducts, infiltration of a few circumductal neutrophils, and centrilobular cholestasis are most often seen. In drug cholestasis, the findings are variable, but usually the inflammatory changes in and around the small bile ducts are absent. Simple centrilobular bile stasis is seen in some forms of drug jaundice, occasionally in heart failure, and in some instances of metastatic carcinoma of the liver.

A centrilobular type of zonal necrosis may follow exposure to halothane anesthesia, ingestion of carbon tetrachloride, or drug therapy and is occasionally seen in a needle biopsy. Peripherolobular change due to phosphorus or to eclampsia is extremely rare. In a small percentage of biopsies, occasional foci of cellular dropout marked by a few round cells are present, usually with mild Kupffer cell hyperplasia. An increase of round cells in the triads is often present. These biopsies are taken, as a rule, in febrile patients who have minimal or no laboratory evidence of liver disease. No etiologic factors have been established.

Because of the small size of a needle biopsy, the diagnosis of cirrhosis should be made with care, unless unequivocal septa and nodules are seen. The diagnosis of specific types of cirrhosis may or may not be possible. In alcoholic liver disease, the fatty change and sclerosis of the centrilobular area are the most helpful criteria. In chronic active hepatitis, the diffuse round cell infiltrate, continuing focal necrosis, and areas of collapse are the chief indicators. Septa and nodules composed of fairly normal hepatocytes without infiltrate suggest cryptogenic cirrhosis. In primary biliary cirrhosis, the lack of bile ducts and peripherolobular cholestasis accompanied by penetration of the lobules by proliferation of connective tissue should be kept in mind. Biopsies on patients with cirrhosis often contain only fragments of pseudolobules, apparently because the needle fails to penetrate thick septa. These fragments are often larger than normal lobules and contain no bile ducts. A few islands of liver cell cancer present among cirrhotic nodules on a biopsy is easy to overlook.

Granulomas were seen in about 4% of our specimens. Occasionally, there is only a solitary lesion, best seen in only one fragment. An acid-fast stain and PAS stains should always be done.

Increased quantities of intracytoplasmic pigment may pose a diagnostic problem. Since it is not always possible to distinguish parenchymal cell iron from lipochrome, an iron stain should be performed. Iron deposition is usually greatest in the periportal zones. Lipochrome predominates in the centrilobular areas. A large quantity of fine brown pigment is usually lipochrome and of no diagnostic concern, but occasionally such pigment is seen in patients who have ingested large quantities of analgesic compounds containing phenacetin, salicylate, and caffeine. The chronic use of cascara compounds also may cause a pigmented liver. Large globules of pigment are seen in Dubin-Johnson syndrome (Fig. 28-37). Recently, lipofuscinosis of the liver was reported in patients with a specific central nervous system disease.[410]

Mild degrees of passive congestion, indicated by dilatation of the central veins and sinusoids, should always be reported. Needle biopsies rarely are performed on patients with advanced passive congestion. Massive congestion with disappearance of liver cells and conversion of large portions of the lobules to blood channels is seen in Budd-Chiari syndrome and radiation damage of the liver. An unusually intense congestion with preservation of cord pattern occasionally is observed in sickle cell disease. The sickled cells form sludged clumps and apparently are unable to move through the sinusoids in a normal manner.

In reporting biopsies, when all structures appear normal, a diagnosis of "needle biopsy of liver, apparently normal" can be made. This does not mean, however, that a few centimeters from the location where the specimen was taken that a local lesion such as a neoplasm or abscess might not be present.

Any abnormalities noted in the specimen should be carefully described and reported to the clinician, along with the pathologist's interpretation. Some lesions are specific and involve only a single microscopic subunit, such as Gaucher's disease and periarteritis nodosa. Others, such as neoplasms and amyloidosis, have identifiable features that allow a positive diagnosis. However, in most diseases seen on biopsy, there is more than one microscopic alteration, so that a discussion of the diagnostic probabilities is in order. Such suggestions are often helpful to the clinician.

REFERENCES
General

1 Schiff, L., editor: Diseases of the liver, ed. 3, Philadelphia, 1969, J. B. Lippincott Co.
2 Sherlock, S.: Diseases of the liver and biliary system, ed. 4, Philadelphia, 1968, F. A. Davis Co.
3 Tanikawa, K.: Ultrastructural aspects of the liver and its disorders, Berlin/Heidelberg/New York, 1968, Springer-Verlag.

Structure and circulation

4 Bhathal, P. S., and Christie, G. S.: Lab. Invest. 20:472-487, 1969 (fluorescence microscopy of terminal and subterminal portions of biliary tree).
5 Hales, M. R., Allan, J. S., and Hall, E. M.: Amer. J. Path. 35:909-941, 1959 (injection corrosion studies of normal and cirrhotic livers).
6 Ham, A. W.: Histology, ed. 6, Philadelphia, 1968, J. B. Lippincott Co.
7 Heath, T., and Wissig, S. L.: Amer. J. Anat. 119:97-127, 1966 (fine structure of surface of mouse hepatic cells).
8 McCuskey, R. S.: Amer. J. Anat. 119:455-477, 1966 (study of hepatic arterioles and sphincters).
9 Michels, N. A.: Amer. J. Surg. 112:337-347, 1966 (variant blood supply and collateral circulation of liver).
10 Mills, D. M., and Zucker-Franklin, D.: Amer. J. Path. 54:147-166, 1969 (electron microscopic study of isolated Kupffer cells).
11 Palmer, E. D.: U. S. Armed Forces Med. J. 9:1685-1690, 1958 (palpability of liver edge in healthy adults).
12 Rappaport, A. M., Borowy, Z. J., Lougheed, W. M., and Lotto, W. N.: Anat. Rec. 119:11-33, 1954 (structural and functional units; hepatic physiology and pathology).
13 Steiner, J. W., and Carruthers, J. S.: Amer. J. Path. 38:639-661, 1961 (structure of terminal branches of biliary tree; morphology of normal bile canaliculi, bile preductules and bile ductules).
14 Tygstrup, N., Winkler, K., Mellemgaard, K., and Andreassen, M.: J. Clin. Invest. 41:447-454, 1962 (hepatic arterial blood flow and oxygen supply during surgery).
15 Zamboni, L.: J. Ultrastruct. Res. 12:509-524, 1965 (ultrastructure of fetal liver).
16 Zamboni, L.: J. Ultrastruct. Res. 12:525-541, 1965 (hemopoietic activity of fetal liver).

Function and laboratory diagnosis

17 Alfidi, R. J., Rastogi, H., Buonocore, E., and Brown, C. H.: Radiology 90:1136-1142, 1968 (hepatic arteriography).
18 Arias, I. M.: Ann. Rev. Med. 17:257-274, 1966 (hepatic aspects of bilirubin metabolism).
19 Barnhart, M. I.: J. Histochem. Cytochem. 13:740-751, 1965 (prothrombin synthesis).
20 Bevan, G., Taswell, H. F., and Gleich, G. J.: J.A.M.A. 203:38-40, 1968 (serum immunoglobulin levels in blood donors implicated in transmission of hepatitis).
21 Bouvier, C. A., and Maurice, P. A.: In Rouiller, C., editor: The liver, New York, 1964, Academic Press, Inc. (liver and blood coagulation).
22 Boyd, J. W.: Biochem. J. 81:434-441, 1961 (intracellular distribution, latency and electrophoretic mobility of L-glutamate-oxaloacetate transaminase).
23 Boyd, J. W.: Clin. Chim. Acta 7:424-431, 1962 (glutamate-oxaloacetate transaminase isoenzymes).
24 Boyde, T. R. C., and Latner, A. L.: Biochem. J. 82:51P, 1962 (starch-gel electrophoresis of transaminases).
25 Carbone, J. V., Grodsky, G. M., and Fanska, R.: J. Clin. Invest. 38:994, 1959 (abstract—chemical and clinical studies in BSP metabolites).
26 Colowick, S. P., and Kaplan, N. D.: Methods in enzymology, vol. 2, New York, 1955, Academic Press, Inc.
27 Deykin, D.: J. Clin. Invest. 45:256-263, 1966 (role of liver in serum-induced thrombosis).
28 Edmondson, H. A., and Peters, R. L.: In Pathology annual, vol. 2 (S. C. Sommers, editor), New York, 1967, Appleton-Century-Crofts (diagnostic problems in liver biopsies).
29 Feizi, T.: Gut 9:193-198, 1968 (immunoglobulin in chronic liver disease).
30 Fleisher, G. A., and Wakim, K. G.: Proc. Soc. Exp. Biol. Med. 106:283-286, 1961 (presence of two glutamic-oxalacetic transaminases).
31 Fleisher, G. A., Potter, C. S., and Wakim, K. G.: Proc. Soc. Exp. Biol. Med. 103:229-231, 1960 (separation of 2 glutamic-oxalacetic transaminases).
32 Gartner, L. M., and Arias, I. M.: New Eng. J. Med. 280:1339-1345, 1969 (formation, transport, metabolism, and excretion of bilirubin).
33 Hargreaves, T.: The liver and bile metabolism, New York, 1968, Appleton-Century-Crofts, chap. 3 (bilirubin metabolism).
34 Krugman, S., Giles, J. P., and Hammond, J.: J.A.M.A. 200:365-373, 1967 (infectious hepatitis—two distinctive types).
35 Leevy, C. M.: Progr. Liver Dis. 1:174-186, 1961 (dye extraction by liver).
36 Lester, R.: In Taylor, W.: editor: The biliary system, Oxford, 1965, Blackwell Scientific Publications (why conjugation is necessary for excretion).
37 Levi, A. J., Gatmaitan, Z., and Arias, I. M.: J. Clin. Invest. 48:2156-2167, 1969 (hepatic cytoplasmic protein fractions Y and Z, their possible role in hepatic uptake of bilirubin, sulfobromophthalein, and other anions).
38 Levitt, M., Schacter, B. A., Zipursky, A., and Israils, L. G.: J. Clin. Invest. 47:1281-1294, 1968 (nonerythropoietic component of bilirubin).
39 Manganiello, V. C., and Phillips, A. H.: J. Biol. Chem. 240:3951-3959, 1965 (relationship between ribosomes and endoplasmic reticulum during protein synthesis).
40 Mlecko, L. M., Rodriguez-Antunez, A., Filson, E. J., and Brown, C. H.: Amer. J. Dig. Dis. 12:499-508, 1967 (scintigrams in diagnosis of hepatic neoplasm).
41 Müller, A. F., and Leuthardt, F.: Helv. Chim. Acta 33:268-273, 1950 (conversion of glutamic acid to aspartic acid in liver mitochondria).
42 Peters, R. L., and Ashcavai, M.: Amer. J.

Clin. Path. 54:102-109, 1970 (immunoglobulin levels in detection of viral hepatitis).

43 Robinson, S. H.: New Eng. J. Med. 279:143-149, 1968 (origins of bilirubin).

44 Rowsell, E. V.: Biochem. J. 64:235-245, 1956 (transaminations with L-glutamate and L-oxoglutarate).

45 Scheuer, P. J.: Liver biopsy interpretation, London, 1968, Baillière, Tindall & Cassell.

46 Schmid, R.: In Taylor, W., editor: The biliary system, Oxford, 1965, Blackwell Scientific Publications (studies of congenital nonhemolytic jaundice with 14C-bilirubin).

47 Schmid, R., and Hammaker, L.: J. Clin. Invest. 42:1720-1734, 1963 (metabolism and disposition of C14 bilirubin in congenital nonhemolytic jaundice).

48 Walker, G., and Doniach, D.: Gut 9:266-269, 1968 (antibodies and immunoglobulins in liver disease).

Necrosis

49 Bearcroft, W. G. C.: J. Path. Bact. 80:19-31, 421-426, 1960 (yellow fever).

50 Biava, C.: Lab. Invest. 13:301-320, 1964 (Mallory alcoholic hyalin).

51 Fletcher, G. F., and Galambos, J. T.: Arch. Intern. Med. (Chicago) 112:846-852, 1963 (phosphorus poisoning).

52 Goldberg, L. I.: J.A.M.A. 190:456-462, 1964 (monoamine oxidase inhibitors).

53 Harinasuta, U., and Zimmerman, H. J.: J.A.M.A. 203:1015-1018, 1968 (diphenylhydantoin sodium hepatitis).

54 Recknagel, R. O., and Ghoshal, A. K.: Lab. Invest. 15:132-148, 1966 (lipoperoxidation as vector in carbon tetrachloride hepatotoxicity).

55 Salfelder, K., Seelkopf, C., and Inglessis, G.: Zbl. Allg. Path. 108:524-529, 1966 (phosphorus poisoning).

56 Schaffner, R., Loebel, A., Weiner, H. A., and Barka, T.: J.A.M.A. 183:343-346, 1963 (hepatocellular cytoplasmic changes in acute alcoholic hepatitis).

57 Smetana, H. F.: Ann. N. Y. Acad. Sci. 104:821-846, 1963 (histopathology of drug-induced liver disease).

58 Smuckler, E. A.: Lab. Invest. 15:157-166, 1966 (studies on carbon tetrachloride on liver slides and isolated organelles in vitro).

59 Trump, B. F., Goldblatt, P. J., and Stowell, R. E.: Lab. Invest. 14:1946-1968, 1965 (studies of necrosis in vitro of mouse hepatic parenchymal cells).

Viral hepatitis

60 Adams, R. D., and Foley, J. M.: Ass. Res. Nerv. Ment. Dis., Proc. (1952) 32:198-237, 1953 (neurologic disorders associated with liver disease).

61 Allen, J. G., Sykes, C., Enerson, D. M., Moulder, P. V., Elghammer, R. M., Grossman, B. J., McKeen, C. L., and Galluzzi, N. J.: J.A.M.A. 144:1069-1074, 1950 (homologous serum jaundice).

62 Almed, M. N., Huang, S., and Spence, L.: Arch. Path. (Chicago) 92:66-72, 1971 (Australia antigen and hepatitis).

63 Almeida, J. D., and Waterson, A. P.: Lancet 2:983-986, 1969 (immune complexes in hepatitis).

64 Alter, H. J., Holland, P. V., and Schmidt, P. J.: Lancet 2:142-143, 1970 (hepatitis-associated antigen).

65 Ashcavai, M. and Peters, R. L.: Amer. J. Clin. Path. 55:262-268, 1971 (hepatitis-associated antigen; improved sensitivity in detection).

66 Atchley, F. O., and Kimbrough, R. D.: Lab. Invest. 15:1520-1527, 1966 (infectious hepatitis in chimpanzees).

67 Babudieri, B., Fiaschi, E., Naccarato, R., and Scuro, L. A.: J. Clin. Path. 19:577-582, 1966 (viruslike bodies in liver cells of patients with infectious hepatitis).

68 Becker, M. D., Scheuer, P. J., Baptista, A., and Sherlock, S.: Lancet 1:53-57, 1970 (prognosis of chronic persistent hepatitis).

69 Biava, C., and Mukhlova-Montiel, M.: Amer. J. Path. 46:775-802, 1965 (electron microscopic observations on Councilman-like acidophilic bodies).

70 Blumberg, B. S., Alter, H. J., and Visnich, S.: J.A.M.A. 191:541-546, 1965 ("new" antigen in leukemia sera).

71 Blumberg, B. S., Sutnick, A. I., and London, W. T.: Bull. N. Y. Acad. Med. 44:1566-1586, 1968 (hepatitis and leukemia: their relation to Australia antigen).

72 Boeve, N. R., Winterscheid, L. C., and Merendino, K. A.: Ann. Surg. 170:833-838, 1969 (fibrinogen-transmitted hepatitis in surgical patient).

73 Boyer, J. L., and Klatskin, G.: New Eng. J. Med. 283:1063-1071, 1970 (pattern of necrosis in acute viral hepatitis—prognostic value of bridging).

74 Bucher, N. L. R., Swaffield, M. N., and DiTroia, J. F.: Cancer Res. 24:509-512, 1964 (incorporation of thymidine-2-C14 into DNA of regenerating rat liver).

75 Carver, D. H., and Seto, D. S. Y.: Science 172:1265-1267, 1971 (production of hemadsorption—negative areas by serums containing Australia antigen).

76 Chang, L. W., and O'Brien, T. F.: Lancet 2:59-61, 1970 (Australia antigen serology in Holy Cross football team hepatitis outbreak).

77 Child, P. L., and Ruiz, A.: Arch. Path. (Chicago) 85:45-50, 1968 (acidophilic bodies).

78 Chung, W. K., Moon, S.-K., and Popper, H.: Gastroenterology 48:1-11, 1965 (anicteric hepatitis in Korea).

79 Cohen, S. N., and Dougherty, W. J.: J.A.M.A. 203:427-429, 1968 (transfusion hepatitis arising from addict blood donors).

80 Cooper, W. C., Gershon, R. K., Sun, S.-C., and Fresh, J. W.: New Eng. J. Med. 274:585-595, 1966 (anicteric viral hepatitis in Taiwan).

81 Cossart, Y. E., and Field, A. M.: Lancet 1:848, 1970 (viruslike particles in serum of patients with Australia-antigen–associated hepatitis).

82 Councilman, W. T.: In Sternberg, G. M.: U. S. Marine Hosp. Pub. Health Bull. 2:151-153, 1890 (acidophilic bodies).

83 Cross, G. F., Waugh, M., Ferris, A. A., Gust, I. D., and Kaldor, J.: Aust. J. Exp. Biol. Med.

Sci. **49**:1-9, 1971 (viruslike particles associated with faecal antigen from hepatitis patients and with Australia antigen).

84 Dane, D. S., Cameron, C. H., and Briggs, M.: Lancet **1**:695-698, 1970 (viruslike particles in serum of patients with Australia-antigen–associated hepatitis).

85 Davidson, C. S., and Gabuzda, G. J.: In Schiff, L., editor: Diseases of the liver, ed. 3, Philadelphia, 1969, J. B. Lippincott Co. (hepatic coma).

86 Davis, M. A., Peters, R. L., Redeker, A. G., and Reynolds, T. B.: New Eng. J. Med. **278**:1248-1253, 1968 (appraisal of mortality in acute fulminant viral hepatitis).

87 DeGroote, J., Desmet, V. J., Gedigk, P., Korb, G., Popper, H., Poulsen, H., Scheuer, P., Schmid, M., Thaler, H., Uehlinger, E., and Wepler, W.: Lancet **2**:626-628, 1968 (classification of chronic hepatitis).

88 Deller, J. J., Jr., Cirksena, W. J., and Marcarelli, J.: New Eng. J. Med. **266**:297-299, 1962 (fatal pancytopenia associated with viral hepatitis).

89 Del Prete, S., Constantino, D., Doglia, M., Graziina, A., Ajdukiewicz, A., Dudley F. J., Fox, R. A., and Sherlock, S.: Lancet **2**:579-583, 1970 (detection of new serum-antigen in three epidemics of short-incubation hepatitis).

90 Dougherty, W. J., and Altman, R.: Amer. J. Med. **32**:704-716, 1962 (viral hepatitis in New Jersey 1960-1961).

91 Dubin, I. N., Sullivan, B. H., Jr., LeGolvan, P. C., and Murphy, L. C.: Amer. J. Med. **29**:55-72, 1960 (cholestatic form of viral hepatitis).

92 Findlay, G. M., and MacCallum, F. O.: Trans. Roy. Soc. Trop. Med. Hyg. **31**:297-308, 1937 (acute hepatitis and yellow fever immunization).

93 Gabuzda, G. J.: Gastroenterology **53**:806-810 1967 (ammonium metabolism and hepatic coma).

94 Gauld, R. L.: Amer. J. Hyg. **43**:248-254, 1946 (epidemiologic field studies).

95 Giles, J. P., McCollum, R. W., Berndtson, L. W., and Krugman, S.: New Eng. J. Med. **281**:119-122, 1969 (viral hepatitis: relation of Australia SH antigen to Willowbrook MS-2 strain).

96 Gocke, D. J., and Kavey, N. B.: Lancet **1**:1055-1059, 1969 (hepatitis antigen: correlation with disease and infectivity of blood donors).

97 Gocke, D. J., Greenberg, H. B., and Kavey, N. B.: J.A.M.A. **212**:877-879, 1970 (correlation of Australia antigen with posttransfusion hepatitis).

98 Gocke, D. J., Hsu, K., Morgan, G., Bombardieri, S., Lockshin, M., and Christian, C. L.: Lancet **2**:1149-1153, 1970 (association between polyarteritis and Australia antigen).

99 Grady, G.: J.A.M.A. **214**:140-142, 1970 (prevention of posttransfusion hepatitis by gamma globulin).

100 Gueft, B.: Arch. Path. (Chicago) **72**:61-69, 1962 (viral hepatitis under electron microscope).

101 Gust, I. D., Cross, G., Kaldor, J., and Ferris, A. A.: Lancet **1**:953, 1970 (viruslike particles in Australia-antigen–associated hepatitis).

102 Hersey, D. F., and Shaw, E. D.: Lab. Invest. **19**:558-572, 1968 (viral agents in hepatitis).

103 Hillis, W. D.: Amer. J. Hyg. **73**:316-328, 1961 (infectious hepatitis among chimpanzee handlers).

104 Kim, C. Y., and Tillis, J. G.: J. Infect. Dis. **123**:618-628, 1971 (immunologic and electrophoretic heterogeneity of hepatitis-associated antigen).

105 Kliman, A.: New Eng. J. Med. **284**:109, 1971 (Australia antigen in volunteer and paid blood donors).

106 Klion, F. M., and Schaffner, F.: Amer. J. Path. **48**:755-767, 1966 (ultrastructure of acidophilic "Councilman-like" bodies in the liver).

107 Krugman, S., Giles, J. P., and Hammond, J.: J.A.M.A. **200**:365-373, 1967 (infectious hepatitis).

108 Krugman, S., Giles, J. P., and Hammond, J.: J.A.M.A. **217**:41-45, 1971 (viral hepatitis, type B—MS-2 strain: studies on active immunization).

109 Krugman, S., Ward, R., and Giles, J. P.: Amer. J. Med. **32**:717-728, 1962 (natural history of infectious hepatitis).

110 LeBouvier, G. L.: J. Infect. Dis. **123**:671-675, 1971 (heterogeneity of Australia antigen).

111 Levine, R. A., and Payne, M. A.: Ann. Intern. Med. **53**:164-178, 1960 (homologous serum hepatitis in youthful heroin users).

112 London, W. T., DiFiglia, M., Sutnick, A. I., and Blumberg, B. S.: New Eng. J. Med. **281**:571-578, 1969 (hepatitis in hemodialysis unit: Australia antigen and host response).

113 Lurman, A.: Berlin Klin. Wschr. **22**:20-23, 1885; cited by Smetana, H.: In Schiff, L., editor: Diseases of the liver, ed. 2, Philadelphia, 1963, J. B. Lippincott Co. (eine icterus epidemie).

114 McDermott, W. V., Jr., Barnes, B. A., Nardi, G. L., and Ackroyd, F. W.: Surg. Gynec. Obstet. **126**:585-590, 1968 (postshunt encephalopathy).

115 MacNalty, A. S.: Annual report, Chief Medical Officer, Ministry of Health, 1937, London, 1938, Her Majesty's Stationery Office.

116 Mosley, J. W., and Galambos, J. T.: In Schiff, L., editor: Diseases of the liver, ed. 3, Philadelphia, 1969, J. B. Lippincott Co. (viral hepatitis).

117 Murray, R., and Ratner, F.: Proc. Soc. Exp. Biol. Med. **83**:554-555, 1953 (safety of immune serum globulin).

118 Paul, J. R.: Bull. N. Y. Acad. Med. **22**:204-216, 1946 (infectious hepatitis).

119 Potter, H. P., Cohen, N. N., and Norris, R. F.: J.A.M.A. **174**:2049-2051, 1960 (chronic hepatic dysfunction in heroin addicts).

120 Prince, A. M., and Trepo, C.: Lancet **1**:1309-1312, 1971 (role of immune complexes involving SH antigen in pathogenesis of chronic active hepatitis and polyarteritis nodosa).

121 Propert, S. A.: Brit. Med. J. **2**:677-678, 1938 (hepatitis after prophylactic serum).

122 Read, A. E., McCarthy, C. F., Ajdukiewicz,

A. B., and Brown, G. J. A.: Lancet 2:999-1001, 1968 (encephalopathy after portacaval anastomosis).

123 Redeker, A., and Carpio, N.: In Diller, J. J., editor: Present concepts in internal medicine, vol. 2, San Francisco, 1969, Letterman General Hospital, pp. 107-112 (hippie hepatitis).

124 Redeker, A. G., Hopkins, C. E., Jackson, B., and Peck, P.: Transfusion 8:60-64, 1968 (controlled study of safety of pooled plasma).

125 Rogers, J. A.: Milit. Surg. 91:386-393, 1942 (outbreak of jaundice in Army).

126 Rubin, E., Gottlieb, C., and Vogel, P.: Amer. J. Med. 45:88-97, 1968 (syndrome of hepatitis and aplastic anemia).

127 Schweitzer, I. L., and Spear, R. L.: New Eng. J. Med. 283:570-572, 1970 (hepatitis-associated antigen in mother and infant).

128 Shulman, N. R., and Barker, L. F.: Science 165:304-306, 1969 (viruslike antigen, antibody, and antigen-antibody complexes in hepatitis).

129 Smetana, H. F.: Lab. Invest. 14:1366-1374, 1965 (viral hepatitis in primates).

130 Soper, F. L., and Smith, H. H.: Amer. J. Trop. Med. 18:111-134, 1938 (yellow fever vaccination).

131 Steinitz, H.: Klin. Wschr. 10:698-699, 1931 (frequent occurrence of icterus in diabetics).

132 Stokes, J. H., Ruedemann, R., Jr., and Lemon, W. S.: Arch. Intern. Med. (Chicago) 26:521-543, 1920 (epidemic infectious jaundice and its relation to therapy of syphilis).

133 Sutnick, A. I., London, W. T., Gerstley, J. S., Cronlund, M. M., and Blumberg, B. S.: J.A.M.A. 205:670-674, 1968 (anicteric hepatitis associated with Australia antigen—occurrence in patients with Down's syndrome).

134 Taswell, H. F., Shorter, R., Poncelet, T. K., and Maxwell, N. G.: J.A.M.A. 214:142-144, 1970 (hepatitis-associated antigen in blood donor populations).

135 Teodori, U., Gentilini, P., and Surrenti, C.: Gastroenterologia (Basel) 108:105-120, 1967 (electron microscope observations of forms of viral hepatitis).

136 Tobe, B. A., Zalan, E., Hamvas, J. J., Kuderewko, O., and Labzoffsky, N. A.: Gastroenterology 60:180, 1971 (abst.) (acute hepatitis associated with Australia antigen and an unusual viruslike particle).

137 Tong, M. J., Sun, S., Schaeffer, B. T., Lo, K., Chang, N., and Peters, R.: Ann. Intern. Med. (in press) (hepatitis-associated antigen in patients with hepatocellular carcinoma in Taiwan).

138 Vlahzevic, C. R.: Med. College of Va. Quart. 4:32-37, 1968 (pathogenesis of hepatic encephalopathy).

139 Wilbert, R., and Delorme, M.: Ann. Inst. Pasteur 41:1139-1155, 1927 (icterohemorrhagic spirochetosis of chimpanzee transmissible to man).

140 Yasuzumi, G., Tsubo, I., Okada, K., Terawaki, A., and Enomoto, Y.: J. Ultrastruct. Res. 23:321-332, 1968 (intranuclear inclusion bodies in hepatic parenchymal cells in serum hepatitis).

Chemical and drug injury

141 Bassi, M.: Exp. Cell Res. 20:313-323, 1960 (electron microscopy of rat liver after carbon tetrachloride).

142 Breitenbucher, R., and Crowley, L.: Minn. Med. 53:949-955, 1970 (hepatorenal toxicity of tetracycline).

143 Emond, M., Erlinger, S., Berthelot, P., Benhamou, J.-P., and Fauvert, R.: Canad. Med. Ass. J. 94:900-904, 1966 (effect of novobiocin on liver function).

144 Fulkerson, L. L., Husen, L. A., Lieberman, P., and Stein, E.: New York J. Med. 69:3045-3046, 1969 (tuberculosis treatment with para-aminosalicylic acid).

145 Hargreaves, T.: Nature (London) 206:154-156, 1965 (cholestatic drugs and bilirubin metabolism).

146 Klatskin, G.: In Schiff, L., editor: Diseases of the liver, ed. 3, Philadelphia, 1969, J. B. Lippincott Co., (toxic and drug-induced hepatitis).

147 Pannekoek, J. H.: In Meyler, L., and Herxheimer, A., editors: Side effects of drugs, vol. 6, Baltimore, 1968, The Williams & Wilkins Co. (oral antidiabetic drugs).

148 Panner, B. J., and Hanss, R. J.: Arch. Path. (Chicago) 87:35-45, 1969 (hepatic injury in mushroom poisoning).

149 Peters, R. L., Edmondson, H. A., Mikkelsen, W. P., and Tatter, D.: Amer. J. Surg. 113:622-632, 1967 (tetracycline-induced fatty liver in nonpregnant patients).

150 Peters, R. L., Edmondson, H. A., Reynolds, T. B., Meister, J. C., and Curphey, T. J.: Amer. J. Med. 47:748-764, 1969 (hepatic necrosis associated with halothane anesthesia).

151 Rehder, K., Forbes, J., Alter, H., Hessler, O., and Stier, A.: Anesthesiology 28:711-715, 1967 (halothane biotransformation—quantitative study).

152 Reynolds, T. B., Peters, R. L. and Yamada, S.: New Eng. J. Med. (in press) (chronic active and lupoid hepatitis caused by laxative oxyphenisatin).

153 Reynolds, T. B., Lapin, A. C., Peters, R. L., and Yamahiro, H. S.: J.A.M.A. 211:86-90, 1970 (puzzling jaundice: probable relationship to laxative ingestion).

154 Rothwell-Jackson, R. L.: Brit. Med. J. 1:252, 1968 (letter to editor—Budd-Chiari syndrome after oral contraceptives).

155 Rubin, E., and Lieber, C. S.: Ann. Intern. Med. 69:1063-1067, 1968 (editorial—alcohol, other drugs, and liver).

156 Rubin, E., and Lieber, C. S.: Science 162:690-691, 1968 (hepatic microsomal enzymes in man and rat).

157 Schaffner, F.: J.A.M.A. 198:1019-1021, 1966 (effect of oral contraceptives on liver).

158 Smuckler, E. A., Iseri, O. A., and Benditt, E. P.: J. Exp. Med. 116:55-72, 1962 (intracellular defect in protein synthesis induced by CCl_4).

159 Van Dyke, R. A., and Chenoweth, M. B.: Anesthesiology 26:348-357, 1965 (metabolism of volatile anesthetics).

160 Walker, C. O., and Combes, B.: Gastro-

enterology **51**:631-640, 1966 (biliary cirrhosis induced by chlorpromazine).

161 Zimmerman, H. J.: Amer. J. Gastroent. **49:** 39-56, 1968 (toxic hepatopathy).

Radiation injury

162 Hendee, W. R., Alders, M. A., and Garciga, C. E.: Amer. J. Roentgen. **105**:147-151, 1969 (development of ultrastructural radiation injury).

163 Reed, G. B., Jr., and Cox, A. J., Jr.: Amer. J. Path. **48**:597-611, 1966 (human liver after radiation injury).

Chronic active hepatitis

164 Bearn, A. G., Kunkel, H. G., and Slater, R. J.: Amer. J. Med. **21**:3-15, 1956 (chronic liver disease in young women).

165 Bettley, F. R.: Lancet **2**:724, 1955 (LE cell phenomenon in active chronic hepatitis).

166 Bulkley, B. H., Heizer, W. D., Goldfinger, S. E., Isselbacher, K. J., and Shulman, N. R.: Lancet **2**:1323-1326, 1970 (distinctions in chronic active hepatitis based on circulating hepatitis-associated antigen).

167 Dudley, F. J., Fox, R. A., Sherlock, S.: Lancet **2**:2-5, 1971 (relationship of HAA to acute and chronic liver disease).

168 Gitnick, G. L., Gleich, G. J., Schoenfield, L. J., Baggenstoss, A. H., Sutnick, A. I., Blumberg, B. S., London, W. T., Summerskill, W. H. J.: Lancet **2**:285-288, 1969 (Australia antigen in chronic active liver disease with cirrhosis).

169 Goldstein, L., Reynolds, T., Redeker, A., Schweitzer, I., and Peters, R. L.: Calif. Med. **114**:26-35, 1971 (chronic liver disease from viral hepatitis).

170 Heller, P., Zimmerman, H. J., Rozenvaig, S., and Singer, K.: New Eng. J. Med. **254**:1160-1165, 1956 (LE cell phenomenon in chronic hepatic disease).

171 Joske, R. A., and King, W. E.: Lancet **2**:477-480, 1955 (LE cell phenomenon in active chronic viral hepatitis).

172 Kunkel, H. G., Ahrens, E. H., Jr., Eisenmenger, W. J., Bongiovanni, A. M., and Slater, R. J.: J. Clin. Invest. **30**:654, 1951 (abstract—hypergammaglobulinemia in young women).

173 Mackay, I. R., Weiden, S., and Hasker, J.: Ann. N. Y. Acad. Sci. **124**:767-780, 1955 (autoimmune hepatitis).

174 MacLachlan, M. J., Rodnan, G. P., Cooper, W. N., and Fennell, R. H.: Ann. Intern. Med. **62**:425-462, 1965 (chronic active "lupoid" hepatitis).

175 Reynolds, T. B., Edmondson, H. A., Peters, R. L., and Redeker, A. G.: Ann. Intern. Med. **61**:650-666, 1964 (lupoid hepatitis).

176 Tisdale, W. A.: New Eng. J. Med. **268**:85-89, 138-142, 1963 (subacute hepatitis).

177 Whittingham, S., Irwin, J., Mackey, I. R., and Smalley, M.: Gastroenterology **51**:499-505, 1966 (smooth muscle autoantibody in "autoimmune" hepatitis).

178 Wright, R., McCollum, R. W., and Klatskin, G.: Lancet **2**:117-121, 1969 (Australia antigen in acute and chronic liver disease).

Acute biliary obstruction

179 Biava, C. G.: Lab. Invest. **13**:840-864, 1964 (fine structure of normal human bile canaliculi).

180 Gall, E. A., and Dobrogorski, O.: Amer. J. Clin. Path. **41**:126-139, 1964 (obstructive jaundice).

181 Schoenfield, L. J., Sjövall, J., and Perman, E.: Nature (London) **212**:93-94, 1967 (bile acids on skin of patients with pruritic hepatobiliary disease).

182 Scott, A. J., and Khan, G. A.: Lancet **2**: 790-792, 1967 (origin of bacteria in bile duct bile).

Cirrhosis

183 Adson, M. A., and Wychulis, A. R.: Arch. Surg. (Chicago) **96**:604-612, 1968 (portal hypertension in secondary biliary cirrhosis).

184 Ahrens, E. H., Payne, M. A., Kunkel, H. G., Eisenmenger, W. J., and Blondheim, S. H.: Medicine (Balt.) **29**:299-364, 1950 (primary biliary cirrhosis).

185 Alpert, L. I., Strauss, L., and Hirschhorn, K.: New Eng. J. Med. **280**:16-20, 1969 (neonatal hepatitis and biliary atresia associated with trisomy 17-18 syndrome).

186 Althausen, T. L., and Sborov, V. M.: In Schiff, L., editor: Diseases of the liver, ed. 3, Philadelphia, 1969, J. B. Lippincott Co. (hemochromatosis).

187 Baggenstoss, A. H., Foulk, W. T., Butt, H. R., and Bahn, R. C.: Amer. J. Clin. Path. **42**: 259-276, 1964 (pathology of primary biliary cirrhosis).

188 Banerjee, D., Bhattacharya, M. C., and Behenan, T.: Indian Pediat. **4**:277-280, 1967 (infantile cirrhosis of liver).

189 Bartholomew, L. G., Cain, J. C., Winkelmann, R. K., and Baggenstoss, A. H.: Amer. J. Dig. Dis. **9**:43-55, 1964 (liver disease in scleroderma).

190 Bateman, J. R., Peters, R. L., Hazen, J. G., and Steinfeld, J. L.: Chemother. Rep. **50**:675-682, 1966 (methyl-methane sulfonate in phase I).

191 Bean, W. B.: Amer. Heart J. **25**:463-477, 1943 (vascular "spiders" and palmar erythema).

192 Bearn, A. G.: Ann. Hum. Genet. **24**:33-43, 1960 (genetic analysis of 30 families with Wilson's disease).

193 Becker, W. B., Kipps, A., and McKenzie, D.: Amer. J. Dis. Child. **115**:1-8, 1968 (disseminated herpes simplex virus infection).

194 Bennett, H. S., Baggenstoss, A. H., and Butt, H. R.: Amer. J. Clin. Path. **20**:814-828, 1950 (testis, breast, and prostate of men who die of cirrhosis of liver).

195 Berg, P. A., Doniach, D., and Roitt, I. M.: J. Exp. Med. **126**:277-290, 1967 (mitochondrial antibodies in primary biliary cirrhosis).

196 Berthelot, P., Walker, J. G., Sherlock, S., and Reid, L.: New Eng. J. Med. **274**:291-298, 1966 (arterial changes in lungs in cirrhosis of liver).

197 Beutler, E., Baluda, M. C., Sturgeon, P., and Day, R. W.: J. Lab. Clin. Med. **68**:646-658, 1966 (genetics of galactose-1-phosphate uridyl transferase deficiency).

198 Bothwell, T. H., and Isaacson, C.: Brit. Med. J. 1:522-524, 1962 (siderosis in Bantu).

199 Bradford, W. D., Elchlepp, J. G., Arstila, A. U., Trump, B. F., and Kinney, T. D.: Amer. J. Path. 56:201-228, 1969 (iron metabolism and cell membrane).

200 Bras, G., Jelliffe, D. B., and Stuart, K. L.: Arch. Path. (Chicago) 57:285-300, 1954 (veno-occlusive disease of liver).

201 Butt, E. M., Nusbaum, R. E., Gilmour, T. C., and DiDio, S. L.: Amer. J. Clin. Path. 26: 225-242, 1956 (hemochromatosis and refractory anemia).

202 Butt, E. M., Nusbaum, R. E., Gilmour, T. C., and DiDio, S. L.: In Seven, M. J., and Johnson, L. A., editors: Metal binding in medicine, Philadelphia, 1960, J. B. Lippincott Co. (proceedings of a symposium sponsored by Hahnemann Medical College and Hospital, Philadelphia—trace metal patterns in disease states; Laennec's cirrhosis and chronic alcoholism).

203 Calabresi, P., and Abelmann, W. H.: J. Clin. Invest. 36:1257-1265, 1957 (portopulmonary anastomoses).

204 Callahan, W. P., and Lorincz, A. E.: Amer. J. Path. 48:277-298, 1966 (hepatic ultrastructure in Hurler syndrome).

205 Cohen, S., Kaplan, M., Gottlieb, L., and Patterson, J.: Gastroenterology 60:237-245, 1971 (liver disease and gallstones in regional enteritis).

206 Craig, J. M., Gellis, S. S., and Hsia, D. Y.-Y.: Amer. J. Dis. Child. 90:299-322, 1955 (cirrhosis of liver in infants and children).

207 Doberneck, R. C., Nunn, D. B., Johnson, D. G., and Chun, B. K.: Arch. Surg. (Chicago) 87:751-756, 1963 (iron metabolism and portacaval shunt in dogs).

208 Dohan, F. C., Richardson, E. M., Bluemle, L. W., Jr., and Gyorgy, P.: J. Clin. Invest. 31:481-498, 1952 (hormone excretion in liver disease).

209 Editorial: J.A.M.A. 209:855, 1969 (phenobarbital halts rise in bilirubin).

210 Edmondson, H. A.: In Proceedings of the Thirty-third seminar of the American Society of Clinical Pathologists, Chicago, 1968, American Society of Clinical Pathologists (galactosemia).

211 Edmondson, H. A., Peters, R. L., Frankel, H. H., and Borowsky, S.: Medicine (Balt.) 46:119-129, 1967 (early stage of liver injury in alcoholics).

212 Edmondson, H. A., Peters, R. L., Reynolds, T. B., and Kuzma, O. T.: Ann. Intern. Med. 59:646-673, 1963 (sclerosing hyaline necrosis).

213 Eisenmenger, W. J.: Ann. Intern. Med. 37: 261-272, 1952 (ascites in patients with cirrhosis).

214 Esterly, J. R., Slusser, R. J., and Ruebner, B. H.: J. Pediat. 71:676-685, 1967 (hepatic lesions in congenital rubella syndrome).

215 Gajdusek, D. C.: Arch. Intern. Med. (Chicago) 101:9-46, 1958 ("autoimmune" reaction against human tissue antigens).

216 Gall, E. A., and Landing, B. H.: Amer. J. Clin. Path. 26:1398-1426, 1956 (hepatic cirrhosis and hereditary disorders of metabolism).

217 Gentz, J., Jagenburg, R., and Zetterström, R.: J. Pediat. 66:670-696, 1965 (tyrosinemia).

218 Glenn, F.: Geriatrics 24:98-103, 1969 (indications for operation in biliary tract disease among elderly).

219 Golden, B., Bell, W. E., and McKee, A. P.: J.A.M.A. 209:1219-1221, 1969 (disseminated herpes simplex with encephalitis in neonate).

220 Goldfischer, S., and Sternlieb, I.: Amer. J. Path. 53:883-901, 1968 (changes in distribution of hepatic copper in relation to progression of Wilson's disease).

221 Grace, N. D., and Balint, J. A.: Amer. J. Dig. Dis. 11:351-358, 1966 (hemochromatosis associated with end-to-end portacaval anastomosis).

222 Grahn, E. P., Dietz, A. A., Stefani, S. S., and Donnelly, W. J.: Amer. J. Med. 45:78-87, 1968 (burr cells, hemolytic anemia and cirrhosis).

223 Halvorsen, S., Pande, H., Løken, A. C., and Gjessing, L. R.: Arch. Dis. Child. 41:238-249, 1966 (tyrosinosis).

224 Hansen, R. G.: J.A.M.A. 208:2077-2082, 1969 (hereditary galactosemia).

225 Harries, J. T., Seakins, J. W. T., Ersser, R. S., and Lloyd, J. K.: Arch. Dis. Child. 44: 258-267, 1969 (recovery after dietary treatment of infant with features of tyrosinosis).

226 Hashem, M.: J. Egypt. Med. Ass. 22:319-354, 1939 (etiology and pathology of types of liver cirrhosis in Egyptian children).

227 Herbert, V.: Progr. Liver Dis. 2:57-68, 1965 (hematopoietic factors in liver diseases).

228 Hoenig, V., Brodanova, M. R., and Kordac, V.: Scand. J. Gastroent. 3:334-338, 1968 (effect of ethanol on iron tolerance).

229 Hug, G., Garancis, J. C., Schubert, W. K., and Kaplan, S.: Amer. J. Dis. Child. 111: 457-474, 1966 (glycogen storage disease).

230 Hug, G., Krill, C. E., Jr., Perrin, E. V., and Guest, G. M.: New Eng. J. Med. 268:113-120, 1963 (Cori's disease).

231 Israel, S. L., Meranze, D. R., and Johnston, C. G.: Amer. J. Med. Sci. 194:835-843, 1937 (inactivation of estrogen by liver).

232 Joffe, N.: Brit. J. Radiol. 37:200-209, 1964 (siderosis in South African Bantu).

233 Jolliffe, N., and Jellinek, E. M.: Quart. J. Stud. Alcohol 2:544-583, 1941 (alcoholic cirrhosis).

234 Jones, W. A., Rao, D. R. G., and Braunstein, H.: Amer. J. Path. 39:393-404, 1961 (renal glomerulus in cirrhosis of liver).

235 Kallai, L.: Rheumatism 20:20-26, 1964 (liver changes in rheumatoid arthritis).

236 Kantor, F. S., and Klatskin, G.: Trans. Ass. Amer. Physicians 80:267-274, 1967 (serologic diagnosis of primary biliary cirrhosis).

237 Kelty, R. H., Baggenstoss, A. H., and Butt, H. R.: Gastroenterology 15:285-295, 1950 (portal hypertension).

238 Kent, G., and Popper, H.: Arch. Path. (Chicago) 70:623-639, 1960 (secondary hemochromatosis and its association with anemia).

239 Kent, G., and Popper, H.: Amer. J. Med. 44: 837-841, 1968 (editorial—liver biopsy in diagnosis of hemochromatosis).

240 Kerr, D. N. S., Harrison, C. V., Sherlock, S.,

and Walker, R. M.: Quart. J. Med. 30:91-117, 1961 (congenital hepatic fibrosis).

241 Kibrick, S., and Benirschke, K.: Pediatrics 22:857-874, 1958 (severe generalized disease in newborn infant due to infection with coxsackievirus, group B).

242 Klatskin, G.: J.A.M.A. 170:1671-1676, 1959 (alcoholic cirrhosis).

243 Klatskin, G.: In Schiff, L., editor: Diseases of the liver, ed. 3, Philadelphia, 1969, J. B. Lippincott Co. (hepatitis associated with systemic infections).

244 Krebs, H. A.: Advances Enzym. Regulat. 6:467-480, 1968 (effects of ethanol on metabolic activities of liver).

245 Lester, R., and Troxler, R. F.: New Eng. J. Med. 280:779-780, 1969 (new light on neonatal jaundice).

246 Levi, A. J., Sherlock, S., Scheuer, P. J., and Cumings, J. N.: Lancet 2:575-579, 1967 (presymptomatic Wilson's disease).

247 Levine, R. A., Briggs, G. W., and Lowell, D. M.: Gastroenterology 50:665-670, 1966 (chronic chlorpromazine cholangiolitic hepatitis).

248 Lieber, C. S.: Advances Intern. Med. 14:151-199, 1968 (metabolic effects produced by alcohol in liver and other tissues).

249 Lieber, C. S., and DeCarli, L. M.: Science 162:917-918, 1968 (ethanol oxidation by hepatic microsomes).

250 Lieberman, F. L., Ito, S., and Reynolds, T. B.: J. Clin. Invest. 48:975-981, 1969 (effective plasma volume in sclerosis of ascites).

251 Liebowitz, H. R.: New York J. Med. 69:2012-2014, 1969 (pathogenesis of ascites in cirrhosis of liver).

252 Lopez, M., and Mazzanti, L.: J. Path. Bact. 69:243-250, 1955 (experimental investigations on alpha-naphthyl-iso-thiocyanate as hyperplastic agent of biliary ducts in rat).

253 Luke, C. G., Davis, P. S., and Deller, D. J.: Lancet 2:1392, 1968 (gastric iron-binding in haemochromatosis).

254 MacDonald, R. A.: Nature (London) 199:922, 1963 (wine as source of iron in hemochromatosis).

255 McIntyre, N., Clink, H. M., Levi, A. J., Cumings, J. N., and Sherlock, S.: New Eng. J. Med. 276:439-444, 1967 (hemolytic anemia in Wilson's disease).

256 McKenzie, D., Hansen, J. D. L., and Becker, W.: Arch. Dis. Child 34:250-256, 1959 (herpes simplex virus infection).

257 McKusick, V. A.: Heritable disorders of connective tissue, ed. 3, St. Louis, 1966, The C. V. Mosby Co., chap. 9.

258 Mikkelsen, W. P., Turrill, F. L., and Pattison, A. C.: Amer. J. Surg. 104:204-215, 1962 (portacaval shunt in cirrhosis of liver).

259 Mikkelsen, W. P., Edmondson, H. A., Peters, R. L., Redeker, A. G., and Reynolds, T. B.: Ann. Surg. 162:602-620, 1965 (hepatoportal sclerosis).

260 Mistilis, S. P.: In Schiff, L., editor: Diseases of the liver, ed. 3, Philadelphia, 1969, J. B. Lippincott Co., pp. 1051-1063 (diseases of liver associated with ulcerative colitis).

261 Mohan, M., Bhargava, S. K., Sobti, J. C., and Tanijo, P. N.: Indian Pediat. 4:125-131, 1967 (Indian childhood cirrhosis).

262 Moschcowitz, E.: Arch. Intern. Med. (Chicago) 78:497-530, 1947 (cirrhosis with toxic goiter).

263 Mullane, J. F., and Gliedman, M. L.: Surgery 59:1135-1146, 1966 (elevation of pressure in inferior vena cava).

264 Nathan, M., and Batsakis, J. G.: Surg. Gynec. Obstet. 128:1033-1041, 1969 (congenital hepatic fibrosis).

265 Nelson, R. S., and Sears, M. E.: Amer. J. Dig. Dis. 13:95-106, 1968 (massive sarcoidosis of liver).

266 Oliver, R. A. M.: J. Path. Bact. 77:171-194, 1959 (siderosis following transfusions of blood).

267 Orloff, M. J., Ross, T. H., Baddeley, R. M., Nutting, R. O., Spitz, B. R., Sloop, R. D., Neesby, T., and Halasz, N. A.: Surgery 56:83-98, 1964 (experimental ascites).

268 Palmer, E. D.: Progr. Liver Dis. 1:329-337, 1961 (management of esophageal varices).

269 Papper, S.: Medicine (Balt.) 37:299-316, 1958 (role of kidney in Laennec's cirrhosis).

270 Patek, A. J., Jr.: In Schiff, L., editor: Diseases of the liver, ed. 3, Philadelphia, 1969, J. B. Lippincott Co. (portal cirrhosis—Laennec's cirrhosis).

271 Patrizi, G., Middelkamp, J. N., and Reed, C. A.: Amer. J. Clin. Path. 49:325-341, 1969 (fine structure of herpes simplex hepatoadrenal necrosis in newborn).

272 Phillips, M. J., Little, J. A., and Ptak, T. W.: Amer. J. Med. 44:910-921, 1968 (subcellular pathology of hereditary fructose intolerance).

273 Porta, E. A., Koch, O. R., and Hartroft, W. S.: Lab. Invest. 20:562-572, 1969 (new experimental approach in study of chronic alcoholism).

274 Powell, L. W.: Quart. J. Med. 34:427-442, 1968 (iron storage in relatives of patients with haemachromatosis and in relatives of patients with alcoholic cirrhosis).

275 Ramboer, C., Thompson, R. P. H., and Williams, R.: Lancet 1:966-968, 1969 (controlled trials of phenobarbitone in neonatal jaundice).

276 Randolph, M., and Gelfman, N. A.: Amer. J. Dis. Child. 116:303-307, 1968 (acute encephalopathy in children).

277 Ratnoff, O. D.: Med. Clin. N. Amer. 47:721-736, 1963 (hemostatic mechanisms in liver disease).

278 Reppart, J. T., Peters, R. L., Edmondson, H. A., and Baker, R. F.: Lab. Invest. 12:1138-1153, 1963 (electron and light microscopy of sclerosing hyaline necrosis).

279 Reynolds, T. B.: In Schiff, L., editor: Diseases of the liver, ed. 3, Philadelphia, 1969, J. B. Lippincott Co. (portal hypertension).

280 Reynolds, T. B., and Redeker, A. G.: In McIntyre, N., and Sherlock, S., editors: Therapeutic agents and the liver, Oxford, 1965, Blackwell Scientific Publications (role of alcohol in pathogenesis of alcoholic cirrhosis).

281 Reynolds, T. B., Redeker, A. G., and Geller, H. M.: Amer. J. Med. 22:341-350, 1957 (wedged hepatic pressure).

282 Reynolds, T. B., Hidemura, R., Michel, H.,

and Peters, R.: Ann. Intern. Med. **70:**497-506, 1969 (portal hypertension without cirrhosis in alcoholic liver disease).

283 Reynolds, T. B., Denison, E. K., Frankl, H. D., Lieberman, F. L., and Peters, R. L.: Gastroenterology **58:**290, 1970 (combination primary biliary cirrhosis, scleroderma, and hereditary hemorrhagic telangiectasia).

284 Rolleston, H. D.: Diseases of the liver, gallbladder, and bile-ducts, Philadelphia, 1905, W. B. Saunders Co.

285 Rubin, E., and Lieber, C. S.: New Eng. J. Med. **278:**869-876, 1968 (alcohol-induced hepatic injury in nonalcoholic volunteers).

286 Ruebner, B. H., and Miyai, K.: Ann. N. Y. Acad. Sci. **111:**375-391, 1963 (neonatal hepatitis and biliary atresia; hemopoiesis and hemosiderin deposition).

287 Ruggieri, B. A., Baggenstoss, A. H., and Logan, G. B.: J. Dis. Child. **94:**64-76, 1957 (juvenile cirrhosis).

288 Rupp, J., Cantarow, A., Rakoff, A. E., and Paschkis, K. E.: J. Clin. Endocr. **11:**688-699, 1951 (hormone excretion in liver disease and in gynecomastia).

289 Satran, L., Sharp, H. L., Schenken, J. R., and Krivit, W.: J. Pediat. **75:**39-46, 1969 (fatal neonatal hepatic steatosis).

290 Saxoni, F., Lapatsanis, P., and Pantelakis, S. N.: Clin. Pediat. (Phila.) **6:**687-691, 1967 (congenital syphilis).

291 Sedgwick, P. E., and Pultzan, A.: Portal hypertension, Boston, 1967, Little, Brown and Co.

292 Selzer, G., and Parker, R. G. F.: Amer. J. Path. **27:**885-907, 1951 (*Senecio* poisoning).

293 Sharp, H. L., Bridges, R. A., Krivit, W., and Freier, E. F.: J. Lab. Clin. Med. **73:**934-939, 1969 (cirrhosis associated with alpha-1-antitrypsin deficiency).

294 Sherlock, S.: Progr. Liver Dis. **1:**145-161, 1961 (portal hypertension).

295 Sherlock, S.: In Schiff, L., editor: Diseases of the liver, ed. 3, Philadelphia, 1969, J. B. Lippincott Co. (liver in circulatory failure).

296 Shier, K. J., and Horn, R. C., Jr.: Canad. Med. Ass. J. **89:**645-651, 1963 (liver cirrhosis in patients with cystic fibrosis of pancreas).

297 Shorter, R. G., and Baggenstoss, A. H.: Amer. J. Clin. Path. **32:**10-17, 1959 (biliary cirrhosis).

298 Silber, R., Amorosi, E., Lhowe, J., and Kayden, H. J.: New Eng. J. Med. **275:**639-643, 1966 (spur-shaped erythrocytes in Laennec's cirrhosis).

299 Smetana, H. F.: and Olen, E.: Amer. J. Clin. Path. **38:**3-25, 1962 (hereditary galactose disease).

300 Smetana, H. F., Edlow, J. B., and Glunz, P. R.: Arch. Path. (Chicago) **80:**553-574, 1965 (neonatal jaundice).

301 Smith, H. L., Amick, L. D., and Sidbury, J. B., Jr.: Amer. J. Dis. Child. **111:**475-481, 1966 (type II glycogenosis).

302 Song, Y. S.: Amer. J. Path. **33:**331-351, 1957 (hepatic lesions in sickle cell anemia).

303 Starzl, T. E., Porter, K. A., Brettschneider, L., Penn, I., Bell, P., Purnam, C. W., and McGuire, R. L.: Surg. Gynec. Obstet. **128:**327-339, 1969 (orthotopic transplantation of human liver).

304 Sternlieb, I.: Gastroenterology **55:**354-367, 1968 (mitochondrial and fatty changes).

305 Stirling, G. A., Bras, G., and Urquhart, A. E.: Arch. Dis. Child. **37:**535-538, 1962 (early lesion in veno-occlusive disease of liver).

306 Strauss, L., and Bernstein, J.: Arch. Path. (Chicago) **86:**317-327, 1968 (neonatal hepatitis in congenital rubella).

307 Symmers, D., and Spain, D. M.: Arch. Path. (Chicago) **42:**64-68, 1946 (hepar lobatum).

308 Takada, A., Hartroft, W. S., and Porta, E. A.: Recent Advances Gastroent. **3:**498-501, 1967 (progression and regression of cirrhosis in choline-deficient rats).

309 Tauxe, W. N., Goldstein, N. P., Randall, R. V., and Gross, J. B.: Amer. J. Med. **41:**375-380, 1966 (radiocopper studies in patients with Wilson's disease and their relatives).

310 Terris, M.: Amer. J. Public Health **57:**2076-2088, 1967 (epidemiology of cirrhosis of liver).

311 Thaler, M. M.: Pediatrics **33:**721-734, 1964 (fatal neonatal cirrhosis).

312 Thaler, M. M., and Gellis, S. S.: Amer. J. Dis. Child. **116:**271-279, 1968 (progression and regression of cirrhosis in biliary atresia).

313 Thaler, M. M., and Gellis, S. S.: Amer. J. Dis. Child. **116:**280-284, 1968 (studies in neonatal hepatitis and biliary atresia).

314 Theron, J. J., Hawtrey, A. O., Liebenberg, N., and Schirren, V.: Amer. J. Path. **43:**73-91, 1963 (experimental dietary siderosis).

315 Toghill, P. J., Bailey, M. E., Williams, R., Zeegen, R., and Bown, R.: Lancet **1:**1351-1354, 1967 (cytomegalovirus hepatitis in adult).

316 Tolstrup, N.: Scand. J. Clin. Lab. Invest. **18** (suppl. 92):148-155, 1966 (clinical and biochemical aspects of galactosemia).

317 Walker, J. G., Doniach, D., Roitt, I. M., and Sherlock, S.: Lancet **1:**827-831, 1965 (serologic tests in diagnosis of primary biliary cirrhosis).

318 Walshe, J. M.: In Schiff, L., editor: Diseases of the liver, ed. 3, Philadelphia, 1969, J. B. Lippincott Co. (liver in hepatolenticular degeneration).

319 Wooles, W. R., and Weymouth, R. J.: Lab. Invest. **18:**709-714, 1968 (prevention of ethanol-induced fatty liver).

320 Worwood, M., Taylor, D. M., and Hunt, A. H.: Brit. Med. J. **3:**344-346, 1968 (copper and manganese concentrations in biliary cirrhosis).

321 Zelasco, J. F., Guido, J. J., Capdevielle, I. S., and Rodriguez, M. D.: Rev. Asoc. Med. Argent. **82:**208-213, 1968 (primary biliary cirrhosis and primary cutaneous amyloidosis).

322 Zuelzer, W. W., and Brough, A. J.: In Schiff, L., editor: Diseases of the liver, ed. 3, Philadelphia, 1969, J. B. Lippincott Co. (liver disease in infancy and childhood).

Disease in pregnancy

323 Crawford, G., Cope, I., and Christie, A.: Med. J. Aust. **2:**49-55, 1960 (liver failure in late pregnancy).

324 Mistilis, S. P.: Aust. Ann. Med. **17:**248-260, 1968 (liver disease in pregnancy).

325 Mokotoff, R., Weiss, L. S., Brandon, L. H., and Camillo, M. F.: Arch. Intern. Med. (Chicago) **119:**375-380, 1967 (liver rupture complicating toxemia of pregnancy).

326 Sheehan, H. L.: J. Obstet. Gynaec. Brit. Emp. **47:**49-62, 1940 (yellow atrophy; chloroform poisoning).

327 Yip, R. L., and Pine, D. K.: Obstet. Gynec. **28:**70-72, 1966 (spontaneous rupture of liver).

Diseases of intrahepatic bile ducts

328 Grua, O. E., and McMurrin, J. A.: Amer. J. Surg. **116:**659-663, 1968 (sclerosing cholangitis).

329 Hunter, F. M., Akdamar, K., Sparks, R. D., Reed, R. J., and Brown, C. L., Jr.: Amer. J. Med. **40:**188-194, 1966 (congenital dilation of intrahepatic bile ducts).

330 McSherry, C. K., Stubenbord, W. T., and Glenn, F.: Surg. Gynec. Obstet. **128:**49-61, 1969 (significance of air in biliary system and liver).

331 Mage, S., and Morel, A. S.: Ann. Surg. **162:**187-190, 1965 (surgical experience with cholangiohepatitis).

332 Mistilis, S. P.: Ann. Intern. Med. **63:**1-16, 1965 (pericholangitis and ulcerative colitis).

333 Thorpe, M. E. C., Scheuer, P. J., and Sherlock, S.: Gut **8:**435-448, 1967 (primary sclerosing cholangitis).

Regeneration; transplantation

334 Bengmark, S., Engevik, L., and Rosengren, K.: Surgery **65:**590-596, 1969 (angiography of regenerating human liver after extensive resection).

335 Bucher, N. L. R.: Int. Rev. Cytol. **15:**245-300, 1963 (regeneration of mammalian liver).

336 Donovan, A. J., Turrill, F. L., and Facey, F. L.: Surg. Clin. N. Amer. **48:**1313-1335, 1968 (hepatic trauma).

337 Flute, P. T., Rake, M. O., Williams, R., Seaman, M. J., and Calne, R. Y.: Brit. Med. J. **3:**20-23, 1969 (liver transplantation in man).

338 King, C. D., and Van Lancker, J. L.: Arch. Biochem. **129:**603-608, 1969 (molecular mechanisms of liver regeneration).

339 Lane, B. P., and Becker, F. F.: Amer. J. Path. **50:**435-445, 1967 (regeneration of mammalian liver).

340 Lee, S., and Edgington, T. S.: Amer. J. Path. **52:**649-669, 1968 (heterotopic liver transplantation—rats).

341 Moolten, F. L., and Bucher, N. L. R.: Science **158:**272-274, 1967 (regeneration of rat liver).

342 Williams, R., et al.: Brit. Med. J. **3:**12-19, 1969 (liver transplantation in man).

Degenerations

343 Bondar, G. F., and Pisesky, W.: Arch. Surg. (Chicago) **94:**707-716, 1967 (complications following small intestinal short-circuiting operations for obesity).

344 Editorial: J.A.M.A. **200:**638, 1967 (complications of intestinal bypass for obesity).

345 Farber, E., Lombardi, B., and Castillo, A. E.: Lab. Invest. **12:**873-883, 1963 (prevention by

adenosine triphosphate of fatty liver induced by ethionine).

346 Graham, R. L.: Bull. Johns Hopkins Hosp. **74:**16-25, 1944 (sudden death and associated fatty liver).

347 Karras, B. G., Cannon, A. H., and Zanon, B., Jr.: Acta Radiol. (Stockholm) **57:**458-468, 1962 (hepatic calcification).

348 Levine, R. A.: Amer. J. Med. **33:**349-357, 1962 (amyloid disease of liver).

349 Maxwell, J. G., Richards, R. C., and Albo, D., Jr.: Amer. J. Surg. **116:**648-652, 1968 (fatty degeneration of liver after intestinal bypass for obesity).

350 Miele, A. J., and Edmonds, H. W.: Radiology **80:**779-785, 1963 (calcified liver metastases).

351 Sidransky, H., and Clark, S.: Arch. Path. (Chicago) **72:**468-479, 1961 (chemical pathology of acute amino acid deficiencies).

352 deSilva, C. C.: Advances Pediat. **13:**213-264, 1964 (common nutritional disorders of childhood in tropics).

353 Theron, J. J., and Liebenberg, N.: J. Path. Bact. **86:**109-112, 1963 (fine cytology of parenchymal liver cells in kwashiorkor patients).

Congenital and acquired abnormalities of form and position

354 Johnstone, G.: Arch. Dis. Child. **40:**541-544, 1965 (accessory lobe of liver).

Traumatic injury

355 Charif, P.: Clin. Pediat. (Phila.) **3:**428-431, 1964 (subcapsular hemorrhage of liver in newborn).

356 Richardson, R. E., Gumbert, J. L., and Gale, S. A.: Arch. Surg. (Chicago) **95:**940-943, 1967 (traumatic intrahepatic hematoma).

357 Ryan, K. C., and Lorber, S. H.: New Eng. J. Med. **279:**1215-1216, 1968 (traumatic fistula between hepatic artery and portal vein).

358 Wilkinson, G. M., Mikkelsen, W. P., and Berne, C. J.: Surg. Clin. N. Amer. **48:**1337-1346, 1968 (treatment of post-traumatic hemobilia).

Hereditary hyperbilirubinemia

359 Black, M., and Billing, B. H.: New Eng. J. Med. **280:**1266-1271, 1969 (hepatic bilirubin UDP-glucuronyl transferase activity).

360 Butt, H. R., Anderson, V. E., Foulk, W. T., Baggenstoss, A. H., Schoenfield, L. J., and Dickson, E. R.: Gastroenterology **51:**619-630, 1966 (studies of chronic idiopathic jaundice).

361 Callahan, E. W., Jr., and Schmid, R.: Gastroenterology **57:**134-137, 1969 (excretion of unconjugated bilirubin in bile of Gunn rats).

362 Carbone, J. V., and Grodsky, G. M.: Proc. Soc. Exp. Biol. Med. **94:**461-463, 1957 (constitutional nonhemolytic hyperbilirubinemia in rat).

363 Cornelius, C. E., and Arias, I. M.: Amer. J. Med. **40:**165-169, 1966 (editorial—biomedical models in veterinary medicine).

364 Cornelius, C. E., Arias, I. M., and Osburn, B.: J. Amer. Vet. Med. Ass. **146:**709-713, 1965 (syndrome in Corriedale sheep resembling Dubin-Johnson).

365 Essner, E., and Novikoff, A. B.: J. Ultrastruct. Res. **3:**374-391, 1960 (human hepatocellular pigments and lysosomes).

366 Fleischner, G., and Arias, I. M.: Amer. J. Med. **49:**576-589, 1970 (bilirubin metabolism, hyperbilirubinemias).

367 Herman, J. D., Cooper, E. B., Takeuchi, A., and Sprinz, H.: Amer. J. Dig. Dis. **9:**160-169, 1964 (constitutional hyperbilirubinemia with unconjugated bilirubin—serum and pigment deposition in liver).

Circulatory disturbances

368 Boler, R. K., and Bibighaus, A. J., III: Lab. Invest. **17:**537-561, 1967 (ultrastructural alterations of dog livers during endotoxin shock).

369 Boyer, J. L., Sen Gupta, K. P., Biswas, S. K., Pal, N. C., Basu Mallick, K. C., Iber, F. L., and Basu, A. K.: Ann. Intern. Med. **66:**41-68, 1967 (idiopathic portal hypertension).

370 Donovan, A. J., Reynolds, T. B., Mikkelsen, W. P., and Peters, R. L.: Surgery **66:**474-482, 1969 (systemic portal arteriovenous fistulas).

371 Editorial: J.A.M.A. **201:**693-695, 1967 (Guido Banti—1852-1925).

372 Imanaga, H., Yamamoto, S., and Kuroyanagi, Y.: Ann. Surg. **155:**42-50, 1962 (surgical treatment of portal hypertension).

373 Ludwick, J. R., Markel, S. F., and Child, C. G., III: Arch. Surg. (Chicago) **91:**697-704, 1965 (Chiari's disease).

374 Luna, A., Meister, H. P., and Szanto, P.: Amer. J. Clin. Path. **49:**710-717, 1968 (esophageal varices in absence of cirrhosis).

375 Mallory, T. B.: J. Mount Sinai Hosp. N. Y. **16:**137-148, 1949 (systemic pathology consequent to traumatic shock).

376 Michaeli, D., Ben-Bassat, I., Miller, H. I., and Deutsch, V.: Gastroenterology **54:**929-932, 1968 (hepatic telangiectases and portosystemic encephalopathy in Osler-Weber-Rendu disease).

377 Mikkelsen, W. P., Edmondson, H. A., Peters, R. L., Redeker, A. G., and Reynolds, T. B.: Ann. Surg. **162:**602-620, 1965 (extrahepatic and intrahepatic portal hypertension without cirrhosis).

378 Myers, J. D., and Hickam, J. B.: J. Clin. Invest. **27:**620-627, 1948 (hepatic blood flow and splanchnic oxygen consumption in heart failure).

379 Ravenna, P.: Arch. Intern. Med. (Chicago) **66:**879-892, 1940 (Banti syndrome).

380 Rousselot, L. M.: J.A.M.A. **107:**1788-1793, 1936 (role of congestion—portal hypertension —in so-called Banti's syndrome).

381 Safran, A. P., and Schaffner, F.: Amer. J. Path. **50:**447-463, 1967 (chronic passive congestion of liver in man).

382 Schumer, W., and Sperling, R.: J.A.M.A. **205:**215-219, 1968 (shock and its effect on cell).

383 Seneviratne, R. D.: Quart. J. Exp. Physiol. **35:**77-110, 1949 (physiologic and pathologic responses in blood vessels of liver).

384 Sherlock, S.: In Schiff, L., editor: Diseases of the liver, ed. 3, Philadelphia, 1969, J. B. Lippincott Co. (liver in circulatory failure).

385 Tisdale, W. A., Klatskin, G., and Glenn, W. W.: New Eng. J. Med. **261:**209-218, 1959 (portal hypertension in bleeding esophageal varices).

386 Weil, M. H., and Spink, W. W.: Arch. Intern. Med. (Chicago) **101:**184-193, 1958 (shock syndrome associated with bacteremia).

Chronic infections and liver abscesses

387 Bernstein, M., Edmondson, H. A., and Barbour, B. H.: Arch. Intern. Med. (Chicago) **116:**491-498, 1965 (liver lesion in Q fever).

388 Block, M. A., Schuman, B. M., Eyler, W. R., Truant, J. P., and DuSault, L. A.: Arch. Surg. (Chicago) **88:**602-610, 1964 (surgery of liver abscesses).

389 Böhm, W., and Willnow, U.: Z. Kinderheilk. **88:**215-225, 1963 (Granulomartige Hepatitis bei konnataler Toxoplasmose).

390 Case records of Massachusetts General Hospital, New Eng. J. Med. **279:**932-940, 1968 (subacute bacterial endocarditis, aortic insufficiency, renal and hepatic polycystic disease).

391 Dehner, L. P., and Kissane, J. M.: J. Pediat. **74:**763-773, 1969 (pyogenic hepatic abscesses in infancy and childhood).

392 Guckian, J. C., and Perry, J. E.: Amer. J. Med. **44:**207-215, 1968 (granulomatous hepatitis of unknown etiology).

393 Holt, J. M., and Spry, C. J. F.: Lancet **2:**198-200, 1966 (solitary pyogenic liver abscess in patients with diabetes mellitus).

394 Kramarsky, B., Edmondson, H. A., Peters R. L., and Reynolds, T. B.: Arch. Path. (Chicago) **85:**516-531, 1968 (lepromatous leprosy in reaction).

395 Kuzemko, J. A.: Arch. Dis. Child. **41:**221-222, 1966 (toxocariasis).

396 May, R. P., Lehmann, J. D., and Sanford, J. P.: Arch. Intern. Med. (Chicago) **119:**69-74, 1967 (defects in differentiating amebic from pyogenic liver abscess).

397 Sheehy, T. W., Parmley, L. F., Jr., Johnston, G. S., and Boyce, H. W.: Gastroenterology **55:**26-34, 1968 (resolution time of an amebic liver abscess).

398 Spink, W. W.: Amer. J. Med. Sci. **247:**129-136, 1964 (host-parasite relationship in human brucellosis).

399 Woodruff, A. W., and Thacker, C. K.: Brit. Med. J. **1:**1001-1005, 1964 (infection with animal helminths).

Cysts

400 Melnick, P. J.: Arch. Path. (Chicago) **59:**162-172, 1955 (polycystic liver).

401 Sanders, D. M., II, and Garrett, J. M.: Southern Med. J. **61:**256-261, 1968 (solitary hepatic cyst).

Tumors

402 Alpert, M. E., and Davidson, C. S.: Amer. J. Med. **46:**325-329, 1969 (mycotoxins).

403 Alpert, M. E., Uriel, J., and Nechaud, B. de: New Eng. J. Med. **278:**984-986, 1968 (alpha-1 fetoglobulin in diagnosis of human hepatoma).

404 Bergs, V. V., and Scotti, T. M.: Science **158:**377-378, 1967 (virus-induced peliosis hepatis in rats).

405 Dolan, M. F., and Janovski, N. A.: Arch.

Path. (Chicago) **86:**22-24, 1968 (adrenal dystopia).

406 Edmondson, H. A.: Amer. J. Dis. Child. **91:** 168-186, 1956 (tumors and tumorlike lesions in infancy and childhood).

407 Edmondson, H. A.: In Atlas of Tumor Pathology, Sect. VII, Fasc. 25, Washintgon, D. C., 1958, Armed Forces Institute of Pathology (tumors of liver and intrahepatic bile ducts).

408 Edmondson, H. A., and Steiner, P. E.: Cancer **7:**462-503, 1954 (primary cancer).

409 Elkington, S. G., McBrien, D. J., and Spencer, H.: Brit. Med. J. **2:**1501-1503, 1963 (hepatoma in cirrhosis).

410 Feldman, R. G., Iseri, O. A., Gottlieb, L. S., and Greenberg, J. P.: Neurology (Minneap.) **19:**503-509, 1969 (familial intention tremor, ataxia, and lipofuscinosis).

411 Fraumeni, J. F., Miller, R. W., and Hill, J. A.: J. Nat. Cancer Inst. **40:**1087-1099, 1968 (primary carcinoma of liver in childhood).

412 Gillman, J., and Payet, M.: Acta Un. Int. Cancr. **13:**860-868, 1957 (primary cancer of liver).

413 Goldberg, S. J., and Fonkalsrud, E.: J.A.M.A. **208:**2473-2474, 1969 (successful treatment of hepatic hemangioma with corticosteroids).

414 Gordon, B. S., Wolf, J., Krause, T., and Shai, F.: Amer. J. Clin. Path. **33:**156-165, 1960 (peliosis hepatis and cholestasis following administration of norethandrolone).

415 Homer, L. W., White, H. J., and Read, R. C.: J. Path. Bact. **96:**499-502, 1968 (neoplastic transformation of von Meyenberg complexes of liver).

416 Houck, J. C., and Patel, Y. M.: Nature (London) **206:**158-160, 1965 (proposed mode of action of corticosteroids on connective tissue).

417 Ishak, K. G., and Glunz, P. R.: Cancer **20:** 396-422, 1967 (hepatoblastoma and hepatocarcinoma in infancy and childhood).

418 Ishida, M., Tsuchida, Y., Saito, S., and Sawaguchi, S.: Ann. Surg. **164:**175-182, 1966 (mesenchymal hamartoma of liver).

419 Ito, J., and Johnson, W. W.: Arch. Path. (Chicago) **87:**259-266, 1969 (hepatoblastoma and hepatoma in infancy and childhood).

420 Jaffe, B. M., Donegan, W. L., Watson, F., and Spratt, J. S., Jr.: Surg. Gynec. Obstet. **127:** 1-11, 1968 (factors influencing survival in patients with untreated hepatic metastases).

421 Keller, R. T., Goldschneider, I., and Lafferty, F. W.: J.A.M.A. **192:**782-784, 1965 (hypercalcemia secondary to a primary hepatoma).

422 Kraybill, H. F.: Environ. Res. **2:**231-246, 1969 (food contaminants and gastrointestinal or liver neoplasia).

423 Lancaster, M. C.: Cancer Res. **28:**2288-2292, 1968 (aflatoxin-induced hepatic tumors).

424 Lin, T.-Y, Chen, C.-C., and Liu, W.-P.: Surgery **60:**1275-1281, 1966 (primary carcinoma of liver in infancy and childhood).

425 McFadzean, A. J. S., and Yeung, R. T. T.: Amer. J. Med. **47:**220-235, 1969 (observations on hypoglycemia).

426 Martin, L. W., and Woodman, K. S.: Arch. Surg. (Chicago) **98:**1-7, 1969 (hepatic lobectomy for hepatoblastoma).

427 More, J. R. S.: J. Clin. Path. **19:**470-474, 1966 (cystadenocarcinoma of liver).

428 Morris, H. P.: Advances Cancer Res. **9:**228-296, 1965 (studies on development, biochemistry, and biology of experimental hepatomas).

429 Moseley, R. V.: Surgery **61:**674-686, 1967. (primary malignant tumors of liver)

430 Muehlbauer, M. A., and Farber, M. G.: Amer. J. Gastroent. **45:**355-365, 1966 (hemangioma of liver).

431 Nakao, K., Kimura, K., Miura, Y., and Takaku, F.: Amer. J. Med. Sci. **251:**161-165, 1966 (erythrocytosis associated with carcinoma of liver).

432 Norkin, S. A., and Campagna-Pinto, D.: Arch. Path. (Chicago) **86:**25-32, 1968 (cytoplasmic hyaline inclusions in hepatoma).

433 Person, D. A., Sargent, T., and Isaac, E.: Arch. Surg. (Chicago) **88:**503-510, 1964 (Thorotrast-induced carcinoma of liver).

434 Plachta, A.: Angiology **16:**594-599, 1965 (triad syndrome inherent to calcified cavernous hemangioma of liver).

435 Rankin, J. G., Skyring, A. P., and Goulston, S. J. M.: Gut **7:**433-437, 1966 (liver in ulcerative colitis—bile duct carcinoma).

436 Reddy, J., and Svoboda, D.: Lab. Invest. **19:** 132-145, 1968 (relationship of nucleolar segregation to ribonucleic acid synthesis following administration of selected hepatocarcinogens).

437 Regelson, W., Kim, U., Ospina, J., and Holland, J. F.: Cancer **21:**514-522, 1968 (hemangioendothelial sarcoma of liver).

438 Sanders, C. F.: Clin. Radiol. (Stockholm) **19:** 341-346, 1968 (plain chest radiograph in seventy-five cases of primary carcinoma of liver).

439 Satterlee, R. C.: U. S. Naval Med. Bull. **40:** 133-136, 1942 (metastatic).

440 Schoental, R.: Cancer Res. **28:**2237-2246, 1968 (pyrrolizidine alkaloids).

441 Shorter, R. G., Baggenstoss, A. H., Logan, G. B., and Hallenbeck, G. A.: Pediatrics **25:**191-203, 1960 (primary carcinoma of liver in infancy and childhood).

442 Steiner, P.: Acta Un. Int. Cancr. **13:**628-645, 1957.

443 Steiner, P., and Higginson, J.: Cancer **12:** 753-759, 1959 (cholangiocellular carcinoma of liver).

444 Stephens, C. L., and Jenevein, E. P., Jr.: Arch. Path. (Chicago) **80:**413-414, 1965 (mesenchymal hamartoma of liver).

445 Tull, J. C.: J. Path. Bact. **35:**557-562, 1932 (primary carcinoma in Orientals).

446 Vogel, C. L., Anthony, P. P., Mody, N., and Barker, L. F.: Lancet **2:**622-624, 1970 (hepatitis-associated antigen in Ugandan patients with hepatocellular carcinoma).

447 von Felten, A., Straub, P. W., and Frick, P. G.: New Eng. J. Med. **280:**405-409, 1969 (dysfibrinogenemia in patient with primary hepatoma).

448 Voûte, P. A., Jr., and Wadman, S. K.: Clin. Chim. Acta **22:**373-378, 1968 (cystathioninuria in hepatoblastoma).

449 Warren, S., and Drake, W. L., Jr.: Amer. J. Path. **27:**573-609, 1951 (hepatic carcinoma in hemochromatosis).

450 Yanoff, M., and Rawson, A. J.: Arch. Path. (Chicago) **77:**159-165, 1964 (peliosis hepatis).

Chapter 29

Gallbladder and biliary ducts

Béla Halpert

STRUCTURE AND FUNCTION

The right and left hepatic ducts as they reach the porta hepatis join at an obtuse angle to form the common hepatic duct. This continues as the common bile duct after giving off the cystic duct at an acute angle. The cystic duct gradually widens into the S-shaped neck of the gallbladder, while the common bile duct terminates in the duodenum at the papilla of Vater.

The biliary ducts, as well as the gallbladder, are lined by tall columnar epithelium. Acinar glands producing a mucinous secretion open into the ducts and into the neck of the gallbladder but are absent in its body and fundus. Beneath the epithelium, the lamina propria is delicate and contains the capillaries. The mucosal surface of the gallbladder is immensely enlarged by deep polygonal spaces bordered by ridges of varying heights. Microscopically, the ridges are richly branching, delicate, connective tissue stalks covered by tall columnar cells (Fig. 29-1). External to the lamina propria is a fairly dense, fibrous connective tissue making up the wall of the extrahepatic biliary ducts. In the gallbladder external to the lamina propria are smooth muscle bundles arranged longitudinally and then obliquely or circularly. The muscular coat is surrounded by the perimuscular layer composed of a loose narrow zone of connective tissue, sometimes interspersed with adipose tissue cells. Serosa covers the perimuscular layer over the peritoneal surface of the gallbladder. The opposite surface is attached to the liver. Particularly on the surface toward the liver, aberrant bile ducts (Luschka ducts) frequently occur in the perimuscular layer.[41]

The closeness of the lining epithelium to the muscular layer and the absence of a submucosa suggest that the muscular coat of the gallbladder is genetically a muscularis mucosae. This is further supported by the observation that the glands in the neck of the gallbladder penetrate the muscular coat just as Brunner's glands traverse the muscularis mucosae of the duodenum.[20] Furthermore, in the course of development, the muscular coat of the gallbladder appears simultaneously with that of the muscularis mucosae and later than the muscular coats of the intestine.[30] This derivation of the muscular coat would explain why direct mechanical, chemical, and electrical stimuli that cause an immediate and powerful contraction of the intestines have no demonstrable effect on the gallbladder.

The blood for the extrahepatic biliary ducts is derived from the hepatic arteries, the right supplying the cystic artery to the gallbladder. The common bile duct receives its main blood supply from the retroduodenal artery, a branch of the gastroduodenal artery.[28, 33] The return from the gallbladder is through the cystic vein that empties into the portal vein.

The network of lymph channels in the wall of the gallbladder drains into the lymph node at the neck of the viscus. From here, the flow is toward the porta hepatis and to the peripancreatic lymph nodes. Enlargement of the nodes within the hepatoduodenal ligament may impede or obstruct the flow of bile through the common bile duct.

The nerve supply is parasympathetic and sympathetic. Whether the pattern of distribution in the gallbladder is that of the myenteric plexus (Auerbach's) or that of the submucous plexus (Meissner's) is as yet undetermined.

The function of the extrahepatic biliary ducts is to provide passage of bile into the duodenum. Bile is the product of the liver cells and is a complex liquid. It apparently is produced continually, with its quantity and composition subject to wide variations.[38] According to a conservative estimate, about 0.6 ml of bile is produced per hour per kilogram of body weight in man,[37] and about 3 ml in rabbits.[23] Bile contains an average of 3% sol-

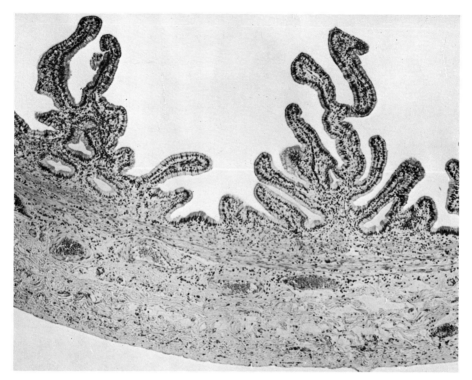

Fig. 29-1 Normal gallbladder (33-year-old woman). In cross section of midportion, delicate connective tissue stalks are covered by tall columnar epithelium. Beneath tunica propria is muscular coat with smooth muscle bundles arranged longitudinally and then obliquely or circularly. External to muscular coat is perimuscular layer. (×40.)

ids. The rest is water.[14] The substances it contains are alkali salts of the bile acids, bile pigments, cholesterol, mucoprotein, and the electrolytes common to all body fluids: sodium, calcium, potassium, and magnesium, as chlorides, bicarbonates, carbonates, and phosphates.[37] The pH of the bile is between 7.1 and 7.3.[35] In the bile from the gallbladder, the range may be between 5.79 and 7.55.[18]

A mechanism at the choledochoduodenal junction regulates the flow of bile into the duodenum. It has long been postulated that an anatomic sphincter exists here and that it has a reciprocal innervation with the gallbladder so that, when the sphincter relaxes, the gallbladder contracts and evacuates its content.[32] Clinical tests assuming the existence of this mechanism are still in use.[31] It is, however, not fully established that an *anatomic sphincter* exists at the choledochoduodenal junction.[16, 22] There is also doubt whether the anatomic arrangement of the biliary ducts and the gallbladder and the distribution and strength of the muscular coat of the viscus permit complete evacuation of the gallbladder by muscle contraction. Occasionally in man

and frequently in animals (rhesus monkey), the gallbladder is completely or almost completely embedded in the liver, without obvious interference with its function.[21]

The function of the gallbladder is to receive and dispose of the overflow of bile while its passage into the duodenum is being negotiated. The bile reaches the gallbladder through the funnel-shaped cystic duct that widens toward the gallbladder. The course of the duct appears somewhat twisted because its lumen is ridged by a series of folds, the valves of Heister.[21] The last of these narrows the lumen toward the gallbladder, offering interference to the flow of bile from the gallbladder. The main force driving the bile into the gallbladder is the pressure on the liver during inspiration.[24] The muscular coat of the gallbladder adjusts the size of the viscus to the change in its content.[25, 34] Overdistention is prevented by ability of the gallbladder to resorb half the volume of its content per hour.[27] According to one concept, mainly water is resorbed,[29, 36] whereas another contends that the mucosa of the gallbladder can resorb all constituents of the bile. Accordingly, the increased concentration of bile in the gallbladder is due to variation in the rate of resorption, some constituents being resorbed more slowly than others.

Certain substances when injected intravenously or given by mouth appear in the bile and reach the gallbladder.[19] Some substances so administered accumulate in the gallbladder in concentrations not attained in the bile coming from the liver.[24] Cholecystography, the visualization of the gallbladder roentgenographically, is based on this selective resorbing ability of the gallbladder. Radiopaque substances (sodium tetraiodophenolphthalein, Priodax,[17] Telepaque,[13] and others) after reaching the gallbladder are resorbed more slowly than the bile, eventually attaining a concentration sufficient to cast a shadow on an x-ray film. The shadow becomes smaller following a fatty meal.[15] This has been interpreted as being due to evacuation of the viscus. Diminution of the shadow may as well be accomplished by selective resorption of the content.[26]

LESIONS

Inflammations, concretions, neoplasms, and anomalies are the important lesions affecting the extrahepatic biliary ducts and the gallbladder. Acute cholecystitis, chronic cholecystitis, and acute cholecystitis superimposed on a chronic cholecystitis are the common inflammatory processes involving the gallbladder. Tuberculous, syphilitic, actinomycotic, and parasitic[44] lesions, when encountered, usually are associated with similar changes in the intrahepatic biliary ducts and in the liver.

Inflammations

Acute cholecystitis. Acute cholecystitis is a nonspecific inflammation caused by streptococci, staphylococci, or the enteric groups of microorganisms. These may reach the viscus in the bile, in the blood, through the lymphatics, or by direct extension from neighboring organs. In the latter instance, the process extends from the outer layers inward and may barely reach the mucosa—pericholecystitis. A temporary increase in bile salt content in the gallbladder also may cause acute cholecystitis, as has been shown experimentally.[46] Enzyme action from reflux of pancreatic secretion into the gallbladder may induce inflammation of the viscus.[40] The gallbladder may become involved in an inflammatory process as a part of an allergic reaction, in polyarteritis nodosa, in endarteritis obliterans, and in terminal uremia. Chemical, enzymatic, and perhaps allergic factors probably excite or play a contributory role in exciting cholecystitis more often than suspected. Vascular obstruction may result in hemorrhagic infarction of the gallbladder, with subsequent acute cholecystitis, and may terminate in acute diffuse peritonitis. The exact mechanism by which acute inflammation of the gallbladder is initiated is, as yet, unknown. However, in acute cholecystitis from whatever cause, the involvement usually starts within the mucosa and extends outward.

In acute cholecystitis, the viscus is enlarged, firm, and discolored reddish brown, with an increase in thickness of its wall up to tenfold. This is caused by spreading of the tissue elements and filling of the spaces with edema fluid and extravasated blood. The lumen usually contains a mixture of bile, blood, and pus. Gallstones usually are not present.

Microscopically, the epithelium may be preserved over extensive areas. Elsewhere it is either shed or missing. All the layers are spread apart and are densely infiltrated with erythrocytes and neutrophilic granulocytes in fibrin or in an amorphous pink substance. In the distended capillaries, margination of white blood cells is conspicuous. The changes are more marked about blood vessels and involve all the layers, including the perimuscular layer and the serosa.

Commensurate with the intensity of the inflammatory process, the clinical signs and symptoms, too, are severe. There is intense pain in the right upper abdomen radiating toward the right shoulder, associated with abdominal rigidity, malaise, nausea, and other signs of beginning peritonitis. The acute process is usually progressive and may end in perforation of the gallbladder with focal abscess or diffuse peritonitis. In rare instances, the inflammation may subside.

Chronic cholecystitis. Various conditions may induce chronic cholecystitis. It usually is assumed to be the sequel of an acute inflammation of the gallbladder (i.e., the healing state of subsiding acute cholecystitis). In other instances, the chronic cholecystitis is due to the presence in the viscus of pure gallstones or of the mulberry-shaped mixed gallstones. Chronic cholecystitis also may be induced by intermittent or continuous abnormal composition of the bile. Attenuated or usually nonpathogenic enteric organisms also may produce chronic cholecystitis. Since so many variables operate in the production of the chronic inflammatory reaction, practically

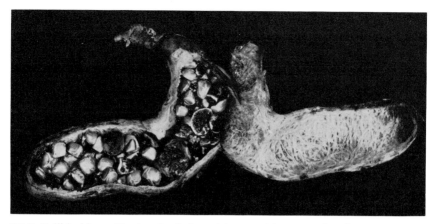

Fig. **29-2** Gallbladder with chronic cholecystitis containing mixed gallstones (40-year-old man). Marked trabeculations on mucosal surface. Calculi faceted and yellow with brown centers.

no two gallbladders with chronic cholecystitis are exactly alike, although they have certain features in common. The most important of these is the almost invariable presence of gallstones. In some instances the gallstones are the cause of and in others the sequel to the chronic inflammatory state of the gallbladder. Familiarity with the chemical composition and structure of gallstones aids, therefore, in interpreting their role in the inflammatory process.

The wall of the gallbladder with chronic cholecystitis is increased to several times its usual thickness. The mucosal folds are coarse and in advanced stages are obliterated or absent, with the surface trabeculated (Fig. 29-2). Occasionally, the wall may become impregnated with calcium (Fig. 29-3) so that a crackling sound (porcelain gallbladder) may be elicited on touch. The lumen of the cystic duct is invariably increased to several times its usual diameter, permitting the passage of calculi into the common bile duct.

Microscopically, the epithelium is usually intact and is mounted on coarse folds. At intervals, it dips to line outpouchings of the mucosa toward the external layers. These outpouchings, the Rokitansky-Aschoff sinuses,[41] usually form along blood vessels and penetrate the thickened muscular coat to varying depths. Their fundi frequently reach the perimuscular layer (Fig. 29-4). They are more numerous in the body and fundus than about the neck of the viscus. The muscular coat is hypertrophied, being increased to several times its usual thickness.[43] The perimuscular layer becomes dense with many coarse collagenous bundles. It may increase to a thickness greater than that of the entire wall of

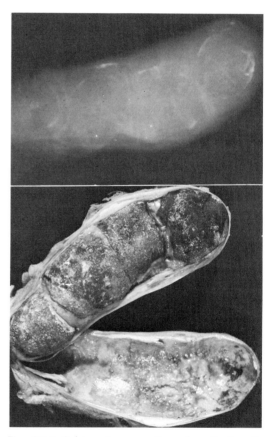

Fig. **29-3** Calcium impregnation of wall of gallbladder (73-year-old black man). Combined calculi with articulating faceted surfaces fill lumen. (Courtesy Dr. William R. Schmalhorst.)

the normal gallbladder. There is also an increase of connective tissue in the lamina propria and between the muscle bundles. All the connective tissue is infiltrated with lymphocytes, plasma cells, large mononuclear

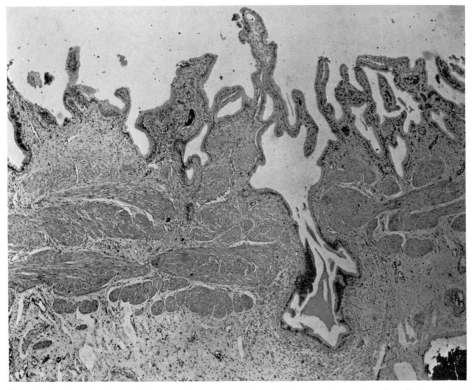

Fig. 29-4 Gallbladder with chronic cholecystitis which contained mixed gallstones (57-year-old woman). In longitudinal section from body of viscus, folds of mucosa are coarse or delicate. Rokitansky-Aschoff sinus extends through entire thickness of markedly hypertrophied muscular coat. Increase in connective tissue in tunica propria and between muscle bundles. Perimuscular layer broad. In all layers, slight infiltration with lymphocytes, plasma cells, large mononuclear cells, and some eosinophilic granulocytes. (×32.)

cells, and eosinophilic granulocytes. Rarely, there is prominence of lymphocytic infiltration in all the layers, with the formation of lymph follicles with large germinal centers—cholecystitis lymph-follicularis[39] (Fig. 29-5). Sometimes, the *Salmonella* group of organisms appears to be responsible[45]; at other times, the cause remains uncertain.

Chronic cholecystitis usually produces vague right upper abdominal distress and distaste for fatty foods. The calculous content of the viscus may occasionally be felt by bimanual palpation. Usually, the gallstones may be visualized roentgenographically. The presence of biliary calculi within the viscus lends clinical importance to chronic cholecystitis. Gallstones may pass through the dilated cystic duct and obstruct the common bile duct, producing jaundice. They also predispose to the development of acute cholecystitis that becomes grafted on the chronic process.

Chronic cholecystitis with superimposed acute cholecystitis. Acute cholecystitis more frequently occurs in a gallbladder with

chronic cholecystitis containing biliary calculi than in an intact gallbladder. Occurrence of chronic and acute cholecystitis in the same gallbladder often is referred to as acute exacerbation of the chronic process, although actually the acute inflammation is superimposed on the chronic inflammatory process.

Grossly, such a gallbladder differs little from one with acute cholecystitis except for the presence of calculi within the viscus. Red, brown, or creamy pus fills the lumen. The calculi may be of any variety, although mixed gallstones of the faceted type are most common. The mucosa is angry red, velvety, and ragged, with frequent erosions. The water-logged wall is many times the usual thickness, and the serosa is discolored red and brown, with flakes of fibrin giving the peritoneal surface a ground glass opacity.

Microscopically, the mucosal folds are coarse, low, or absent. The epithelium varies in height. Rokitansky-Aschoff sinuses are numerous. The muscular coat is markedly hypertrophied with an increase of the inter-

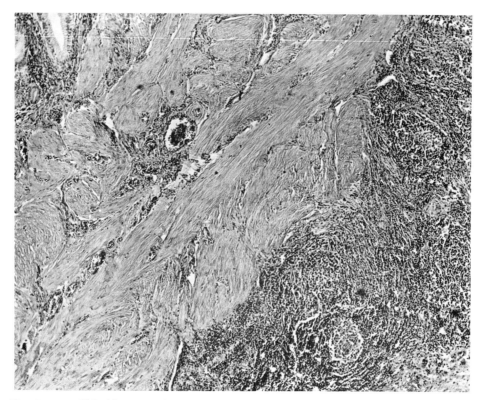

Fig. 29-5 Gallbladder with cholecystitis lymphfollicularis, cholelithiasis (calcium bilirubinate calculi), and acute cholecystitis (52-year-old man). Dense lymphocytic infiltration with formation of lymph follicles having germinal centers. Lymphocytic infiltration mostly in intermuscular connective tissue and in perimuscular layer. Superimposed are edema, extravasation of erythrocytes, and infiltrations with neutrophilic granulocytes. (×60.)

Table 29-1 Classification of gallstones

Type	Composition	Appearance	Factors in origin	Changes in gallbladder
Pure gallstones (10%)	Cholesterol (crystalline)	Solitary; crystalline surface	Increased cholesterol content in bile	Cholesterolosis
	Calcium bilirubinate	Multiple; jet black; crystalline or amorphous	Increased pigment content in bile	No change
	Calcium carbonate	Grayish white; amorphous	Unknown	No change
Mixed gallstones (80%)	Cholesterol and calcium bilirubinate	Multiple, faceted or lobulated, laminated, and crystalline on cut surfaces; hue depends on content: cholesterol, yellow; calcium bilirubinate, black; calcium carbonate, white	Chronic cholecystitis plus increased content in bile of cholesterol, calcium bilirubinate, or calcium carbonate	Chronic cholecystitis
	Cholesterol and calcium carbonate			
	Calcium bilirubinate and calcium carbonate			
	Cholesterol, calcium bilirubinate, and calcium carbonate			
Combined gallstones (10%)	Pure gallstone nucleus with mixed gallstone shell	Largest of gallstones, when single; hue depends on composition of shell	As in pure gallstones, followed by chronic cholecystitis	Chronic cholecystitis
	Mixed gallstone nucleus with pure gallstone shell		As in mixed gallstones, followed by increased content in bile of cholesterol, calcium bilirubinate, or calcium carbonate	Chronic cholecystitis

muscular connective tissue and thickening of the perimuscular layer. In all the layers there is a scattering of lymphocytes, plasma cells, and large mononuclear cells. In addition, a hemorrhagic fibrinopurulent exudate covers denuded areas of the mucosa. All the layers are markedly spread apart by inflammatory edema and infiltrated with freshly extravasated erythrocytes and neutrophilic granulocytes. The serosal surface is covered by fibrin.

Chronic cholecystitis with superimposed acute cholecystitis is a well-known entity. This is the lesion that most commonly necessitates surgical intervention and removal of the gallbladder.[42] The clinical signs and symptoms are those of acute cholecystitis. Because of the presence of biliary calculi, obstruction of the common bile duct may occur, and jaundice may accompany the process. In acute cholecystitis without cholelithiasis, jaundice does not occur unless there is concomitant hepatitis or cholangitis. Perforation of the gallbladder, with subsequent focal or diffuse peritonitis, is a common sequel of acute cholecystitis superimposed on chronic cholecystitis with cholelithiasis.

Concretions

Gallstones usually form in the gallbladder and only occasionally in the biliary ducts. The presence of biliary calculi or gallstones in the gallbladder or in the biliary ducts is called cholelithiasis. The roles played in the formation of gallstones by faulty composition of the bile, stagnation of bile in the gallbladder, and inflammation of the gallbladder and biliary ducts are, as yet, not definitely determined.[47] Gallstones are best grouped according to their composition. Chemical analysis or infrared spectroscopy[52] reveals that three normal constituents of the bile—cholesterol, calcium bilirubinate, and calcium carbonate—are the principal stone-forming substances.[53] Gallstones may be composed almost entirely of one of these substances (pure gallstones), of a mixture of them in varying proportions (mixed gallstones), or of a combination in which one kind of gallstone forms the nucleus and another the shell (combined gallstones) (Table 29-1).

Pure gallstones. About 10% of biliary calculi in surgically removed gallbladders are pure gallstones. Pure gallstones form when the bile contains intermittently or continually an excess of one of the stone-forming substances. This excess is due to disturbances of metabolism or of liver function rather than to an inflammatory reaction of the gallbladder or of the biliary ducts. Pure gallstones are composed almost entirely of cholesterol or of calcium bilirubinate and, rarely, of calcium carbonate.

The *crystalline cholesterol stone* is the most common and is always solitary and remains so as long as its surface is crystalline (Fig. 29-6). It may vary from 0.5 cm to 5 cm in diameter. The smaller ones are spherical, and the larger ones ovoid. Eventually, the crystalline surface becomes obscured, the crevices are filled in, and the entire calculus becomes permeated with calcium carbonate so as to cast a faint radiographic shadow. Yet, the cut surfaces remain crystalline with a glistening radiating pattern. A metabolic disturbance causing an increased cholesterol content of the bile results in the formation of the crystalline cholesterol stone.[48] The gallbladder containing such a stone may present no other change in the mucosa than a delicate network of yellowish white lines corresponding to the slightly broadened ridges of the pri-

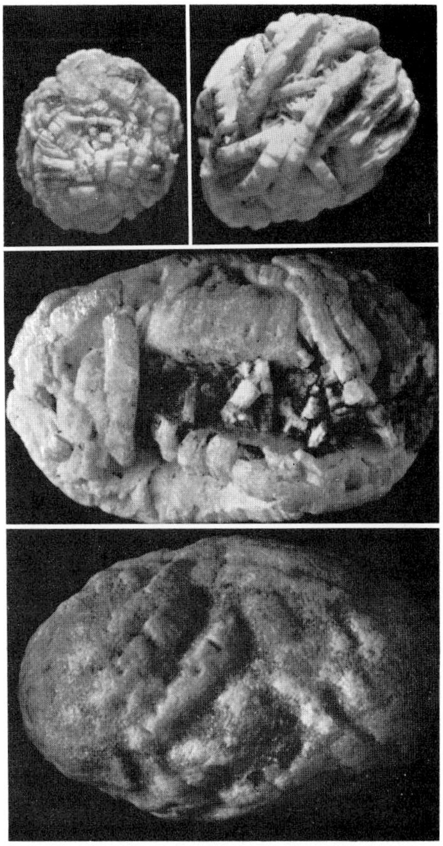

Fig. 29-6 Crystalline cholesterol stones of varying sizes, each from a different gallbladder. (×2; courtesy Dr. Malcolm A. Hyman.)

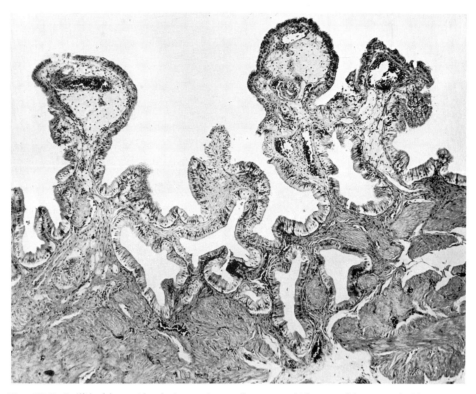

Fig. 29-7 Gallbladder with cholesterolosis of mucosa (46-year-old woman). Viscus contained crystalline cholesterol stone. In cross section from near neck, folds are enlarged and rounded. Connective tissue stalks contain many large mononuclear cells with light-stained cytoplasm and eccentric nuclei. These cells contain anisotropic lipoid substances that can be demonstrated by fat stains. (×60.)

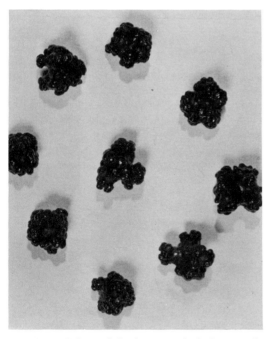

Fig. 29-8 Calcium bilirubinate calculi from gallbladder (78-year-old black man).

mary and secondary folds. Microscopically (Fig. 29-7), in the connective tissue stalks of the folds are many large mononuclear cells with doubly refractile lipoid substances (cholesterol esters) in their cytoplasm (cholesterolosis, p. 1270).

The *calcium bilirubinate stones* are encountered less frequently than the crystalline cholesterol stone. Usually, they are mutiple, jet black, with the shape of jackstones, and rarely are over 1 cm in diameter (Fig. 29-8). Some are firm and preserve their shape. Others are fragile and readily crumble into small fragments. Their calcium content renders them radiopaque. The principal factor in the production of calcium bilirubinate calculi appears to be an intermittent or continuous increase in the bilirubin content of the blood serum due to hemolysis from whatever cause.[55] Hereditary defects in the erythrocytes such as are assumed to occur in hemolytic icterus and sickle cell anemia[63] probably play a role in some instances. In others, hemolysis may be due to hemolysins (antibodies or chemicals) or to infections (malaria).

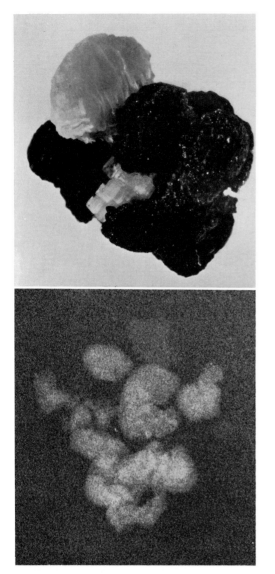

Fig. 29-9 "Paired" pure gallstone from gallbladder (41-year-old woman). Calculus 0.9 cm in diameter. Attached to black calcium bilirubinate concretion are clusters of crystalline cholesterol. Calcium bilirubinate portion radiopaque. (Courtesy Dr. Malcolm A. Hyman.)

A "paired" pure gallstone composed of calcium bilirubinate and crystalline cholesterol has been observed (Fig. 29-9).

The *calcium carbonate stone* is the rarest of the pure gallstones (Fig. 29-10). It is usually grayish white and amorphous.[49] The source of the calcium is undetermined, and the appearance of such calculous material in the bile is not related to any known disturbance of calcium metabolism. Its precipitation may be due to changes in the pH of the gallbladder content. The relation between the

amorphous calcium carbonate calculus and the precipitation of a paste of lime salts, "milk of calcium bile,"[59] still remains to be investigated.

Mixed gallstones. About 80% of the biliary calculi in surgically removed gallbladders are mixed gallstones—i.e., they are composed in varying proportions of all three of the stone-forming constituents of the bile. They form when the function of the gallbladder is so altered that the solvents (bile acids) are resorbed faster than the stone-forming substances they hold in solution. This creates opportunities in the gallbladder for further concentration, precipitation, and crystallization of these substances. Mixed gallstones have the greatest variety in size, number, external appearance, and structure. They vary from 0.1 cm to 2 cm in diameter and are always multiple. When they are small, several thousands of them may be contained in a single gallbladder.[62] Their surfaces usually are faceted, with adjacent stones articulating (Fig. 29-11). Some mixed gallstones have a lobulated surface with the contour of a mulberry. These are twisted, petrified, and broken-off polypoid projections of the gallbladder mucosa that contained lipoid substances (Fig. 29-12). They usually are about 0.5 cm in diameter and rarely reach the size of 1 cm.

The appearance and structure of mixed gallstones depend largely on their chemical composition. Cholesterol lends a yellow hue, calcium bilirubinate a black hue, and calcium carbonate a white hue. Predominance of the color is a fair indication of the chemical composition. Accordingly, mixed gallstones may be grouped as having a predominant content of cholesterol and calcium bilirubinate (yellow-black hue), cholesterol and calcium carbonate (yellow-white hue), calcium bilirubinate and calcium carbonate (gray-black hue), cholesterol, calcium bilirubinate, and calcium carbonate (yellow-black-white hue).

Radiopacity of mixed gallstones depends on their calcium content in the form of calcium bilirubinate, calcium carbonate, or both. When the calcium content is high and the calculi are large enough or numerous enough, they cast a shadow without the aid of cholecystography.

The mode of the formation of mixed gallstones appears to be more complicated than that of pure gallstones. It seems certain that disturbance of the resorptive activity of the gallbladder plays a leading part. Whether this disturbance that allows resorption of the sol-

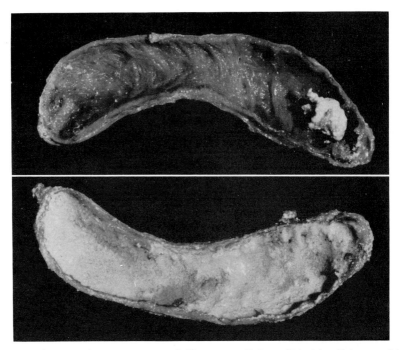

Fig. 29-10 Calcium carbonate stone and "lime paste" in gallbladder (34-year-old man).

vents faster than that of the stone-forming constituents is alone responsible for the formation of mixed gallstones is uncertain. A coincidental increase in stone-forming substances in the bile would certainly accelerate the formation of mixed gallstones and would determine the relative amounts of the various components. It is also uncertain whether the process causing the mixed gallstones to form is also the cause of the chronic cholecystitis that is almost always observed in a gallbladder containing mixed gallstones. It is, however, more likely that chronic cholecystitis itself is the principal cause of the formation of mixed gallstones.

Combined gallstones. About 10% of the biliary calculi in surgically removed gallbladders are combined gallstones—i.e., they are composed of a combination of the ingredients of pure and mixed gallstones, with the one forming the nucleus and the other the shell. They form when the two principal conditions favorable to the formation of gallstones prevail in one or the other sequence. Most commonly, the combined gallstone is solitary, and its nucleus is a pure cholesterol stone; the shell, any one of the mixed gallstones. In some instances, in addition to the large combined stone, a crop of smaller mixed gallstones having the same composition as the shell of the large stone is present in the same

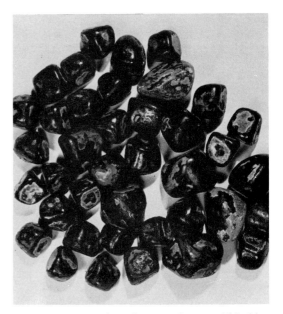

Fig. 29-11 Mixed gallstones from gallbladder (68-year-old black man). Calculi of almost equal size with articulating faceted surfaces. Black with lighter black-brown centers.

gallbladder. Calcium bilirubinate stones may acquire a shell of mixed stone. Conversely, mixed gallstones may acquire shells composed of cholesterol or of calcium bilirubinate or of calcium carbonate. A solitary combined gallstone attains the largest size, sometimes fill-

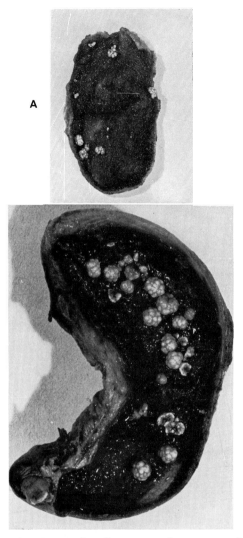

Fig. 29-12 Mixed gallstones, mulberry type. **A,** Gallbladder (46-year-old man). Petrified polypoid projections attached to mucosa (natural size). **B,** Gallbladder (42-year-old man). Calculi have same appearance and composition as polypoid projections in **A.**

ing the entire lumen of the viscus. The gallbladder containing a combined gallstone or combined gallstones always discloses evidences of chronic cholecystitis, not unlike gallbladders containing mixed gallstones.

Incidence. Cholelithiasis rarely is observed in the first and second decades of life.[60] Mixed gallstones occur about four times more frequently in women than in men. The childbearing period in its second half appears to predispose to cholelithiasis. Combined gallstones occur more frequently in the older age groups.[54]

Effects. Calculi within the gallbladder need

not produce clinical manifestations. This is true particularly of pure gallstones (viz. the crystalline cholesterol stone and the calcium bilirubinate stones). Their presence, however, may induce chronic cholecystitis, or there may occur in such a gallbladder acute cholecystitis with appropriate clinical signs and symptoms.

A solitary cholesterol stone in the gallbladder may float in the bile and become imprisoned in the neck between the folds of Heister. This situation cannot develop until the cystic duct has become dilated to at least five times its usual diameter. This dilatation is brought about by intermittently, prolonged closure of the opening of the common bile duct into the duodenum. After the extrahepatic biliary ducts have reached a state of distention, the valvelike action of the stone permits the bile to enter the gallbladder. Because of increased pressure in the biliary ducts, white bile that contains little or no coloring matter is intermittently produced and fills the distended, thin-walled gallbladder (hydrops of the gallbladder). A predisposition to the formation of white bile exists in a patient whose cystic duct has a low insertion and whose common bile duct therefore is short. A pure gallstone imprisoned in the neck of the gallbladder, producing intermittent distention of the viscus by its ball-valve action, may cause only transient discomfort in the right upper abdomen. Later, a chronic inflammatory reaction develops, interfering with the resorptive function of the viscus. Thereafter, three clinical courses are possible: the gallbladder becomes nonfunctioning and no signs and symptoms of cholecystic disease appear; or signs and symptoms of chronic cholecystitis develop; or, if bacterial invasion occurs, empyema of the gallbladder develops.

Calcium bilirubinate stones and calcium carbonate precipitates are usually silent—i.e., they produce no clinical manifestations whatsoever.[61]

Mixed gallstones are contained in gallbladders with chronic cholecystitis. The cystic duct of such a gallbladder is always enlarged to several times its usual diameter. This occurs because of intermittently increased intravesical pressure. As a result of this intravesical hypertension, there develops hypertrophy of the muscular coat, with outpouchings of the mucosa toward the external layers producing the Rokitansky-Aschoff sinuses.[43] The dilatation of the cystic duct with eventual incompetence of its folds at times allows passage of the mixed calculi from the gallbladder into the common bile duct, causing obstruction of the flow of bile into the duodenum. The clinical manifestations produced by the passage of gallstones are intense pain in the right upper abdomen, often radiating to the right shoulder, and sometimes associated mild fever and leukocytosis. A gradually deepening jaundice with clay-colored stools follows obstruction of the common bile duct.

Combined gallstone or gallstones, like mixed gallstones, are contained in gallbladders with chronic cholecystitis. A gallbladder with a large combined gallstone may become fused with the duodenum or with the transverse colon, causing a communication between the gallbladder and the duodenum or the colon. Through a cholecystoduodenal fistula, the calculus may pass from the gallbladder into the duodenum and onward through the jejunum; and, if of sufficient size, it may cause obstruction in the narrow portion of the ileum.[50, 51] Communication with the colon opens a way for retrograde infection of the gallbladder and biliary ducts.

The presence of gallstones in the gallbladder, although silent at times, constitutes an indication for surgical removal of the viscus. Mixed and combined gallstones are a pending threat, in that they predispose to cholecystitis and also to passage of the calculi, resulting in obstruction either of the common bile duct or of the small intestine.

Cholesterolosis. When the cholesterol content of the bile is within physiologic limits, resorption of the cholesterol apparently leaves no demonstrable trace in the mucosa of the gallbladder. When there is an increased cholesterol content, the folds of the mucosa of the gallbladder become streaked with yellow, suggesting the pattern of the surface of a ripe strawberry ("strawberry gallbladder").[56, 64] This condition precedes and is usually concomitant with the presence of the crystalline cholesterol stone and also is observed with mixed gallstones having high cholesterol content. This cholesterolosis may be seen in otherwise normal gallbladders containing no calculi, in gallbladders containing a crystalline cholesterol stone, and in gallbladders with chronic cholecystitis containing mixed or combined gallstones. Up to 20% of all gallbladders removed surgically disclose some degree of cholesterolosis.

Cholecystography. Visualization of the gallbladder by means of radiopaque substances may reveal whether the resorptive function of the viscus is intact or impaired. Occasionally, the Rokitansky-Aschoff sinuses may be visualized.[57] Cholecystography also may disclose anomalies in the shape and position of the gallbladder and the presence of gallstones and occasionally of neoplasms.[58, 72, 74]

Among the biliary calculi, the crystalline cholesterol stone is nonopaque. It may occasionally visualize as a negative shadow in the opaque medium filling the viscus. Calcium bilirubinate stones are radiopaque and, if of sufficient size and number, may cast a shadow without any contrast medium. The radiopacity of mixed gallstones depends on their calcium content. Their visualization with the aid of a contrast medium may be unsuccessful because of the usually impaired resorptive function of the gallbladder. Combined gallstones usually visualize without the aid of cholecystography (scout film).

Neoplasms

In the extrahepatic biliary ducts, neoplasms are rarely encountered.[68a] They are more frequent in the gallbladder.

Papilloma, adenoma, and adenomyoma

Soft projections on the mucosa of the gallbladder, papillomas,[65, 71, 75] may occur singly or in groups or may be scattered over a large part of the surface. The cauliflower-like or seaweedlike, readily movable projection is composed microscopically of delicate or coarse connective tissue stalks covered by columnar epithelium like that of the rest of the mucosa. In the connective tissue stalks, there may be infiltrations with large mononuclear cells filled with doubly refractile lipoid substances. Sometimes these projections may become inspissated, petrified, twisted, or broken off and form the center or framework of berrylike mixed calculi. The papillomas are not precursors of, nor do they predispose to, carcinoma of the gallbladder. However, the possibility of malignant change in a preexisting neoplasm cannot be entirely dismissed.[74]

Adenoma is a low, flat elevation on the mucosal surface, usually of the body of the gallbladder, causing some thickening of the wall. Microscopically, acinar tubular structures lined by cuboidal or columnar epithelium are within a scanty connective tissue stroma. Some of the acini may open into the lumen of the viscus. They do not usually extend into the muscular coat. An adenoma is not a precursor of a carcinoma.

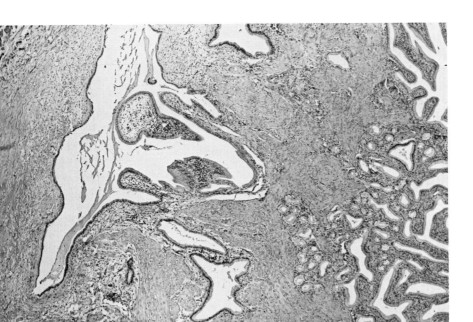

Fig. 29-13 Adenomyoma of gallbladder (56-year-old woman). System of acinar tubular structures lined by cuboidal or columnar cells in scanty connective tissue stroma between interlacing smooth muscle bundles. (×32; courtesy Dr. Malcolm A. Hyman.)

Adenomyoma occurs on or near the fundus, causing slight thickening in that region.[65] Microscopically, there is a system of acinar tubular structures lined by cuboidal or columnar cells in a scanty connective tissue stroma between interlacing smooth muscle bundles (Fig. 29-13). Adenomyomas are malformations rather than neoplasms. They probably represent the anlage either of a part of the fundus that did not develop or of the fundus of an undeveloped bifid or bilobed gallbladder.

Carcinoma

Carcinoma of the extrahepatic biliary ducts usually arises in either of the hepatic ducts, near their junction, or in the common hepatic or common bile ducts, where the cystic duct branches off, or at the papilla of Vater.[76] When the carcinoma involves the intraduodenal portion of the common bile duct, it is frequently difficult or impossible to determine whether the growth originated in the common bile duct, in the papilla of Vater, in the pancreas, or in the duodenum proper.[69] While carcinoma of the head of the pancreas usually obstructs the common bile duct, possible origin of the carcinoma in the other sites is to be considered. Carcinomas of the biliary ducts produce a local stiffening, thick-

ening, distortion of the wall, and gradual obstruction of the lumen of the duct without necessarily involving its entire circumference. The growth usually enlarges by direct extension and spreads to regional lymph nodes. After obstruction of the common bile duct occurs, jaundice appears. When the obstruction is gradual, the proximal tributaries, including the intrahepatic biliary ducts, become dilated, with the eventual production of "white bile" (hydrohepatosis).[67] While still small, these carcinomas cause obstruction, and the patient develops jaundice early and usually dies with cachexia. Practically all carcinomas of the extrahepatic biliary ducts, like those of the intrahepatic biliary ducts, are columnar cell carcinomas.[68] They exhibit considerable variation in the height of the cells lining the acinar tubular structures or covering papillary projections (Fig. 29-14). The degree of differentiation of the cells, the number of cells in a state of division, and the amount and character of the stroma also vary in the individual growths.

Carcinoma of the gallbladder[66, 70, 73] usually originates in the fundus or neck of the viscus and occasionally in the cystic duct. It infiltrates the viscus locally, causing thickening and stiffening of the wall at the site of

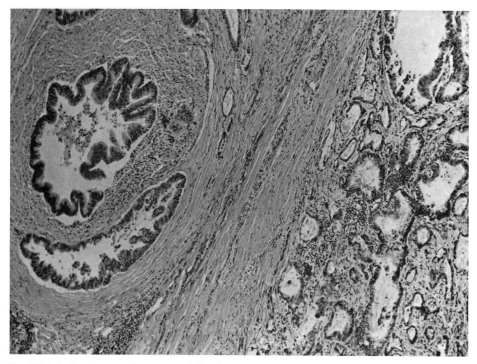

Fig. 29-14 Carcinoma of common bile duct (83-year-old man). Neoplastic cuboidal and columnar cells form acinar tubular structures or are mounted on delicate connective tissue stalks. Neoplastic cells are within sheath of nerve. There was complete obstruction of common bile duct, but no involvement of regional lymph nodes and no distant metastasis. (×60.)

involvement. It may involve the entire gall-bladder (Fig. 29-15, *A*). Some growths protrude into the lumen as irregular, small or bulky, firm or soft masses. More frequently, the growth infiltrates the entire viscus and by direct extension involves the liver about the fossa of the gallbladder, forming a crust, several centimeters thick, of solid neoplastic tissue (Fig. 29-15, *B*). In rare instances in which the entire wall is diffusely involved with multiple areas of ulceration in the mucosa, the extension of the growth is toward the porta hepatis and down the course of the common bile duct, involving the pancreas and duodenum as well. It is estimated that in about 90% of carcinomas of the gallbladder there is cholelithiasis. This has led to the assertion that cholelithiasis predisposes to the development of carcinoma of the gallbladder.

Microscopically, over 90% of carcinomas of the gallbladder are columnar cell carcinomas. Their pattern and structure are similar to those of carcinomas that occur in the biliary ducts. Neoplastic columnar cells of varying heights are mounted on delicate connective tissue stalks or form acinar tubular structures in a scanty or more abundant, loose or dense, fibrous connective tissue stroma (Fig. 29-16). Occasionally, the columnar cells produce mucin in abundance. In rare instances, the mucin-producing cells have a signet-ring appearance. Occasionally, a squamous cell carcinoma is encountered in the gallbladder and, quite rarely, the growth may be a columnar cell and squamous cell carcinoma (adenoacanthoma).

Anomalies

Some of the anomalies of the extrahepatic biliary ducts[80, 82] are incompatible with extra-uterine existence. Anomalies of the gallbladder usually do not interfere with its function. Hypoplasia to the degree of stenosis or atresia of the lumen of the common bile duct is sometimes seen in newborn infants. A large cystlike outpouching of the common bile duct (idiopathic cyst) has been observed and, in some instances, successfully removed.[81] Variations occur in the number of the hepatic ducts and in the manner of their junction with one another and with the cystic duct. Variations occur also in the manner of distribution of the arteries.[79]

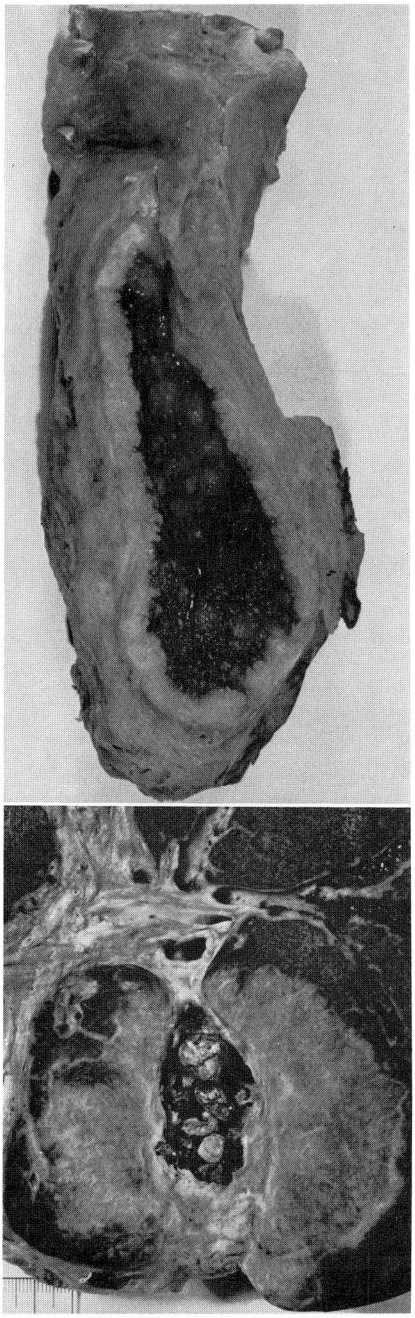

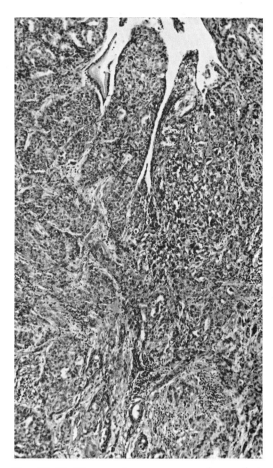

Fig. 29-15 Carcinoma of gallbladder. **A,** Entire wall diffusely involved with multiple areas of ulceration in mucosa. Viscus contained no calculi (39-year-old man). **B,** Lumen filled with mixed gallstones that are faceted. Wall of viscus blends with neoplastic tissue that forms crust several centimeters thick about gallbladder (55-year-old man).

A

B

Fig. 29-16 Microscopic appearance of growth in gallbladder shown in Fig. 29-15, A. Sheets of neoplastic epithelial cells permeate entire thickness of wall. (×60.)

There may be no anlage for the gallbladder, resulting in absence (agenesis) of the viscus, or there may be a double anlage, resulting in partial or complete duplication. Both conditions are rare. Bilobed, double, and septate fundi appear in man but are more common in animals, particularly cats.[77] A "stocking cap" reflection with a septum protruding into the lumen is observed in about 5% of gallbladders. Sometimes, the sep-

tum is near the center, giving the viscus the shape of a dumbbell. Variations in form, size, and peritoneal relations are frequent. The gallbladder may be small and end several centimeters short of the inferior margin of the liver—hypoplasia. In such instances, the cystic duct is usually short, while the common bile duct is long. The reverse is usually true of large gallbladders. The cystic duct runs parallel with the common bile duct, sometimes for a distance of several centimeters, and is fused with it, being separated only by a septum. Usually, about half of the surface of the human gallbladder is covered by peritoneum. Rarely, the entire circumference is surrounded by liver tissue. Occasionally, the viscus is covered by peritoneum with a mesentery-like peritoneal attachment. All transitions between these two extremes may be observed. In rare instances, a small accessory lobe completely detached from the liver is encountered on the surface of the gallbladder.[78] It has been inferred that there was a relation between such an accessory lobe of liver and aberrant bile ducts (Luschka ducts)[41] in the perimuscular layer of the gallbladder. Other heterotopic structures, such as pancreatic tissue or gastric and intestinal epithelium, also have been observed.[83]

REFERENCES
General

1 Aschoff, L., and Bacmeister, A.: Die Cholelithiasis, Jena, 1909, Gustav Fischer.
2 Bockus, H. L.: Gastroenterology, Philadelphia, 1946, W. B. Saunders Co.
3 Graham, E. A., Cole, W. H., Copher, G. H., and Moore, S.: Diseases of the gallbladder and bile ducts, Philadelphia, 1928, Lea & Febiger.
4 Hargreaves, T.: The liver and bile metabolism, New York, 1968, Appleton-Century-Crofts.
5 Lichtman, S. S.: Diseases of the liver, gallbladder and bile ducts, ed. 3, Philadelphia, 1953, Lea & Febiger.
6 Michels, N. A.: Blood supply and anatomy of the upper abdominal organs, Philadelphia, 1955, J. B. Lippincott Co.
7 Popper, H., and Schaffner, F.: Liver structure and function, New York, 1957, McGraw-Hill Book Co.
8 Rolleston, H. D., and McNee, J. W.: Diseases of the liver, gallbladder and bile-ducts, ed. 3, London, 1929, The Macmillan Co.
9 Sherlock, S.: Diseases of the liver and biliary system, ed. 4, Oxford, 1968, Blackwell Scientific Publications.
10 Walters, W., and Snell, A. M.: Diseases of the gallbladder and bile ducts, Philadelphia, 1940, W. B. Saunders Co.
11 Weiss, S.: Diseases of the liver, gall bladder, ducts and pancreas, New York, 1935, Paul B. Hoeber, Inc.
12 With, T. K.: Bile pigments: chemical, biological, and clinical aspects (translated by J. P. Kennedy), New York/London, 1968, Academic Press, Inc.

Structure and function

13 Berti, A. D., and Posse, D. R.: Amer. J. Roentgen. 75:354-359, 1956 (visualization of biliary ducts).
14 Bollman, J. L.: In Walters, W., and Snell, A. M., editors: Diseases of the gallbladder and bile ducts, Philadelphia, 1940, W. B. Saunders Co.

15 Boyden, E. A.: Anat. Rec. 40:147-191, 1928 (reaction of gallbladder to food).
16 Boyden, E. A.: Surgery 1:25-37, 1937 (sphincter of Oddi).
17 Einsel, I. H., and Einsel, T. H.: Amer. J. Dig. Dis. 10:206-208, 1943 (roentgenologic examination).
18 Gilleland, J. L., Gast, J. H., and Halpert, B.: Proc. Soc. Exp. Biol. Med. 94:118-119, 1957.
19 Graham, E. A., and Cole, W. T.: J.A.M.A. 82: 613-614, 1924 (roentgenologic examination).
20 Halpert, B.: Bull. Johns Hopkins Hosp. 40: 390-408, 1927.
21 Halpert, B.: Arch. Surg. (Chicago) 19:1037-1060, 1929.
22 Halpert, B.: Anat. Rec. 53:83-102, 1932 (choledochoduodenal junction).
23 Halpert, B.: Proc. Soc. Exp. Biol. Med. 39: 115-119, 1938 (rate of bile flow).
24 Halpert, B., and Hanke, M. T.: Amer. J. Physiol. 88:351-361, 1929.
25 Halpert, B., and Lewis, J. H.: Amer. J. Physiol. 93:506-520, 1930.
26 Halpert, B., Russo, P. E., and Cushing, V. D.: Proc. Soc. Exp. Biol. Med. 63:102-104, 1946 (roentgenologic studies).
27 Halpert, B., Thompson, W. R., and Marting, F. L.: Amer. J. Physiol. 111:31-34, 1935 (resorption).
28 Henley, F. A.: Brit. J. Surg. 43:75-80, 1955 (blood supply of common bile duct).
29 Ivy, A. C., and Goldman, L.: J.A.M.A. 113: 2413-2417, 1939 (function).
30 Lee, H., and Halpert, B.: Anat. Rec. 54:29-43, 1932 (development).
31 Lyon, B. B. V.: Non-surgical drainage of gall tract, Philadelphia, 1923, Lea & Febiger.
32 Meltzer, S. J.: Amer. J. Med. Sci. 153:469-477, 1917.
33 Parke, W. W., Michels, N. A., and Ghosh, G. M.: Surg. Gynec. Obstet. 117:47-55, 1963.
34 Ravdin, I. S., and Morrison, J. L.: Arch. Surg. (Chicago) 22:810-828, 1931 (function).
35 Reinhold, J. G., and Ferguson, L. K.: J. Exp. Med. 49:681-694, 1929 (reaction of bile).
36 Rous, P., and McMaster, P. D.: J. Exp. Med. 34:47-73, 1921 (concentrating activity).
37 Sobotka, H.: Physiological chemistry of the bile, Baltimore, 1937, The Williams & Wilkins Co.
38 Thureborn, E.: Acta Chir. Scand. suppl. 303, pp. 1-63, 1962 (composition of human bile).

Lesions
Inflammations

39 Anderson, W. A. D.: Personal communication.
40 Bisgard, J. D., and Baker, C. P.: Ann. Surg. 112:1006-1034, 1940 (pathogenesis).
41 Halpert, B.: Bull. Johns Hopkins Hosp. 41: 77-103, 1927 (morphologic studies).
42 Halpert, B.: Surgery 33:444-445, 1953.
43 Halpert, B.: Amer. J. Gastroent. 35:534-539, 1961 (significance of Rokitansky-Aschoff sinuses).
44 Hou, P. C.: J. Path. Bact. 70:53-64, 1955 (Clonorchis sinensis infestation).
45 Mallory, T. B., and Lawson, G. M., Jr.: Amer. J. Path. 7:71-76, 1931 (typhoid cholecystitis).
46 Womack, N. A., and Bricker, E. M.: Arch.

Surg. (Chicago) **44:**658-676, 1942 (pathogenesis).

Concretions

47 Andrews, E., Schoenheimer, R., and Hrdina, L.: Arch. Surg. (Chicago) **25:**796-810, 1932 (etiology).

48 Aschoff, L.: Lectures on pathology, New York, 1924, Paul B. Hoeber, Inc.

49 Báron, J.: Radiology **35:**741-742, 1940.

50 Buetow, G. W., and Crampton, R. S.: Arch. Surg. (Chicago) **86:**504-511, 1963.

51 Coffey, R. J., and Wilcox, G. D.: Amer. Surg. **18:**286-296, 1952 (gallstone obstruction of intestinal tract).

52 Edwards, J. D., Jr., Adams, W. D., and Halpert, B.: Amer. J. Clin. Path. **29:**236-238, 1958 (infrared spectrums).

53 Halpert, B.: Arch. Path. (Chicago) **6:**623-631, 1928 (classification).

54 Halpert, B., and Lawrence, K. B.: Surg. Gynec. Obstet. **62:**43-49, 1936.

54a Höra, F., and Schulz, H.: Beitr. Path. Anat. **141:**195-212, 1970 (strawberry gallbladder, ultrastructure).

55 Illingworth, C. F. W.: Edinburgh Med. J. **43:**481-497, 1936 (pathogenesis).

56 Mackey, W. A.: Brit. J. Surg. **28:**462-467, 1941 (cholesterolosis).

57 March, H. C.: Amer. J. Roentgen. **59:**197-203, 1948 (visualization of Rokitansky-Aschoff sinuses).

58 Moore, R. D.: Amer. J. Roentgen. **75:**360-365, 1956.

59 Phemister, D. B., Day, L., and Hastings, A. B.: Ann. Surg. **96:**595-614, 1932.

60 Potter, A. H.: Surg. Gynec. Obstet. **66:**604-610, 1938 (young subjects).

61 Robertson, H. E.: Gastroenterology **5:**345-372, 1945.

62 Schenken, J. R., and Coleman, F. C.: Gastroenterology **4:**344-346, 1945.

63 Weens, H. S.: Ann. Intern. Med. **22:**182-191, 1945 (in sickle cell anemia).

64 Womack, N. A., and Haffner, H.: Ann. Surg. **119:**391-410, 1944 (cholesterolosis).

Neoplasms

65 Bricker, D. L., and Halpert, B.: Surgery **53:**615-620, 1963.

66 Cooper, W. A.: Arch. Surg. (Chicago) **35:**431-448, 1937 (carcinoma).

67 Counseller, V. S., and McIndoe, A. H.: Surg. Gynec. Obstet. **43:**729-740, 1926.

68 D'Aunoy, R., Ogden, M. A., and Halpert, B.: Surgery **3:**670-678, 1938 (carcinoma).

68a Gray, G. F., and McDivitt, R. W.: Path. Ann. **4:**231-251, 1969.

69 Heaney, J. P., Wise, R. A., and Halpert, B.: Cancer **4:**737-744, 1951.

70 Illingworth, C. F. W.: Brit. J. Surg. **23:**4-18, 1935 (carcinoma).

71 Kane, C. F., Brown, C. H., and Hoerr, S. O.: Amer. J. Surg. **83:**161-164, 1952 (papilloma of gallbladder).

72 Kirklin, B. R.: Amer. J. Roentgen. **29:**8-16, 1933 (roentgenologic examination).

73 Kirschbaum, J. D., and Kozoll, D. D.: Surg. Gynec. Obstet. **73:**740-754, 1941 (carcinoma).

74 Ochsner, S., and Carrera, G. M.: Gastroenterology **31:**266-273, 1956.

75 Shepard, V. D., Walters, W., and Dockerty, M. B.: Arch. Surg. (Chicago) **45:**1-18, 1942.

76 Thorbjarnarson, B.: Cancer **12:**708-713, 1959 (carcinoma of bile ducts).

Anomalies

77 Boyden, E. A.: Amer. J. Anat. **38:**177-222, 1926.

78 Cullen, T. S.: Arch. Surg. (Chicago) **11:**718-764, 1925.

79 Grant, J. C. B.: An atlas of anatomy, ed. 5, Baltimore, 1962, The Williams & Wilkins Co.

80 Ladd, W. E.: Ann. Surg. **102:**742-751, 1935.

81 McWhorter, G. L.: Arch. Surg. (Chicago) **38:**397-411, 1939.

82 Redo, S. F.: Arch. Surg. (Chicago) **69:**886-897, 1954.

83 Williams, M. J., and Humm, J. J.: Surgery **34:**133-139, 1953.

Chapter 30

Pancreas and diabetes mellitus

Paul E. Lacy and John M. Kissane

NORMAL FORM AND DEVELOPMENT

The pancreas is an elongated gland that extends transversely across the posterior abdominal wall from the concavity of the duodenal loop. In the adult, it measures 12 cm to 15 cm in length and weighs 60 gm to 100 gm.

The pancreas is subdivided into angular lobes and lobules by delicate connective tissue septa in which are found blood and lymphatic vessels, nerves, and ducts. The acini within the lobules are formed by pyramid-shaped acinar cells that contain numerous zymogen granules at their apices. Enzymes such as chymotrypsin, carboxypeptidase, and elastase have been demonstrated within individual zymogen granules by the fluorescent antibody technique. The basal portions of the acinar cells are basophilic and free of zymogen granules.

With electron microscopy, the zymogen granules appear as dense round structures encased within smooth membranous sacs. The basal portions of the cells are filled with a lamellar type of ergastoplasm with numerous ribonucleoprotein granules attached to the membranes. The ergastoplasm is responsible for the basophilic reaction of these cells. Recent electron microscopic and biochemical studies indicate that the zymogen granules are formed within the ergastoplasmic sacs, are subsequently transmitted to the Golgi zone where they apparently undergo further maturation, and finally move to the apical portion of the cell. Following stimulation, the zymogen granules with their encompassing sacs move to the apical surface of the cell; the membranous sacs fuse with the plasma membrane and rupture, and the zymogen granules are liberated into the lumina of the acini. The acinar and ductal cells are firmly attached by distinct desmosomes that prevent the enzymes within the zymogen granules from passing into the interstitial tissue. The precise intracellular metabolic changes that initiate the migration and liberation of the zymogen granules are unknown.

Development. Among several segmental diverticula of the foregut that appear in 3 mm to 4 mm embryos, two persist and give rise to the definitive pancreas. The larger *dorsal pancreatic diverticulum* arises from the foregut just cephalad to the hepatic diverticulum and elongates to the left in the retroperitoneal space. The smaller *ventral pancreatic diverticulum* arises in the angle between the hepatic diverticulum and foregut and, after more rapid growth of the hepatic diverticulum, comes to arise from that structure. Differential growth rotates the developing duodenum to the right and shifts the ventral pancreatic anlage into the dorsal mesentery, where it fuses with the dorsal anlage and contributes the uncinate process to the definitive organ.

Each pancreatic anlage possesses an axial duct. The distal end of the duct of the ventral pancreas ordinarily anastomoses with the duct of the dorsal pancreas and, as the duct of Wirsung, provides the major drainage for pancreatic secretions into the duodenum at the major duodenal papilla (of Vater). Distal to the point of anastomosis with the duct of Wirsung, the duct of the dorsal pancreas persists in about half of all individuals and, as the duct of Santorini, enters the duodenum at the minor duodenal papilla cephalad to the major papilla. In about 10% of individuals, the duct of the ventral pancreas regresses, and the duct of Santorini provides the entire drainage into the duodenum. These relationships are important in the pathogenesis of acute pancreatitis (see below).

Pancreatic acini appear initially as buds

from the ducts and subsequently differentiate into acinar cells containing zymogen granules. Lumina of the acini retain communication with the centroacinar ducts that converge and form a passageway for exocrine secretions of the pancreas into the duodenum. The islets of Langerhans also develop from the outer surfaces of the ultimate radicals of the pancreatic ducts. Solid masses of islet cells detach from the ducts and are vascularized by capillary sprouts. The first islets to be formed, primary islets, contain specific granules of beta cells as well as of delta cells. Insulin and several pancreatic enzymes have been identified very early in the primordial pancreas of rat embryos.[3] During the last six months of embryonic development, the primary islets undergo degeneration, and a second generation of islet tissue originates from the ductal cells. Both primary and secondary islets arise from ductal tissue, not from acinar cells.

ABNORMALITIES OF FORM AND DEVELOPMENT
Annular pancreas

Annular pancreas results from failure of rotation of the ventral pancreas. When the ventral pancreas fuses with the dorsal, it therefore forms a ring of pancreatic tissue that envelops the second portion of the duodenum. Usually the encirclement is complete, but occasionally a gap may be found anteriorly. In children, an annular pancreas may be associated with atresia or stenosis of the duodenum that results in intestinal obstruction.[7] In adults, an annular pancreas usually produces no symptoms, although in some instances duodenal obstruction, peptic ulceration, and pancreatitis may be present. The relationship of annular pancreas to these symptoms is not clearly understood.

Ectopic pancreas

Pancreatic tissue may be found in the gastrointestinal tract in loci other than its normal anatomic area. The most common locations of ectopic pancreas are the duodenum, stomach, jejunum, and Meckel's diverticulum. Usually, nodules of ectopic pancreatic tissue are small, less than 1 cm in diameter, located in the submucosa as circumscribed, mobile masses of firm yellow-white lobular tissue superficially suggesting a neoplasm. Microscopically, the masses consist of normal-appearing pancreatic tissue, often including islets of Langerhans. Usually, pancreatic heterotopias are asymptomatic. Rarely, such masses may produce pyloric or duodenal obstruction, lead an intussusception, ulcerate and bleed, or serve as the site for an ectopic islet cell neoplasm.

Fibrocystic disease

Fibrocystic disease of the pancreas is a hereditary disorder characterized by increased viscosity of mucous secretions, including those of the pancreas, intestinal glands, tracheal and bronchial glands, and mucous salivary glands and by increased concentrations of electrolytes, especially sodium and chloride, in secretions of other glands, notably eccrine sweat glands and also parotid salivary glands. The disease is transmitted as a mendelian recessive trait with clinical consequences only in homozygotes. The frequency of heterozygous carriers in most white populations must range between 2% and 5%. Factors that contribute toward maintaining this very high gene frequency in spite of the virtually lethal aspect of the homozygous state may include an as yet uncharacterized reproductive advantage in heterozygotes. Fibrocystic disease has been referred to as the commonest hereditary disease in white populations.[18] The disease is very rare in blacks and almost unknown in Orientals. It is responsible for approximately 5% of all deaths in infants and children who are born alive. Although meticulous clinical management has conspicuously improved the length of survival, few affected children reach adulthood.

The nature of the basic biologic defect in fibrocystic disease is not known. The initially attractive hypothesis that the essential disorder consists of increased viscosity of mucous secretions gave rise to the early designation "mucoviscidosis" but could not be supported when more widespread disturbances, including those of eccrine sweat glands and serous glands such as parotid salivary glands, were discovered. Lines of investigation of the basic defect in fibrocystic disease are currently directed in four, not necessarily exclusive, directions.

Biochemical composition of mucous secretions

Although results are not unanimous, the consensus is that mucous secretions of many origins from patients with fibrocystic disease are higher in the ratio of fucose to sialic acid than are secretions of normal individuals. Further information regarding a defect in biosynthesis of mucoid secretions is not available.

Autonomic function

Many of the deviations from normal in the eccrine secretions of patients with fibrocystic disease resemble those that result from exhaustive parasympathetic stimulation of normal secretory mechanisms. Such nonsecretory autonomic mechanisms as the speed of pupillary mydriasis in the dark appear to be impaired in patients with fibrocystic disease.[29]

Electrolyte concentrating mechanism

In the normal formation of sweat, a solution with composition essentially that of an ultrafiltrate of plasma accumulates in the coiled portions of eccrine sweat glands. Preferential absorption of sodium and chloride in excess of water from the duct results in the excretion of the normally hypotonic sweat. Micropuncture studies[26] suggest that primary secretion in the coil is normal in those with fibrocystic disease and that defective absorption of solute from the duct results in hypertonicity of the sweat. Recently, diminished resorption of sodium and chloride has been demonstrated in rat parotid glands perfused with sweat from patients with fibrocystic disease.[26] Sweat from normal children had no effect on the absorptive mechanism.

Effect on ciliary motility

Recently, asynchronous and uncoordinated ciliary motility has been observed in cultured explants of rat tracheal mucosa exposed to serum from patients with fibrocystic disease. The factor responsible for this disturbance in ciliary motility is heat labile and nondialyzable. Similar effects were produced by sera from some parents of patients with fibrocystic disease.[31]

Metachromasia in cultured fibroblasts

Recent studies have demonstrated that cultured fibroblasts from patients with fibrocystic disease elaborate metachromatic material either as discrete cytoplasmic granules or as diffuse cytoplasmic metachromasia. Cultured fibroblasts from parents and other relatives of patients showed the same type of metachromasia.[18] These results are important not only as a possible means of detecting asymptomatic heterozygous carriers of the gene for fibrocystic disease, but also for the suggestion that fibrocystic disease may not be a homogeneous entity but may result from homozygosity at two distinct loci.

Clinical features

Clinical features of fibrocystic disease are highly variable, even among affected siblings. From 10% to 15% of affected individuals present in the newborn period with intestinal, usually distal ileal, obstruction by chalky masses of inspissated intestinal contents, *meconium ileus.* The frequency of associated ileal atresia supports an acquired mechanism for intestinal atresia. Intestinal perforation *in utero* with production of sterile meconium peritonitis may occur. Acute or episodic intestinal obstruction beyond infancy is increasingly reported as "meconium ileus equivalent."

Failure to gain weight in spite of adequate appetite, nonspecific feeding problems, steatorrhea, or other manifestations of intestinal malabsorption characterize one-fourth to one-third of all patients with fibrocystic disease. Rectal prolapse occurs in as many as one-sixth of all patients. Heat prostration may be an early manifestation. In older children, ascites, bleeding from esophageal varices, or unexplained splenomegaly may be the first symptoms of fibrocystic disease.

Beyond infancy, respiratory complications are by far the commonest manifestations of fibrocystic disease and comprise its chief threat to life. Recurrent bouts of pneumonia, bronchiolitis, or bronchitis are usual but not invariable manifestations of the disease. Signs and symptoms of chronic respiratory insufficiency or of right ventricular failure occasionally may precede any indication of infection of the lower respiratory tract. The finding of inflammatory nasal polyps in the upper respiratory tract of a prepubertal child compels consideration of the diagnosis of fibrocystic disease.

Pathologic changes

Most pathologic changes in fibrocystic disease are interpretable as secondary to obstruction by abnormally viscid mucus in a variety of viscera.

Pancreas. The pancreas is probably never normal in fibrocystic disease, although the degree of pancreatic involvement varies widely from case to case and correlates only crudely with age. Grossly, especially in infancy, the pancreas may appear deceptively normal (Fig. 30-1). Close examination even then, however, may disclose an almost too tidy demarcation of lobules and an increase in consistency. Later, pancreatic lobules come to assume an ovoid rather than a rhomboidal or polyhedral contour and to bulge from the cut surface.

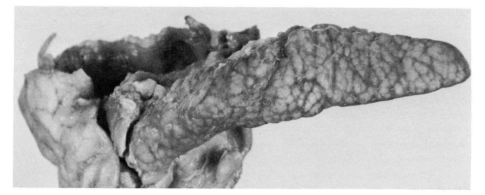

Fig. 30-1 Pancreas from child with fibrocystic disease showing accentuation of lobules but general preservation of size and contour of organ. (From Kissane, J. M., and Smith, M. G.: Pathology of infancy and childhood, The C. V. Mosby Co.)

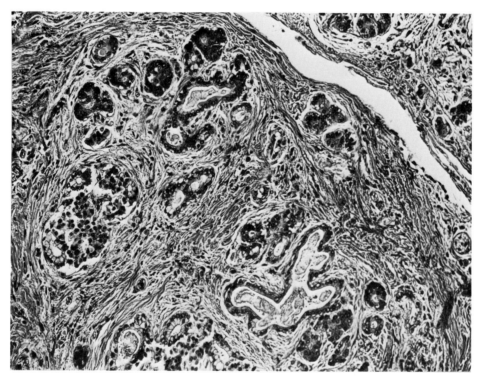

Fig. 30-2 Pancreas in fibrocystic disease showing dilated centrilobular ducts containing laminated concretions. Acini almost totally replaced by fibrous tissue that still reflects lobular pattern of organ.

Ultimately, the pancreas, still preserving relatively normal size and contour, represents gross fatty replacement of parenchyma. Fibrosis is rarely pronounced grossly, and macroscopic cysts are rarely discernible.

Microscopically, acinar atrophy and interlobular fibrosis are far out of proportion to the gross abnormality. Centroacinar ducts frequently contain laminated, eosinophilic concretions, and distal to these, acini are conspicuously atrophic although stromal recapitulation of lobular architecture may be well preserved (Fig. 30-2). Islets persist until late in the evolution of the disease. Inflammation, fat necrosis, and pseudocyst formation are rarely prominent.

Intestine. In 12% to 15% of patients with fibrocystic disease, intestinal obstruction occurs in the newborn period. The obstructing lesion in *meconium ileus* is a plug of chalky, inspissated meconium in the distal ileum. Ileal atresia, volvulus, or perforation with the development of meconium peritonitis may occur secondarily, and total intestinal length usually is shortened. The occurrence of meconium ileus correlates more with dilatation of intestinal glands by inspissated mucus secretions than with the extent of pancreatic lesions.

Attention has been called to the occurrence of peptic ulcers in patients with fibrocystic disease.[15] Above normal frequency of peptic ulcer in parents of patients with fibrocystic disease has been claimed.

Respiratory tract. In a typical case, the lungs present gross compensatory overexpansion anteriorly, alternating posteriorly with areas of atelectasis and overt consolidation. Bronchi are dilated and contain inspissated mucopurulent exudate. Dilated small bronchi containing similar material usually can be appreciated in the centers of consolidated pulmonary lobules. Microscopically, the pulmonary lesion is a purulent bronchitis and bronchiolitis with resulting bronchiectasis and bronchiolectasis accompanied by a limited peribronchiolar pneumonia. Parenchymatous purulent necrosis with abscess formation is distinctly unusual.

Larynx, trachea, and major bronchi show chronic inflammation, often with foci of squamous metaplasia. Submucous glands are distended with inspissated secretions. In the upper respiratory tract, inflammatory nasal polyps may be found.

Liver. The liver is usually of normal size. Significant fatty metamorphosis is not common. Focal stellate areas of portal fibrosis and ductular proliferation may be seen, occasionally sufficiently extensive to justify the designation *focal biliary cirrhosis*. The lesion may produce portal hypertension with its consequences—ascites, congestive splenomegaly, and gastroesophageal varices (see p. 1225).

Sweat glands. In view of the constancy and diagnostic importance of hypersecretion of sodium and chloride in the sweat, microscopic alterations in sweat glands are disappointingly scanty. Munger et al.[27] described diminished vacuolation of mucoid cells.

Reproductive system. The frequent finding of azoospermia in postpubertal males with fibrocystic disease has recently been attributed to absence of vasa deferentia.[24] There is no anatomic correlate for the high maternal mortality among pregnant women with fibrocystic disease.

PANCREATITIS

Inflammation of the pancreas constitutes a spectrum of disorders that ranges from acute hemorrhagic pancreatitis, a prostrating, catastrophic disease with a high mortality rate, to chronic relapsing pancreatitis, a disorder marked by recurring episodes of upper abdominal pain and eventual pancreatic insufficiency.

Acute hemorrhagic pancreatitis

Acute hemorrhagic pancreatitis is almost entirely a disease of adults between 40 and 70 years of age, slightly commoner in females than in males. The onset is abrupt and calamitous, often following a heavy meal or an alcoholic debauch. Severe epigastric pain, especially radiating to the back, nausea, vomiting, and shock are prominent clinical features. Peculiar ecchymotic mottling of the skin of the flanks, Grey-Turner spots, may be seen in severe cases. Early in the disease, pancreatic enzymes are liberated into the blood stream, and increased levels of amylase and lipase in the serum are important in establishing the diagnosis. The mortality rate, even with vigorous supportive measures, is between 15% and 25%.

Pathologic changes. In the first few days, the pancreas is swollen and edematous. After a day or two, friable foci of necrosis appear, followed by interstitial hemorrhage that varies from reddish reticulation between pancreatic lobules to obliteration of grossly recognizable pancreatic tissue in a massive retroperitoneal hematoma. Foci of fat necrosis in the peripancreatic tissue, mesentery, and omentum

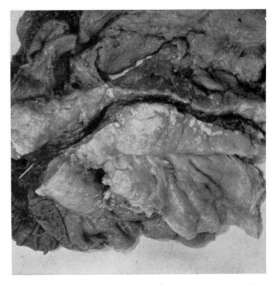

Fig. 30-3 Fat necrosis and acute pancreatitis. White opaque areas represent fat necrosis. Small white rod is in duct opening into duodenum.

appear rapidly as small ovoid yellow-white nodules of pasty, gritty material (Fig. 30-3). The peritoneal cavity usually contains a moderate effusion of turbid rusty fluid with high amylase activity. Rarely, remote adipose tissues such as subcutaneous fat and fatty marrow may contain foci of necrosis attributable to lipolysis by enzymes borne in the plasma.

Very early in the disease, the pancreas microscopically shows only interstitial edema. Later, the pancreas contains patches of coagulative necrosis rimmed by infiltrates of polymorphonuclear leukocytes (Fig. 30-4). Still later, necrosis of arteries and arterioles is responsible for gross hemorrhages. Veins often are thrombosed. Eventually, as bacteria lodge in the necrotic pancreas, either via the ducts or the bloodstream, frank suppuration may occur.

A late complication of acute pancreatitis is the occasional development of a pseudocyst—an accumulation of enzyme-rich fluid, necrotic debris, and altered blood confined, not by an epithelial capsule, but by retroperitoneal connective tissue, adherent upper abdominal viscera, and the peritoneal components of the lesser omental sac. Pancreatic pseudocysts also may follow blunt trauma to the abdomen.

Pathogenesis. The destructive changes that occur in the pancreas can be attributed to the liberation and activation of the proteolytic

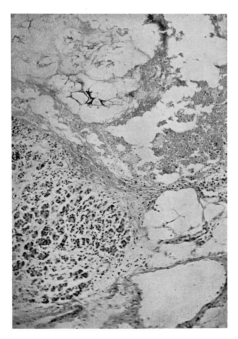

Fig. 30-4 Fat necrosis of pancreas.

and lipolytic enzymes normally secreted by this organ. Active proteolytic enzymes such as trypsin and elastase produce necrosis of blood vessels, with resultant thrombosis and hemorrhage. Lipase liberated into the interstitial tissue causes necrosis of adipose tissue and the breakdown of triglycerides into fatty acids. Fatty acids combine with calcium in the interstitial tissue to form insoluble calcium soaps. This may produce a significant decrease in the level of serum calcium and lead to symptoms of hypocalcemia.

The pathogenesis of this sequence of events is not entirely clear. Experimentally, pancreatitis can be produced by injecting bile into the pancreatic duct at a pressure sufficient to rupture the ductal system. Opie's early report[43] of acute pancreatitis resulting from impaction of a gallstone in the ampula of Vater directed perhaps undue attention toward the necessity for a "common channel" for biliary and pancreatic secretions to provide anatomically possible regurgitation of bile into the pancreatic duct. Detailed anatomic studies show that the configuration of the pancreatic ducts and common bile duct allows regurgitation of bile into the pancreatic duct in about 90% of specimens.[2]

Even in the presence of an anatomic "common channel," measurements of pressures in the pancreatic duct and in the common bile duct indicate that the higher pressure in the pancreatic duct normally prevents the reflux of bile into the pancreatic duct. Increased pancreatic secretory pressure is clearly an important factor. The frequent association of chronic alcoholism with pancreatitis suggests that alcohol functions not only by producing edema and partial obstruction of the sphincter of Oddi but also by stimulating pancreatic secretion.

Vascular ischemia has been implicated in the production of hemorrhagic pancreatitis, since it has been demonstrated experimentally that the pancreatic edema that follows ligation of the pancreatic duct in the dog can be transformed into acute hemorrhagic pancreatitis by the production of temporary ischemia in the pancreas. This factor alone is apparently not sufficient to produce the sequence of events, since vascular necroses in the pancreas in malignant hypertension are accompanied by only focal areas of necrosis, not a fulminating hemorrhagic pancreatitis.

Trauma also has been implicated as an etiologic factor. Acute pancreatitis is a recognized complication of closed abdominal trauma such as may result from "steering wheel" injuries to the abdomen. Acute pancreatitis also may complicate extensive surgery in the gastroduodenal area. On historical grounds, trauma can be excluded as a pathogenic mechanism in most cases.

Circulating antibodies to pancreatic tissue have been demonstrated in the bloodstream of patients with pancreatitis. It is not clear whether these antibodies have an etiologic role in the production of pancreatitis or whether they are simply immunologic by-products following pancreatic necrosis due to other factors.

The central themes that underlie most of the numerous suggested etiologic factors are partial or complete pancreatic ductal obstruction and increased pancreatic secretion. Further detailed studies of experimental models and of the human disease are needed to clarify the etiology of acute hemorrhagic pancreatitis.

Chronic pancreatitis

Chronic pancreatitis produces progressive destruction of the pancreas as the result of

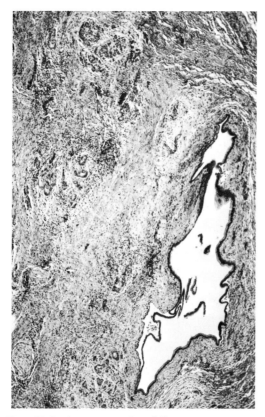

Fig. 30-5 Acinar atrophy following pancreatic duct obstruction.

repeated episodes of necrosis of the parenchyma. Approximately one-third of all patients who survive an episode of acute pancreatitis sustain subsequent acute episodes that ultimately progress to chronic pancreatitis. Some patients arrive at the stage of pancreatic insufficiency without sustaining a documented attack of acute pancreatitis. Chronic pancreatitis is a recognized manifestation of hyperparathyroidism and of a hereditary metabolic disorder usually, but not always, accompanied by aminoaciduria. These latter account for only a small percentage of cases of chronic pancreatitis. Chronic relapsing pancreatitis occurs most frequently in the fourth or fifth decade. The disease is frequently associated with biliary tract disease or alcoholism.

Pathologic changes in the pancreas depend upon the stage of the development of the disease. In acute exacerbations, diffuse edema, local areas of necrosis, and peripancreatic inflammation may be present. After the acute attacks, the pancreas will be firm and nodular, with areas of dense fibrosis, loss of acinar and islet tissue (Fig. 30-5), calcification in the interstitial tissue and pancreatic ducts, infiltration with plasma cells and lymphocytes, and formation of pseudocysts. The destruction of the pancreas eventually results in exocrine pancreatic insufficiency and, ultimately, diabetes mellitus.

Hereditary pancreatitis is a form of chronic pancreatitis that is transmitted as a mendelian dominant autosomal gene. In contrast to sporadic chronic pancreatitis, hereditary pancreaatitis begins in childhood, and there is a relative infrequency of alcoholism and chronic biliary disease.[39]

PANCREATIC LESIONS IN SYSTEMIC DISEASE

Dilatation of acini and ducts of the pancreas occurs in approximately 40% to 50% of patients with uremia. The dilated structures contain eosinophilic inspissated material. In some instances, the individual lobules are separated by edematous tissue with a mild infiltrate of neutrophils.

Histologic changes in the acinar cells of the pancreatic lobules may be present in chronic congestive heart failure. Peripheral acinar cells in the pancreatic lobules appear atrophic, with diminished zymogen granules and decreased basophilia of their cytoplasm, whereas cells adjacent to islets retain their normal appearance. These histologic changes are apparently related to increased venous pressure and vascular stasis within the pancreatic venous circulation.

NEOPLASMS OF EXOCRINE PANCREAS
Cystadenoma

Cystadenomas of the pancreas are rare, slow-growing neoplasms that arise from ductal epithelium. They occur more commonly in females and usually are located in the tail of the pancreas. The tumor appears as a round, coarsely lobulated mass comprised of multilocular cysts (Fig. 30-6). The cystic spaces are filled with fluid that may be clear, hemorrhagic, or gelatinous. The multilocu-

lated cysts are lined by a cuboidal or flattened epithelium. Papillary projections may be present. A rare malignant counterpart, cystadenocarcinoma, has been described.

Carcinoma

Carcinoma of the pancreas ranks fourth in frequency among fatal neoplastic diseases in the United States and is responsible for approximately 6% of all deaths due to cancer. As a cause of death in the United States, carcinoma of the pancreas now exceeds such neoplastic diseases as carcinoma of the stomach, malignant lymphoma of all types, carcinoma of the prostate, and carcinoma of the cervix. Carcinoma of the pancreas is extremely rare

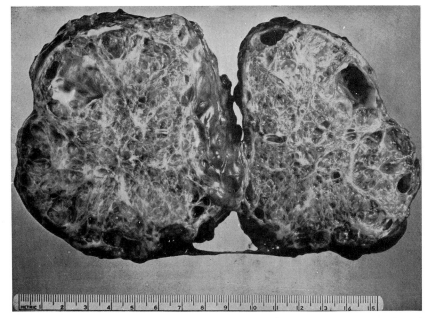

Fig. 30-6 Cystadenoma of pancreas. Coarse porous surface is typical. (From Brunschwig, A.: Surgery of pancreatic tumors, The C. V. Mosby Co.)

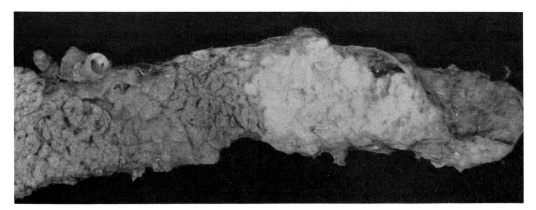

Fig. 30-7 Carcinoma of body and tail of pancreas. (Courtesy Dr. B. Halpert.)

before 40 years of age. Approximately two-thirds of patients are over the age of 60 years.

Clinical symptoms of carcinoma of the pancreas depend upon the site of the origin of the tumor. If it arises in the head of the pancreas, obstruction of the common bile duct occurs early, producing obstructive jaundice. Clinical recognition of carcinoma of the body and tail (Fig. 30-7) is difficult because of the paucity of distinctive signs and symptoms. Pain is the most common initial symptom of carcinoma of the pancreas, regardless of its location. Symptoms that appear later in the disease include anorexia, weight loss, cachexia, and weakness. The great majority of patients with carcinoma of the pancreas are dead within a year after the onset of symptoms. Approximately one-half of the deaths occur within three months of the onset of symptoms. Among selected patients with carcinoma of the pancreas who are subjected to radical pancreaticoduodenectomy, some 12% survive longer than five years.[61] This figure approaches 40% in cases of (usually well-differentiated) ampullary carcinoma, a lesion that should be distinguished from pancreatic carcinoma.

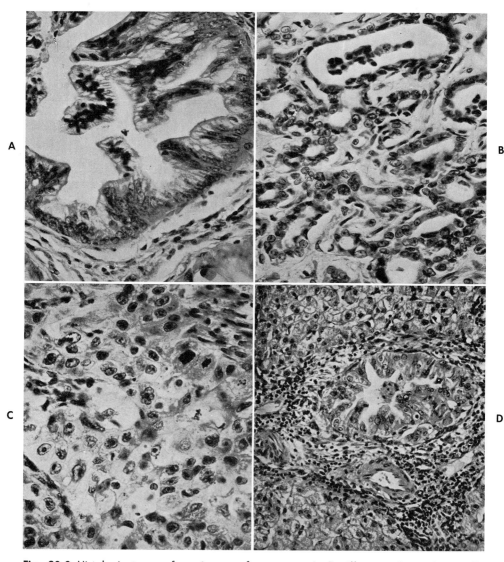

Fig. 30-8 Histologic types of carcinoma of pancreas. **A,** Papillary cystic carcinoma. **B,** Adenocarcinoma, reproducing small ducts. **C,** Medullary carcinoma, composed of large anaplastic cells. **D,** Metastatic duct cell carcinoma of pancreas in liver. (From Brunschwig, A.: Surgery of pancreatic tumors, The C. V. Mosby Co.)

Approximately 70% of carcinomas of the pancreas occur in the head of the organ. The close proximity of the neoplasm to the common bile duct results in neoplastic invasion of the wall of the duct, producing obstruction and dilatation. Obstruction of the common bile duct also occurs in cases of carcinoma of the body and tail of the pancreas. However, this is usually a late complication.

Carcinomas of the body and tail of the pancreas are, on the average, larger than those of the head. Metastases occur most frequently in the regional lymph nodes, liver, lungs, peritoneum, and adrenal glands. The incidence of metastases is higher in cases of carcinoma of the body and tail than of the head of the pancreas.

Grossly, the neoplasm is an ill-defined, firm expansion of a portion of the pancreas, with no sharp line of demarcation between the neoplasm and the surrounding parenchyma. The most common neoplasm is adenocarcinoma that originates from the ducts of the pancreas. Histologically, adenocarcinomas are composed of ductlike structures lined by one or several layers of neoplastic cells supported by a dense fibrous stroma. The degree of differentiation varies from neoplasms with well-defined ductal structures to those with anaplastic undifferentiated cells (Fig. 30-8). In some instances, the tumor may appear as a mucinous adenocarcinoma. A rare type of tumor originating from the ducts is epidermoid carcinoma. Acinic carcinoma is a rare neoplasm that recapitulates the pattern of acini of the normal pancreas and may contain zymogen granules.

Adenocarcinoma of the pancreas frequently invades the perineural lymphatics. This invasion of the nerves accounts for the frequency of abdominal pain in these patients. Multiple venous thromboses may be associated with carcinoma of the pancreas and occur more frequently when the neoplasm is in the body or tail of the pancreas. The veins most frequently involved are the iliac and femoral. The mechanism of thrombosis is not clearly defined.

ENDOCRINE PANCREAS
Diabetes mellitus

Diabetes mellitus is a hereditary disease with a time of onset extending from a few months after birth to eight or nine decades later. At the present time, the only known clinical elements that serve to characterize the disease are hyperglycemia and glycosuria.

Based upon the time of onset of diabetes mellitus, the disease can be subdivided into juvenile and maturity-onset diabetes. There is obvious overlap between these subclassifications. However, the classic juvenile diabetic patient has a low insulin reserve in the pancreas and is not responsive to sulfonylurea therapy, whereas the maturity-onset diabetic patient may have a relatively normal insulin reserve and insulin is released from the pancreas following sulfonylurea administration. In recent years, a new clinical entity has been introduced which is termed prediabetes. In this instance, the prediabetic individual is the offspring of a diabetic mother and father, and it is presumed that these individuals will subsequently develop diabetes.

The hyperglycemia and glycosuria that occur in the diabetic individual are probably secondary to a genetic defect or defects, and intensive investigations are in progress in order to elucidate the genetic abnormality. Studies on the basement membranes of peripheral capillaries in muscle indicate that thickening of the basement membrane may be present in the prediabetic person, as well as in the individual with overt diabetes. Recent investigations indicate an absence of an initial insulin release from the pancreas occurring within four to six minutes after the administration of glucose. This same initial response is missing in the prediabetic individual.

In searching for the etiology of diabetes mellitus, abnormalities of the islets of Langerhans were believed initially to be the cause of the disease process and as insulin therapy was developed and utilized, attention turned to possible insulin inhibitors in the bloodstream of diabetic individuals. The pendulum has now swung back and the islets of Langerhans are again believed to contain the pathologic lesions that would explain the etiology of diabetes mellitus. In order to establish even a working hypothesis as to the cause of diabetes mellitus in which the islets were not functioning properly, it is essential that basic information be made available on the normal mechanisms by which the beta cells of the islets form, store, and release insulin into the bloodstream.

Structure and function of beta cells

The islets of Langerhans comprise about 1% to 3% of the weight of the pancreas, and the concentration of islets is greater in the tail than in the head or body of the pancreas. By the use of special stains, the islet cells can

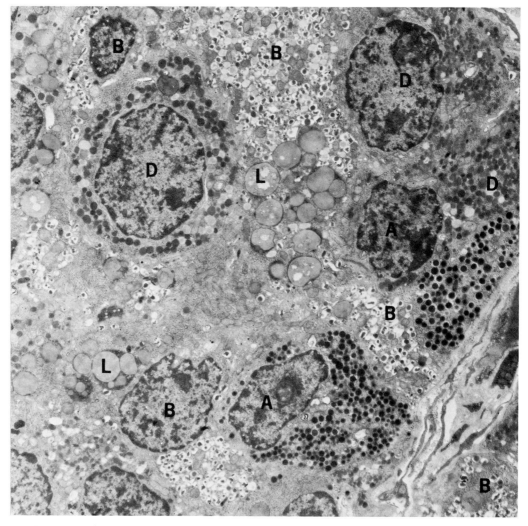

Fig. 30-9 Electron micrograph of islet cells of normal human pancreas. **A,** Alpha cell. **B,** Beta cell. **D,** Delta cell. Lipochrome pigment, **L,** present in cells. (Courtesy Dr. M. Greider.)

be subclassified into alpha, beta, and delta cells. The beta cells comprise 60% to 70% of the islet cell population; alpha cells, 20% to 30%; and delta cells, 2% to 8%.

Beta granules. Insulin is stored in the beta cell in the form of beta granules as evidenced by the correlation of the degree of beta granulation with the insulin content of the pancreas in normal and diabetic individuals, electron microscopic immunochemical demonstration of insulin in the granules using peroxidase-labeled antiinsulin serum, and demonstration of insulin in secretory granules isolated by differential centrifugation from islet homogenates. Beta granules also contain zinc and possibly the C peptide fragment of proinsulin.

Electron microscopic studies indicate that the beta granules may have a crystalline structure with a remarkable variability in the ultrastructural appearance of the granules in different species. In man, the granules have a rectangular profile, with repeating lines of periodicity demonstrable in the core of the granule. This feature makes it possible to differentiate a beta cell from other types of islet cells in the human pancreas (Fig. 30-9). The granules are surrounded by a smooth, membranous sac and thus are separated from the cytoplasm by this limiting membrane.

Beta granule formation. The development of the collagenase technique for the isolation of intact islets from the normal pancreas has made it feasible to accomplish *in vitro* studies on the direct effect of agents on the formation and release of insulin from islets maintained

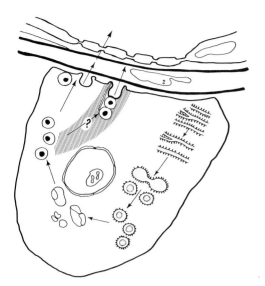

Fig. 30-10 Schematic representation of mechanism of beta cell secretion. Proinsulin apparently formed in endoplasmic reticulum and transferred to Golgi complex. Mature beta granules containing insulin originate from Golgi complex and are released from beta cell by emiocytosis. Shaded area represents hypothesis of emiocytosis involving microtubular system of beta cell.

under controlled conditions. Electron microscopic autoradiographic studies of rat islets incubated *in vitro* in the presence of a pulse-label of tritiated leucine indicate that beta granule formation occurs initially within the endoplasmic reticulum and that the label subsequently is transferred to the Golgi complex (Fig. 30-10). Ultrastructural studies of the islets under experimental conditions *in vivo* reveal an amorphous material in the endoplasmic reticulum that is probably the precursor of the beta granule.

The remarkable discovery of proinsulin in isolated islets has provided a biochemical explanation as to the mode of formation of the A and B chains of insulin. Proinsulin consists of the A and B chains linked by a connecting peptide segment that is termed the C chain, and it has little or no biologic activity. However, treatment of the material with trypsin will remove the C peptide fragment, and biologically active insulin will be produced. Studies on subcellular fractions of islets incubated *in vitro* indicate that proinsulin is predominantly in the microsomal fraction, whereas insulin is present in the beta granules. It is presumed that the site of transformation of proinsulin to insulin occurs within the Golgi complex. However, definitive evidence for this is lacking at the present time.

Studies are in progress to determine whether proinsulin is present in significant quantities in the bloodstream of diabetic individuals, since this agent does not produce hypoglycemia. Thus, the secretion of proinsulin instead of insulin could produce diabetes. The validity of this hypothesis can be tested when specific antibodies to human proinsulin are obtained and measurements of proinsulin in the normal and in diabetic individuals are accomplished.

Biochemical studies on the islets indicate that beta cells are freely permeable to glucose, and initiation of insulin synthesis by beta cells requires phosphorylation of glucose. Apparently, insulin synthesis is initiated in the further metabolism of glucose-6-phosphate. However, the precise events or precise metabolites produced that initiate synthesis has not been determined. Tolbutamide, a sulfonylurea compound, stimulates the release of insulin from the beta cell *in vivo* and *in vitro* but does not increase synthesis, whereas glucose stimulates both synthesis and release of insulin.

Beta granule release. Secretion of beta granules occurs by the simple process of emiocytosis. Stimulation of the beta cells by either hyperglycemia or sulfonylurea compounds causes the beta granules enclosed in their smooth, membranous sacs to move to the cell surface. The sacs fuse with the plasma membrane and rupture, and the granules are liberated into the extracellular space, where they undergo dissolution. The sacs encasing the granules apparently become a part of the plasma membrane, and depressions can be observed on the cell surface where the granules have been ejected.

Electron microscopic studies indicate that beta granules are probably liberated in tandem at specific loci on the cell membrane with resultant production of deep concavities in the cell surface and the formation of microvilli that project from the cell. These cytoplasmic projections on the surface of beta cells recently have been demonstrated by scanning electron microscopy (Fig. 30-11).

The biochemical events that initiate the secretion of insulin are not clearly defined. The adenyl cyclase system may play a role in initiating secretion, since glucagon stimulates insulin release and the accumulation of cyclic 3,5-AMP in beta cells. Theophylline stimulates insulin secretion presumably through inhibition of phosphodiesterase, which is an enzyme that breaks down cyclic

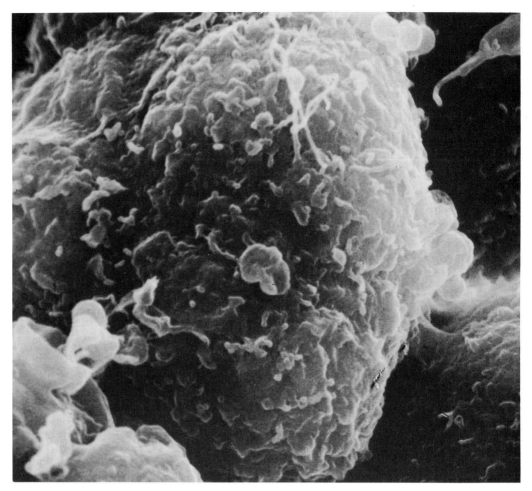

Fig. 30-11 Scanning electron micrograph of surface of stimulated beta cell of rat. Numerous microvilli evident on surface of cell.

AMP, and the addition of cyclic AMP to islets *in vitro* produces direct stimulation of insulin release. Thus, the adenyl cyclase system apparently plays a role in insulin secretion under the foregoing conditions. However, it is unknown if this system is involved with the physiologic stimulus—glucose. Calcium ions are required for the stimulatory effect of all agents on the islets. A biochemical difference in the mechanism of action of tolbutamide and glucose is evident, since mannoheptulose and diazoxide blocks insulin secretion by glucose but has no effect on insulin release with tolbutamide, whereas epinephrine blocks the stimulatory action of both glucose and tolbutamide. These interesting and provocative clues form the basis for future intensive investigations to delineate the biochemical events of insulin secretion.

A working hypothesis has been proposed as to the mechanism by which beta granules are transported in tandem to the cell surface for release. This hypothesis involves the microtubular system that is present within beta cells and postulates that the sacs encasing the granules are associated or possibly attached to the microtubules and that with glucose stimulation the microtubules contract and convey the granules to the cell membrane, where they are liberated by emiocytosis. This working hypothesis would provide an explanation for two compartments of insulin within the beta cell, with one available for immediate release and the second requiring attachment to the microtubular system for release at a later interval. Such a model could explain the absence of immediate release of insulin from the beta cells of prediabetic and diabetic individuals based upon abnormalities of the microtubular system or the relationship of the system to the granules.

Insulin released from the solubilized beta

granules in the extracellular space traverses a basement membrane associated with the beta cell, a second basement membrane associated with the endothelium, and, finally, the plasma membranes and cytoplasm of the endothelium prior to entering the bloodstream. Accumulation of amyloid between these two basement membranes occurs in some maturity-onset diabetic patients. This accumulation undoubtedly impairs secretion in the affected islets. However, the number of islets containing amyloid within the pancreas of a diabetic individual is insufficient to explain the diabetic course. Thickening of the basement membranes of the islets has been suggested as a possible cause of impaired release of insulin in the individual with diabetes. However, the rate of glucagon secretion from the pancreas of a diabetic patient is apparently normal, and no information is available as to whether a thickened basement membrane actually impairs insulin transport.

Pathologic changes in islets

The specific, pathologic lesion or lesions that would explain the etiology and pathogenesis of diabetes mellitus have not been elucidated. In spite of this, a number of pathologic changes do occur in the islets in association with diabetes. These include degranulation of beta cells, amyloidosis, glycogenosis, and leukocytic infiltration. Beta cell degranulation occurs as a result of the hyperglycemia in the individuals and can be produced experimentally by many different procedures.

Distinct differences in the pathologic changes are present in the pancreases of individuals with classic juvenile and maturity-onset diabetes. In juvenile diabetes, the number of islets is usually reduced, degranulation of beta cells and fibrosis may be present, and, in occasional instances, lymphocytic infiltration is observed. In maturity-onset diabetes, the number of islets may be normal, the degree of beta cell degranulation may be normal or moderately reduced, and amyloidosis may be present within the islets. In approximately 20% of patients with maturity-onset diabetes, no distinct light microscopic changes can be observed in the islets.

Amyloidosis of islets. By light microscopy, amyloid appears as an eosinophilic, amorphous material deposited around the capillaries of the islets, compressing and displacing the islet cells (Fig. 30-12). The change was

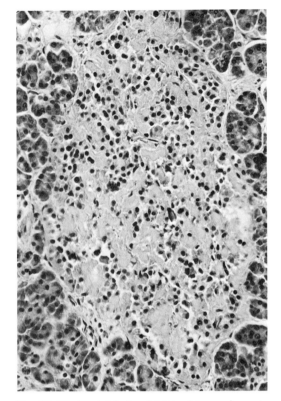

Fig. 30-12 Amyloidosis of islet of Langerhans in diabetic patient.

previously called hyalinization of the islets of Langerhans and was one of the earlier morphologic findings observed in diabetic patients.

By electron microscopy, the amyloid has a fibrillar appearance and is deposited between the two basement membranes, separating the islet cells from the capillaries. Amyloidosis does not involve all the islets within a single pancreas but has a patchy distribution. Thus, it is unlikely that this pathologic change has any significant role in the etiology of the diabetic state.

No information is available as to the reason for the deposition of the amyloid in the islets. Amyloidosis of the islets is not limited to diabetic patients but has been found, to a minor degree, in about 2% of nondiabetic individuals over 40 years of age.

Glycogenosis of islets. Glycogen is deposited in beta cells of the islets when there is a persistent hyperglycemia for a period of time. This lesion previously was called hydropic degeneration of beta cells and occurs in human beings with diabetes as well as in experimental diabetes (Fig. 30-13). It is now an unusual finding at autopsy due to im-

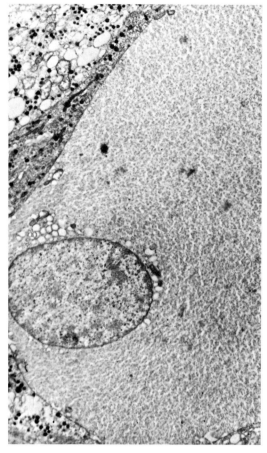

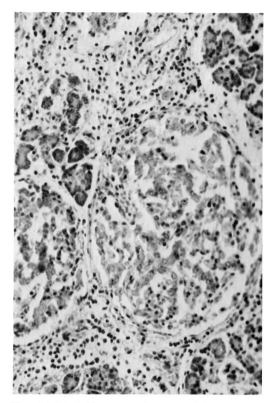

Fig. 30-14 Infiltration of eosinophils in peri-insular tissue of newborn infant of diabetic mother.

Fig. 30-13 Electron micrograph of beta cell containing massive accumulation of glycogen in diabetic hamster. Glycogen accumulation presents appearance of hydropic degeneration in ordinary microscopic preparations.

proved therapy of the diabetic state and the rarity of expiration of a patient in diabetic acidosis. However, it undoubtedly occurs *in vivo* during periods of prolonged hyperglycemia.

The deposition of glycogen apparently is due to a change in the intracellular metabolism of glucose. Electron microscopic studies indicate that glycogen accumulates first as small focal masses within the beta cell and that, as the hyperglycemic state becomes more severe, the masses increase in size and displace the normal intracellular organelles. In addition to the biochemical abnormalities that must exist in these cells, the mere presence of the mass of glycogen would interfere with the organized production of insulin by the endoplasmic reticulum, thus increasing the severity of the diabetic state. Glycogenosis of the beta cell is apparently a reversible change, since the glycogen disappears follow-

ing treatment with insulin and production of normoglycemia. The role of this reversible lesion in the pathogenesis of diabetes is difficult to understand, since it is presumed that continued hyperglycemia in the diabetic individual will result in destruction of beta cells. In addition, permanent diabetes has been produced in the cat simply by repeated injections of glucose and in the dog by injections of glucose and growth hormone.

Recent electron microscopic studies have revealed a second pathologic change in beta cells of dogs with experimental diabetes. This lesion was called "ballooning degeneration," since multiple vacuoles were present in the cytoplasm that were devoid of glycogen and the cells appeared to be undergoing degeneration. Glycogenosis was evident in other beta cells of the islets. This degenerative change separate from glycogenosis may represent the initial stages in the destruction of beta cells during prolonged hyperglycemia.

Lymphocytic and eosinophilic infiltration of islets. Lymphocytic infiltration of the islets of Langerhans may be observed rarely in juvenile diabetes. It is particularly evident in those patients who come to autopsy within days or weeks after the onset of the disease process. Similar lymphocytic infiltration of the islets can be produced experimentally by repeated administration of beef insulin to cattle and to rabbits. In both instances, antibodies to beef insulin are produced and, in the case of the rabbit, a permanent diabetic state has been induced in some of the animals.

Infiltration of eosinophils and lymphocytes within and around the islets and in the interstitial tissue of the pancreas is observed in approximately 25% of infants who are born to diabetic mothers and who expire within one to two weeks after birth (Fig. 30-14). This infiltration is invariably associated with islet hypertrophy and hyperplasia and is diagnostic of diabetes mellitus in the mother. The occurrence of eosinophilic infiltration is not related to the severity of the diabetes or the form of therapy received by the mother and, in some instances, she has no clinical evidence of diabetes during pregnancy and may become diabetic within a period of months or years subsequently. Experimentally, a morphologic counterpart of this lesion has been produced by the acute injection of anti-insulin serum into rats. In these animals, a severe diabetic state is produced and an infiltration of eosinophils and lymphocytes is present in the interstitial tissue and peri-insular area of the pancreas. This allergic reaction is apparently the result of an interaction of antibody with endogenous insulin in the islets.

The production of an allergic type of inflammatory response in the pancreas of experimental animals by injection of anti-insulin serum, the establishment of diabetes in the rabbit by immunization with insulin, and the morphologic similarity of the experimental lesions with those observed rarely in juvenile diabetic patients and in the newborn infants of diabetic mothers could be interpreted as suggestive of an autoimmune mechanism in diabetes in man. Further immunologic evidence is needed in studies of diabetic mothers and juvenile diabetic patients before such a hypothesis could be given serious consideration.

Hemochromatosis

Hemosiderin may be evident within acinar and beta cells of the pancreas in hemochromatosis. The alpha cells are greatly reduced in number and do not contain hemosiderin. Atrophy of the acinar cells and interstitial fibrosis are usually present. The term "bronze diabetes" is sometimes used, since increased pigmentation of the skin, diabetes mellitus, and cirrhosis of the liver may be present in hemochromatosis.

Diabetic microangiopathy

Light and electron microscopic studies indicate diffuse involvement of small blood vessels and capillaries in patients with diabetes mellitus. Pathologic changes have been observed in peripheral capillaries of the skin, muscle, kidney, peripheral nerves, and eye. The common denominator of these lesions is a distinct and definitive thickening of the basement membrane of the capillaries. Sufficient material has now been examined to indicate that the increased thickness of the basement membrane in muscle capillaries is specific for diabetes mellitus (Fig. 30-15). A major difference between the capillaries of skeletal muscle and the glomerulus is that the basement membrane of the glomerulus progressively thickens with the duration of diabetes, whereas basement membrane thickness in muscle capillaries is unrelated to the duration of the disease. It is unknown if the thickening occurs as the result of increased production or decreased removal of basement membrane.

A basic question related to the basement membrane changes in the capillaries is whether this lesion is a complication of the diabetic state or is due to a separate genetic abnormality that is associated with diabetes mellitus. Significant increase in the thickness of the basement membrane of muscle capillaries has been demonstrated in prediabetic individuals who have no clinical or chemical evidence of diabetes mellitus at the time of observation. Two cases have been observed in adults with no family history of diabetes and no clinical or chemical evidence of the disease. However, biopsies of the kidney and skeletal muscle revealed nodular lesions of intercapillary glomerulosclerosis and significant thickening of the basement membranes of muscle capillaries. Initial studies have indicated that in patients with acromegaly and diabetes mellitus, with no family history of diabetes, the basement membrane thickness of muscle capillaries is within the normal range for patients of similar age and sex. These initial observations are suggestive of the presence of a separate genetic abnormality affecting the basement membrane.

The functional impairment that may result from the thickened basement membranes is

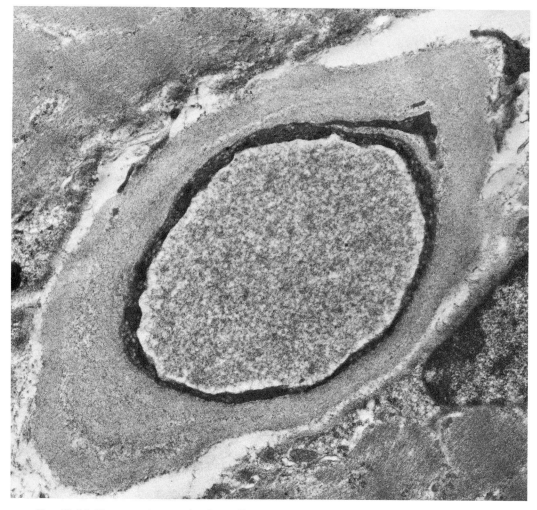

Fig. 30-15 Electron micrograph of capillary in skeletal muscle of diabetic patient. Basement membrane surrounding capillary tremendously thickened. (Courtesy Dr. J. R. Williamson.)

not clearly defined. From the standpoint of morphology, the thickened basement membrane around the capillaries could interfere with the rate of transfer of nutrients and inflammatory cells from the bloodstream to the surrounding tissues. This could impair the resistance of the skin to secondary infections and delay the rate of healing following injuries. Both of these phenomena are observed in patients with diabetes mellitus, but no quantitative information is available on either the rate of emigration of leukocytes or the physicochemical binding properties of the basement membrane in diabetic patients.

Kidney in diabetes

The nodular lesions of the glomeruli described by Kimmelstiel and Wilson[71] are characteristic pathologic changes found in the kidney in diabetes mellitus. This lesion is apparently the result of focal thickening of the basement membrane and, in some way, may be associated with the mesangial cells (p. 793). Marked hyalinization of the afferent and efferent arterioles also is found with diabetic glomerulosclerosis.

Vacuolization of the pars recta of the proximal convoluted tubules at the corticomedullary junction may be observed in patients dying with uncontrolled diabetes and severe hyperglycemia. These vacuoles represent areas of glycogen deposition within the tubules that disappear when the diabetic state is treated. This condition is called the Armanni-Ebstein lesion of the kidney.

Necrotizing renal papillitis is a rare but serious complication of diabetes mellitus. This condition is not limited to diabetic patients but also may occur in nondiabetic individuals with obstructive lesions of the urinary tract. The condition is characterized clinically in the diabetic patient by the rapid onset of uremia and subsequent death due to infarction and sloughing of the renal papillae (p. 805).

Eye in diabetes

The characteristic pathologic changes in diabetic retinopathy are microaneurysms of the retinal vessels and intraretinal hemorrhages. The basement membranes of the retinal vessels are thickened and may be reduplicated. A pericapillary cell is found embedded in the basement membrane around the capillaries in muscle, skin, and eye. In the skin and muscle, these cells are called pericytes, whereas in the eye, they are called mural cells. It is probable that the mesangial cell of the glomerulus is a corresponding analogue of these pericapillary cells. Their function, with respect to basement membrane formation or destruction, is unknown at the present time.

Evidence is available that the mural cells in the retinal capillaries may undergo degeneration and disappear in diabetes mellitus. It is postulated that the loss of these cells affects the capillary hydrodynamics within the retina, producing large vascular shunts that may develop aneurysms, with degeneration of adjacent capillary beds (p. 1041).

Peripheral nerves in diabetes

Peripheral neuropathy is particularly prone to occur in the older diabetic patient, with approximately 30% to 50% of the patients showing minor reflex changes and evanescent pains in the extremities. Diffuse and patchy areas of demyelination have been observed within the peripheral nerves. It is probable that the changes within the nerve are due to involvement of the small vessels supplying these different areas or that the abnormal state of carbohydrate metabolism in patients with diabetes may have a direct effect on the nerves, resulting in degenerative changes.

Arteries in diabetes

From a clinical standpoint, the impression is gained that arteriosclerosis is a complication of diabetes mellitus, for it apparently occurs earlier and with a higher incidence than in the general population. Controlled clinical studies have been in progress in several institutions for the past few years in order to obtain factual information on this point. The two major areas involved in the diabetic patient are the coronary vessels, resulting in myocardial infarction, and the vessels of the lower extremities, producing gangrene of the toes and feet.

The precipitating causes of gangrene of the lower extremities are usually mechanical, thermal, or chemical trauma to the extremities resulting in ulceration, infection, and subsequent gangrene. Comparison of the ultrastructure of dermal capillaries of the toes in amputated specimens from diabetic and nondiabetic individuals indicates that thickening of the basement membrane of the capillaries is limited to the diabetic group. The marked thickening in the basement membranes in diabetic patients may play some role in the inception and complication of the vascular insufficiency of the lower extremities, possibly by interfering with nutrition and response of the tissues to injury.

NEOPLASMS OF PANCREATIC ISLETS
Beta cell tumors

Functioning beta cell neoplasms retain the capacity to form, store, and release insulin into the bloodstream. The neoplastic beta cells differ from the normal in that they are no longer responsive to the normal control mechanisms affecting insulin release and thus will release insulin at an uncontrolled rate, resulting in repeated attacks of hypoglycemia. Measurements of insulin levels in the bloodstream during these hypoglycemic episodes indicate marked increases in its concentration. Stimulation of insulin release from these neoplasms can be produced by the administration of tolbutamide and arginine. Diazoxide, which inhibits insulin secretion by normal beta cells, also will diminish the release of insulin from the neoplastic beta cells.

The most common sites for these neoplasms is in the body and tail of the pancreas. Grossly, the tumors are usually encapsulated and well circumscribed, varying from 5 mm to 10 cm in diameter. They have a homogeneous color and increased consistency, thus making it possible to delineate them from the surrounding normal pancreas.

Microscopically, the beta cell tumors may appear as ribbons or cords of cells passing between vascular sinusoids. It is extremely difficult to assess the degree of malignancy of these neoplasms based upon the presence of anaplasia and hyperchromatism of the nuclei, since these changes may be present in a circumscribed adenoma or in one that has metastasized. The degree of beta granulation within the neoplasms may vary from a few scattered granules to an intense degree of granulation similar to the normal beta cell. Measurements of insulin in microdissected neoplastic cells from frozen-dried sections confirm this marked variability in insulin content of the cells. Electron microscopically, the neoplastic cells contain the typical crystalline, rectangular granules that are present in normal beta cells, and the number of these vary markedly within different neoplasms. Amyloid frequently is observed between the two basement membranes separating the neoplastic cells from the capillaries and, in some instances, calcification may be present in this area.

Fluorescein-labeled antibodies to insulin have been used to study the endogenous insulin of neoplastic beta cells. Insulin in the neoplastic cells does not react with the labeled antibodies, whereas normal beta cells give a positive reaction. This indicates that insulin in the secretory granules of the neoplasms is stored in a form that is immunologically unreactive with the labeled antibodies. Studies on the amino acid composition of insulin from neoplastic beta cells have been accomplished, and the composition was found to be the same as that of normal human insulin. Thus, the lack of immunologic reactivity of endogenous insulin in the neoplasms may be due to a difference in the macromolecular structure of the insulin in the beta granules of the neoplastic cells.

Glucagonoma

An alpha cell carcinoma has been described recently which contained glucagon. Because of the present state of confusion over possible subtypes of alpha cells, it appears appropriate to call this neoplasm a glucagonoma. The level of glucagon in the plasma of the patient was significantly above normal values, and the individual had diabetes mellitus. The possible interrelationship of the diabetic state and the glucagonoma is unknown. Electron microscopically, the neoplastic cells had the ultrastructural appearance of normal alpha cells and contained numerous secretory granules.

This is a rare lesion, but now that it has been identified, undoubtedly additional cases will be reported. This interesting neoplasm clearly indicates the need for a combined light microscopic, electron microscopic, and hormonal assay examination of certain endocrine tumors in order to delineate the type of neoplasm present.

Zollinger-Ellison syndrome

Zollinger and Ellison[102] described a diagnostic triad that consists of:

1 A fulminating peptic ulcer diathesis persisting despite medical therapy or other radical procedures
2 Marked gastric acid hypersecretion
3 The presence of a nonbeta cell tumor in the pancreas

Approximately one-third of the ulcers observed in the patients have been found in unusual locations, such as the esophageal, postbulbar, and jejunal areas. The tumors most frequently occur in the body and tail of the pancreas and, in a few instances, the neoplasm was found in the wall of the duodenum, apparently originating in heterotopic foci of pancreatic tissue. Multiple adenomas involving the pituitary, adrenal, and parathyroid glands and islets of Langerhans have been found in approximately one-third of the patients.

Histologically, the neoplastic cells have neither the tinctorial properties nor the ultrastructural characteristics of beta or alpha cells but are most similar to delta cells. Gastrin has been isolated from these tumors and from metastases. Excessive and uncontrolled release of gastrin would obviously produce hypersecretion of acid from the stomach and could result in a fulminating peptic ulcer diathesis. Recently, the fluorescent antibody technique has been utilized to localize gastrin in the stomach and in the pancreas. These investigations indicate that gastrin-containing cells are present within the islets in a low percentage, and presumably these are delta cells. Thus, it would appear that the cell of origin of the tumors in this syndrome are the delta cells present in the normal islet and that with neoplastic change the cells release gastrin at an uncontrolled rate.

In some of the patients diagnosed as having the Zollinger-Ellison syndrome, watery diarrhea was a predominant clinical symptom. As further cases were reported, it became apparent that a separate entity existed that was characterized clinically by the presence of watery diarrhea, hypokalemia, and achlorhydria in association with a nonbeta cell tumor of the pancreas. Gastrin was absent in the tumor and metastases, and suggestive evidence is available that the neoplasms contain a secretin-like hormone. If it is established that the neoplasm in these cases contains secretin, then it raises the question of the possible presence of a cell within the islet which normally secretes secretin.

REFERENCES
Normal form and development

1 Liu, H. M., and Potter, E. L.: Arch. Path. (Chicago) **74:**439-452, 1962.
2 Millbourn, E.: Acta Anat. (Basel) **9:**1-34, 1950.
3 Rutter, W. J., Clark, W. R., Kemp, J. D., Bradshaw, W. S., Sanders, T. G., and Ball, W. D.: Epithelial-mesenchymal interactions, Baltimore, 1968, The Williams & Wilkins Co.
4 Wessells, N. K., and Cohen, J. H.: Develop. Biol. **15:**237-270, 1967.
5 Wessells, N. K., and Evans, J.: Develop. Biol. **17:**413-446, 1968.

Abnormalities of form and development

6 Barbosa, J. J. de C., Dockerty, M. B., and Waugh, J. M.: Surg. Gynec. Obstet. **82:**527-542, 1946 (ectopic pancreas).
7 Elliott, G. B., Kliman, M. R., and Elliott, K. A.: Canad. J. Surg. **11:**357-364, 1968.
8 Feldman, M., and Weinberg, T.: J.A.M.A. **148:**893-898, 1952 (ectopic pancreas).
9 Huebner, G. D., and Reed, P. A.: Amer. J. Surg. **104:**869-873, 1962 (annular pancreas).
10 Lundquist, G.: Acta Chir. Scand. **117:**451-454, 1959 (annular pancreas).
11 Pearson, S.: Arch. Surg. (Chicago) **63:**168-184, 1951 (ectopic pancreas).
12 Van Der Horst, L. F.: Arch. Surg. (Chicago) **83:**249-252, 1961 (annular pancreas).

Fibrocystic disease

13 Andersen, D. H.: Amer. J. Dis. Child. **56:**344-399, 1938.
14 Andersen, D. H.: Amer. J. Dis. Child. **63:**643-658, 1942.
15 Aterman, K.: Amer. J. Dis. Child. **101:**210-215, 1961.
16 Bodian, M.: Fibrocystic disease of the pancreas, New York, 1953, Grune & Stratton, Inc.
17 Clarke, J. T., Elian, E., and Shwachman, H.: Amer. J. Dis. Child. **101:**490-500, 1961.
18 Danes, B. S., and Bearn, A. G.: J. Exp. Med. **129:**775-793, 1969.
19 di Sant'Agnese, P. A., and Lepore, M. J.: Gastroenterology **40:**64-74, 1961.
20 di Sant'Agnese, P. A., and Talamo, R. C.: New Eng. J. Med. **277:**1287-1294, 1344-1352, 1399-1408, 1967.
21 Dische, Z., di Sant'Agnese, P. A., Pallavicini, C., and Youlos, J.: Pediatrics **24:**74-91, 1959.
22 Farber, S.: Arch. Path. (Chicago) **37:**238-250, 1944.
23 Farber, S.: J. Pediat.. **24:**387-392, 1944.
24 Kaplan, E., Shwachman, H., Perlmutter, A. D., Rule, A., Khow, K.-T., and Holsclaw, D. S.: New Eng. J. Med. **279:**65-69, 1968.
25 Macdonald, J. A., and Trusler, G. A.: Canad. Med. Ass. J. **83:**881-885, 1960.

26 Mangos, J. A., and McSherry, N. R.: Science **158:**135-136, 1967.
27 Munger, B. L., Brusilow, S. W., and Cooke, R. E.: J. Pediat. **59:**497-511, 1961.
28 Roberts, G. B.: Ann. Hum. Genet. **24:**127-135, 1960.
29 Rubin, L. S., Barbero, G. J., Chernick, W. S., and Sibinga, M. S.: J. Pediat. **63:**1120-1129, 1963.
30 Smoller, M., and Hsia, D. Y.: Amer. J. Dis. Child. **98:**277-292, 1959.
31 Spock, A., Heick, H. M. C., Cress, H., and Logan, W.: Mod. Probl. Pediat. **10:**200-206, 1967.

Pancreatitis

32 Baggenstoss, A. H.: Amer. J. Path. **24:**1003-1017, 1948 (acinar ectasia).
33 Blumenthal, H. G., and Probstein, J. G.: Pancreatitis, Springfield, Ill., 1959, Charles C Thomas, Publisher.
34 Ciba Foundation Symposium: The exocrine pancreas, Boston, 1961, Little, Brown and Co.
35 Dreiling, D. A.: J. Mount Sinai Hosp. N. Y. **36:**388-407, 1969.
36 Edmonson, H. A., and Berne, C. J.: Surg. Gynec. Obstet. **79:**240-244, 1944 (calcium changes in pancreatic necrosis).
37 Elliott, D. W., Williams, R. D., and Zollinger, R. M.: Ann. Surg. **146:**669-682, 1957.
38 Gross, J. B., and Comfort, M. W.: Amer. J. Med. **21:**596-617, 1956 (chronic pancreatitis).
39 Gross, J. B., Gambill, E. E., and Ulrich, J. A.: Amer. J. Med. **33:**358-364, 1962 (hereditary pancreatitis).
40 Hanna, W. A.: Brit. J. Surg. **47:**495-498, 1960 (rupture of pseudocysts).
41 Hranilovich, G. T., and Baggenstoss, A. H.: Arch. Path. (Chicago) **55:**443-456, 1953.
42 Murphy, R. F., and Hinkamp, J. F.: Arch. Surg. (Chicago) **81:**564-568, 1960 (pseudocysts).
43 Opie, E. L.: Bull. Johns Hopkins Hosp. **12:**182-188, 1901 (common channel).
44 Ponka, J. L., Landrum, S. E., and Chaikof, L.: Arch. Surg. (Chicago) **83:**475-490, 1961 (postoperative pancreatitis).
45 Popper, H. L., Necheles, H., and Russell, K. C.: Surg. Gynec. Obstet. **87:**79-82, 1948 (ischemia).
46 Rich, A. R., and Duff, G. L.: Bull. Johns Hopkins Hosp. **58:**212-259, 1936 (role of pancreatic duct obstruction).
47 Szymanski, F. J., and Bluefarb, S. M.: Arch. Derm. (Chicago) **83:**224-229, 1961 (cutaneous fat necrosis).
48 Thal, A. P.: Surg. Forum **11:**367-369, 1960 (pancreatic antibodies).
49 Tumen, H. J.: Amer. J. Dig. Dis. **6:**435-440, 1961 (pathogenesis).

Tumors of exocrine pancreas

50 Auger, C.: Arch. Path. (Chicago) **43:**400-405, 1947 (fat necrosis with carcinoma).
51 Bell, E. T.: Amer. J. Path. **33:**499-523, 1957 (carcinoma).
52 Cornes, J. S., and Azzopardi, J. C.: Brit. J. Surg. **47:**139-144, 1959 (cystadenocarcinoma).

53 Frantz, V. K.: In Atlas of tumor pathology, Sect. VII, Fascs. 27 and 28, Washington, D. C., 1959, Armed Forces Institute of Pathology (tumors of pancreas).

54 Kaplan, N., and Angrist, A.: Surg. Gynec. Obstet. **77**:199-204, 1943 (mechanism of jaundice with carcinoma).

55 Kenney, W. E.: Surgery **14**:600-609, 1943 (venous thrombi with pancreatic carcinoma).

56 Lafler, C. J., and Hinerman, D. L.: Cancer **14**:944-952, 1961 (venous thrombi with pancreatic carcinoma).

57 Mikal, S., and Campbell, A. J. A.: Surgery **28**:963-969, 1950 (carcinoma).

58 Miller, J. R., Baggenstoss, A. H., and Comfort, M. W.: Cancer **4**:233-241, 1951 (cancer).

59 Piper, C. E., Jr., Remine, W. H., and Priestley, J. T.: J.A.M.A. **180**:648-652, 1962 (cystadenoma).

60 Probstein, J. G., and Blumenthal, H. T.: Arch. Surg. (Chicago) **81**:683-689, 1960 (malignant transformation of cystadenoma).

61 Warren, K. W., Braasch, J. W., and Thum, C. W.: Surg. Clin. N. Amer. **48**:601-618, 1968.

62 Weinstein, J. J.: Amer. J. Gastroent. **37**:629-641, 1962 (carcinoma in periampullary area).

Diabetes mellitus

63 Aagenaes, O., and Moe, H.: Diabetes **10**:253-259, 1961 (electron microscopy of dermal capillaries).

64 Allen, A. C.: Arch. Path. (Chicago) **32**:33-51, 1941 (diabetic glomerulosclerosis).

65 Banson, B. B., and Lacy, P. E.: Amer. J. Path. **45**:41-58, 1964 (basement membrane in diabetic gangrene).

66 Bloodworth, J. M., Jr.: Diabetes **12**:99-114, 1963 (microangiopathy).

67 Cerasi, E., and Luft, R.: Acta Endocr. (Kobenhavn) **55**:278-304, 1967 (absent initial peak insulin release in diabetes).

68 Cogan, D. G., and Kuwabara, T.: Diabetes **12**:293-300, 1963 (mural cells of retina).

69 Ehrlich, J. C., and Ratner, I. M.: Amer. J. Path. **38**:49-59, 1961 (amyloidosis of islets).

70 Howell, S. L., Kostianovsky, M., and Lacy, P. E.: J. Cell Biol. **42**:695-705, 1969 (autoradiography of beta granule formation).

71 Kimmelstiel, P., and Wilson, C.: Amer. J. Path. **12**:83-97, 1936.

72 Lacy, P. E.: New Eng. J. Med. **276**:187-195, 1967 (review—structure and function of islet cells).

73 Lacy, P. E., and Kostianovsky, M.: Diabetes **16**:35-39, 1967 (collagenase isolation of islets).

74 Lacy, P. E., and Wright, P. H.: Diabetes **14**:634-642, 1965 (experimental eosinophil infiltration of islets).

75 Lacy, P. E., Howell, S. L., Young, D. A., and Fink, C. J.: Nature (London) **219**:1177-1179, 1968 (hypothesis of insulin secretion).

76 Lazarus, S. S., and Volk, B. W.: The pancreas in human and experimental diabetes, New York, 1962, Grune & Stratton, Inc.

77 McGavran, M. H., and Hartroft, W. S.: Amer. J. Path. **32**:631, 1956 (hemochromatosis).

78 Nagler, W., and Taylor, H.: J.A.M.A. **184**:723-725, 1963 (lymphocytic infiltration of islets).

79 Silverman, J. L.: Diabetes **12**:528-537, 1963 (eosinophilic infiltration of islets).

80 Siperstein, M. D., Unger, R. H., and Madison, L. L.: J. Clin. Invest. **47**:1973-1999, 1968 (basement membrane in diabetes).

81 Steiner, D. F., Cunningham, D. D., Spigelman, L., and Aten, B.: Science **157**:697-700, 1967 (proinsulin).

82 Toreson, W. E.: Amer. J. Path. **27**:327-347, 1951 (glycogen and hydropic change).

83 Toreson, W. E., Lee, J. C., and Grodsky, G. M.: Amer. J. Path. **52**:1099-1115, 1968 (immune diabetes in rabbits).

84 Volk, B. W., and Lazarus, S. S.: Lab. Invest. **12**:697-711, 1963 (ballooning degeneration of beta cells).

85 Warren, S., and LeCompte, P. M.: The pathology of diabetes mellitus, Philadelphia, 1966, Lea & Febiger.

86 Williams, R. H., editor: Diabetes, New York, 1960, Hoeber Medical Division, Harper & Row, Publishers.

87 Williamson, J. R.: Diabetes **9**:471-480, 1960 (electron microscopy of glycogen in beta cells).

88 Zacks, S. I., Pegues, J. J., and Elliott, F. A.: Metabolism **11**:381-393, 1962 (electron microscopy of muscle capillaries).

Neoplasms of pancreatic islets
Beta cell tumors

89 Duff, G. L.: Amer. J. Med. Sci. **203**:437-451, 1942.

90 Frantz, V. K.: Ann. Surg. **112**:161-176, 1940.

91 Howard, J. M., Moss, N. H., and Rhoads, J. E.: Int. Abst. Surg. **90**:417-455, 1950.

92 Laidlaw, G. F.: Amer. J. Path. **14**:125-134, 1938.

93 Markowitz, A. M., Slanetz, C. A., Jr., and Frantz, V. K.: Ann. Surg. **154**:877-884, 1961.

94 Porta, E. A., Yerry, R., and Scott, R. F.: Amer. J. Path. **41**:623-631, 1962.

95 Scholz, D. A., Remine, W. H., and Priestley, J. T.: Proc. Mayo Clin. **35**:545-550, 1960.

96 Sieracki, J., Marshall, R. B., and Horn, R. C., Jr.: Cancer **13**:347-357, 1960.

Glucagonoma; Zollinger-Ellison syndrome

97 Gregory, R. A., Tracy, H. J., French, J. M., and Sircus, W.: Lancet **1**:1045-1048, 1960.

98 Hallenbeck, G. A., Code, C. F., and Kennedy, J. C.: Gastroenterology **44**:631-636, 1963.

99 Lomsky, R., Langr, F., and Vortel, V.: Nature (London) **223**:618-619, 1969 (immunochemical localization of gastrin in islets).

100 McGavran, M. H., Unger, R. H., Recant, L., Polk, H. C., Kilo, C., and Levin, M. E.: New Eng. J. Med. **274**:1408-1413, 1966 (glucagonoma).

101 Zollinger, R. M., and Craig, T. V.: Amer. J. Surg. **99**:424-432, 1960.

102 Zollinger, R. M., and Ellison, E. H.: Ann. Surg. **142**:709-728, 1955.

103 Zollinger, R. M., Tompkins, R. K., Amerson, J. R., Endahl, G. L., Kraft, A. R., and Moore, F. T.: Ann. Surg. **168**:502-521, 1968 (diarrheogenic non-beta islet cell tumor).

Chapter 31

Hemopoietic system: reticuloendothelium, spleen, lymph nodes, blood, and bone marrow

John B. Miale

The hemopoietic and reticuloendothelial system is a physiologic and pathophysiologic unit rather than an anatomic entity. Traditionally, some of its discrete anatomic subunits (spleen, lymph nodes, bone marrow) receive separate discussion. However, aside from some differences in anatomic location or in special physiologic functions, most of the functions of the system and the cellular changes accompanying benign and malignant proliferation are the same regardless of location. It is preferable, therefore, to discuss first the function and cellular changes common to the entire reticuloendothelial system. When, for convenience, the anatomic subunits are considered separately, the student will appreciate the physiologic common denominators and the interrelationship between the subunits.

■ Reticuloendothelial system

DEFINITION AND TERMINOLOGY

The term "reticuloendothelial system" (RES) was coined by Aschoff and Kiyono[1] to cover, by an inclusive term, a system of cells found within and outside of organs and characterized functionally by (1) phagocytosis, (2) staining by vital dyes, and (3) anatomically, by juxtaposition to the reticulum of connective tissues and to the lining membrane of blood vessels. They thus recognized and labeled the common biologic and functional nature of cells seemingly of diverse nature, such as the clasmatocytes of Ranvier, the adventitial cells of Marchand, the fixed histiocytes of Maximow, the endothelial sinusoidal cells in lymph nodes, bone marrow,

adrenal cortex, hypophysis, and spleen, and the Kupffer cells in the liver. The presence of fibrils demonstrable as an argentophilic reticulum (reticulin, Ranvier and Bizzozero) led to the assumption that the stellate, supravitally staining "reticulum cells" were one-half of the reticuloendothelial system, the other half being the argentophilic reticulum supporting the tissue and endothelial cells.

As long as it was assumed that reticulum cells formed the argentophilic reticulum, it seemed possible for all to agree on what was meant by the term "reticulum cell." However, it then became apparent, chiefly due to the histochemical studies of Hortega, that the glial cells in the brain have argentophilic cytoplasm and cytoplasmic processes and that, in an inflammatory reaction, these cells become rounded up (the compound granular corpuscles) and actively phagocytic and stain with vital dyes. Using Hortega's techniques, it was then shown that cells similar in structure and metamorphosis can be found in the spleen and other extracerebral sites.

It seems that the cellular components of the reticuloendothelial system need not be in close association with reticulum fibrils. A close association to reticulum fibers is found in lymph nodes, tonsils, spleen, bone marrow, thymus, lymphoid nodules in the intestines, sinuses of the liver, perivascular connective tissue, pituitary gland, adrenal cortex, and alveolar walls of the lung. A lack of reticulum is characteristic of glial cells, omentum, and serous membrane. This has given rise to polemics over nomenclature, and criticism of the term reticulum cell has extended into recent years. Most recently, Gall[4a] has indicated

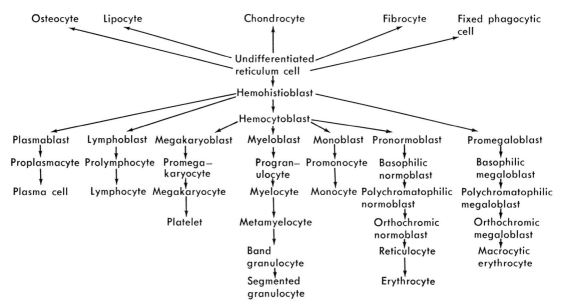

Fig. 31-1 Reticuloendothelial system from standpoint of its multipotentiality. According to this scheme, the most primitive and still undifferentiated cell is called "undifferentiated reticulum cell." This cell is neither phagocytic nor stainable with vital dyes. It is capable of differentiating into various types of connective tissue cells (osteocytes, lipocytes, chondrocytes, and fibrocytes) as well as into "classic" cell of reticuloendothelial system— fixed phagocytic cell. It is also able to differentiate in hemopoietic direction, at which time it may be considered to be hemopoietic reticulum cell in general sense, or, more specifically, hemohistioblast or hemocytoblast. Undifferentiated reticulum cell, hemocytoblast, and hemohistioblast cannot be distinguished from one another on morphologic criteria alone. (From Miale, J. B.: Laboratory medicine—hematology, The C. V. Mosby Co.)

the inexactness of the term "reticulum cell" and prefers to use "histiocyte" instead. Note, however, that the validity of this and other arguments is diminished when it is based on purely morphologic criteria, for what a cell is and is capable of becoming cannot be determined accurately by morphology alone. In fact, the importance of the reticuloendothelial system is in the concept of its biologic role in hemopoiesis, reaction to injury, antibody formation, and neoplasia, as discussed below, and not in its morphologic composition.

Furthermore, a very important cellular component of the reticuloendothelial system is a primitive mesenchymal cell that is neither phagocytic nor stainable with vital dyes. This, in our opinion, occupies the central position in the many functions and transformations of the system, for it is multipotential and able to differentiate into phagocytic and non-phagocytic histiocytes, into fibroblasts, and into precursors of lymphocytes and other blood and tissue hemopoietic cells.

Provided that this multipotentiality is appreciated, it matters little which nomenclature is used. The scheme and nomenclature used in this chapter is shown in Fig. 31-1.

PATHOPHYSIOLOGY

The functions of the reticuloendothelial system in the broad sense—the reticulum cell, its cellular derivatives, and, in the anatomic sense, the organs and specialized tissues that contain them (spleen, liver, lymph nodes, thymus, bone marrow)—can be classified as follows:

1 Hemopoiesis, the production and maintenance at physiologic levels of the cells of the blood and bone marrow
2 Phagocytosis, of senescent blood cells, cellular breakdown products and other particulate matter, bacteria, fungi, and parasites, and storage and clearance from the blood and interstitial tissues of certain chemical by-products of normal and abnormal metabolism (hemoglobin, hemosiderin, bilirubin, lipids, glycogen)
3 The production of antibodies
4 Benign and malignant proliferation (hyperplasia and neoplasia)

Hemopoiesis

In the embryo, the mesenchymal stem cells of the yolk sac differentiate into groups of cells characterized by a large nucleus contain-

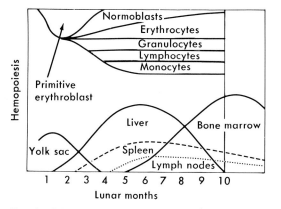

Fig. 31-2 Hemopoietic sequences in fetus. Degree and site of hemopoietic activity (lower portion) and appearance of blood cells in peripheral blood (upper portion). (From Miale, J. B.: Laboratory medicine—hematology, The C. V. Mosby Co.)

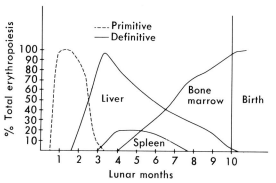

Fig. 31-3 Erythropoiesis in fetus. Comparison of primitive and definitive erythroid precursors and estimate of relative contribution of liver, spleen, and bone marrow. (From Miale, J. B.: Laboratory medicine—hematology, The C. V. Mosby Co.)

ing spongy chromatin, one or two nucleolar chromatin condensations, and a deeply basophilic cytoplasm. This primitive cell is committed by differentiation to form blood cells, becoming a hemopoietic reticulum cell. As shown in Fig. 31-1, this is the *hemohistioblast,* normally giving rise to the plasma cell and lymphocyte series and to megaloblasts in the abnormal erythropoiesis of pernicious anemia and other megaloblastic dysplasias. In the early hemopoiesis of the yolk sac phase (Fig. 31-2), only a primitive type of nucleated erythrocyte precursor is formed, the *primitive erythroblast.* These do not survive beyond a few weeks, being replaced by the definitive type of erythroid precursor, the *normoblast.* In the yolk sac of a 9-week-old embryo, half of the cells are primitive erythroblasts while the other half are definitive normoblasts.

By the third month of fetal life, *mesoblastic* (yolk sac) hemopoiesis has gradually ceased and the liver has become the chief site of blood cell formation. This second phase is referred to as the period of *hepatic hemopoiesis.* It reaches peak activity during the fifth to sixth month and remains active until shortly before birth. Only a few hemopoietic foci are normally present in the liver of full-term infants. However, many are present in the liver of the premature infant. Although about four-fifths of the hemopoietic activity in the liver is related to the production of erythrocytes (erythropoiesis) (Fig. 31-3), there is also production of leukocytes (leukopoiesis) and platelets (thrombocytopoiesis). There is also, during the middle and last third of fetal life, hemopoiesis in the spleen,

thymus, and lymph nodes. The spleen is at first active in the production of all three types of blood cells, but later it is primarily a site for erythropoiesis and lymphopoiesis. The lymph nodes are essentially sites for lymphopoiesis, although an occasional granulocyte can be seen.

From birth on, the bone marrow is the chief hemopoietic organ. It becomes increasingly active during the later months of gestation, during which time the marrow cavities (sternum, vertebrae, pelvis, ribs, skull, and proximal portions of the long bones) enlarge to accommodate more and more bone marrow cells. During the same period, the hemopoietic activity in the liver diminishes, so that at birth the bone marrow accounts for all of the erythrocytes, all of the granulocytes, all of the platelets, most of the plasma cells, and a significant number of lymphocytes. This, then, is the situation in the normal adult: the bone marrow is the chief hemopoietic tissue, the hemopoietic activity outside of the bone marrow being limited to lymphocytopoiesis in the spleen, lymph nodes, and other lymphoid tissue.

It is of great interest to note that the sequence of events in the development of fetal and adult hemopoiesis is recapitulated and exaggerated in some hematologic diseases in the adult. When hemopoietic activity ceases in the liver and spleen of the fetus, the primitive mesenchymal cells remain in a dormant state. At any later time, these can be stimulated again to form blood cells, at which time we see the phenomenon of *extramedullary hemopoiesis*—i.e., hemopoiesis outside of the normal adult hemopoietic organ, the bone marrow. When this occurs, the liver, spleen, and whatever other tissue involved becomes very much enlarged and, when studied under the microscope, much of the enlargement is seen to be due to proliferating blood cells. This situation is seen in both benign (the so-called myeloproliferative syndromes) and malignant (leukemic and lymphomatous) proliferation.

Phagocytosis, storage, and clearance

The second function of the reticuloendothelial system (phagocytosis, storage, and clearance) is involved in several important physiologic activities. For example, phagocytosis of senescent erythrocytes and other blood cells eliminates those cells that are no longer useful or functioning. When an erythrocyte is "worn out" at the end of its normal life span of about 120 days, it is disposed of by the phagocytic cells of the reticuloendothelial system. Since there are many phagocytes in the spleen and also in the liver, most of the phagocytic activity occurs in these organs. When disintegrating erythrocytes are removed from the blood by phagocytic cells in the spleen, the hemoglobin is broken down into the pigment moiety (bilirubin), the protein moiety (globin), and iron (Fig. 31-4).

While this is a function common to all phagocytic reticuloendothelial cells regardless of location, it is difficult for us to ascribe such important activities to a diffuse, anatomically indistinct tissue. It is more comfortable to ascribe these functions to specific organs such as the spleen, for example, for this has the respectability of a distinct organ, can be palpated at the bedside to the accompaniment of the medical student's admiring murmurs, and is subject to excision by the surgeon. Thus, when it seems that there is an accelerated destruction of blood cells, it is tempting to visualize this as occurring in the spleen and then to avail one's self of the term "hypersplenism." Nevertheless, there is justification for the term, for the anatomic structure of the spleen is such that there is a sluggish flow of blood through the complex of sinuses and, because of this, erythrocytes particularly are exposed in a semistagnant situation to the lytic and other functions of this organ.

In some situations, the phagocytic and cytolytic role of the spleen is striking. In congenital spherocytic hemolytic anemia, for example, the erythrocytes are spherocytic

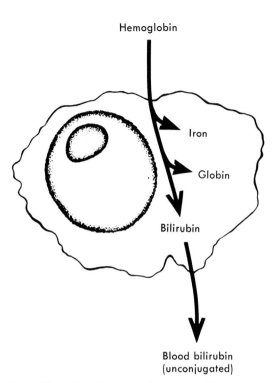

Fig. 31-4 Breakdown of hemoglobin within phagocytic reticuloendothelial cell (splenic macrophage, Kupffer cell in liver, alveolar macrophage of lung, etc.). Hemoglobin iron in form of hemosiderin is stored in phagocyte to various degrees, depending on body's need for iron, and is in equilibrium with plasma iron pool. Globin passes into plasma protein pool, while unconjugated bilirubin liberated into blood will be cleared and conjugated in parenchymal cells of liver.

rather than biconcave discs, and this aberration in shape is recognized by the spleen, which promptly destroys them. The slow passage through the splenic sinusoids is a major factor in the apparent localization of this destructive activity in that organ and, indeed, splenectomy in such cases is dramatically beneficial. One more example will suffice. It was noted, some years ago, (Knutti and Hawkins[7]) that splenectomized dogs often succumb to an overwhelming infection with bartonella, an organism previously tolerated as long as the spleen destroyed the infected erythrocytes in numbers sufficient to keep the infection under control.

Production of antibodies

The third function of the reticuloendothelial system, the production of antibodies, is without doubt of primary importance. The reticuloendothelial system is concerned with immune phenomena and immune reactions that may be helpful (protective) or harmful

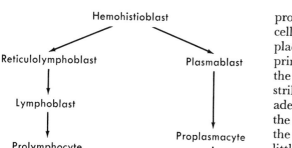

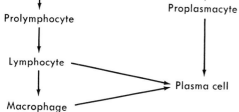

Fig. 31-5 Transformation of antibody-producing cells of reticuloendothelial system in reactive states.

(pathogenic) to the host. Diseases related to immunologic competence or incompetence are discussed in another chapter. For the purpose of this general introduction, it is sufficient to note that we are dealing with those cells, and derivative cells, of the reticuloendothelial system shown in Fig. 31-5. It should be noted that cells given a certain morphologic identity (i.e., lymphocytes and plasma cells) are probably heterogeneous from the standpoint of derivation and function.

It is now recognized that circulating lymphocytes can recognize a foreign antigen and initiate an immunologic reaction against it. However, the total immune response probably requires the participation of all lymphoid tissue, and this may represent at least two distinct lines of lymphocytes, each with different functions. In the chicken, the lymphoid system is made up of two separate anatomic and functional units: the thymus, from which originate lymphocytes involved in homograft and delayed hypersensitivity reactions, and the bursa of Fabricius, which is responsible for the germinal centers and plasma cells in lymph nodes and spleen and for immunoglobulin production. In man there is also, most probably, a heterogeneous population of lymphocytes and lymphoid structures.

Benign and malignant proliferation

It was previously (p. 1299) noted that primitive and resting reticuloendothelial cells are capable of being again stimulated to produce blood cells at sites where they have been dormant. In a way, this is a model of the proliferative capacity of the reticuloendothelial cells. First, the site where proliferation takes place is determined by the presence there of primitive cells capable of proliferating. When the proliferation is primarily lymphocytic, a striking enlargement of lymph nodes (lymphadenopathy) and moderate enlargement of the spleen (splenomegaly) are seen. When the proliferation is primarily granulocytic, little lymphadenopathy but striking splenomegaly are seen. Second, the proliferative reaction may be either benign or malignant. Benign proliferative reactions often involve single cell types—e.g., lymphocytes and lymphoid tissue in viral infections, granulocytes in the bone marrow and spleen in bacterial infection, and the erythrocyte precursors in the bone marrow in hypoxia and hemolytic anemia. The same is true of malignant proliferations, the lymphomas and lymphocytic leukemias affecting chiefly the lymph nodes and other lymphoid tissue and granulocytic leukemia affecting the bone marrow and spleen.

It should be noted also that while the foregoing generalizations are valid, the process of proliferation, particularly the malignant type, can take place wherever there are primitive reticuloendothelial cells having the appropriate ability to proliferate, so that these diseases are usually multicentric. For example, leukemias and lymphomas may involve lymph nodes throughout the body, and sometimes organs and tissues, such as heart, meninges, etc., that might seem to be involved by metastasis.

The general scheme of the proliferative capabilties of the reticuloendothelial system is shown in Fig. 31-6.

Summary

The reticuloendothelial system is a system of cells that, while present in large numbers in the spleen, liver, and lymph nodes, are in fact present in many tissues and organs in the body. Not only do these cells have specialized functions, but the primitive reticuloendothelial cell also is capable of differentiating along many lines. The derivative cells are then specialized to perform the various functions of phagocytosis, to produce immunoglobulins, and to serve the body's needs for blood cells. Misguided and uncontrolled proliferation leads to lymphoma or leukemia. These neoplasms may appear to be localized in those organs richest in reticuloendothelial cells (lymph nodes, spleen, liver, bone mar-

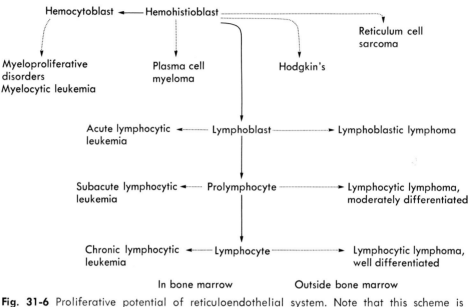

"Myeloproliferation" • "Lymphoproliferation"

Hemocytoblast ◄── Hemohistioblast ·································▼ Reticulum cell
                                                                        sarcoma

Myeloproliferative   Plasma cell   Hodgkin's
disorders   myeloma
Myelocytic leukemia

Acute lymphocytic ◄········ Lymphoblast ········► Lymphoblastic lymphoma
leukemia

Subacute lymphocytic ◄······· Prolymphocyte ········► Lymphocytic lymphoma,
leukemia   moderately differentiated

Chronic lymphocytic ◄········ Lymphocyte ········► Lymphocytic lymphoma,
leukemia   well differentiated

In bone marrow   Outside bone marrow

Fig. 31-6 Proliferative potential of reticuloendothelial system. Note that this scheme is concerned primarily with neoplastic proliferation. Benign proliferations (granulocytes, lymphocytes, plasma cells, etc.) differ only in that they are usually not life-threatening. Definition of myeloproliferative syndromes given on p. 1360. (From Miale, J. B.: Laboratory medicine—hematology, The C. V. Mosby Co.)

row) but may be found in any organ or tissue in the body. Because of the frequently striking involvement of the spleen, lymph nodes, and bone marrow, it is traditional to describe the anatomic pathology of these individual organs. It should be obvious, however, aside from special and individual characteristics of these organs, that the common denominator is their content of reticuloendothelial cells.

■ Spleen

STRUCTURE

The spleen comprises the largest single collection of lymphocytes and reticuloendothelial cells in the body. However, it is supplied by arterial blood by the splenic artery and is therefore in the vascular rather than the lymphatic system. It is roughly ovoid, with a convex upper surface and a concave surface below where the hilar vessels enter the organ. It lies beneath the ninth, tenth, and eleventh ribs, its long axis is parallel to them, and in the adult it weighs about 140 gm (range 100 gm to 170 gm). The capsule consists of a thin band of connective tissue with elastic fibers, covered by serous mesothelium. In man, there

is little, if any, smooth muscle in the capsule and thus, unlike in some animal species, there is no intrinsic contractile capability.

Grossly, the surface is purple and the consistency friable. The cut surface shows tiny gray-white islands of *white pulp* scattered throughout the soft red-purple *red pulp* that makes up the bulk of splenic tissue. Scraping the normal surface with the edge of a knife yields a moderate amount of bloody cellular material.

The tiny nodules of the white pulp are collections of small lymphocytes that form a sheath around arterioles of about 0.2 mm diameter and usually extend around even smaller arterioles. The lymphoid nodules are often called malpighian corpuscles. They may or may not show germinal centers as in the lymph nodes. When the spleen shows reaction to acute inflammation ("acute splenic tumor," "acute splenic hyperplasia," or "acute splenitis"), germinal centers are prominent and contain young lymphocytes and phagocytic histiocytes.

The red pulp as usually seen under the microscope does not seem particularly exciting, for the sinusoids are collapsed and one sees only many erythrocytes scattered, among

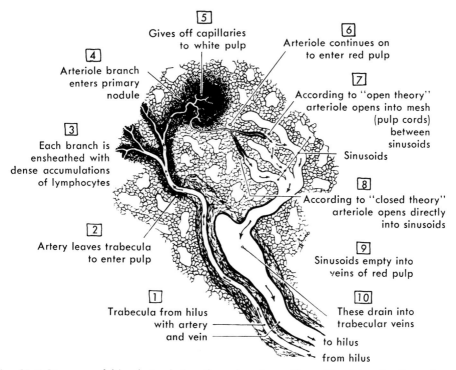

5 | Gives off capillaries to white pulp

6 | Arteriole continues on to enter red pulp

4 | Arteriole branch enters primary nodule

7 | According to "open theory" arteriole opens into mesh (pulp cords) between sinusoids

3 | Each branch is ensheathed with dense accumulations of lymphocytes

Sinusoids

8 | According to "closed theory" arteriole opens directly into sinusoids

2 | Artery leaves trabecula to enter pulp

9 | Sinusoids empty into veins of red pulp

1 | Trabecula from hilus with artery and vein

10 | These drain into trabecular veins

to hilus
from hilus

Fig. 31-7 Diagram of blood circulation through spleen. (From Blaustein, A.: The spleen; copyrighted by McGraw-Hill Book Co.; used with permission.)

which are a few neutrophils and phagocytic histiocytes. If the spleen is distended by injecting fixative through the splenic vein, however, the true structure is revealed. The framework of the organ consists of a mesh of argentophilic reticulum fibers that are continuous with the collagen fibers of the capsule and trabeculae. Supported by this framework are many sinusoids lined with long narrow endothelial cells. The cells of the red pulp, chiefly erythrocytes but also phagocytic reticulum cells and some granulocytes and plasma cells, fill the areas between adjacent sinusoids. This cellular component has been thought of as consisting of cords of cells (hence the term "cords of Billroth"), but, in fact, there is no cordlike structure in the three-dimensional model.

The vascular system of the spleen (Fig. 31-7) is not like that in any other organ. Characteristic is the system of sinusoids that permits slow passage of blood cells through the organ and thus allows time for phagocytosis and other functions that will be discussed later. The splenic artery usually divides into several branches, these entering the organ at different points along the hilus. Each arterial branch enters the spleen within one of the large trabeculae of the capsule. When

it leaves the trabecula, it becomes ensheathed with nodular collections of lymphocytes. The nodules of periarterial lymphocytes have been described previously as the "white pulp" of the spleen. The artery and arterioles within the white pulp are called "follicular arteries." These leave the white pulp and enter the red pulp as straight arterioles called "penicillar arteries."

There are several opinions as to the nature of the transition between the arterial and the venous vessels. It is agreed that between the two lie the sinusoids, but one opinion is that the penicillar arteries open directly into the sinusoids (the "closed" theory), whereas others think that the artery opens into the pulp cords from which the blood enters the sinusoids through a discontinuous endothelial lining (the "open" theory). Knisely[27] describes yet another system (in other species) made up of two portions: the arteriole empties directly into the sinusoid and a capillary shunt connects arterioles and venules. The veins leave the spleen at the hilus in association with the arteries that enter it. It is agreed that the blood flow through the sinusoids and through the red pulp is sluggish and that it is here that the cellular changes take place.

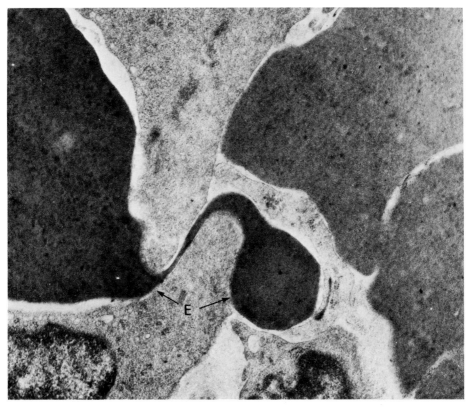

Fig. 31-8 Erythrocyte, **E,** lying partially within (smaller portion) and partially outside sinusoid. Spleen, hemoglobin H disease, electron microphotograph. (From Wennberg, E., and Weiss, L.: Blood **31:**778-790, 1968; by permission.)

The structure of the sinusoids deserve special mention. They do not have a basement membrane. They have been likened to a barrel, the endothelial cells being arranged longitudinally, touching but not cemented together, with "ring fibers" running at right angles and binding them together. The ring fibers have cytochemical characteristics similar to those of the basement membrane of the renal glomerulus and have been shown by King et al.[26] not to have the properties of reticulum in the classic sense. It has been suggested that the absence of a basement membrane makes the sinusoidal wall discontinuous, allowing blood cells to pass through the spaces between the endothelial cells (Fig. 31-8).

The extent of the lymphatics in the spleen has been debated for many years. Goldberg,[22] on the basis of the location of tumor metastases, has presented evidence that lymphatic vessels do indeed extend deeply into the splenic parenchyma and that they are present in the adventitia of arteries and arterioles and in the subintima of veins.

FUNCTION

The functions of the spleen can be classified under two general headings: (1) those that reflect the functions of the reticuloendothelial system and (2) special functions characteristic of the organ.

A Functions related to the spleen as an organ of the reticuloendothelial system
  1 Production of lymphocytes and plasma cells
  2 Production of antibodies
  3 Storage of iron
  4 Storage of other metabolites
B Functions characteristic of the organ
  1 Related to erythrocytes
    a Maturation of the surface of the erythrocytes
    b Reservoir function
    c "Culling" function
    d "Pitting" function
    e Disposal of senescent or abnormal erythrocytes
  2 Related to platelet life span
  3 Related to leukocyte life span

The production of cells capable of making antibodies (lymphocytes and plasma cells) and the role of the spleen as an immunologic organ go hand in hand, although it should be understood that antibodies also are made at other sites. Because the spleen represents the largest localization of lymphoid and reticuloendothelial tissue, and also because it is surgically accessible, this organ is sometimes excised when it is suspected to be hyperactive in the production of antibodies. Splenectomy per se has no effect on antibody production. For example, if an adult who has had a splenectomy for nonhematologic reasons (i.e., traumatic rupture) is challenged with a variety of antigens, it is found that he forms antibodies in no lesser titer than a normal person with an intact spleen. Supposedly, the antibody-producing role is assumed by other immunologically competent tissues. However, this is not true in children. Smith et al.[76] presented nineteen cases of severe and often fulminating infection in children who had been subjected to splenectomy. In two children, the splenectomy was performed for traumatic ruptures. In the others, the spleen was excised because of various hematologic disorders. Baumgartner[39] explains the different susceptibility to infection to "serologic immaturity" in infants, whereas in the adult the entire immunologic system has matured and is capable of assuming the additional stress of splenectomy. Most authors also agree that hematologic disorders that are often indications for splenectomy are accompanied by an underlying immunologic deficiency or abnormality and that in this group the incidence of postoperative infection is high.

Phagocytosis of erythrocytes and breakdown of the hemoglobin occurs in the entire reticuloendothelial system, but roughly half of this catabolic activity is localized in the normal spleen. In splenomegaly, the major portion of hemoglobin breakdown occurs in the spleen. The iron that is liberated is stored in the splenic phagocytes. These can be seen to be markedly engorged with hemosiderin when erythrocyte destruction is accelerated, as in the hemolytic anemias. When there is a marked increase in stored iron, the spleen is said to be "siderotic." Iron stored in the spleen can be used again for the synthesis of hemoglobin.

In addition to storing iron, the spleen participates in the "storage diseases" such as Gaucher's and Niemann-Pick disease (see discussion on retinculoendothelioses). Abnormal lipid metabolites accumulate in all phagocytic reticuloendothelial cells but may so involve the many phagocytes in the spleen as to produce huge splenomegaly.

The functions of the spleen that are characteristic of this organ relate primarily to the circulation of erythrocytes through it. In a normal person, the spleen contains only about 20 ml to 30 ml of erythrocytes, but in splenomegaly the reservoir function is increased markedly and the abnormally enlarged spleen contains many times this volume of red blood cells. The transit time is then lengthened, and the erythrocytes are subject to lytic effects for a long time. In part, stasis causes consumption of glucose, upon which the erythrocyte is dependent for the maintenance of normal metabolism, and the erythrocyte is destroyed. Selective destruction of abnormal erythrocytes is also accelerated by the splenic pooling.

As erythrocytes pass through the spleen, the organ inspects them for imperfections and destroys those that it recognizes as abnormal or senescent. This is called the "culling" function. Even more remarkable is the "pitting" function, by which the spleen removes granular inclusions (Howell-Jolly bodies, siderotic granules, etc.) without destroying the erythrocyte. This normal function of the spleen keeps the number of circulating erythrocytes with inclusions to a minimum. By the same token, after splenectomy the peripheral blood reflects the loss of the pitting effect. Thus, the postsplenectomy peripheral blood film shows Howell-Jolly bodies, siderotic granules, and flat target cells. The last is a consequence of the loss of normal surface membrane maturation, for the spleen is responsible for the rearrangement of lipid molecules at the surface of the erythrocyte to form the adult surface membrane.

The spleen also pools platelets in large numbers. The entry of platelets into the splenic pool and their return to the circulation is extensive. In splenomegaly, the splenic pool may be so large as to produce thrombocytopenia. This lowering of the platelet count in splenomegaly has been erroneously interpreted as increased destruction of platelets in the spleen. Sequestration of leukoctyes in the enlarged spleen in similar fashion may produce leukopenia.

The concept of *hypersplenism,* then, is that in some cases the sequestering effect on one or more of the three types of circulating blood cells (erythrocytes, granulocytes, and platelets) is so striking as to reduce the content of these cells in the peripheral blood. This sequestering effect can be demonstrated by the finding that isotope-labeled erythrocytes and platelets accumulate in the enlarged spleen, as evidenced by increased radioactivity of the organ.

CONGENITAL ANOMALIES

Congenital absence of the spleen *(asplenia; agenesis of the spleen)* is rare and, by itself, causes no difficulties. Quite often, however, asplenia is associated with congenital heart disease (defects or absence of the atrial or ventricular septum, persistent common atrioventricular canal, pulmonary stenosis or atresia, transposition of the great vessels, anomalous connections of the pulmonary veins, presence of both superior venae cavae with absent coronary sinus). These abnormalities usually produce cyanotic disease in the young infant but are seldom amenable to surgical

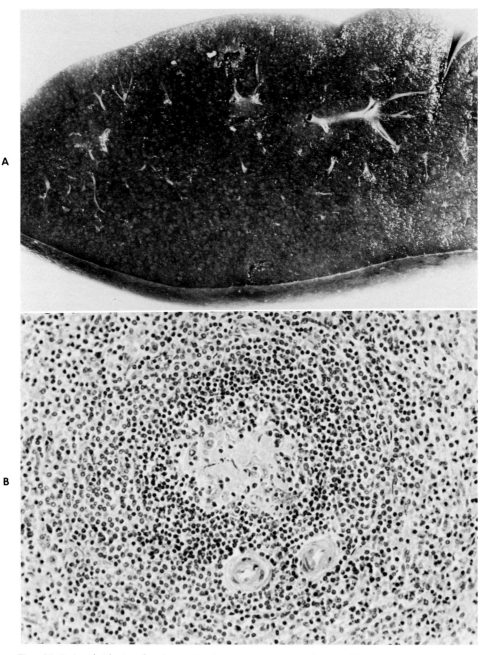

Fig. 31-9 Amyloidosis of spleen. **A,** Gross appearance. **B,** Paraffin section. Note deposit of amyloid in wall of arterioles and in center of follicle. (**B,** Hematoxylin-eosin; ×125.)

correction, in contradistinction to other types of congenital heart disease where the spleen is normally present. The combination of cyanotic heart disease and a peripheral blood picture characteristic of asplenia (Howell-Jolly bodies, target cells, and siderocytes) makes this an easily detected syndrome.

A more common congenital anomaly is the occurrence of accessory spleens. In one series of necropsies (Halpert and Györkey[85]), accessory spleens were found in about 10% of the cases. One of every six accessory spleens is located in the tail of the pancreas. Lesions affecting the main spleen usually affect the accessory spleen as well.

The least common congenital anomaly is fusion of the spleen and gonads.

REGRESSIVE CHANGES
Hyalinization

Hyaline degeneration of the arterial wall may be found in persons of any age, even the very young, and is nonspecific in nature. In young persons, hyaline thickening often accompanies hypertension. This degenerative change is most prominent in the sheathed arterioles of the lymphoid follicles.

Amyloidosis

Amyloid is deposited in the spleen under the same conditions as in other organs and is therefore found mainly when amyloid occurs in other sites. In systemic diseases leading to amyloidosis, the spleen is the organ most frequently involved.

The spleen may be normal in size, or it may be markedly enlarged, depending on the amount and distribution of amyloid. Two types of involvement are seen: nodular and diffuse.

In the nodular or *sago* type, amyloid is found in the walls of the sheathed arteries and within the follicles (Fig. 31-9) but not in the red pulp. When so distributed, the nodules of amyloid are prominent on cut surface, and their waxy translucent appearance suggests the appearance of sago grains—hence the term "sago spleen."

In the diffuse type, the follicles are not involved, the red pulp is prominently involved, the spleen is usually greatly enlarged and firm, and the cut surface is characteristically waxy and translucent.

Atrophy

Atrophy of the spleen (50 gm to 70 gm) is not uncommon in elderly individuals. It also may occur in wasting diseases. In chronic hemolytic anemias, particularly sickle cell anemia, there is progressive loss of pulp, increasing fibrosis, scarring from multiple infarcts, and incrustation with iron and calcium deposits (Fig. 31-10, *A*). In the final stage of atrophy, the spleen may be so small as to be hardly recognizable (Fig. 31-10, *B*). Advanced atrophy sometimes is referred to as *autosplenectomy*.

Pigmentation

The pigments found in the spleen are (1) hemosiderin and hematoidin, derived from hemoglobin, (2) malarial pigment, and (3) anthracotic pigment.

Hemosiderin is the pigment form of excess iron, whether this is derived from endogenous or exogenous sources. It is seen readily in tissue sections as coarse golden brown granules within phagocytic cells. It gives a positive Prussian blue reaction and therefore contains ferric iron. Large amounts of hemosiderin are deposited in all phagocytic cells of the reticuloendothelial system when there is iron excess, as in chronic hemolytic anemia or after many blood transfusions. Deposition of hemosiderin iron in the spleen in abnormally large amounts is called *siderosis* or *hemosiderosis* of the spleen (Fig. 31-11). The same descriptive terms are used for other organs. In moderate amounts, hemosiderin produces little reaction in the tissues. In large amounts, it stimulates proliferation of fibrous tissue. Siderosis sometimes has been called secondary hemochromatosis to distinguish it from primary hemochromatosis, a primary metabolic defect in iron utilization and storage, but siderosis is the preferred term.

The nature of the pigment called *hematoidin* is largely unknown. It is not related to iron metabolism in the same way as hemosiderin, in that it is not deposited as a consequence of systemic iron overload. Rather, it is formed in areas of hemorrhage or infarction, possibly in an hypoxic environment. It appears as golden brown burrlike or crystalline masses and does not give the Prussian blue reaction for ferric iron but gives a positive Gmelin reaction for bile pigments. From this it must be concluded for the present that hematoidin is a noniron-containing breakdown product of hemoglobin. The Gmelin reaction, positive with various bile pigments, does not help better to define this pigment.

In malaria, the black pigment imparts a dark brown color to the pulp of the spleen.

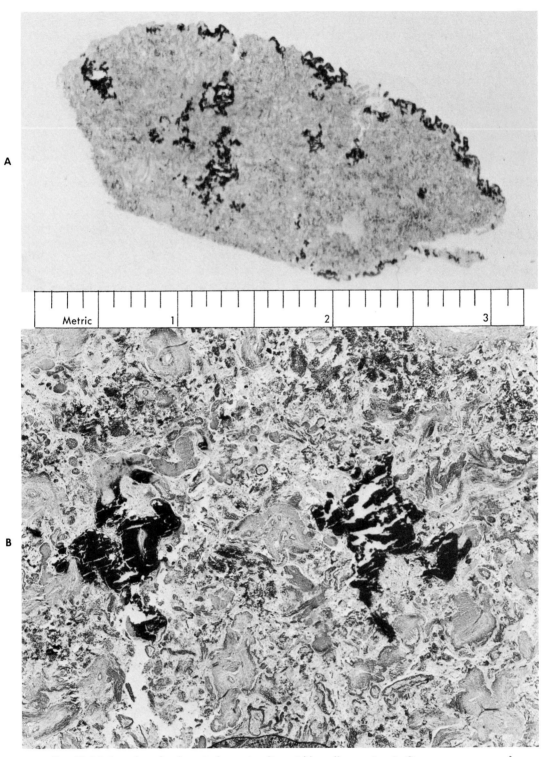

Fig. 31-10 Atrophy of spleen in long-standing sickle cell anemia. **A,** Gross appearance of bisected organ showing actual size of spleen bisected along its greatest dimension. **B,** Paraffin section. Note complete loss of normal architecture and replacement by fibrous tissue, pigment, and calcium deposits. (**B,** Hematoxylin-eosin; ×25.)

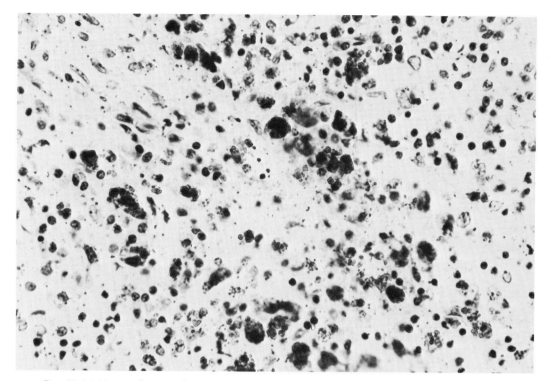

Fig. 31-11 Hemosiderosis of spleen. Most of hemosiderin lies within phagocytic histiocytes. (Hematoxylin-eosin; ×125.)

The pigment is of the hematin type and is found within phagocytes.

Anthracotic pigmentation of the spleen is rare. Askanazy[92] describes finding anthracotic pigment in the bone marrow, liver, and spleen ("Kohlenmetastase") in necropsy studies of anthracosis. The spread from the respiratory system is probably hematogenous.

Rupture

Rupture of a normal spleen may result from severe blunt trauma to the abdomen. An enlarged soft spleen, such as that seen in infectious mononucleosis, leukemia, malaria, or typhoid fever, ruptures easily with minimal trauma. The trauma may be so slight that the rupture is thought to be "spontaneous." It is not unusual for such a spleen to be ruptured as the result of enthusiastic palpation maneuvers by the physician, straining at stool, or even violent retching. In some cases, rupture is delayed for some days after the trauma.

One consequence of splenic rupture is autoimplantation of splenic tissue on the peritoneal surfaces, forming multiple implants (splenosis).

CIRCULATORY DISTURBANCES
Active hyperemia

Active hyperemia accompanies the reaction in the spleen to acute systemic infections. This is called *septic splenitis, acute splenic tumor,* or *acute reactive hyperplasia of the spleen* (p. 1312). The spleen is moderately enlarged, the capsule is tense even though the organ is soft, and the cut surface is dark red and bulging, and its architecture is obscured by the bulging, cellular, bloody pulp.

Passive hyperemia

Passive hyperemia (chronic passive congestion) is caused by interference with the venous return through the portal circulation. This may be caused by an increase in systemic venous pressure, as in cardiac decompensation, or to increased pressure in the portal circulation alone.

In passive hyperemia due to cardiac disease, the spleen is only moderately enlarged, very firm, and rubbery. The cut surface is dry, the cut edges are sharp, and the trabecular markings are increased. In long-standing cases, the spleen is smaller than normal and there is thickening of the trabeculae, fibro-

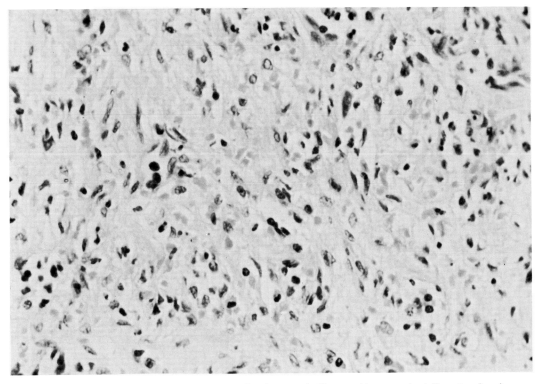

Fig. 31-12 Chronic passive congestion of spleen with fibrosis. Note marked fibrosis of red pulp. (Hematoxylin-eosin; ×125.)

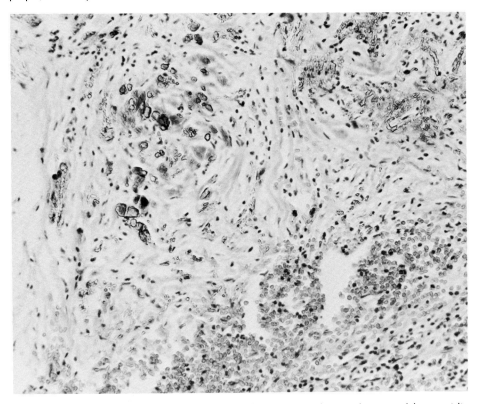

Fig. 31-13 Gamna-Gandy body consisting of fibrous tissue, hemosiderin, and hematoidin. (Hematoxylin-eosin; ×125.)

sis of the red pulp (Fig. 31-12), and atrophy of lymphoid tissue.

When congestion occurs as a result of increased portal pressure, the gross appearance of the spleen is similar to that in passive hyperemia, although the organ is often enlarged to 500 gm or more. In distinguishing this type of congestion from passive congestion, two points deserve special mention: the causes of portal hypertension and the relationship of this type of splenomegaly to the so-called Banti's disease or Banti's syndrome.

Portal hypertension has many causes. The most frequent is cirrhosis of the liver, which is accompanied by splenomegaly in about 80% of the cases. Here, the obstruction to blood flow is intrahepatic. The obstruction may be essentially extrahepatic as in (1) the right-sided heart failure of tricuspid insufficiency, pulmonary disease, or constrictive pericarditis, (2) splenic vein sclerosis or thrombosis, (3) portal vein thrombosis, or (4) idiopathic portal hypertension where neither intrahepatic nor extrahepatic obstruction is demonstrable.

The term "Banti's disease" is now only of historical interest, although some authors cannot bear to discard it. As originally described by Banti, the syndrome begins with splenomegaly and anemia (the term "splenic anemia" was used) and is followed by cirrhosis of the liver and ascites. He attributed the syndrome to an infectious process in the spleen and splenic vein, with subsequent involvement of the liver. Without reviewing many years of controversy over the identity of such a syndrome and the pathogenesis postulated for it, suffice it to say that we now feel that the cases described as Banti's disease in the past are merely instances of congestive splenomegaly on the basis of portal hypertension. The one special feature is evidence of splenic hyperactivity (hypersplenism) as manifested in anemia and, occasionally, leukopenia. These features of hypersplenism in splenomegaly are discussed earlier in this chapter. The only real mystery remaining is why hypersplenism accompanies some, but not all, cases of congestive splenomegaly. Perhaps minor degrees are missed.

Much has also been written about the gross and microscopic pathology of the spleen in "Banti's disease." This also can be resolved into two components. The first is the splenomegaly, prominent trabeculae, and fibrosis of the red pulp common to all passively congested spleens. The second is referable to the

pooling of erythrocytes in the enlarged spleen, a pooling that can be interpreted as "hemorrhage." Subsequent involution is accompanied by deposition of iron and calcium salts that become encrusted on connective tissue fibers to form the "siderotic nodules" or "Gamna-Gandy bodies" (Fig. 31-13). Such lesions may be formed wherever there is hemorrhage within the pulp of the spleen.

Infarction

Infarction results from occlusion of the splenic artery or branches. Occlusion may be due to thrombosis, to localized occlusion on the basis of sclerosis, to subendothelial infiltration with leukemic cells in chronic myelocytic leukemia, or to sludging and thrombosis in sickle cell anemia, sickle cell trait, and sickle cell–hemoglobin C disease. Occlusion on the basis of emboli is most commonly seen in heart disease, either from mural thrombi in the left auricle or ventricle or vegetations on the valves on the left side of the heart. Occasionally, infarcts are found at necropsy without apparent cause for thrombosis and embolism.

Infarcts are sometimes conical, with the base at the capsular surface, and sometimes irregular in shape. Although they are classified as anemic or hemorrhagic on the basis of gross appearance (pale or red, respectively), most are hemorrhagic at first. Later, dehemoglobinization occurs and the infarcted area becomes pale, gray-white with a hyperemic border (Fig. 31-14). Later still, the center undergoes ischemic necrosis and the necrotic tissue is replaced by scarring with contraction.

If the embolus contains bacteria, as from

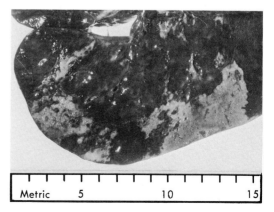

Fig. 31-14 Multiple infarcts of spleen. (From Rezek, P. R., and Millard, M.: Autopsy pathology, Charles C Thomas, Publisher.)

vegetative endocarditis of the mitral or aortic valve, the infarct undergoes rapid softening and suppuration as the bacteria multiply. This is called a *septic infarct.*

A special type of ischemic necrosis was described by Feitis as a terminal event in uremia. The necrotic areas are white or yellowish and of varied sizes and irregular shapes, central as well as peripheral. The diffuseness of the necrosis gives the cut surface a spotted appearance—hence the term "Fleckmilz" (spotted spleen). While not uncommon in uremia, this distribution of necrotic areas also is seen in systemic infections, with or without vascular occlusion. The term is thus purely descriptive.

SPLEEN IN SYSTEMIC INFECTIONS
General features

Enlargement of the spleen (250 gm to 350 gm) is common in acute systemic infections. The enlarged, soft, even diffluent, cellular organ is then said to show *acute reactive hyperplasia.* Other terms used are *acute inflammatory splenomegaly, septic splenitis,* or *acute splenic tumor.*

The splenomegaly is caused in part by a true reactive hyperplasia of the myeloid and lymphoid cells of the pulp and in part by congestion with erythrocytes. The reaction may be to pathogenic organisms, but most often it is to the products of inflammation, substances responsible for the mobilization of neutrophils, lymphocytes, and eosinophils (Gordon et al.[113]). The spleen also can react to foreign substances not the product of inflammation, such as foreign protein or a distant focus of necrotic tissue. The spleen is never enlarged in bacterial peritonitis.

Acute reactive hyperplasia is characterized by an increase in the cells of the red pulp. Grossly, the cut surface is purple-red, and the gray follicles are prominent. Microscopically, neutrophils are found without difficulty, and some may be of intermediate maturity. There is also an increase in phagocytic cells, both of the mononuclear type and of the fixed histiocyte type. These contain ingested debris from dead leukocytes and erythrocytes and sometimes bacteria and other organisms. A number of plasma cells also can be found. The lymphoid follicles are usually hyperplastic, although the lymphoid hyperplasia may be obscured by the marked congestion of the red pulp. Sometimes, the follicles have large reactive centers showing much phagocytic activity.

These general features are modified slightly in various infectious diseases but usually not sufficiently to enable one to make an etiologic diagnosis solely on the basis of morphologic changes.

Bacteremia and septicemia

In typhoid fever, the spleen is markedly enlarged, soft, and congested. Infiltration with granulocytes is minimal, but mononuclear cells are numerous. There is much phagocytic activity. Focal necrosis, hemorrhage, and rupture are not uncommon.

In the septicemia of *Clostridium welchii,* there is intense hyperemia and congestion of the red pulp, the sinusoids are collapsed, and there is evidence of extensive hemolysis of erythrocytes.

In streptococcal septicemia (whether acute or of the subacute type), as in subacute bacterial endocarditis, the spleen is large and extremely soft and flabby. In subacute bacterial endocarditis, infarcts (both bland and septic) are not uncommon.

Infectious mononucleosis

As mentioned earlier, the large soft spleen in infectious mononucleosis is easily subject to rupture. This complication, necessitating splenectomy, has provided most of the material studied.[118] The spleen is enlarged to three or four times the normal size. Characteristic changes are as follows:

1 Large numbers of atypical lymphocytes (virocytes) like those found in the peripheral blood, bone marrow, and lymph nodes are seen in the red pulp and in the sinusoids.
2 The follicles are usually not hyperplastic.
3 The virocytes usually infiltrate the capsule, trabeculae, adventitia of the arteries, and subintima of the veins and sinusoids.

It is thought that the cellular infiltration and edema of the capsule account for the high incidence of rupture.

Chronic granulomatous inflammation

There are few features of chronic granulomatous inflammation of the spleen that are not common to a given granulomatous inflammation in another organ or tissue. The spleen is normal in size or unusually enlarged, depending on the extent of the infection. A few special features deserve mention.

In fibrocaseous *tuberculosis* of the lungs,

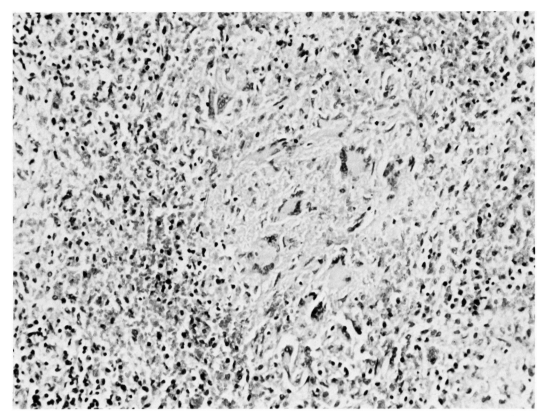

Fig. 31-15 Miliary tuberculosis of spleen. Tubercle is composed of epithelial cells and Langhans' giant cells, and there is no caseous necrosis. (Hematoxylin-eosin; ×125.)

the spleen is usually normal, but in tuberculous pneumonitis, it may be hyperplastic as part of the generalized reaction to severe acute infection. In miliary tuberculosis, the spleen is involved almost always (Fig. 31-15). The tubercles may be few or very numerous, minute or readily visible. In either case, splenomegaly is slight. When numerous, the tubercles can be readily seen on cut surface or through the capsule. Occasionally, a large tumorlike *tuberculoma,* usually single and measuring several centimeters in diameter, is the only lesion found (see chapter on lung, pleura, and mediastinum).

The lesions in *syphilis* depend on the stage of the disease. In congenital syphilis, there is splenomegaly with hyperplastic changes in the red pulp that contains an increased number of granulocytes, plasma cells, and phagocytic histiocytes. Spirochetes are very numerous and easily demonstrated by special staining technics. In the acquired disease, the spleen is normal during the primary stage. In the secondary stage, it is enlarged and shows follicular hyperplasia and many plasma cells in the red pulp. In the tertiary stage, it is

generally normal except for the rare occurrence of the large spheroid lesions, called *gummas,* characteristic of tertiary syphilis. Occasionally, splenomegaly in tertiary syphilis is secondary to syphilitic cirrhosis of the liver with obstruction of the portal blood flow.

In *sarcoidosis,* the spleen is involved quite often as part of the generalized disease, but occasionally the splenic involvement is so severe in proportion to lesions in other organs as to appear primary. The lesions vary from microscopic to grossly nodular. In the former, they may be merely nodular aggregates of epithelioid cells. In the latter, they show the noncaseating type of granulomatous inflammation characteristic of sarcoidosis. It must be noted that sarcoidlike lesions (i.e., noncaseating granulomas) may be found in a variety of conditions: leprosy, tularemia, histoplasmosis, brucellosis, berylliosis, splenic deposition of silica, lipid storage diseases, and some reactions to parasites. To be distinguished from sarcoidosis are the rare cases of tuberculosis in which the tubercles fail to show central caseation. In granulomatous inflammation, calcification is common only in chronic brucellosis.

PARASITIC INFECTION

Enlargement of the spleen is so common in malaria that this physical sign is used as presumptive evidence of infection when epidemiologists survey inhabitants of endemic areas. In the acute stages of malaria, the febrile episodes are accompanied by reactive hyperplasia of the spleen. In chronic malaria, the spleen is markedly enlarged, even up to 6,000 gm, in spite of fibrosis. It is firm, the capsule usually is studded with pearly white thickenings (the "ague cake spleen"), and the cut surface is slate gray due to large amounts of malarial pigment (hematin). Under the microscope, one sees malarial parasites and hematin in the sinus endothelium and the phagocytic cells of the red pulp. This pigment gives a negative reaction when stained for ferric iron. Fibrosis is prominent in infection of long duration. Rupture is not uncommon.

The spleen also enlarges in *leishmaniasis* (kala-azar). Except for the absence of pigmentation, the spleen is the same as described for malaria. Definitive diagnosis is based on identifying the many parasites *(Leishmania donovani)* in phagocytic cells.

Splenomegaly in schistosomiasis is secondary to cirrhosis of the liver and portal hypertension. Only rarely are parasites to be found in the red pulp. Then, pseudotubercles are formed. Occasionally, there is hemorrhage in the red pulp and, in the later stages of resolution, siderotic nodules are formed.

SPLEEN IN HEMOLYTIC ANEMIA

Hemolytic anemia is the general term applied to anemia referable to decreased life span of the erythrocytes. When the rate of destruction is greater than can be compensated for by the bone marrow, then anemia results. When there is accelerated destruction of erythrocytes, the spleen's normal role in disposing of damaged erythrocytes is exaggerated and so, in that sense, the spleen plays an important role in hemolytic disease. However, study of the pathologic anatomy of the spleen in hemolytic diseases contributes relatively little to an understanding of their pathogenesis, just as a study of the city's garbage disposal plant provides only a superficial impression of contemporary society.

Hemolytic anemia is a complex subject that cannot be covered here. For details, the student is referred to standard texts in hematol-

ogy. Some generalizations, however, can be made.

Decreased erythrocyte survival is the result of one of two abnormal situations: the erythrocyte is itself abnormal, an *intrinsic* defect, and therefore not able to survive normally, or there is an *extrinsic* influence that damages an otherwise normal erythrocyte and shortens its life span. In either case, the spleen seems to dispose of the defective erythrocytes, but especially when the erythrocytes are intrinsically abnormal.

In *congenital spherocytic hemolytic anemia (hereditary spherocytosis)*, an intrinsic abnormality of the erythrocytes gives rise to erythrocytes that are small and spheroid rather than the normal flattened biconcave discs. Although there is evidence that intracellular glycolysis and phosphorylation are abnormal, the nature of the intrinsic defect is not known. The two components of the disease are the production by the bone marrow of spherocytic erythrocytes and increased destruction of these cells in the spleen. The spleen destroys spherocytes selectively, as shown by the following observations:

1 Normal erythrocytes transfused into a person having hereditary spherocytosis survive for a normal time.

2 Erythrocytes from hereditary spherocytosis transfused into a normal recipient are rapidly destroyed.

3 Erythrocytes from hereditary spherocytosis transfused into a recipient previously subjected to splenectomy survive for a normal time.

4 In hereditary spherocytosis, splenectomy cures completely the hemolytic disease, even though the bone marrow continues to make spherocytes and the appearance of the peripheral blood smear is unchanged.

The spleen is always enlarged, and weights of 500 gm to 1,000 gm are not uncommon. The cut surface is deep red and hemorrhagic. The microscopic features (Fig. 31-16) that are characteristic are as follows:

1 Marked congestion of the red pulp, possibly because the spheroid erythrocytes do not pass readily through the sinusoidal walls

2 Hyperplasia of the endothelial cells lining the sinusoids

3 Relatively empty sinusoids

4 Little or no hemosiderin, in contrast to many other hemolytic anemias

If accessory spleens are present, they not

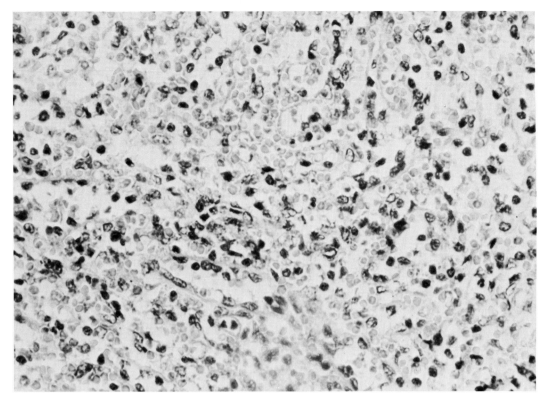

Fig. 31-16 Spleen in congenital spherocytosis. Note congestion of red pulp and hyperplasia of endothelial cells lining sinusoids. (Hematoxylin-eosin; ×125.)

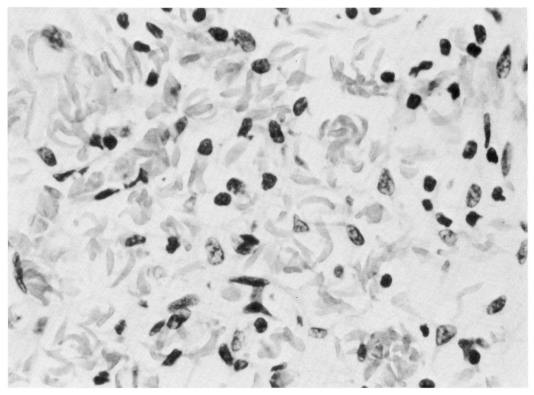

Fig. 31-17 Sickled erythrocytes in spleen in sickle cell anemia. (Hematoxylin-eosin; ×450.)

only show the same morphology but, if not excised along with the principal spleen, will take over the destructive function and the original splenectomy will be ineffective.

In *sickle cell disease,* as well as in some severe variants such as hemoglobin S, hemoglobin C, or hemoglobin S thalassemia combinations, the spleen is severely involved. The changes are progressive and are most severe in long-standing cases. As in hereditary spherocytosis, the defect in the erythrocytes is intrinsic, the content of hemoglobin S causing them to assume rigid, bizarre, sicklelike shapes under hypoxic conditions. The rigidity and peculiar shape of the erythrocytes cause them to plug up small blood vessels, and most of the clinical findings can be explained on the basis of microthrombi. In the spleen, they do not pass out of the red pulp, so that this is markedly congested and contains many sickled erythrocytes (Fig. 31-17). Later, the spleen shows the effect of repeated hemorrhages and infarcts, the hemorrhages leading to diffuse fibrosis with scattered siderotic nodules, whereas repeated infarction produces many large depressed scars. The most severe degree of fibrosis and atrophy has already been discussed and illustrated (p. 1309 and Fig. 31-12).

The microscopic features that distinguish the spleen in sickle cell disease are as follows:

1 The sickled erythrocytes, always prominent in formalin-fixed tissue

2 The large amount of hemosiderin (as opposed to the spleen in congenital spherocytosis)

3 Progressive fibrosis

4 Numerous infarcts

It should be noted that some sickled erythrocytes are seen in any hemoglobulinopathy in which hemoglobin S is one of the hemoglobins. Thus, they may be seen in sickle cell trait (hemoglobin S plus hemoglobin A). Here, however, the spleen is relatively normal.

The spleen also is severely involved in *thalassemia* (Cooley's anemia; Mediterranean anemia). This hemoglobinopathy differs from the others in that an abnormal molecular form of hemoglobin is not present. Rather, there is a suppression of synthesis of beta polypeptide chains (beta thalassemia) or alpha polypeptide chains (alpha thalassemia)

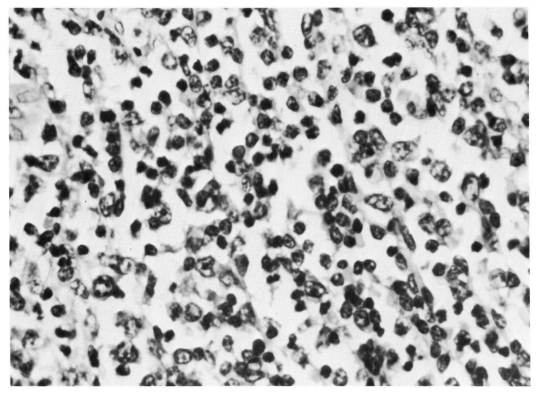

Fig. 31-18 Spleen in thalassemia. There are numerous large hyperplastic reticulum cells and some normoblasts. (Hematoxylin-eosin; ×250.)

resulting in deficient synthesis of normal hemoglobin. Suppression of normal hemoglobin synthesis is accompanied by increased amounts of hemoglobin A_2 or hemoglobin F. The erythrocytes are not only deficient in normal hemoglobin (hypochromic) but are also abnormal in shape, many being target cells, whereas the others vary markedly in size and shape. Their life span is short because they are destroyed in large number by the spleen.

The disease ranges in severity from mild to very severe. The changes in the spleen are greatest in the severe form called thalassemia major. The spleen is very large, often seeming to fill the abdominal cavity. The organ is firm and the capsule often thickened. The cut surface is dark red. Microscopically, there is marked congestion, fibrosis, and hyperplasia of reticuloendothelial cells (Fig. 31-18). The one feature that is characteristic is the presence of foci of blood cell formation, extramedullary hemopoiesis. Also characteristic, but not so frequent, is the presence of foam cells in the red pulp. These are large and show a foamy cytoplasm that contains PAS-positive mucopolysaccharide. Siderotic nodules sometimes are found, but these are seen also in other hemolytic anemias.

SPLEEN IN OTHER DISEASES OF BLOOD AND BLOOD-FORMING ORGANS

The spleen, as one organ of the reticuloendothelial system, seldom escapes being involved in proliferative reactions that, classically, are described as having their genesis in other organs, such as lymph nodes or bone marrow. Thus, in addition to the conditions already discussed, which may be considered to involve primarily some special splenic function, splenomegaly is found in hematologic disorders involving granulocytopoiesis, lymphopoiesis, erythropoiesis, and proliferation of other cell types (see accompanying classification). For convenience, the involvement of the spleen in these diseases will be discussed in subsequent sections (granulocytic leukemia, p. 1371; lymphocytic leukemia, p. 1372; myeloproliferative syndromes, p. 1360; and lymphomas, p. 1336).

Splenomegaly due primarily to hemopoietic activity
A Granulocytopoiesis
  1 Reactive hyperplasia to acute and chronic infections
    a "Acute splenic tumor" of various acute infections
    b Tuberculosis
    c Congenital syphilis
    d Malaria
    e Trypanosomiasis
    f Histoplasmosis
    g Schistosomiasis
    h Leishmaniasis
    i Echinococcosis
  2 Myeloproliferative syndromes
  3 Granulocytic leukemia
B Lymphopoiesis
  1 Generalized lymphocytic reactions
    a Infectious mononucleosis
    b Other viral infections
    c Hyperthyroidism
  2 Lymphocytic leukemia
  3 Lymphocytic lymphomas
C Erythropoiesis
  1 Hemolytic anemias
  2 Myeloproliferative syndromes including polycythemia vera
  3 Erythroleukemia
D Other cell types
  1 Plasmocytosis, reactive
  2 Multiple myeloma
  3 Monocytic leukemia

Splenomegaly due primarily to destructive activity
A Hemolytic anemias
B Thrombocytopenic purpura
C Splenic neutropenia

Splenomegaly due to reticuloendothelial hyperactivity
A Reticuloendothelial hyperplasia in acute and chronic infections
B Disseminated lupus erythematosus
C Rheumatoid arthritis
D Felty's syndrome
E Hemochromatosis and hemosiderosis
F Gaucher's disease
G Niemann-Pick disease
H Amyloidosis
I Diabetes mellitus
J Gargoylism
K Reticulum cell sarcoma

Splenomegaly due to vascular factors (congestive splenomegaly)
A Cirrhosis of liver
B Portal vein blockage
C Splenic vein thrombosis and other obstructions
D Cardiac failure
E Infarction

Splenomegaly due to nonspecific afflictions
A Primary neoplasms and cysts
B Metastatic neoplasms
C Macrosomia

PRIMARY TUMORS

The spleen is only rarely the site of primary tumor in the strict sense of the word. Thus, most of the leukemias and lymphomas, being multicentric in origin, are excluded as being primary splenic tumors. Very rarely, lymphoma of varying cell types seems to originate in the spleen and nowhere else. These have been called primary lymphomas of the

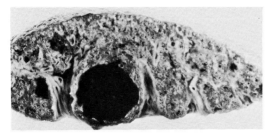

Fig. 31-19 Hemangioma of spleen with fibrosis.

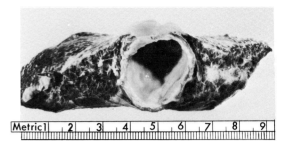

Fig. 31-21 Dermoid cyst of spleen.

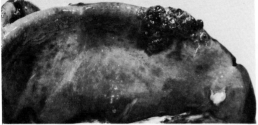

Fig. 31-20 Lymphangioma of spleen.

spleen, but in the few cases I have seen that seem to fall into this category a careful search revealed that there was also, although less obvious, involvement of the lymph nodes and bone marrow. A review of the literature on supposedly primary lymphomas of the spleen reveals that this diagnosis is not supported by negative lymphangiographic studies.

The most common primary tumor is the cavernous hemangioma. These are sometimes only a few millimeters in diameter, more often measuring 1 cm or 2 cm and occasionally are so large as to cause splenomegaly (Fig. 31-19). Next in frequency are the lymphangiomas. These may also be very large and may present as multicystic lesions (Fig. 31-20). Other benign tumors (fibroma, chondroma, osteoma) are extremely rare. Also rare are malignant endotheliomas.

METASTATIC TUMORS

The frequency of involvement of the spleen by metastatic tumor ranges from rare to 50% in the various series reported. The higher values probably reflect the true incidence of metastases, for the more care taken to examine all portions of the spleen, both grossly and microscopically, the higher the incidence of metastatic tumor.

Metastases occur late in the course of the primary cancer and are not found in the absence of metastases to other organs. The primary tumors that metastasize to the spleen are many. The most common types, in order of decreasing frequency, are lung, breast, prostate gland, colon, and stomach. Metastases may be either nodular or diffuse. Most represent hematogenous spread from the primary lesion, but some of the metastases are undoubtedly by lymphatic dissemination. Spleens showing only microscopic metastases range in weight from 60 gm to 400 gm. Those showing large nodules of metastatic tumor range from 70 gm to 1,100 gm. Those showing diffuse gross involvement range from 100 gm to 3,000 gm.

CYSTS

Cysts of the spleen are rare. They include parasitic cysts, of which those due to *Taenia echinococcus* are the most frequent, and neoplastic (benign) cysts, which are usually cystic lymphangiomas, cavernous hemangiomas, or dermoid cysts (Fig. 31-21). The latter may contain sebum and hair and may be lined with well-preserved squamous epithelium and sebaceous glands. Non-neoplastic cysts (pseudocysts) are the result of degeneration and cyst formation in an area of hemorrhage or infarction.

SPLEEN IN AUTOIMMUNE DISEASES

The concept of "autoimmune disease," a direct and noxious attack by specific immunologic agents against cells and tissues, is based on firm experimental evidence. For example, allergic encephalomyelitis and thyroiditis can be produced by injecting organ extracts into animals, whereas graft-versus-host reactions may involve such evidence of generalized disease as Coombs-positive hemolytic anemia, polyarthritis, myocarditis, nephritis, etc. While the experimental autoimmune diseases usually are characterized by the presence of tissue-specific antibodies in the blood, it does not necessarily follow that autoimmune antibodies

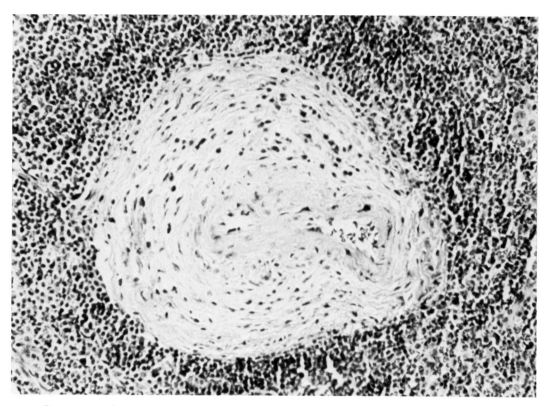

Fig. 31-22 Spleen in disseminated lupus erythematosus. Note "onion skin" appearance of arteriolar wall. (Hematoxylin-eosin; ×125.)

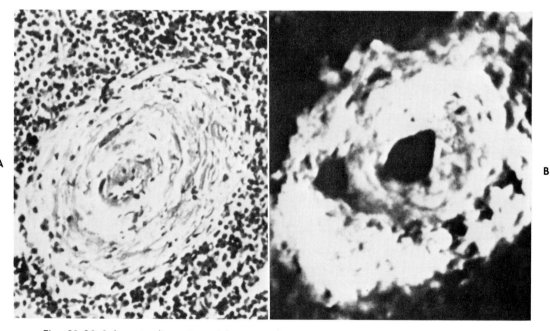

Fig. 31-23 Spleen in disseminated lupus erythematosus. **A,** Typical "onion skin" appearance of arteriole. **B,** Immunofluorescence reaction with antigamma globulin serum showing deposition of gamma globulin. (From Miescher, P. A., and Muller-Eberhard, H. J.: Textbook of immunopathology, Grune & Stratton, Inc.; by permission.)

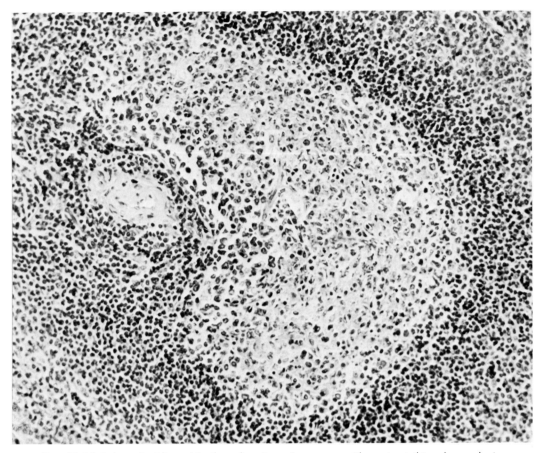

Fig. 31-24 Spleen in idiopathic thrombocytopenic purpura. There is striking hyperplasia of lymphoid follicle. (Hematoxylin-eosin; ×125.)

in the blood in human diseases are in every instance directly toxic on cells and tissues. Nevertheless, it would seem that a common denominator in these diseases is the reaction of connective tissue. Since the spleen often is involved, the pathologic changes in this organ deserve brief mention.

Splenomegaly, with or without characteristic histologic alterations, is common to the entire group. In *rheumatoid arthritis,* for example, the spleen usually is enlarged but presents no characteristic histologic changes. On the other hand, the spleen in *systemic lupus erythematosus* usually shows foci of degenerating collagen in the capsule and the characteristic periarterial "onion skin" lesion (Fig. 31-22) that affects the central and penicillar arteries. By immunofluorescence, gamma globulin (Fig. 31-23), complement, and fibrinogen can be demonstrated in the laminae of the lesion.

There are two types of thrombocytopenic purpura in which the spleen shows recogniz-

able involvement. In *idiopathic thrombocytopenic purpura,* an immunologic thrombocytopenia, the spleen is usually unremarkable. Occasionally, the lymphoid follicles are hyperplastic (Fig. 31-24), megakaryocytes may be found in the red pulp, and there may also be occasional foamy histiocytes. *Thrombotic thrombocytopenic purpura,* on the other hand, is thought not to be caused by an immunologic reaction. There is diffuse thrombosis of small blood vessels, once thought to be due to platelet thrombi, but we have come to appreciate that the occlusion is caused by intravascular deposition of fibrin with secondary entrapment of platelets. The lesions can be found in the spleen as well as in most other organs.

SPLEEN IN RETICULOENDOTHELIOSES

The term "reticuloendotheliosis" applies to a heterogeneous group of disorders in which there is evidence of reticuloendothelial cell proliferation plus various degrees of lipid stor-

Table 31-1 Typical findings in reticuloendothelioses*

Disease	Age group	Clinical features	Hematologic findings	Roentgenologic findings	Diagnostic features
Gaucher's	All ages; 50% of cases under 8 yr; 17% under 1 yr	Chronic course; splenomegaly; pingueculae; skin pigmentation; bone pain	Anemia; leukopenia; leukocytosis; thrombocytopenia; monocytosis	Rarefaction of distal shafts; swelling; erosion of cortex	Gaucher cells in bone marrow and splenic tissue; lipid is glucose cerebroside
Niemann-Pick	Infants, predominantly girls	Rapidly fatal: hepatomegaly; digestive disturbances; lymphadenopathy	Anemia; leukopenia; thrombocytopenia	Generalized osteoporosis	Niemann-Pick cells in bone marrow and splenic tissue; lipid is sphingomyelin
Letterer-Siwe	Below 2 yr	Rapidly fatal: hepatosplenomegaly; fever; pulmonary involvement	Severe anemia; thrombocytopenia	Osteolytic lesions of skull	Histologic diagnosis of tissue obtained by surgical biopsy; lipid is cholesterol
Hand-Schüller-Christian	Over 2 yr	Chronic course; exophthalmos; diabetes insipidus; moderate hepatosplenomegaly	Minimal; anemia may or may not be present	Cystic lesions of skull, particularly base of skull and hypophyseal region	Histologic diagnosis of tissue obtained by surgical biopsy; lipid is cholesterol
Eosinophilic granuloma	Adolescents and young adults	Limited to localized bone pain; course chronic and benign	Leukocytosis; eosinophilia	Radiolucent areas; cortical expansion; pathologic fracture	Histologic diagnosis of tissue obtained by surgical biopsy; lipid is cholesterol

*From Miale, J. B.: Laboratory medicine—hematology, ed. 3, St. Louis, 1967, The C. V. Mosby Co.

age in phagocytes. Some authors divide the reticuloendothelioses into two types, lipid and nonlipid, but this is not sound since, to various degrees, they all have an element of lipid deposition. On the other hand, to lump them all together under the term "lipidoses" implies that common to all is a primary disorder of lipid metabolism. This is almost certainly not true. Those diseases characterized by massive lipid storage (Gaucher's and Niemann-Pick disease) are classified as primary lipidoses, whereas Letterer-Siwe disease, Hand-Schüller-Christian disease, and eosinophilic granuloma are called "inflammatory histiocytoses." The truth is that our knowledge of the pathogenesis of these diseases is too limited as yet to allow a satisfactory classification. It does seem likely that, in some at least, the basic metabolic defect is the lack of specific glycoprotein-splitting enzymes in the cells, leading to an accumulation of lipid material. The chief features of the diseases in this group are given in Table 31-1.

It must be emphasized again that involvement of the spleen in these disorders occurs as part of a generalized reaction of the reticuloendothelial system. In all of them, other tissues (bone marrow and lymph nodes) usually are involved. Nevertheless, the splenic involvement is often the most striking.

Splenomegaly may be the first sign of *Gaucher's disease*. The spleen is markedly enlarged, sometimes up to one hundred times its normal weight. The organ is firm and the cut surface red-gray and greasy. Microscopically, there is diffuse and nodular infiltration with Gaucher cells (Fig. 31-25). These are histiocytes whose cytoplasm is engorged with lipids of the cerebroside type, composed of sphingosine, fatty acid, and either glucose or galactose. The cerebroside in Gaucher's disease has been called "kerasin," but it should be called "glucose cerebroside." The typical Gaucher cell (Fig. 31-26) is 20μ to 80μ, has a relatively small nucleus with coarsely clumped chromatin, and the cytoplasm is filled with

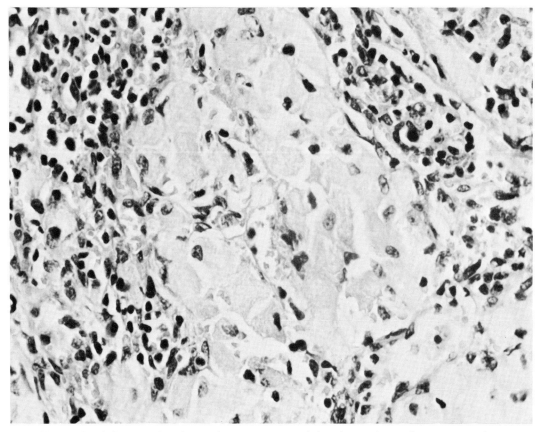

Fig. 31-25 Spleen in Gaucher's disease. Note nodule of Gaucher cells. (Hematoxylin-eosin; ×250.)

fibrillar pale-staining lipid. The cytoplasm is PAS positive. The cytoplasmic arrangement of the lipid is beautifully seen by electron microscopy (Fig. 31-27). The lipid does not stain with the usual lipid stains.

Gaucher's disease is usually discovered in childhood, 50% of the cases before the age of 8 years. Symptoms may be absent for a long time, and splenomegaly is often the first sign. There is a strongly familial tendency, thought to be caused by the inheritance of an autosomal recessive gene that produces in a homozygous person the absence of glucose cerebroside–splitting enzyme and thereby the accumulation of the material intracellularly. There are, in the later stages, various abnormalities of blood cell production and destruction. Some of these (thrombocytopenia, anemia, leukopenia) are the result of increased splenic sequestration of these cells.

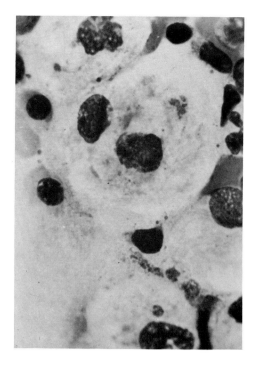

Fig. 31-26 Gaucher cell. (Spleen imprint; Wright's stain; ×950; from Miale, J. B.: Laboratory medicine—hematology, The C. V. Mosby Co.)

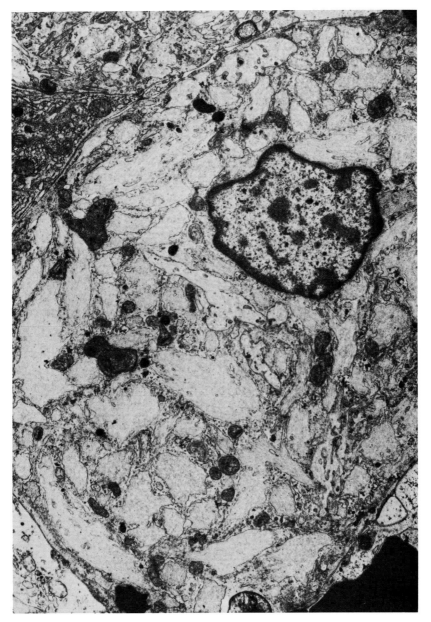

Fig. 31-27 Gaucher cell as seen by electron microscopy. Nucleus is irregular body in upper right area. Remainder is cytoplasm which contains lipid. (From Miale, J. B.: Laboratory medicine—hematology, The C. V. Mosby Co.)

Niemann-Pick disease is seen only in infants. The clinical and hematologic findings are not unlike those in Gaucher's disease. However, the hepatomegaly is more striking than the splenomegaly. The spleen and bone marrow contain cells similar to the Gaucher cell but with a honeycombed vacuolated cytoplasm. The lipid material is a phosphatide, sphingomyelin, which stains with Sudan III and other fat stains.

In Letterer-Siwe disease, sometimes called nonlipid reticuloendotheliosis, there is proliferation of reticuloendothelial cells in all tissues but particularly in spleen, lymph nodes, and bone marrow. There may be diffuse or nodular infiltration with large mononuclear cells and occasional multinucleated giant cells (Fig. 31-28). These cells are smaller than those in Gaucher's or Niemann-Pick disease and are only occasionally foamy and then contain cholesterol. Usually, the spleen is only moderately enlarged, but it may be very large

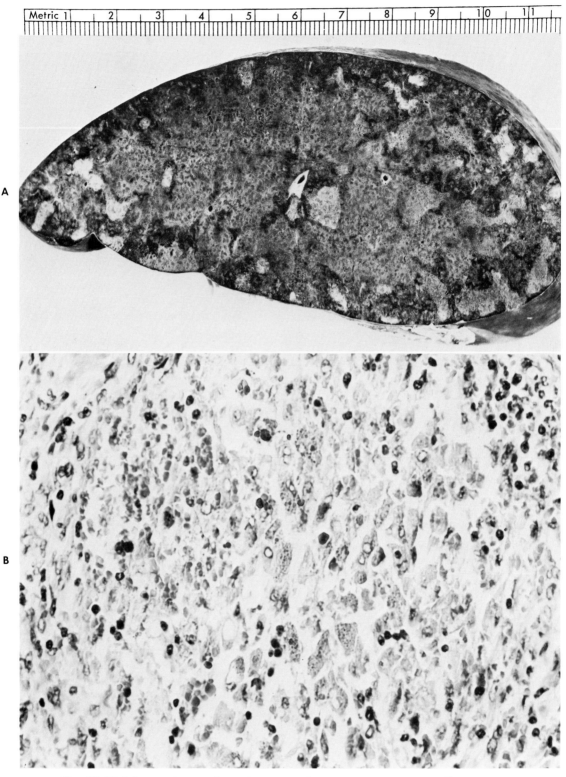

Fig. 31-28 Spleen in Letterer-Siwe disease. **A,** Gross appearance. **B,** Paraffin section. (**B,** Hematoxylin-eosin; ×250.)

in affected older infants. Thrombocytopenia and purpura on the basis of hypersplenism is not uncommon. A characteristic rash, papular and sometimes hemorrhagic, may be the first sign of the disease. This disease is usually fatal within a few weeks or months.

Hand-Schüller-Christian disease, on the other hand, is benign and chronic in spite of many features similar to Letterer-Siwe disease. The most severely affected tissue is bone, and radiologic evidence of destruction and pathologic features usually overshadow the relatively slight involvement of the spleen and lymph nodes. The bone marrow is usually normal. The histologic picture varies with the stage of the disease, the earliest lesions showing only eosinophilia and proliferation of lipid-filled histiocytes that contain cholesterol (Fig. 31-29).

It should be noted that finding some "foam cells" or "lipid-filled" histiocytes does not, of itself, always indicate the presence of one of the lipid-storage diseases. Such cells may be

encountered, admittedly in small number, in diabetes mellitus, in thrombocytopenic purpura, in thalassemia, and in chronic myelocytic leukemia.

■ Lymph nodes

STRUCTURE
Normal structure—histologic

Lymph nodes are discrete nodules of lymphoid tissue located at anatomically constant points along the course of lymphatic vessels. Lymphoid tissue is not found exclusively in lymph nodes, for lymphoid aggregates are present in the submucosa of the intestinal tract and bronchi, in normal bone marrow, in the spleen, and diffusely in the thymus. However, as in the case of the spleen, lymph nodes represent circumscribed and identifiable structures whose enlargement is easily discovered by palpation. As discrete structures, they can be excised and subjected to

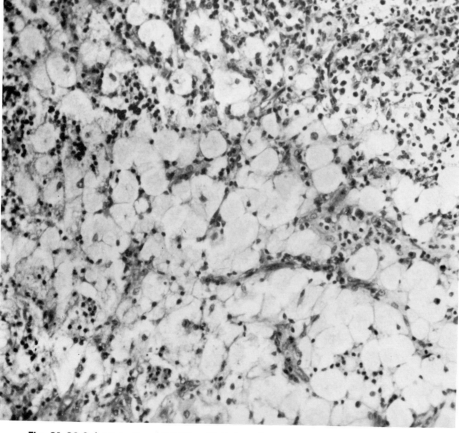

Fig. 31-29 Spleen in Hand-Schüller-Christian disease. (Hematoxylin-eosin; ×250.)

detailed bacteriologic, cytologic, and histologic study.

Lymph nodes have a fibrous capsule from which connective tissue trabeculae extend into the node in a roughly radial arrangement. The connective tissue framework between the trabeculae consists of a network of reticulum fibers, and this stroma supports primitive reticuloendothelial cells, scattered phagocytic histiocytes, and the predominant lymphocytes. In the central or *medullary* portion of the lymph node, the small lymphocytes are packed tightly in sheets and cords. In the peripheral or cortical portion, the lymphocytes are condensed into roughly spherical *lymphoid nodules*. These may consist entirely of small lymphocytes when the lymph node is in a completely resting or nonreactive state. When stimulated, the primary lymphoid nodules develop *germinal* or *reactive* centers that consist of medium and large lymphocytes, some in mitosis, scattered reticulum cells that may or may not be phagocytic, and some plasma cells. The proliferating germinal *center* is usually pale-staining and sharply circumscribed by the crowded dark-staining small lymphocytes at the periphery that form a *corona* around the reactive center.

When studied in serial sections, the germinal centers can be shown to be spheroidal with two poles. The superficial hemisphere, adjacent to the marginal sinus in a lymph node or epithelium in the intestine, is directed toward the nearest source of antigen and stains lightly because the cells are larger and have a more abundant cytoplasm. The deep hemisphere stains dark because the cells have scantier cytoplasm, and the corona of small lymphocytes is usually less distinct than at the upper pole. The polar structure corresponds to immunologic reactions, for it has been shown (Nossal et al.[192]) that bacterial antigens injected intravenously localize first in the perifollicular region and then migrate to the superficial or light area of the reactive center.

Lymph enters the node through afferent vessels and empties into a subcapsular sinus that is continuous with sinuses running along the trabeculae. These ultimately form efferent lymphatics that leave the node at the hilus. The sinuses are lined by flat *littoral* or *lining* cells sometimes called endothelial, but littoral and endothelial cells are quite different when studied by electron microscopy (Bernhard and Leplus[168]). The chief difference is that littoral cells are phagocytic, and, as such, they are

Table 31-2 Differential counts from normal lymph node imprints*

Cell	%
Reticulum cells	0-0.1
Mast cells	0-0.5
Lymphoblasts	0.1-0.9
Prolymphocytes	5.3-16.4
Lymphocytes	67.8-90.0
Monoblasts	0-0.5
Promonocytes	0-0.5
Monocytes	0.2-7.4
Plasmoblasts	0-0.1
Proplasmocytes	0-0.5
Plasma cells	0-4.7
Neutrophils	0-2.2
Eosinophils	0-0.3
Basophils	0-0.2

*Slightly modified from Lucas, P. F.: Blood **10**:1030-1054, 1955; by permission; from Miale, J. B.: Laboratory medicine—hematology, The C. V. Mosby Co.

active in performing a housecleaning function on the lymph. Under pathologic conditions, these cells hypertrophy, multiply, and become detached as free phagocytes in the lymph sinus, the "Sinuskatarr" of German authors.

Normal structure—cytologic

Study of the morphology of individual cells, as seen in imprints from the freshly cut surface of a lymph node or from smears of aspirated material, is a useful adjunct to the histopathologic appearance. Histologic sections are essential for determining the relationship of cells to each other and to the architecture of the tissue, but cellular details are partially obscured by fixation and by the thickness of the section. On the other hand, imprints make possible a study of individual cells, as in a blood smear, and often reveal details of morphology that, in combination with the histologic appearance, are extremely useful in arriving at the correct diagnosis.

Imprints of a normal node show a predominance of small lymphocytes, a few less mature lymphoid cells, and scattered cells of other types (Table 31-2). When the node is abnormal, quantitative and qualitative abnormalities will be found. Some of these will be illustrated in later discussions.

FUNCTION

The functions of the lymph nodes are three: (1) formation of lymphocytes, (2) production of antibodies, and (3) filtration of the lymph.

The lymph nodes are responsible for a portion of the total lymphocyte-producing capacity of lymphoid tissue. There is as yet no information on how many lymphocytes enter the total lymphocyte pool from lymph nodes and how many are produced elsewhere. On the basis of weight, lymph nodes contain about 100 gm of lymphoid tissue as compared to 70 gm in the bone marrow and 1,300 gm scattered throughout other tissues. Lymphocytes originating in lymph nodes enter the lymph channels on the efferent side. Some enter the bloodstream directly by passing through the walls of capillary vessels. According to modern concepts of lymphocytopoiesis and immunology, the lymphoid system is divided into a "central" portion, consisting of lymphoid tissue in Peyer's patches, appendix, and tonsils plus the lymphoid tissue in the thymus, and a "peripheral" portion consisting of spleen and lymph nodes. The spleen and lymph nodes not only generate new lymphocytes, but also are populated by lymphocytes originating in the central tissues.

The role of the lymphocytes in the production of antibodies has already been mentioned (p. 1300). In lymph nodes, immunologic activity is a property of the lymphoid nodules: the small lymphocytes in the corona are responsible for cellular immunity (homograft rejection, delayed hypersensitivity, and graft vs. host reactivity), whereas the plasma and other cells in the reactive center are responsible for humoral immunity (production of immunoglobulins and specific antibodies).

Lymph nodes play an obvious but relatively unimportant role as filters of particulate matter (anthracotic pigment, cellular debris, bacteria). Tumor cells carried by the lymph from the primary site to regional lymph nodes may implant and grow to form metastases.

LYMPHADENITIS

Since primary tumors other than lymphomas or leukemias are never found in lymph nodes (with the possible exception of primary Kaposi's sarcoma), the pathologist examining a stained section of a node usually must decide whether the histologic changes represent a nonspecific or specific inflammatory reaction, a lymphoma or leukemia, or metastatic neoplasm. In most instances, an enlarged lymph node is excised for pathologic examination in order to rule out a lymphomatous process or metastatic involvement.

Acute lymphadenitis

Since the lymphatic drainage from a sinus area to the regional lymph nodes varies but little, an acute pyogenic inflammatory reaction in a lymph node is accompanied by inflammation in the area it drains. When the primary infection is caused by a pyogenic organism such as staphylococcus or streptococcus, the regional lymph node is enlarged and tender, and the pulp between follicles is hyperemic and infiltrated with neutrophilic leukocytes. Later, there is an exudation of monocytes and phagocytes, the latter containing ingested cellular debris. When bacteria have been carried to the node, they may multiply and produce hemorrhage and abscesses.

Chronic lymphadenitis

The chronic inflammatory response is characterized by a predominance of monocytes and phagocytic histiocytes, some plasma cells, and a relative scarcity of neutrophil leukocytes. The medullary tissue between sinuses may contain so many histiocytes, sometimes in nodular aggregates, as to suggest a more serious lesion. However, regardless of the intensity of the histiocytic response, the normal architecture of the node is preserved, as contrasted to lymphomatous or leukemic proliferation. The lymphoid follicles usually are hypertrophied with large clear reactive centers that also contain phagocytic histiocytes and may show young lymphocytes in mitosis (Fig. 31-30). The lymph sinus characteristically contains many desquamated macrophages, and the dilated sinus sometimes is seen to extend into the medulla of the node along the trabeculae. Diffuse fibrosis of the medullary zone may be seen in chronic lymphadenitis of long duration.

These changes are "nonspecific" in the sense that they are caused by a variety of toxic agents and products of inflammation draining to the lymph node. In some specific inflammatory reactions, the histologic appearance will be more characteristic. For example, in chronic *brucellosis,* the reticuloendothelial cell hyperplasia may be so striking as to suggest Hodgkin's disease, particularly when there is formation of atypical multinucleated cells. In lymphogranuloma, the node often shows microabscesses surrounded by mononuclear cells rather than polymorphonuclear neutrophils.

INFECTIOUS MONONUCLEOSIS

Infectious mononucleosis is a viral infection characterized by a reaction of lymphoid tissue with the formation of "atypical" lymphocytes

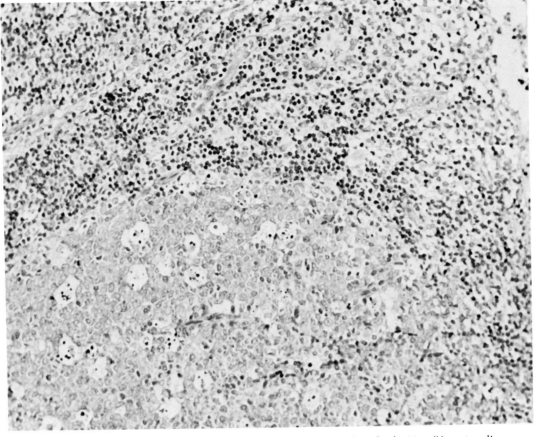

Fig. 31-30 Lymph node. Reactive hyperplasia in chronic lymphadenitis. (Hematoxylin-eosin; ×125.)

that have been called infectious mononucleosis cells. More properly, these are called *virocytes*, for similar cells are produced by a variety of viral infections or even stress. The virocyte appears in the peripheral blood and is found in the lymph nodes from which it originates. Generalized or cervical lymphadenopathy is a characteristic presenting sign. Histologically, there is moderate hyperplasia of reticulum cells and diffuse infiltration with the characteristic virocytes. These are large cells with a round or ovoid nucleus and a foamy or basophilic cytoplasm. Their typical morphology as seen in peripheral blood films can be seen very well in imprints from the lymph node (Fig. 31-31). At times, the diffuse hyperplasia of reticulum cells, the presence of atypical lymphocytes, and a moderately obscured architecture may create difficulties in diagnosis. When the histologic picture is interpreted with the help of all available clinical and hematologic data, the diagnosis usually is obvious. It is a reckless pathologist indeed who does not take advantage of all available data when examining any tissue, particularly lymph nodes.

Somewhat similar changes are sometimes found in lymph nodes enlarged in other viral infections. In the prodromal stage of measles, one finds multinucleated giant cells in the lymphoid follicles. These cells are called Warthin-Finkeldey giant cells.

TUBERCULOUS LYMPHADENITIS

Tuberculous involvement of lymph nodes presents the entire spectrum of the histopathology of tuberculosis, from the typical small tubercle to caseous necrosis, fibrosis, and calcification (Fig. 31-32). Lymph node involvement is usually secondary to drainage from a primary site, as in involvement of hilar and peribronchial lymph nodes in pulmonary tuberculosis. Even when the lesion is typical, with caseous necrosis and giant cells, it is well to confirm the diagnosis by bacteriologic culture of homogenized tissue. It should be noted that the demonstration of acid-fast bacilli in paraffin-embedded tissue is usually dis-

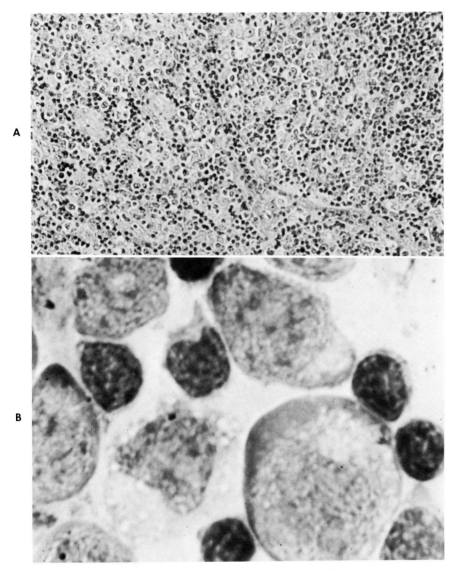

Fig. 31-31 Lymph node in infectious mononucleosis. **A,** Paraffin section. **B,** Imprint. (**A,** Hematoxylin-eosin; ×100; **B,** Wright's stain; ×1080; **A** and **B,** courtesy Dr. J. C. Sieracki.)

appointing. Furthermore, bacteriologic studies are necessary to identify the mycobacterium as being the typical *Mycobacterium tuberculosis* or one of the atypical varieties (see chapter on lung, pleura, and mediastinum).

SARCOIDOSIS

The lymph nodes are involved in sarcoidosis as part of the generalized disease. Characteristically, the lesions are granulomatous and noncaseous and, in the later stages, fibrotic. The early granuloma is composed of epithelioid cells and may contain giant cells of the Langhans type (Fig. 31-33). At this stage, it may not be possible to determine the

nature of the granuloma, for similar lesions are sometimes found in fungal infections, in berylliosis, in leprosy, in toxoplasmosis, in early noncaseous tuberculosis, and even in nodes draining a carcinomatous area (Fig. 31-34). Special mention should be made of the not uncommon occurrence of sarcoidlike lesions in scalene lymph nodes (lower deep jugular) draining a primary carcinoma of the lung.

Sarcoid lesions may contain foreign body formations (Schaumann's bodies, Fig. 31-35, and asteroids) that are not diagnostic of sarcoidosis, since they may be found in berylliosis as well. Furthermore, sarcoid lesions do, at times, undergo central necrosis. It will be

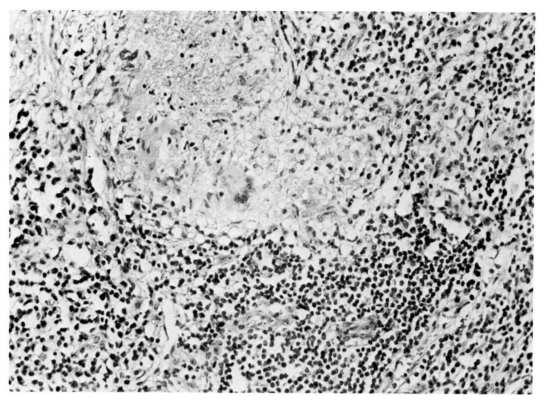

Fig. 31-32 Lymph node in tuberculosis. (Hematoxylin-eosin; ×125.)

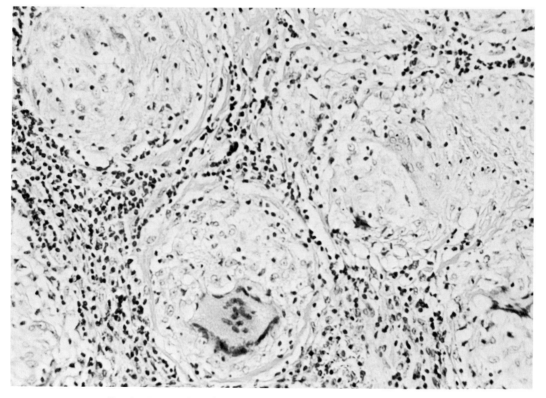

Fig. 31-33 Lymph node in sarcoidosis. (Hematoxylin-eosin; ×125.)

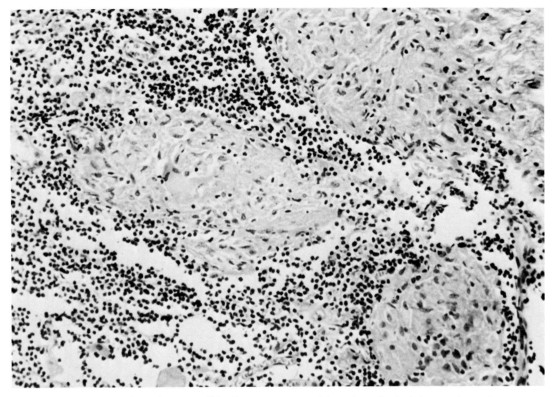

Fig. 31-34 Lymph node. Sarcoidlike lesions in cervical lymph node draining carcinomatous area. (Hematoxylin-eosin; ×125.)

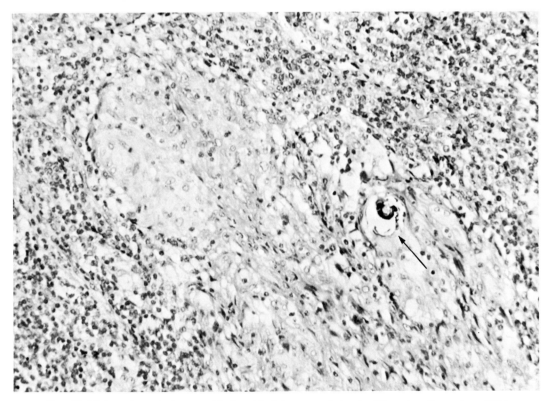

Fig. 31-35 Lymph node in sarcoidosis with Schaumann's body. (Hematoxylin-eosin; ×125.)

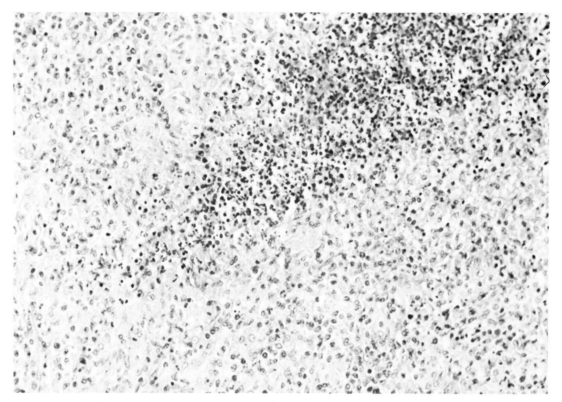

Fig. 31-36 Lymph node in cat-scratch disease. (Hematoxylin-eosin; ×125.)

seen that the specific diagnosis of granulomatous inflammation is, at times, difficult and requires the correlation of clinical and laboratory data with the histologic appearance of the lesion.

CAT-SCRATCH DISEASE

Cat-scratch disease is one of the causes of enlargement of regional lymph nodes. The causative agent is unknown, but the two most likely suggestions are an atypical mycobacterium or a virus of the psittacosis-lymphogranuloma group. In any case, it is almost certainly caused by an infectious agent inoculated percutaneously by a cat-scratch (60% of the cases), a cat bite (10%), or various injuries such as from splinters, thorns, pins, fishhooks, rabbit claws, and porcupine quills (5%), whereas in about one-fourth of the cases there is no known skin injury, although most of the patients are known to have had a cat in the household.

Since regional lymphadenopathy is the cardinal sign of cat-scratch disease, this disease must be considered in the differential diagnosis of lymphadenopathy. The histologic appearance of the lymph node is that of epithelioid granulomas in the early cases, characteristically surrounded by palisading reticulum cells, progressing to microabscesses suggesting acute bacterial lymphadenitis (Fig. 31-36) and still later to caseous necrosis. Giant cells of the Langhans type have been described. This sequence of changes may suggest a variety of diagnoses such as sarcoidosis, brucellosis, tularemia, lymphogranuloma venereum, and caseous tuberculous lymphadenitis (see also p. 397).

DERMATOPATHIC LYMPHADENITIS

Sometimes called *lipomelanotic reticulosis,* dermatopathic lymphadenitis also is associated with lesions of the skin but is thought not to be caused by an infectious agent. It is characterized by reticuloendothelial cell hyperplasia with the deposition of melanin (and sometimes hemosiderin) in phagocytic histiocytes (Fig. 31-37). Extensive skin involvement, particularly when there is severe scaling and itching, plus the presence of pigment in the lymph nodes should clarify what might otherwise seem to be a difficult problem.

POSTLYMPHANGIOGRAPHY LYMPHADENITIS

The angiographic contrast media used for studying the roentgenographic morphology of superficial and deep lymph nodes (lym-

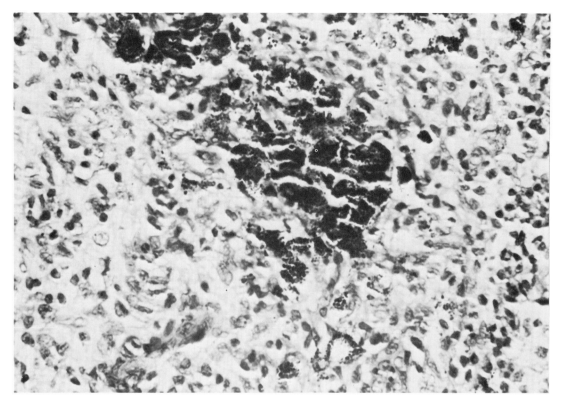

Fig. 31-37 Lymph node in dermatopathic lymphadenitis. (Hematoxylin-eosin; ×250.)

phangiography) produces characteristic histologic changes.[217] They range from the early reaction consisting of exudation of neutrophils, eosinophils, and a few plasma cells through the chronic reaction characterized by marked foreign body giant cells surrounding droplets of contrast medium plus plasma cell infiltration.

PSEUDOLYMPHOMATOUS LYMPHADENITIS

Between reactive lymphadenitis on one hand and the malignant lymphomas on the other are found some benign reactive lesions that mimic the histopathology of lymphoma. Four lesions resemble lymphoma so closely that they truly deserve to be called pseudolymphomatous: (1) pseudolymphomatous lymphadenitis secondary to ingestion of anticonvulsant drugs, (2) postvaccinal lymphadenitis,[231] (3) "sinus histocytosis with lymphadenopathy,"[240] and (4) "chronic pseudolymphomatous lymphadenopathy."[227]

Pseudolymphomatous lymphadenitis secondary to ingestion of anticonvulsant drugs

Ingestion of anticonvulsant drugs (used in the treatment of epilepsy) sometimes pro-

duces an illness resembling malignant lymphoma both in the hematologic picture and in the histologic changes in lymph nodes and skin. One or more of the following may occur at any time after one week to many months of therapy: morbilliform skin rash, lymphadenopathy, fever, hepatosplenomegaly, and painful joints. Eosinophilia in the peripheral blood is not uncommon. The commonest offending drugs are diphenylhydantoin (Dilantin) and mephenytoin (Mesantoin), but several other drugs of the same type also have been implicated (see also p. 190).

The histologic appearance of the lymph nodes shows many features suggesting lymphoma. There is moderate to complete loss of normal architecture, diffuse hyperplasia of reticulum cells having pleomorphic nuclei and prominent nucleoli, and diffuse infiltration with eosinophils, neutrophils, and plasma cells (Fig. 31-38). Mitotic figures are found, and infiltration of the capsule is common. One of the most common features is focal areas of necrosis accompanied by phagocytosis of nuclear debris.

In the differentiation of this lesion from the lymphomas, the clinical history is most important. It has been estimated that there are one million epileptic patients in the

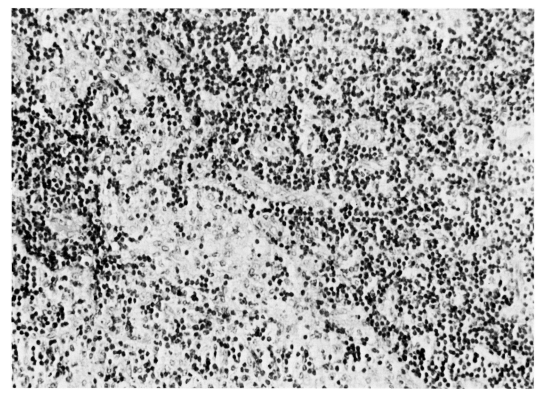

Fig. 31-38 Lymph node in pseudolymphomatous lymphadenitis secondary to ingestion of anticonvulsant drug. (Hematoxylin-eosin; ×125.)

United States. Most of these are receiving anticonvulsive therapy, so that pseudolymphomatous lymphadenitis may challenge the pathologist at any time. It also must be noted that an individual with epilepsy under treatment can develop, independent of other circumstances, a true lymphoma. It has been suggested, indeed, that the incidence of lymphoma is higher in epileptic patients under treatment than in the general population, but this is not based on good statistical evidence.

Postvaccinal lymphadenitis

Hartsock[230] (see also Lukes et al.[236] and Rappaport[238]) has shown that the lymph nodes draining the site of smallpox vaccination undergo an intensive reaction that might, if not recognized, lead to an erroneous diagnosis of lymphoma. While there should be no reason to excise for biopsy a node draining a vaccination site, the history of vaccination may be overlooked. Of the twenty cases reviewed by Hartsock,[230] nine had been diagnosed as lymphoma, and in fourteen the history of vaccination had been overlooked.

Histologically, such a node shows (1)

nodular or diffuse hyperplasia, (2) an increased number of reticular lymphoblasts, (3) vascular and sinusoidal changes, and (4) a mixed cellular response. The hyperplasia involves primarily a proliferation of reticular lymphoblasts which, interspersed among other lymphocytes, produce a mottled appearance under low magnification. The reticular lymphoblasts have a single nucleus and one or more irregularly shaped acidophilic nucleoli but lack the strict characteristics of Sternberg-Reed cells (multinuclear with single large nucleoli). The inconstant findings of focal dilation of lymph sinuses, a mixed cellular response with scattered eosinophils, neutrophils, and plasma cells, and hypertrophy and hyperplasia of endothelial cells are not seen in lymphoma.

"Sinus histiocytosis with lymphadenopathy"

Rosai and Dorfman[240] have described a benign disease characterized clinically by massive lymphadenopathy, fever, and leukocytosis. The lymph nodes show marked dilatation of the subcapsular and medullary sinuses. These are filled with proliferating sinus histiocytes and, in advanced cases, there is total loss of normal architecture so that the lesion mimics a lymphoma. The authors feel that phagocytosis of lymphocytes by the proliferating histiocytes is one of the features that distinguishes this lesion from others that show histiocytic proliferation.

The lymphadenopathy usually persists for months or years, but the clinical course is entirely benign. These cases have been mistaken for "malignant reticuloendotheliosis," a term which, at best, has little pathologic specificity.

"Chronic pseudolymphomatous lymphadenopathy"

A syndrome described by Canale and Smith,[227] "chronic pseudolymphomatous lymphadenopathy" is also a benign lymphadenopathy but has a characteristic set of clinical and pathologic features: lymphadenopathy and hepatosplenomegaly with onset in childhood, anemia, thrombocytopenia, and evidence of an immunologic disease such as a positive antiglobulin (Coombs') test, hypergammaglobulinemia, and response to immunosuppressive drugs. Histologically, the normal architecture of the lymph node is distorted by infiltration with large lymphocytes, histiocytes, and other mononuclear cells.

BENIGN HAMARTOMATOUS LYMPHOID MASSES

In 1954, Castleman and Towne[228] reported a case of a large lymphoid mass in the mediastinum which, because of certain histologic characteristics, they called "benign lymph node hyperplasia resembling thymoma." Since then, more than fifty cases have been reported. The majority occur in the mediastinum or other intrathoracic sites, but, because they also may be found intramuscularly, subcutaneously, in the maxillary antrum, retroorbitally, and in other locations in which lymph nodes do not occur normally, Lattes and Pachter[233] suggest that the lymphoid masses are not hyperplastic lymph nodes but rather hamartomatous or choristomatous (a developmental anomaly of lymphoid tissue at an unusual site). They give five histologic criteria for this lesion:

1 A nodular or follicular architecture
2 The presence of epithelioid-like cells in the follicle centers, arranged to mimic a Hassall's corpuscle
3 Absence of the subcapsular and medullary sinuses found in normal lymph nodes
4 A distinctive vascular pattern, with prominent arterioles in the center of lymphoid follicles and prominent vascularity of the interfollicular tissue
5 A population of entirely normal lymphocytes

METASTATIC NEOPLASMS

Since lymph drains from the site of a primary neoplasm to the regional lymph nodes, the latter are frequently the site of metastases. The tumor tissue in the lymph node usually, but not always, reproduces the cellular and architectural features of the primary tumor. Tumor cells or small nodules are first found in the subcapsular or paratrabecular lymph sinuses (Fig. 31-39). When there is extensive involvement, the normal architecture of the lymph node is completely destroyed.

When the surgeon excises a primary neoplasm, he also is concerned with this potential involvement of the regional lymph nodes. In some circumstances, however, a lymph node may be excised and examined histologically in order to establish whether a primary neoplasm exists in the area or organ it drains. For example, intra-abdominal carcinoma, particularly carcinoma of the stomach, sometimes metastasizes to the left supraclavicular lymph nodes by way of the thoracic duct. An enlarged supraclavicular node containing tumor tissue sometimes is called *"Virchow's node."* Another example is involvement of the scalene lymph nodes in intrathoracic tumors. Since biopsy of these nodes is being done with increasing frequency, it deserves special mention.

The scalene (lower deep jugular) lymph nodes in the neck lie within the scalene fat pad deep to the prevertebral fascia and lateral to the internal jugular veins. They receive lymphatic drainage from the lung and, on the left side, from the intra-abdominal organs as well. The percentage of positive biopsies is dependent on several factors:

1 When one or more of the scalene nodes is grossly enlarged, pathologic examination will reveal an abnormality in 80% to 90% of the cases. When there is no gross change, the yield is 30% or less.
2 If both the left and the right scalene nodes are studied, the yield is higher than if only one side is excised.
3 The more painstaking the pathologist's examination, the higher the percentage of abnormal findings.

In most of the series reported, the most

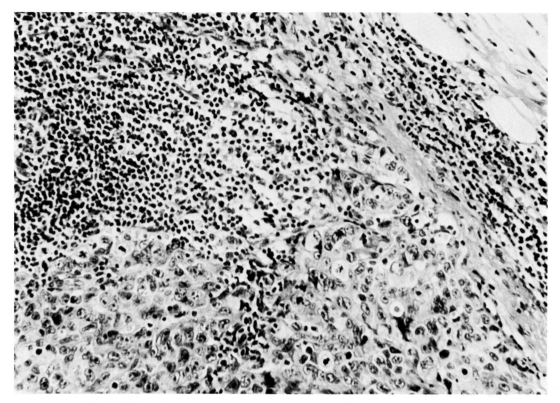

Fig. 31-39 Lymph node with metastatic carcinoma. (Hematoxylin-eosin; ×125.)

frequent diagnosis made has been that of carcinoma of the lung or sarcoidosis, but extrapulmonary tumor, tuberculosis, and other granulomas may be found.

LYMPHOMA

With the exception of very rare cases of primary Kaposi's sarcoma,[262, 263, 265] the primary neoplasms of the lymph nodes are malignant proliferations of the reticuloendothelial and lymphoid elements that are normally found there. Although they vary greatly in degree of malignancy, the lymphomas are considered to be malignant neoplasms and usually are referred to as malignant lymphomas.

Fig. 31-6 shows that the lymphocytic leukemias and lymphomas are "lymphoproliferative" diseases distinguished somewhat arbitrarily by the site of maximum or most obvious involvement. Thus, although leukemia usually involves the lymph nodes, the outpouring of leukemic cells into the peripheral blood is from leukemic proliferation in the bone marrow. Likewise, lymphoma not infrequently involves the bone marrow, and there also may be a release of malignant cells into the peripheral blood, but usually the major involvement is of lymphoid tissue outside the bone marrow. The distinction between leukemia and lymphoma is sharper if one considers myelocytic rather than lymphocytic leukemia, but we should note that in this case the proliferating cell (granulocyte) is normally an inhabitant of the bone marrow and not the lymph node, so that this geographic accident does not, of itself, indicate a fundamental difference between the leukemias and the lymphomas. In fact, there are many more similarities than differences, and the more advanced the disease, the more difficult it is to decide that it is one rather than the other.

Classification

The classification of the lymphomas has undergone a series of changes over the years. The one included in Table 31-3 was proposed by Rappaport et al. but, although it is widely used and we have recommended it, it has not been adopted by all. Uniformity of nomenclature is always desirable, particularly in the case of the lymphomas. As has been done so well by Lukes[307] for Hodgkin's disease, the correlation of classification, staging, and prognosis, needs to be done for the other lymphomas.

Table 31-3 Classification of lymphomas*

Nodular	Diffuse

I Lymphocytic lymphoma
  1 Poorly differentiated
  2 Moderately differentiated
  3 Well differentiated
	I Lymphocytic lymphoma
	  1 Poorly differentiated
	  2 Moderately differentiated
	  3 Well differentiated

II Lymphoma, mixed cell type	II Lymphoma, mixed cell type
III Reticulum cell sarcoma (histiocytic lymphoma, Gall)	III Reticulum cell sarcoma (histiocytic lymphoma, Gall)
IV Hodgkin's disease (see Table 31-4)	IV Hodgkin's disease (see Table 31-4)

*After Rappaport, H., Winter, W. J., and Hicks, E. B.: Cancer **9:**792-821, 1956.

The not inconsiderable literature is almost impossible to interpret, for statistics on the result of treatment are, in most cases, based on vague or otherwise undesirable terminologies. For example, one of the most complete studies of survival in lymphoma was reported by Gall and Mallory[291] in 1942 in their classic paper, which first brought some order out of the chaos of the terminology of that time. However, as recently as 1960 and 1961, there continued to be reported extensive series of cases of "lymphosarcoma," a term that includes most of the lymphocytic lymphomas, nodular and diffuse, undifferentiated or differentiated, and even those having a mixed population of cells. Not only are statistics on survival of limited significance, but without an exact classification, it is very difficult to judge the benefits of treatment or to compare one therapeutic regimen to another.

Gross appearance

Lymphomatous lymph nodes are enlarged and firm. Not uncommonly, several enlarged nodes are matted together into a large, firm nodular mass, which, on cut surface, shows the outline of the fused nodes. The cut surface is gray-cream in color, and the tissue has been likened to fish flesh. Rarely, there are small foci of liquefaction.

Histopathology
General features

The first, and most important, decision the pathologist must make when examining a section of a lymph node is whether the histologic changes represent a reactive process or a lymphoma. Some general features can be outlined which, although not always present, help in making the distinction.

The most common feature of lymphoma is the effacement of the normal architecture of the node. The sinusoids, particularly the sub-capsular, are no longer seen. There is no longer a distinction between the cortex of the node, with regularly spaced and clearly defined lymphoid nodules, and the medulla. Reticulum stains may be helpful in demonstrating loss of the normal pattern. In the diffuse types of lymphoma, lymphoid follicles may be completely replaced by neoplastic lymphoid or reticulum cells so that, regardless of whether one looks at the cortical or medullary area, there is a monotonous sameness to every microscopic field. In the nodular lymphomas, the nodules are large, of about the same size, and tend to touch, with very little medullary tissue between them. Also, the nodules are composed of only one cell type and do not show the variety of cell types that are found in reactive follicles. Whereas reactive follicles are sharply outlined by a corona of densely packed small lymphocytes often having the appearance of concentric rings around the reactive center, the follicles in nodular lymphoma are poorly demarcated and fade into the surrounding tissue. In most of the lymphomas, there is infiltration of the capsule and pericapsular fat by neoplastic cells. Infiltration of the capsule by normal lymphocytes sometimes is seen in reactive lymphadenitis, but the infiltration is seldom severe and the infiltrating cells are normal lymphocytes.

When sections are studied under high magnification, it is noted that the population of cells in lymphoma varies, according to the disease, from well-differentiated lymphocytes to highly pleomorphic and obviously malignant cells. The cell population in a reactive lymphadenitis is made up of small and large lymphocytes, histiocytes, neutrophil leukocytes, and some plasma cells. Of the lymphomas, only the mixed type of Hodgkin's disease shows eosinophils, neutrophils, and plasma cells. The final differential feature is the

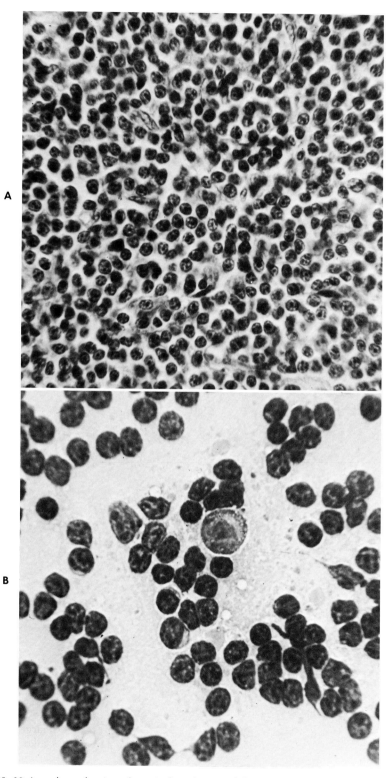

Fig. 31-40 Lymph node. Lymphocytic lymphoma, diffuse, well differentiated. Note how well maturity of cells is shown in imprint preparation, **B.** (**A,** Hematoxylin-eosin; ×450; **B,** Wright's stain; ×1080; **A** and **B,** courtesy Dr. J. C. Sieracki.)

type of involvement of blood vessels. In lymphoma (and leukemia), the vessel wall is often infiltrated by neoplastic cells, whereas in benign hyperplasia, there is no infiltration but frequently there is hyperplasia of endothelial cells.

Reference to Table 31-3 shows that each type of lymphoma can also be classified as either diffuse or nodular. This refers to whether a nodular architecture is seen under low magnification. Nodular lymphomas may transform into the diffuse type, but diffuse lymphomas do not become nodular. In either case, the cytologic characteristics remain the same. Accordingly, there is no place in the modern classification for the terms "Brill-Symmers disease" and "giant follicular lymphoblastoma," terms that have been used for nodular lymphomas of various cell types. The old term "lymphosarcoma" also should be

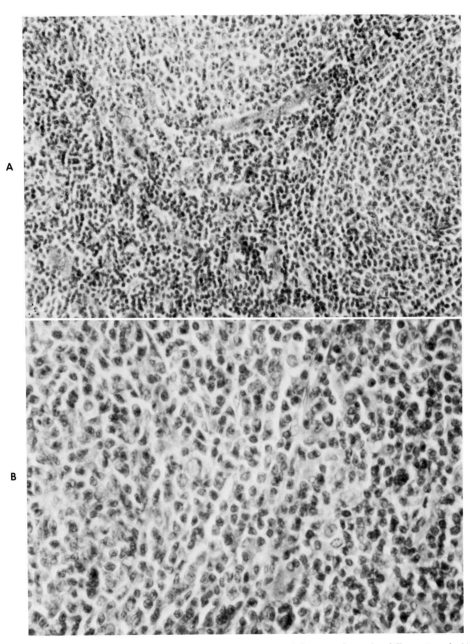

Fig. 31-41 Lymph node. Lymphocytic lymphoma, nodular, moderately differentiated. (**A,** Hematoxylin-eosin; ×125; **B,** hematoxylin-eosin; ×250.)

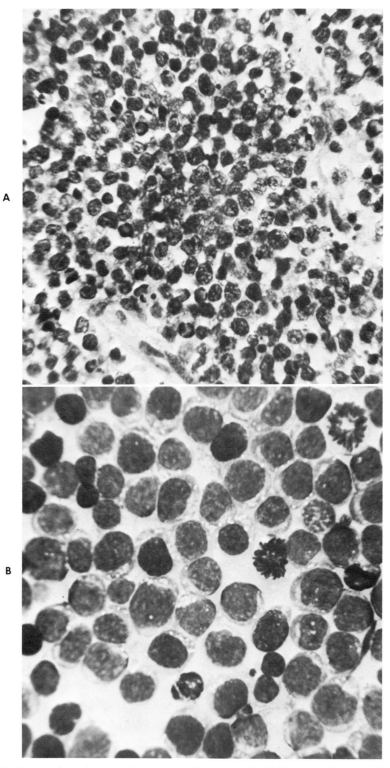

Fig. 31-42 Lymph node. Lymphocytic lymphoma, poorly differentiated. Note obvious immaturity of lymphocytes in imprint preparation, **B**. (**A**, Hematoxylin-eosin; ×450; **B**, Wright's stain; ×950; **A** and **B**, courtesy Dr. J. C. Sieracki.)

dropped and be replaced by "lymphocytic lymphoma," further defined according to cell type and architecture.

Finally, lymph nodes should be sectioned at a thickness no greater than 4μ. Poor fixation of the tissue, too thick a section, and poor staining can make what is always a difficult problem one that cannot be resolved. We also feel, strongly, that when a lymph node is excised for biopsy, it should be sent to the surgical pathology laboratory promptly and nonfixed. The pathologist, in turn, should in each case make imprints from the freshly cut surface and, whenever possible, freeze half or a portion of the node for culture should this be indicated.

Lymphocytic lymphoma

Lymphocytic lymphoma—well differentiated. In well-differentiated lymphocytic lym-

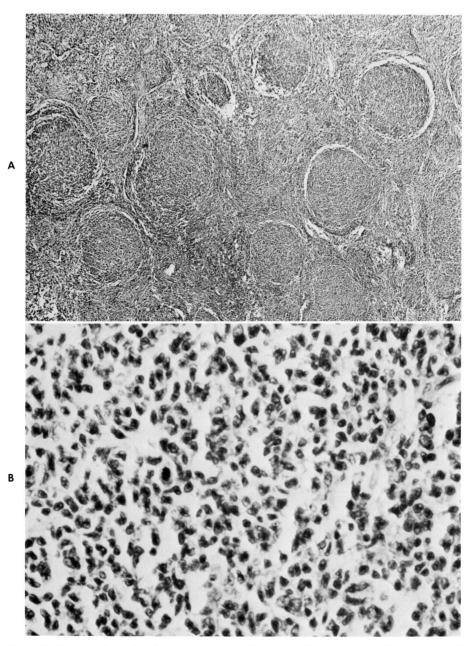

Fig. 31-43 Lymph node. Lymphocytic lymphoma, nodular, poorly differentiated. (**A,** Hematoxylin-eosin; ×100; **B,** hematoxylin-eosin; ×250.)

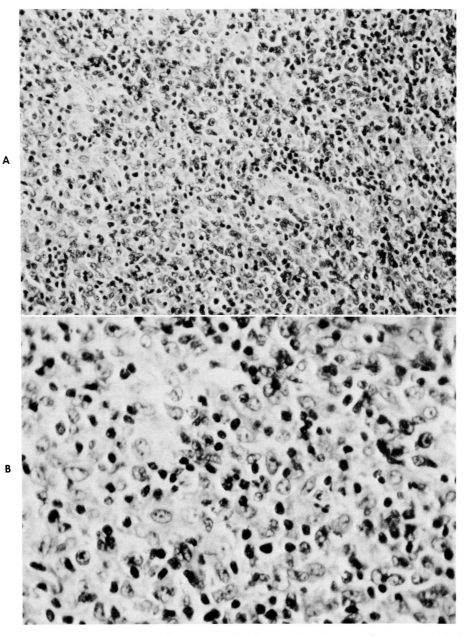

Fig. 31-44 Lymph node. Lymphoma, mixed cell type. (**A,** Hematoxylin-eosin; ×100; **B,** hematoxylin-eosin; ×250.)

phoma, the normal lymph node architecture is effaced by a sheet of mature small lymphocytes (Fig. 31-40). The infiltration is either diffuse or nodular. There may be infiltration of the capsule and pericapsular tissue by lymphocytes like those infiltrating the entire node. There is no evidence of a reactive process. In chronic lymphocytic leukemia, the histologic appearance of the lymph nodes is that of lymphocytic lymphoma, diffuse, well differentiated.

Lymphocytic lymphoma—moderately differentiated. In moderately differentiated lymphocytic lymphoma, the infiltrating cells are intermediate between lymphoblasts and the mature lymphocytes of well-differentiated lymphocytic lymphoma (Fig. 31-41).

Lymphocytic lymphoma—poorly differentiated. In poorly differentiated lymphocytic lymphoma, the infiltrating cell is the lymphoblast (Fig. 31-42). Note that in this example of the nodular type (Fig. 31-43), the atypical

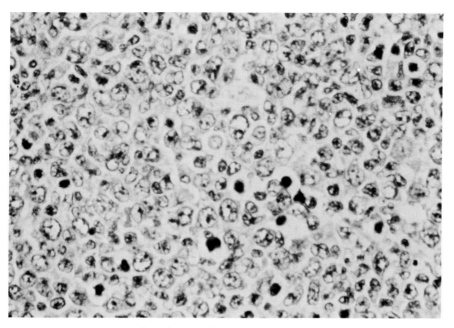

Fig. 31-45 Lymph node. Reticulum cell sarcoma, nodular. (×250.)

follicles are packed closely together and lack the clear dense corona of normal follicles. Note also the "cracking" phenomenon, the circular or semicircular separation of the nodule from the surrounding tissue. Although this is a fixation artifact, it is seen frequently in nodular lymphomas and never in benign hyperplasias.

Lymphocytic lymphoma—mixed cell type. In lymphocytic lymphoma of the mixed cell type, the architecture is destroyed by an infiltrate composed of lymphoblasts and reticulum cells (Fig. 31-44). Occasionally, especially in the nodular type, small lymphocytes also are present but are not numerous. The reticulum cells show considerable variation in in size and shape as well as in the structure of the nuclear chromatin. This atypicality of the reticulum cells and the absence of phagocytosis helps to differentiate lymphoma of the mixed cell type from severe degrees of reactive hyperplasia. (Note, however, that the histiocytes in Burkitt's lymphoma, p. 1354, often show phagocytosis.)

Reticulum cell sarcoma

In reticulum cell sarcoma (Gall[290] prefers the term histiocytic lymphoma; p. 1337), the infiltrating cells are reticulum cells (Figs. 31-45 and 31-46) and no other cell type is present in significant number. The reticulum cells vary in size, shape, and nuclear structure so as to present the pleomorphic picture of ma-

lignant cells. Occasionally, the pleomorphism is extreme, and large atypical reticulum cells are seen that resemble Sternberg-Reed cells but do not fulfill the strict criteria for these cells. In other instances, the cells are very primitive and not so pleomorphic, having the appearance of stem cells, and this variant is called the stem cell type of reticulum cell sarcoma (Fig. 31-47).

Hodgkin's disease

Classification. The lymphoma that bears his name was described by Thomas Hodgkin in 1832 in a communication entitled *"On some morbid appearances of the absorbant glands and spleen."* This communication attracted little attention but, in 1856, Wilks rediscovered the disease and suggested the eponym "Hodgkin's disease." The first useful classification was proposed by Jackson and Parker[302] in 1944. They classified Hodgkin's disease into three groups: paragranuloma, granuloma, and sarcoma. In 1966, Lukes et al.[309] proposed a new classification based on the histologic characteristics and showed that the new grouping related very well to prognosis and survival. At about the same time (September, 1965), a Conference on Hodgkin's Disease was held in Rye, N. Y., and, unfortunately, a committee on nomenclature recommended a slightly different nomenclature, an abridgement of that proposed by Lukes and associates. There are many instances, in medical history, where the results of com-

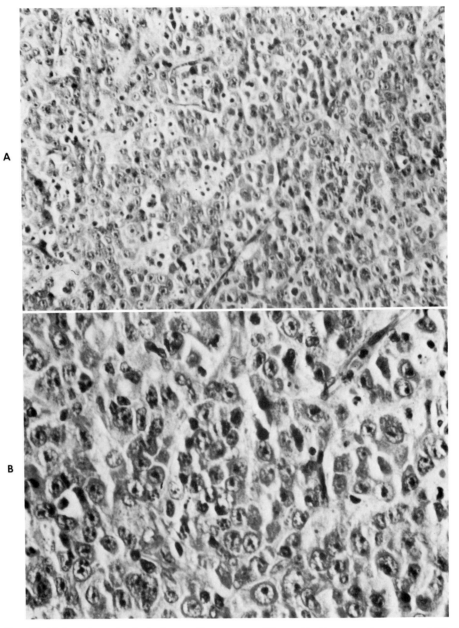

Fig. 31-46 Lymph node. Reticulum cell sarcoma, diffuse. (**A,** Hematoxylin-eosin; ×125; **B,** hematoxylin-eosin; ×250.)

mittee deliberations on nomenclatures leave much to be desired and this may be another example. The nomenclatures are summarized in Table 31-4. I believe that the original classification proposed by Lukes and co-workers is more descriptive and useful. Since the lymphocytic and histiocytic nodular group shows a significantly better survival than the lymphocytic and histiocytic diffuse group (43% vs. 27% fifteen-year survival), the two should not be lumped into the same category.

The features of the histologic types described by Lukes et al.[309] are summarized in Table 31-5.

Sternberg-Reed cell. Sternberg-Reed cells represent a transformation of reticulum cells to a neoplastic variant having a characteristic appearance. Since the diagnosis of Hodgkin's disease depends on the presence of these cells, the criteria that a cell must meet to be called a Sternberg-Reed cell are strict. The cell is multinucleated, binucleated, or bilobed,

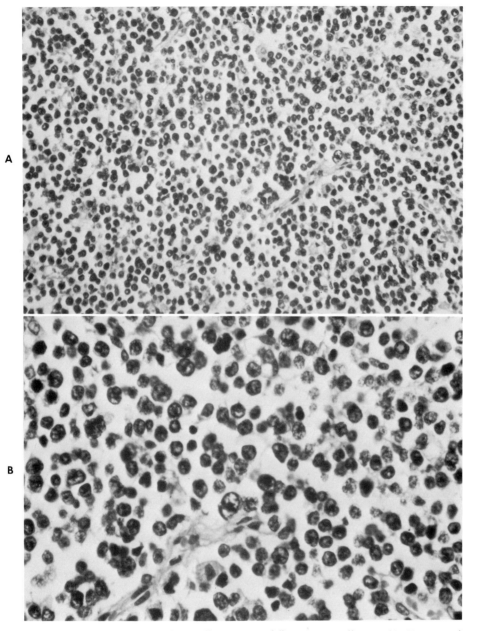

Fig. 31-47 Lymph node. Reticulum cell sarcoma, diffuse, stem cell type. (**A**, Hematoxylin-eosin; ×125; **B**, hematoxylin-eosin; ×250.)

the nuclear membrane is thick, and the cytoplasm is abundant, slightly eosinophilic, or amphophilic. The nucleoli in each nucleus or lobe are large, round, or oval, eosinophilic, and surrounded by a clear perinucleolar halo (Fig. 31-48).

Cells having a single nucleus and characteristic nucleolus may be encountered. These undoubtedly represent an earlier stage of development, but the search for typical, multinucleated cells should be continued until one

is found. Sternberg-Reed cells may be very scarce in some types of Hodgkin's disease, such as the lymphocytic and histiocytic and nodular sclerosis, and many sections may be necessary before a typical cell is found. They are most common in the reticular type, where they are often very pleomorphic.

Lymphocytic and histiocytic—diffuse type. The infiltrate is predominantly lymphocytic and histiocytic, the relative number of cells varying from predominantly lymphocytic (Fig.

Table 31-4 Histologic types of Hodgkin's disease—comparison of old nomenclature, that proposed by Lukes et al. in 1966, and modified Lukes et al. classfication recommended at the Conference of Hodgkin's Disease, Rye, N. Y., September, 1965*

Old terminology	Lukes et al., 1966†	Conference on Hodgkin's Disease, 1965‡
	I Lymphocytic and histiocytic	**I** Hodgkin's disease, lymphocytic predominance
Hodgkin's paragranuloma Lymphoreticular medullary reticulosis Benign Hodgkin's disease Reticular lymphoma	**A** Diffuse (lymphocytes predominant)	
Follicular lymphoma, Hodgkin's type	**B** Nodular (lymphocytes predominant)	
Hodgkin's granuloma Lymphocytic Hodgkin's	**C** Nodular or diffuse (histiocytes predominant)	
Hodgkin's granuloma Fibromyeloid medullary reticulosis	**II** Mixed	**II** Hodgkin's disease, mixed type
Hodgkin's granuloma with sclerosis	**III** Nodular sclerosis	**III** Hodgkin's disease, nodular sclerosis type
	IV Diffuse fibrosis	**IV** Hodgkin's disease, lymphocytic depletion type
Hodgkin's granuloma	**V** Reticular **A** With nonpleomorphic Reed-Sternberg cells	
Hodgkin's sarcoma	**B** With pleomorphic Reed-Sternberg cells	

*From Miale, J. B.: Laboratory medicine—hematology, The C. V. Mosby Co.
†Slightly modified from Lukes, R. J., Butler, J. J., and Hicks, E. B.: Cancer **19:**317-344, 1966.
‡From Lukes, R. J., et al.: Cancer Res. **26:**1311, 1966.

Table 31-5 Schematic representation of variation in morphologic features in histologic types of Hodgkin's disease*

Histologic groups	Lymphocyte	Histiocytes	Eosinophils	Plasma cells	Fibrillar reticulum	Collagen	Sternberg-Reed cells
Lymphocytic and histiocytic							
Nodular	++++ ++++	+	0	0	0	0	+
Diffuse	++++++	+++	0	0	0	0	+
Nodular sclerosis	+ to ++++	+ to ++	+	+	+	+ to ++++	+
Mixed	+	+++	++	+	++	0	++
Diffuse fibrosis	0	+	+	+	+++++	0	++
Reticular	+	0	++	+	+	0	+++++

*From Lukes, R. J., Butler, J. J., and Hicks, E. B.: Cancer **19:**317-344, 1966.

31-49) through an equal mixture (Fig. 31-50) to predominantly histiocytic. Eosinophils and plasma cells are rare or absent. There is no fibrosis or necrosis. Sternberg-Reed cells are rare. The pale-staining histiocytes of the infiltrate should not be mistaken for Sternberg-Reed cells, even when the nucleus is polyploid.

Lymphocytic and histiocytic—nodular type. The cytologic features in the nodular type are the same as those of the diffuse type except that predominantly lymphocytic prolif-

eration is most common. The nodular character of the lesion is not always obvious but is clearly evident when the section is stained for reticulum.

Mixed type. In the mixed type of Hodgkin's disease, a wide variety of cell types are found: reactive histiocytes, lymphocytes, eosinophils, and plasma cells (Fig. 31-51). Sternberg-Reed cells are usually numerous. There is slight fibrosis, and small foci of necrosis may be present.

Nodular sclerosis. Characteristically, inter-

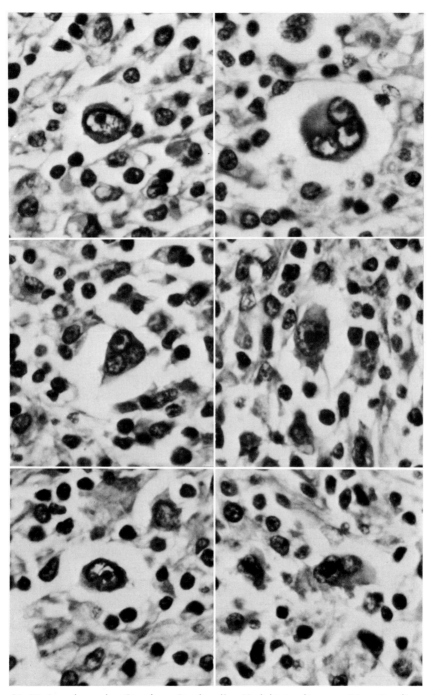

Fig. 31-48 Lymph node. Sternberg-Reed cells, Hodgkin's disease. (Hematoxylin-eosin; ×450.)

connecting bands of collagenous connective tissue circumscribe nodules of abnormal lymphoid tissue (Fig. 31-52). The cellular infiltrate varies depending on the stage of development. In the early lesion, the cells are mostly lymphocytes with clusters of reactive and hyperlobated histiocytes and typical Sternberg-Reed cells. At a more advanced stage, eosinophils and neutrophils are found and the collagen is denser. Later still, the collagen is very heavy, and with advanced sclerosis, the tissue is hypocellular.

Diffuse fibrosis. Diffuse fibrosis represents the stage of cellular depletion and re-

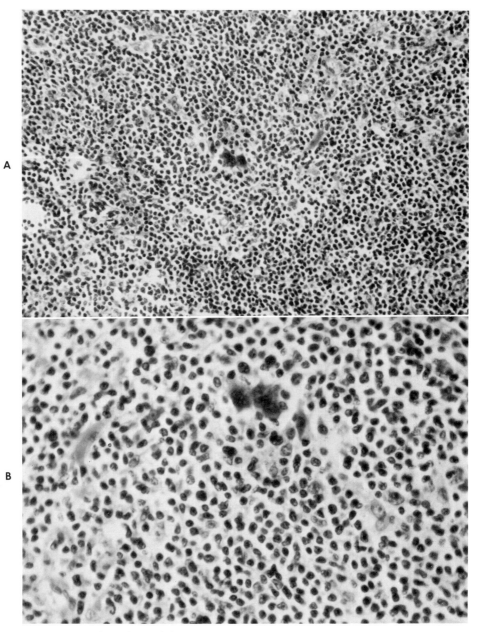

Fig. 31-49 Lymph node. Hodgkin's disease, lymphocytic and histiocytic, diffuse type. (**A,** Hematoxylin-eosin; ×125; **B,** hematoxylin-eosin; ×250.)

placement with diffuse and disorderly collagen (Fig. 31-53). It may represent the final histologic expression of the disease, for it characterizes terminal untreated Hodgkin's disease. There is no formation of collagen bands, and the collagen is not birefringent by polarized light. Focal necrosis is common. Although relatively hypocellular, islands of lymphocytes remain and Sternberg-Reed cells are numerous.

Reticular type. In the reticular type, the

Sternberg-Reed cell is the predominant component. There is a relative depletion of lymphocytes. The Sternberg-Reed cells may be typical or markedly pleomorphic (Fig. 31-54), the latter being the "sarcoma" of Jackson and Parker.[302, 303]

Clinical correlations

Accurate histologic classification of neoplasms is essential for meaningful clinical correlation: clinical staging, prognosis and

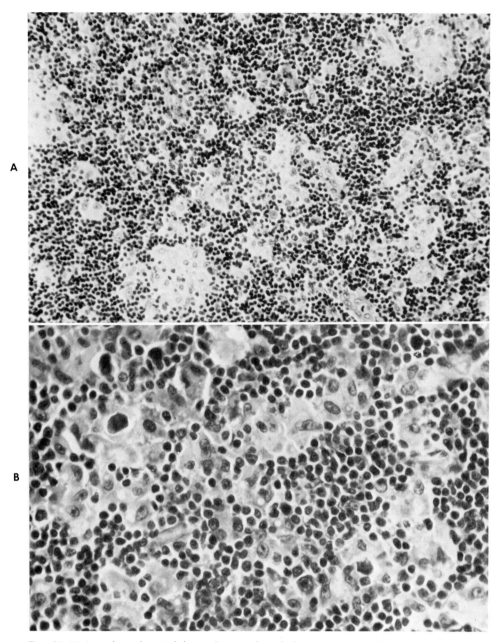

Fig. 31-50 Lymph node. Hodgkin's disease, lymphohistiocytic type. (**A,** Hematoxylin-eosin; ×125; **B,** hematoxylin-eosin; ×250.)

survival, and evaluation of treatment programs. This is particularly applicable to the lymphomas, in which the variety of histologic expression does indeed reflect prognosis.

The data on survival for the lymphomas other than Hodgkin's disease are unsatisfactory, due primarily to the various nomenclatures used. Nevertheless, some generalizations are possible.[307-309]

1 The more differentiated the cells, the better the survival. Thus, the patients with lymphocytic lymphomas with well-differentiated lymphocytes have a longer survival than those with poorly differentiated lymphocytes.

2 The poorest survival is in patients having lymphoma of the mixed type and those having reticulum cell sarcoma.

3 For patients with Hodgkin's disease, survival is strikingly related to the histologic group.

The student interested in detailed survival

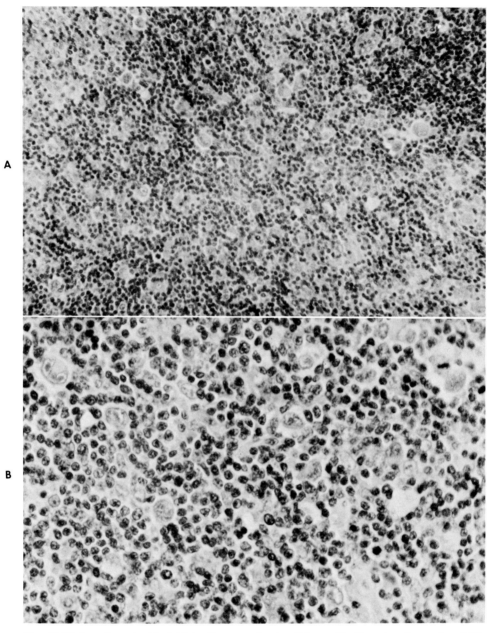

Fig. 31-51 Lymph node. Hodgkin's disease, mixed cell type. (**A,** Hematoxylin-eosin; ×125; **B,** hematoxylin-eosin; ×250.)

figures is referred to the references at the end of the chapter. In reading and interpreting the literature, some points must be kept in mind constantly. Lymphomas usually are classified under at least five categories:

1 The histologic classification of the lymphoma (hopefully, this would be exact and based on the classification given in Table 31-3)
2 Classification according to clinical "staging"—i.e., whether the disease is localized or involves other nodes and distant organs (this should be based on lymphangiography and spleen and bone marrow scans with radioisotopes, for without these staging is unreliable)
3 Interval between onset of signs or symptoms and diagnosis
4 Type and intensity of treatment used
5 Survival at five, ten, and fifteen years after diagnosis or treatment

To my knowledge definitive data based on

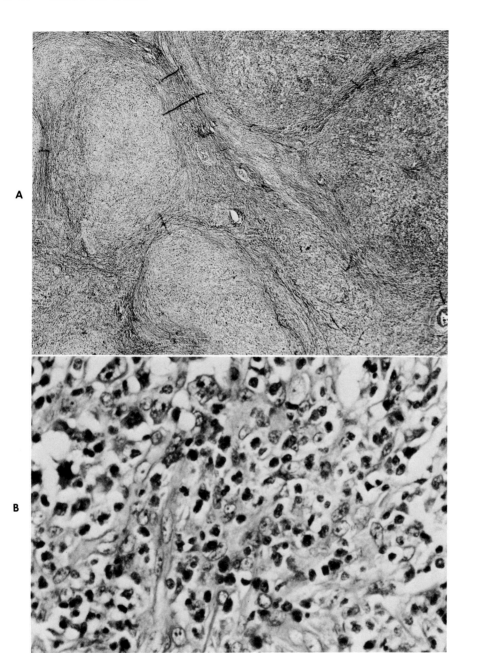

Fig. 31-52 Lymph node. Hodgkin's disease, sclerosing, nodular. (**A,** Hematoxylin-eosin; ×90; **B,** hematoxylin-eosin; ×250.)

these criteria are not available for the first three categories of lymphoma listed in Table 31-3. Accurate classification is certainly the greatest weakness. For example, some authors regrettably call all lymphomas showing a nodular or follicular structure "giant follicular lymphoma" or "Brill's disease," whereas others call all types of lymphoma "lymphosarcoma."

These criticisms generally do not apply to the survival statistics for Hodgkin's disease, thanks mostly to the classic papers of Lukes and associates.[307-309] Lukes et al.[309] studied 377 cases of Hodgkin's disease in persons in Army service; 97% occurred in the age group of 18-39 years, and 98% were in men. These figures reflect that this was a nonrepresentative group both as to age and sex distribution. In the general population, the age distribution is broader and the ratio of men to women about 1.5:1.

It can be seen from Table 31-6 that the

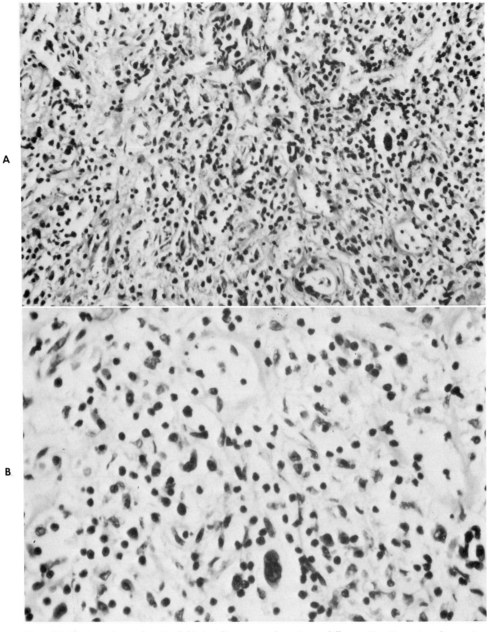

Fig. 31-53 Lymph node. Hodgkin's disease, sclerosing, diffuse. (**A,** Hematoxylin-eosin; ×125; **B,** hematoxylin-eosin; ×250.)

lymphocyte depletion types (diffuse fibrosis and reticular) have the shortest survival. The high incidence of the nodular sclerosis type is noteworthy, particularly since this type has the best prognosis. The majority of 155 cases of Hodgkin's disease in which the patients survived more than ten years have been shown to be of the nodular sclerosis type. As expected, survival of all patients in clinical stage I is better than for those in stage II,

and these, in turn, have a better survival than those in stage III. Thus, there are two important prognostic indices: the histologic type and the clinical stage. Since the aggressiveness of the disease, as well as its long-term response to therapy, is related to the histologic type, the prognosis can be estimated as follows: quiescent disease is expressed histologically by the lymphocytic and histiocytic types in clinical stage I, whereas progressive

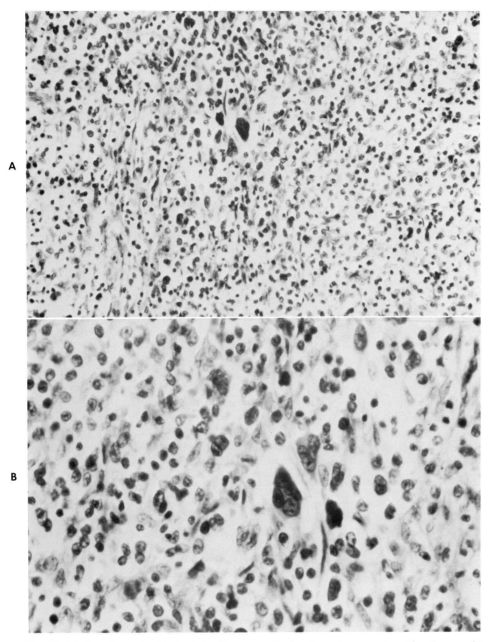

Fig. 31-54 Lymph node. Hodgkin's disease, reticular type (sarcoma), with pleomorphic Sternberg-Reed cells. (**A,** Hematoxylin-eosin; ×125; **B,** hematoxylin-eosin; ×250.)

disease is expressed histologically by the lymphocytic depletion types in clinical stages II and III and with systemic symptoms; the mixed type and stages II and III reflect changing disease. Reticular Hodgkin's disease is usually stage II or III and progressive.

Immunologically, any of the lymphomas may show severe abnormalities. In Hodgkin's disease, the expression of immunologic deficiency is seen as delayed hypersensitivity to common antigens, delayed hypersensitivity after transfer of cells from sensitized donors, rejection of skin allografts, development of contact sensitivity to dinitrochlorobenzene or dinitrofluorobenzene, and depletion of lymphocytes in skin window preparations. There is, however, a normal response to pneumococcal polysaccharide and other bacterial antigens. Thus, the anergy seems limited to the delayed hypersensitivity reaction. In most

Table 31-6 Distribution of histologic groups and survival data for Hodgkin's disease*

Histologic group	Cases	Clinical stage† (%)			Median survival (yr)		
		I	II	III	Stage I	Stage II	Stage III
Lymphocytic and histiocytic							
Nodular	23	78	9	13	16.0	12.0	4.3
Diffuse	40	65	27	8	9.5	4.8	5.5
Nodular sclerosis	149	36	36	28	11.0	3.2	1.8
Mixed	97	37	40	23	4.8	2.5	1.2
Diffuse fibrosis	47	11	27	62	1.1	3.2	0.4
Reticular	21	19	38	43	5.7	2.7	0.6
Totals	377	38	34	28	Av. 9.1	Av. 3.2	Av. 1.3

*Data from Lukes, R. J., Butler, J. J., and Hicks, E. B.: Cancer **19:**317-344, 1966.
†In this series, clinical staging was not based on lymphangiography. Stage criteria are as follows: stage I, involvement of a single lymph node or a single lesion; stage II, involvement of two or more adjacent nodes, either upper or lower trunk; stage III, involvement of two or more nodes in both upper and lower trunks.

cases, there is no immunoglobulin deficit or excess, even when there is lymphocyte depletion, but data correlating the immunologic deficiencies and histologic type are lacking. Autoimmune hemolytic anemia may occur but is rare, and the etiology of the anemia frequently seen in advanced Hodgkin's disease is still unknown.

In patients with lymphoma other than Hodgkin's disease, there is a significant incidence of hypogammaglobulinemia, hypergammaglobulinemia, or acquired autoimmune hemolytic anemia, but again the literature gives a confused picture due to lack of correlation with exact histologic type.

The different expressions of immunologic incompetence among lymphoproliferative diseases, as well as the different peak age distributions, have led Miller[313] to make the intriguing suggestion that lymphoma, leukemia, and Hodgkin's disease involve proliferation of lymphocytes of diverse origin. It has been suggested that Hodgkin's disease reflects the proliferation of thymus-dependent lymphocytes, whereas other lymphomas and lymphocytic leukemia involve nonthymus-dependent lymphocytes. This suggestion provides an interesting explanation for the high incidence of Hodgkin's disease during years of relative immune deficiency for tuberculin-type sensitivity and the high incidence of other lymphomas and lymphocytic leukemia during years of relative deficiency of production of circulating antibody.

Partly because of the abnormal immu-

nologic status, patients with lymphoma are subject to severe, sometimes overwhelming, infection with bacteria, fungi, and viruses. Chemotherapy, radiation therapy, and administration of corticosteroids can further alter the patient's immunologic responsiveness. In general, patients having Hodgkin's disease are most susceptible to mycobacterial or cryptococcal infection, while those with other lymphomas and with leukemia are more subject to bacterial and viral disease. It has been shown[281] that these infections are relatively uncommon early in the course of these diseases and that they frequently are terminal episodes in the late stages.

Lymphoma in African children (Burkitt's lymphoma)

Burkitt,[278] in 1958, and Burkitt and O'Conor[279] and Burkitt et al.[280] in subsequent years have reported the high incidence of childhood lymphoma in Central Africa that now is known as Burkitt's tumor or Burkitt's lymphoma. It is a clinically disfiguring tumor with a predilection for the jaw and facial bones of children. The age distribution (Fig. 31-55) is characteristic and different from that in leukemia and other lymphomas. In fact, the disease is prevalent in areas in which leukemia is rare and transition from lymphoma to leukemia does not occur. Although a few cases fulfilling the criteria for this lymphoma have been reported from many other countries, including the United States, the high incidence in Central Africa and New

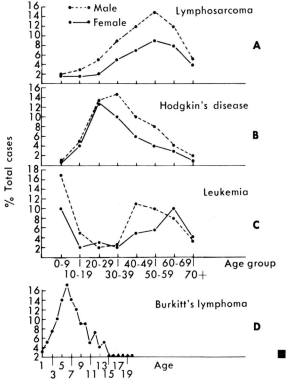

Fig. 31-55 Age distributions of patients with lymphosarcoma, **A,** Hodgkin's disease, **B,** leukemia, **C,** and Burkitt's lymphoma, **D.** (A to C, Data from Razis, D. V., Diamond, H. D., and Craver, L. F.: Ann. Intern. Med. **51:**933-971, 1959; **D,** data from Wright, D. H.: Cancer Res. **27:**2424-2438, 1967.)

Guinea suggests that local environmental factors come into play in the high incidence areas. The working hypothesis at this time is that (1) an infectious agent is involved, probably viral, (2) the infectious agent is a common one of which the tumor is an uncommon manifestation, and (3) the infectious agent is mosquito borne.

Although the involvement of the jaw and facial bones is a spectacular feature of this lymphoma, only 40% of the patients present with facial involvement. Another 40% present with primary abdominal involvement, particularly bilateral ovarian tumor and kidney involvement, and the remaining 20% have primary involvement of other sites. It has been suggested that those cases in which involvement is extrafacial are similar to cases of lymphosarcoma of children seen in nonendemic areas.

Histologically, most of the tumors of the Burkitt's type are classified as lymphocytic lymphomas, poorly differentiated (lymphosar-

coma in old terminology). One feature found in almost all cases is the presence of large phagocytic histiocytes that give the tissue a "starry sky" pattern. The remaining cells are lymphoblasts. Occasional tumors of histiocytic or mixed type have been reported.

Rappaport et al.[321] recommend using a combination of clinical and histologic criteria for the diagnosis of Burkitt's lymphoma:

1 Histologic: lymphoblasts with with scattered phagocytic histiocytes giving a "starry sky" pattern
2 Clinical:
   a Presentation with jaw tumors, abdominal masses, or extranodal tumors in unusual locations such as thyroid gland and salivary gland
   b Absence of leukemic cells in the peripheral blood
   c Occurrence in children
   d Peripheral lymph nodes, mediastinal lymph nodes, and spleen usually not involved

■ Bone marrow

FUNCTION

We have already discussed two of the three identifiable morphologic entities in the reticuloendothelial system, the spleen and the lymph nodes. The third, the bone marrow, also has some functions that are common to other tissues rich in reticuloendothelial cells (p. 1298). Also like the others, it has a special function, in this case to serve as the chief site of blood cell formation in the normal adult. This is medullary hemopoiesis. It is sometimes said that medullary hemopoiesis is involved in the production of erythrocytes, granulocytes, and platelets, whereas lymphocytes and monocytes are formed outside the marrow. However, as shown in Table 31-7, the lymphocytic and monocytic population in the bone marrow is considerable. Note that there is thirteen times as much lymphoid tissue outside as there is within lymph nodes and spleen.

As discussed on p. 1299, the spleen and liver are active sites of normal hemopoiesis in the fetus. Hemopoietic activity in the liver stops by the end of full-term gestation; in the spleen it is markedly reduced. However, these organs retain their content of primitive mesenchymal cells capable of differentiating, when stimulated to do so, into hemopoietic cells. In the adult, therefore, certain hematologic disorders are characterized by formation

Table 31-7 Number and distribution of blood cells in normal person weighing 70 kg*

	In hemopoietic organs		Outside hemopoietic organs			
Cell type	Bone marrow (gm)	Lymphoid tissue and spleen (gm)	In peripheral blood and hemopoietic organs (gm)	Outside peripheral blood and hemopoietic organs (gm)	Ratio of cells within blood to cells outside blood	Total blood cells in body (gm)
Erythrocytic	100	0	2,500	0		2,600
Granulocytic	900	0	10	600	1:60	1,500
Lymphocytic	100	100	3	1,300	1:433	1,500
Monocytic, plasmocytic, thrombocytic, and disintegrated cells	200	200	1	400	1:400	800

*Slightly modified from Osgood, E. E.: Blood **9**:1141-1154, 1954; by permission; from Miale, J. B.: Laboratory medicine—hematology, The C. V. Mosby Co.

of blood cells at sites outside of the bone marrow. This is *extramedullary hemopoiesis*. A consequence of hepatic and splenic involvement in extramedullary hemopoietic activity is hepatomegaly and splenomegaly.

STRUCTURE

At birth, all possible bone cavities contain active red marrow. By the age of 4 years, there is beginning replacement of red marrow by fatty marrow, and at the age of 20 years red marrow is found only in the skull, clavicles, scapulae, sternum, ribs, pelvis, and proximal ends of the long bones, while the distal portions of the long bones contain only fatty marrow. In the normal adult, the ratio of red to fatty marrow is 1:1. Ellis[332] gives the total amount of active red marrow in a man weighing 70 kg as 1,459 gm, about equal to the weight of the liver, and gives data for distribution in various bones (Table 31-8). When marrow volume and cellularity are determined by means of radioisotopes of iron and gold, the values for the normal distribution are not changed appreciably, but these methods give interesting data in hematologic abnormalities.

The vascular bed of the bone marrow is unusual in several respects. For one thing, the rigid cortical bone that encases it makes in the marrow an unyielding hydrostatic system unlike that in any other organ. The arteries entering the marrow cavity have a normal structure (Fig. 31-56, *A*), but soon after entering the marrow, the thick-walled arteries change abruptly into thin-walled arteries (Fig. 31-56, *B*), the wall of which consists of a flattened thin media and flat endothelium. The thin-walled arteries in turn open into large sinuses. The sinus walls are not

Table 31-8 Distribution of red marrow by weight in bones of normal 40-year-old man*

	Weight of red marrow (gm)	% Total red marrow
Cranium and mandible	136.6	13.1
Humeri, scapulae, and clavicles	86.7	8.3
Sternum	23.4	2.3
Ribs	82.6	7.9
Vertebrae	297.8	28.4
Pelvis	418.6	40.0

*Slightly modified from Ellis, R. E.: Phys. Med. Biol. **5**:255-258, 1961; from Miale, J. B.: Laboratory medicine—hematology, The C. V. Mosby Co.

easily distinguished in routine sections but by electron microscopy they can be seen to consist of lining endothelium, basement membrane, and adventitial cells. Furthermore, the sinus walls appear not to be continuous, and there are long segments in which the absence of a complete sinus wall permits open communication with the hemopoietic tissue of the marrow.

The combination of a rigidly enclosed system and discontinuous sinus walls is ideally suited to free exchange of cells and plasma between the sinuses and the hemopoietic tissue. This, plus the inherent motility of some of the blood cells, accounts for the entrance of newly formed cells into the systemic circulation. The patency of the system is illustrated by the finding that materials injected into the bone marrow (colloidal thorium dioxide, [22]sodium chloride, ^{131}I albumin, ^{131}I hippuran) are dispersed throughout the marrow in a few minutes, whereas the isotopically labeled materials are detectable in the systemic circulation in a matter of seconds.

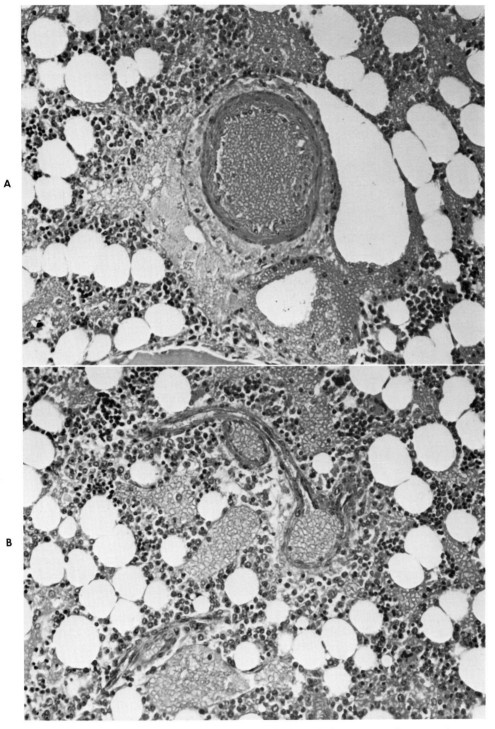

Fig. 31-56 Arterial supply of bone marrow. **A,** Thick-walled artery. **B,** Thin-walled artery. (Hematoxylin-eosin; ×125.)

METHODS OF STUDY
Biopsy

Biopsy of bone marrow is performed most commonly by aspiration. The sternum, anterior and posterior iliac crests, and the vertebral spinous processes all give representative specimens. After the marrow is entered, a small sample (0.2 ml) of marrow is aspirated into the syringe, and this is used to prepare thin smears. A second sample of several milliliters is then aspirated into a fresh syringe. Marrow particles are harvested from this sample, fixed, and sectioned. Routine sections are cut at 5μ and stained with hematoxylin and eosin. Special stains such as the Giemsa stain can be used, but cellular morphology is best studied in the thin smears stained with Wright's stain.

If aspiration biopsy is unsuccessful, a core of bone marrow can be obtained by trephine with a modified Vim-Silverman needle. Details of biopsy techniques are given by Miale.[10] A particle of bone marrow should be teased out of the core and used for a crush smear. The remainder of the specimen is fixed and used for routine sections.

It is sometimes necessary to obtain bone marrow by open surgical biopsy. The sample obtained in this case usually consists of cortical bone and bone marrow and requires decalcification. Since decalcification often produces cytologic alterations, it is recommended that before the specimen is processed particles of marrow be teased out for smears and, if possible, sectioned without decalcification.

At necropsy

Bone marrow cells undergo degeneration soon after death. There is no relationship between rate of degeneration and age, sex, storage temperature, and mode of death, although some investigators believe that cellular damage is more rapid when death is due to an infectious disease. Within the first three hours after death, the marrow cells are well preserved and can be identified easily in smears from aspirated material. After three hours, there is progressive degeneration of the cells, the oldest cells such as mature granulocytes and mature normoblasts degenerating earlier than immature cells, lymphocytes, and plasma cells. After fifteen or more hours from the time of death, cellular damage is so far advanced that aspirated material is practically worthless.

The degenerative change usually is called autolysis of the cells, but this may not be an accurate definition of what happens. For one thing, routine sections of paraffin-embedded marrow do not show marked loss of cellular detail even when the tissue is obtained many hours after death. Also, it has been shown that if marrow is suspended in 5% bovine albumin and then smeared, the cells are well preserved and easily identified many hours after death. It would seem, then, that the postmortem change is not a true autolysis, which would be irreversible, but rather an increased fragility of the cytoplasm and possibly of the nucleus as well.

RELATION TO PERIPHERAL BLOOD

The cellular population of the peripheral blood reflects the net of several effects: (1) rate of hemopoiesis in the bone marrow, (2) rate of release of cells from the bone marrow, and (3) rate of survival of cells in the peripheral blood. Hematologic diagnosis is based on making full use of all data that are pertinent to these basic mechanisms.

The hemopoietic activity of the bone marrow can be determined from the cellularity of the tissue sections and from the distribution of cells, according to type and degree of maturation, in the thin smears. It should be noted that the bone marrow in infants and young children is normally rich in cells and poor in fat, that in normal adults the distribution is half cells and half fat, and that in normal elderly persons the distribution is about one-third cells and two-thirds fat.

The rate of release of blood cells from the bone marrow into the peripheral blood is more difficult to establish. The presence in the blood of immature granulocytes indicates that leukocytic release is normal. Likewise, the presence of reticulocytes in normal number indicates normal release of erythrocytes. When the reticulocyte count is high, we can conclude that more young erythrocytes are being released than normal, and in this case the marrow will show hyperplasia of erythrocyte precursors. In special situations, such as the "aplastic crisis" of hemolytic anemia, the peripheral blood contains no reticulocytes, and we know that either the marrow maturation is arrested or that no new cells are being released. It is not always possible to distinguish maturation arrest from lack of release. In pernicious anemia, for example, the marrow is hyperplastic, but the peripheral blood shows anemia and a low reticulocyte count. It can be shown that in this example the failure is partially in the release mechanism, for the marrow is full of reticulocytes that are not liberated into the blood. When vitamin B_{12} is given, one of the effects is to unblock the release mechanism and induce a shower of reticulocytes into the peripheral blood.

Finally, the rate of survival of erythrocytes can be established accurately by a variety of radioisotope methods; these also detect whether a decreased life span is due to an intrinsic defect in the erythrocytes or to extracorpuscular hemolytic mechanisms. Thus, hemolytic disease is related to shortened life span of the erythrocytes and can be classified into two major categories, one related to intrinsic abnormality of the erythrocyte (hemoglobinopathy, enzyme deficiency, etc.) and the other to extracorpuscular factors (autoantibodies, isoantibodies, etc.). Life span of platelets is determined with only fair accuracy. Life span of leukocytes has so far defied an exact and direct definition. Unlike the erythrocytes, which once in the peripheral blood do not normally leave it except when they die, leukocytes wander in and out of the blood, spending variable time in organs such as the spleen, liver, and lungs. To further complicate the problem, each type of white blood cell has a cycle and history different from the others.

HYPOPLASIA, APLASIA, AND HYPERPLASIA

The bone marrow can be hypoplastic or aplastic as the result of a variety of toxic and suppressive effects:

I Bone marrow injury caused by physical or chemical agent
  A Ionizing radiation
  B Chemical agents (partial list)
    1 Aminopyrine
    2 Arsenicals, organic
    3 Atabrine
    4 Benzol
    5 Bismuth salts
    6 Chloramphenicol
    7 Chlorpromazine
    8 Colchicine
    9 Dinitrophenol
    10 Diphenylhydantoin sodium
    11 Folic acid antagonists
    12 Gold salts
    13 Mepazine
    14 Mercury salts
    15 Methimazole
    16 Methyl-ethyl-phenyl hydantoin
    17 Naphthalene
    18 Nitrogen mustard and derivatives
    19 Paraphenylenediamine (hair dyes)
    20 Perphenazine
    21 Phenindione
    22 Phenylbutazone
    23 Prochlorperazine
    24 Promazine
    25 Promethazine
    26 Pyrimethamine
    27 Quinacrine
    28 Quinidine
    29 Ristocetin
    30 Sulfonamides
    31 Streptomycin
    32 Stoddard's solvent
    33 Thiouracils
    34 Triflupromazine
    35 Trimethadione
    36 Trinitrotoluene
    37 Tripelennamine HCl
II Congenital aplastic anemia (Diamond-Blackfan type)
III Familial aplastic anemia
  A Associated with developmental anomalies (Fanconi type)
  B Without developmental anomalies (Estren and Dameshek type)
IV Chronic erythrocytic hypoplasia in adults
V Aplastic anemia associated with thymoma
VI Metabolic inhibition of bone marrow
  A Malignancy
  B Infection
  C Renal failure
  D Endocrinopathies
  E Chronic liver disease
  F Allergy
  G Pancreatic insufficiency
VII Erythroid hypoplasia of bone marrow in hemolytic disease
VIII Idiopathic aplastic anemia
IX Aplastic anemia in myeloproliferative disorders (myelophthisic anemia)

Sectioned tissue shows a markedly hypocellular marrow (Fig. 31-57) with a preponderance of fat. The remaining cells are lymphocytes and reticulum cells. When the tissue section shows such a severe degree of hemopoietic failure, one is justified in calling the marrow aplastic. It should be noted, however, that representative sections from many sites may still fail to reveal some remaining foci of hemopoietic activity, and it is probable that complete aplasia of the entire bone marrow is a very rare occurrence.

Hypoplasia can affect only one or two cell types, particularly when the offending agent is a myelotoxic drug. Such selective hypoplasia is reflected in the peripheral blood by a reduction of the corresponding circulating cells. Thus, the peripheral blood may show leukopenia with neutropenia, or thrombocytopenia, or anemia, or combinations of these. The term "aplastic anemia" refers specifically to the anemia secondary to bone marrow depression but is sometimes used loosely to refer to aplasia of the marrow and suppression of all cell types in the peripheral blood (pan-

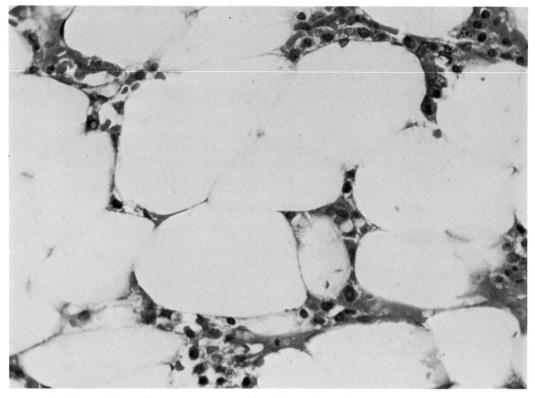

Fig. 31-57 Aplastic bone marrow caused by chloramphenicol. (Hematoxylin-eosin; ×125.)

cytopenia). We know, however, that the pancytopenia in some cases is accompanied by hyperplasia of the bone marrow. This anomalous finding is one of the situations that brought about a reconsideration of the pathophysiology of the "myeloproliferative syndromes."

Hyperplasia of the bone marrow may be selective or generalized. In most instances, the hyperplasia is the result of a specific stimulation of one type of cell and is therefore selective. In anemia of whatever etiology, there is hyperplasia of erythroid cells to compensate for the anemia.

A special type of erythroid hyperplasia is seen in those anemias caused by a deficiency of folic acid or vitamin B_{12}. Instead of the usual normoblastic maturation, there is a profound abnormality of maturation that affects all cell types, a *dyspoiesis*. The erythroid cells are large and atypical, resembling reticulum cells, and are called megaloblasts (Fig. 31-58, *A* and *B*). There is also abnormal maturation of granulocytes, and the metamyelocytes and bands are two or three times normal size (Fig. 31-58, *C*). Megakaryocytes are even more bizarre than usual. In infectious diseases characterized by leukocytosis, there is granu-

locytic hyperplasia. Hyperplasia of all cell types usually is seen in the myeloproliferative syndromes, although even in these, one series may be more hyperplastic than the others.

MYELOPROLIFERATIVE SYNDROMES

The concept of the "myeloproliferative syndromes" was expressed in 1951 by Dameshek,[374] who speculated on the possibility of a common etiologic agent for myelocytic leukemia, polycythemia vera, agnogenic myeloid metaplasia, thrombocythemia, megakaryocytic leukemia, and erythroleukemia. His suggestion that these diseases have a common myeloproliferative stimulus, hormonal or steroid, remains only a speculation and, in fact, an unlikely possibility. However, the concept that apparently dissimilar diseases are related insofar as each is a manifestation of abnormal hemopoietic proliferation has deepened our understanding of the clinical and hematologic findings.

Previously, pathologists and hematologists had focused attention on criteria to distinguish among and identify diseases showing in various combinations features such as (1) leukocytosis or leukopenia with immature cells (myeloid or erythroid) in the peripheral

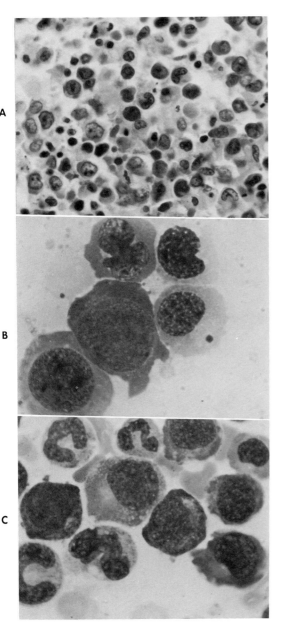

Fig. 31-58 Megaloblastic dyspoiesis in bone marrow. **A,** Paraffin section. **B,** Smear. All cells are megaloblasts. **C,** Smear. Note giant neutrophil metamyelocytes and stab cells. (**A,** Hematoxylineosin; ×400; **B** and **C,** Wright's stain; ×950.)

blood, (2) bone marrow that might be aplastic, sclerotic, hyperplastic, infiltrated with tumor cells, or normal, (3) various degrees of splenomegaly and hepatomegaly, (4) anemia, and (5) polycythemia. The question of leukemia versus a benign process was always a serious concern.

The terms to be found in the literature for the various "diseases" showing one or several

of these abnormalities reflect the most striking presenting finding and the principal concern of the investigator with the "atypical" nature of these diseases. These may be grouped as follows:*

Differentiation from leukemia

Pseudoleukemia
Aleukemic myelosis
Chronic nonleukemic myelosis
Atypical myelosis
Megakaryocytic myelosis
Aleukemic megakaryocytic myelosis
Myeloid megakaryocytic myelosis

Splenomegaly and hepatomegaly

Agnogenic myeloid metaplasia of spleen
Splenomegaly with myeloid transformation
Splenomegaly with sclerosis of bone marrow
Splenomegaly with anemia
Myelophthisic splenomegaly
Splenomegaly with anemia and myelemia
Myeloid splenomegaly without myelocythemia
Aleukemic hepatosplenic myelosis
Myeloid megakaryocytic hepatosplenomegaly

Abnormalities in peripheral blood

Leukanemia
Myeloid splenic anemia
Leukoerythroblastic anemia
Leukoerythroblastosis
Osteosclerotic anemia
Polycythemia vera
Thrombocythemia
Leukemoid reaction
Pancytopenia
Erythroleukemia
Erythremic myelosis
Di Guglielmo's disease

Abnormalities in bone marrow

Myelosclerosis
Myelofibrosis
Osteosclerosis
Atypical aplastic anemia
Myelophthisic anemia
Myelopathic anemia
Panmyelophthisis

This impressive list could be extended into a meaningless triumph of descriptive pathology by combining several of the features of a given disease. In any case, there is implicit in any list of "diseases" or "syndromes" the supposition that each disease can be characterized by a set of features that distinguish it from the others. Experience has shown that this usually is impossible. The final blow to the concept of individual and characteristic diseases is dealt by the realization that, when one has the opportunity to follow the course

*From Miale, J. B.: Laboratory medicine—hematology, St. Louis, The C. V. Mosby Co.

Text continued on p. 1366.

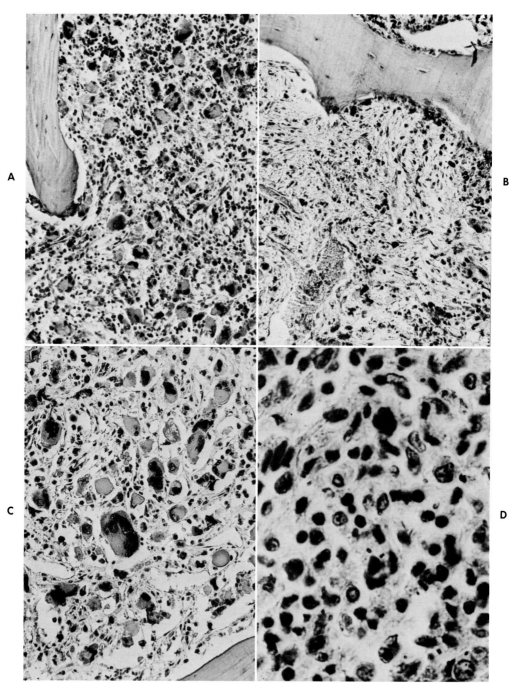

Fig. 31-59 Myelosclerosis with megakaryocytic myelosis of spleen in 61-year-old white man. Onset occurred six months before death, with pancytopenia, fatigue, and weight loss. There was progressive pancytopenia, and death was due to thrombocytopenia and hemorrhage. Bone marrow was fibrotic, with striking megakaryocytic proliferation. Spleen was small, weighing 60 gm, but showed striking megakaryocytic myelosis. **A** to **C**, Bone marrow. **D**, Spleen. (**A** and **B**, Hematoxylin-eosin; ×130; **C**, hematoxylin-eosin; ×350; **D**, hematoxylin-eosin; ×585.)

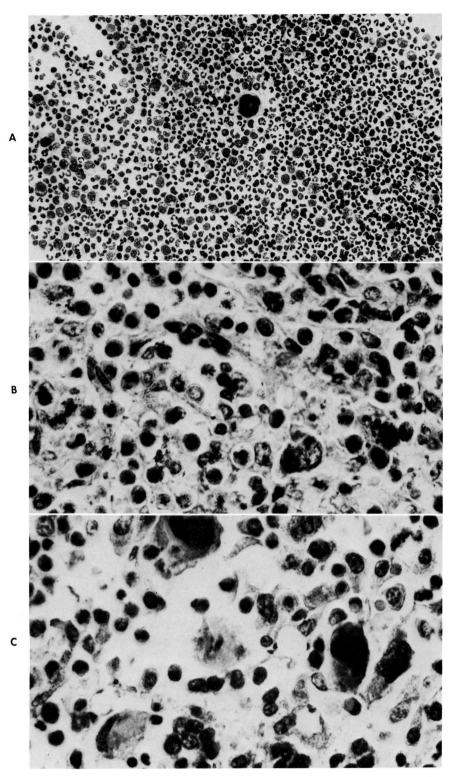

Fig. 31-60 Leukemoid reaction with hepatosplenomegaly and megakaryocytic myelosis of spleen in 71-year-old white man. Patient admitted to hospital because of mental confusion and leukocytosis one year before death. Leukocyte count at admission was 74,000 per cubic millimeter, and there was shift to left with immature granulocytes. Bone marrow during life was hyperplastic. There was striking splenomegaly. Necropsy revealed glioblastoma multiforme of right frontal lobe, splenomegaly (960 gm), and cardiac failure. **A,** Antemortem bone marrow aspiration. **B** and **C,** Paraffin sections of spleen. (**A,** Wright's stain; ×130; **B,** hematoxylin-eosin; ×450; **C,** hematoxylin-eosin; ×585.)

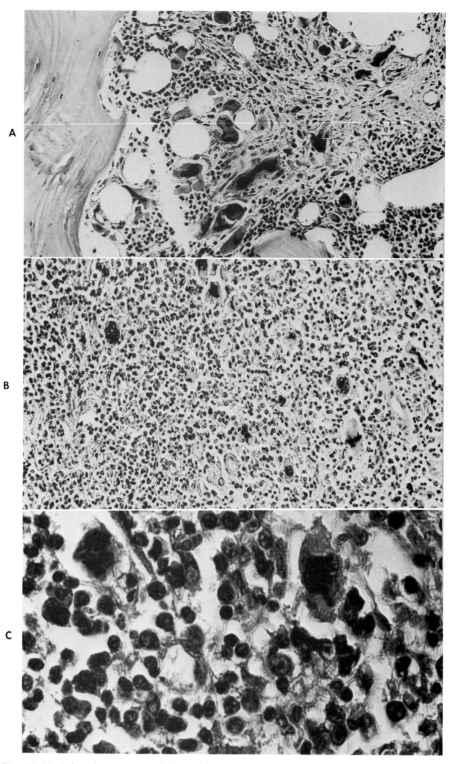

Fig. 31-61 Polycythemia vera followed by myelofibrosis and megakaryocytic myelosis in 77-year-old white man. Diagnosis of polycythemia vera was established seven years before death and patient treated with P³². Five years later, white blood cell count rose to 45,000 per cubic millimeter and peripheral blood picture was leukemoid. One year later, peripheral blood picture changed again to leukoerythroblastic form with many immature leukocytes and 17% normoblasts. During last year of life, patient developed progressive anemia characterized by markedly decreased Cr⁵¹-erythrocyte survival. Splenectomy was performed. Death occurred postoperatively. **A,** Postmortem bone marrow. **B** and **C,** Antemortem spleen. (**A,** Hematoxylin-eosin; ×130; **B,** hematoxylin-eosin; ×130; **C,** hematoxylin-eosin; ×585.)

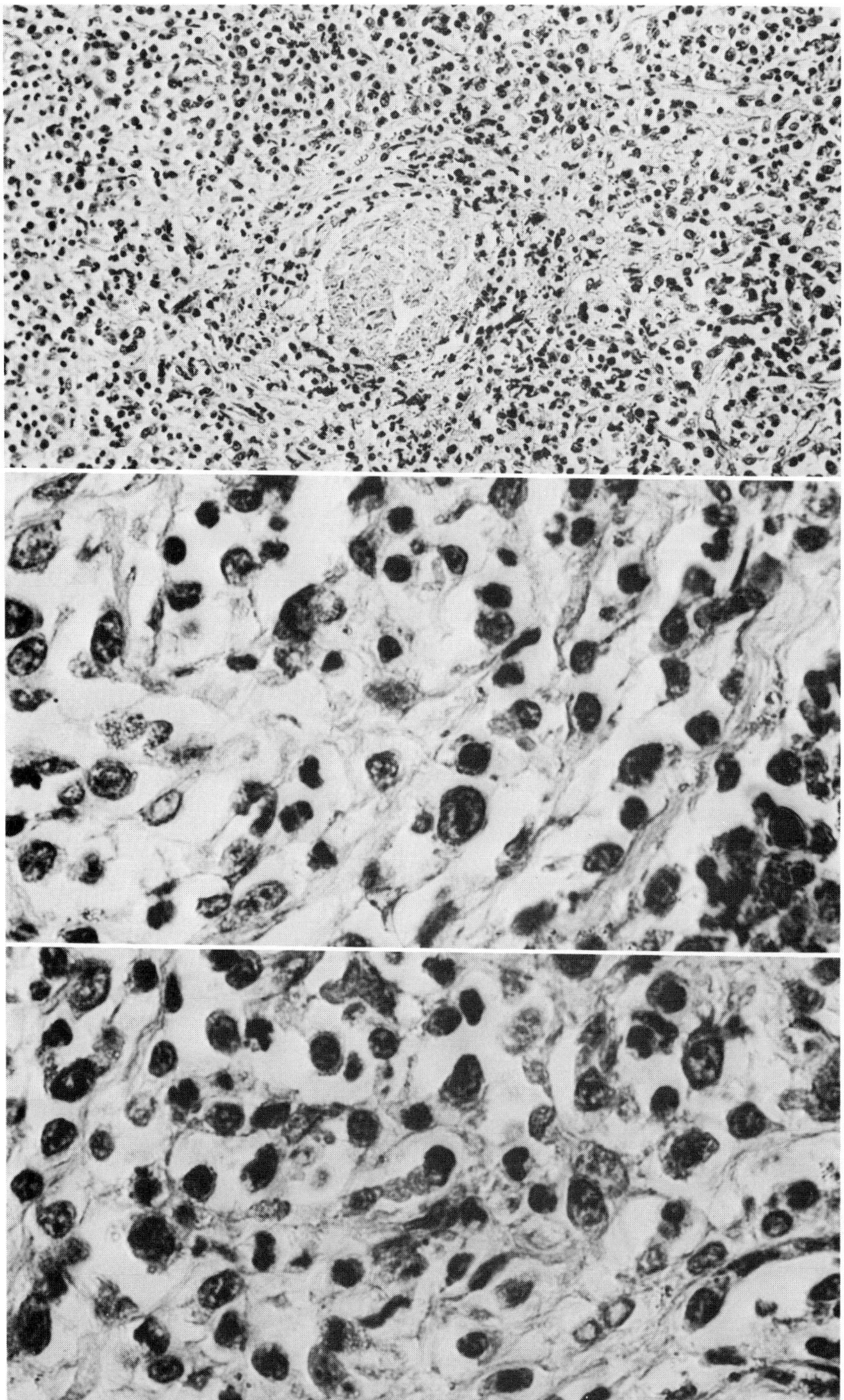

Fig. 31-62 Chronic myelocytic leukemia (?) with hypersplenism in 38-year-old white man. There was eleven-year history of leukocytosis before gastrectomy for peptic ulcer. At operation, spleen found to be moderately enlarged but was not removed. White cell count at that time was 49,700. Differential count showed 2% blasts, 24.5% myelocytes, 13% metamyelocytes, 40% segmented neutrophils, and 2% normoblasts. One year before death (four years postgastrectomy), patient treated with cobalt irradiation, following which he developed pancytopenia. Simultaneously, there was sudden enlargement of spleen. Although leukopenic, differential count on peripheral blood showed 20% blasts. Cr^{51}-erythrocyte survival was very short (half-life of seven days). Splenectomy was performed. Death occurred from staphylococcus septicemia. Spleen weighed 3,300 gm. Necropsy did not reveal typical histopathologic lesions of leukemia. **A** to **C**, Spleen. Note siderosis in **B** and **C**. (**A**, Hematoxylin-eosin; ×130; **B** and **C**, hematoxylin-eosin; ×585.)

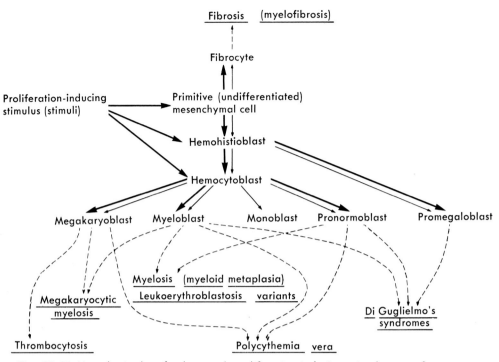

Fig. 31-63 Hypothesis that fundamental proliferation-inducing stimulus acts first on undifferentiated mesenchymal cells and, through these, to other cell lines to produce various myeloproliferative syndromes. (From Miale, J. B.: Laboratory medicine—hematology, The C. V. Mosby Co.)

of these patients over a period of time, the disease often progresses through a series of clinical and morphologic variants. At any given time, the diagnostic term that is applicable may well be different from that used a year previously or a year hence (Figs. 31-59 to 31-62).

What, then, is the common denominator and how does one face the problem of diagnosis?

We have postulated that a proliferation-inducing stimulus (or stimuli with selective effects) acts on undifferentiated mesenchymal cells and their immediate derivatives to produce medullary and extramedullary hemopoietic and connective tissue proliferation (Fig. 31-63). Proliferation and differentiation along one or several lines would account for the many variants observed, the changing patterns as the disease progresses, and the concomitant occurrence of fibrosis and hemopoietic proliferation. This last is, in my opinion, a strong point in favor of the hypothesis. Otherwise, how can we explain the simultaneous proliferation of connective tissue and blood cells in the bone marrow in acute leukemia. Support for the hypothesis also can be derived from noncontroversial reactions

that are accepted by all. For example, when the stimulus is of known infectious origin, stimulation of the marrow may result in such a striking increase in the number of circulating leukocytes, and a shift toward immature forms as well, as to mimic leukemia (hence, *leukemoid* reaction). In chronic myelocytic leukemia we have an example of involvement of more than one cell type at the same time: granulocytes (leukocytosis) and platelets (thrombocytosis). We know also that hypoxia, as from a prolonged sojourn at high altitudes, cyanotic heart disease, etc., is a specific stimulus for proliferation of erythroid cells with resultant secondary polycythemia.

The splenomegaly and hepatomegaly seen so frequently in the myeloproliferative disorders are not "compensatory," as is sometimes said. If this were the case, then massive splenomegaly and hepatomegaly should be seen in cases of complete marrow aplasia, as in chloramphenicol toxicity. In fact, extramedullary hemopoiesis does not occur in such cases. Rather, hepatosplenomegaly (extramedullary hemopoiesis also may occur in other tissues) reflects the stimulation of primitive mesenchymal cells dormant in the adult organ (p. 1299). It should be noted that in

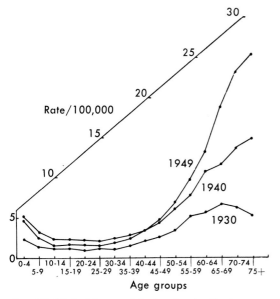

Fig. 31-64 Incidence of leukemia deaths by age in 1930, 1940, and 1949. (From Cooke, J. V.: Blood **9**:340-347, 1954; by permission.)

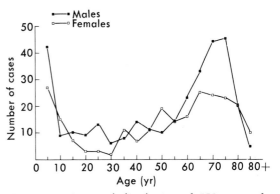

Fig. 31-65 Age and distribution of 553 cases of leukemia. (Data from Gunz, F. W., and Hough, R. F.: Blood **11**:882-901, 1956; from Miale, J. B.: Laboratory medicine—hematology, The C. V. Mosby Co.)

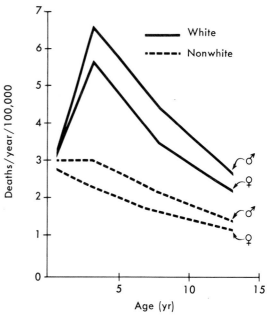

Fig. 31-66 Death rate from acute leukemia in white and black children, 1950-1959. (Data from Ederer, F., Miller, R. W., and Scotto, J.: J.A.M.A. **192**:593-596, 1965; from Miale, J. B.: Laboratory medicine—hematology, The C. V. Mosby Co.)

rare cases, the spleen is not enlarged, even though all the histologic features of extramedullary hemopoiesis are present (Fig. 31-59).

We might speculate a little on the nature of the proliferation-inducing stimulus or stimuli. Many of the myeloproliferative syndromes mimic leukemia, and, in fact, many have a terminal leukemic phase. In experimental animals, variants of leukomogenic viruses produce nonleukemic myeloproliferative disease. If human leukemia is caused by viruses as many think, then it is tempting to postulate that, at least in some of the myeloproliferative syndromes, we see either an attenuated viral stimulus or an altered host response to a leukemogenic virus.

LEUKEMIA

Leukemia is a neoplastic disease characterized by the proliferation of hemopoietic cells in the bone marrow and other organs. By definition, the term leukemia refers to the appearance of these cells in the peripheral blood. The disease is uniformly fatal. There are some very few cases on record of suppressed spontaneous cure. Most of these can be attributed to the original diagnosis being in error. Since spontaneous cures of other malignant tumors have been seen, we can accept that one or two cases of leukemia (usually chronic lymphocytic) may fall into this category.

Incidence

The incidence of leukemia has shown a steady increase during the past forty years (Fig. 31-64). In the United States, the mortality from leukemia has risen from 3.9 per 100,000 in 1940 to 6.5 per 100,000 in 1954 and to 8 per 100,000 in 1964. An upward trend is seen in other countries as well. Perhaps a portion of the increase can be ascribed to better diagnosis but, even when allowance is made for this and other factors, there remains what appears to be a true increase in incidence. There has been a proportionately greater increase in incidence in the older age groups. Only a small fraction of this can be ascribed to greater longevity. The remarkable figures for improved longevity given by the biostatisticians reflect almost entirely improved neonatal and childhood survival, and the life expectancy for the middle-aged has improved only a little. In any case, if the incidence of all leukemias is plotted according to age (Fig. 31-65), two peaks are noted: one between the third and fourth year and one between the ages of 70 and 80 years. In the older age group, the incidence in men is significantly higher than in women. In the younger age group, the incidence in white children is significantly greater than in black children (Fig. 31-66).

Although any type of leukemia can occur at any age, a consistent pattern is found in most large series. Acute leukemia is more common than chronic leukemia at all ages and is most frequent in children and in elderly persons. Chronic myelocytic leukemia is rare in childhood, becoming increasingly more frequent in older age groups. Chronic lymphocytic leukemia is rare before the age of 35 years but is the most common type in elderly individuals. The overall distribution by type in the United States is as follows: chronic lymphocytic, 25%; chronic myelocytic, 22%; chronic myelomonocytic, 3%; acute lymphocytic, 20%; acute myelocytic, 20%; and acute myelomonocytic leukemia, 10%. Chronic lymphocytic leukemia is rare in China, Japan, and India. In children, almost all leukemias are acute lymphocytic (225 of 258 cases, with thirteen acute myelocytic, thirteen acute monocytic, four blast cell, and three chronic myelocytic leukemia).

Etiology and epidemiology

The etiology of leukemia is not known. There are four partially overlapping approaches to the investigation of etiology: epidemiologic, the leukemogenic effect of ionizing radiation, the role of viruses, and the genetic (chromosomal) determinants.

Epidemiology. The epidemiology of leukemia shows some interesting but unexplained features. We know that there are some true differences in incidence among special groups:

1 The incidence in black children is lower than in whites and does not peak at 3 to 4 years of age.

2 The incidence of leukemia in Japan is about half of that in the United States, due partly to a lower incidence in middle-aged persons and partly to the rarity of chronic lymphocytic leukemia in older Japanese.

3 African children have the lowest incidence of leukemia, even though the incidence of Burkitt's lymphoma is high.

4 There are occasional families with a high incidence of leukemia; it is noteworthy however that in these families the leukemia is sometimes of the same type (chronic lymphocytic) and sometimes of different types (the next most frequent association is chronic lymphocytic and chronic myelocytic leukemia).

5 The incidence of leukemia in both identical and nonidentical twins may be higher than in only one of the twins.

Leukemogenic effect of ionizing radiation. There is no longer doubt that ionizing radiation is leukemogenic. Among survivors of the atomic explosion over Hiroshima, the first cases of leukemia appeared eighteen months later and the peak incidence occurred five years later. The highest incidence was in those receiving the greatest dose of radiation. Of great interest is the finding that, in line with the low incidence of chronic lymphocytic leukemia in the Japanese, no case of chronic lymphocytic leukemia developed in the survivors. Therapeutic and diagnostic x-radia-

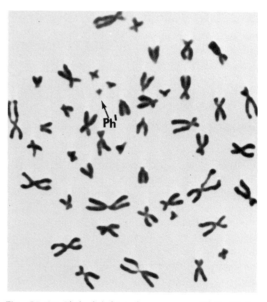

Fig. 31-67 Philadelphia chromosome (Ph¹). Metaphase of diploid marrow cell in chronic myelocytic leukemia. (Courtesy Dr. J. Whang and Dr. J. H. Tjio.)

tion also can be leukemogenic. The mechanism by which irradiation induces leukemia is not known.

Role of viruses. The induction by viruses of leukemia in fowls has been studied for over a half century. In 1951, Gross[424] showed that mouse leukemia can be transmitted to newborn mice by cell-free filtrates. A viral etiology for human leukemia remains a likely possibility, but as yet no proof has been forthcoming. Direct transfusion of leukemic blood into normal recipients does not transmit leukemia. If a viral etiology is operative in human leukemia, it must be supposed that there are other interacting factors such as genetic predisposition, ionizing radiation, and the latency of the virus until activated by intrinsic or extrinsic factors.

Chromosomal abnormalities. The association of chromosomal abnormalities with leukemia is well established. The most constant and characteristic change involves chromosome 21. In chronic myelocytic leukemia, a characteristic small chromosome, called the Philadelphia or Ph[1] chromosome (Fig. 31-67), is formed by deletion or translocation of portions of the normal 21 chromosome. This abnormal chromosome is not found in normal persons or in those with nonleukemic myelo-proliferative syndromes. Some cases of chronic myelocytic leukemia without the Ph[1] chromosome also have been found. The high incidence of leukemia in mongoloids (seventeen times greater than in normal children) also suggests that abnormalities of chromosome 21 (mongoloids have trisomy 21) is related to the development of leukemia.

Classification

Leukemia is classified according to (1) clinical duration of the disease, (2) cell type in the blood and bone marrow, and (3) leukocyte count in the peripheral blood.

On the basis of duration, *acute* leukemia has a short life expectancy (twelve months or more). The term *subacute* is used by some for cases of intermediate duration and by others for cases in transition between chronic and acute. The use of chemotherapy and improved supportive therapy makes this clinical classification a retrospective one.

Classification of leukemia on the basis of cell type is as follows:

I Blast cell leukemia (acute)*
II Lymphocytic leukemia

*Predominant cell is a blast that cannot be otherwise identified at the time; "stem cell leukemia."

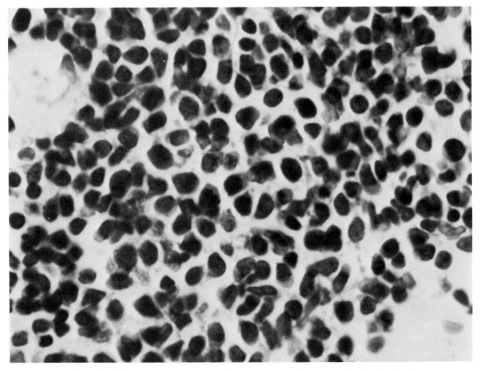

Fig. 31-68 Bone marrow in acute leukemia. (Courtesy Dr. A. Rywlin.)

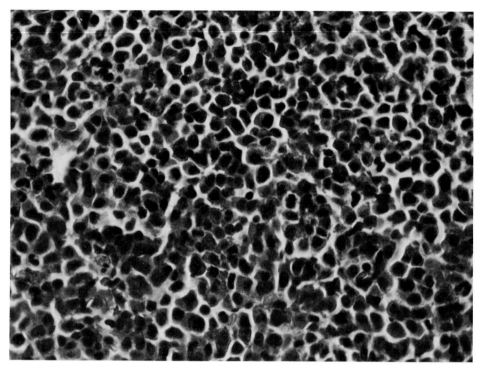

Fig. 31-69 Bone marrow in chronic myelocytic leukemia. (Courtesy Dr. A. Rywlin.)

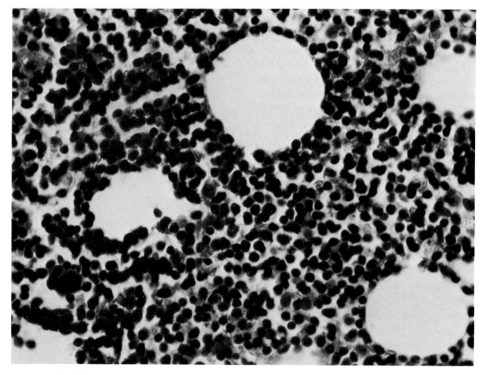

Fig. 31-70 Bone marrow in chronic lymphocytic leukemia. (Courtesy Dr. A. Rywlin.)

III Myelocytic leukemia*
IV Monocytic leukemia
  A Myelomonocytic (Naegeli type)†
  B Histiocytic (Schilling type)
V Plasmacytic leukemia and multiple myeloma
VI Erythroleukemia
VII Mast cell leukemia

Generally the more immature the cells the more acute the clinical course.

On the basis of the leukocyte count in the peripheral blood, leukemia is classified as *leukemic* (high leukocyte count), *subleukemic* (low leukocyte count but abnormal cells present), and *aleukemic* (low leukocyte count with no abnormal cells). It is improbable that truly aleukemic cases exist. Abnormal cells usually can be found if smears of the buffy coat of centrifuged blood are examined.

Acute leukemia

Morphologically, acute leukemia is characterized by the preponderance of immature cells classified as blasts (Fig. 31-68). These may belong to one or another of the cell types and therefore can be subclassified as acute lymphocytic leukemia, acute myelocytic leukemia, etc. Sometimes the cells are so immature that they cannot be classified, and then the term "stem cell" leukemia is applied. In most cases, however, cell identification is possible on morphologic grounds or from the presence of other more mature cells.

Clinically, the onset is marked by one or several of the following: pallor, fever, purpura, malaise, bone pain, splenomegaly, lymphadenopathy, and central nervous system involvement. Lymphadenopathy is common in acute lymphocytic leukemia and uncommon in acute myelocytic leukemia. Splenomegaly may be present in any type but is most common in acute lymphocytic leukemia.

The leukocyte count is moderately or strikingly elevated, and thrombocytopenia is common. Anemia is sometimes severe. When the leukocyte count is not elevated, the onset may mimic idiopathic thrombocytopenia purpura or aplastic anemia.

Chronic myelocytic leukemia

Most cases of chronic myelocytic leukemia occur in adults. Splenomegaly, sometimes with the spleen so large as to seemingly fill

---

*Includes neutrophilic, eosinophilic, and basophilic types that are variants and need not be classified separately.
†Some classify this under myelocytic leukemia.

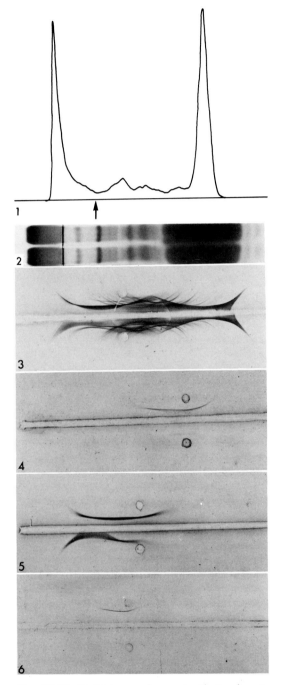

Fig. 31-71 Multiple myeloma. 1, Electrophoretic pattern showing abnormal gamma peak. 2, Starch gel electrophoresis showing abnormal gamma band. 3 to 6, Immunoelectrophoresis: control subject, top; patient, bottom. 3, Polyvalent antiserum showing abnormal gamma components. 4, Anti-IgA serum showing reduction of IgA. 5, Anti-IgG serum showing abnormal and increased IgG component. 6, Anti-IgM serum showing decreased IgM. (From Miale, J. B.: Laboratory medicine—hematology, The C. V. Mosby Co.)

the abdomen, is the most striking clinical finding. Lymphadenopathy is rare.

The leukocyte count usually is very high, and the differential count shows many immature granulocytes (metamyelocytes, myelocytes, and progranulocytes) and only a slight increase in myeloblasts. Characteristically many basophils are present, but this also may be seen in myeloproliferative syndromes. The leukocytes show reduced alkaline phosphatase activity. In myeloproliferative syndromes, alkaline phosphatase is high except when in transition to the leukemic phase. Thrombocytosis is common. The bone marrow is hypercellular and contains a proponderance of myeloid cells (Fig. 31-69).

Chronic lymphocytic leukemia

Chronic lymphocytic leukemia is usually so benign as to raise the question of whether it is a true leukemia. It is often discovered when a routine blood count is done in a person who is asymptomatic. Sometimes, usually late in the disease, there is lymphadenopathy and splenomegaly. Death is quite often due to some other disease.

The leukocyte count in the peripheral blood is moderately to strikingly elevated—from 40,000 to several hundred thousand per cubic millimeter. The differential count shows a preponderance of small lymphocytes. Characteristically, there are many "smudge" or degenerated cells. Anemia is not common and, when present, is of the acquired autoimmune type. The bone marrow shows solid sheets of small lymphocytes as the predominant cell (Fig. 31-70). The histopathology of the lymph nodes is that of a diffuse well-differentiated lymphocytic lymphoma.

Monocytic leukemias

Monocytic leukemia occurs in two basically unrelated forms. The more common, myelomonocytic leukemia (Naegeli type) is thought by some to be a variant of myelocytic leukemia, but we believe it to be a morphologic and clinical entity. Morphologically, the myelocytes and progranulocytes show a delicate, folded nucleus unlike that of a typical myeloid cell. The granules in the cytoplasm are not unusual. True *monocytic* leukemia or *histiocytic* leukemia (Schilling type) is very

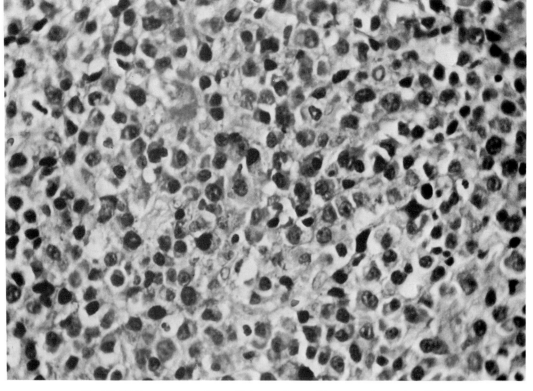

Fig. 31-72 Bone marrow in multiple myeloma. (Hematoxylin-eosin; ×250.)

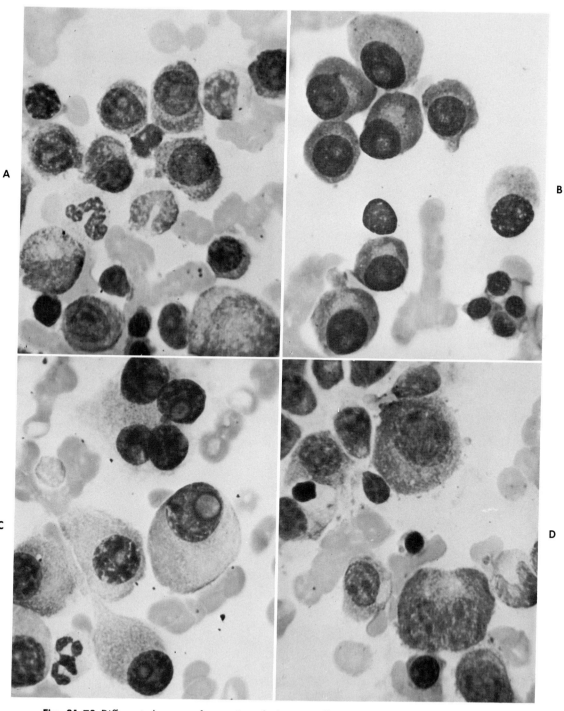

Fig. 31-73 Different degrees of maturity of plasma cells in multiple myeloma. Bone marrow smears. **A,** Most mature. **D,** Least mature. (**A** to **D,** Wright's stain; ×950; from Miale, J. B.: Laboratory medicine—hematology, The C. V. Mosby Co.)

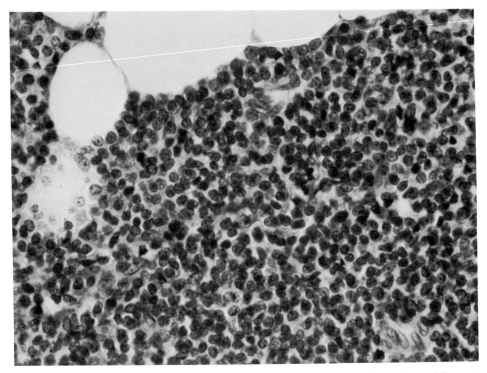

Fig. 31-74 Bone marrow infiltrated by lymphocytic lymphoma, moderately undifferentiated. (Hematoxylin-eosin; ×250; courtesy Dr. A. Rywlin.)

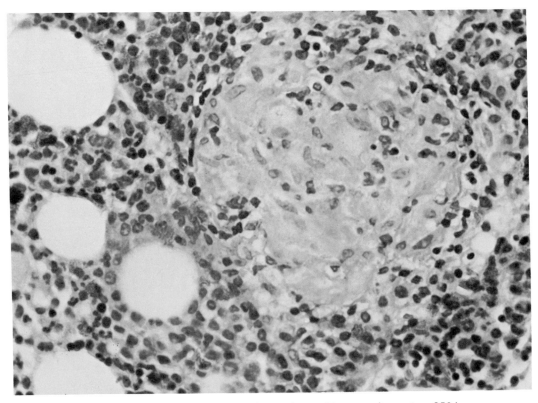

Fig. 31-75 Bone marrow in sarcoid granuloma. (Hematoxylin-eosin; ×250.)

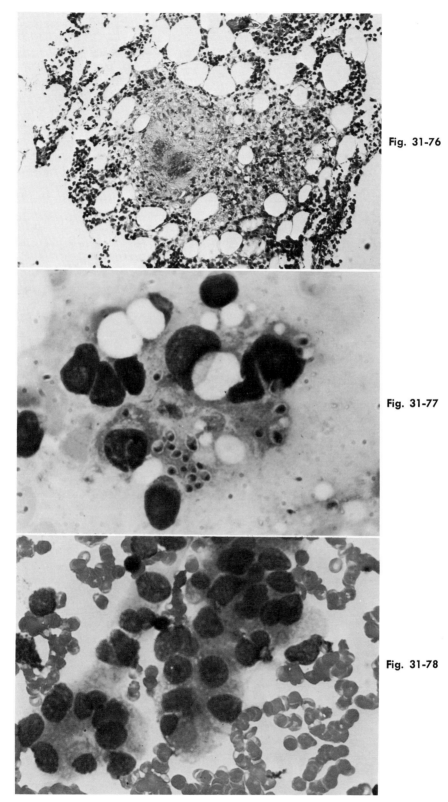

Fig. 31-76

Fig. 31-77

Fig. 31-78

Fig. 31-76 Bone marrow in miliary tuberculosis. (Hematoxylin-eosin; ×120.)
Fig. 31-77 Bone marrow in histoplasmosis. Smear. (Wright's stain; ×950.)
Fig. 31-78 Bone marrow in metastatic carcinoma of prostate. Smear. (Wright's stain; ×950.)

rare. The cells have a true monocytic nucleus, and the granules in the cytoplasm are of the pink monocytic type.

Mast cell leukemia

Mast cell leukemia is the rarest of the leukemias and was described relatively recently.[414] The leukemic cell is the tissue mast cell, and the release of histamine from these cells gives symptoms of flushing, palpitation, nausea, vomiting, and diarrhea. The clinical course is acute.

MULTIPLE MYELOMA

Myelomas are neoplasms of proliferating plasma cells. They may present as solitary tumors involving bone or other tissues, the *solitary myeloma,* or as neoplasms involving the bone marrow and other organs, *multiple myeloma.* Solitary myeloma may remain localized or may change into multiple myeloma. Multiple myeloma may show a terminal leukemic phase, *plasma cell leukemia.* Multiple myeloma can be classified either as a leukemia or a lymphoma (see also p. 1749).

Proliferation of plasma cells at extramedullary sites accounts for splenomegaly (present in about 10% of the patients) and hepatomegaly (present in about 30% of the patients). Hyperproteinemia accounts for the characteristic renal lesion, the *myeloma kidney,* consisting of tubular degeneration with proteinaceous casts. Atypical amyloid deposits (paramyloidosis) are formed by a combination of protein and polysaccharide. Proliferation of plasma cells in the bone marrow produces destruction of cortical bone. This results in pain, swelling, deformity, or pathologic fracture. Roentgenographic evidence of bone destruction can be found in about 80% of the patients, the ribs, sternum, and vertebral bodies being involved most commonly.

Abnormal protein metabolism is characteristic of multiple myeloma. The laboratory evidence for protein abnormalities is one or more of the following:

1 Hyperproteinemia
2 Hyperglobulinemia
3 Electrophoretic evidence of an abnormal protein component in the serum
4 Bence Jones protein in the urine
5 Electrophoretic evidence of an abnormal globulin component in the urine with or without Bence Jones protein
6 Cryoglobulinemia
7 Pyroglobulinemia
8 Macroglobulinemia
9 Identification and quantitation of the excess globulin by immunoelectrophoresis (Fig. 31-71)

Multiple myeloma is one of the diseases having an abnormal globulin component that, because of its relation to antibody globulin, now falls into the group called *immunoglobulins.* In addition to myeloma, there are other diseases (Waldenström's macroglobulinemia is one) in which there is an immunoglobulin abnormality. There are now five known classes of immunoglobulins: IgG, IgA, IgM, IgD, and IgE. Most commonly, multiple myeloma shows an increase in IgA or IgG, but other types have been described. Rarely, in about 1% of all patients with myelomas, there is no demonstrable immunoglobulin increase in either the serum or the urine.

Morphologically, from aspiration biopsy of the bone marrow, spleen, or a lesion identified by roentgenography, the diagnosis is made on the basis of the tissue being infiltrated by plasma cells (Fig. 31-72). These are sometimes essentially normal in appearance. Sometimes they are immature (plasmablasts) and, characteristically, have a very large pale-staining nucleolus (Fig. 31-73).

MISCELLANEOUS ABNORMALITIES

Tissue from the bone marrow may show a number of other abnormalities. These include involvement by lymphomas (Fig. 31-74), sarcoidosis (Fig. 31-75), tuberculosis (Fig. 31-76), histoplasmosis (Fig. 31-77), and metastatic tumor (Fig. 31-78). Since the morphology of these lesions is not different from that in other tissues, they are not discussed further.

REFERENCES
Reticuloendothelial system

1 Aschoff, L., and Kiyono: Folia Haemat. (Frankfurt) 15:383-390, 1913.
2 Bolande, R. P.: Cellular aspects of developmental pathology, Philadelphia, 1967, Lea & Febiger.
3 Fidalgo, B. V., and Najjar, V. A.: Biochemistry (Wash.) 6:3386-3392, 1967 (leukokinin).
4 Gabrieli, E. R., Yeostros, S. J., Doganer, Y., and Snell, F. M.: Arch. Path. (Chicago) 80:24-29, 1965.
4a Gall, E. A.: Ann. N. Y. Acad. Sci. 73:120-130, 1958.
5 Green, I.: J. Exp. Med. 128:729-751, 1968 (antibody-forming cells).
6 Halpern, B. N., Benacerraf, B., and Delafresnaye, J. F., editors: Physiopathology of the reticulo-endothelial system; a symposium organized by The Council for International Organizations of Medical Societies, Springfield, Ill., 1957, Charles C Thomas, Publisher.

7 Knutti, R. E., and Hawkins, W. B.: J. Exp. Med. 61:115-125, 1935 (Bartonella).

8 Ling, N. R.: Lymphocyte stimulation, New York, 1968, John Wiley & Sons, Inc.

9 Marshall, A. H. E.: An outline of the cytology and pathology of the reticular tissue, London, 1956, Oliver & Boyd, Ltd.

10 Miale, J. B.: Laboratory medicine—hematology, ed. 3, St. Louis, 1967, The C. V. Mosby Co.

11 Miescher, P. A., and Muller-Eberhard, H. J.: Textbook of immunopathology, vol. 1, New York, 1968, Grune & Stratton, Inc.

12 Miescher, P. A., and Muller-Eberhard, H. J.: Textbook of immunopathology, vol. 2, New York, 1969, Grune & Stratton, Inc.

13 Najjar, V. A., Robinson, J. P., Lawton, A. R., and Fidalgo, B. V.: Johns Hopkins Med. J. 120:63-77, 1967 (antibody-antigen reaction).

14 Samter, M., and Alexander, H. L.: Immunological diseases, Boston, 1965, Little, Brown and Co.

15 Trubowitz, S., and Masek, B.: Blood 32:610-628, 1968.

Spleen
Structure

16 Bjorkman, S. E.: Acta Med. Scand. suppl. 191, pp. 1-89, 1947 (splenic circulation).

17 Blaustein, A.: The spleen, New York, 1963, McGraw-Hill Book Co.

18 Boles, E. T., Baxter, C. F., and Newton, W. A., Jr.: Clin. Pediat. (Phila.) 2:161-168, 1963 (splenomegaly in childhood).

19 Foot, N. C.: Anat. Rec. 36:79-86, 1927 (reticulum of spleen).

20 Foot, N. C.: Anat. Rec. 36:91-102, 1927 (endothelium of venous sinuses).

21 Galindo, B., and Freeman, J. A.: Anat. Rec. 147:25-41, 1963 (fine structure of splenic pulp).

22 Goldberg, G. M.: Lab. Invest. 6:383-388, 1957.

23 Goldberg, G. M.: Amer. J. Clin. Path. 35:328-337, 1961.

24 Goldberg, G. M., and Saphir, O.: Amer. J. Path. 34:1123-1137, 1958 (follicular lipidosis of spleen).

25 Goldberg, G. M., and Ungar, H.: Lab. Invest. 7:146-151, 1958 (lymphatics).

26 King, J. T., Puchtler, H., and Sweat, F.: Arch. Path. (Chicago) 85:237-245, 1968 (ring fibers).

27 Knisely, M. H.: Anat. Rec. 65:23-50, 1936 (circulation).

28 Koyama, S., Aoki, S., and Deguchi, K.: Mie Med. J. 14:143-188, 1964 (splenic pulp).

29 Lillie, R. D.: Amer. J. Clin. Path. 21:484-488, 1951 (allochrome procedure).

30 McCormick, W. F., and Kashgarian, M.: Amer. J. Clin. Path. 43:332-333, 1965 (weight).

31 Marymont, J. H., Jr., and Gross, S.: Amer. J. Clin. Path. 40:58-66, 1963 (metastatic cancer).

32 Mollier, S.: Arch. Mikr. Anat. 76:608-657, 1911.

33 Palade, G. E.: J. Biophys. Biochem. Cytol. 2(suppl.):85-98, 1956 (endoplasmic reticulum).

34 Weiss, L.: Amer. J. Anat. 111:131-179, 1962 (arterial vessels).

35 Weiss, L.: Amer. J. Anat. 113:51-91, 1963 (vascular structure).

36 Wennberg, E., and Weiss, L.: Blood 31:778-790, 1968 (hemoglobin H disease).

Function

37 Argyris, B. F.: J. Exp. Med. 128:459-467, 1968 (macrophages).

38 Ashby, W. B., and Balliger, W. F., II: Arch. Surg. (Chicago) 85:913-927, 1962 (indications for splenectomy).

39 Baumgartner, L.: Yale J. Biol. Med. 6:403-434, 1934 (age and immunologic reactions).

40 Bell, W. N., and Alton, H. G.: Acta Haemat. (Basel) 13:1-7, 1955 (platelets).

41 Boveri, R. M.: Guy Hosp. Rep. 91:81-90, 1942 (Howell-Jolly bodies).

42 Cantrell, W., and Elko, E. E.: J. Infect. Dis. 116:429-438, 1966.

43 Crosby, W. H.: Blood 7:261-274, 1952 (spherocytes and leptocytes).

44 Crosby, W. H.: Blood 12:165-170, 1957 (siderocytes).

45 Crosby, W. H.: Blood 14:399-408, 1959.

46 Crosby, W. H.: Ann. Rev. Med. 13:127-146, 1962 (hypersplenism).

47 Crosby, W. H., and Estren, S.: The spleen and hypersplenism, New York, 1947, Grune & Stratton, Inc.

48 Cruchaud, A.: Lab. Invest. 19:15-24, 1968 (antibody formation).

49 Cunningham, A. J., Smith, J. B., and Mercer, E. H.: J. Exp. Med. 124:701-714, 1966 (antibody formation).

50 Fidalgo, B. V., and Najjar, V. A.: Biochemistry (Wash.) 6:3386-3392, 1967 (leukokinin).

51 Fliedner, T. M.: In Yoffey, J. M., editor: The lymphocyte in immunology and haemopoiesis, London, 1966, Edward Arnold (Publishers) Ltd.

52 Gabuzda, T. G.: Blood 27:568-579, 1966 (hemoglobin H).

53 Goldberg, G. M.: Lab. Invest. 6:383-388, 1957 (metastatic carcinoma).

54 Goldberg, G. M.: J. Anat. 92:310-314, 1958 (lymphatics).

55 Green, I.: J. Exp. Med. 128:729-751, 1968 (antibody-forming cells).

56 Halpern, B. N., Benacerraf, B., and Delafresnaye, J. F., editors: Physiopathology of the reticulo-endothelial system; a symposium organized by The Council for International Organizations of Medical Societies, Springfield, Ill., 1957, Charles C Thomas, Publisher.

57 Hayhoe, F. G. J., and Whitby, L.: Quart. J. Med. 24:365-391, 1955 (splenectomy).

58 Hummeler, K., Harris, T. N., Tomassini, N., Hechtel, M., and Farber, M. B.: J. Exp. Med. 124:255-262, 1966 (antibody-producing cells).

59 Humphrey, J. H., Parrott, D. M., and East, J.: Immunology 7:419-439, 1964 (antibody production).

60 Jandl, J. H., and Aster, R. H.: Amer. J. Med. Sci. 253:383-398, 1967 (hypersplenism).

61 Jandl, J. H., Jacob, H. S., and Daland, G. A.: New Eng. J. Med. 264:1063-1071, 1961 (hypersplenism).

62 Knutti, R. E., and Hawkins, W. B.: J. Exp. Med. **61**:115-125, 1935 (Bartonella).

63 Koyama, S., Aoki, S., and Deguchi, K.: Mie Med. J. **14**:143-188, 1964.

64 La Via, M. F., Vatter, A. E., Claman, H. N., and Brunstetter, F. H.: Lab. Invest. **18**:763-770, 1968.

65 Lipson, R. L., Bayrd, E. D., and Watkins, C. H.: Amer. J. Clin. Path. **32**:526-532, 1959 (postsplenectomy blood picture).

66 Lucas, R. V., and Krivit, W.: J. Pediat. **57**:185-191, 1960 (infection following splenectomy).

67 McKinnon, W. M. P., Boley, S. J., and Manpel, J.: Amer. J. Dis. Child. **98**:710-712, 1959 (infection following splenectomy).

68 Marshall, A. H. E.: An outline of the cytology and pathology of the reticular tissue, London, 1956, Oliver & Boyd, Ltd.

69 Miescher, P. A., and Muller-Eberhard, H. J.: Textbook of immunopathology, vol. 1, New York, 1968, Grune & Stratton, Inc.

70 Miescher, P. A., and Muller-Eberhard, H. J.: Textbook of immunopathology, vol. 2, New York, 1969, Grune & Stratton, Inc.

71 Miller, E. B., Singer, K., and Dameshek, W.: Proc. Soc. Exp. Biol. Med. **49**:42-45, 1942 (target cells).

72 Najjar, V. A., Fidalgo, B. V., and Stitt, E.: Biochemistry (Wash.) **7**:2376-2379, 1968 (leukokinin).

73 Najjar, V. A., Robinson, J. P., Lawton, A. R., and Fidalgo, B. V.: Johns Hopkins Med. J. **120**:63-77, 1967 (antibody-antigen reaction).

74 Samter, M., and Alexander, H. L.: Immunological diseases, Boston, 1965, Little, Brown and Co.

75 Saslaw, S., Bouroncle, B. A., Wall, R. L., and Doan, C. A.: New Eng. J. Med. **261**:120-125, 1959 (antibody response after splenectomy).

76 Smith, C. H., Erlandson, M., Schulman, I., and Stern, G.: Amer. J. Med. **22**:390-404, 1957 (infection after splenectomy).

77 Thurman, W. G.: Amer. J. Dis. Child. **105**:138-145, 1963 (splenectomy and immunity).

78 Von Haam, E., and Awny, A. J.: Amer. J. Clin. Path. **18**:313-322, 1948 (pathology of hypersplenism).

79 Wennberg, E., and Weiss, L.: Blood **31**:778-790, 1968 (hemoglobin H disease).

Congenital anomalies

80 Adler, N. N., and Van Slyke, E. J.: J. Pediat. **42**:471-473, 1953 (absence).

81 Aguilar, M. J., Stephens, H. B., and Crane, J. T.: Circulation **14**:520-531, 1956 (absence).

82 Bush, J. A., and Ainger, L. E.: Pediatrics **15**:93-99, 1955 (absence).

83 Evans, T. S., Spinner, S., Piccolo, P., Swirsky, M., White, R., and Kiesewetter, W.: Acta Haemat. (Basel) **10**:350-359, 1953 (accessory spleen).

84 Glen, J. E.: J. Urol. **73**:1057-1058, 1955 (accessory spleen).

85 Halpert, B., and Györkey, F.: Amer. J. Clin. Path. **32**:165-168, 1959 (accessory spleen).

86 Ivemark, B. I.: Acta Paediat. Scand. suppl. 104, pp. 1-110, 1955 (agenesis and cardiac malformations).

87 Kevy, S. V., Tefft, M., Vawter, G. F., and Rosen, F. S.: Pediatrics **42**:752-757, 1968 (hypoplasia).

88 Lucas, R. V., Jr., Neufeld, H. N., Lester, R. G., and Edwards, J. E.: Circulation **25**:973-975, 1962 (roentgen sign of asplenia).

89 Polhemus, D. W., and Schafer, W. B.: Pediatrics **9**:696-708, 1952 (absence and cardiac malformation).

90 Roberts, W. C., Berry, W. B., and Morrow, A. G.: Circulation **26**:1251-1253, 1962 (asplenia and cardiac malformation).

91 Ruttenberg, H. D., Neufeld, H. N., Lucas, R. V., Jr., Carey, L. S., Adams, P., Jr., Anderson, R. C., and Edwards, J. E.: Amer. J. Cardiol. **13**:387-406, 1964 (asplenia and cardiac malformation).

Regressive changes

92 Askanazy, M.: In Henke, F., and Lubarsch, O., editors: Handbuch der speziellen pathologischen Anatomie und Histologie, vol. 1, Berlin, 1927, Julius Springer.

93 Davis, C., Jr., Alexander, R. W., and DeYoung, H. D.: Arch. Surg. (Chicago) **86**:523-533, 1963 (rupture).

94 Husni, E. A., and Turell, D.: Arch. Surg. (Chicago) **83**:286-290, 1961 (rupture).

95 Lubitz, J. M.: Blood **4**:1168-1176, 1949 (rupture).

96 McCann, W. J.: Brit. Med. J. **1**:1271-1272, 1956 (splenosis).

97 MacDonald, R. A., and Mallory, G. K.: Arch. Intern. Med. (Chicago) **105**:686-700, 1960 (hemochromatosis).

98 Miller, D.: Blood **14**:1350-1353, 1959 (bone marrow anthracosis).

99 Slotkowski, E. L., and Hand, A. M.: Pediatrics **4**:296-300, 1949 (rupture).

100 Strassman, G. S.: Amer. J. Clin. Path. **24**:453-471, 1954 (iron deposits).

101 Waugh, R. L.: New Eng. J. Med. **234**:621-625, 1946 (splenosis).

Circulatory disturbances

102 Ball, M. J., and Silver, M. D.: Canad. Med. Ass. J. **99**:1239-1245, 1968 (arteriolosclerosis).

103 Bedford, P. D., and Lodge, B.: Gut **1**:312-320, 1960 (aneurysm).

104 Goldberg, G. M., and Saphir, O.: Arch. Path. (Chicago) **71**:222-228, 1961 (pseudoemboli).

105 Kelsey, M. P., Robertson, H. E., and Giffin, H. Z.: Surg. Gynec. Obstet. **85**:289-293, 1947 (splenic anemia).

106 Leevy, C. M., Cherrick, G. R., and Davidson, C. S.: New Eng. J. Med. **262**:397-403, 451-456, 1960 (portal hypertension).

107 Moschcowitz, E.: Medicine (Balt.) **27**:187-221, 1948 (congestive splenomegaly).

108 Rabson, S. M., and Richter, M. N.: Amer. J. Clin. Path. **37**:597-607, 1962 (multiple necroses).

109 Whipple, A. O.: Ann. Surg. **122**:449-475, 1945 (portal hypertension).

Spleen in systemic infections

110 Ash, J. E., and Spitz, S.: Pathology of tropical diseases, Philadelphia, 1945, W. B. Saunders Co.

111 Beswick, I. P.: J. Path. Bact. **70**:407-414, 1955 (glandular fever).

112 Frankel, A., Ashkari, H., Dreiling, D. A., and Kark, A. E.: J. Mount Sinai Hosp. **33**:404-413, 1966 (abscess).

113 Gordon, A. S., Handler, E. S., Siegel, C. D., Dornfest, B. S., and LoBue, J.: Ann. N. Y. Acad. Sci. **113**:766-789, 1964.

114 Harmos, O., and Myers, M. E.: Amer. J. Clin. Path. **21**:737-742, 1951 (syphilitic splenomegaly).

115 Pfischner, W. C. E., Jr., Ishak, K. G., Neptune, E. M., Jr., Fox, S. M., III, Farid, Z., and Nor el Din, G.: Amer. J. Med. **22**: 915-929, 1957 (brucellosis).

116 Rabson, S. M.: Amer. J. Clin. Path. **9**:604-614, 1939 (brucellosis).

117 Rich, A. R.: Proc. Soc. Exp. Biol. Med. **32**: 1349-1351, 1935 (splenitis).

118 Smith, E. B., and Custer, R. P.: Blood **1**:317-333, 1946 (infectious mononucleosis).

119 Watson, C. J.: Arch. Path. (Chicago) **8**:224-229, 1929 (congenital syphilis).

120 Yow, E. M., Brennan, J. C., Nathan, M. H., and Israel, L.: Ann. Intern. Med. **55**:307-313, 1961 (granuloma).

Spleen in hemolytic anemia

121 Beet, E. A.: E. Afr. Med. J. **26**:180-186, 1949 (sickle cell disease).

122 Diggs, L. W.: J.A.M.A. **104**:538-541, 1935 (sickle cell anemia).

123 Diggs, L. W., and Vorder Bruegge, C. F.: J. Nat. Med. Ass. **46**:46-49, 1954 (sickle cell disease).

124 Greig, H. B. W., and Metz, J.: S. Afr. J. Med. Sci. **22**:7-12, 1957 (thalassemia).

125 Jensen, W. N., Schoefield, R. A., and Agner, R.: Blood **12**:74-83, 1957 (hemoglobin C disease).

126 Kimmelstiel, P.: Amer. J. Med. Sci. **216**:11-19, 1948 (sickle cell disease).

127 Mukherjee, A. M., Sen Gupta, P. C., and Chatterjea, J. B.: J. Indian Med. Ass. **33**:451-459, 1959 (thalassemia).

128 Sen Gupta, P. C., Chatterjea, J. B., Mukherjee, A. M., and Chatterji, A.: Blood **16**:1039-1044, 1960 (thalassemia).

129 Smith, C. H., Schulman, I., Ando, R. E., and Stern, G.: Blood **10**:582-599, 1955 (Cooley's anemia).

130 Smith, E. W., and Conley, C. L.: Bull. Johns Hopkins Hosp. **96**:35-41, 1955 (sicklemia and flying).

131 Stock, A. E.: Ann. Intern. Med. **44**:554-556, 1956 (sicklemia and flying).

132 Watson, R. J., Lichtman, H. C., and Shapiro, H. D.: Amer. J. Med. **20**:196-206, 1956 (splenomegaly in sickle anemia).

133 Whipple, G. H., and Bradford, W. L.: J. Pediat. **9**:279-311, 1936 (Cooley's anemia).

134 Wiland, O. K., and Smith, E. B.: Amer. J. Clin. Path. **26**:619-629, 1956 (hereditary spherocytosis).

Primary tumors; metastatic tumors

135 Ahmann, D. L., Kiely, J. M., Harrison, E. G., Jr., and Payne, W. S.: Cancer **19**:461-469, 1966 (lymphoma).

136 Bauer, D. deF., and Stanford, W. R.: Arch. Path. (Chicago) **41**:668-673, 1946 (hemangiosarcoma).

137 Pratt-Thomas, H. R., and Switzer, P. K.: Arch. Path. (Chicago) **49**:159-162, 1950 (cyst).

138 Snyder, J. W., and Rezek, P. R.: Southern Med. J. **36**:263-268, 1943 (cyst).

139 Tasker, R. G.: J. Clin. Path. **11**:142-145, 1958 (hemangioendothelioma).

140 Weinstein, M., Roberts, M., Reynolds, B., and Marshall, P.: Ann. Surg. **148**:851-854, 1958 (dermoid cyst).

141 Willis, R. A.: Med. J. Aust. **2**:258-265, 1941 (metastases).

Spleen in autoimmune disease

142 Bowman, H. E., Pettit, V. D., Caldwell, F. T., and Smith, E. B.: Lab Invest. **4**:206-216, 1955 (thrombocytopenic purpura).

143 Craig, J. M., and Gitlin, D.: Amer. J. Path. **33**:251-265, 1957 (thrombocytopenic purpura).

144 Crawford, T., and Woolf, N.: J. Path. Bact. **79**:221-225, 1960 (arteriosclerosis).

145 Klemperer, P., Pollack, A. D., and Baehr, G.: Arch. Path. (Chicago) **32**:569-631, 1941 (lupus erythematosus).

146 Moore, R. D., and Schoenberg, M. D.: Blood **15**:511-516, 1960 (thrombocytopenic purpura).

147 Nickerson, D. A., and Sunderland, D. A.: Amer. J. Path. **13**:463-489, 1937 (thrombocytopenic purpura).

Spleen in reticuloendothelioses

148 Balint, J. A., Nyhan, W. L., Lietman, P., and Turner, D. A.: J. Lab. Clin. Med. **58**:548-558, 1961 (Niemann-Pick disease).

149 Burdick, C. O.: Arch. Path. (Chicago) **79**: 583-587, 1965 (lipidosis).

150 Crocker, A. C., and Farber, S.: Medicine (Balt.) **37**:1-95, 1958 (Niemann-Pick disease).

151 Dollberg, L., Casper, J., Djaldetti, M., Klibansky, C., and De Vries, A.: Amer. J. Clin. Path. **43**:16-25, 1965 (thrombocytopenic purpura).

152 Fleischmajer, R.: The dyslipidoses, Springfield, Ill. 1960, Charles C Thomas, Publisher.

153 Foot, N. C., and Olcott, C. T.: Amer. J. Path. **10**:81-95, 1934 (nonlipoid histiocytosis).

154 Franklin, S. M.: Proc. Roy. Soc. Med. **30**:711, 1937 (lipemia).

155 Harslöf, E.: Acta Med. Scand. **130**:140-155, 1948 (familial hyperlipemia).

156 Hill, J. M., Speer, R. J., and Gedikoglu, H.: Amer. J. Clin. Path. **39**:607-615, 1963 (secondary lipidosis).

157 Medoff, A. S., and Bayrd, E. D.: Ann. Intern. Med. **40**:481-492, 1954 (Gaucher's disease).

158 Oberman, H. A.: Pediatrics **28**:307-327, 1961 (eosinophilic granuloma).

159 Pick, L.: Amer. J. Med. Sci. **185**:601-616, 1933 (xanthomatosis).

160 Schettler, G., editor: Lipids and lipidoses, New York, 1967, Springer-Verlag.

161 Terry, R. D., Sperry, W. M., and Brodoff, B.: Amer. J. Path. **30**:263-285, 1954 (adult lipidosis).

162 Uzman, L. L.: Arch. Path. (Chicago) **51**:329-339, 1951 (Gaucher's disease).
163 Uzman, L. L.: Arch. Path. (Chicago) **65**:331-339, 1958 (lipidoses).
164 Varga, C., Richter, M. N., and DeSanctis, A. G.: Amer. J. Dis. Child. **75**:376-384, 1948 (Letterer-Siwe disease).
165 Warren, S., and Root, H. F.: Amer. J. Path. **2**:69-80, 1926 (lipemia).
166 Wiland, O. K., and Smith, E. B.: Arch. Path. (Chicago) **64**:623-628, 1957 (lipid globules).

Lymph nodes
Structure; function

167 Berman, L.: Blood **21**:246-249, 1963 ("immunocytes").
168 Bernhard, W., and Leplus, R.: Fine structure of the normal and malignant human lymph node, New York, 1964, The Macmillan Co.
169 Bierring, F.: Acta Anat. (Basel) **55**:9-15, 1963 (lymphocyte content of bone marrow).
170 Billingham, R. E., and Silvers, W. K.: In Defendi, V., and Metcalf, D., editors: The thymus, Wistar Institute Symposium Monograph No. 2, Philadelphia, 1964, Wistar Institute Press, pp. 41-51, (some biological differences between thymocytes and lymphoid cells).
171 Brody, J. I., and Beizer, L. H.: Ann. Intern. Med. **64**:1237-1245, 1966 (leukemia).
172 Burnet, F. M.: Aust. Ann. Med. **11**:79-91, 1962 (thymus and immunity).
173 Cardozo, P. L.: Acta Cytol. (Balt.) **8**:194-205, 1964 (cytologic diagnosis of lymph node).
174 Cronkite, E. P., Jansen, C. R., Cottier, H., Rai, K., and Sipe, C. R.: Ann. N. Y. Acad. Sci. **113**:566-577, 1964 (lymphocyte production).
175 Daniels, J. C., Ritzman, S. E., and Levin, W. C.: Texas Rep. Biol. Med. **26**:5-93, 1968 (lymphocytes—review).
176 Drinker, C. K., and Yoffey, J. M.: Lymphatics, lymph, and lymphoid tissue, Cambridge, Mass., 1941, Harvard University Press.
177 Elves, M. W.: The lymphocytes, London, 1966, Lloyd-Luke (Medical Books) Ltd.
178 Everett, N. B., Caffrey, R. W., and Ricke, W. O.: Ann. N. Y. Acad. Sci. **113**:887-897, 1964 (recirculation of lymphocytes).
179 Fisher, B., and Fisher, E. R.: Cancer **20**:1907-1913, 1914-1919, 1967 (barrier function of lymph node).
180 Ford, C. E., and Micklem, H. S.: Lancet **1**:359-362, 1963 (radiation).
181 Gall, E. A.: Ann. N. Y. Acad. Sci. **73**:120-130, 1958 (mesenchymal cells of lymphoid tissue).
182 Gowans, J. L.: Brit. Med. Bull. **21**:106-110, 1965 (lymphocytes in destruction of homographs).
183 Hall, J. G., and Morris, B.: Lancet **1**:1077-1080, 1964 (radiation).
184 Holman, R. L.: Southern Med. J. **48**:1311-1317, 1955 (structure and function of lymph nodes).
185 Lucas, P. F.: Postgrad. Med. J. **30**:544-548, 1954 (lymph node aspiration).
186 Lucas, P. F.: Blood **10**:1030-1054, 1955 (lymph node smears).

187 Maximow, A. A., and Bloom, W.: A textbook of histology, ed. 6, Philadelphia, 1952, W. B. Saunders Company.
188 Millikin, P. D.: Arch. Path. (Chicago) **82**:499-505, 1966 (germinal centers).
189 Moore, R. D., and Reagen, J. W.: Cancer **6**:606-618, 1953 (lymph node imprints).
190 Morrison, M., Samwick, A. A., Rubinstein, J., Stich, M., and Loewe, L.: Amer. J. Clin. Path. **22**:255-262, 1952 (lymph node aspiration).
191 Nossal, G. J. V.: Ann. N. Y. Acad. Sci. **120**:171-181, 1964 (lymphocytes from thymus).
192 Nossal, G. J. V., Austin, C. M., Pye, J., and Mitchell, J.: Int. Arch. Allerg. **29**:368-383, 1966 (antigens in spleen).
193 Osgood, E. E.: Blood **9**:1141-1154, 1954 (hemic cells).
194 Pavlovsky, A.: Acta Haemat. (Basel) **36**:296-312, 1966 (cytology).
195 Sarles, H. E., Smith, G. H., Fish, J. C., and Remmers, A. R., Jr.: Texas Rep. Biol. Med. **25**:573-583, 1967 (lymph diversion).
196 Söderström, N.: Scand. J. Haemat. **5**:138-152, 1968 (lymphoglandular bodies).
197 Stich, M. H.: Amer. J. Med. Sci. **243**:1-12, 1962 (lymph node aspiration).
198 Turk, J. L., and Stone, S. H.: In Amos, B., and Koprowski, H.: Cell-bound antibodies, Philadelphia, 1963, Wistar Institute Press (implications of cellular changes in lymph nodes during development and inhibition of delayed type hypersensitivity).
199 Ultmann, J. E., Koprowska, I., and Engle, R. L., Jr.: Cancer **11**:507-524, 1958 (lymph node imprints).
200 Yoffey, J. M.: Ann. Rev. Med. **15**:125-148, 1964 (lymphocyte).
201 Yoffey, J. M., and Courtice, F. C.: Lymphatics, lymph and lymphoid tissue, Cambridge, Mass., 1956, Harvard University Press.
202 Zacharski, L. R., Hill, R. W., and Maldonado, J. E.: Mayo Clin. Proc. **42**:431-451, 1967 (lymphocyte).

Lymphadenitis

203 Black, M. M., and Speer, F. D.: Surg. Gynec. Obstet. **110**:477-487, 1960 (cancer).
204 Cummer, C. L.: Amer. J. Syph. **12**:13-40, 1928 (syphilis).
205 Debré, R., and Job, J.-C.: Acta Paediat. Scand. **43**(suppl. 96):1-86, 1954.
206 Evans, N.: Arch. Path. (Chicago) **37**:175-179, 1944 (syphilis).
207 Fox, R. A., and Rosahn, P. D.: Amer. J. Path. **19**:73-99, 1943 (lupus erythematosus).
208 Gall, E. A., and Stout, H. A.: Amer. J. Path. **16**:433-448, 1940 (infectious mononucleosis).
209 Hurwitt, E. S.: J. Invest. Derm. **5**:197-204, 1942 (dermatopathic lymphadenitis).
210 Kalter, S. S.: Ann. Intern. Med. **55**:903-910, 1961 (cat-scratch disease).
211 Manning, J. D., and Reid, J. D.: Amer. J. Clin. Path. **29**:430-432, 1958 (cat-scratch disease).
212 Meleney, H. E.: Amer. J. Trop. Med. **20**:603-616, 1940 (histoplasmosis).
213 Moore, R. D., Weisberger, A. S., and Bower-

find, E. S., Jr.: Arch. Intern. Med. (Chicago) **99**:751-759, 1957 (lymphadenopathy).

214 Naji, A. F., Carbonell, F., and Barker, H. J.: Amer. J. Clin. Path. **38**:513-521, 1962 (cat-scratch disease).

215 Rabson, S. M.: Amer. J. Clin. Path. **9**:604-614, 1939 (brucellosis).

216 Randerath, E.: Virchow Arch. Path. Anat. **312**:165, 1944 (tularemia).

217 Ravel, R.: Amer. J. Clin. Path. **46**:335-340, 1966 (lymphangiography).

218 Saxén, E., and Saxén, L.: Lab. Invest. **8**:386-394, 1959 (toxoplasmosis).

219 Towers, R. P.: J. Clin. Path. **10**:175-177, 1957 (polyvinylpyrrolidone).

220 Warwick, W. J.: Lab. Anim. Care **14**:420-432, 1964 (cat-scratch disease).

221 Warwick, W. J., and Good, R. A.: Amer. J. Dis. Child. **100**:241-247, 1960 (cat-scratch disease).

222 Winship, T.: Amer. J. Clin. Path. **23**:1012-1018, 1953 (cat-scratch disease).

**Pseudolymphomatous lymphadenitis;
benign hamartomatous lymphoid masses**

223 Bajoghli, M.: Pediatrics **28**:943-945, 1961.

224 Best, W. R., and Paul, J. T.: Amer. J. Med. **8**:124-130, 1950.

225 Bodart, F.: Wien. Z. Inn. Med. **34**:375-379, 1953.

226 Braverman, I. M., and Levin, J.: Amer. J. Med. **35**:418-422, 1963 (Dilantin).

227 Canale, V. C., and Smith, C. H.: J. Pediat. **70**:891-899, 1967.

228 Castleman, B., and Towne, V. W.: New Eng. J. Med. **250**:26-30, 1954.

229 Gropper, A. L.: New Eng. J. Med. **254**:522-523, 1956 (diphenylhydantoin).

230 Hartsock, R. J.: Cancer **21**:632-649, 1968 (postvaccinal lymphadenitis).

231 Hartsock, R. J., and Bellanti, J. A.: Fed. Proc. **25**:534, 1966 (postvaccinal lymphadenitis).

232 Hyman, G. A., and Sommers, S. C.: Blood **28**:416-427, 1966.

233 Lattes, R., and Pachter, M. R.: Cancer **15**:197-214, 1962 (hamartoma).

234 LeVan, P., and Bierman, S. M.: Arch. Derm. (Chicago) **86**:254-256, 1962 (Dilantin).

235 Lindqvist, T.: Acta Med. Scand. **158**:131-138, 1957 (Mesantoin).

236 Lukes, R. J., Butler, J. J., and Hicks, B. B.: Cancer **19**:317-344, 1966 (Hodgkin's disease).

237 Peremans, J. M., and Nijs, P. H. J:. Acta Clin. Belg. **20**:425-430, 1965 (hyperplasia).

238 Rappaport, H.: In Atlas of tumor pathology, Sec. III, Fasc. 8, Washington, D. C., 1966, Armed Forces Institute of Pathology, (tumors of hematopoietic system).

239 Ringertz, N., and Adamson, C. A.: Acta Path. Microbiol. Scand. suppl. 86, pp. 1-69, 1950 (antigens).

240 Rosai, J., and Dorfman, R. F.: Arch. Path. (Chicago) **87**:63-70, 1969 (sinus histiocytosis).

241 Rosenfeld, S., Swiller, A. I., Shenoy, Y. M., and Morrison, A. N.: J.A.M.A. **176**:491-493, 1961 (diphenylhydantoin).

242 Saltzstein, S. L., and Ackerman, L. V.: Cancer **12**:164-182, 1959 (lymphadenopathy from anticonvulsive drugs).

243 Saltzstein, S. L., Jaudon, J. C., Luse, S. A., and Ackerman, L. V.: J.A.M.A. **167**:1618-1620, 1958 (ethotoin).

244 Schreiber, M. M., and McGregor, J. G.: Arch. Derm. (Chicago) **97**:297-300, 1968 (anticonvulsant drugs).

245 Steinberg, S. H.: Med. Ann. D. C. **22**:600-603, 638, 1953 (hydantoin).

Metastatic neoplasms

246 Bennett, W. A., and Carr, D. T.: Amer. Rev. Tuberc. **76**:503-505, 1957 (scalene lymphadenopathy).

247 Downs, A. R., and McMorris, L. S.: Canad. J. Surg. **2**:276-278, 1959 (scalene node biopsy).

248 Gondos, B., and Reingold, I. M.: J. Thorac. Cardiovasc. Surg. **47**:430-437, 1964 (scalene nodes).

249 Gondos, B., and Reingold, I. M.: Cancer **18**:84-88, 1965 (scalene nodes).

250 Hoffman, L., Cohn, J. E., and Gaensler, E. A.: New Eng. J. Med. **267**:577-589, 1962 (eosinophilic granuloma).

251 Lillington, G. A., and Jamplis, R. W.: Ann. Intern. Med. **59**:101-110, 1963 (scalene nodes).

252 Maloney, J. V., Jr., Franks, R., Makoff, D., and Sherman, P. H.: J. Thorac. Cardiovasc. Surg. **47**:438-445, 1964 (scalene nodes).

253 Mazur, B. K., and Brinkman, G. L.: Henry Ford Hosp. Med. Bull. **10**:433-438, 1962 (scalene nodes).

254 Moertel, C. G., Woolner, L. B., and Bernatz, P. E.: Proc. Mayo Clin. **34**:152-157, 1959 (pulmonary alveolar proteinosis).

255 Moore, R. D., Weisberger, A. S., and Bowerfind, E. S., Jr.: Arch. Intern. Med. (Chicago) **99**:751-759, 1957 (lymphadenopathy in systemic disease).

256 Morgan, S. W., and Scott, S. M.: J. Thorac. Cardiovasc. Surg. **43**:548-551, 1962 (scalene biopsy).

257 Nadeau, P. J., Ellis, F. H., Jr., Harrison, E. G., Jr., and Fontana, R. S.: Dis. Chest **37**:325-339, 1960 (histiocytosis X).

258 Onuigbo, W. I. B.: Thorax **17**:201-204, 1962 (cervical node metastases).

259 Ten Seldam, R. E. J.: Med. J. Aust. **1**:916-919, 1956 (sarcoid-like lesions).

260 Umiker, W. O.: Dis. Chest. **37**:82-90, 1960 (scalene node biopsy).

261 Wolf, P. L., Lewis, B., and McCormick, G. R.: Arch. Intern. Med. (Chicago) **112**:397-400, 1963 (scalene node "sarcoidosis").

Primary neoplasms
Nonlymphomatous

262 Dutz, W., and Stout, A. P.: Cancer **13**:684-694, 1960 (Kaposi's sarcoma).

263 Ecklund, R. E., and Valaitis, J.: Arch. Path. (Chicago) **74**:224-229, 1962 (Kaposi's sarcoma).

264 Lazarus, J. A., and Marks, M. S.: Amer. J. Surg. **71**:479-490, 1946 (endotheliomas).

265 Lee, S. C. H., and Moore, O. S.: Arch. Path. (Chicago) **80**:651-654, 1965 (Kaposi's sarcoma).

266 Melnick, P. J.: Arch. Path. (Chicago) **20**: 760-766, 1935 (angiosarcomatosis).

Lymphoma

267 Aisenberg, A. C.: New Eng. J. Med. **270**: 508-514, 565-570, 617-622, 1964 (Hodgkin's disease).

268 Aisenberg, A. C.: Cancer **19**:385-394, 1966 (Hodgkin's disease).

269 Aisenberg, A. C., and Leskowitz, S.: New Eng. J. Med. **282**:1269-1272, 1963 (Hodgkin's disease).

270 Anderson, R. E., and Ishida, K.: Ann. Intern. Med. **61**:853-862, 1964 (lymphoma in survivors of atomic bomb).

271 Andrial, M.: Oncologia (Basel) **15**:3-17, 1962 (leukemia).

272 Baumgarten, A., Curtain, C. C., and Whiteside, M. G.: Aust. Ann. Med. **14**:125-129, 1965 (cryomacroglobulins in lymphoma).

273 Berman, L.: Blood **8**:195-210, 1953 (classification).

274 Bierman, H. R., Marshall, G. J., and Winer, M. L.: J.A.M.A. **186**:185-192, 1963 (lymphoma).

275 Blaylock, W. K., Clendenning, W. E., Carbone, P. P., and Van Scott, E. J.: Cancer **19**:233-236, 1966 (mycosis fungoides).

276 Blumenberg, R. M., Olson, K. B., Stein, A. A., and Hawkins, T. L.: Amer. J. Med. **35**:832-841, 1963 (giant follicle lymphoma).

277 Bryan, W. R.: Cancer Res. **27**:2507-2509, 1967 (Burkitt's tumor).

278 Burkitt, D.: Brit. J. Surg. **46**:218-223, 1958.

279 Burkitt, D., and O'Conor, G. T.: Cancer **14**: 258-269, 1961 (African lymphoma).

280 Burkitt, D., Hutt, M. S., and Wright, D. H.: Cancer **18**:399-410, 1965 (African lymphoma).

281 Casazza, A. R., Duvall, C. P., and Carbone, P. P.: J.A.M.A. **197**:710-716, 1966 (infection).

282 Cook, J. C., Krabbenhoft, K. L., and Leucutia, T.: Amer. J. Roentgen. **84**:656-665, 1960 (radiation therapy).

283 Craig, L., and Seidman, H.: Blood **17**:319-327, 1961 (mortality).

284 Custer, R. P., and Bernhard, W. G.: Amer. J. Med. Sci. **216**:625-642, 1948 (Hodgkin's disease).

285 Dent, P. B., Gabrielsen, A. E., Cooper, M. D., Peterson, R. D. A., and Good, R. A.: In Miescher, P. A., and Muller-Eberhard, H. J.: Textbook of immunopathology, vol. II, New York, 1969, Grune & Stratton, Inc., (secondary immunologic deficiency diseases associated with lymphoproliferative disorders).

286 Desai, P. B., Meher-Homji, D. R., and Paymaster, J. C.: Cancer **18**:25-33, 1965.

287 Dorfman, R. F.: Cancer **18**:418-430, 1965 (childhood lymphosarcoma).

288 Firat, D., Stutzman, L., Studenski, E. R., and Pickren, J.: Amer. J. Med. **39**:252-259, 1965 (follicular lymphoma).

289 Franssila, K. O., Kalima, T. V., and Voutlainen, A.: Cancer **20**:1594-1601, 1967 (Hodgkin's disease).

290 Gall, E. A.: Ann. N. Y. Acad. Sci. **73**:120-130, 1958 (mesenchymal cells).

291 Gall, E. A., and Mallory, T. B.: Amer. J. Path. **18**:381-429, 1942.

292 Goldberg, G. M., and Emanuel, B.: Cancer **17**:277-287, 1964.

293 Goldman, J. M., and Hobbs, J. R.: Immunology **13**:421-431, 1967 (Hodgkin's disease).

294 Hanson, T. A. S.: Cancer **17**:1595-1603, 1964 (Hodgkin's disease).

295 Hauswirth, L., Rosenow, G., and Lansman, W.: Acta Haemat. (Basel) **1**:45-54, 1948 (lymphosarcoma cell leukemia).

296 Heath, C. W., Jr.: Cancer Res. **27**:2439-2440, 1967 (Burkitt's tumor).

297 Hersh, E. M., Bodey, G. P., Nies, B. A., and Freireich, E. J.: J.A.M.A. **193**:105-109, 1965 (acute leukemia).

298 Hurst, D. W., and Meyer, O. O.: Cancer **14**: 753-778, 1961 (follicular lymphoma).

299 Hutter, R. V. P., and Collins, H. S.: Lab. Invest. **11**:1035-1045, 1962 (fungus infections in cancer).

300 Hutter, R. V. P., Lieberman, P. H., and Collins, H. S.: Cancer **17**:747-756, 1964 (aspergillosis in cancer).

301 Irving, W. R., Jr., Maré, A., and Miale, J. B.: Southern Med. J. **58**:891-895, 1965 (infections).

302 Jackson, H., Jr., and Parker, F., Jr.: New Eng. J. Med. **231**:35-44, 1944 (Hodgkin's disease).

303 Jackson, H., Jr., and Parker, F., Jr.: Hodgkin's disease and allied disorders, New York, 1947, Oxford University Press.

304 James, A. H.: Quart. J. Med. **29**:47-66, 1960 (Hodgkin's disease).

305 James, D. G., Sharma, O. P., and Bradstreet, P.: Lancet **2**:1274-1275, 1967 (Kveim-Siltzbach test).

306 Klein, G., Klein, E., and Clifford, P.: Cancer Res. **27**:2510-2520, 1967 (Burkitt's tumor).

307 Lukes, R. J.: Amer. J. Roentgen. **90**:944-955, 1963 (Hodgkin's disease).

308 Lukes, R. J., and Butler, J. J.: Cancer Res. **26**:1063-1083, 1966 (Hodgkin's disease).

309 Lukes, R. J., Butler, J. J., and Hicks, E. B.: Cancer **19**:317-344, 1966 (Hodgkin's disease).

310 MacMahon, B.: Cancer **21**:558-561, 1968 (Burkitt's tumor).

311 Meighan, S. S., and Ramsay, J. D.: Brit. J. Cancer **17**:24-36, 1963 (Hodgkin's disease).

312 Metcalf, D.: Med. J. Aust. **1**:225-230, 1965 (thymus in carcinogenesis).

313 Miller, D. G.: Cancer **20**:579-588, 1967.

314 O'Conor, G. T.: Cancer **14**:270-283, 1961 (African lymphoma).

315 O'Conor, G. T.: Cancer Res. **23**:1514-1518, 1963 (African lymphoma).

316 Oettgen, H. F., Aoki, T., Geering, G., Boyse, E. A., and Old, L. J.: Cancer Res. **27**:2532-2534, 1967 (Burkitt's lymphoma).

317 Pavlovsky, A.: Acta Haemat. (Basel) **36**:296-312, 1966 (cytology).

318 Peters, M. V., Alison, R., and Bush, R. S.: Cancer **19**:308-316, 1966 (Hodgkin's disease).

319 Peterson, R. D. A., Cooper, M. D., and Good, R. A.: Amer. J. Med. **38**:579-604, 1965 (immunologic deficiency).

320 Rappaport, H., Winter, W. J., and Hicks, E. B.: Cancer **9**:792-821, 1956 (follicular lymphoma).

321 Rappaport, H., Wright, D. H., and Dorfman, R. F.: Cancer Res. **27:**2632, 1967 (Burkitt's tumor).
322 Rosenberg, S. A.: Cancer Chemother. Rep. 52:213-228, 1968 (lymphangiography).
323 Solowey, A. C., and Rapaport, F. T.: Surg. Gynec. Obstet **121:**756-760, 1965 (immunology).
324 Spiers, A. S. D., and Baikie, A. G.: Lancet **1:** 506-509, 1966 (cytology).
325 Ultmann, J. E.: Cancer **19:**297-307, 1966 (Hodgkin's disease).
326 Ultmann, J. E., Fish, W., Osserman, E., and Gellhorn, A.: Ann. Intern. Med. **51:**501-516, 1959 (hypogammaglobulinemia).
327 Wright, D. H.: Cancer Res. **27:**2424-2438, 1967 (Burkitt's tumor).
328 Zeffren, J. L., and Ultmann, J. E.: Blood **15:** 277-284, 1960 (reticulum cell sarcoma).

Bone marrow
Structure and function

329 Brånemark, P.-I.: Angiology **12:**293-306, 1961 (microcirculation).
330 Calvo, W.: Amer. J. Anat. **123:**315-328, 1968 (innervation).
331 Edwards, C. L., Andrews, G. A., Sitterson, B. W., and Kniseley, R. M.: Blood **23:**741-756, 1964 (scanning).
332 Ellis, R. E.: Phys. Med. Biol. **5:**255-258, 1961 (distribution).
333 Harrison, W. J.: J. Clin. Path. **15:**254-259, 1962 (total cellularity).
334 Haschen, R. J.: Acta Haemat. (Basel) **16:**235-246, 1956.
335 Hudson, G.: Brit. J. Haemat. **11:**446-452, 1965 (volume).
336 Petrakis, N. L., Masouredis, S. P., and Miller, P.: J. Clin. Invest. **32:**952-963, 1953 (blood flow).
337 Rohr, K. L.: Das menschliche Knochenmark: seine Anatomie, Physiologie und Pathologie nach Ergebnissen der intravitalen Markpunktion, Stuttgart, 1949, Georg Thieme Verlag.
338 Russell, W. J., Yoshinaga, H., Antoku, S., and Mizuno, M.: Brit. J. Radiol. **39:**735-739, 1966 (distribution).
339 Trubowitz, S., Strauss, H., and Small, M. J.: J. Nucl. Med. **5:**864-870, 1964 (circulation).
340 Van Dyke, D.: Clin. Orthop. **52:**37-51, 1967 (blood flow).
341 Van Dyke, D., Anger, H. O., Yano, Y., and Bozzini, C.: Amer. J. Physiol. **209:**65-70, 1965 (blood flow).
342 Weiss, L.: J. Morph. **117:**467-537, 1965 (structure).
343 Weiss, L.: Clin. Orthop. **52:**13-23, 1967 (histophysiology).
344 Yoffey, J. M.: J. Anat. **96:**425, 1962 (arteries).
345 Zamboni, L., and Pease, D. C.: J. Ultrastruct. Res. **5:**65-85, 1961 (vascular bed).

Methods of study

346 Agress, H.: Amer. J. Clin. Path. **27:**282-299, 1957.
347 Astaldi, G., Lacroix, G., and Sacchetti, C.: Minerva Medicoleg. **70:**144-146, 1950.
348 Berenbaum, M. C.: J. Clin. Path. **9:**381-383, 1956.

349 Berman, L., and Axelrod, A. R.: Amer. J. Clin. Path. **17:**61-66, 1947 (aspiration).
350 Hoffman, S. B., Morrow, G. W., Jr., Pease, G. L., and Stroebel, C. F.: Amer. J. Clin. Path. **41:**281-286, 1964 (autolysis).
351 Krumbhaar, E. B.: Ann. Med. Hist. **8:**232-235, 1936.
352 Rickert, R. R., and Vidone, R. A.: Blood **31:** 74-80, 1968.
353 Rohr, K., and Hafter, E.: Folia Haemat. (Leipzig) **58:**38-50, 1937.

Hypoplasia, aplasia, and hyperplasia

354 Arakawa, E. T.: New Eng. J. Med. **263:**488-493, 1960 (atomic bomb survivors).
355 Diggs, L. W., and Hewlett, J. S.: Blood **3:** 1090-1104, 1948 (purpura).
356 Edwards, C. L., Andrews, G. A., Sitterson, B. W., and Kniseley, R. M.: Blood **23:**741-756, 1964 (scanning).
357 Erslev, A. J.: Clin. Orthop. **52:**25-36, 1967 (blood formation).
358 Ervin, F. R., Glazier, J. B., Aronow, S., Nathan, D., Coleman, R., Avery, N., Shohet, S., and Leeman, C.: New Eng. J. Med. **266:** 1127-1137, 1962 (atomic radiation).
359 Evans, T. C.: Radiol. Clin. N. Amer. **3:**219-226, 1965 (radiation).
360 Harrison, W. J.: J. Clin. Path. **15:**254-259, 1962 (cellularity).
361 Heck, F. J.: Med. Clin. N. Amer. **40:**1077-1090, 1956 (drugs).
362 Hudson, G.: Brit. J. Haemat. **11:**446-452, 1965 (volume).
363 Lange, R. D., Wright, S. W., Tomonaga, M., Kurasaki, H., Matsuoke, S., and Matsunaga, H.: Blood **10:**312-324, 1955 (atomic radiation).
364 McCurdy, P. R.: J.A.M.A. **176:**588-593, 1961 (chloramphenicol).
365 Van Dyke, D., and Anger, H. O.: J. Nucl. Med. **6:**109-120, 1965.
366 Van Swaay, H.: Lancet **2:**225-227, 1955 (irradiation).
367 Wald, N., Thoma, G. E., Jr. and Broun, G. O., Jr.: Progr. Hemat. **3:**1-52, 1962 (hematologic manifestations of radiation exposure in man).
268 Worobec, T.: Dis. Chest **47:**208-217, 1965 (chemotherapy).

Myeloproliferative syndromes

369 Abildgaard, C. F., Cornet, J. A., and Schulman, I.: J. Pediat. **63:**1072-1080, 1963 (erythrocytes).
370 Bouroncle, B. A., and Doan, C. A.: Amer. J. Med. Sci. **243:**697-715, 1962 (myelofibrosis).
371 Brody, J. I., Beizer, L. H., and Schwartz, S.: Amer. J. Med. **36:**315-319, 1964 (myeloma).
372 Calabresi, P.: Blood **13:**642-651, 1958 (leukemia).
373 Chen, H. P., and Walz, D. V.: Amer. J. Clin. Path. **29:**345-349, 1958 (leukemoid reaction).
374 Dameshek, W.: Blood **6:**372-375, 1951.
375 Dameshek, W., and Baldini, M.: Blood **13:** 192-194, 1958 (Di Guglielmo syndrome).
376 Engel, A. G., and Stickney, J. M.: Arch. Intern. Med. (Chicago) **109:**168-175, 1962 (polycythemia vera).

377 Forsberg, S. A.: Acta Med. Scand. **171:**209-221, 1962 (polycythemia vera).

378 Hansen-Pruss, O. C., and Goodman, E. G.: N. Carolina Med. J. **4:**254-258, 1943 (polycythemia vera).

379 Heller, E. L., Lewisohn, M. G., and Palin, W. E.: Amer. J. Path. **23:**327-365, 1947 (aleukemia myelosis).

380 Hutt, M. S. R., Pinniger, J. L., and Wetherley-Mein, G.: Blood **8:**295-314, 1953 (myelofibrosis).

381 Lobdell, D. H., and Europa, D. L.: Lab. Invest. **11:**58-64, 1962 (megakaryocytes).

382 Lopas, H., and Josephson, A. M.: Arch. Intern. Med. (Chicago) **114:**754-759, 1964 (polycythemia vera).

383 Martin, W. J., and Bayrd, E. D.: Blood **9:**321-339, 1954 (erythroleukemia).

384 Merskey, C.: Clin. Proc. **8:**150-162, 1949 (polycythemia and leukemia).

385 Mitus, W. J., Mednicoff, I. B., and Dameshek, W.: New Eng. J. Med. **260:**1131-1133, 1959 (phosphatase).

386 Mitus, W. J., Bergna, L. J., Mednicoff, I. B., and Dameshek, W.: Amer. J. Clin. Path. **30:**285-294, 1958 (phosphatase).

387 Pitcock, J. A., Reinhard, E. H., Justus, B. W., and Mendelsohn, R. S.: Ann. Intern. Med. **57:**73-84, 1962

388 Rado, J. P., and Hammer, S.: Blood **14:**1143-1150, 1959 (polycythemia vera).

389 Randall, D. L., Reiquam, C. W., Githens, J. H., and Robinson, A.: Amer. J. Dis. Child. **110:**479-500, 1965 (familial myeloproliferative disease).

390 Roath, S., and Israëls, M. C. G.: Lancet **2:**1140-1143, 1962 (erythremic myelosis).

391 Sandberg, A. A., Ishihara, T., Crosswhite, L., H., and Hauschka, T. S.: Blood **20:**393-423, 1962 (chromosomes).

392 Scott, R. B., Ellison, R. R., and Ley, A. B.: Amer. J. Med. **37:**162-171, 1964 (Di Guglielmo's syndrome).

393 Spaet, T. H., Bauer, S., and Melamed, S.: Arch. Intern. Med. (Chicago) **98:**377-383, 1956 (thrombocythemia).

394 Spickard, A.: Bull. Johns Hopkins Hosp. **107:**234-240, 1960 (myeloma).

395 Upton, A. C., and Furth, J.: Acta Haemat. (Basel) **13:**65-76, 1955 (in mice).

396 Zarafonetis, C. J. D., Overman, R. L., and Molthan, L.: Blood **12:**1011-1015, 1957.

Leukemia

397 Adams, A., Fitzgerald, P. H., and Gunz, F. W.: Brit. Med. J. **2:**1474-1476, 1961 (chromosome abnormality).

398 Ager, E. A., Schuman, L. M., Wallace, H. M., Rosenfield, A. B., and Gullen, W. H.: J. Chronic Dis. **18:**113-132, 1965 (childhood).

399 Anderson, R. C.: Amer. J. Dis. Child. **81:**313-322, 1951 (familial).

400 Anderson, R. C., and Hermann, H. W.: J.A.M.A. **158:**652-654, 1955 (in twins).

401 Asboe-Hansen, G., and Kaalund-Jorgensen, O.: Acta Haemat. (Basel) **16:**273-279, 1956 (mast cell).

402 Baikie, A. G., Jacobs, P. A., McBride, J. A., and Tough, I. M.: Brit. Med. J. **1:**1564-1571, 1961 (cytogenetic studies).

403 Bentley, H. P., Jr., Reardon, A. E., Knoedler, J. P., and Krivit, W.: Amer. J. Med. **30:**310-322, 1961 (eosinophilic).

404 Berenblum, I., and Trainin, N.: Science **132:**40-41, 1960 (experimental leukemogenesis).

405 Brescia, M. A., Santora, E., and Sarnataro, V. F.: J. Pediat. **55:**35-41, 1959 (congenital).

406 Brill, A. B., Tomonaga, M., and Heyssel, R. M.: Ann. Intern. Med. **56:**590-609, 1962 (atomic radiation).

407 Buckton, K. E., Harnden, D. G., Baikie, A. G., and Woods, G. E.: Lancet **1:**171-172, 1961 (mongolism and leukemia).

408 Burch, P. R. J.: Proc. Roy. Soc. Biol. **162:**223-239, 240-263, 1965 (radiation).

409 Chang, I. W.: Amer. J. Obstet. Gynec. **86:**903-908, 1963 (phosphatase).

410 Court-Brown, W. M.: Acta Haemat. (Basel) **20:**44-48, 1958 (radiation leukemogenesis).

411 Craig, L., and Seidman, H.: Blood **17:**319-327, 1961 (radiation).

412 Cronkite, E. P.: Blood **18:**370-376, 1961 (radiation).

413 Cronkite, E. P., Moloney, W., and Bond, V. P.: Amer. J. Med. **28:**673-682, 1960 (radiation).

414 Efrati, P., Klajman, A., and Spitz, H.: Blood **12:**869-882, 1957 (mast cell).

415 Evans, A. E.: Cancer **17:**256-258, 1963 (nervous system).

416 Fitzgerald, P. H., and Adams, A.: J. Nat. Cancer Inst. **34:**827-839, 1965 (chromosome studies).

417 Fitzgerald, P. H., Adams, A., and Gunz, F. W.: Blood **21:**183-196, 1963 (Philadelphia chromosome).

418 Freireich, E. J., Thomas, L. B., Frei, E., III, Fritz, R. D., and Forkner, C. E., Jr.: Cancer **13:**146-154, 1960 (intracerebral hemorrhage).

419 Goh, K., and Swisher, S. N.: Arch. Intern. Med. (Chicago) **115:**475-478, 1965 (in twins).

420 Goh, K., Swisher, S. N., and Rosenberg, C. A.: Ann. Intern. Med. **62:**80-86, 1965 (eosinophilic leukemia).

421 Goldberg, G. M., and Saphir, O.: Arch. Path. (Chicago) **71:**222-228, 1961 (spleen).

422 Goldberg, G. M., Rubenstone, A. I., and Saphir, O.: Cancer **14:**30-35, 1961 (histologic criteria).

423 Gonnella, J. S., and Lipsey, A. I.: New Eng. J. Med. **271:**533-535, 1964 (mastocytosis).

424 Gross, L.: Proc. Soc. Exp. Biol. Med. **76:**27-32, 1951 (in mice).

425 Gruenwald, H., Kiossoglou, K. A., Mitus, W. J., and Dameshek, W.: Amer. J. Med. **39:**1003-1010, 1965 (Philadelphia chromosome).

426 Gunz, F. W., Fitzgerald, P. H., and Adams, A.: Brit. Med. J. **2:**1097-1099, 1962 (chromosomes).

427 Heath, C. W., Jr., and Moloney, W. C.: Blood **26:**471-478, 1965 (Philadelphia chromosome).

428 Heyssel, R. M., Brill, A. B., Woodbury, L. A., Nishimura, E. T., Ghose, T., Hoshino, T., and Yamasaki, M.: Blood **15:**313-331, 1960 (atomic radiation).

429 Jackson, I. M. D., and Clark, R. M.: Amer. J. Med. Sci. **249:**72-74, 1965 (neutrophilic).

430 Jackson, W. L.: J. Lancet 85:25-29, 1965 (epidemiology).
431 Koprowski, H.: Amer. J. Med. 38:716-725, 1965 (virus-induced).
432 Krauss, S., Sokal, J. E., and Sandberg, A. A.: Ann. Intern. Med. 61:625-635, 1964 (chromosomes).
433 Lawrence, J. S.: J.A.M.A. 190:1049-1054, 1964 (irradiation leukemogenesis).
434 Lewis, E. B.: Science 142:1492-1494, 1963 (in radiologists).
435 McClure, P. D., Thaler, M. M., and Conen, P. E.: Arch. Intern. Med. (Chicago) 115:697-703, 1965 (chromosomes).
436 Makino, S., and Sasaki, M. S.: Lancet 1:851-852, 1964 (chromosomes).
437 March, H. C.: Amer. J. Med. Sci. 242:137-149, 1961 (in radiologists).
438 Moloney, W. C.: New Eng. J. Med. 253:88-90, 1955 (atomic radiation).
439 Moore, E. W., Thomas, L. B., Shaw, R. K., and Freireich, E. J.: Arch. Intern. Med. (Chicago) 105:451-468, 1960 (nervous system).
440 Pearson, H. A., Grello, F. W., and Cone, T. E., Jr.: New Eng. J. Med. 268:1151-1156, 1963 (in twins).
441 Reich, C.: J.A.M.A. 170:169-171, 1959 (remission).
442 Rosenthal, R. L.: Blood 21:495-508, 1963 (promyelocytic).
443 Sandberg, A. A., Ishihara, T., Crosswhite, L. H., and Hauschka, T. S.: Blood 20:393-423, 1962 (chromosomes).
444 Schwartz, S. O., Greenspan, I., and Brown, E. R.: J.A.M.A. 186:106-108, 1963 (leukemia cluster).
445 Scott, R. B., Ellison, R. R., and Ley, A. B.: Amer. J. Med. 37:162-171, 1964 (Di Guglielmo's syndrome).
446 Southam, C. M.: J. Pediat. 63:138-157, 1963 (viruses).
447 Stutzman, L., Zsoldos, S., Ambrus, J. L., and Asboe-Hansen, G.: Amer. J. Med. 29:894-901, 1960 (mast cell).
448 Syverton, J. T., and Ross, J. D.: Amer. J. Med. 28:683-698, 1960 (viruses).
449 Szweda, J. A., Abraham, J. P., Fine, G., Nixon, R. K., and Rupe, C. E.: Amer. J. Med. 32:227-239, 1962 (mast cell).
450 Warkany, J., Schubert, W. K., and Thompson, J. N.: New Eng. J. Med. 268:1-4, 1963 (mongolism).
451 Watkins, C. H., and Hall, B. E.: Amer. J. Clin. Path. 10:387-396, 1940 (monocytic).
452 Wells, R., and Lau, K. S.: Brit. Med. J. 1:759-763, 1960 (incidence in Chinese).
453 Whang, J., Frei, E., III, Tjio, J. H., Carbone, P. P., and Brecher, G.: Blood 22:664-673, 1963 (Philadelphia chromosome).

Multiple myeloma

454 Argani, I., and Kipkie, G. F.: Amer. J. Med. 36:151-157, 1964 (macroglobulinemia of Waldenström).
455 Bayrd, E. D.: Blood 3:987-1018, 1948.
456 Berlin, N. I., Merwin, R., Potter, M., Fahey, J. L., Carbone, P. P., and Cline, M. J.: Ann. Intern. Med. 58:1017-1036, 1963.
457 Bernier, G. M., and Putnam, F. W.: Progr. Hemat. 4:160-186, 1964, (proteins and macroglobulins).
458 Bessis, M.: Lab. Invest. 10:1041-1067, 1961 (ultrastructure).
459 Best, W. R.: J.A.M.A. 188:741-745, 1964.
460 Brody, J. I., Beizer, L. H., and Schwartz, S.: Amer. J. Med. 36:315-319, 1964.
461 Carson, C. P., Ackerman, L. V., and Maltby, J. D.: Amer. J. Clin. Path. 25:849-888, 1955.
462 Cohen, S., and Porter, R. R.: Advances Immun. 4:287-349, 1964 (immunoglobulins).
463 Cone, L. A., and Uhr, J. W.: J. Clin. Invest. 42:925, 1963 (immunologic deficiency).
464 Diggs, L. W., and Sirridge, M. S.: J. Lab. Clin. Med. 32:167-177, 1947.
465 Edelman, G. M., and Gally, J. A.: J. Exp. Med. 116:207-227, 1962 (Bence Jones proteins).
466 Fadem, R. S., and McBirnie, J. E.: Blood 5:191-200, 1950 (plasmacytosis).
467 Fahey, J. L.: J. Clin. Invest. 42:111-123, 1963 (proteins).
468 Fahey, J. L.: J.A.M.A. 194:71-74, 1965 (immunoglobulins).
469 Fahey, J. L.: J.A.M.A. 194:255-258, 1965 (immunoglobulins).
470 Fahey, J. L., and Goodman, H.: Science 143:588-590, 1963 (immunoglobulins).
471 Franklin, E. C.: Arthritis Rheum. 6:381-385, 1963 (immune globulins).
472 Franklin, E. C.: Progr. Allerg. 8:58-148, 1964 (immune globulins).
473 Franklin, E. C., Lowenstein, J., Bigelow, B., and Meltzer, M.: Amer. J. Med. 37:332-350, 1964 (heavy chain disease).
474 Ginsberg, D. M.: Ann. Intern. Med. 57:843-846, 1962 (circulating plasma cells).
475 Good, R. A.: J. Lab. Clin. Med. 46:167-181, 1955 (agammaglobulinemia).
476 Hamre, L., and Bruland, H.: Acta Path. Microbiol. Scand. 49:21-29, 1960 (plasmocytoma).
477 Harley, B. J. S., Kemp, T. A., and Abdullah, A. D.: Lancet 2:527-528, 1955.
478 Klein, H., and Block, M.: Blood 8:1034-1041, 1953 (bone marrow plasmocytosis).
479 Kobernick, S. D., and Whiteside, J. H.: Lab. Invest. 6:478-485, 1957 (renal glomeruli).
480 McCall, J. W., and Bailey, C. H.: Ann. Otol. 69:906-917, 1960 (extramedullary plasmacytoma).
481 Martin, N. H.: Lancet 1:237-239, 1961 (incidence).
482 Osserman, E. F.: Amer. J. Med. 31:671-675, 1961 (plasmocytic dyscrasias).
483 Osserman, E. F., and Lawlor, D. P.: Ann. N. Y. Acad. Sci. 94:93-109, 1961 (Waldenström's macroglobulinemia).
484 Osserman, E. F., and Takatsuki, K.: Medicine (Balt.) 42:357-384, 1963 (Franklin's disease).
485 Rosen, F. S.: New Eng. J. Med. 267:491-497, 546-550, 1962 (macroglobulins).
486 Rowe, D. S., and Fahey, J. L.: J. Exp. Med. 121:171-184, 1965 (myeloma protein).
487 Spickard, A.: Bull. Johns Hopkins Hosp. 107:234-240, 1960 (myelofibrosis).
488 Vander, J. B., and Johnson, H. A.: Ann. Intern. Med. 53:1052-1059, 1960 (leukemia).
489 Waldenström, J.: Progr. Hemat. 3:266-293,

1962 (hypergammaglobulinemia as clinical hematologic problem: study in gammopathies).

490 Waldenström, J., Paraskevas, F., and Heremans, J.: Lancet 1:1147, 1961 (cytology).

Miscellaneous abnormalities

491 Alyea, E. P., and Rundles, R. W.: J. Urol. 62:332-339, 1949 (carcinoma of prostate).

492 Aust, C. H., and Smith, E. B.: Amer. J. Clin. Path. 37:66-74, 1962 (Whipple's disease).

493 Bayrd, E. D., Paulson, G. S., and Hargraves, M. M.: Blood 9:46-56, 1954 (Hodgkin's disease).

494 Berkheiser, S. W.: Cancer 8:958-960, 1955 (malignant cells).

495 Bussi, L., and Bottura, C.: Acta Haemat. (Basel) 19:269-277, 1958 (Weber-Christian disease).

496 Conn, R. B., Jr., and Sundberg, R. D.: Amer. J. Path. 38:61-71, 1961 (amyloid).

497 Cooper, T., Stickney, J. M., Pease, G. L., and Bennett, W. A.: Amer. J. Med. 13:374-383, 1952 (purpura).

498 Cooperberg, A. A., and Schwartz, J.: Ann. Intern. Med. 61:289-295, 1964 (histoplasmosis).

499 Fisher, B.: Acta Haemat. (Basel) 6:31-37, 1951 (brucellosis).

500 Foldes, J.: Amer. J. Clin. Path. 23:918-920, 1953 (trichinosis).

501 Franklin, J. W., Zavala, D. C., and Radcliffe, C. E.: Blood 7:934-941, 1952 (melanoma).

502 Gaffney, P. C., Hansman, C. F., and Fetterman, G. H.: Amer. J. Clin. Path. 31:213-221, 1959 (neuroblastoma).

503 Groen, J., and Garrer, A. H.: Blood 3:1221-1237, 1948 (Gaucher's disease).

504 Hosley, H. F., Scharfman, W. B., and Propp, S.: New York J. Med. 61:73-82, 1961 (malignancy).

505 Hovde, R. F., and Sundberg, R. D.: Blood 5:209-232, 1950 (granulomas).

506 Jacobson, B. M., and Russell, H. K.: U. S. Naval Med. Bull. 45:429-432, 1945 (malaria).

507 Jaimet, C. H., and Amy, H. E.: Ann. Intern. Med. 44:617-629, 1956 (malignancy).

508 Kennedy, A. C.: Glasgow Med. J. 31:10-18, 1950 (sarcoidosis).

509 Limarzi, L. R., and Paul, J. T.: Amer. J. Clin. Path. 19:929-961, 1949 (Hodgkin's disease).

510 Miller, D.: Blood 14:1350-1353, 1959 (anthracosis).

511 Motulsky, A. G., and Rohn, R. J.: J. Lab. Clin. Med. 41:526-533, 1953 (melanoma).

512 Pease, G. L.: Amer. J. Clin. Path. 25:654-678, 1955 (hemopoietic disorders).

513 Pease, G. L.: Blood 11:720-734, 1956 (granulomas).

514 Pettet, J. D., Pease, G. L., and Cooper, T.: Blood 10:820-830, 1955 (lymphoma).

Chapter 32

Thymus

Stanley B. Smith

STRUCTURE AND FUNCTION

The thymus is a lymphoepithelial organ located in the anterior portion of the mediastinum. Morphologic differences between thymus and lymph nodes are outlined in Table 32-1. The thymus is divided into two lobes covered by a capsule of loose connective tissue. Septa from the capsule divide the lobes into lobules, which measure approximately 1 mm to 2 mm in diameter. Each lobule is composed of a peripheral cortex and a central medulla. The medullary area is connected to a central stalk. The cortical layer is composed almost entirely of closely packed small lymphocytes, which have been termed thymocytes. Small numbers of scattered larger mononuclear cells also are found in the cortex and appear particularly prominent during acute episodes of thymic involution, when they ingest lymphocytes and show abundant pale-staining cytoplasm. These larger phagocytic cells have been termed reticular cells, but their origin is uncertain. The medulla contains fewer lymphocytes, which are scattered among many reticular cells. Although the reticular cells in the medulla bear many similarities to those in the cortex, it is not certain whether their derivation and function are similar. Hassall's corpuscles, found in the medulla, are spherical structures 30μ to 100μ in diameter composed of concentric layers of epithelial cells that may be seen to form keratin. Hassall's corpuscles frequently undergo cystic degeneration and calcification. Eosinophils, neutrophils, and lymphocytes are found within Hassall's corpuscles from time to time. Although generally believed of epithelial origin, some consider Hassall's corpuscles to be of vascular origin. Their function is not clear.

The thymus is derived embryologically from the third and sometimes the fourth branchial pouches in association with the parathyroid glands. The parathyroid glands normally remain in the neck as the thymus migrates downward into the anterior part of the mediastinum. Sometimes, residual thymic tissue remains in the neck in close association with parathyroid tissue, or parathyroid tissue may be found in the mediastinum.

The thymus is prominent in infancy and childhood but begins to atrophy after puberty, which has long suggested that it plays a role in developmental biology. Largely by extirpating the thymus in the neonatal period, and then restoring function with thymic grafts, it has been shown that the thymus plays an essential role in the development of cellular immunity (delayed hypersensitivity).[2, 8, 11]

According to current concepts,[3, 10] there are two general types of lymphoid tissue: central and peripheral. The central lymphoid tissue is composed of the thymus and the mucosal gastrointestinal lymphoid tissue. The peripheral lymphoid tissue is composed of lymph nodes and spleen. The two types are functionally related in that precursor lymphoid cells are thought to originate in the bone marrow and migrate to either the thymus or the mucosal-related gastrointestinal lymphoid tissue, where they are induced to develop their genetic potential into particular cell lines. Cells derived from the thymus, after distribution to the periphery, express the thymic-dependent function of cellular immunity. Examples of this form of immune response are delayed hypersensitivity, graft-versus-host reactivity, homograft rejection, tumor rejection, and resistance to certain viral and fungal diseases and to tuberculosis. Children with a thymic deficiency show increased susceptibility to these infections.

The gastrointestinal mucosa-related central lymphoid tissue has been termed "bursal-derived" system. This term came into use after the discovery by Glick et al.[5] that the bursa of Fabricius in birds, a mucosal-related

Table 32-1 Morphologic differences between thymus and lymph nodes*

Characteristics	Normal thymus	Normal lymph node
Histogenesis	Foregut endoderm	Mesoderm
Histologic maturity attained	First trimester	Childhood
Growth rate at maximum	During gestation	After birth
Age involution	Depletion of all cell types Fatty and fibrous replacement Increase in PAS positive cells Increase in spindled cells	Depletion of cortical lymphocytes only
Lymphatic channels	Efferent only, of uncertain significance	Afferent and efferent united by sinusoids
Connective tissue	Scanty Enters from septa and capsule Isolated from parenchyma	Abundant Radiates from a hilum In continuity with parenchyma
Hassall's corpuscles	Unique to thymus	None
Stem cell	Reticular epithelial Possibly secretory as well as phagocytic	Reticulum cells of mesenchyme Phagocytic
Lymphocytes	Form mast cells readily High glycogen content	Form mast cells less readily High protein content
Morphologic behavior	Suppressed maximally by steroids No specific change on antigenic stimulation Exceptionally high mitotic rate and DNA incorporation	Suppressed maximally by radiation Germinal center formation on antigenic stimulation Less mitotic activity

*From Chatten, J.: Amer. J. Med. Sci. **248:**715-727, 1964.

lymphoid organ, was necessary for the development of lymphoid cells capable of producing antibodies. They found that removal of the bursa from a newborn chicken resulted in its failure to develop circulating immunoglobulins in a normal manner. Peyer's patches, vermiform appendix, and pharyngeal tonsils all have been considered as possible bursal equivalents in man.

The deep cortical areas of peripheral lymph nodes are the thymic-dependent areas. The outer cortex, germinal centers, and medullary cords are dependent for their development upon the mammalian bursal equivalent. Fig. 32-1 shows that absence or abnormality of bone marrow–derived stem cells can result in a defect of both immunoglobulin production and cellular sensitivity. Absence or abnormality of the thymus results in a defect in cellular sensitivity, but, in general, production of immunoglobulins remains normal. On the other hand, an individual with a normal thymus and a defective or absent bursal-derived system has a defect involving only production of immunoglobulins. It also should be realized that any congenital or acquired defect involving recognition of antigen, engulfment of antigen, or processing of antigen or a defect in one of the steps involved in subsequent production of the immune response would lead to deficiency of one or more classes of the immune response.

Three mechanisms to explain how the thymus exerts its functions have been suggested:

"1 Inductive influence on immigrant lymphoid stem cells of hemopoietic origin within the thymus establishes a line of differentiation and sets the stage for further differentiation of these cells along specific lines.

"2 Cells are induced to proliferate and emigrate to the peripheral lymphoid tissues, giving rise to a population of immunocompetent cells.

"3 The thymic stroma exerts a humoral inductive influence that may act within the thymus or in the periphery to expand and differentiate the thymus-dependent lymphoid population."*

Similar activities are postulated for the bursal equivalent tissue.

Lesions of the thymus have been reported in many so-called autoimmune diseases. An autoimmune disease may be viewed as one in which there is a loss of immunologic tolerance[4, 7, 9, 13] to antigens present in one's own body constituents (i.e., to one's own "self" antigens). In the normal individual there is neither a humoral nor a cellular immune response to self-antigens. This failure of an im-

*From Meuwissen, H. J., Stutman, O., and Good, R. A.: Seminars Hemat. **6:**28-66, 1969; by permission.

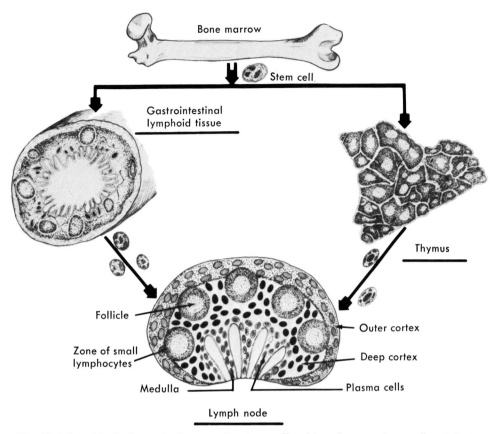

Lymph node

Fig. 32-1 Simplified schematic diagram showing traffic of lymphocytes. Stem cells originate in bone marrow and migrate to thymus or gastrointestinal lymphoid tissue. Thymic-derived cells migrate chiefly to deep cortical areas of lymph nodes. Outer cortex, mantle zone around germinal centers, and medulla of lymph node are dependent upon functioning gastrointestinal lymphoid system. Some cells may migrate directly from bone marrow to lymph nodes.

mune response to self-antigens is known as self-tolerance. The variation in pathologic findings and symptomatology in autoimmune diseases is dependent upon the type and location of antigen to which there is a loss of tolerance, as well as to the type of immune response mounted against the individual's own tissue.[12] For example, if an individual develops humoral antibodies against antigens present in his own erythrocytes, there results an autoimmune hemolytic anemia. The lesions found in encephalomyelitis following rabies vaccination and in chronic thyroiditis are histologically compatible with those of the cellular or delayed sensitivity type. The variety of location of lesions and type of tissue damage inflicted in autoimmune diseases depend upon location and type of antigen and type of immune response. Experimental findings indicate that the thymus has a role in some forms of immune tolerance[6] (see also p. 489).

Table 32-2 Weight of thymus*

Age (yr)	Weight (gm)		
	Minimum	Average	Maximum
Newborn	7.3	15.2	25.5
1-5	8.0	25.7	48.0
5-10	13.0	29.4	48.0
10-15	19.0	29.4	43.3
15-20	15.9	26.2	49.7
21-25	9.5	21.0	51.0
26-30	8.3	19.5	51.5
31-35	9.0	20.2	37.0
36-43	5.9	19.0	36.0
47-55	6.0	17.3	45.0
56-65	2.1	14.3	27.0
66-90	3.0	14.0	31.0

*According to Hammar, J. A.: Die Menschenthymus in Gesundheit und Krankheit, Leipzig, 1926, Akademische Verlagsgesellschaft; from Fisher, E. R.: Pathology of the thymus and its relation to human disease. In Good, R. A., and Gabrielsen, A. E., editors: The thymus in immunobiology, New York, 1964, Hoeber Medical Division, Harper & Row, Publishers.

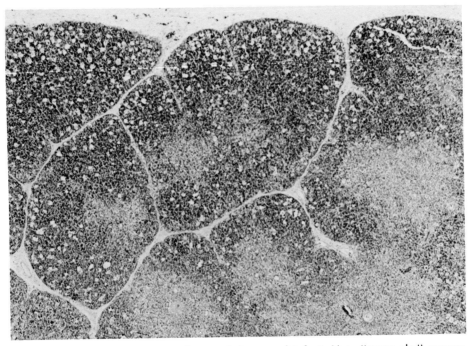

Fig. 32-2 Acute or accidental involution of thymus of infant. Note "starry sky" appearance in cortex and lack of chronic involution. Except for this acute stress reaction, gland is normal. (×55.)

INVOLUTION

There is a considerable variation in weight of the thymus according to age, and a relatively large variation occurs within each age group. For this reason, there is difficulty in defining thymic hyperplasia or hypertrophy solely in terms of weight (Table 32-2).

The thymus increases in weight until puberty, at which time it begins to decrease in size (physiologic involution). Decrease in size secondary to stress, such as occurs in infection, is termed accidental thymic involution (Figs. 32-2 and 32-3), and a striking decrease in thymic size as observed by roentgenogram of the chest may occur within twelve hours of onset of severe stress.[14] Caution should be used in interpreting a roentgenogram showing a small thymus in an acutely ill child suspected of having an immunologic deficiency disorder.

In physiologic involution,[16] the thymic parenchyma gradually decreases in size, cortical lymphocytes are scanty, and the lobules are separated by adipose tissue. Epithelial elements of the medulla may have a fusiform or spindle shape. In occasional glands, epithelial rosettes are seen. Hassall's corpuscles vary in number, sometimes are closely packed,

and occasionally appear partially calcified or cystic. The thymus in adults, particularly those of advanced age, often contains cysts ranging in size up to about 1 cm and is lined by flat cells. It is presumed that some of these are the end stage of cystic Hassall's corpuscles (Figs. 32-4 and 32-5).

In accidental involution,[17] the early changes include clumping and fragmentation of lymphocytes and phagocytosis of lymphocytes by large cortical cells, sometimes giving the so-called "starry sky" appearance (Fig. 32-2). These cortical phagocytes accumulate nuclear debris, PAS-positive material, phospholipid, and neutral lipid, all probably the result of cellular breakdown. The lympholysis is accompanied by depletion of lymphocytes from the cortex of the gland. There is an early increase in plasma cells and mast cells, followed by a later decrease in these elements. Accidental involution also is characterized by progressive collapse of the reticulin lobular network and fibrosis (Fig. 32-6). In the final stage, the lobule is completely collapsed and surrounded by fibrous septa. The extent of the capacity for regeneration may decrease with the degree of collapse and fibrosis (Fig. 32-7).

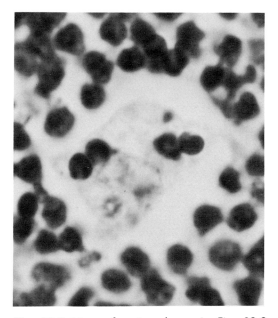

Fig. 32-3 View of cortex shown in Fig. 32-2. Lymphocytes within large cortical mononuclear cell. It is not known whether this results from phagocytosis or lymphocytic migration into mononuclear cell. (×1,890.)

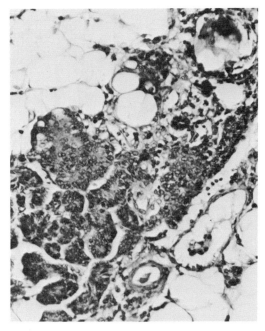

Fig. 32-4 Chronic involution of thymus with rosettes and microcysts. (×207.)

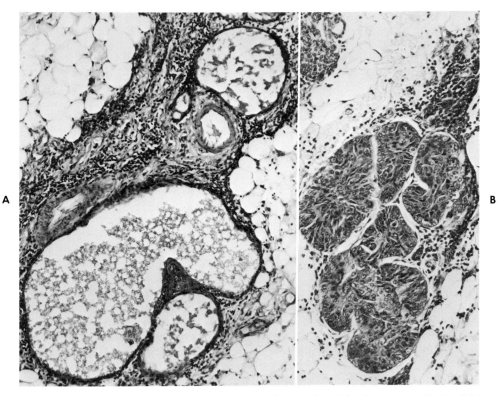

Fig. 32-5 Chronic involution of thymus. **A,** With cysts lined by flattened cells. **B,** With prominent rosettes similar to those seen in some thymomas. Patient had no known immunologic abnormalities, and there was no evidence of primary carcinoma. (**A and B,** ×165.)

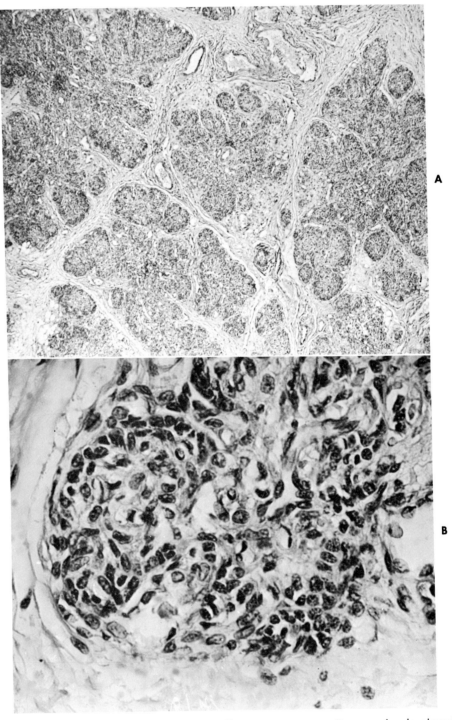

Fig. 32-6 Thymic alymphoplasia showing fibrous septa separating poorly developed lobules and absence of small lymphocytes and Hassall's bodies. (**A**, ×52; **B**, ×486; courtesy Dr. David Gitlin and Dr. John M. Craig.)

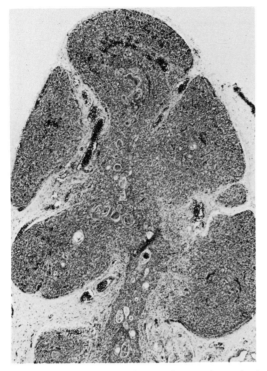

Fig. 32-7 Thymus of newborn infant with marked depletion of cortical lymphocytes in acute involution probably secondary to infection in utero. Presence of Hassall's corpuscles distinguishes this from thymic alymphoplasia. (×60.)

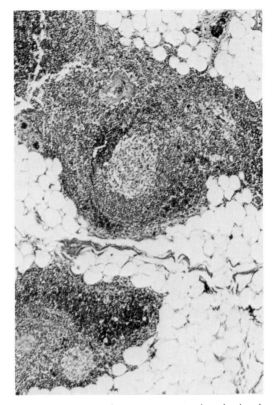

Fig. 32-8 Germinal centers in involuted gland. This can be viewed as hyperplasia in atrophic gland. Patient had myasthenia gravis.

HYPERPLASIA

Hyperplasia of the thymus cannot be defined using weight as the only criterion. The presence of germinal centers in the medulla has been considered to be histologic evidence of thymic hyperplasia (Fig. 32-8). The presence of lymph follicles in the medulla frequently have been reported in association with various diseases in which there is an immunologic abnormality such as myasthenia gravis, systemic lupus erythematosus, Hashimoto's disease, thyrotoxicosis, chronic glomerulonephritis, etc. Although thymic germinal centers have been considered suggestive of an autoimmune disorder,[19] their occurrence in cases of accidental death[18] indicates that their presence is not diagnostic.

IMMUNOLOGIC DEFICIENCIES WITH THYMIC ABNORMALITIES

Thymoma with agammaglobulinemia (Good's syndrome)[36]

In thymoma with agammaglobulinemia, there is epithelial cell or spindle cell type of thymoma and an associated decrease or absence of plasma cells. The number of circulating lymphocytes is low. Immunoglobulins are reduced, and there is a deficiency of humoral antibody production to all antigens as well as a deficient response of cell-mediated immunity to all antigens. Eosinophils are absent or decreased in the blood and bone marrow. Some cases have also an associated pure red cell aplasia.

Ataxia-telangiectasia (Louis-Bar syndrome)[20, 41, 42, 44, 45]

Ataxia-telangiectasia is transmitted as an autosomal recessive trait. The infant appears normal at birth, but at about 2 years of age the child is noted to have ataxia and prominent oculocutaneous blood vessels. By the age of 16 years, the patient is generally confined to a wheelchair. By that time, telangiectases, which at first involved only bulbar conjunctivae, extend to the butterfly area of face, ears, antecubital fossae, and neck. The chief finding in the brain is degeneration of Purkinje cells in the cerebellum. Gonadal dysgenesis is a commonly associated defect. There is an increased incidence of malignancies in these patients (tumors of the lymphoid system, ovarian dysgerminomas, cerebellar medulloblastoma, and frontal lobe gliomas). Many of the children develop sinopulmonary infections, progressive bronchiectasis, respiratory insufficiency, and pneumonia.

The condition is accompanied by an embryonic type of thymus that is small and lacks cortical and medullary organization. Hassall's corpuscles have been lacking in all but one reported case. Lymphocytes are deficient in the thymic-dependent areas of the lymph nodes in most cases. In a few cases, the lymph nodes appear relatively normal, but in others consist almost entirely of stromal cells with an absence of follicles and lymphocytes. The number of circulating lymphocytes tends to be slightly decreased. As would be expected from these pathologic findings, the cell-mediated responses are constantly deficient. Blast transformation of lymphocytes exposed in vitro to phytohemagglutinin, which is thought to be associated with cell-mediated immune responses, is reduced in these patients.[38, 40] Attempts to transfer cell-mediated immunity with cells from previously sensitized normal donors to these patients has failed. This suggests that there may be a defect in the effector-mechanism in addition to the presumed defect in the development of delayed hypersensitivity.[26, 43, 48]

An immunoglobulin deficit usually is present. A deficiency in IgA is most common. IgG may be low, normal, or elevated. IgM is usually normal, occasionally high, and rarely low. The number of plasma cells in the tissues is variable.

Thymic aplasia (Di George's syndrome; congenital absence of thymus and parathyroid glands)[21, 24, 25, 37]

Thymic aplasia is characterized by a failure of development of both the third and fourth pharyngeal pouches with resulting absence of both thymus and parathyroid glands. Anomalies of the aortic arch, which originate in the fourth branchial arch, also have been seen in this syndrome. There is an absence of lymphocytes in the thymic-dependent areas (Fig. 32-9). Germinal centers are present. Circulating lymphocytes are usually low but may sometimes be in the normal range. Plasma cells are present, and immunoglobulins are normal. In some patients, responses are deficient in the production of humoral antibodies to a variety of antigens, but in others the humoral response is normal. All mediated immune responses to all antigens are absent. Infants with this syndrome usually present with signs

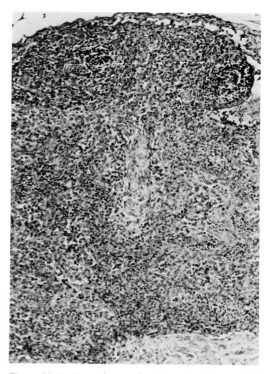

Fig. 32-9 Lymph node in thymic aplasia (DiGeorge's syndrome). Note absence of lymphocytes in deep cortical areas and small germinal centers with thin mantle zone of lymphocytes. (×165.)

of tetany in the newborn period. No genetic abnormality has been described. Cleveland et al.[21] have described and are following a single patient in whom thymic function has apparently been restored by implantation of a fetal thymus.

Hereditary lymphopenic immunologic deficiency[29, 34]

Hereditary lymphopenic immunologic deficiency is a sex-linked disease affecting males. The children often die of viral or fungal infection in early childhood. The thymus is hypoplastic and lacks corticomedullary differentiation and Hassall's corpuscles (Fig. 32-6). Rosettes and whorls are seen in this condition. There is gross depletion of lymphocytes in the tissues, but occasional small perivascular nests of lymphocytes are found in the gastrointestinal tract, lymph nodes, and spleen. The number of circulating lymphocytes is low but shows some variation. Plasma cells in the tissues are variable but usually are decreased. Immunoglobulins are decreased but show some variation of degree among the different classes. Cell-mediated immune responses are deficient.

Autosomal recessive alymphocytic agammaglobulinemia (Glanzmann and Riniker's lymphocytophthisis; Swiss-type agammaglobulinemia)[30, 33, 51]

Autosomal recessive alymphocytic agammaglobulinemia is a severe autosomal recessive deficiency disease in which the patient does not survive infancy. It is characterized by an absence of plasma cells in the tissues, accompanied by an extreme deficiency of all classes of immunoglobulins and lack of antibody production to all antigens. The thymus is vestigal, lacks both Hassall's corpuscles and lymphocytes, and is composed of epithelial cells. Epithelial rosettes are uncommon in contrast to the hereditary lymphopenic immunologic deficiency. Lymphoid follicles and germinal centers are not seen. Lymphocytes are not found in lymph nodes, gastrointestinal tract, or spleen. Cell-mediated immune responses to all antigens are deficient. This condition could result from either a defect in the stem cell or from defective development of both thymic and gastrointestinal lymphoid tissues.[20]

Autosomal recessive lymphopenia with normal plasma cells and immunoglobulins (Nezelof's syndrome; pure alymphocytosis)[28, 39]

Autosomal recessive lymphopenia with normal plasma cells and immunoglobulins is a familial and probably an autosomal recessive disorder in which plasma cells are present and immunoglobulin levels are normal. Humoral antibody responses are present but may be decreased. The thymus is hypoplastic and does not contain lymphoid cells or Hassall's corpuscles. Lymphoid follicles and germinal centers are not present in lymph nodes. A few scattered lymphocytes are present in the submucosa of the intestine and appendix, but Peyer's patches are not seen. Germinal centers are absent from the spleen. An unproved speculation is that this entity may be the same as autosomal recessive alymphocytic agammaglobulinemia with the addition of chimerism from a maternal fetal cellular transfer. The lack of evidence of a graft-versus-host response in these patients fails to support this concept.

IMMUNOLOGIC DEFICIENCIES WITHOUT PRIMARY THYMIC ABNORMALITY
Infantile sex-linked agammaglobulinemia (Bruton's disease)[31]

Infantile sex-linked agammaglobulinemia occurs in males and is characterized by recur-rent infections, particularly with pyogenic organisms. There is a normal thymus, as well as normality in the number of circulating lymphocytes in the blood, the thymic-dependent areas of the lymph nodes, and the bone marrow lymphocytes. Functionally, the patients have normal cell-mediated responses. Plasma cells are absent in the tissues even after stimulation by potent antigens. The lymphoid tissue shows an absence of plasma cells and germinal centers. Tonsils are small, with absence of germinal centers and poorly developed crypts. Peyer's patches are poorly developed and lack follicles. Plasma cells are not seen in the lamina propria of the intestinal tract. There is marked deficiency in all classes of immunoglobulins, as well as an extremely deficient production of antibodies to all antigens.

Selective immunoglobulin deficiency[32, 46, 50, 52, 53]

Selective deficiencies for IgM, IgG, IgD, and IgE are not yet described. Some individuals with a selective IgA deficiency remain well, whereas others are subject to sinusitis, bronchitis, and exudative enteropathy. All of the histologic and laboratory parameters mentioned in the other deficiency diseases are normal except for an absence of IgA-producing plasma cells and IgA in both the serum and the secretions. The genetics are unknown.

Transient hypogammaglobulinemia of infancy[35, 49]

In transient hypogammaglobulinemia of infancy, there is deficiency of plasma cells and IgG. Humoral antibody responses are decreased or absent. All other parameters of the immune response are normal. The patients may have low normal or low IgG later in life.

Nonsex-linked primary immunoglobulin deficiency of variable onset and expression[22, 27, 47]

Nonsex-linked primary immunoglobulin deficiency of variable onset and expression, including the so-called congenital nonsex-linked and acquired primary deficiencies and dysgammaglobulinemias, probably consists of several entities and may be subclassified as more information becomes available. The pathologic characteristics of the thymus are unknown. Plasma cells usually are decreased. There may be reticulum hyperplasia of lymphoid tissue and hyperplasia of the tonsils, and occasionally giant follicle hyperplasia is seen in the spleen and lymph nodes. The number of circulating lymphocytes is normal. Cell-mediated immune responses to some antigens may be deficient. Immunoglobulin deficiencies are present but vary in regard to the class of immunoglobulin involved. Humoral antibody responses to most, but not all, antigens are reduced. The genetics are unknown but are thought to be an autosomal recessive trait or, in some cases, it has been speculated that multiple factors may be involved.

Immune deficiency with thrombocytopenia and eczema (Wiskott-Aldrich syndrome)[23]

Immune deficiency with thrombocytopenia and eczema is a sex-linked genetic disease in which male children develop thrombocytopenia, eczema, and frequent infections. The cause of death usually is due to either infection or hemorrhage, but some patients have developed malignant reticuloendotheliosis. An immunoglobulin deficiency is present. The most common pattern is a decreased IgM level and a normal or even an elevated level of IgA. Commonly, there is a deficiency in the ability to produce isohemagglutinins or to produce antibodies to carbohydrate antigens. Plasma cells are present. In some individuals, the thymus has been normal, but in others, there is a decrease in thymic lymphocytes, an indistinct corticomedullary relationship, and numerous Hassall's corpuscles. This constellation of histologic findings is characteristic of involutional atrophy of the thymus. The number of circulating lymphocytes is usually low, and cellular immunity usually is impaired. Reticulum cell hyperplasia is a frequent finding in the lymphoreticular tissue.

Reticuloendothelial insufficiency is probably not the basis for the susceptibility to infections, and complement levels have been found to be normal.[23] Also normal is the ability of peripheral blood leukocytes to phagocytize and digest bacteria and the inflammatory response in the skin to a nonspecific stimulus.[23] Cooper et al.[23] speculate that the primary defect may be proximal to the site of actual induction of antibody synthesis to polysaccharide antigens, so that it may be a genetic defect of the afferent limb of immunity that relates to an essential step in the preparation of polysaccharide antigens for induction of the immune response.

RELATIONSHIP OF THYMUS TO MYASTHENIA GRAVIS[69]

Myasthenia gravis is characterized clinically by weakness and easy fatigability of voluntary muscle. The symptoms are aggravated by exercise and are ameliorated by rest. Since the first description of a thymic tumor in association with myasthenia gravis in 1901 by Laquer and Weigert, numerous examples have been recorded. Later, the presence of germinal centers in the thymus in myasthenia gravis was noted.[54, 67] Early descriptions of a lymphocytic infiltrate in skeletal muscle (lymphorrhages), together with other degenerative muscle changes, are recorded.[56] The similarity of the clinical state to curare poisoning suggested a mechanism of neuromuscular block.[81] Thymectomy has been reported to be of some therapeutic benefit, particularly in young female patients who are found to have germinal centers in the thymus.[77, 78] A relationship between myasthenia gravis and autoimmunity has been suggested and numerous similarities pointed out between myasthenia gravis and systemic lupus erythematosus with regard to age, sex, clinical course, and symptomatology.[65, 66, 77-80] Serum from myasthenic patients has been shown to have twice the normal incidence of lytic activity on frog muscle.[63]

Fluctuations of serum complement levels in myasthenic patients correlated with their clinical state.[63] Reciprocal absorption studies and complement fixation have shown that two types of antibody are present, an "S" antibody, which fixes complement and reacts with antigenic determinants present only in skeletal muscle, and an "SH" antibody, which reacts with antigen present in both skeletal muscle and thymus and which does not fix complement.[55, 68] More recently, it has been shown that the antibody localizes with the I bands of the skeletal muscle, and it has been suggested that the antigens may be tropomyosin and troponin.[70] It has been shown that ribonucleoprotein-rich fractions and microsomal fractions will absorb antistriated muscle antibodies that have been found by immunofluorescence.[61, 62] The interpretation of these findings is not yet clear. The presence of germinal centers in the thymus in myasthenia gravis, together with the experimental production of lesions composed of perivascular collections of plasma cells and lymphoid nodules with germinal centers,[59, 60] supported the idea that the immunologic reaction in myasthenia gravis originated within the thymus—i.e., that there may be a selective loss of immunologic tolerance to an antigen present in the thymus. The rediscovery of the thymic myoid cells[75] caused speculation that these may be the source of antigen. In considering these ideas, one should keep in mind that thymic hyperplasia (i.e., the presence of germinal centers within thymus) is found three to five times more frequently in myasthenia gravis than is thymoma. In some cases of myasthenia gravis, the thymus may contain both a thymoma and germinal center formation.

At the present time, the antimuscle antibodies are thought to represent indicators of the disease but not believed to initiate the neuromuscular blockage. It has been speculated that the as yet undiscovered neuromuscular blocking agent may be released by damaged thymic tissue. It should be noted that in twelve of fifty-one patients with thymoma, but without myasthenia gravis, antibodies against thymus and muscle were found[71, 73] and, further, that in female patients with myasthenia gravis, whose children exhibited transient neonatal myasthenia, circulating antibodies against muscle or thymic tissue usually were not demonstrated.[64, 74] Only 30% of myasthenic patients without thymoma show antimuscle or antithymus antibodies.

Immunization of guinea pigs with saline extracts of thymus has been reported to produce a dense lymphocytic infiltrate around Hassall's corpuscles.[57, 58] This lesion has been termed autoimmune thymitis. Confirmation of this finding is lacking.[76]

STATUS THYMICOLYMPHATICUS[82-86]

According to the concept of status thymicolymphaticus, there is a constitutional abnormality in certain persons (usually infants and children) characterized by generalized lymphoid hyperplasia, hypoplasia of the aorta, atrophy of the adrenal glands, and underdevelopment of the gonads. Such children supposedly are subject to sudden death as a result of some trivial stimulus. It is now recognized that such sudden deaths in most cases are due to respiratory infection. The concept is now discredited (p. 1469).

TUMORS
Thymoma

Tumors of the thymus are uncommon lesions. In one-third of the patients, the tumors are asymptomatic and are discovered on a routine chest roentgenogram.[103] In one-third, the symptoms present as an anterior mediastinal mass, such as cough, dysphagia, dyspnea, retrosternal pain, or signs of compression of the superior vena cava. In one-third, the tumors are found in association with myasthenia gravis.

Gross features. Most thymic tumors are lobulated or multinodular and appear well encapsulated, although some are nonencapsulated and appear to extend by local invasion. There is considerable variation in size, ranging from 1 cm to 20 cm in diameter. The cut surfaces show varying colors of pink, gray, or yellow and show fibrous septa. Cystic degeneration is seen occasionally in larger tumors.

Histologic classification. Lattes and Jonas[104] proposed a classification of thymomas into four major groups according to the predominant cell: lymphoid, spindle cell, epithelial, and rosette-forming types (Fig. 32-10).

The most common is the lymphoid type, which shows thymic lymphocytes separated into lobules by fibrous septa. Follicles and germinal centers are not seen within the tumor. Epithelial cells are singly scattered or are present in small islands of spindle-shaped or squamoid-type cells.

The spindle cell type is the second most common variety. It is generally held that these cells are of epithelial origin. The cells are plump with oval vesicular nuclei. Cytoplasmic boundaries frequently are indistinct. The cells may be arranged in whorls or elongated bundles and show areas of pseudorosette formation. In some areas, there may be a cribriform or microcystic appearance. These areas also have been described as lymphangiomatous. Spindle cell thymomas are more likely to show calcification, cyst formation, and fibrosis than are the other histologic types. Reticulin stains usually fail to show reticulin fibers between individual cells. Spindle cell tumors are associated infrequently with myasthenia gravis.[91, 103]

In the epithelial type of thymoma, the cells are arranged in sheets. Occasional areas of palisading are seen. Individual cells are squamoid or cuboidal and frequently have clear cytoplasm. There is an inconstant mixture of epithelial cells and lymphocytes (Fig. 32-11). Sometimes, there is a suggestion of Hassall's corpuscles. Occasionally, the cells, in part, may be arranged in an organoid pattern.

The pseudorosette type is the least common pattern. In this variety, the epithelial cells

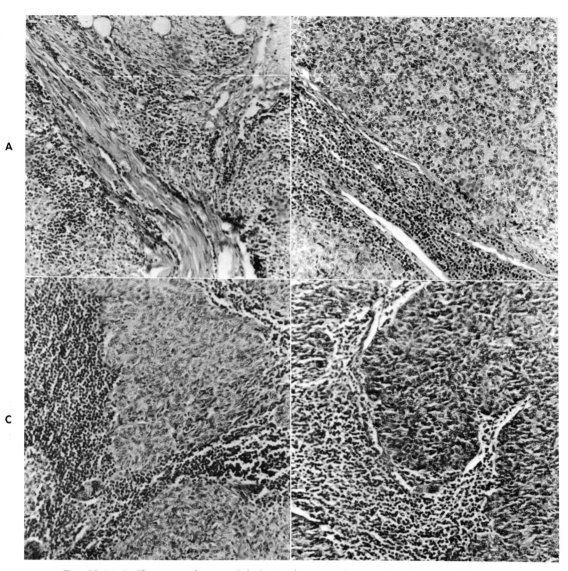

Fig. 32-10 A, Thymoma showing lobulation by stromal connective tissue proliferation. **B,** Thymoma showing rosette-forming area. **C,** Thymoma with lymphoid and epithelial-appearing areas. **D,** Thymoma with lymphoid areas and spindle cell masses.

appear to be arranged in clusters surrounding a central area without a true lumen.

The term "granulomatous thymoma" has been applied to tumors involving the thymus, but not mediastinal or peripheral lymph nodes, in which there is participation of thymic epithelium with production of sheets of squamoid cells with or without cysts. The granulomatous component resembles the nodular sclerosing form of Hodgkin's disease except that the Sternberg-Reed cells are not typical and often contain PAS-positive material. Hassall's corpuscles often are seen in the midst of the nodular sclerosing areas. These tumors are now generally considered to

represent Hodgkin's disease involving the thymus. Typical Hodgkin's disease has developed in a number of these patients.[93, 98]

Thymic tumors have been found in association with numerous diseases which, in addition to myasthenia gravis, include multiple myeloma,[88, 106] hypogammaglobulinemia,[95] Cushing's syndrome,[111] pure erythroid hypoplasia,[87, 97, 108, 110, 111] myositis and granulomatous myocarditis,[94, 101, 112] meningoencephalitis,[100] generalized cutaneous candidiasis,[107] systemic lupus erythematosus,[102] dermatomyositis,[99] scleroderma, and Sjögren's syndrome.

The prognosis of patients with thymoma in association with myasthenia gravis depends,

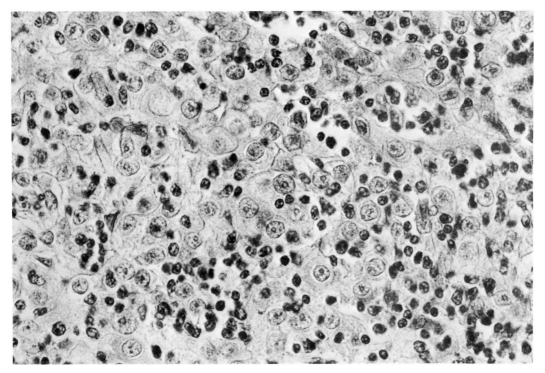

Fig. 32-11 Predominantly epithelial type of thymoma. (×585.)

in general, upon the course of the myasthenia. Prognosis in nonmyasthenic patients with thymoma seems to depend more on the gross characteristics of the tumor than on the histologic pattern. Those patients in whom the tumor is nonencapsulated at the time of surgery have a poorer prognosis than those with an encapsulated tumor that does not show signs of local invasion. Both surgery[103, 109] and radiation have been favored in therapy. In the series of Wilkins et al.,[113] the ten-year cumulative survival rate for patients with thymoma but without myasthenia gravis is 67%, but only 32% when thymoma is complicated by myasthenia gravis. They also report a 100% ten-year survival of patients with encapsulated thymomas without myasthenia gravis. None of the patients with both evidence of invasion and myasthenia gravis survived ten years.

Seminoma

A few seminoma-like tumors of the thymus have been reported[92] that histologically resemble seminomas of the testis or dysgerminomas of the ovary and also have been termed pseudoseminoma, seminoma-like thymoma, germinoma, or gonocytoma. The origin of this tumor is unknown. The tumors usually are lobulated, with the lobules being separated by thin fibrous septa. Histologically, they are composed of large numbers of round or polygonal cells with either clear or eosinophilic cytoplasm. The nuclei tend to be large, round, and hyperchromatic. Sometimes, nucleoli are prominent. In some tumors, nonspecific granulomatous foci are seen. Areas of thymic tissue are identifiable. Cystic degeneration may occur.

Thymolipoma (lipothymoma)[89, 90, 105]

The thymolipoma is a rare benign tumor that is generally curable by local excision. The majority of reported cases have been in men. They are composed mostly of mature fatty tissue separated into distinct lobules by bands of fibrous tissue, with only a few foci of thymic tissue. Some tumors are composed chiefly of lobules of thymic tissue with preservation of corticomedullary architecture and numerous Hassall's corpuscles. No association with other diseases has been described, but long-term follow-ups have not been reported.

Cysts

Cysts of the thymus large enough to produce symptoms are rare (Fig. 32-12). Cystic degeneration of Hassall's corpuscles is common particularly in infections. A recent review of

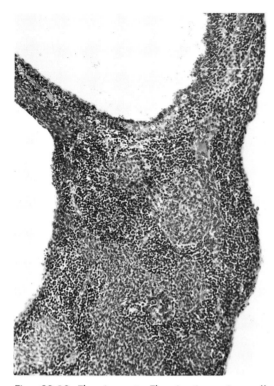

Fig. 32-12 Thymic cyst. Thymic tissue in wall shows lymphoid tissue and Hassall's bodies. (×125; courtesy Dr. S. E. Gould.)

anterior mediastinal fat pads in several hundred autopsies revealed that small cysts measuring up to 5 mm in diameter are common (an incidence of approximately 3% in adults over 50 years of age). Since these have atrophic thymic tissue in their wall, they probably should be classified as thymic cysts (see Chapter 23 for further discussion of thymic cysts and mediastinal cysts).

REFERENCES
General

1 Goldstein, G., and Mackay, I. R.: The human thymus, St. Louis, 1969, Warren H. Green, Inc.

Structure and function

2 Arnason, B. G., Jankovic, B. D., Waksman, B. H., and Wennersten, C.: J. Exp. Med. 116: 177-186, 1962.
3 Cooper, M. D., Perey, D. Y., Peterson, R. D. A., Gabrielsen, A. E., and Good, R. A.: Birth Defects: Original Article Series IV(1):7-16, 1968; The National Foundation, New York.
4 Dresser, D. W., and Mitchison, N. A.: Advances Immun. 8:129-181, 1968.
5 Glick, B., Chang, T. S. and Jaap, R. G.: Poult. Sci. 35:224-225, 1956.
6 Horiuchi, A., and Waksman, B. H.: J. Immun. 101:1322-1332, 1968 (role of thymus in immune tolerance).
7 Hraba, T.: Monographs in allergy, vol. 3, Basel/New York, 1968, S. Karger, p. 1, (mechanism and role of immunologic tolerance).
8 Jankovic, B. D., Waksman, B. H. and Arnason, B. G.: J. Exp. Med. 116:159-176, 1962.
9 Landy, M., and Braun, W.: Immunologic tolerance, New York/London, 1969, Academic Press, Inc.
10 Meuwissen, H. J., Stutman, O., and Good, R. A.: Seminars Hemat. 6:28-66, 1969 (functions of lymphocyte).
11 Miller, J. F. A. P.: Lancet 2:748-749, 1961.
12 Waksman, B. H.: Medicine (Balt.) 41:93-141, 1962.
13 Weigle, W. O.: Natural and acquired immunologic unresponsiveness, Cleveland/New York, 1967, World Publishing Co.

Involution

14 Davis, J. H., Reiss, E., Artz, C. P., and Amspacher, W. H.: Armed Forces Med. J. 5: 545-548, 1954 (involution after burns).
15 Fisher, E. R.: Pathology of the thymus and its relation to human disease. In Good, R. A., and Gabrielsen, A. E., editors: The thymus in immunobiology, New York, 1964, Hoeber Medical Division, Harper & Row, Publishers.
16 Henry, L.: J. Path. Bact. 93:661-671, 1967 (involution).
17 Henry, L.: J. Path. Bact. 96:337-343, 1968 (accidental involution).

Hyperplasia

18 Middleton, G.: Aust. J. Exp. Biol. Med. Sci. 45:189-199, 1967.
19 Okabe, H.: Acta Path. Jap. 16:109-130, 1966.

Immunologic deficiencies with thymic abnormalities

20 Boder, E., and Sedgwick, R. P.: Pediatrics 21:526-554, 1958.
21 Cleveland, W. W., Fogel, B. J., and Kay, H. E.: J. Clin. Invest. 47:20a-21a, 1968.
22 Comings, D. E.: Arch. Intern. Med. (Chicago) 115:79-87, 1965.
23 Cooper, M. D., Chase, H. P., Lowman, J. T., Krivit, W., and Good, R. A.: Birth Defects Original Article Series IV(1):378-387, 1968; The National Foundation, New York.
24 DiGeorge, A. M.: Discussion of Cooper, M. D., Peterson, R. D. A., and Good, R. A.: J. Pediat. 67:907-908, 1965.
25 DiGeorge, A. M.: Birth Defects Original Article Series IV(1):116-123, 1968; The National Foundation, New York.
26 Eisen, A. H., Karpati, G., Laszlo, T., Andermann, F., Robb, J. P., and Bacal H. L.: New Eng. J. Med. 272:18-22, 1965.
27 Fudenberg, H. H., Kamin, R., Salmon, S. and Tormey, D. C.: In Killander, J. editor: The gamma globulins, Nobel Symposium III, Stockholm, 1967, Almqvist & Wiksells, Publishers.
27a Fudenberg, H. H., Good, R. A., Goodman, H. C., Hitzig, W., Kunkel, H. G., Roitt, I. M.,

Rosen, F. S., Rowe, D. S., Seligmann, M., and Soothill, J. R.: Pediatrics **47**:927-946, 1971 (primary immune deficiencies).

28 Fulginiti, V. A., Hathaway, W. E., Pearlman, D. S., Blackburn, W. R., Reiquam, C. W., Githens, J. H., Clamand, H. N., and Kempe, C. H.: Lancet **2**:5-8, 1966.

29 Gitlin, D., and Craig, J. M.: Pediatrics **32**:517-530, 1963.

30 Glanzmann, E. von, and Riniker, P.: Ann. Paediat. **175**:1-32, 1950.

31 Good, R. A., Peterson, R. D. A., Perey, D. Y., Finstad, J., and Cooper, M. D.: Birth Defects Original Article Series **IV**(1):17-39, 1968; The National Foundation, New York.

32 Hanson, L. A.: Birth Defects Original Article Series **IV**(1):292-297, 1968; The National Foundation, New York.

33 Hitzig, W. H., and Willi, H.: Schweiz. Med. Wschr. **91**:1625-1633, 1961.

34 Hoyer, J. R., Cooper, M. D., Gabrielsen, A. E., and Good, R. A.: Birth Defects Original Article Series **IV**(1):91-103, 1968; The National Foundation, New York.

35 Janeway, C. A., and Gitlin, D.: Advances Pediat. **9**:65-136, 1957.

36 Jeunet, F. S., and Good, R. A.: Birth Defects Original Article Series **IV**(1):192-206, 1968; The National Foundation, New York.

37 Kretschmer, R., Burhan, S., Brown, D. and Rosen, F. S.: New Eng. J. Med. **279**:1295-1301, 1968.

38 Leikin, S. L., Bazelon, M., and Parks, K. H.: J. Pediat. **68**:477-479, 1966.

39 Nezelof, C., Jammet, M.-L., Lortholary, P., Labrune, B., and Lamy, M.: Arch. Franc. Pediat. **21**:897-920, 1964.

40 Oppenheim, J. J., Barlow, M., Waldmann, T. A., and Block, J. B.: Brit. Med. J. **2**:330-333, 1966.

41 Peterson, R. D. A., and Good, R. A.: Birth Defects Original Article Series **IV**(1):370-377, 1968; The National Foundation, New York.

42 Peterson, R. D. A., Cooper, M. D., and Good, R. A.: Amer. J. Med. **41**:342-359, 1966.

43 Peterson, R. D. A., Kelly, W. D., and Good, R. A.: Lancet **1**:1189-1193, 1964.

44 Pump, K. K., Dunn, H. G., and Meuwissen, H.: Dis. Chest **47**:473-486, 1965.

45 Reed, W. B., Epstein, W. L., Boder, E., and Sedgwick, R.: J.A.M.A. **195**:746-753, 1966.

46 Rockey, J. H., Hanson, L. A., Heremans, J. F., and Kunkel, H. G.: J. Lab. Clin. Med. **63**:205-212, 1964.

47 Rosen, F. S., and Janeway, C. A.: New Eng. J. Med. **275**:709-715, 769-775, 1966.

48 Rosenthal, I. M., Markowitz, A. S., and Medenis, R.: Amer. J. Dis. Child. **110**:69-75, 1965.

49 Soothill, J. F., Hayes, K., and Dudgeon, J. A.: Lancet **1**:1385-1388, 1966.

50 South, M. A., Cooper, M. D., Hong, R., Wollheim, F. A., and Good, R. A.: Birth Defects Original Article Series **IV**(1):283-291, 1968; The National Foundation, New York.

51 Tobler, R., and Cottier, H.: Helv. Paediat. Acta **13**:313-338, 1958.

52 Tomasi, T. B., Jr., and Czerwinski, D. S.: Birth Defects Original Article Series **IV**(1): 270-282, 1968; The National Foundation, New York.

53 West, C. D., Hong, R., and Holland, N. H.: J. Clin. Invest. **41**:2054-2064, 1962.

Relationship of thymus and myasthenia gravis

54 Barton, F. E., and Branch, C. F.: J.A.M.A. **109**:2044-2048, 1937.

55 Beutner, E. H., Witebsky, E., Ricken, D., and Adler, R. H.: J.A.M.A. **182**:46-58, 1962.

56 Buzzard, E. F.: Brain **28**:438-483, 1905.

57 Goldstein, G., and Whittingham, S.: Lancet **2**:315-318, 1966.

58 Goldstein, G., and Whittingham, S.: Clin. Exp. Immun. **2**:257-268, 1967.

59 Marshall, A. H. E., and White, R. G.: Brit. J. Exp. Path. **42**:379-385, 1961.

60 Marshall, A. H. E., and White, R. G.: Lancet **1**:1030-1031, 1961.

61 Namba, T., and Grob, D.: Ann. N. Y. Acad. Sci. **135**:606-630, 1966.

62 Namba, T., Himei, H., and Grob, D. J.: Lab. Clin. Med. **70**:258-272, 1967.

63 Nastuk, W. L., Plescia, O. J., and Osserman, K. E.: Proc. Soc. Exp. Biol. Med. **105**:177-184, 1960.

64 Oosterhuis, H. J.: Lancet **2**:1226-1227, 1966.

65 Perlo, V. P., Poskanzer, D. C., Schwab, R. S., Viets, H. R., Osserman, K. E., and Genkins, G.: Neurology (Minneap.) **16**:431-439, 1966.

66 Simpson, J. A.: Scot. Med. J. **5**:419-436, 1960.

67 Sloan, H. E., Jr.: Surgery **13**:154-174, 1943.

68 Strauss, A. J. L.: Lancet **2**:351-352, 1962.

69 Strauss, A. J. L.: Advances Intern. Med. **14**:241-280, 1968.

70 Strauss, A. J. L., and Kemp, P. G., Jr.: J. Immun. **99**:945-953, 1967.

71 Strauss, A. J. L., and van der Geld, H. W. R.: In Wolstenholme, G. E. W., and Porter, R.: editors: The thymus: experimental and clinical studies, Boston, 1966, Little, Brown and Co.

72 Strauss, A. J. L., Seegal, B. C., Hsu, K. C., Burkholder, P. M., Nastuk, W. L., and Osserman, K. E.: Proc. Soc. Exp. Biol. Med. **105**:184-191, 1960.

73 Strauss, A. J. L., Smith, C. W., Cage, G. W., van der Geld, H. W. R., McFarlin, D. E., and Barlow, M.: Ann. N. Y. Acad. Sci. **135**:557-579, 1966.

74 van der Geld, H. W. R., and Strauss, A. J. L.: Lancet **1**:57-60, 1966.

75 Van de Velde, R. L., and Friedman, N. B.: J.A.M.A. **198**:287-288, 1966.

76 Vetters, J. M., Simpson, J. A., and Folkarde, A.: Lancet **2**:28-31, 1969.

77 Viets, H.: J.A.M.A. **153**:1273-1280, 1953.

78 Viets, H.: Amer. J. Med. **19**:658-660, 1955.

79 Viets, H.: Med. Hist. **9**:184-186, 1965.

80 Viets, H. R., and Schwab, R. S.: Thymectomy for myasthenia gravis, Springfield, Ill., 1960, Charles C Thomas, Publisher.

81 Walker, M. B.: Lancet **1**:1200-1201, 1934.

Status thymicolymphaticus

82 Conti, E. A., Patton, G. D., Conti, J. E., and Hempelmann, L. H.: Radiology **74**:386-391, 1960.

83 Friedlander, A.: Arch. Pediat. **24**:490-501, 1907.

84 Saenger, E. L., Silverman, F. N., Sterling, T. D., and Turner, M. E.: Radiology 74:889-904, 1960.

85 Simpson, C. L., and Hempelmann, L. H.: Cancer 10:42-56, 1957.

86 Simpson, C. L., Hempelmann, L. H., and Fuller, L. M.: Radiology 64:840-845, 1955.

Tumors

87 Andersen, S. B., and Ladefoged, J.: Acta Haemat. (Basel) 30:319-325, 1963.

88 Anderson, E. T., and Vye, M. V.: Ann. Intern. Med. 66:141-149, 1967.

89 Bernstein, A., Klosk, E., Simon, F., and Brodkin, H. A.: Circulation 3:508-513, 1951.

90 Boetsch, C. H., Swoyer, G. B., Adams, A., and Walker, J. H.: Dis. Chest 50:539-543, 1966.

91 Castleman, B.: In Atlas of tumor pathology, Sec. V, Fasc. 19, Washington, D. C., 1955, Armed Forces Institute of Pathology.

92 Edland, R. W., Levine, S., Serfas, L. S., and Flair, R. C.: Amer. J. Roentgen. 103:25-31, 1968.

93 Fechner, R. E.: Cancer 23:16-23, 1969.

94 Funkhouser, J. W.: New Eng. J. Med. 264:34-36, 1961.

95 Good, R. A.: Bull. Univ. Minn. Hosp. 26:1-19, 1954.

96 Hale, J. F., and Scowen, E. F.: Thymic tumors—their association with myasthenia gravis and their treatment by radiotherapy, London, 1967, Lloyd-Luke (Medical Books) Ltd.

97 Hirst, E., and Robertson, T. I.: Medicine (Balt.) 46:225-264, 1967.

98 Katz, A., and Lattes, R.: Cancer 23:1-15, 1969.

99 Klein, J. J., Gottlieb, A. J., Mones, R. J., Oppel, S. H., and Osserman, K. E.: Arch. Intern. Med. (Chicago) 113:142-152, 1964.

100 Lambie, J. A., and Pilot, R.: J. Lancet 88:315-318, 1968.

101 Langston, J. D., Wagman, G. F., and Dickenman, R. C.: Arch. Path. (Chicago) 68:367-373, 1959.

102 Larsson, O.: Lancet 2:655-656, 1963.

103 Lattes, R.: Cancer 15:1224-1260, 1962.

104 Lattes, R., and Jonas, S.: Bull. N. Y. Acad. Med. 33:145-147, 1957.

105 Levine, S., Labiche, H., and Chandor, S.: Amer. Rev. Resp. Dis. 98:875-878, 1968.

106 Lindstrom, F. D., Williams, R. C., and Brunning, R. D.: Arch. Intern. Med. (Chicago) 122:526-531, 1968.

107 Montes, L. F., Carter, E., Moreland, N., and Aballos, R.: J.A.M.A. 204:351-354, 1968.

108 Murray, W. D., and Webb, J. N.: Amer. J. Med. 41:974-980, 1966 (thymoma, hypogammaglobulinemia, and pure red cell aplasia).

109 Sawyers, J. L., and Foster, J. H.: Arch. Surg. (Chicago) 96:814-817, 1968.

110 Schmid, J. R., Kiely, J. M., Harrison, E. G., Jr., Bayrd, G. L., and Peas, G. L.: Cancer 18:216-230, 1965.

111 Scholz, D. A., and Bahn, R. C.: Mayo Clin. Proc. 34:433-441, 1959.

112 Waller, J. V., Shapiro, M., and Paltauf, R.: Amer. Heart. J. 53:479-484, 1957.

113 Wilkins, E. W., Jr., Edmunds, L. H., and Castleman, B.: J. Thorac. Cardiovasc. Surg. 52:322-330, 1966.

Chapter 33

Pituitary gland

A. R. Currie

STRUCTURE AND FUNCTION OF NORMAL HYPOPHYSIS
Embryology

The epithelial parts of the hypophysis, consisting of the pars anterior, the pars intermedia, and the pars tuberalis, develop from Rathke's pouch, which is a midline ectodermal outgrowth of the oral cavity. It is doubtful if the pars intermedia of the lower vertebrates is present in the human adult, but there is an intermediate zone that contains, in variable degree, colloid-filled cysts, the remnants of Rathke's pouch, and basophil cells that invade the pars nervosa. With the growth of the fundus of Rathke's pouch, the neck elongates and becomes a solid stalk, the craniopharyngeal stalk, which usually has disappeared by the tenth week of intrauterine life. The pharyngeal pituitary, which is constantly present in the roof of the nasopharynx, is derived from the buccal end of the stalk. Epithelial remnants rarely are found in a craniopharyngeal canal traversing the body of the sphenoid bone. The fundus of Rathke's pouch proliferates to form the adenohypophysis. The infundibulum and neurohypophysis are derived from a downgrowth of the floor of the forebrain, and their development depends on contact with the buccal part.

It seems that the human fetal adenohypophysis begins to produce its hormones about the twelfth to fourteenth week of pregnancy. Growth hormone has been detected at this time with an immunofluorescence system[27] (Fig. 33-1). It is not yet known, however, if the hormones produced by the pituitary gland at this stage are secreted and play a part in fetal growth and development.

The following residual structures may persist in or around the hypophysis and may give rise to tumors or cysts: (1) juxtahypophyseal epithelial residues, (2) remnants of Rathke's cleft, (3) the pharyngeal pituitary, and (4) intrasphenoidal remnants of the craniopharyngeal stalk.

Anatomy

General aspects. In the human adult, the pituitary gland weighs from 0.5 gm to 0.9 gm. The *adenohypophysis* (anterior lobe, including the pars distalis and anterior hypophysis) forms the greater part of the gland and is prolonged over the stalk toward the base of the brain as the pars tuberalis (Fig. 33-2). The posterior lobe (pars nervosa and intermediate zone) is directly continuous with the neural tissues of the pituitary stalk and forms part of the *neurohypophysis,* which also includes the median eminence, the infundibular stem, and the infundibular process. In midhorizontal cut section, the normal adult anterior lobe is kidney-shaped; the anterior pole and central parts are reddish in color, whereas the lateral expansions are opaque and yellow. There are often one or more cysts of pinhead size between the anterior and posterior lobes in the adult. In early life, a wide cleft, filled with gelatinous material, usually separates the lobes. This is the persistent cavity of Rathke's pouch that is usually obliterated in later years. On cut section, the posterior lobe is soft, gray, and semitranslucent. As age advances, there is a progressive tendency for the accumulation of brown pigment throughout the lobe.

Neural connections. The continuity of the posterior lobe with the base of the brain is of prime functional importance, since the pituitary stalk carries the main tractus hypophyseus (paraventriculo-supraoptico-hypophyseal tract). The innervation of this region is derived from the supraoptic and paraventricular nuclei, from the tuberoinfundibular nuclei, and perhaps from other nuclear regions of the hypothalamus. The fibers ramify through the posterior lobe and end near the

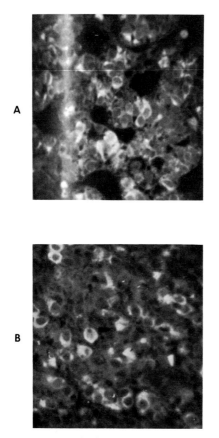

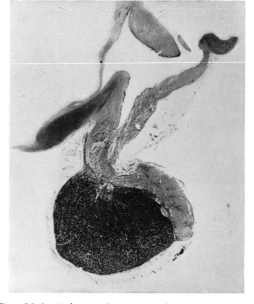

Fig. 33-2 Midsagittal section of pituitary gland to show neural attachments. (Hematoxylin-eosin; ×4; courtesy Dr. Dorothy S. Russell.)

Fig. 33-1 Growth hormone–containing cells in fetal human adenohypophysis. **A,** Fifteen-week fetus. **B,** Twenty-three-week fetus. Note increase in amount of cytoplasm with increasing age and compare with Fig. 33-5. (**A** and **B,** Indirect immunofluorescence technique; ×400; from Ellis, S. T., Beck, J. S., and Currie, A. R.: J. Path. Bact. **92:**179-183, 1966.)

walls of the blood vessels—it is not accepted that any fibers pass from the hypothalamus to the anterior lobe. It is believed that the hormones of the posterior lobe are produced in the neurons of the hypothalamic nuclei mentioned[37] and that the secretion travels in some way in the nerve fibers of the tractus hypophyseus to the posterior lobe: the posterior lobe acts as a store or reservoir for these hormones.

Vascular supply. The complicated and complex vascular supply of the pituitary gland has been studied intensively in recent years,[91, 97] and it now seems clear that the main blood supply of the anterior lobe comes from the anterior and lateral superior hypophyseal arteries, while the inferior hypophyseal arteries nourish the posterior lobe. A branch from the inferior capsular artery sup-

plies the lateral poles of the anterior lobe, and it may have a tenuous anastomosis with the lower end of the artery of the fibrous core (a branch of the loral artery, which is given off the anterior superior artery). There is a variable anastomotic supply from the inferior hypophyseal circle. The adenohypophysis also receives a large portal supply which consists of large, thin-walled vessels that convey blood from capillary networks in the median eminence and in the stalk.

Histology and histochemistry
Adenohypophysis

The anterior lobe is composed of groups of several types of polygonal epithelial cells, supported by connective tissue and the capillary sinusoids (Fig. 33-3). On the basis of histologic stains such as Mallory's trichrome technique, the cells traditionally have been classed in three main groups:

1 Acidophil (alpha or eosinophil) cells, about 40% of the total, which are large, well defined, and contain strongly eosinophilic granules
2 Basophil (beta) cells, about 10% of the total, whose granules stain with hematoxylin and aniline blue
3 Chromophobe cells, about 50% of the total, which are small and have a scanty and nongranular cytoplasm.

There has been much interest shown in

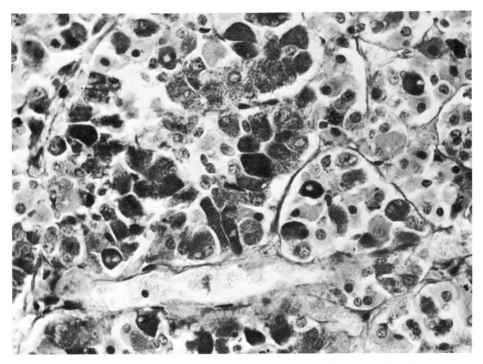

Fig. 33-3 Normal adult adenohypophysis showing groups of epithelial cells supported by connective tissue and sinusoids. "Dark" cells are basophils. (PAS-trichrome; ×500.)

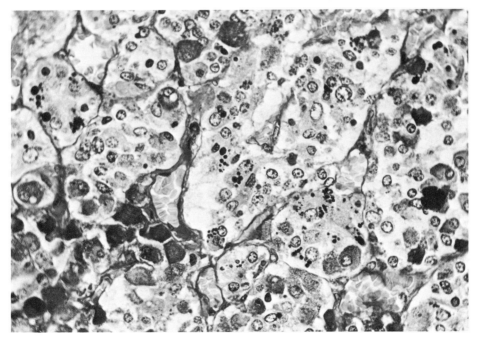

Fig. 33-4 Vesiculate chromophobe cells in adenohypophysis of patient with myxedema. Note variation in size of the PAS-positive granules. (PAS-trichrome; ×500.)

recent years in the cells of the adenohypophysis. The types of cells demonstrable in the optical microscope depend on the fixative, the preliminary use of oxidizing agents in some cases, the chemical nature of the hormones (which may show species variations), and the staining methods employed. There has been considerable confusion about the nomenclature of the cells and the cellular localization of the hormones. Several names have been applied to functionally similar cells and, on occasions, one name, usually a letter of the Greek alphabet, has been given to two types of cells of quite different properties. An excellent account of the situation has been written by Purves.[74] The International Committee for Nomenclature of the Adenohypophysis recommended in 1963 that a functional terminology should be used whenever possible.[102]

Basophils. Almost twenty years ago, Pearse[71, 72] reported that the basophils in man stained with the periodic acid–Schiff (PAS) technique, suggesting that they contain a glycoprotein. In addition, some cells that stain as chromophobes with Mallory's trichrome technique and other methods are also PAS positive. Pearse called all these PAS-positive cells mucoid cells and listed the following types: maximal (heavily granulated), intermediate (lightly granulated), vesiculate chromophobe (Fig. 33-4), disperse, and punctate. Basophils of intermediate lobe origin in human glands may be demonstrated with the aldehyde thionine–PAS–orange G technique.[70] They are large, often irregular in shape, and PAS positive. Other types of basophils can be differentiated by size and shape and are stained purple with aldehyde thionine. After performic acid oxidation, the intermediate lobe basophils are PAS positive ("R" cells), whereas other basophils do not retain PAS and can be stained with alcian blue ("S" cells). This difference is used in the PAS–performic acid–alcian blue technique of Adams and Pearse[1] and Adams and Swettenham.[2] The "S" cells contain a cystine-rich protein and because of the sulfur content of this amino acid were given their name. The sulfur in cystine is oxidized by performic acid to sulfonate, which combines with alcian blue to give blue-stained granules. By contrast, the protein of the "R" cells, which are poor in cystine, is resistant to extraction with performic acid and the granules of these "R" cells when subsequently counterstained with PAS are reddish-purple in color.

A short, useful, and critical account of other staining methods and their value has been written recently by Russfield.[85]

Since thyrotropin and the gonadotropins are glycoproteins and are known to have a high carbohydrate content, it is virtually certain that they stain with the PAS technique. Nevertheless, it must be emphasized that we cannot develop *hormone-specific* histochemical methods until we know more about the chemistry of the pituitary hormones and the chemical state in which they are stored in the cells.

With immunofluorescence systems, it has been claimed that corticotropin is localized in some basophils in man,[49] and luteinizing hormone in basophils that do not stain with aldehyde thionine.[79]

Acidophils. Two types of acidophil are readily demonstrated in the human adenohypophysis with Herlant's tetrachrome method,[39] and it has been claimed that the somatotropic cells stain with orange G, whereas the prolactin cells take up red erythrosin. The only specific method for the demonstration of

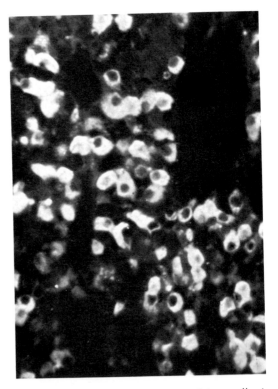

Fig. 33-5 Growth hormone-containing cells in adult human adenohypophysis. (Indirect immunofluorescence technique; ×400; from Porteous, I. B., Beck, J. S., and Currie, A. R.: J. Path. Bact. **91:** 539-543, 1966.)

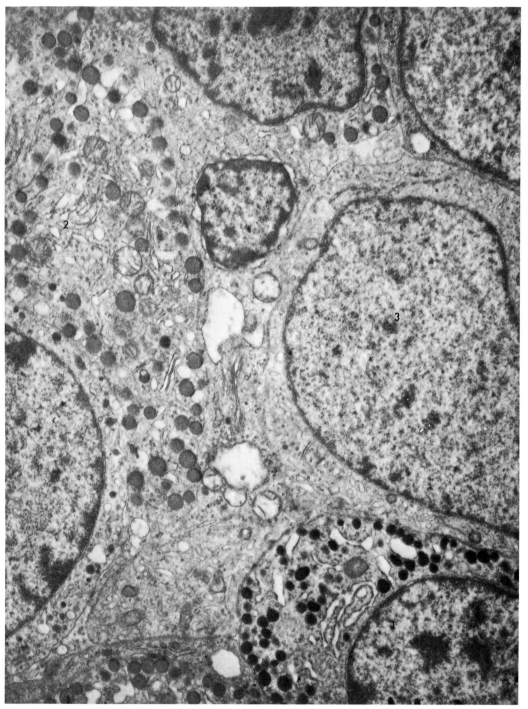

Fig. 33-6 Electron micrograph of eighteen-week fetal human adenohypophysis showing granular cells and one agranular cell. Granules vary in size from cell to cell and within one cell. **1,** Granule size approximately 280 mμ—basophil. **2,** Granule size approximately 500 mμ—acidophil. **3,** Agranular—chromophobe. (Glutaraldehyde and Palade; Karnovsky; ×12,600; from Ellis, S. T.: Ph.D. thesis, University of Aberdeen.)

growth hormone in the human pituitary gland, however, is an immunofluorescence system[7] (Figs. 33-1 and 33-5). This has shown that growth hormone is present in about 97% of the acidophils, 5% of the chromophobes, and about 3% of the mucoid cells. These findings must raise the question of the functional validity of the orthodox cytologic classification of the adenohypophysis and stimulate caution in assigning functional significance to preparations stained with methods that are not hormone specific. It is perhaps necessary, too, to emphasize that in the localization of cell antigens with an immunofluorescence system, the serologic testing of the antisera must be thorough to ensure immunologic specificity.

Most of the attempts to assign a precise functional significance to the various cell types in the human adenohypophysis have been largely speculative and have been based upon observations in various endocrine disturbances. Some of these are discussed later in this chapter.

Chromophobes. With the optical microscope, about 50% of the cells of the pars distalis appear to be chromophobes, but a few secretory granules usually can be demonstrated in them with the electron microscope.

Cellular localization of hormones. There is little doubt that basophil cells produce follicle-stimulating hormone, luteinizing hormone, thyrotropin, and corticotropin, while the acidophil cells produce somatotropin and prolactin. Corticotropin also may be produced by some anterior lobe chromophobes. It is perhaps premature to use the terms thyrotroph, gonadotroph, corticotroph, somatotroph, and mammotroph for cells in the human adenohypophysis. When truly specific methods are available for the demonstration of all the pituitary hormones, we shall be in a much stronger position to classify the cells and use functional terminology, and it will be of interest to discover whether a particular cell type is responsible for the production, storage, and secretion of more than one of the hormones.

Cell ultrastructure. In experimental animals, it is possible to distinguish some of the functional cell types by the morphology of the cytoplasmic granules in the electron microscope. In man, the acidophils are easily recognized because of the osmiophilia and large size of their secretion granules (400 mμ to 700 mμ in diameter) (Fig. 33-6). To date, there is no specific method available for

demonstrating any of the protein hormones in the electron microscope.

Neurohypophysis

Since the neurohypophysis is an extension of the brain, the interstitial tissue is composed of cells of the neural type, the pituicytes. They are elongated slender cells that occupy the interstices between the numerous anastomosing blood vessels. They also are present in the pituitary stalk and in the expanded lower end of the neurohypophysis, interdigitating with the fine nerve fiber terminals of the tractus hypophyseus. These nerve terminals contain the so-called neurosecretory material that also can be demonstrated in smaller amounts in occasional fibers of the tractus hypophyseus, in cell bodies of the supraoptic nuclei, and in the large cell component of the paraventricular nuclei.[5, 94] This neurosecretory material may be stained with the aldehyde-fuchsin method or, more specifically, with the performic acid–alcian blue technique.[83]

The posterior lobe, then, is composed of pituicytes and nerve fibers. Both alkaline and acid phosphatase are demonstrable in the neurohypophyseal vessels, and phosphamidase is found in some of the nerve fibers.[29] At one time, it was believed that the pituicytes produced the hormones they contain, but now it is thought that they are synthesized by neurons of the hypothalamohypophyseal system. Some days after section of the pituitary stalk, neurosecretory material accumulates proximal to the site of section.[96] The amount of neurosecretory material stored varies with the functional state of the gland: the store is diminished if there is increased secretion of antidiuretic hormone. It has been shown with histochemical techniques that the neurosecretory material is rich in cystine,[93] and so are the hormones. Sloper[95] has written a detailed account of the histochemistry of the neurohypophysis.

Hormones of adenohypophysis

The hormones of the adenohypophysis are protein and polypeptide in nature. The amino acid composition and sequence of some of these have been determined. We still have much to learn about their chemical state of storage in the cells of the pituitary gland, their mode of transport in the blood, and, as Li has indicated, "the *actual* nature of protein or peptide hormones as they occur in the body in their role of physiologically active catalysts."* It may be that the hormone extracted by the chemist is a prohormone and that it must be converted to its active biologic form by the enzymes of the cells of the target organ. Following are the hormones of the adenohypophysis:

1 Adrenocorticotropic hormone (corticotropin; ACTH)
2 Thyrotropic hormone (thyrotropin; thyroid-stimulating hormone; TSH)
3 Follicle-stimulating hormone (FSH)
4 Luteinizing hormone (LH; interstitial cell–stimulating hormone; ICSH)
5 Luteotropic hormone (prolactin; lactogenic hormone)
6 Growth hormone (somatotropic hormone; somatotropin; STH; GH)

Their probable *cellular localization* in the adenohypophysis is given on p. 1408.

Assay

Apart from the measurement of gonadotropins in urine, there are no *routine* methods yet available for concentrating and assaying the pituitary hormones in the body fluids. The methods currently used are described and critically evaluated by Loraine and Bell,[55] who also review the application of these techniques and the results of investigation of clinical problems.

Adrenocorticotropic hormone

Chemistry. The chemistry of corticotropin has been reviewed by Engel and Lebovitz.[28] ACTH is a polypeptide of about 4,500 molecular weight with thirty-nine amino acid residues, the first twenty-four and the last seven from the N terminus (positions 1 to 24 and 33 to 39) are identical in the human being, pig, cattle, and sheep preparations, but there are slight species differences in composition and sequence in positions 25 to 32.

Either a portion or the whole of the ACTH molecule has been synthesized by various groups of workers, and synthetic ACTH has been shown to be biologically active in the human subject. The biologic activity of synthetic ACTH preparations is in the molecule with twenty-four amino acid residues, and the biologic role of the "inessential" part of the molecule is not yet known. It has been suggested that it may shield the active part

of the molecule from enzymes or that it may have biologic functions still to be discovered.

Biologic actions. In addition to controlling the secretory activity of the adrenal cortex, ACTH has a number of extra-adrenal effects that also have been reviewed by Engel and Lebovitz[28]: adipokinetic effects *in vivo*, effects on carbohydrate metabolism *in vivo*, metabolic effects on adipose tissue *in vitro*, and a number of "miscellaneous" actions, including melanocyte stimulation. It is of interest that the melanophore-stimulating hormone isolated from the posterior lobe of the porcine gland consists of 18 amino acids and that a portion of the amino acid sequence is identical with a sequence found in corticotropin. Li[50] has suggested that this may account for the melanocyte-stimulating activity of pure corticotropin preparations.

Assay. There are several methods available for assaying ACTH in body fluids and in tissues, and these have been reviewed by Vernikos-Danellis.[103] Most of the techniques, which have so far been described, are not sufficiently sensitive to detect the hormone in body fluids, and there is relatively little quantitative information available on ACTH levels in health and disease. Assays in hypophysectomized animals are more precise and more specific than those conducted in animals with intact pituitary glands. One of the most satisfactory is the measurement of the in vivo secretion of corticosterone by the rat adrenal gland.[54] Radioimmunologic assay methods, such as that of Yalow et al.,[107] are claimed to be sufficiently sensitive to detect the hormone in human plasma.

Storage in pituitary gland. The adult human pituitary gland contains about 20 to 25 IU of corticotropin, and there is some evidence that the hormone is stored in two forms: a "free" compound of low molecular weight and a protein or protein-bound form.[17] Corticotropic activity has been detected in the fetal pituitary gland at about the sixteenth week of gestation.[101]

Thyrotropic hormone

Chemistry. Purified preparations of TSH are not yet completely homogeneous as judged by criteria involving electrophoresis and ultracentrifugation. The molecular weight of bovine TSH has been estimated to be of the order of 28,000.

Biologic actions. TSH controls the activity of the thyroid gland, and it has extrathyroid effects on skin and connective tissues. The

---

*From Li, C. H.: Advances Protein Chem. **11**:101-190, 1956; copyrighted by Academic Press, Inc.

"exophthalmos-producing substance" is chemically different from TSH.

Assay. Of the many bioassay methods available for the assay of TSH, Loraine and Bell[55] recommend in vitro methods that depend on the maintenance of weight of thyroid slices or on the release of iodine[131] from guinea pig thyroid tissue. These bioassay methods have a high degree of sensitivity, but it seems likely that they will be replaced in the near future by radioimmunologic techniques. The serum of a proportion of thyrotoxic patients contains long-acting thyroid stimulator (LATS), which produces an abnormal response in certain biologic assays for TSH (p. 1436).

Storage in pituitary gland. The adult human pituitary gland contains about 2 IU of TSH.

Gonadotropins[55]—follicle-stimulating hormone; luteinizing hormone; luteotropic hormone

Chemistry. Three substances with gonadotropic activity are elaborated by the adenohypophysis: follicle-stimulating, luteinizing, and luteotropic hormones. The molecular weight of human LH has been estimated to be 26,000, but similar information is not available for FSH. Both hormones are believed to be glycoproteins. Human urinary FSH has not yet been completely separated from urinary LH.

Biologic actions. FSH promotes Graafian follicle maturation in the ovary and spermatogenesis in the testis. LH causes luteinization of the ovarian follicles and stimulates the interstitial cells in the testis.

Assay. The majority of the many assay methods available are not sufficiently sensitive to detect FSH and LH activity in the blood with regularity, and most studies have been made on urine that has been extracted and concentrated by a variety of methods. There is not yet a highly sensitive method for assaying FSH activity. Changes in the weight of the ovaries of immature rats that have been primed with human chorionic gonadotropin may be used to estimate FSH. LH activity may be assessed by measuring the enlargement of the ventral lobe of the prostate of immature hypophysectomized rats. A new assay method for LH, based on ovarian cholesterol depletion in rats, has been developed by Bell et al.,[8] who claim that it is more sensitive than other available techniques and may be used for measuring LH activity in blood as well as in urine. Increase

in uterine weight in intact mice frequently is used as a measure of total urinary gonadotropic activity. It is likely that radioimmunologic methods will be developed in the course of time for FSH and LH.

Storage in pituitary gland. The yield of gonadotropins from the human adult pituitary gland is somewhat higher in the female than in the male and increases with age.[18]

Growth hormone

Chemistry. Highly purified preparations of human growth hormone have been made by several groups of workers, and the amino acid composition has been established. The molecular weight is believed to be about 21,500 on the basis of both equilibrium ultracentrifugation studies and amino acid analysis.[51, 52]

Biologic actions. Growth hormone preparations from animal pituitary glands have little, if any, anabolic action in man, whereas human preparations are generally highly active. The hormone causes accelerated mobilization of fat and may cause diminished fat formation. It is concerned with cartilage and bone growth (p. 1422).

Assay. The increase in width of the proximal epiphyseal cartilage of the tibia of the hypophysectomized rat is a sensitive bioassay method for growth hormone. Immunologic rather than biologic methods should now be used for the assay of growth hormone in body fluids and, at the present time, the method of choice is the radioimmunologic procedure of Hunter and Greenwood.[42] The hemagglutination-inhibition methods lack specificity and should not be used in clinical work.[55]

Storage in pituitary gland. The average yield of growth hormone from human glands is high, up to 15.4 mg. per gland,[33] and it has been reported that it does not vary with age.

Prolactin

Chemistry. It has been claimed by some that human pituitary prolactin is identical with human growth hormone,[9] whereas others believe that it is a separate entity.[3] There seems to be general agreement that these hormones do exist as separate entities in animal glands, and the molecular weight of sheep prolactin is approximately 23,000.

Biologic action. Prolactin is believed to be essential for the initiation and probably also for the maintenance of lactation. It also has luteotropic properties.

Assay. The activity of prolactin may be

measured by the increase it causes in the weight of the crop gland in the immature pigeon.

Storage in pituitary gland. The yield of prolactin from the human pituitary gland tends to increase with advancing age.[18]

Control of secretion of adenohypophyseal hormones

This complex and difficult field can only be briefly and summarily dealt with in this chapter. Most of the functions of the anterior pituitary gland are controlled by release factors (RF) and inhibitory factors that are produced in the hypothalamus.[91]

The probable sites of the centers that secrete the various *release factors* are as follows:

Corticotropin RF	Anterior and middle parts of median eminence
Follicle-stimulating hormone RF Luteinizing hormone RF	Median eminence behind the infundibulum; LH possibly also in preoptic area
Thyrotropin RF	Preoptic area between optic chiasma and paraventricular nuclei
Growth hormone RF	Anterior part of median eminence

It is generally accepted that the release factors are produced in the nerve cells and pass down the nerve fibers to the infundibulum and pituitary stalk, as does vasopressin neurosecretory material from the supraoptic and paraventricular nuclei. It seems, however, that these two processes are separate and distinct and, at present, it is generally believed that the release factor system is not part of the standard neurosecretion system.[91] Although injection of vasopressin into the hypothalamus does produce secretion of ACTH, it is thought to be due to release of endogenous corticotropin release factor. The centers that secrete release factors do not correspond with any of the standard anatomic nuclei, and they are probably made up of the small nerve cells in the undifferentiated gray matter. From the infundibulum and pituitary stalk, the release factors are carried by the portal blood vessels to the adenohypophysis.

For many years, it has been known that there is an inverse relationship between the blood levels of the hormones of the "target" endocrine organs and the blood levels of the pituitary tropic hormones. This is believed to result from a *negative feedback mechanism—*

e.g., an increase in the blood cortisol level causes a decrease in the output of corticotropin. The general principles of this negative feedback mechanism suggest that the production of the release factors is controlled by *receptor centers,* which are sensitive to the peripheral hormones. Some of these are also sensitive to the pituitary tropic hormones. The location of these centers is at present being mapped out, and it is probable that there also may be receptor centers in parts of the brain above the hypothalamus.

Hormones of neurohypophysis

The neurohypophyseal hormones, vasopressin (antidiuretic hormone) and oxytocin, are stored mainly in the posterior lobe of the pituitary gland but, in most species, including man, 1% to 3% of the total is found in the hypothalamus and infundibular stalk. These hormones or their precursors are linked with about thirty times their weight of the van Dyke carrier protein, and the complex is the "neurosecretory material" or "neurosecretion."

The hormones are produced in the neurons of the supraoptic and paraventricular nuclei and pass down the hypothalamohypophyseal tract to the posterior lobe, where they are discharged from the nerve endings into the pericapillary spaces and then into the general circulation. It is not known in what form the hormones reach the circulation, and it is possible that they also may be released directly into the bloodstream from the hypothalamus.

Chemistry. Three mammalian neurohypophyseal hormones (oxytocin, arginine-vasopressin, and lysine-vasopressin) have been isolated and characterized.[26] They are octapeptides. The amino acid sequence of oxytocin is as follows:

Cys.-Tyr.-Ileu.-Glu.-NH₂Asp.-NH₂Cys.-Pro.-Leu.-Gly.-NH₂

Arginine-vasopressin is formed by man, and its amino acid sequence is as follows:

Cys.-Tyr.-Phc.-Glu.-NH₂Cys.-Pro.-Arg.-Gly.-NH₂

Biologic actions. *Vasopressin* regulates the reabsorption of free water in the kidneys. If it is deficient, there is uncontrolled loss of water through the kidneys, and diabetes insipidus (p. 1424) results. It has yet to be shown that its vasopressor action is important in man. Vasopressin stimulates the release of corticotropin, but it now seems that the principal corticotropin release factor is a related but not identical polypeptide.

Oxytocin stimulates the myoepithelium of the lactating mammary gland, and, at term, small amounts given intravenously cause contraction of the human uterus.

Assay. There is no *routine* method yet available for the measurement of vasopressin and oxytocin in body fluids. Biologic assay methods for vasopressin depend on its vasopressor effect on the rat and on its antidiuretic effect in the dog. The increase in pressure within the lactating mammary gland of the rabbit is used as a bioassay method for oxytocin. It seems that these methods soon will be replaced by radioimmunologic assay techniques.

Storage in posterior lobe of pituitary gland. About 15 units of vasopressin are stored in the posterior lobe of the pituitary gland. In man, vasopressin and oxytocin are not stored bound in fixed proportions to protein.[20]

Control of secretion. The release of *vasopressin* depends mainly on changes in the osmotic pressure of the plasma, especially on an increase or decrease due to sodium and chloride—a rise in the osmotic pressure stimulates release of the hormone. The volume of the plasma and extracellular fluid also is concerned in the control of secretion of vasopressin.

During lactation, *oxytocin* is released by reflex action—the afferent pathway arises in the richly innervated nipple. Release also is influenced by stimuli from above the hypothalamus that act on the supraoptic and paraventricular nuclei.

Physiologic changes

Age. As age advances, basophils of the intermediate lobe type invade the posterior lobe of the pituitary gland, which often becomes deeply pigmented. There is an irregular, mainly extracellular, deposition of granules of this brownish pigment in the neural tissue. The chemical nature of the pigment is not known.

In middle-aged or elderly subjects, small rests of squamous cells are frequently seen in relation to the glandular epithelial cells. They often are present near the junction of the stalk with the anterior lobe and in the pars tuberalis. It is now generally believed that these are foci of squamous metaplasia and not embryonic rests.

With decline in sexual activity, the number of the basophil cells in the anterior lobe increases and many of them show cytoplasmic vacuolation. The "castration cells" seen in lower vertebrates are not found in man.

The stored amounts of some of the hypophyseal hormones change as age advances (p. 1409).

Pregnancy. As pregnancy advances, the adenohypophysis increases in size, and with repeated pregnancies, it may become permanently enlarged—due to an increase in the number of cells in the gland. It is claimed that one type of basophil decreases sharply and that the stored amount of gonadotropin in the gland is much reduced. There is a striking increase in the number of so-called pregnancy cells: wedge-shaped cells with a rather indistinct cytoplasmic outline. The cytoplasm contains few granules, which are usually faintly orange G positive. It has been suggested that these cells are actively synthesizing and secreting prolactin. In recent immunofluorescence studies with antisera to human growth hormone and human placental lactogen, Haugen and Beck[38] reported that the majority of the pregnancy cells did not stain: the cells do not contain significant quantities of growth hormone or of other cross-reacting antigens. If "pregnancy cells" do indeed contain prolactin, then this hormone would appear to be antigenically different from growth hormone.

It is, of course, difficult to analyse the function of the endocrine glands during pregnancy, since the placenta produces large quantities of placental lactogen, chorionic gonadotropin, and steroid hormones. The changes in the adenohypophysis in pregnancy may be secondary to placental hormone secretion.

DEVELOPMENTAL ANOMALIES
Pharyngeal pituitary gland

The pharyngeal pituitary gland is a small embryologic remnant constantly present in man in the submucosa of the nasopharynx[35, 65] (p. 1403). It is oval, about 3 mm to 4 mm in length, and situated in the midline under the periosteum between the sphenoid bone and the vomer. It usually is composed of small chromophobes (Fig. 33-7), among which there are often occasional acidophils but seldom basophils. Some of the acidophils contain growth hormone,[61] and McGrath has reported that pooled pharyngeal pituitary glands contain significant amounts of prolactin and growth hormone.[60] Both "S" and "R" basophils are present, and it has been claimed that ACTH

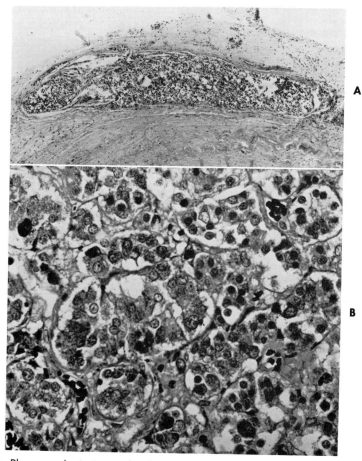

Fig. 33-7 A, Pharyngeal pituitary gland. **B,** Pharyngeal pituitary gland showing mainly chromophobe cells. (**A,** Hematoxylin-eosin; ×44; **B,** acid fuchsin-aniline blue; ×350; **A** and **B,** courtesy Dr. Dorothy S. Russell.)

is present in the "R" cells.[36] Increased chromophil differentiation and enlargement of the pharyngeal pituitary gland has been reported in some individuals with congenital deformities affecting the function of the pars distalis and in some who have had surgical hypophysectomies.[67, 68] It has been suggested that the pharyngeal pituitary gland may take over some of the functions of the adenohypophysis in circumstances such as these, but this has still to be proved. It has been claimed that the pharyngeal pituitary gland rarely may give rise to adenomas.

Pars distalis

The two major developmental anomalies of the pars distalis are aplasia, in which there is defective formation of Rathke's pouch, and anencephaly.

In *aplasia,* there may be no detectable adenohypophyseal tissue, or small nodules of cells may be found on the pituitary stalk or in the region of the pharyngeal pituitary gland. The posterior lobe also may be absent. If the infant survives, there is evidence of severe deficiency of all the tropic hormones.

In *anencephaly,* the neurohypophysis often is absent, and the anterior lobe may be very small or may be deformed because of the malformation of the skull. Most of the gland consists of chromophobes and acidophils with few basophils. Neurosecretory material that normally appears in the fifth month of fetal life is not demonstrable. The adrenal hypoplasia (p. 1466) is due to the absence of the fetal zone and usually is ascribed to pituitary insufficiency. In this connection, it is of interest that the gonads and thyroid gland show no abnormality of note.

Dystopia is a rare condition in which the neurohypophysis is arrested in its downward development in fetal life.

INFLAMMATORY DISEASES
Acute inflammation

Acute inflammation may be a diffuse acute purulent lesion or a localized abscess that can occur in the course of a blood-borne pyogenic infection. It is of interest that either lesion may be associated with ascending purulent urinary infections without detectable pyemic abscesses in other organs. The anterior lobe of the pituitary gland is affected more often than the posterior lobe. Purulent inflammation also may result from direct spread from the leptomeninges and adjacent sinuses or bone.

Chronic inflammation and granulomas

Giant cell granuloma. A rare lesion, giant cell granuloma arises usually in the anterior lobe of the pituitary gland and occurs mostly in middle-aged or elderly women. Its size is variable. There may be much destruction of the anterior lobe with consequent hypopituitarism (p. 1422), or it may be a chance finding on microscopy. The histologic appearances are similar to those of Boeck's sarcoid, but the multinucleate giant cells are more numerous than in the latter and the reticulin pattern is different. The parenchyma between the granulomatous foci is infiltrated by lymphocytes, plasma cells, and eosinophils. It has been suggested that this is a degenerative process and that the epithelioid and giant cells are altered granular cells, but clearly this theory cannot be extended to cases in which the posterior lobe and stalk are involved. Doniach[25] has proposed the view that giant cell granuloma represents an autoimmune process, and he remarked on the concurrent presence of similar granulomas in the atrophic adrenal glands in the patients with associated hypopituitarism.

Boeck's sarcoid. The hypothalamus and the pituitary gland may be involved in sarcoidosis, and in some patients diabetes insipidus may result. In these, there may be a tumorlike mass in the tuber cinereum and the pituitary stalk, or the infiltration may be diffuse.

Tuberculosis. Miliary tubercles are not uncommonly present in either the anterior or the posterior lobe of the pituitary gland in patients with generalized miliary tuberculosis. The pituitary gland also may be involved by direct extension from basal tuberculous meningitis.

Syphilis. In congenital syphilis, there may be interstitial inflammation of the anterior lobe of the pituitary gland, and a gumma is a rare finding in the tertiary stage of the acquired disease.

Mycotic infections. Actinomycosis and other fungal infections rarely involve the pituitary gland.

INFILTRATIONS AND METABOLIC DISORDERS

Amyloid. The pituitary gland frequently is affected in generalized secondary amyloidosis (Fig. 33-8). There is a variable degree of amyloid deposition in the walls of arteries, arterioles, and sinusoids of the anterior lobe, but there is usually little, if any, destruction of the epithelial cells.

Hunter-Hurler disease (gargoylism). The adenohypophysis is consistently involved in gargoylism, which is now regarded as a generalized metabolic disturbance in which there is an accumulation of large amounts of mucopolysaccharides in the cells of many tissues and organs. Many cells of the adenohypophysis are involved. They are pale, swollen, and vacuolated in routine histologic preparations.

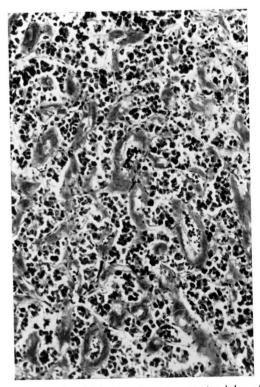

Fig. 33-8 Amyloid deposition in anterior lobe of pituitary gland. (Hematoxylin-eosin; ×140; courtesy Dr. Dorothy S. Russell.)

Xanthomatosis. In Hand-Schüller-Christian disease, with the classic triad of diabetes insipidus, proptosis, and radiologic evidence of bone destruction, the bone and dura around the pituitary gland are infiltrated with lipid-filled macrophages. The posterior lobe and the pituitary stalk also may be affected, but the anterior lobe is not involved.

VASCULAR DISTURBANCES

Hemorrhage. There may be bleeding into the pituitary gland in traumatic lesions of the base of the skull. Hemorrhage may occur into tumors of the gland.

Infarction. Small foci of necrosis are not uncommon in the pituitary gland, and the pathogenesis is not always clear. More extensive infarction may be associated with atherosclerosis of the internal carotid artery or the hypophyseal arteries and with cavernous sinus thrombosis. Rarely, emboli from the heart or from an aortic mural thrombus are the cause. Necrosis also is found in some cases of diabetes mellitus, temporal arteritis, basal meningitis, ascending suppurative pyelonephritis, after section of the lower end of the pituitary stalk,[82] and as a complication of intracranial neoplasms.

Most cases of massive necrosis of the anterior lobe are caused by puerperal circulatory collapse, usually after severe hemorrhage at parturition[90] (p. 1422). There is thrombosis in the sinusoids ventral to the attachment of the stalk to the gland and ischemic or hemorrhagic infarction of the anterior lobe. The central parts are affected, and there is survival of a narrow peripheral rim which is widest in the area adjoining the posterior lobe because of the collateral circulation in this region (Fig. 33-15). The neurohypophysis also may be affected.[91] If the patient survives the acute episode, postnecrotic scarring of the gland results (Fig. 33-15), and calcification, and even ossification, may develop in the scar tissue.

TUMORS
Tumors arising in developmental anomalies

Cysts and tumors of parapituitary epithelial residues.[104] Parapituitary epithelial residues are small epithelial islands frequently found on the upper surface of the adenohypophysis and especially around the infundibulum of the adult gland, and cysts or tumors may arise from them. The cysts almost invariably are lined by stratified squamous epithelium. The tumors may be of squamous type, but many show an ameloblastoma-like structure. They are slowly growing and locally malignant.

Intrapituitary cysts arising from remnants of Rathke's pouch. Large cysts lined wholly or in part by ciliated epithelium may arise from remnants of Rathke's pouch.

Teratoma. Well-differentiated pituitary teratomas are very rare. Less rarely, the posterior lobe, pituitary stalk, and tuber cinereum are the sites of the ectopic pinealoma, a malignant tumor that has been claimed to be an undifferentiated or atypical teratoma.[81] The tumor, which generally occurs in young subjects, forms a solid, grayish, diffusely infiltrating mass. Microscopically, it consists of solid groups of large polygonal or spheroidal cells with eosinophilic cytoplasm and a centrally placed vesiculated nucleus with a conspicuous nucleolus. Many small lymphocytes are characteristically present in the stroma (Fig. 33-9). Diabetes insipidus is frequently present.

Craniopharyngioma. It is generally believed that craniopharyngiomas arise from displaced

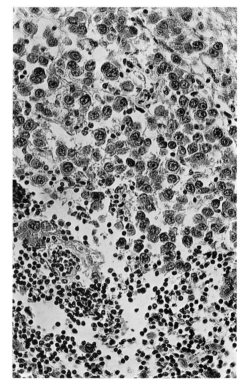

Fig. 33-9 Atypical teratoma ("ectopic pinealoma") of pituitary stalk and posterior lobe of pituitary gland. (Hematoxylin-eosin; ×260; courtesy Dr. Dorothy S. Russell.)

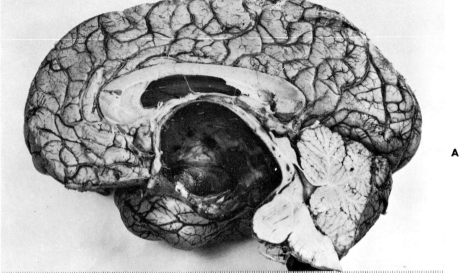

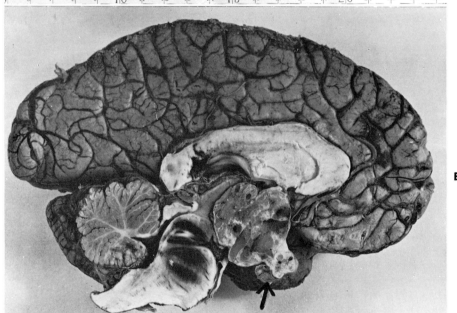

Fig. 33-10 A, Cystic suprasellar craniopharyngioma. **B,** Solid and cystic suprasellar cranio-pharyngioma. Pituitary gland indicated by arrow. (Courtesy Dr. Dorothy S. Russell.)

remnants of the embryonic hypophyseal duct (p. 1403). They are almost always suprasellar but may occur within the sella. The suprasellar type forms about 3% of all intracranial tumors and usually presents in childhood and adolescence.

The tumors may be cystic or cystic and solid (Fig. 33-10). The cysts, which usually contain straw-colored or turbid brown fluid and cholesterol crystals, are lined by stratified squamous epithelium, and the solid areas consist of large trabecular masses of squamous cells in loose connective tissue. At the periphery of these solid areas, the cells are frequently columnar and resemble basal cells (Fig. 33-11), and tumors of this pattern are often inappropriately called adamantinoma.

The clinical effects, of course, depend on

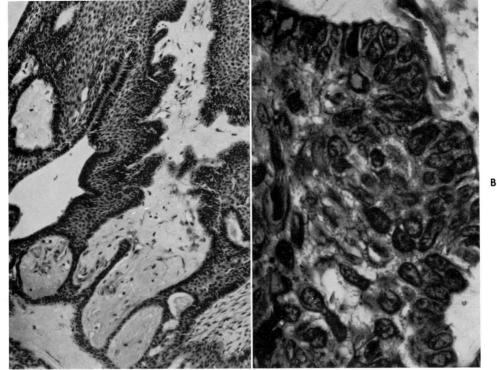

Fig. 33-11 Craniopharyngioma. **A,** Solid anastomosing trabeculae of cells. **B,** Surface cells of basal type and squamous cells. (**A,** Hematoxylin-eosin; ×140; **B,** phosphotungstic acid–hematoxylin; ×850; courtesy Dr. Dorothy S. Russell.)

the size and site of the tumor. There may be the symptoms and signs of an intracranial space-occupying lesion or of pressure on the pituitary gland and destruction of hypothalamic nuclei, causing, for example, pituitary dwarfism or diabetes insipidus. Optic atrophy may result from involvement of the optic chiasma. Calcification commonly is found in the tumor, and this may be of radiodiagnostic value.

Lymphomas

Lymphomas consist of reticular tissue and have a predilection for the infundibulum and the posterior lobe of the pituitary gland and may therefore cause diabetes insipidus. There also may be involvement of other sites elsewhere in the body.

Histologically, the appearances may be those of lymphosarcoma, reticulum cell sarcoma, microgliomatosis, and, rarely, Hodgkin's disease.

Glandular tumors of adenohypophysis[43]
Adenomas

Adenomas are classified according to the nature of the predominant cell type as (1)

chromophobe adenoma, (2) acidophil adenoma, or (3) basophil adenoma, but in many cases there is a mixture of cell types. Adenomas may arise in any part of the anterior lobe of the pituitary gland, and it also has been claimed that they may originate in the pharyngeal pituitary gland or in an embryonic rest of the craniopharyngeal duct. As a general rule, the tumors grow slowly, and Willis has suggested that they begin as areas of focal hyperplasia[105]: single or multiple microscopic foci of hyperplasia frequently are found in the pituitary glands of older persons. The tumors may cause enlargement of the pituitary fossa and, if large, may go through the diaphragma sellae into the cranial cavity and press on the optic chiasma and tracts, on the hypothalamus or midbrain, and even on the ventroposterior part of a frontal lobe or laterally on a temporal lobe.

In addition to the mechanical effects of space-occupying lesions, the tumors may cause endocrine effects resulting from secretion by the tumor cells or from replacement of normal pituitary tissue with consequent hypofunction of the gland.

Chromophobe adenoma. Chromophobe ad-

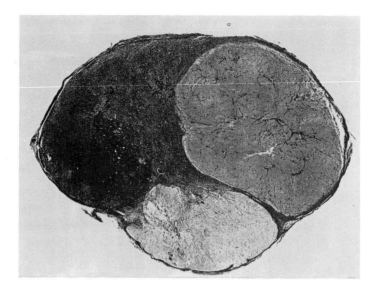

Fig. 33-12 Small chromophobe adenoma of anterior lobe of pituitary gland. Clinically silent. (Acid fuchsin–aniline blue; ×6; courtesy Dr. Dorothy S. Russell.)

enomas account for about two-thirds of all pituitary adenomas, and they tend to attain a large size (Figs. 33-12 and 33-13). They arise in adults, usually in those between 30 and 50 years of age, and even quite large tumors (Fig. 33-12) may be found incidentally at necropsy. Larger chromophobe adenomas cause clinical disturbances because of pressure effects on adjacent structures and, in a small proportion of patients, there may be remote effects due to adenohypophyseal hypofunction. The most frequent manifestation of the latter is hypogonadism.

Microscopically, the appearances vary from case to case and even in different parts of an individual tumor. Some of the tumors are composed of polyhedral cells, with intervening stroma and blood vessels, and present an appearance like that of the normal gland. Most of the tumors either are of a diffuse type or have a papillary structure. Others show a reticular pattern or have a conspicuous perivascular arrangement (Fig. 33-14).

Acidophil adenoma. About 30% of pituitary adenomas consist in whole or in part of acidophils. They are generally smaller than the chromophobe adenomas and usually are confined to the sella turcica. Tumors large enough to be easily visible are relatively uncommon and traditionally are associated with acromegaly or gigantism (p. 1421). The tumors usually are well circumscribed and consist of compact masses of polygonal cells whose cytoplasm contains fine or coarse acidophil granules. It has been shown, with

the fluorescence-antibody technique, that these cells contain growth hormone.[48]

Basophil adenoma. Microscopic foci of basophil cell hyperplasia occasionally are found incidentally in the anterior lobe of the pituitary gland, but larger masses, that merit the term adenoma, are rare. Cushing[22, 23] considered that the basophil adenoma was the cause of the syndrome now commonly named after him, but subsequent experience has shown that this tumor is found in only a small proportion of cases (p. 1474).

Microscopically, the cells of the tumor are well defined, polygonal in shape, and variable in size. It has been reported[45] that they consist of PAS-positive cells of the "R" type. The tumor cells do not usually show Crooke's hyaline change, which may be marked in the basophils of the surrounding glandular tissue of the adenohypophysis. ACTH has been demonstrated in the tumor cells with an immunofluorescence system.[45, 49]

In many patients with adrenal hyperactivity, pituitary adenomas, basophil or chromophobe, have become clinically manifest and may have arisen after bilateral adrenalectomy.[69] It is not yet known whether adrenalectomy is responsible for the initiation of tumor growth or if it results in the stimulation of a preexisting microscopic lesion.

Invasive adenomas and primary carcinoma. As we have already seen, adenomas may show considerable invasive properties, but metastasis by the bloodstream is extremely rare. Secondary deposits may develop in the

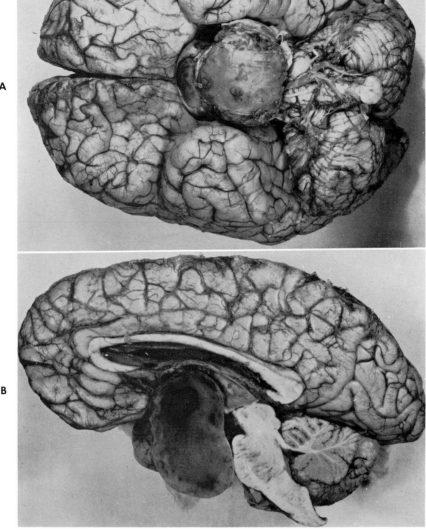

Fig. 33-13 A, Basal view of intrasellar part of large chromophobe adenoma. Note distortion of optic chiasm. **B,** Midsaggital view of same specimen shown in **A.** (Courtesy Dr. Dorothy S. Russell.)

meninges as a result of dissemination in the cerebrospinal fluid.

Pluriglandular adenomatosis. Pluriglandular adenomatosis is a curious and rare syndrome[63, 66] in which the anterior lobe of the pituitary gland, the pancreatic islets of Langerhans, and the parathyroid glands are the site of adenomas or of adenomatoid hyperplasia. The pituitary adenoma may be either chromophobe or acidophil, the islet tumors single or multiple, and one or more of the parathyroid

glands show hyperplasia or contain an adenoma. The clinical effects may be referable to one or all of these lesions. Acromegaly frequently is present. Duodenal or gastric ulcers have developed in some patients.

Tumors of neurohypophysis

Primary tumors of the posterior lobe of the pituitary gland are very rare. Apart from atypical teratomas (p. 1415) and lymphomas

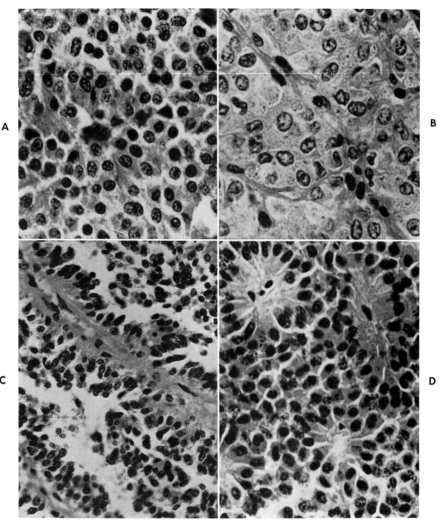

Fig. 33-14 Chromophobe adenoma. **A,** Diffuse type. **B,** Diffuse type with larger cells containing fine cytoplasmic granules. **C** and **D,** Perisinusoidal arrangement of cells. (**A,** Hematoxylin-eosin; ×490; **B,** acid fuchsin–aniline blue; ×620; **C,** hematoxylin-eosin; ×350; **D,** hematoxylin-eosin; ×540; courtesy Dr. Dorothy S. Russell.)

(p. 1417), gliomas and choristomas may arise in the posterior lobe but are extremely rare.

Secondary neoplasms of pituitary gland

Direct spread from a neighboring primary tumor may displace the pituitary gland, but the gland generally tends to resist invasion. Carcinomas of the nasopharynx may infiltrate the pituitary gland, especially the posterior lobe. Blood-borne deposits of secondary carcinoma are not uncommon. The posterior lobe is involved much more frequently than the anterior lobe, but the tumor may spread from the posterior into the anterior lobe. Luft[57] has drawn attention to the high incidence of metastatic deposits in the pituitary gland when the gland is examined histologically after hypophysectomy in patients with disseminated breast cancer.

Experimental pituitary tumors

Over thirty years ago, there were three independent reports[14, 59, 110] of pituitary tumors developing in rodents after prolonged administration of naturally occurring estrogens. The numbers of animals were small and few specimens were examined, and it now seems possible that some of the lesions were hyperplastic rather than neoplastic. Since stilbestrol was synthesized and became easily available, it has been used almost invariably in investigative work involving estrogens.

The pathologic effects of the naturally occurring estrogens, some of which are readily available, have been inadequately studied. Stevens and Helfenstein[98] have reported that the administration of estrone, estriol, 16-epiestriol, or equilenin prevents the appearance of the castration changes in the basophils of the ovariectomized rat but that, of these, only estrone caused tumor formation.

Functioning transplantable pituitary tumors have been induced in rodents by chronic thyroid deficiency and by x-irradiation. Furth and Clifton[32] have shown that irradiation-induced pituitary tumors occur much more commonly in female than in male mice and that most of these tumors produce mammotropin.[32] Adrenotropin-secreting and thyrotropin-secreting tumors also have been produced.[13] Ovariectomy after irradiation reduces the incidence both of mammotropin-secreting tumors and of mammary tumors.[32] Most of the estrogen-induced mammotropin-secreting tumors were at first transplantable only in estrogenized animals, whereas all the radiation-induced tumors of this type were autonomous neoplasms. The "mammatrope cell" is a lightly granulated acidophil, and the "adrenotrope cell" is a chromophobe.

DISORDERS OF PITUITARY FUNCTION
Hypersecretion of hormones
Acromegaly

Our knowledge of pituitary function probably started in 1886 with the description of acromegaly by Pierre Marie.[62] The word "acromegaly" is descriptive of one of the most striking clinical features of the disease—enlargement of the extremities. This rare condition is caused by excessive secretion of growth hormone, which affects virtually all organs and tissues, and, in most cases, is due to an acidophil adenoma of the pituitary gland. Most of the specific features of the disease are due to the effects of growth hormone on connective tissue, cartilage, and bone (see also p. 1718).

Clinical features. Patients are usually over the age of 30 years at the time of diagnosis, and the disease occurs with almost equal frequency in men and women. The hands have been aptly described as spadelike. The feet, too, are increased in size, especially in width. This enlargement of the extremities is mainly due to a gross increase in the soft tissues, which also affects the face, nose, lips, tongue, and skin. There is hypertrophy of the costal cartilages, and hypertrophy of nasal and aural cartilage accounts for part of the enlargement of the nose and ears. There may be arthritis and, late in the disease, kyphosis occurs due to osteoporosis, and there is muscle weakness. There is overgrowth of the supraorbital ridge and of the maxilla. The mandible protrudes, and the lower teeth project beyond those of the maxilla, with consequent malocclusion. The long bones thicken and become massive, but since almost all cases of acromegaly occur after normal ossification has been completed, there is generally no increase in height.

In the early stages of the disease, there may be diabetes mellitus, presumably a result of the diabetogenic action of growth hormone, but in the later stages, increased sugar tolerance may develop. Randle has reported a marked increase in plasma insulin activity,[76] and it has been suggested that this is due to the stimulation of insulin secretion by growth hormone. The serum level of growth hormone is raised.[78]

In addition to these features, which are attributable to excessive growth hormone secretion, there are others that may be due to excess or deficiency of other pituitary hormones. Hypogonadism (impotence in the male and amenorrhea in the female), galactorrhea, pigmentation, thyroid enlargement, adrenal hyperplasia, and virilization may occur. Death often is due to congestive cardiac failure.

Tissue pathology. Most, although not all, patients with acromegaly have a pituitary adenoma (p. 1417) which is often surprisingly small. It usually is composed predominantly of acidophils, but there is no doubt that acromegaly can occur in patients with tumors that appear to be chromophobe by optical microscopy.[108]

There are now several reports of the *ultrastructure* of the pituitary tumors of patients with acromegaly.[12, 34, 58, 87, 88] Some have described a range of granule size from 100 mμ to 500 mμ, whereas one worker considers that the tumor cells, regardless of their appearance at the optical microscope level, contain typical 300 mμ acidophil secretion granules.[87, 88]

There is splanchnomegaly. The abdominal organs are greatly enlarged. There may be gross cardiomegaly, enlargement of the thyroid due to multiple colloid adenomas, and enlargement of other internal organs. These changes usually are attributed to the excessive secretion of growth hormone, but this may not be the whole explanation in all instances.

Evidence has been presented that the pituitary tumors of some patients with acromegaly may secrete corticotropin as well as growth hormone, and this could account for the adrenal hyperplasia that is common in acromegaly.[64]

The bone changes result from rather uneven osteoblastic activity. There is a sclerosing osteoporosis with giant bony trabeculae. In the later stages, the bone changes resemble those found in osteitis deformans.

Gigantism

Excessive secretion of growth hormone, beginning before ossification is completed, is an important cause of gigantism. There may be an acidophil adenoma of the pituitary gland, but in some cases, acidophil hyperplasia has been reported. Skeletal growth is precocious, excessive but proportionate—a height of about 8 ft may be attained. In some cases, there may be features of acromegaly. Late in the course of the disease, there may be evidence of hypogonadism.

"Stress"

In "stress," there is increased secretion of corticotropin, and the histologic changes in the adenohypophysis have been described. There is a relative increase in the number of lightly granulated mucoid cells,[19] and "S" cells are present in large numbers.[1] These pituitary changes are associated with the increased secretion of corticotropin in corticosteroids. There are lipid depletion of the adrenal cortex and an increase in the ribonucleic acid and enzyme content of the zona fasciculata. There does not appear to be any correlation of the pituitary findings with changes in the total stored amounts of any pituitary hormone.[18, 20, 21] However, there is some evidence to suggest that in acute "stress," corticotropin is released from the cells in a low molecular weight form, although most of it seems to be stored in a protein or protein-bound form.[21] It is of particular interest that there is no correlation between "stress" and the yield of vasopressin from the posterior lobe of the pituitary gland.[20]

Hyposecretion of hormones
Pituitary insufficiency (adenohypophyseal failure)

Destruction of the pituitary gland may be caused by many pathologic conditions. *Acute insufficiency* is generally due to necrosis (p. 1415), and the most noteworthy cause of this is severe and prolonged puerperal circulatory collapse.[90] There are many *chronic lesions* that may result in clinical pituitary insufficiency[92]—e.g., chromophobe adenoma of the pituitary gland, "scarring of uncertain cause," intrasellar cysts, extrasellar tumors and cysts such as craniopharyngioma, gliomas of the hypothalamus, suprasellar meningiomas, angiomas of the pituitary stalk, and tumors of the sphenoid bone. In many of these cases, there is thrombosis of the portal vessels. Low division of the pituitary stalk with section of the loral arteries arrests the blood supply to the anterior lobe (via the artery of the fibrous core) and results in almost complete necrosis of the lobe.[82]

The *local cause* of postpartum necrosis of the anterior lobe (Sheehan's syndrome) is an occlusive spasm of all the arteries that supply it. This develops at about the point of entry of the arteries into the lobe.[91] This cuts off the blood flow up the long stalk arteries and therefore interferes with the main source of the portal blood supply. Within a matter of two to three hours, the arterial spasm passes off, but by this time the anterior lobe has undergone ischemic necrosis. The blood again flows through the vessels of the anterior lobe and stalk, but since they have suffered severe ischemic damage, they become dilated and thrombosed. Vascular lesions are found commonly in the stalk but are very rare and quite trivial in the posterior lobe.

Significant functional effects are not produced unless more than 50% of the gland is destroyed.

Clinical effects. *Acute pituitary insufficiency* occurs if pituitary necrosis is acute and massive. Death is likely to ensue within two weeks of the onset of symptoms. The patient is pale and lethargic and gradually lapses into "pituitary coma."

In *chronic pituitary insufficiency (Simmonds' disease)*, Sheehan[90, 92] often has emphasized that marked wasting is not common and that the most noteworthy external sign is the loss of axillary and pubic hair. The patient may complain of weakness, loss of energy, loss of libido, failure to sweat, and amenorrhea. The complexion is pale or sallow, the skin is smooth and dry, and the facies is myxedematous. Both the blood pressure and the basal metabolic rate tend to be lowered, and anemia, usually hypochromic or normochromic, may be a feature. Urinary gonadotropins and corticosteroids are decreased. Rarely, diabetes insipidus occurs. The response of growth hormone to induced hypoglycemia may be lost in

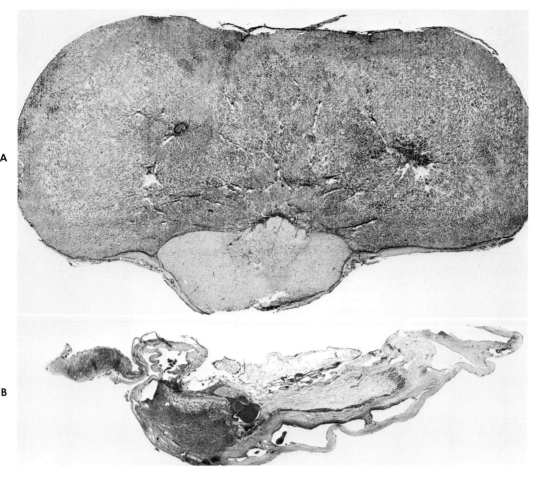

Fig. 33-15 Postpartum necrosis of pituitary gland. **A,** Most of anterior lobe affected. **B,** Gland shrivelled and deformed. Patient survived for many years. (**A** and **B,** Hematoxylin-eosin; ×10; sections courtesy Prof. H. L. Sheehan.)

hypopituitarism even before the gonadotropins disappear.

The earliest and most frequent manifestations are the result of failure of growth hormone and gonadotropin secretion. Secondary gonadal failure usually is followed by evidence of thyroid deficiency and later by adrenocortical deficiency. The physician is faced with the problem of distinguishing between pituitary insufficiency and primary gonadal, thyroid, or adrenal failure.

Histopathology. The changes in the adenohypophysis associated with postpartum necrosis already have been described (p. 1415) (Fig. 33-15). If the patient survives the acute phase of illness, the necrotic tissue is absorbed, the anterior lobe becomes shriveled and deformed, and postnecrotic fibrous scarring results. Calcification and ossification may develop in the fibrous scar tissue. The loss of

anterior lobe tissue is considerable. In a series of patients who died of hypopituitarism many years later, over one-third had less than 1% of the parenchyma, nearly one-third had 1% to 2%, nearly one-fourth had 2% to 5%, and the remainder less than 11%.[91]

In patients who survive for some years, the stalk is virtually normal but the *posterior lobe* shows various gross changes, which are found only when the necrosis involves at least 95% of the anterior lobe. They include subcapsular atrophy (which may be severe), uniform atrophy, and subgenual and genual scarring.

Significant abnormalities of the *hypothalamus* are not present during the first few weeks but, later on, changes are found in the subventricular nucleus and in the supraoptic and paraventricular nuclei.[91] There is gross hypertrophy of the subventricular nucleus in about two-thirds of the women who have suffered from postpartum hypopituitarism for many years. This finding seems to be associated with absence of estrogen secretion. These same patients often have atrophy of the supraoptic nucleus and, to a lesser degree, of the paraventricular nucleus.

There is atrophy of the other *endocrine organs.* The thyroid gland may be much reduced in weight and show acinar atrophy, lymphoid infiltration, and sometimes severe fibrosis. The adrenal glands are small due to cortical atrophy, and the gonads and genital tract also are atrophied. The other *viscera,* such as heart, spleen, liver, and kidneys, also show atrophic changes.

Pituitary dwarfism

Stunted growth may be found in various chronic diseases, such as primary gonadal dysgenesis, glomerulonephritis, and pituitary insufficiency. Dwarfism of pituitary or Lorain-Levi type is rare and may be associated with tumors of the anterior lobe or intrasellar cysts arising in childhood, although dwarfism is not a common result of such lesions. Failure to grow in these individuals may be accompanied by thyroid, adrenocortical, and gonadal insufficiency. The pituitary dwarf is characteristically of normal body proportions and has slender extremities. The epiphyses remain open.

Children with hypothalamic lesions, who survive to adult life, often grow normally, although some with craniopharyngiomas are dwarfed. This probably is caused by pressure on the pituitary gland rather than by interference with the center for release factors of growth hormone.

There have been few adequate studies of the pathology of the pituitary gland in cases of primary growth hormone failure. Some normally proportioned dwarfs seem to have an isolated growth hormone deficiency and have normal adrenal, thyroid, and sexual function.[85] This type of dwarfism seems to be due to a genetically transmitted recessive characteristic.

Fröhlich's syndrome

First described by Fröhlich in 1901 as dystrophia adiposogenitalis,[31] Fröhlich's syndrome is characterized by marked obesity of the eunuchoid type and is associated with gonadal failure. Boys are affected more often than girls. The most common causes are craniopharyngioma (p. 1415) and chromophobe adenoma (p. 1417), but it also may occur in

association with lesions of the hypothalamus and the floor of the third ventricle. The obesity may be due to damage of the satiety center in the hypothalamus.[91] The child is often mentally alert, but some with extensive lesions may have diabetes insipidus and somnolence.

Hormone-induced hypopituitarism

Administration of thyroid, gonadal, or adrenocortical hormones causes pituitary hypofunction because of reduction in the rate of synthesis and release of the respective tropic hormones. Prolonged suppression of ovulation by oral contraceptive pills is followed by normal menstrual cycles about one or two months after treatment is stopped. Pituitary-adrenal suppression after long-term administration of corticosteroids is often of great clinical importance. Corticotropin secretion is reduced, the basophil cells show Crooke's hyaline change (p. 1427), and adrenal atrophy results. The patient may have a "cushingoid facies," and his ability to respond to "stress" is seriously impaired. If treatment is stopped, abruptly or gradually, the patient may develop the so-called steroid withdrawal syndrome.

Neurohypophyseal failure— diabetes insipidus

It is customary to subdivide cases of diabetes insipidus into two categories: true diabetes insipidus due to deficiency of vasopressin (antidiuretic hormone) and false diabetes insipidus or psychogenic polydipsia. In true diabetes insipidus, the polyuria is primary and the polydipsia is secondary, whereas the reverse holds in psychogenic polydipsia. Although most cases presenting with these symptoms fall into one or other category, there are some of an intermediate kind.

The normal stimulus for release of vasopressin is an increase in the osmotic concentration of the serum. If the neurohypophysis fails to function, and there are many possible causes of this, the appropriate stimulus does not provoke release of vasopressin. Diabetes insipidus, therefore, may occur in any condition that damages the neurohypophyseal system, and it may be caused by the interruption of the nonmyelinated fibers of the tractus hypophyseus at any level from the floor of the third ventricle downward. It would appear that the anterior lobe of the pituitary gland must function normally if persistent diabetes insipidus is to develop. Surgical hypophysectomy and low section of the pituitary stalk with resultant necrosis of the anterior lobe are followed by hypopituitarism without persistent diabetes insipidus. In Blotner's[10] series, idiopathic cases made up the largest group (45%), primary brain tumors accounted for 29%, and syphilis for 6%, whereas head injuries (2.4%) and deposits of metastatic cancer (2.4%) were relatively infrequent. This contrasts with the experience of Leaf.[47]

Clinical features. The salient symptoms are polyuria and polydipsia. The patient excretes between 5 liters and 10 liters of urine in twenty-four hours, and the specific gravity is usually around 1.002. Water deprivation results in only a moderate reduction of urine volume, and the urine is still hypotonic in relation to the plasma. Some patients are unable to sweat, and, rarely, the thirst center also is affected. The urine volume falls sharply on treatment with vasopressin, but is unaffected by nicotine,[91] which normally causes antidiuresis by stimulating the secretion of vasopressin.

Diabetes mellitus, chronic nephritis, and potassium-losing nephritis are other important causes of polyuria and polydipsia.

EFFECTS OF HYPOPHYSECTOMY IN MAN

Hypophysectomy, either surgical or by irradiation, has been used in the treatment of patients with certain endocrine diseases or with certain types of disseminated cancer, since it became possible to give them adequate hormonal replacement by therapy with cortisone, thyroid hormone, and gonadal steroids.[30, 57, 77] Indeed, the main results of hypophysectomy in man—amenorrhea, atrophy of testes, sparse axillary and pubic hair, marked reduction in urinary gonadotropins, estrogens, and corticosteroids, and clinical evidence of thyroid hypofunction—are attributable to hypofunction of the adrenal cortex, the thyroid gland, and the gonads. Aldosterone is the only adrenocortical hormone that continues to be produced in comparatively normal amounts.

Whether diabetes insipidus develops apparently depends on the degree of damage to the hypothalamoneurohypophyseal system: with high stalk section, moderately severe diabetes insipidus almost always occurs, whereas with section of the pituitary stalk close to the diaphragma sellae, there is only minimal evidence of altered renal function.

In patients with mild diabetes mellitus, insulin may no longer be required, whereas in those with severe disease, less insulin is needed than before hypophysectomy. Significant improvement in diabetic retinopathy has been found after hypophysectomy.

The hypophysectomized patient on adequate hormonal replacement therapy has a normal appearance. Tanning of the skin occurs normally after exposure to sunlight. The absence of corticotropin has no obvious effect on the skin. Callus formation may follow regression of secondary carcinomatous osteolytic deposits. Bone repair does not seem to be hindered by hypophysectomy in these patients.

■ ■ ■

In general, **section of the pituitary stalk** in man has the same clinical effects as hypophysectomy, but these do depend on whether the section is high or low. Neurosecretion accumulates above the cut end of the stalk within a few days of section, and this also has been shown to occur in the tractus hypophyseus and in the supraoptic and paraventricular nuclei.[96] If the patient lives for a few months after the operation, there is a great diminution in the number of neurons in the supraoptic nuclei and in the rostral halves of the paraventricular nuclei.[96] Some of the surviving neurons in these nuclei contain neurosecretion.

HYPOPHYSIS AND CANCER

In 1896, Beatson[6] of Glasgow, Scotland, described regression of disseminated breast cancer following ovariectomy. Almost fifty years later, Charles Huggins[40] reported that castration resulted in remission of human prostatic cancer and subsequently did his pioneer work on the endocrine aspects of breast cancer. Huggins' findings stimulated the interest of many research workers throughout the world in this important field.

It had often been suggested that hypophysectomy should be tried in the treatment of breast cancer. It was argued that removal of growth hormone would depress the growth of the cancer cells. It was not until cortisone became available, however, that this became a practicable proposition. Luft et al.,[56] in Sweden, showed that there was objective improvement in some patients with disseminated breast cancer treated by hypophysectomy. Since then, there have been many reports of treating breast cancer by pituitary ablation and, by and large, it results in remission of the disease for an average period of fifteen months.[4] In general, if a tumor regresses for a time after ovariectomy and subsequently recurs, it will respond to adrenalectomy or to ablation of the pituitary gland by surgical removal, stalk section, or irradiation. It is not known whether the response to pituitary ablation is due to the direct effect of the loss of one or more of the pituitary hormones or to an indirect effect through the depression of ovarian and adrenal activity.

Patients with carcinoma of the prostate gland, whose disease has relapsed under other treatment, may benefit from hypophysectomy but, again, it is not known whether this is a direct or an indirect effect. Treatment with thyroid hormone leads to remission in some patients with well-differentiated carcinoma of the thyroid gland. This is probably attributable to the depression of thyrotropin. ACTH and cortisone may have a beneficial effect, albeit temporary, in patients with lymphoid tumors and leukemia.

As a general rule, the cancers that respond to alteration of the hormonal environment arise from organs normally under hormonal influence. It is not known why some respond to endocrine ablative procedures whereas others do not. The pituitary and adrenal glands from cancer patients do not differ histologically from those of patients who have died of other diseases.[100]

Experimental pituitary-hormone-dependent tumors

The great majority of spontaneous mammary tumors in the mouse do not respond to additive or ablative endocrine therapy. The most satisfactory experimental model system for studying many of the endocrine aspects of breast cancer is the tumor induced in the Sprague-Dawley rat by 3-methylcholanthrene or by 7,12-dimethylbenz(a)anthracene (DMBA).[41, 99] One large dose of DMBA given intravenously or intragastrically induces mammary tumors in most of the rats within two to three months. The tumors that continue to grow (some remain static and others regress spontaneously) have a histologic appearance very similar to that of well-differentiated human breast cancer, and most of those are hormone dependent: regression occurs after ovariectomy and hypophysectomy. The cellular changes associated with regression are hydropic degeneration, focal cytoplasmic degradation, and atrophy.[89] The hypophysectomized animal will not develop these carcinogen-induced mammary tumors unless sub-

stitution hormone therapy—estrogen, progesterone, and growth hormone—is given.[109] To date, this experimental tumor is the best available for studying some of the problems of hormone-dependent breast cancer.

PITUITARY GLAND IN DISTURBANCES OF OTHER ENDOCRINE GLANDS

Because of the functional relationship of the pituitary gland to the other endocrine glands, it is not perhaps unexpected that it may show changes when there are primary disturbances of the thyroid gland, the adrenal glands, or of the gonads.

Thyroid gland

It seems likely that thyrotropin is produced and secreted by rather large, coarsely granulated basophil cells, but it is not yet known whether the thyrotropin-producing basophil in man, which is thought to make up approximately 6% of the cell population of the normal gland, has only this function.

In *primary untreated hypothyroidism*,[85] there is increased production of thyrotropin, and the pituitary gland may be of normal size or be significantly enlarged due to cell proliferation in the adenohypophysis. There is a reduction in the number and granularity of the acidophils as well as a marked increase in the number of vesiculate chromophobes (Fig. 33-4) and of sparsely granulated basophils. Whereas the changes in the basophils presumably are associated with increased production and secretion of thyrotropin, those in the acidophils are believed to be related to disturbance of the biosynthesis of growth hormone. In the rat, a minimum quantity of circulating thyroid hormone is needed for the synthesis of growth hormone by the acidophils.[75] This growth hormone deficiency, along with the deficiency of thyroid hormone, explains the poor somatic growth of thyroid-deficient children.

In some hypothyroid female children, with sellar enlargement, there is increased secretion not only of thyrotropin but apparently also of other tropic hormones. Galactorrhea may occur, and this suggests excess secretion of prolactin. Precocious puberty also has been reported, and this is almost certainly due to increased secretion of gonadotropin.

Treatment with *thyroid hormone* results in an increased percentage of "somatotropic acidophils" and an apparent decrease in "thyrotropin basophils."[85]

In *hyperthyroidism*, normal numbers of

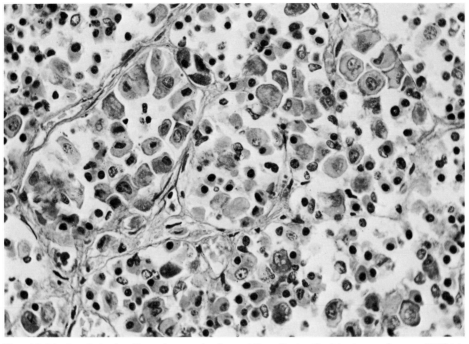

Fig. 33-16 Crooke's hyaline change in basophil cells in Cushing's syndrome. (PAS-tri-chrome; ×500.)

"thyrotropin basophils" are found, but many of them are shrunken.[85] There may be an increase in the number of acidophils. After treatment with antithyroid drugs, the histologic picture of the pituitary gland is similar to that already described for hypothyroidism.

Gonads

Recent studies have shown that the small round basophils believed to be concerned with gonadotropin production are scarce in young children.[85] The changes occurring in the pituitary gland in pregnancy (p. 1412) and aging (p. 1412) already have been described. Hyperplasia of lightly granulated mucoid cells has been observed following surgical castration[86] and in Klinefelter's syndrome.[11] Heavily granulated basophils may be markedly increased in number in some cells of the Laurence-Moon-Biedl syndrome.[80] The pituitary changes accompanying administration of pharmacologic doses of estrogens in the rat are described on p. 1410.

Adrenal cortex

It is possible that corticotropin is produced by two different cell types: the large basophil cells of probable intermediate lobe origin ("R" type) and chromophobe cells of anterior lobe origin.

Adrenocortical hyperfunction. In a relatively small proportion of patients with Cushing's syndrome (about 10%[85]), there is a basophil or a chromophobe adenoma of the pituitary gland (p. 1418). The only constant finding in the hypophysis in the adrenal hyperactivity of Cushing's syndrome is the presence of Crooke's hyaline cells[15] (Fig. 33-16) with the proportion of cells affected varying from case to case. This hyaline cytoplasmic change occurs in the basophil cells that are believed to produce corticotropin. The basophil cells that invade the pars nervosa and the cells of a basophil adenoma usually are not affected. The hyaline material accumulates first around the nucleus or in a position intermediate between the nucleus and the periphery of the cell and then spreads throughout the cytoplasm. Electron microscopic studies of the hyaline cytoplasm of Crooke's cell show that it is composed of very fine filaments through which occasional secretion granules, ribosomes, and lysosomes may be scattered.[73] Immunofluorescence studies have shown that the corticotropin is present in the granular areas of Crooke's cells but is absent from the hyaline portions.[44] The pituitary gland in patients with Cushing's syndrome, in whom the basophils show Crooke's hyaline change and an adenoma is not present, apparently stores subnormal amounts of corticotropin, but all the detectable hormone is in the low molecular weight form.[21]

The functional significance of hyaline change is not yet known. It may represent activity[72] or inactivity[106] of the cells. It is of interest in this connection that there have been several reports of raised blood levels of corticotropin in Cushing's syndrome.[24, 53] Since cytoplasmic hyalinization of the basophils occurs in other forms of adrenocortical hyperactivity, such as in virilism and in some cases of precocious puberty, and as a result of therapeutic administration of corticotropin or cortisone,[46] there is little doubt that it is secondary to the presence of excessive amounts of adrenocortical hormones. It also may be seen rarely in patients with bronchial carcinoma and some other cancers, and, in these, there are other features of Cushing's syndrome.

It is possible, too, that some basophil adenomas may represent a secondary change. In many patients with adrenocortical hyperfunction, pituitary tumors first become clinically manifest after bilateral adrenalectomy.[69] It is not yet known whether adrenalectomy precipitates or initiates tumor growth or whether it stimulates active growth of a preexisting microscopic lesion. These postadrenalectomy tumors may be of either basophil or chromophobe type[85] (see also pp. 1476 and 1719).

Adrenocortical hypofunction. In Addison's disease, whatever its cause (p. 1471), there is a reduction in the percentage of acidophils, a conspicuous decrease in the mature granulated basophil cells, and a marked increase in sparsely granulated PAS-positive basophils (Crooke-Russell cells[16]). It seems that these Crooke-Russell cells are of the "R" type and that they are concerned in the active secretion of corticotropin. Raised blood levels of corticotropin have been recorded in Addison's disease, and the abnormal pigmentation of the skin and mucosae is believed to be due to the melanocyte-stimulating activity of this hormone. The posterior lobe of the pituitary gland is normal. Adequate treatment with glucocorticoids restores the pituitary cell count to about normal values.[84]

REFERENCES

1 Adams, C. W. M., and Pearse, A. G. E.: J. Endocr. **18**:147-153, 1959.

2 Adams, C. W. M., and Swettenham, K. V.: J. Path. Bact. **75**:95-103, 1958.

3 Apostolakis, M.: Acta Endocr. (Kobenhavn) **49**:1-16, 1965.

4 Baker, W. H.: In Astwood, E. B., editor: Clinical endocrinology, vol. 1, New York, 1960, Grune & Stratton, Inc., p. 571.

5 Bargmann, W., and Scharrer, E.: Amer. Sci. **39**:255-259, 1951.

6 Beatson, G. T:. Lancet **2**:104-107, 162, 1896.

7 Beck, J. S., Ellis, S. T., Legge, J., Porteous, I. B., Currie, A. R., and Read, C.: J. Path. Bact. **91**:531-538, 1966.

8 Bell, E. T., Mukerji, S., and Loraine, J. A.: J. Endocr. **28**:321-328, 1964.

9 Berson, S. A., and Yalow, R. S.: In Pincus, G., Thimann, K. V., and Astwood, E. B., editors: The hormones, vol. 4, New York, 1964, Academic Press, Inc., p. 557.

10 Blotner, H.: Metabolism **7**:191-200, 1958.

11 Burt, A. S., Reiner, L., Cohen, R. B., and Sniffen, R. C.: J. Clin. Endocr. **14**:719-728, 1954.

12 Cardell, R. R., Jr., and Knighton, R. S.: Trans. Amer. Micr. Soc. **85**:58-78, 1966.

13 Clifton, K. H.: Cancer Res. **19**:2-22, 1959.

14 Cramer, W., and Horning, E. S.: Lancet **1**: 247-249, 1936.

15 Crooke, A. C.: J. Path. Bact. **41**:339-349, 1935.

16 Crooke, A. C., and Russell, D. S.: J. Path. Bact. **40**:255-283, 1935.

17 Currie, A. R., and Davies, B. M. A.: Acta Endocr. (Kobenhavn) **42**:69-84, 1963.

18 Currie, A. R., and Dekanski, J. B.: Acta Endocr. (Kobenhavn) **36**:185-196, 1961.

19 Currie, A. R., and Symington, T.: Ciba Foundation Colloquia on Endocrinology, vol. 8, (G. E. W. Wolstenholme and M. P. Cameron, editors), Boston, 1955, Little, Brown and Co., p. 396.

20 Currie, A. R., Adamsons, K., and van Dyke, H. B.: J. Clin. Endocr. **20**:947-951, 1960.

21 Currie, A. R., Davies, B. M. A., and Symington, T.: Acta Endocr. (Kobenhavn) **43**: 255-263, 1963.

22 Cushing, H.: Bull. Johns Hopkins Hosp. **50**: 137-195, 1932.

23 Cushing, H.: Arch. Intern. Med. (Chicago) **51**:487-557, 1933.

24 Davies, B. M. A.: In Currie, A. R., Symington, T. and Grant, J. K., editors: The human adrenal cortex, Edinburgh, 1962, E. & S. Livingstone, Ltd., p. 468.

25 Doniach, I.: In Harrison, C. V., editor: Recent advances in pathology, ed. 7, London, 1960, J. & A. Churchill, Ltd., p. 211.

26 Du Vigneaud, V.: Harvey Lect. **50**:1-26, 1954-1955.

27 Ellis, S. T., Beck, J. S., and Currie, A. R.: J. Path. Bact. **92**:179-183, 1966.

28 Engel, F. L., and Lebovitz, H. E.: Amer. J. Med. **35**:721-726, 1963.

29 Fand, S. B.: J. Clin. Endocr. **15**:685-692, 1955.

30 Forrest, A. P. M., Blair, D. W., Morris, S. R., Peebles Brown, D. A., Sandison, A. T., Valentine, J. S. and Illingworth, C. F. W.: In Currie, A. R., editor: Endocrine aspects of breast cancer, Edinburgh, 1958, E. & S. Livingstone, Ltd., p. 46.

31 Frölich, A.: Wien. Klin. Rdsch. **15**:883, 1901.

32 Furth, J., and Clifton, K. H.: In Currie, A. R., editor: Endocrine aspects of breast cancer,

Edinburgh, 1958, E. & S. Livingstone, Ltd., p. 276.

33 Gemzell, C. A., and Li, C. H.: J. Clin. Endocr. **18:**149-157, 1958.

34 Gusek, V. W.: Endokrinologie **42:**257-283, 1962.

35 Haberfeld, W.: Beitr. Path. Anat. **46:**133-232, 1909.

36 Hachmeister, U.: Endokrinologie **51:**145-163, 1967.

37 Harris, G. W.: Neural control of the pituitary gland, London, 1955, Edward Arnold (Publishers) Ltd.

38 Haugen, O. A., and Beck, J. S.: J. Path. **98:** 97-104, 1969.

39 Herlant, M.: Bull. Micr. Appl. (Paris) **10:** 37-44, 1960.

40 Huggins, C.: Ann. Surg. **115:**1192-1200, 1942.

41 Huggins, C., Briziarelli, G., and Sutton, H., Jr.: J. Exp. Med. **109:**25-42, 1959.

42 Hunter, W. M., and Greenwood, F. C.: Biochem. J. **91:**43-56, 1964.

43 Kernohan, J. W., and Sayre, G. P.: In Atlas of tumor pathology, Sect. X, Fasc. 36, Washington, D. C., 1956, Armed Forces Institute of Pathology.

44 Kracht, J., and Hachmeister, U.: Endokrinologie **51:**164-169, 1967.

45 Kracht, J., Zimmermann, H.-D. and Hachmeister, U.: Virchow Arch. Path. Anat. **340:** 270-275, 1966.

46 Laqueur, G. L.: Stanford Med. Bull. **9:**75-87, 1951.

47 Leaf, A.: In Astwood, E. B., editor: Clinical endocrinology, vol. 1, New York, 1960, Grune & Stratton, Inc., p. 73.

48 Leznoff, A., Fishman, J., Goodfriend, L., McGarry, E., Beck, J. C., and Rose, B.: Proc. Soc. Exp. Biol. Med. **104:**232-235, 1960.

49 Leznoff, A., Fishman, J., Talbot, M., McGarry, E. E., Beck, J. C., and Rose, B.: J. Clin. Invest. **41:**1720-1724, 1962.

50 Li, C. H.: Advances Protein Chem. **11:**101-190, 1956.

51 Li, C. H., and Liu, W. K.: Experientia **20:** 169-177, 1964.

52 Li, C. H., and Starman, B.: Biochim. Biophys. Acta **86:**175-176, 1964.

53 Liddle, G. W., and Williams, W. C.: In Currie, A. R., Symington, T., and Grant, J. K., editors: The human adrenal cortex, Edinburgh, 1962, E. & S. Livingstone, Ltd., p. 461.

54 Lipscomb, H. S., and Nelson, D. H.: Endocrinology **71:**13-23, 1962.

55 Loraine, J. A., and Bell, E. T.: Hormone assays and their clinical application, Edinburgh, 1966, E. & S. Livingstone, Ltd.

56 Luft, R., Olivecrona, H., and Sjögren, B.: Nord. Med. **47:**351-354, 1952.

57 Luft, R., Olivecrona, H., Ikkos, D., Nilsson, L. B., and Mossberg, H.: In Currie, A. R., editor: Endocrine aspects of breast cancer, Edinburgh, 1958, E. & S. Livingstone, Ltd., p. 27.

58 Luse, S.: Progr. Exp. Tumor Res. **2:**1-35, 1961.

59 McEuen, C. S., Selye, H., and Collip, J. B.: Lancet **1:**775-776, 1936.

60 McGrath, P.: Aust. New Zeal. J. Surg. **37:** 16-27, 1967.

61 McPhie, J. L., and Beck, J. S.: Nature (London) **219:**625-626, 1968.

62 Marie, P.: Rev. Med. (Paris) **6:**297-333, 1886.

63 Marshall, A. H. E., and Sloper, J. C.: J. Path. Bact. **68:**225-229, 1954.

64 Mautalen, C. A., and Mellinger, R. C.: J. Clin. Endocr. **25:**1423-1428, 1965.

65 Melchionna, R. H., and Moore, R. A.: Amer. J. Path. **14:**763-771, 1938.

66 Moldawer, M. P., Nardi, G. L. and Raker, J. W.: Amer. J. Med. Sci. **228:**190-206, 1944.

67 Müller, W.: Z. Menschl. Vererb. Konstitutionsl. **34:**187-193, 1957.

68 Müller, W.: In Currie, A. R., editor: Endocrine aspects of breast cancer, Edinburgh, 1958, E. & S. Livingstone, Ltd., p. 106.

69 Nelson, D. H., Meakin, J., and Thorn, G. W.: Ann. Intern. Med. **52:**560-569, 1960.

70 Paget, G. E. and Eccleston, E.: Stain Techn. **35:**119-122, 1960.

71 Pearse, A. G. E.: J. Path. Bact. **64:**811-826, 1952.

72 Pearse, A. G. E.: J. Path. Bact. **65:**355-370, 1953.

73 Porcile, E., and Racadot, J.: C. R. Acad. Sci. [D] (Paris) **263:**948-951, 1966.

74 Purves, H. D.: In Harris, G. W., and Donovan, B. T., editors: The pituitary gland, vol. 1, London, 1966, Butterworth & Co. (Publishers) Ltd., p. 147.

75 Purves, H. D., and Griesbach, W. E.: Brit. J. Exp. Path. **27:**294-297, 1946.

76 Randle, P. J.: In Smith, R. W., Baebler, O. H., and Long C. N. H., editors: Hypophyseal growth hormone, nature and actions, New York, 1955, Blakiston Division, McGraw-Hill Book Co., p. 415.

77 Ray, B. S., and Pearson, O. H.: In Currie, A. R., editor: Endocrine aspects of breast cancer, Edinburgh, 1958, E. & S. Livingstone, Ltd., p. 36.

78 Read, C. H., and Bryan, G. T.: Recent Progr. Hormone Res. **16:**187-218, 1960.

79 Robyn, C., Bossaert, Y., Hubinont, P.-O., Pasteels, J.-L., and Herlant, M.: C. R. Acad. Sci. [D] (Paris) **259:**1226-1228, 1964.

80 Ross, C. F., Crome, L., and MacKenzie, D. Y.: J. Path. Bact. **72:**161-172, 1956.

81 Russell, D. S.: J. Path. Bact. **68:**125-129, 1954.

82 Russell, D. S.: Lancet **1:**466-468, 1956.

83 Russell, D. S.: Proc. Roy. Soc. Med. **49:**1018-1019, 1956.

84 Russfield, A. B.: Cancer **8:**523-537, 1955.

85 Russfield, A. B.: In Bloodworth, J. M. B., editor: Endocrine pathology, Baltimore, 1968, The Williams & Wilkins Co., p. 78.

86 Russfield, A. B., and Byrnes, R. L.: Cancer **11:**817-828, 1958.

87 Schelin, U.: Acta Path. Microbiol. Scand. suppl. 154, pp. 89-90, 1962.

88 Schelin, U.: Acta Path. Microbiol. Scand. suppl. 158, pp. 1-80, 1962.

89 Scott, G. B., Christian, H. J., and Currie, A. R.: In Wissler, R. W., Dao, T. L., and Wood, S., editors: Endogenous factors influencing host-tumor balance, Chicago/London, 1967, The University of Chicago Press, p. 99.

90 Sheehan, H. L.: J. Path. Bact. **45:**189-214, 1937.

91 Sheehan, H. L.: In Bloodworth, J. M. B., editor: Endocrine pathology, Baltimore, 1968, The Williams & Wilkins Co., p. 17.

92 Sheehan, H. L., and Summers, V. K.: Quart. J. Med. **18:**319-378, 1949.

93 Sloper, J. C.: J. Anat. **89:**301-316, 1955.

94 Sloper, J. C.: Int. Rev. Cytol. **7:**337-389, 1958.

95 Sloper, J. C.: In Currie, A. R., Symington, T., and Grant, J. K., editors: The human adrenal cortex, Edinburgh, 1962, E. & S. Livingstone, Ltd., p. 230.

96 Sloper, J. C., and Adams, C. W. M.: J. Path. Bact. **72:**587-602, 1956.

97 Stanfield, J. P.: J. Anat. **94:**257-273, 1960.

98 Stevens, E., and Helfenstein, J. E.: Nature (London) **211:**879-880, 1966.

99 Stevens, L., Stevens, E., and Currie, A. R.: J. Path. Bact. **89:**581-589, 1965.

100 Symington, T., and Currie, A. R.: In Currie, A. R., editor: Endocrine aspects of breast cancer, Edinburgh, 1958, E. & S. Livingstone, Ltd., p. 136.

101 Taylor, N. R. W., Loraine, J. A., and Robertson, H. A.: J. Endocr. **9:**334-341, 1953.

102 Van Oordt, P. G. W. J.: Gen. Comp. Endocr. **5:**131-134, 1965.

103 Vernikos-Danellis, J.: Vitamins Hormones (N. Y.) **23:**97-152, 1965.

104 Willis, R. A.: The borderland of embryology and pathology, ed. 2, London, 1962, Butterworth & Co. (Publishers) Ltd., p. 276.

105 Willis, R. A.: Pathology of tumours, ed. 4, London, 1967, Butterworth & Co. (Publishers) Ltd., p. 642.

106 Wilton, A., Thorell, B., and Sundwall, U.: J. Path. Bact. **67:**65-68, 1954.

107 Yalow, R. S., Roth, J., Glick, S. M., and Berson, S. A.: In Proceedings of the Second International Congress on Endocrinology, (S. Taylor, editor), Amsterdam, 1965, Excerpta Medica Foundation, p. 292.

108 Young, D. G., Bahn, R. C. and Randall, R. V.: J. Clin. Endocr. **25:**249-259, 1965.

109 Young, S.: Nature (London) **190:**356-357, 1961.

110 Zondek, B.: Lancet **1:**776-778, 1936.

Chapter 34

Thyroid gland

Sheldon C. Sommers

STRUCTURE AND FUNCTION

Clinicopathologic correlations generally are satisfactory in the human thyroid gland. Also the important lesions are classifiable into a limited number of categories. The normal weight of the adult thyroid gland is 15 gm to 35 gm, or not more than 0.35 gm per kilogram of body weight. In the newborn infant, the normal weight is 1.4 gm to 3.5 gm. The functional unit comprises a main thyroid follicle and satellite follicles which together form lobules. On gross examination, the bilobed thyroid gland, isthmus, and variable pyramidal lobe have a translucent capsule. Sectioning shows homogeneous, moist, tan, slightly gelatinous tissue. Histologically, the normal thyroid gland is composed of uniform, regularly arranged follicles filled with colloid and lined by low cuboidal follicular epithelium with a thin basement membrane. The interfollicular vascular stroma is delicate.

Normally, the circulating free thyroxine (T_4) is maintained at uniform concentrations through fine adjustments required by such factors as temperature changes, blood glucose levels, and circulatory adjustments. These act through the hypothalamic-pituitary axis mediated by thyrotropin-releasing factor, thyroid-stimulating hormone (TSH), and the controlling feedback effects of T_4 and triiodothyronine (T_3). Increased colloid storage of the two major thyroid hormones is reflected by a flattening and secretion by a columnar hypertrophy of the epithelial cells. Their microvilli, secretory or resorptive vacuoles, lysosomes, and other organelles alter with thyroid function.

The thyroid gland preferentially absorbs iodide from the blood and concentrates it forty times or more. By five important enzymatic reactions, the iodide is trapped and organified, iodotyrosines are coupled and deiodinated, and thyroglobulin is formed, to be resorbed subsequently and secreted as T_3 and T_4. Enzymatic defects are the cause of most familial goiters. In the circulation, some 80% of T_4 is attached to the plasma thyroid-binding globulin and thyroid-binding prealbumin. When this globulin is increased, as by estrogens, thyroid gland hypertrophy ensues to maintain the normal plasma concentration of free T_4. The parafollicular or C cells in the human thyroid gland are not identifiable by ordinary light or electron microscopy. Thyrocalcitonin or calcitonin secreted by these cells is a polypeptide hormone of low molecular weight with a hypocalcemic effect that counterbalances parathyroid hormone. Animal thyroid extracts contain much more activity than human material. Despite intensive research, no disease has been correlated clearly with thyrocalcitonin, except for some instances of pseudohypoparathyroidism.

CONGENITAL ABNORMALITIES

Lingual thyroid gland is a persistent undescended embryonic anlage forming a mass at the base of the tongue. Its removal usually renders the patient athyrotic. Normally, the anlage descends in the anterior cervical midline, and incomplete descent results in aberrant subhyoid or intratracheal thyroid tissue. Heterotopic thyroid tissue also has been found in the larynx, pericardium, heart, porta hepatis, and inguinal canal.

Thyroglossal duct cysts are commonly thin walled, are 1 cm to 2 cm in diameter, and contain sticky yellow fluid. The cyst wall is formed either by mature thyroid epithelium or by ciliated columnar or metaplastic stratified squamous epithelium. Because of its propinquity, the hyoid bone also is often removed surgically to prevent recurrent cyst formation. Except for occasional small thyroid follicles in the wall, only the midline location distinguishes most thyroglossal duct cysts from laterally placed branchial cleft cysts.

Substernal thyroid tissue is due to embryologic descent into the anterior mediastinum. Substernal goiters may rise with respiration into the suprasternal notch or become incarcerated there. Lingual and subhyoid thyroid tissue sometimes also forms goiters. Papillary adenomas and carcinomas occur in thyroglossal duct cysts, but few of these cancers have metastasized. "Lateral aberrant thyroid" ordinarily refers to microscopic groups of mature follicles in lymph nodes, cervical strap muscles, or fat located a few millimeters from the thyroid capsule. When larger lateral thyroid masses are removed, practically all prove to be prominent metastases of an unrecognized intrathyroid carcinoma.

Failure of thyroid organogenesis may result in a mixture of ducts, lymphatic nodules, connective tissue, and a few follicles. Abundant fat mingled with mature thyroid tissue is termed adenolipomatosis or hamartomatous thyroid adiposity. Minor malformations of branchial pouch differentiation include intrathyroidal parathyroid glands or portions of thymus. Ducts or squamous cell cysts in otherwise well-formed thyroid glands may represent remnants of the embryonic ultimobranchial body.

Cretinism centers around congenital thyroid deficiency. Cretins typically have a large head, broad nose, wide-set eyes, low forehead, large,

thick tongue, and dry skin. The most serious clinical aspect is failure of central nervous system development. If infantile hypothyroidism is not discovered and treated within six months, irreversible mental retardation may result. Cretins show stunted growth, enamel dysplasia, umbilical hernia, and sexual infantilism, and they may have other defects of the central nervous system, such as deafmutism.

Thyroid aplasia, so-called athyrotic cretinism, is the usual type in the United States. Hypoplasia of either a normally located or ectopic thyroid gland also occurs. Together, these conditions comprise sporadic, nongoitrous cretinism.

GOITER AND ALTERED HORMONAL BIOSYNTHESIS

Goiter means persistent thyroid enlargement. Different terms for thyroid disease are used by clinicians and pathologists, but interpretation is not difficult (Table 34-1). Most goiters weigh over 40 gm, but some are as small as 25 gm.

Simple goiter also is called diffuse or colloid-storage goiter. Adolescent girls and pregnant women and other women exposed to increased estrogens may develop the symmetrical thyroid enlargement and swanlike neck

Table 34-1 Classification of major diseases of the thyroid gland

Clinical diagnosis	Pathologic diagnosis
Euthyroidism with:	
Nontoxic diffuse goiter	Simple or colloid storage goiter
Nontoxic uninodular goiter	Thyroid nodule
Nontoxic multinodular goiter	Nodular goiter
Tumors	
Benign—adenoma or teratoma	Same
Malignant—primary or secondary	See Tables 34-3 and 34-4
Acute thyroiditis	Same
Chronic thyroiditis	Same; see Table 34-2
Degeneration or infiltration	Same; see text
Congenital anomaly	See text
Hyperthyroidism with:	
Toxic diffuse goiter (Graves' disease)	Primary thyroid hyperplasia
Toxic uninodular goiter	Nodular thyroid or adenoma with hyperplasia
Toxic multinodular goiter	Nodular goiter with secondary hyperplasia
Hypothyroidism with:	
Idiopathic myxedema	Thyroid atrophy
Cretinism	
Endemic	See text
Congenital goitrous	Neonatal nodular goiter
Thyrotropin deficiency	Thyroid atrophy
Thyrotropin-releasing factor deficiency	Thyroid atrophy
Thyroid destruction	Thyroid absent; thyroid remnant; fibrosis; radiation reaction
Congenital aplasia	Same

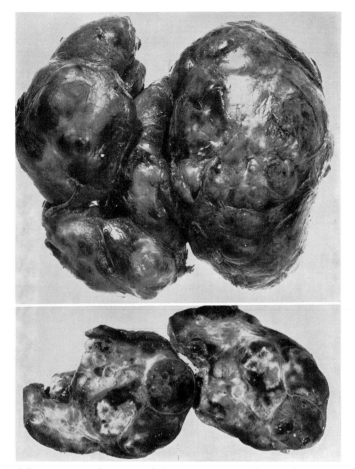

Fig. 34-1 Nodular goiter with areas of degeneration and hemorrhage. (From Anderson, W. A. D.: Synopsis of pathology, The C. V. Mosby Co.)

depicted in Renaissance paintings. Treatment of a euthyroid individual with T_4 rarely produces a simple goiter. Colloid storage goiters ordinarily involute. Grossly, the tissue is homogeneous and notably gelatinous. Microscopically, the follicles generally are enlarged with excessive colloid content, and the lining epithelium is flattened.

Nodular goiter is the most familiar thyroid disease. It also is called, among various names, adenomatous, endemic, nodular colloid, and nontoxic multinodular goiter. The last term implies a correlation of function and structure.

Iodine deficiency is the ordinary cause of nodular goiter. Before the widespread use of iodized salt, iodine-poor diets predisposed to goiter, particularly in such mountainous areas as Switzerland, Tibet, and Mendoza in Argentina or around inland fresh waters like the Great Lakes in the United States. In Southern Austria (Styria) and some areas of the Andes mountains, nodular goiter is still commonplace. Women are affected more than men in a ratio of about 6:1. With iodine deficiency, thyroid extraction of blood iodine is increased and relatively more triiodothyronine (T_3) is secreted. At first, the entire thyroid gland becomes enlarged and more vascular. Follicles shrink, and their epithelium proliferates. An opportunity to see this early diffuse hyperplastic reaction is uncommon except experimentally.

Typical nodular goiters are large, weighing from 60 gm to over 1,000 gm. Grossly and microscopically, they have four characteristics: nodules, hemorrhage, fibrosis, and calcification (Fig. 34-1). The nodules vary in size and colloid content, and some are colored red or brown by recent or old hemorrhage. Histologically, the appearance also is varied, with undemarcated rounded masses of abnormally large colloid-filled follicles compressing the intervening normal-sized or small so-

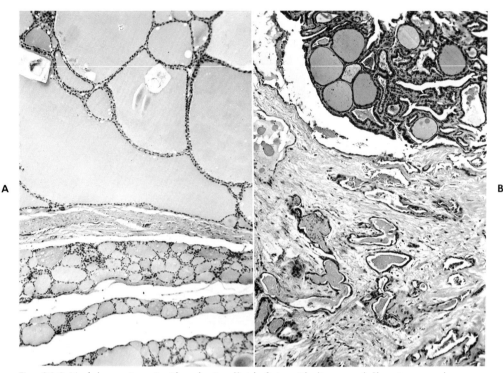

Fig. 34-2 Nodular goiter. **A,** Abundant colloid, flat epithelium, and fibrosis around upper nodule. **B,** Fibrosis and nodule with hyperplasia. (**A** and **B,** ×85; courtesy Dr. S. E. Gould.)

called fetal follicles that contain very little colloid. Practically no unaltered follicles remain. In questionable cases, individual follicles larger than 2 mm in diameter, or four times the upper limit of normal, indicate a nodular goiter. The follicular epithelium is predominantly flat cuboidal. Locally thickened areas, either small polsters or large reticulated epithelial papillary structures protruding into the follicles (Fig. 34-2), are common. These have no known functional importance. Histochemically, the epithelial peroxidase is decreased. The colloid contains PAS-staining granules and is either vacuolated or centrally condensed, suggesting stagnation. The capillary network is reduced. Among the follicles are focal hemorrhages attributable to pressure and ischemic necrosis. Consequences of the necrosis and hemorrhage are interfollicular infiltrates of macrophages, organized hematomas, cholesterol crystals, atheromas, foreign body giant cells, and irregular fibrosis with focal calcification.

In established nodular goiters, the major processes are irregular degeneration and regeneration, hypertrophy, and colloid storage. The characteristic nodules are nonneoplastic and have no known precancerous significance. Nodular goiters usually are removed for diag-

nosis or cosmetic reasons, when the individuals are euthyroid. Two important complications are local hemorrhage with sudden enlargement of the goiter and secondary hyperthyroidism, which is considered later.

Goitrous cretinism classically reflects severe maternal and critical fetal iodine deficiency with a functionally inadequate compensatory embryonic thyroid enlargement. The endemic type has become rarer with the availability of iodized salt. Iodine lack is not the sole cause however, since the presence of goiter with endemic cretinism varies from occasional in Switzerland and Styria to usual in the Himalayas. Older cretins may be euthyroid. Genetic factors contribute to both sporadic and endemic goitrous cretinism. Some cretins represent instances of familial goiter, with the histologic peculiarities described below (Fig. 34-3).

Genetically mutant human beings or animals may lack an enzyme involved in one of the major biosynthetic reactions necessary for the secretion of thyroxine (T_4). The metabolic blocks generally are believed due to autosomal recessive genes. Familial goiter may result, either with euthyroidism or with hypothyroidism. Following are six identified metabolic defects:

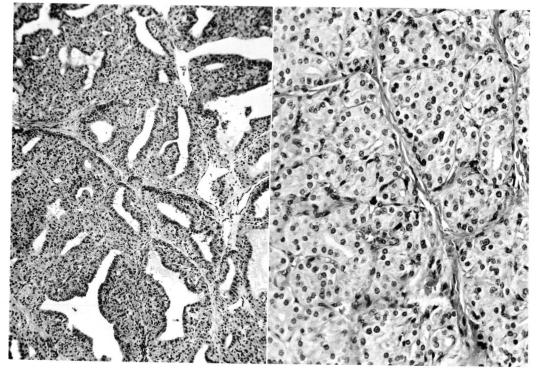

Fig. 34-3 A, Congenital goiter with hyperplastic appearance. **B,** Goiter from cretin with pale and notably hyperplastic epithelium. (**A,** ×85; **B,** ×240; courtesy Dr. S. E. Gould.)

1 Iodide trapping
2 Iodide conversion to organically bound iodine (peroxidase deficiency)
3 Iodide organification, partially like the defect noted in 2, with eighth nerve deafness (Pendred's syndrome)
4 Mono-iodotyrosine and di-iodotyrosine conversions to T_3 and T_4
5 Iodotyrosine deiodination (dehalogenase deficiency)
6 T_4 release in a nonbutanol extractable form

Additional metabolic defects are still unidentified. Peripheral tissue unreactivity to T_4 has also been postulated.

Familial goiters are grossly indistinguishable from other nodular goiters. Microscopically, their recognizable peculiarities occasionally include nodules of bizarre embryonal or fetal appearance and striking cytologic atypia with irregular nuclei or large hydropic cells (Fig. 34-3, *B*). Hyperplastic epithelium occurs unaccompanied by hyperthyroidism. Genuine anaplasia and some features of carcinoma such as calcospherites and local invasion may be present, but the clinical course is ordinarily benign.

Dietary nodular goiters may develop after excessive ingestion of cabbage, which contains cyanates, or turnips, soybeans, and other foods containing goitrogens.

IATROGENIC ABNORMALITIES

Medications such as cyanates, thiocyanates, salicylates, and sulfonylureas may induce nodular goiter formation. Unrelated substances that inhibit oxidative enzymes, including resorcinol, potassium perchlorate, and cobalt chloride, are also sometimes goitrogenic. Treatment with such drugs or with thiouracil compounds during pregnancy may result in the birth of a goitrous cretin infant.

Iodide goiter may be congenital if the mother received considerable potassium iodide or iodopyrine. High plasma iodide levels inhibit the fetal thyroid peroxidase and T_4 secretion, with loss of feedback control of fetal pituitary TSH. The fetus is evidently more sensitive than its mother to the goitrogenic effects of excess iodide. A few adults treated with iodides or iodine-containing compounds also have developed iodide goiter because of an unusual susceptibility to thyroid peroxidase inhibition. After birth, or in adults following the discontinuance of therapy, iodide goiters usually regress, with colloid resorption and a transient epithelial hyperplasia accompanied by hyperfunction. Thyroid hormones administered during pregnancy occasionally may cause an infantile goiter with epithelial hyperplasia. In euthyroid adults, ingestion of desiccated thyroid produces functional changes that include exacerbated thyrotoxicosis but no morphologic effects. At least twenty-five other drugs affect thyroid function tests.

Ionizing radiation has notable effects on the thyroid gland from the fetal stage until adulthood. Thereafter, the thyroid is less radiosensitive, probably because its cell turnover becomes slower. After x-irradiation, atomic irradiation, or exposure to radioactive ^{131}I, histologic evidence of irradiation includes an irregular hyaline fibrosis of interstitial thyroid tissue and vessel walls. Cytologically, the size, arrangement, and staining of its epithelial cells vary, with nuclei of irregular sizes and chromatin content (Fig. 34-4). Post irradiation thyroid regeneration may be nodular. Adenomas or carcinomas may develop. Neonatal or childhood x-irradiation of the

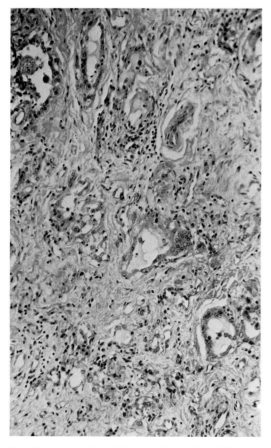

Fig. 34-4 Atrophy of thyroid following ^{131}I therapy. Abnormal epithelial cells at upper left. (×85.)

thyroid area is a major carcinogenic stimulus identified in more than half the children and adolescents who develop thyroid carcinomas.

HYPERPLASIA
Primary hyperplasia

Clinically, Graves' or Basedow's disease is a hypermetabolic state associated with a fine tremor, a vascular bruit over the thyroid lobes, and often exophthalmos. An "exophthalmic goiter" removed surgically usually weighs 35 gm to 60 gm. The thyroid gland is diffusely enlarged, firm, red brown, opaque and nongelatinous. Microscopically, the colloid is depleted. The follicular epithelium is columnar and folded in places to form inward projecting papillae. Typically, the colloid margins are scalloped, an artifact of aqueous fixation that reflects increased proteolysis of the peripheral colloid prior to its accelerated resorption (Fig. 34-5). Histochemically, the thyroid epithelial peroxidase and the cytoplasmic and colloid RNA are increased, and the rich capillary network shows alkaline phosphatase activity.

Hyperthyroidism typically goes through cycles of exacerbation with depletion or disappearance of the stored colloid and increased epithelial height, followed by remission accompanied by decreased epithelial hyperplasia and enhanced colloid storage. In young persons, intrathyroid lymph follicles are common, possibly related to lymphoid cell production of LATS (long-acting thyroid stimulator). This antithyroid immunoglobulin G is increased in about half the individuals with Graves' disease. LATS titers correlate with the presence of exophthalmos and pretibial myxedema. By cell counts or measurements, a good correlation may be achieved between the thyroid activity and its morphology. The epithelial papillae persist permanently even in involuted or hyperinvoluted glands. Recurrent primary thyroid hyperplasia, either untreated or following surgical or medical therapy, manifests an irregular interfollicular fibrosis and nodularity. Postoperatively, follicles may become mingled with the cervical strap muscles. Long-neglected cases merge in appearance with nodular goiter, but the intrafollicular papillae remain to indicate antecedent primary hyperplasia. Thiouracil-type medication produces no distinctive human thyroid alterations. However, since it has been in use, irregularly involuted primary thyroid hyperplasia has become more frequent. Preoperative therapy with thiouracil preparations causes the histologic hyperplasia to remain static, despite the inhibited thyroid hormone secretion.

Thyroid storm or crisis is a life-threatening exacerbated thyrotoxicosis. Psychosis, shock, and death from cardiopulmonary complica-tions may occur. Severe primary thyroid hyperplasia is usually responsible, but rarely it is thyroiditis with hyperplasia. Following trauma or infection, the normal thyroid gland responds subclinically by increased hormone secretion, with localized thickenings of the follicular epithelium (Sanderson polsters) and vacuolization of the overlying colloid. Even glucose infusions increase the thyroid secretory activity cytologically.

Secondary hyperplasia

Nodular goiter complicated by hyper-thyroidism chiefly affects older people, in whom the clinical signs are often atypical. Grossly, red-tan granular thyroid tissue is found either in or between the nodules. Microscopically, nodular goiter with second-ary hyperplasia is characterized by some fol-licles containing peripherally scalloped col-loid and columnar epithelial cells. Papillae formed in secondary hyperplasia are distin-guished by small follicles enclosed in their stroma (Fig. 34-6). In difficult cases, indi-vidual abnormally large follicles and papillae with follicles in their stalks indicate secondary hyperplasia rather than recurrent primary thyroid hyperplasia with irregular involution.

Iodine treatment of a person with nodular goiter may be followed by secondary hyper-thyroidism, called *jodbasedow*.

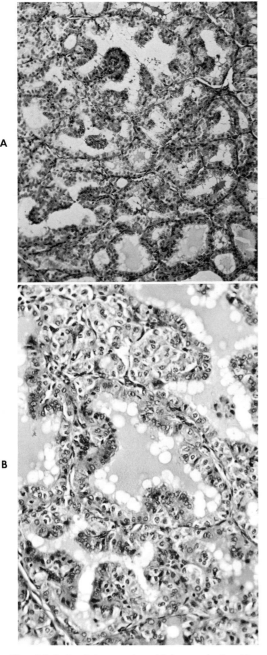

A

B

Fig. 34-5 **A**, Primary thyroid hyperplasia. Note scanty colloid and epithelial papillae. **B**, In pri-mary hyperplasia with Graves' disease, follicular epithelium is tall with papillary infoldings and peripheral vacuolation of colloid. (**A**, ×85; **B**, ×200; courtesy Dr. S. E. Gould.)

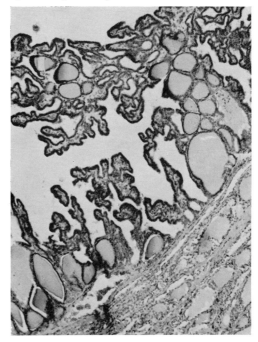

Fig. 34-6 Secondary hyperplasia in nodular goiter, with characteristic follicles in stalks of papillae. (×85; AFIP 59-6958.)

Table 34-2 Clinicopathologic features of noninfective chronic thyroiditis

Type	Sex	Age (yr)	Weight of gland (gm)	Salient histopathology	Eventual hypothyroidism
Lymphocytic	F (90%)	6-35 (av, 31)	Av, 19	Lymphocytes	0-2%
Nonspecific	F (85%)	Av, 40	35-60	Plasma cells	50%
Hashimoto's struma	F (98%)	8-71 (av, 50)	60-225	Lymph follicles; epithelial damage	80%
Granulomatous	F (84%)	20-40	45-60	Foreign body granulomas	6%-20%
Riedel's struma	M = F	20-70	Bulky	Dense local fibrosis	Uncommon

The clinical term "hot nodule" usually refers to a focus of secondary hyperplasia in a nodular goiter that concentrates ^{131}I with or without demonstrable hyperthyroidism. Until surgical removal, it may not be evident that the entire gland is nodular and either enlarged or of normal weight. A genuine follicular adenoma with secondary hyperplasia is uncommon. While clinicians have a tendency to dignify apparently solitary hyperfunctional thyroid nodules as "toxic adenomas," over 90% of these prove pathologically to be merely the dominant nodule of a diffusely nodular thyroid gland. Secondary hyperthyroidism sometimes also complicates a follicular thyroid adenocarcinoma.

THYROIDITIS
Acute thyroiditis

Acute thyroiditis appears often to be a complication of bacterial or viral infection of the oropharynx or salivary glands. The thyroid gland becomes temporarily enlarged and tender but rarely requires operation except for drainage of suppuration. Biopsy specimens show interstitial neutrophils and some follicle degeneration.

Chronic thyroiditis

Chronic thyroiditis represents a more difficult problem, since there is no agreement on its classification or pathogenesis. The distinctive clinicopathologic features of five recognized noninfective types are listed in Table 34-2.

Hashimoto's struma. Hashimoto's struma, or struma lymphomatosa, is characterized by a firm, rubbery, enlarged gland that weighs 60 gm to 225 gm and is covered by an unaltered, thin capsule. On section, the thyroid tissue has a uniform, faintly lobulated, opaque yellow-tan surface unlike the grayish

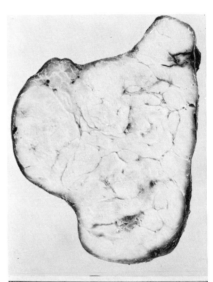

Fig. 34-7 Thyroid gland in Hashimoto's disease. (From Anderson, W. A. D.: Synopsis of pathology, The C. V. Mosby Co.)

pink granularity of cancer (Fig. 34-7). It is often difficult microscopically to recognize thyroid follicles due to a notable lymphocytic infiltrate in sheets and follicles with germinal centers. Remnants of thyroid follicles and epithelial nests persist, often with metaplastic granular eosinophilic cytoplasm, termed Hürthle cells (Fig. 34-8). They are more precisely named Askanazy or oxyphil cells, which are apparently nonfunctional but packed with mitochondria. Hürthle cells are common in Hashimoto's struma but also accompany primary and secondary hyperplasias, nodular goiters, neoplasms, and other types of thyroiditis.

Lymphocytic thyroiditis. Lymphocytic thyroiditis, also called juvenile or adolescent thyroiditis, was recognized relatively recently.

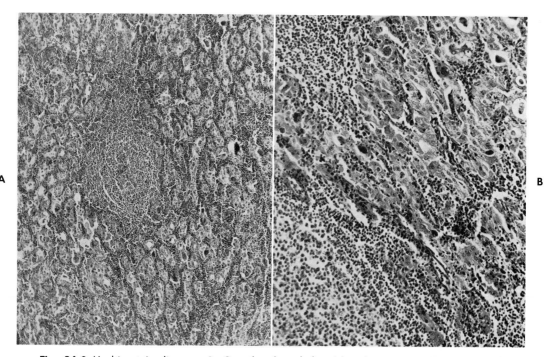

Fig. 34-8 Hashimoto's disease. **A,** Greatly altered thyroid architecture. **B,** Destruction of follicles, lymphocytic infiltrate, and oxyphilic cells characteristic of Hashimoto's struma. (**A,** ×50; **B,** ×150.)

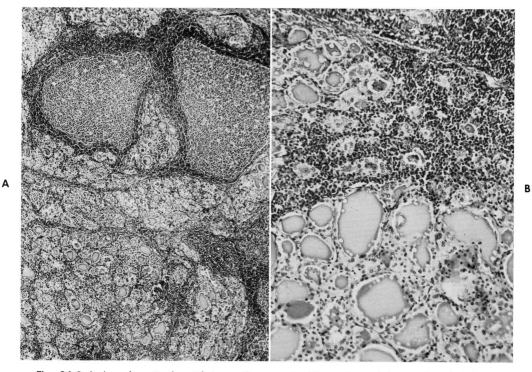

Fig. 34-9 A, Lymphocytic thyroiditis, easily recognizable as thyroid despite lymph follicles with germinal centers. **B,** Some follicles intact and others small and partly degenerated. (**A,** ×50; **B,** ×150.)

The gland is less enlarged than in Hashimoto's struma or of normal weight. Microscopically, the lymphocytic infiltration is less extensive than in Hashimoto's struma, with little or no thyroid epithelial destruction or fibrosis (Fig. 34-9). The follicles may appear unaltered or hyperplastic. Perhaps this condition represents an earlier or milder manifestation of Hashimoto's struma affecting a younger population.

Nonspecific chronic thyroiditis. Nonspecific chronic thyroiditis, also called chronic sclerosing thyroiditis, is the most common type of thyroiditis and often is confused with Hashimoto's struma. However, it differs from the latter in three ways. The gland is smaller, weighing 35 gm to 60 gm. Microscopically, the thyroid parenchyma is easily recognized despite some follicular disruption, mild fibrosis, and infrequent lymph follicles. The most distinctive feature is an abundance of interstitial plasma cells. There also may be focal squamous metaplasia. In brief, an ordinary chronic inflammatory reaction is present, possibly subsequent to an infectious, chemical, immunologic, or vascular injury.

Granulomatous thyroiditis. Granulomatous thyroiditis is synonymous with giant cell, pseudotuberculous, de Quervain's, or so-called subacute thyroiditis. Neither clinically nor pathologically is it subacute. Grossly, the thyroid gland is moderately enlarged, but the tissue is pale and hard like a raw turnip. Histologically, a striking multifocal foreign body giant cell reaction surrounds colloid escaped from disorganized follicles, mingled with granulomas composed of epithelioid macrophages (Fig. 34-10). An intervening chronic inflammatory infiltrate is present, sometimes containing microabscesses and calcium oxalate crystals. One-third of the cases involve the gland asymmetrically.

Riedel's struma. Riedel's struma (struma fibrosa or invasive fibrous thyroiditis) is the rarest type of thyroiditis. It produces a localized hard cervical mass that on resection proves to be a dense fibrous scar involving the thyroid gland and contiguous tissues. Histologically, this appears like an exaggerated fibrous connective tissue response to unilateral injury.

■ ■ ■

Specific types of chronic thyroiditis include sarcoidosis, tuberculosis, syphilis, and echinococcosis, all of which are uncommon.

The clinical diagnosis of chronic thyroiditis

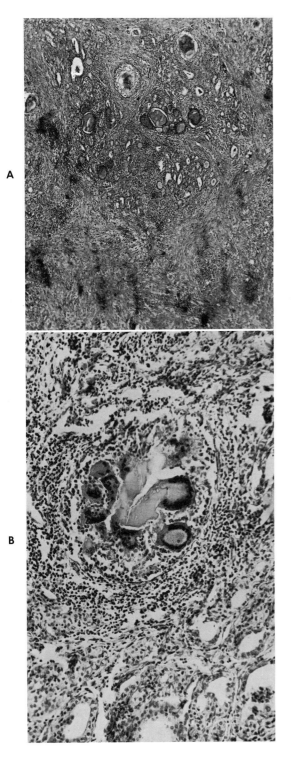

A

B

Fig. 34-10 A, Granulomatous thyroiditis with nodular and fibrotic appearance. **B,** Foreign body giant cell reaction around colloid and granuloma formation. (**A,** ×50; **B,** ×150.)

is assisted by serum antithyroid antibody tests. Whether Hashimoto's struma and the other types are true autoimmune diseases is uncertain. They appear equally likely to be nonimmunologically initiated diseases, which may be perpetuated and exaggerated by immune reactions. Histochemically, basement membrane dissolution is found in early chronic thyroiditis. Chronic thyroiditis produced experimentally in animals resembles the nonspecific type histopathologically more than it does Hashimoto's struma. Further investigations are necessary to understand these lesions.

AGE CHANGES, DEGENERATION, AND ATROPHY

Beyond 50 years of age, about half of normal-sized thyroid glands contain single or multiple nodules with increased colloid storage, mostly clinically impalpable. Irregular colloid repletion and depletion appear responsible. The nodular thyroid gland has no known clinical significance. Mild interstitial fibrosis, calcium oxalate crystals, and medial calcification of the thyroid arteries also are common in elderly persons.

Hyaline interstitial fibrosis and follicle shrinkage represent the most familiar thyroid degeneration. When the hyalin is abundant and partly involves vessel walls, special staining may demonstrate amyloid. Amyloid goiter is a massive deposit predominantly restricted to the thyroid gland (Fig. 34-11).

Cytoplasmic iron-positive pigment is usual in hemochromatosis and occasionally in hemosiderosis. Ochronosis also pigments the thyroid gland.

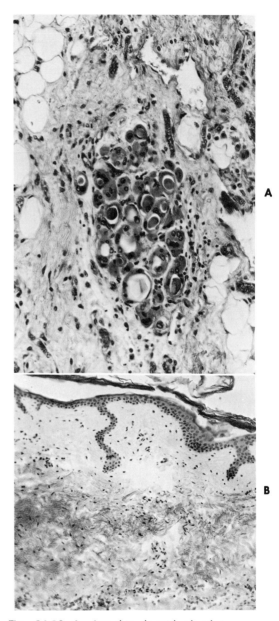

Fig. 34-12 A, Atrophic thyroid gland in myxedema. Few small follicles remain, surrounded by fibroadipose tissue. **B,** Skin in myxedema, with edematous thickening of upper dermis. (**A** and **B,** ×120; **B,** courtesy Dr. S. E. Gould.)

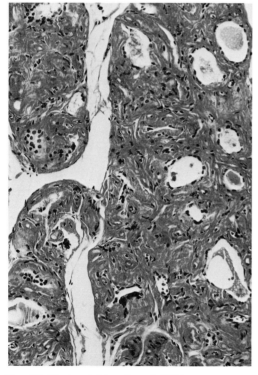

Fig. 34-11 Amyloid goiter. (×120.)

Mild thyroid atrophy with small follicles may accompany aging or chronic systemic diseases. Moderate atrophy reduces the gland weights to 10 gm or 12 gm. In severe atrophy, the thyroid gland weighs only 3.5 gm to 6 gm, representing mostly capsule, vessels, and infiltrative fibroadipose connective tissue. A few miniature follicles or nests of Hürthle cells remain (Fig. 34-12).

Myxedema results from subtotal or total thyroid inactivity. The characteristic facies of myxedema comprise a puffy, pasty complexion, sparse eyebrows, coarse hair, and large tongue. Menorrhagia and increased sensitivity to cold are common. Mental activity is sluggish, frequently with irritability. Deep tendon reflexes are slow. Coma may complicate myxedema, associated with hypothermia, carbon dioxide retention, and hyponatremia. Bradycardia, low-voltage electrocardiograms, cardiac hypertrophy with basophilic myocardial degeneration and circulating thyroid antibodies are common in myxedema. Skin biopsy demonstrates increases in hyaluronic acid and neutral mucoprotein ground substance in the upper dermis.

Usually, myxedema appears due to idiopathic thyroid failure. Fewer cases are secondary to TSH insufficiency or panhypopituitarism, whereas hypothalamic myxedema is rare. In all three situations, the thyroid gland is moderately or severely atrophied. Hypothyroidism or myxedema after thyroid operations or ^{131}I therapy for thyrotoxicosis is not unusual. Chronic thyroiditis also causes hypothyroidism.

Pretibial myxedema is a localized bilateral swelling of the shins due to excessive myxoid dermal connective tissue. Paradoxically, it usually accompanies hyperthyroidism and increased LATS titers.

NEOPLASMS
Benign neoplasms

Thyroid adenomas are true neoplasms, usually solitary and predominating in women, with a sex ratio of 5:1 or 6:1. Thyroid nodules outnumber adenomas at least 10:1, but adenomas require special scrutiny because they are sometimes precancerous. About 10% show invasive characteristics. Five diagnostic criteria of thyroid adenoma are complete fibrous encapsulation, a different architecture inside and outside the capsule, a uniform internal growth pattern, compression of follicles outside the capsule into crescentic shapes, and singleness (Fig. 34-13).

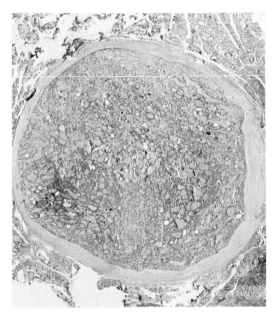

Fig. 34-13 Follicular adenoma. (×50.)

Adenomas

Adenomas are divided most simply into follicular, papillary, and atypical types.

Follicular adenomas. Follicular adenomas have five variants. In order of decreasing frequency, there are fetal, colloid, simple, embryonal, and Hürthle cell types. Grossly, an adenoma usually measures 1.5 cm to 5 cm in diameter, and on section the tan, smooth tissue everts, indicating compression by the fibrous capsule. In the center of larger adenomas may be a dense white fibrous scar. Fetal adenoma is by far the most common. The miniature "fetal" follicles contain small colloid masses and lie closely packed or loosely arranged in an edematous fibrovascular stroma (Fig. 34-14). In embryonal adenoma, the epithelium grows in branching cords with little or no follicle formation. Simple adenomas have follicles of normal adult size. This is the type that, on rare occasions, develops hyperplasia and constitutes the genuine "toxic adenoma." In colloid adenoma, the follicles are unusually large. Hürthle cell adenoma is characterized by large granular oxyphil cells which form cords and follicles containing scanty colloid (Fig. 34-15). Because Hürthle cells are metaplastic, it may be preferable to designate these as follicular adenomas with oxyphilic (Hürthle cell) metaplasia.

Follicular adenomas require careful study of the capsule and the vessels within and outside of it to determine the presence of invasion. Some specialists believe eight to twelve blocks should be examined microscopically for evidence of capsular and blood vessel invasion. Elastic tissue stains simplify the identification of veins. Tumor that penetrates a vessel wall and also occupies its lumen is most clearly acceptable as invasive.

Terminology for designating a follicular adenoma with capsular or vascular invasion varies. Angioinvasive adenoma and encapsulated follicular carcinoma are two related terms. In effect, it is usually an early stage of follicular adenocarcinoma. As such, there

is an excellent chance of cure by a simple excision that includes some extracapsular thyroid tissue. The recurrence rate thereafter is 15% or less after five years. The comparative frequency of invasion and malignant behavior for adenomas of different growth patterns is given in Table 34-3.

Papillary adenoma. Papillary adenoma is grossly distinctive, since on sectioning it typically contains wine-red fluid and a capsule lined by granular gray tissue nodules. Microscopically, few papillary adenomas are completely encapsulated. If this diagnostic criterion is satisfied, only 0.5% of adenomas are papillary. Expert opinion differs on what designation should be applied to papillary adenomas with capsular invasion. Similar disagreements exist on classifying papillary neoplasms of the urinary bladder, ovary, and breast. In the absence of any significant cytologic dysplasia and other evidence of invasive activity, it is not clear that incom-

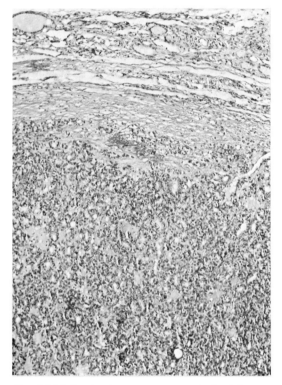

Fig. 34-14 Fetal adenoma composed of miniature follicles and fibrous capsule. (×85.)

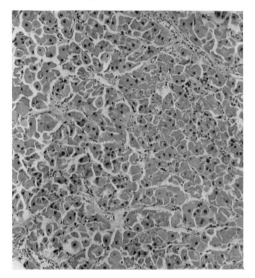

Fig. 34-15 Hürthle cell adenoma with large acidophilic cells. (×100.)

Table 34-3 Adenomas of thyroid gland—invasion, metastasis, and death

Adenoma	Cases	% Invasion	% Metastasis (5 yr)	% Death (10 yr)
Follicular	1,105	5.1	15*	10
Fetal type	459	4.8		
Embryonal type	134	25		
Simple type	204	0	0	0
Colloid type	288	0	0	0
Hürthle cell type	20	5.0	0	0
Atypical	70	4.3	0	0
Papillary	138	46	11	15
Total adenomas	1,313	9.5	14*	11*

*% Metastasis or death from cancer in adenomas with invasion.

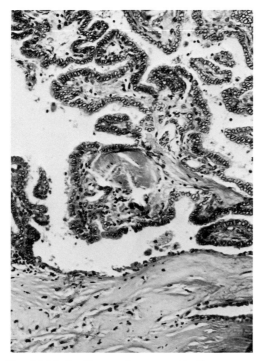

Fig. 34-16 Papillary adenoma with fibrous capsule below. (×120.)

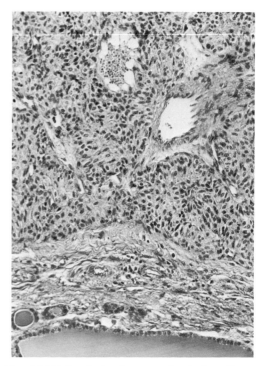

Fig. 34-17 Atypical adenoma of spindle cell pattern. (×120; AFIP 68-9551.)

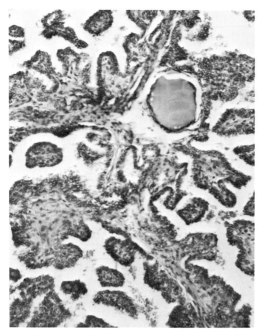

Fig. 34-18 Papillary carcinoma of thyroid gland with atypical layered epithelium. (×85.)

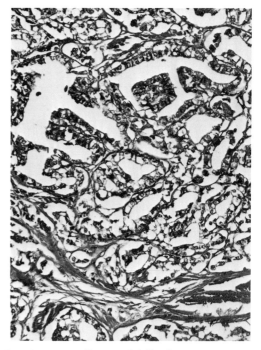

Fig. 34-19 Papillary and follicular carcinoma, including some clear cells. (×120; courtesy Dr. F. R. Skelton.)

plete encapsulation of a papillary adenoma indicates cancer (Fig. 34-16). Statistically, extensive surgery appears unnecessary for well-differentiated papillary adenomas.

Atypical adenoma. Atypical adenoma is a rarity, making up 2% to 5% of the adenomas. Grossly, the tissue is more opaque and grayish pink than in other adenomas. Microscopically, closely packed spindle cells form bundles separated by stromal bands, unlike the usual thyroid patterns (Fig. 34-17). A few atypical adenomas are composed of clear cells or pale follicles resembling parathyroid tissue ("parastruma") or possess bizarre giant nuclei without other indications of carcinoma. Despite the peculiar and somewhat ominous cytology, their course is benign.

Teratoma

Teratoma of the thyroid gland is a curiosity usually affecting newborn infants. Grossly, teratomas are partly cystic with mesodermal components including muscle, glia, and glandular or other epithelial elements of ectodermal and endodermal origin. The benign thyroid teratoma is dangerous chiefly because of its strategic cervical location.

Malignant neoplasms
Carcinoma

Papillary carcinoma. The most common thyroid cancer, papillary carcinoma comprises over 60% of thyroid carcinomas in large series. Generally, it has a long, sluggish natural history, corresponding to grade I carcinomas elsewhere. Most affected children and adolescents have been exposed to ionizing radiation. Grossly, papillary carcinomas may not be discernible. Larger carcinomas are either partly encapsulated or unencapsulated, or the tumor may massively involve the thyroid and adjacent tissues.

Papillary carcinomas of microscopic size usually are discovered by recognizing the more prominent metastases in lateral cervical lymph nodes. After resection of the homolateral thyroid lobe, careful study by multiple or subserial sections reveals the primary carcinoma, which is sometimes less than 2 mm in diameter.

Partly encapsulated papillary carcinomas may originate from papillary adenomas. In carcinomas, anaplastic epithelium is piled up on papillae or growing in solid masses, with clear-cut invasion of the adjacent gland (Fig. 34-18). Unencapsulated papillary carcinomas are histologically identical but show no indi-

cation of an original adenoma. Some are multicentric. Patients with localized varieties of papillary carcinoma survive after treatment as well as the normal population, based on twenty-year to forty-year postoperative follow-up of over 700 cases. Seventeen deaths from thyroid carcinoma (2.3%) were reported by Woolner et al.[143] Metastases are relatively radiosensitive.

Massive papillary carcinoma spreading into the extrathyroid tissues and lymph nodes is lethal in about one-third of patients within twenty years and compares to stage III, grade I carcinomas elsewhere. Peculiar to papillary carcinoma are its notable tendency to lymphatic invasion with metastasis to regional cervical lymph nodes and the calcospherites ("psammoma bodies") found in the stroma. Calcospherites may remain in areas of local tumor regression, and their presence suggests nearby papillary carcinoma.

Papillary carcinoma may grow purely in this pattern, or papillary and follicular carcinoma may be found together in the original site, in metastases, or in both (Fig. 34-19). Sometimes, an apparently pure papillary carcinoma has lymph node metastases with predominant follicular carcinoma. Squamous foci also sometimes are present. No difference in prognosis has been found between these papillary carcinoma variants; this is better than for follicular carcinoma. The stages and grades of papillary and other thyroid carcinomas are summarized in Table 34-4.

Follicular carcinoma. Follicular carcinoma of the thyroid gland is generally comparable to stage II, grade II adenocarcinomas in other tissues. Three varieties of follicular carcinoma are the most favorable:

1 Nonencapsulated sclerosing carcinoma (Hazard-Crile tumor). In a thyroid gland removed for another reason, sectioning shows a minute stellate scar. Histologically, this is a very localized scirrhous adenocarcinoma incidentally discovered and nonrecurrent. Some regard it as a variant of papillary carcinoma.

2 Encapsulated follicular carcinoma. This merges with follicular adenoma manifesting capsular or vascular invasion. Acceptable cases have reasonably apparent cytologic anaplasia. Only about 15% of the patients develop metastases and die of cancer.

3 Langhans' struma is a sluggish tumor that grows in continuity to fill the

Table 34-4 Carcinomas of thyroid gland—pathologic grades and clinical stages*

	Pathologic grade	Clinical stage†	Survival	
			10 yr	15 yr
Follicular adenoma with invasion	0-I	IB		
Papillary adenoma with invasion	0-I	IA or B	For total 694 stage I cases	
Papillary carcinoma	I	IA or B, II or III	89%	83%
Papillary and follicular carcinoma	I or II	IB, II, or III		
Nonencapsulated sclerosing carcinoma	I or II	IA		
Langhans' struma	I or II	III		
Follicular carcinoma	II	IB or II	For total 151 stage II cases	
			54%	42%
Medullary carcinoma	II	I, II, or III	For total 101 stage III cases	
Small cell compact carcinoma	III	III or IV	29%	16%
Small cell diffuse carcinoma	III	II, III, or IV	For total 60 stage IV cases	
			10%	10%
Giant cell carcinoma	III	III or IV		

*Modified from Pub. 8, American Joint Committee for Cancer Staging and End Results Reporting, 1967.
†Stage I tumors are less than 5 cm in diameter, with or without cervical lymph node metastases; A, impalpable; B, palpable. Stage II tumors are 5 cm in diameter or larger, with or without cervical lymph node metastases. Stage III tumors extend directly into adjacent structures. Stage IV tumors have distant metastasis.

anterior part of the neck and finally compromises respiration. Microscopically, its monotonous appearance resembles fetal adenoma but is unconfined. It is too rare to give prognostic figures.

Grossly, a follicular thyroid carcinoma is ordinarily a hard, gritty, grayish pink unencapsulated mass 2 cm or more in diameter, not unlike a breast carcinoma in appearance. Microscopically, it may vary from an obviously anaplastic solid epithelial growth that forms a few follicles to a well-differentiated follicle-forming tumor recognizable as carcinoma by glands with disproportionately large nuclei growing back to back (Fig. 34-20). Sometimes, the best differentiated follicular carcinomas metastasize to lymph nodes, bones, or elsewhere and, focally, are of practically normal thyroid appearance. However, a careful study usually reveals some neoplastic qualities. "Benign metastasizing thyroid" is largely a myth.

Blood vessel invasion, which is not uncommon in follicular carcinoma, contributes to the likelihood of pulmonary and osseous metastases. A few cases concentrate sufficient iodine to make ^{131}I therapy worthwhile. Survival rates are 34% at ten years and 16% at twenty years, according to the data of Woolner et al.[143] One-fifth of follicular carcinomas are of Hürthle cell type, and these have shown no distinctive clinical behavior.

Medullary carcinoma with amyloid stroma. Medullary carcinoma of the thyroid gland with amyloid stroma, also called solid carcinoma, was first distinguished in 1959 by

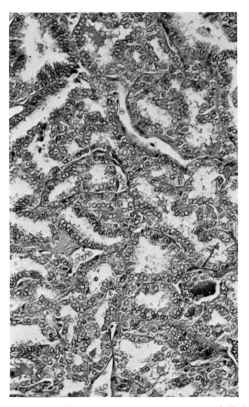

Fig. 34-20 Follicular carcinoma. Only one follicle contains colloid. (×150; AFIP 59-7430.)

Hazard et al.[127] Grossly, medullary carcinoma varies from less than 1.5 cm to massive size. It has a rounded, demarcated outline without encapsulation, and the tumor tissue is gray or white with focal hemorrhages. Microscopically, the structure is solid and cellular

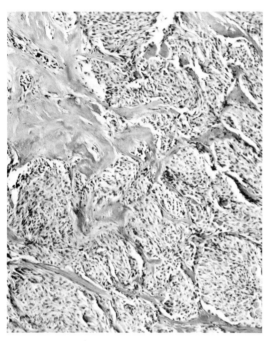

Fig. 34-21 Medullary carcinoma of thyroid gland with amyloid-positive stroma. (×85.)

and, most typically, is composed of spindle cells, unlike any pattern expected in a thyroid neoplasm but sometimes resembling a carcinoid. The stroma is irregularly hyalinized. Special staining regularly demonstrates amyloid, but this often is not diffuse or obvious (Fig. 34-21). Amyloid occurs also in the metastases. Despite the rather undifferentiated appearance of medullary thyroid carcinomas and a tendency to bilaterality, these tumors behave like moderately malignant (grade II) neoplasms. If there are no lymph node metastases, the ten-year and twenty-year survival rates are as good as for the age-matched population without cancer. With metastases, the ten-year survival is reduced to 42%.

Electron microscopy shows that the medullary carcinoma cells contain specialized granules of thyrocalcitonin, indicating the tumor to be a parafollicular cell carcinoma or C cell carcinoma. No clear clinical evidence of thyrocalcitonin excess has been found, although some cases are accompanied by parathyroid hyperplasia.

Several unusual syndromes are related to medullary thyroid carcinoma. These include pheochromocytoma, especially familial or bilateral, and sometimes multiple familial endocrine adenomas. Further, neurofibromatosis, neurofibromas, or multiple mucosal

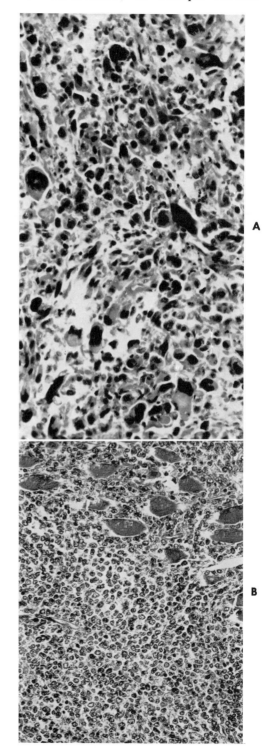

Fig. 34-22 Carcinoma of thyroid gland. **A,** Giant cell carcinoma. **B,** Small cell diffuse carcinoma invading striated muscle at upper right. (**A,** ×150; AFIP 59-6950; **B,** ×150; AFIP 59-6943.)

neuromas, and sometimes Marfan's syndrome are correlated. Lately, cases of diarrhea, the carcinoid syndrome, or Cushing's syndrome attributable to medullary thyroid carcinoma have been recognized. In its aberrant endocrine activities, medullary carcinoma now rivals oat cell lung carcinomas and pancreatic islet tumors, all of which are derived from foregut endoderm.

Undifferentiated carcinoma. Undifferentiated carcinomas also are termed anaplastic. Ordinarily, they are obviously malignant clinically, grossly, and microscopically due to their hard consistency and rapid growth. Older people are affected. Regardless of the histologic type, in the series reported by Woolner et al.,[143] half of the patients were dead of cancer in five months and nearly all by three years. Four of 160 patients lived over five years. Occasionally, a long history begins with an invasive adenoma, progresses to follicular carcinoma, and ends with death from undifferentiated carcinoma twenty-five years or more thereafter. The plasticity of one human thyroid carcinoma has been shown by sequential animal transplants, which grew over several years in most of the major histologic patterns.

Small cell compact undifferentiated carcinoma in some series is the most common grade III variety. Grossly and microscopically, it resembles a scirrhous breast carcinoma except for a few neoplastic follicles. Giant cell carcinoma, also called spindle and giant cell carcinoma or carcinosarcoma, is the other relatively well-known undifferentiated carcinoma. Some arise from adenomas. The bizarre and disorderly neoplastic cells are unrecognizable as thyroid, and tumor giant cells of striking variability are present (Fig. 34-22, *A*).

Small cell diffuse carcinoma is uncommon and not easily distinguished from malignant lymphoma, even in well-prepared sections. Both in the thyroid and nodal metastases, the small cells retain some epithelial characteristics, such as cordlike growth and compression of the preexisting reticulin (Fig. 34-22, *B*).

Rarer and ordinarily lethal carcinomas include adenoacanthoma, squamous cell carcinoma, and mixed carcinoma that includes intermingled components of a moderately differentiated grade II and an undifferentiated grade III carcinoma. Hürthle cell carcinoma is now regarded as a metaplastic alteration of some other neoplasm and not as an entity.

Stromal tumors

Sarcoma of the thyroid gland most often is malignant lymphoma—lymphosarcoma, reticulum cell sarcoma, or Hodgkin's disease. Elderly women usually are the victims of either primary or secondary thyroid lymphomas. The features used to distinguish thyroid lymphoma from carcinoma or thyroiditis are essentially the same as those employed in lymph nodes. Plasmacytoma restricted to the thyroid gland is said to have the same benign course observed in certain other extramedullary sites.

Fibrosarcoma, rhabdomyosarcoma, osteosarcoma, and angiosarcoma have been described in thyroid glands. Benign mesenchymal thyroid tumors include lipoma, hemangioma, neurilemoma, and leiomyoma.

Metastatic cancer

Metastatic cancer of the thyroid gland is fairly common at autopsy with widely disseminated tumors. Breast or lung carcinomas and malignant melanoma are the most common sources of thyroid metastases.

REFERENCES
General

1 Committee on Nomenclature, American Thyroid Association: J. Clin. Endocr. **29:**860-862, 1969.
2 Hazard, J. B., and Smith, D. E., editors: The thyroid, Baltimore, 1964, The Williams & Wilkins Co.
3 Pitt-Rivers, R., and Trotter, W. R., editors: The thyroid gland, vols. 1 and 2, London, 1964, Butterworth & Co. (Publishers) Ltd.
4 Rawson, R. W., Sonenberg, M., and Money, W. L.: In Duncan, G. G., editor: Diseases of metabolism, Philadelphia, 1964, W. B. Saunders Co., Chap. 17.
5 Sommers, S. C.: In Bloodworth, J. M. B., editor: Endocrine pathology, Baltimore, 1968, The Williams & Wilkins Co., chap. 6.

Structure and function

6 Aliapoulios, M. A., and Morain, W. D.: Amer. J. Surg. **117:**554-557, 1969 (thyrocalcitonin).
7 Blizzard, R. M., Chandler, W. W., Landing, B. H., Pettit, M. D., and West, C. D.: New Eng. J. Med. **263:**327-336, 1960 (familial cretinism).
8 Braunstein, H., and Stephens, C. L.: Arch. Path. (Chicago) **86:**659-666, 1968 (parafollicular cells).
9 Copp, D. H., Cockcroft, D. W., Kueh, Y., and Melville, M.: In Calcitonin: proceedings of the symposium on Thyrocalcitonin and C cells, New York, 1968, Springer-Verlag New York Inc., p. 306.
10 Evans, T. C., Kretzschmar, R. M., Hodges, R. E., and Song, C. W.: J. Nucl. Med. **8:**157-165, 1967 (fetal thyroid function).
11 Frantz, V. K., Forsythe, R., Hanford, J. M.,

and Rogers, W. M.: Ann. Surg. 115:161-183, 1942 (embryology).

12 Goldberg, H. M., and Harvey, P:. Brit. J. Surg. 43:565-569, 1956 (squamous cysts).

13 Goormaghtigh, N., and Thomas, F.: Amer. J. Path. 10:713-730, 1934 (cytology).

14 Gross, R. E., and Connerley, M. L.: New Eng. J. Med. 223:616-624, 1940 (thyroglossal duct cysts).

15 Haley, H. L., Dews, G. M., and Sommers, S. C.: Arch. Path. (Chicago) 59:635-640, 1955 (histochemistry).

16 Heimann, P.: Acta Endocr. (Kobenhavn) 53 (suppl. 110):1-102, 1966 (ultrastructure).

16a Jaques, D. A., Chambers, R. G., and Oertel, J. E.: Amer. J. Surg. 120:439-446, 1970 (thyroglossal duct carcinoma).

17 Klopp, C. T., and Kirson, S. M.: Ann. Surg. 163:653-664, 1966 (ectopia).

18 Little, G., Meador, C. K., Cunningham, R., and Pittman, J. A.: J. Clin. Endocr. 25:1529-1536, 1965 (sporadic cretinism).

19 Nolan, L. E.: Arch. Path. (Chicago) 25:1-16, 1938 (size and weight).

20 Roth, L. M.: Cancer 18:105-111, 1965 (inclusions in nodes).

21 Shepard, T. H., Andersen, H., and Andersen, H. J.: Anat. Rec. 149:363-379, 1964 (fetal histochemistry).

22 Sherman, P. H., and Shahbahrami, F.: Amer. Surg. 32:137-142, 1966 (substernal goiter).

23 Stanbury, J. B., and deGroot, L. J.: Clin. Chem. 13:542-553, 1967 (pathophysiology).

24 Tremblay, G.: Lab. Invest. 11:514-517, 1962 (Askanazy cells).

Goiter and altered hormonal biosynthesis

25 Anon.: Brit. Med. J. 1:167, 1962 (goitrous cretinism).

26 Batsakis, J. F., Nishiyama, R. H., and Schmidt, R. W.: Amer. J. Clin. Path. 39:241-251, 1963 (congenital goiter).

27 Coble, Y., Davis, J., Schulert, A., Heta, F., and Awad, A. Y.: Amer. J. Clin. Nutr. 21:277-283, 1968 (Egyptian goiter).

28 Fierro-Benitez, R., Penafiel, W., De Groot, L. J., and Ramirez, I.: New Eng. J. Med. 280:296-302, 1969 (Andean goiter and cretinism).

29 Lupulescu, A., Negoescu, I., Petrovici, A., Nicolae, I., Stoian, M., Balan, M., and Stancu, H.: Acta Anat. (Basel) 66:321-338, 1967 (ultrastructure of goiter in cretin).

30 Marine, D., and Kimball, O. P.: J.A.M.A. 77:1068, 1921 (simple goiter).

31 Miller, J. M., Horn, R. C., and Block, M. A.: J. Clin. Endocr. 27:1264-1274, 1967 (nodules and activity).

32 Moore, G. H.: Arch. Path. (Chicago) 74:35-46, 1962 (familial goitrous cretinism).

33 Silverstein, G. E., Burke, G., and Cogan, R.: Ann. Intern. Med. 67:539-548, 1967 (hyperactive nodules).

34 Stanbury, J. B., Brownell, G. L., Riggs, D. S., Perinetti, H., Itoiz, J., and del Castillo, E. B.: Endemic goiter, Cambridge, Mass., 1954, Harvard University Press.

35 Stanbury, J. B., Wyngaarden, J. B., and Fredrickson, D. S., editors: The metabolic basis of inherited disease, ed. 2, New York, 1966, Blakiston Division, McGraw-Hill Book Co. (familial goiter).

36 Thould, A. K., and Scowen, E. F.: J. Endocr. 30:69-77, 1964 (Pendred's syndrome).

37 Weaver, D. K., Nishiyama, R. H., Burton, W. D., and Batsakis, J. G.: Arch. Surg. (Chicago) 92:796-801, 1966 (nodular goiter).

Iatrogenic abnormalities

38 Anderson, G. S., and Bird, T.: Lancet 2:742-743, 1961 (congenital iodide goiter).

39 Beach, S. A., and Dolphin, G. W.: Phys. Med. Biol. 6:583-598, 1962 (radiation doses and cancer).

40 Dolphin, G. W.: Health Phys. 15:219-228, 1968 (radiation carcinogenesis).

41 Doniach, I., Eadie, D. G. A., and Hope-Stone, H. F.: Brit. J. Surg. 53:681-685, 1966 (postirradiation adenomas).

42 Freiesleben, E., and Kjerulf-Jensen, K.: J. Clin. Endocr. 7:47-51, 1947 (maternal thiouracil and fetal effects).

43 Galina, M. P., Avnet, N. L., and Einhorn, A.: New Eng. J. Med. 267:1124-1127, 1962 (fatal newborn iodide goiter).

44 Greig, W. R., Crooks, J., and Macgregor, A. G.: Proc. Roy. Soc. Med. 59:599-602, 1966 (radiation effects).

45 Guinet, P., Tourniaire, J., and Peyrin, J. O.: Ann. Endocr. (Paris) 28:199-206, 1967 (resorcinol goiter).

46 Oppenheimer, J. H., and McPherson, H. T.: Amer. J. Med. 30:281-288, 1961 (iodide goiter).

47 Pincus, R. A., Reichlin, S., and Hempelmann, L. H.: Ann. Intern. Med. 66:1154-1164, 1967 (x-radiation of infant thyroid).

48 Roy, P. E., Bonenfant, J. L., and Turcot, L.: Amer. J. Clin. Path. 50:234-239, 1968 (cobalt).

49 Schottstaedt, E. S., and Smoller, M.: Ann. Intern. Med. 64:847-849, 1966 (thyroid tablet poisoning).

50 Sheline, G. E., Lindsay, S., McCormack, K. R., and Galante, M.: J. Clin. Endocr. 22:8-18, 1962 (postirradiation nodular regeneration).

51 Winship, T., and Rosvoll, R. V.: Amer. J. Surg. 102:747-752, 1961 (postirradiation carcinoma).

52 Wood, J. W., Tamagaki, H., Neriishi, S., Sato, T., Sheldon, W. F., Archer, P. G., Hamilton, H. B., and Johnson, K. G.: Amer. J. Epidem. 89:4-14, 1969 (atomic radiation carcinoma).

Hyperplasia
Primary hyperplasia

53 Adams, D. D.: Brit. Med. J. 1:1015-1019, 1965 (Graves' disease).

54 Benua, R. S., and Lipsett, M. B.: J. Clin. Endocr. 19:19-27, 1959 (thyroid stimulation).

55 Buckle, R. M., Mason, A. M. S., and Middleton, J. E.: Lancet 1:1128-1130, 1969 (hypercalcemia).

56 Carneiro, L., Dorrington, K. J., and Munro, D. S.: Lancet 2:878-880, 1966 (LATS and hyperplasia).

57 French, G. N.: New Eng. J. Med. 241:299-301, 1949 (pretibial myxedema).

58 Gaan, D.: Brit. Med. J. **3:**415-416, 1967 (myopathy).

59 Goddard, J. W., and Sommers, S. C.: Lab. Invest. **3:**197-210, 1954 (cytologic hyperplasia).

60 Hershman, J. M., Givens, J. R., Cassidy, C. E., and Astwood, E. B.: J. Clin. Endocr. **26:**803-807, 1966 (recurrent hyperthyroidism).

61 Liddle, G. W., Heyssel, R. M., and McKenzie, J. M.: Amer. J. Med. **39:**845-848, 1965 (exophthalmos).

62 Lipman, L. M., Green, D. E., Snyder, N. J., Nelson, J. C., and Solomon, D. H.: Amer. J. Med. **43:**486-498, 1967 (LATS and Graves' disease).

63 Millikan, C. H., and Haines, S. F.: Arch. Intern. Med. (Chicago) **92:**5-39, 1953 (myopathy).

64 Spjut, H. J., Warren, W. D., and Ackerman, L. V.: Amer. J. Clin. Path. **27:**367-392, 1957 (recurrent hyperplasia).

Secondary hyperplasia

65 Greene, R., and Farrau, H. E.: J. Endocr. **33:**537-538, 1965.

66 McKenzie, J. M.: J. Clin. Endocr. **26:**779-781, 1966.

67 Miller, J. M., Horn, R. C., and Block, M. A.: Arch. Intern. Med. (Chicago) **113:**72-88, 1964.

68 Molnar, G. D., Wilbur, R. D., Lee, R. E., Woolner, L. B., and Keating, F. R., Jr.: Mayo Clin. Proc. **40:**665-684, 1965.

69 Shahani, S. N., Ganatra, R. D., Sharma, S. M., Ramanath, P., Bagwe, B. A., Desai, K. B., and Antia, F. P.: Arch. Surg. (Chicago) **96:**798-803, 1968.

70 Taylor, S.: Brit. Med. Bull. **16:**102-105, 1960.

Thyroiditis

71 Anon.: Brit. Med. J. **2:**380-381, 1965 (Hashimoto's disease).

72 Crile, G., Jr., and Rumsey, E. W.: J.A.M.A. **142:**458-462, 1950 (subacute thyroiditis).

73 Doniach, D., Nilsson, L. R., and Roitt, I. M.: Acta Paediat. Scand. **54:**260-274, 1965 (autoimmune lymphocytic thyroiditis).

74 Follis, R. H., Jr.: Proc. Soc. Exp. Biol. Med. **102:**425-429, 1959 (experimental iodine thyroiditis).

75 Hahn, H. B., Jr., Hayles, A. B., and Woolner, L. B.: J. Pediat. **66:**73-78, 1965 (lymphocytic thyroiditis).

76 Hall, R., and Stanbury, J. B.: Clin. Exp. Immun. **2:**719-725, 1967 (familial autoimmune thyroiditis).

77 Hazard, J. B.: Amer. J. Clin. Path. **25:**289-298, 399-426, 1955.

78 Ling, N. R., Acton, A. B., Roitt, I. M., and Doniach, D.: Brit. J. Exp. Path. **46:**348-359, 1965 (lymphocyte effects).

79 Raphael, H. A., Beahrs, O. H., Woolner, L. B., and Scholz, D. A.: Mayo Clin. Proc. **41:**375-382, 1966 (Riedel's struma).

80 Roitt, I. M., and Doniach, D.: Brit. Med. Bull. **16:**152-158, 1960 (autoimmunity).

81 Shane, L. L., Valensi, Q. J., Sobrevilla, L., and Gabrilove, J. L.: Amer. J. Med. Sci. **250:**532-541, 1965 (clinical thyroiditis).

82 Sobel, H. J., and Geller, J.: Amer. J. Path. **46:**149-163, 1965 (experimental thyroiditis).

83 Sommers, S. C., and Meissner, W. A.: Amer. J. Clin. Path. **24:**434-440, 1954 (basement membranes).

84 Stuart, A. E., and Allan, W. S. A.: Lancet **2:**1204-1206, 1958 (basement membranes).

85 Thomas, W. C., Jr., Anderson, R. M., Jurkiewicz, M. J., Arujo, J. D., and Blizzard, R. M.: Ann. Intern. Med. **63:**808-818, 1965.

86 Weigle, W. O.: J. Exp. Med. **122:**1049-1062, 1965 (experimental thyroiditis).

87 Witebsky, E., and Rose, N. R.: New York J. Med. **63:**56-59, 1963 (autoimmunity).

88 Woolner, L. B., McConahey, W. M., and Beahrs, O. H.: J. Clin. Endocr. **19:**53-83, 1959 (thyroiditis—histologic study).

Degeneration and atrophy

89 Becker, C. E.: Calif. Med. **110:**61-69, 1969 (myxedema coma).

90 Bullock, W. K., Hummer, G. J., and Kahler, J. E.: Cancer **5:**966-974, 1952 (squamous metaplasia).

91 Daoud, F. S., Nieman, R. E., and Vilter, R. W.: Amer. J. Med. **43:**604-608, 1967 (amyloid goiter).

92 Dubin, I. N.: Amer. J. Clin. Path. **25:**514-542, 1955 (hemochromatosis and siderosis).

93 Hazard, J. B., and Kaufman, N.: Amer. J. Clin. Path. **22:**860-865, 1952 (nodules).

94 Johnson, W. C., and Helwig, E. B.: Arch. Derm. (Chicago) **93:**13-20, 1966 (pretibial myxedema).

95 Kleckner, M. S., Jr., Baggenstoss, A. H., and Weir, J. F.: Amer. J. Clin. Path. **25:**915-931, 1955 (iron storage).

96 Mortensen, J. D., Woolner, L. B., and Bennett, W. A.: J. Clin. Endocr. **15:**1270-1280, 1955 (nodules).

97 Richter, M. N., and McCarty, K. S.: Amer. J. Path. **30:**545-553, 1954 (oxalate crystals).

98 Roth, S. I., Olen, E., and Hansen, L. S.: Lab. Invest. **11:**933-941, 1962 (Hürthle cells).

99 Watanakunakorn, C., Hodges, R. E., and Evans, T. C.: Arch. Intern. Med. (Chicago) **116:**183-190, 1965 (myxedema).

Neoplasms
General

100 Gardner, L. W.: Arch. Path. (Chicago) **59:**372-381, 1955 (Hürthle cell tumors).

101 Hazard, J. B.: In Young, S., and Inman, D. R., editors: Thyroid neoplasia; proceedings of the second Imperial Cancer Research Fund Symposium, London, April 1967, London/New York, 1968, Academic Press, Inc., pp. 3-37.

102 Hazard, J. B., and Kenyon, R.: Arch. Path. (Chicago) **58:**554-563, 1954 (atypical adenoma).

103 Hazard, J. B., and Kenyon, R.: Amer. J. Clin. Path. **24:**755-766, 1954 (vascular invasion).

104 Horn, R. C., Jr.: Cancer **7:**234-244, 1954 (Hürthle cell tumors).

105 Horn, R. C., Jr.: Arch Path. (Chicago) **69:**481-492, 1960.

106 Hurxthal, L. M., and Heineman, A. C.: New Eng. J. Med. **258:**457-465, 1958.

106a Knowlson, G. T. G.: Brit. J. Surg. **58**:253-254, 1971 (cancer in solitary nodule).

107 Lahey, F. H., and Hare, H. F.: J.A.M.A. **145**: 689-695, 1951.

108 Meissner, W. A., and McManus, R. G.: J. Clin. Endocr. **12**:1474-1479, 1952.

109 Silverberg, S. G., and Vidone, R. A.: Cancer **19**:1053-1062, 1966.

110 Spigelman, M.: Med. J. Aust. **1**:53-54, 1969 (thyroid teratoma).

111 Valenta, L., and Jirasek, J. E.: Arch. Path. (Chicago) **84**:215-223, 1967 (histochemistry).

112 Veith, F. J., Brooks, J. R., Grigsby, W. P., and Selenkow, H. A.: New Eng. J. Med. **270**: 431-436, 1964.

113 Warren, S., and Meissner, W. A.: In Atlas of tumor pathology, Sect. IV, Fasc. 14, Washington, D. C., 1953, Armed Forces Institute of Pathology (tumors of thyroid gland).

114 Winship, T.: In Raven, R. W., editor: Cancer, vol. 2, London, 1958, Butterworth & Co. (Publishers) Ltd., chap. 20.

Carcinoma

115 Batsakis, J. G., Nishiyama, R. H., and Rich, C. R.: Arch. Path. (Chicago) **69**:493-498, 1960 (calcospherites).

116 de Yoanna, G., and McManus, R. G.: Arch. Surg. (Chicago) **60**:1199-1204, 1950 (minute papillary carcinoma).

117 Dobyns, B. M., and Lennon, B.: Cancer **5**: 45-51, 1952 (transplanted carcinoma).

118 Ehrlich, J. C., and Kaneko, M.: J. Mount Sinai Hosp. N. Y. **24**:804-815, 1957.

119 Fetterman, G. H.: Amer. J. Dis. Child. **92**: 581-587, 1956.

120 Fisher, E. R., and Hellstrom, H. R.: Amer. J. Clin. Path. **37**:633-638, 1962 (histochemistry).

121 Frazell, E. L., and Foote, F. W., Jr.: J. Clin. Endocr. **9**:1023-1030, 1949.

122 Frazell, E. L., and Foote, F. W., Jr.: Cancer **11**:895-922, 1958 (papillary carcinoma).

123 Gikas, P. W., Labow, S. S., DiGiulio, W., and Finger, J. E.: Cancer **20**:2100-2104, 1967 (papillary carcinoma).

124 Gorlin, R. J., Sedano, H. O., Vickers, R. A., and Červenka, J.: Cancer **22**:293-299, 1968 (medullary carcinoma).

125 Hamperl, H.: Arch. Path. (Chicago) **49**:563-567, 1950 (Hürthle cell tumors).

126 Hazard, J. B.: Lab. Invest. **9**:86-97, 1960 (sclerosing tumor).

127 Hazard, J. B., Hawk, W. A., and Crile, G., Jr.: J. Clin. Endocr. **19**:152-161, 1959 (medullary carcinoma).

128 Horn, R. C., Jr.: Cancer **4**:697-707, 1951 (small cell compact carcinoma).

129 Hutter, R. V. P., Tollefsen, H. R., DeCosse, J. J., Foote, F. W., Jr., and Frazell, E. L.: Amer. J. Surg. **110**:660-668, 1965 (giant cell carcinoma).

130 Kalderon, A. E., and Cohn, J. D.: Cancer **19**: 839-843, 1966 (in thyroglossal cyst).

131 Klinck, G. H., and Winship, T.: Cancer **8**: 701-706, 1955 (sclerosing tumor).

132 Klinck, G. H., and Winship, T.: Cancer **12**: 656-662, 1959 (calcospherites).

133 Kniseley, R. M., and Andrews, G. A.: Amer. J. Clin. Path. **26**:1427-1438, 1956 (clear cell carcinoma).

134 Meissner, W. A., and Adler, A.: Arch. Path. (Chicago) **66**:518-525, 1958 (papillary carcinoma).

135 Meissner, W. A., and Legg, M. A.: J. Clin. Endocr. **18**:91-98, 1958.

136 Meissner, W. A., and Phillips, M. J.: Arch. Path. (Chicago) **74**:291-297, 1962 (small cell diffuse carcinoma).

137 Mortensen, J. D., Woolner, L. B., and Bennett, W. A.: Cancer **9**:306-309, 1956 (metastases to thyroid).

138 Pollock, W. F., and Juler, G.: Amer. J. Dis. Child. **105**:243-248, 1963.

139 Raventos, A., Horn, R. C., Jr., and Ravdin, I. S.: J. Clin. Endocr. **22**:886-891, 1962.

140 Russell, W. O., Ibanez, M. L., Clark, R. L., and White, E. C.: Cancer **16**:1425-1460, 1963 (mixed carcinomas).

141 Task Force on Carcinoma of Thyroid Gland: Clinical staging system, Chicago, 1967, American Joint Committee for Cancer Staging and End-Results Reporting.

142 Tollefsen, H. R., DeCosse, J. J., and Hutter, R. V. P.: Cancer **17**:1035-1044, 1964.

143 Woolner, L. B., Beahrs, O. H., Black, B. M., McConahey, W. M., and Keating, F. R., Jr.: In Young, S., and Inman, D. R., editors: Thyroid neoplasia; proceedings of the second Imperial Cancer Research Fund Symposium, London, April 1967, London/New York, 1968, Academic Press, Inc.

144 Woolner, L. B., Beahrs, O. H., Black, B. M., McConahey, W. M., and Keating, F. R., Jr.: Amer. J. Surg. **102**:354-387, 1961.

145 Zehbe, M.: Virchow Arch. Path. Anat. **197**: 240-291, 1909 (Langhans struma).

Stromal tumors

146 Cox, M. T.: J. Clin. Path. **17**:591-601, 1964.

147 More, J. R. S., Dawson, D. W., Ralston, A. J., and Craig, I.: J. Clin. Path. **21**:661-667, 1968 (plasmacytoma).

148 Roberts, C.: J. Path. Bact. **95**:537-540, 1968 (sarcoma).

149 Walt, A. J., Woolner, L. B., and Black, B. M.: Cancer **10**:663-677, 1957.

150 Wegmann, W.: Schweiz. Med. Wschr. **92**:39-48, 1962 (sarcoma).

151 Woolner, L. B., McConahey, W. M., Beahrs, O. H., and Black, B. M.: Amer. J. Surg. **111**: 502-523, 1966.

Chapter 35

Parathyroid glands

James E. Oertel and W. A. D. Anderson

The parathyroid glands are important regulators of the metabolism of calcium and phosphorus and act to maintain normal levels of these elements in the blood. The normal serum calcium level is approximately 9 mg to 10.2 mg per 100 ml. About half of this is ionized. Most of the rest is bound to protein. Normal serum inorganic phosphate is 3.0 mg to 4.5 mg per 100 ml in adults.

DEVELOPMENT AND STRUCTURE

The parathyroid glands, usually four in number, are developed from endoderm of the third and fourth branchial pouches, in intimate relationship to portions of the thymus, but quite independent of the thyroid gland.[4-6] The superior pair of glands is derived from the fourth pharyngeal pouches, whereas the inferior pair, derived from the third pouches, outdistances the superior pair and the thyroid gland in caudal migration and hence takes the lower position. Their close connection with the development of the thymus explains the occasional occurrence of one or more parathyroid glands near or even embedded in thymic tissue. This possibility should be borne in mind during search for parathyroid tissue or a parathyroid adenoma by surgical procedures or at autopsy.

Although four parathyroid glands are usually present, variations in number from two to ten have been reported. The superior pair are situated rather constantly on the medial part of the dorsal surface of each lobe of the thyroid gland, about the junction of the middle and upper thirds, and lie close to ascending branches of the inferior thyroid artery. They often are embedded in thyroid substance but separated from it by a connective tissue capsule. The inferior parathyroid glands, more inconstant in position, are found usually on the dorsal surface of the lateral lobes of the thyroid gland, near the lower pole.

The parathyroid glands are brownish yellow, oval, somewhat flattened bodies, each measuring, in the adult, about 1.5 mm × 3.5 mm × 6.5 mm, and having a combined weight of about 120 mg to 130 mg (four glands). The amount of interstitial tissue is quite variable, but the mean weight of parenchymal tissue has been estimated to be about 80 mg to 90 mg (four glands).[7]

Each parathyroid gland possesses a capsule of connective tissue, from which bands pass through the gland. The parenchymal cells may be arranged in solid masses but frequently appear in cords or columns. Acinar or follicular structures may be found, tending to increase in frequency with age. These may contain colloid. Interstitial adipose tissue is present after puberty and tends to increase in proportionate amount with age until the middle of the fifth decade. This interstitial fat is replaced and decreases or disappears when there is hyperplasia or adenomatous growth of the parenchyma.

The parenchymal cells appear in three main forms: chief cells, water-clear cells, and oxyphil cells. Transitional forms occur.

The chief cell (6μ to 8μ in diameter) is the most numerous. Its cytoplasm is weakly acidophilic and often appears vacuolated by light microscopy. Electron microscopy suggests that the inactive chief cell is rich in glycogen and has a small Golgi complex and a few dense secretory granules. The active chief cell has less glycogen, a prominent Golgi complex, and more numerous secretory granules.[10, 11] The water-clear cell is larger (10μ to 15μ), has abundant clear cytoplasm and a relatively small pyknotic nucleus, and has well-defined cell borders, a feature often evident in all varieties of parathyroid cells. This cell is rare in normal glands. Large membrane-limited cytoplasmic vacuoles are the most conspicuous aspect of its fine structure. Dense secretory granules are sparse.

The oxyphil cell is 8μ to 14μ in diameter. Its eosinophilic granular cytoplasm is packed with mitochondria, secretory granules are rare, and glycogen is present in moderate amounts. Before puberty, oxyphil cells are uncommon. They increase in number with age and in certain diseases, such as chronic renal failure.[2]

Lipofuscin pigment and small cysts may be found in parathyroid tissue. Of interest is the marked resistance to radiation injury exhibited by the parathyroid glands.

HORMONES
Parathyroid hormone

Parathyroid hormone is a small polypeptide that acts to elevate serum calcium and reduce serum phosphate.[12] Reduction of serum ionized calcium promptly causes increased secretion of the hormone, whereas elevation of serum calcium results in decreased secretion. Magnesium ions have similar effects. Experimental work suggests that the hormone may stimulate the plasma membrane–bound enzyme adenyl cyclase of the renal cortex to produce 3′,5′-adenosine monophosphate which, in turn, acts in an unknown manner on the tubular cells of the nephrons to inhibit reabsorption of phosphate and to promote absorption of calcium.[15] Parathyroid hormone causes resorption of bone matrix and bone mineral. The adenyl cyclase of bone is also sensitive to parathyroid hormone, suggesting that a similar mechanism mediates the action of the hormone on both kidney and bone. Animal experimental work indicates that parathyroid hormone exerts stimulatory effects on osteoclasts and inhibitory effects on osteoblasts via enhancement and suppression, respectively, of nuclear RNA synthesis.[13] Also, by a slowly acting mechanism, parathyroid hormone enhances the absorption of calcium and phosphate from the small intestine. Hormone inactivation occurs in the kidney.

Calcitonin

Calcitonin is a small polypeptide hormone that has hypocalcemic and hypophosphatemic effects and apparently is produced by cells originating in the ultimobranchial body of the embryo.[16] In many mammals, thyroid parafollicular cells have an ultimobranchial origin. In man, thyroid parafollicular cells are sparse, and similar cells are probably present in the parathyroid glands and thymus.[19] Some medullary thyroid carcinomas produce calcitonin. Elevation of serum calcium causes increased secretion of the hormone, which acts to inhibit bone resorption.

REGULATION OF CALCIUM METABOLISM

The regulation of calcium metabolism is a complex mechanism involving the effects of hormones and ions on bone, the absorption of calcium and phosphate from the small intestine, and the loss of calcium and phosphate in the urine and other external secretions. Parathyroid hormone maintains the calcium level in the blood and other extracellular fluids by promoting calcium reabsorption by the renal tubules, by removing calcium from bone, and by enhancing its absorption from the small intestine. Calcitonin partly counters parathyroid hormone by preventing resorption of bone. It is likely that parathyroid hormone and calcitonin play important roles in the fundamental metabolism of all cells by regulating the influx and efflux of calcium across the plasma membranes.[14]

The uptake and removal of calcium from bone is related to ionic concentrations of calcium and phosphate as well as the hormone balance.[21] Bone resorption is inhibited by increased concentrations of both phosphate and calcium. A high phosphate diet controls some of the manifestations of hyperparathyroidism. Magnesium is necessary for the action of parathyroid hormone on bone and kidney.[18]

Vitamin D is essential in promoting intestinal absorption of calcium (and phosphate), probably by mediating the synthesis of a calcium-binding protein, and is necessary for the action of parathyroid hormone on bone.[78] Excess vitamin D elevates serum calcium and causes bone resorption even in the absence of parathyroid hormone. Deficiency of metabolically active vitamin D is associated with a loss of responsiveness to parathyroid hormone by bone.

Other hormones have effects on calcium metabolism, but their roles are less clear. Triiodothyronine affects the skeleton as a regulator of metabolic rate. Excess thyroid hormone may elevate serum calcium and may cause increased loss in urine and feces. Glucagon lowers serum calcium apparently by enhancing the uptake of calcium by the bone. Glucocorticosteroids in excess reduce calcium absorption, increase renal excretion of calcium, and cause osteoporosis. Estrogens, androgens, and growth hormone also have long-term effects on the skeleton, but their short-term influence on divalent cation metabolism is unknown.

PATHOLOGIC CALCIFICATION

Pathologic calcification is the deposition of calcium salts in tissues not normally calcified as well as in excretory or secretory ducts. Calcium salts occur in some soft tissues quite regularly, however (e.g., the pineal gland after puberty). Calcium phosphate and calcium carbonate are the salts usually found. They are present most often as hydroxyapatite. Calcium oxalate deposits also may be present.

Pathologic calcification usually has been described under four categories: dystrophic calcification, metastatic calcification, calcinosis, and calciphylaxis (see also p. 86).

Dystrophic calcification is the deposition of calcium salts in injured or dead tissue. The systemic chemical balance is normal, but the local environment is altered to encourage precipitation of the salts. Metastatic calcification is the deposition of calcium salts in soft tissue as a result of a systemic disturbance of calcium and phosphate metabolism. Calcinosis is local or generalized calcification in or under the skin, sometimes including muscles, fasciae, nerves, and tendons, and occasionally is associated with scleroderma. Tumoral calcinosis refers to a localized, often cystic, calcific mass in the soft tissue next to a large joint, usually solitary. Calciphylaxis is an experimental process whereby hypercalcemia is produced by a "sensitizing" agent (vitamin D, parathyroid hormone) followed by a "challenging" agent that produces calcification either in the soft tissues at the site of injection or application or in a distant tissue if injected intravenously.

It is likely that these categories of calcification are somewhat artificial. Metastatic calcification associated with vitamin D intoxication, uremia, or hyperparathyroidism, for example, is probably occurring in tissues already damaged by the systemic disease and is therefore related to dystrophic calcification. The possible relationships to Selye's calciphylaxis are also apparent.

Calcification of soft tissues is a complex process that is poorly understood and depends on the local balance of inhibitor substances and of compounds promoting calcification as well as the systemic chemical environment. Major factors promoting calcification include elevation of the calcium-phosphate product Ca $\times$ P in mg/100 ml) resulting from higher levels of calcium or phosphate or both, elevation of pH locally or systemically, and the presence of circulating substances that may cause tissue damage.[78] The local elevation of pH in the eye and kidney (because the cells establish a hydrogen ion gradient across their membranes) may enhance calcification. Whether a similar mechanism occurs in the stomach, lungs, and bursae is controversial.[29] Other possible factors leading to deposition of calcium salts are local increases in calcium or phosphate concentrations as a result of intracellular transport mechanisms, concentration of calcium ions in mucopolysaccharides, removal of inhibiting pyrophosphate by pyrophosphatases, decrease in inhibitor peptides (especially in urine), and the action of collagen and elastin as nucleating substances for crystal formation.

HYPOPARATHYROIDISM

Diminution or absence of circulating parathyroid hormone causes a reduction of serum calcium (to as little as half the normal level) and an elevation of serum phosphate (to as much as three or four times normal levels). Little or no calcium appears in the urine. Tetany and other evidence of neuromuscular irritability are the most important clinical manifestations of hypoparathyroidism. If the disorder begins early in life, the individuals affected may have (in addition to tetany) skin disorders, abnormal nail growth, loss of hair, cataracts, defective teeth, mental retardation, and roentgenographic evidence of increased bone density and calcification in the vessels of the basal ganglia of the brain. Convulsions, papilledema, gastrointestinal disturbances, and *Candida* infections may be present. If hypoparathyroidism begins during adult life, tetany and cataracts are the most conspicuous manifestations. The skeletal, ectodermal, and gastrointestinal abnormalities also may be apparent.

The most common cause of hypoparathyroidism is the removal of all or part of the parathyroid tissue during surgery of the neck, especially during thyroidectomy. If only part of the gland tissue is removed, or if the glands are partially injured by impairment of their blood supply or by postoperative edema, then the hormonal deficiency will be temporary. Complete removal or more severe damage results in permanent impairment of function.

Temporary neonatal hypoparathyroidism may be manifest in infants suffering injury to the neck during birth, in infants subject to a phosphate load in their diet, infants with a low birth weight whose parathyroid function may be immature, and in infants of mothers with hyperparathyroidism or other causes of hypercalcemia.[36]

So-called idiopathic hypoparathyroidism is

a rare disease that is sporadic or familial and, in some instances, may be an autoimmune disorder. The glands are either replaced by fat or cannot be found.[32, 34] Permanent idiopathic hypoparathyroidism developing during the first year of life may be associated with congenital hypoplasia or absence of the parathyroid glands and thymus, and the children usually die.[39] Another type of early-onset hypoparathyroidism occurs predominantly in boys and may be an inherited sex-linked recessive disorder, and the children usually live.[31] Idiopathic hypoparathyroidism developing after the first year of life (and appearing as late as adult life) is sporadic or familial and may or may not be associated with hypoadrenocorticism, pernicious anemia, and *Candida* infections.[38] In some of these individuals circulating autoantibodies to parathyroid, adrenal, and thyroid tissue and to gastric parietal cells have been detected.

Hypoparathyroidism must be distinguished from vitamin D deficiency, chronic renal disease, intestinal malabsorption, familial and sporadic hypophosphatemia, renal tubular acidosis, and pseudohypoparathyroidism.

PSEUDOHYPOPARATHYROIDISM

Pseudohypoparathyroidism and pseudopseudohypoparathyroidism are related disorders and may be called Albright's hereditary osteodystrophy. Pseudohypoparathyroidism is familial with a female predominance and is characterized by clinical and chemical features suggestive of idiopathic hypoparathyroidism: hypocalcemia, hyperphosphatemia, skeletal abnormalities, and mental retardation. Brachydactyly, short stature, round facies, and multiple foci of soft tissue calcification and ossification are additional distinctive features. Renal glomerular function is normal. Pseudopseudohypoparathyroidism is similar, but the serum calcium and phosphate levels are normal.

In these disorders, the parathyroid glands are normal or hyperplastic. Parathyroid function is intact. Circulating parathyroid hormone levels are increased, but when hypercalcemia is induced experimentally, the level of circulating hormone falls. The disease appears to be the result of the inability of the renal tubules and the skeleton to respond to parathyroid hormone, possibly because the enzyme adenyl cyclase normally sensitive to parathyroid hormone is absent or defective.[33] Bone changes suggestive of hyperparathyroidism are sometimes present, perhaps because circulating parathyroid hormone levels are increased and the bone may be less refractory to the hormone than the kidney.

HYPERPARATHYROIDISM

Excessive production of parathyroid hormone results from several different disorders: from a disturbance of calcium and phosphorus metabolism originating elsewhere in the body (renal failure, vitamin D deficiency) and leading to secondary hyperplasia of parathyroid tissue, from autonomous or primary hyperplasia of the parathyroid tissue, from benign and malignant tumors of the parathyroid glands, and, rarely, from a neoplasm not of parathyroid origin, such as carcinoma of the lung or of the kidney.

Hyperparathyroidism may occur at any age but is more likely after the age of 30 years. It is more common in women, and there is evidence that primary hyperparathyroidism is especially likely to occur in women about the time of the menopause.

In some patients, there is no clinical evidence of disease. Laboratory tests reveal the presence of the disorder.[40] A few persons complain only of malaise. The most common signs and symptoms in hyperparathyroidism are those related to urinary calculi. Renal manifestations also include nephrocalcinosis and uremia. Less common are signs and symptoms of skeletal disease, such as pathologic fractures, bone pain, and generalized demineralization of the skeleton. Gastrointestinal disorders occur, including epigastric discomfort, constipation, and vague abdominal complaints. More important, peptic ulcers occur in 10% to 15% of hyperparathyroid patients, especially men, and acute pancreatitis is also fairly common. Central nervous system disturbances may constitute an important part of the clinical picture. These include depressive reactions, confusion, stupor, and personality changes. Additional manifestations of hypercalcemia include weakness, polydipsia, and polyuria. The ophthalmologist may find band keratopathy, a corneal opacity extending across the cornea from within the limbus, and also may note crystals in the conjunctivae. One-fourth to one-half of the patients have hypertension, often the result of renal damage, but in some instances the relationship to kidney disease is unclear because impairment of renal function cannot be demonstrated.[50]

Elevated levels of circulating parathyroid hormone cause increased urinary excretion of inorganic phosphate, decreased serum phosphate, increased serum calcium, and increased urinary excretion of calcium (because the calcium load presented to the tubules exceeds their capacity for reabsorption). Intestinal absorption of calcium rises. If skeletal lesions are present, serum alkaline phosphatase is elevated, and the urinary excretion of hydroxyproline rises (see also p. 1721).

Hyperparathyroidism must be differentiated from other causes of hypercalcemia such as hypervitaminosis D, hyperthyroidism, the milk-alkali syndrome (excessive ingestion of milk and absorbable alkalies leading to hypercalcemia, alkalosis, and azotemia without hypophosphatemia or hypercalciuria), sarcoidosis, multiple myeloma, leukemia, lymphoma, and some other malignant neoplasms with and without metastatic foci in bone. Idiopathic hypercalciuria with normal serum calcium and repeated renal stone formation and the hypercalciuria in renal tubular acidosis are two conditions that also must be distinguished from hyperparathyroidism. The radiographic changes in bone must be differentiated from those of osteoporosis, Paget's disease, fibrous dysplasia, osteogenesis imperfecta, acute bone atrophy due to immobilization, and rickets and osteomalacia (vitamin D deficiency).

Hyperplasia
Secondary hyperplasia

Disturbances in calcium and phosphorus metabolism not primarily involving the parathyroid glands may, in time, cause changes in the glands as they respond to the metabolic abnormalities. Chronic renal glomerular insufficiency resulting in retention of phosphate and depression of intestinal absorption of calcium is the most common cause of compensatory parathyroid hyperfunction and hyperplasia. Very high levels of circulating parathyroid hormone may be present, but the glands are still responsive to changes in serum calcium. Hyperplasia may occur in rickets and osteomalacia due to vitamin D deficiency, with intestinal malabsorption syndromes causing deficiencies of calcium and vitamin D, in primary hypophosphatemia, and in pseudohypoparathyroidism. Hyperplasia has been reported during fluoride ingestion, apparently because the hydroxyapatite crystal is less soluble when fluoride is incorporated in it, thereby lowering serum calcium slightly and causing compensatory parathyroid hyperfunction. Hyperplasia has been associated with extensive skeletal involvement by malignant neoplasms and occasionally with neoplasms not involving bone (mechanism uncertain). The hyperplasia present with some

medullary thyroid carcinomas producing calcitonin may be secondary to the calcitonin excess or may be primary hyperplasia as a part of a multiple endocrine tumor syndrome.

The hyperplastic glands range from normal size to considerably enlarged. Variation in the size of the individual glands in one person may be evident. The lower pair are often larger. The glands are creamy gray, grayish tan, or reddish tan, usually not brown, and distinctly firmer than normal. There is a marked decrease or even absence of stromal fat, and the glands are cellular, composed usually of pale and vacuolated chief cells. Transitional oxyphil or water-clear cells may predominate occasionally. The cells often are arranged in solid masses, but nests, cords, or acinar patterns may occur. Nodules of oxyphil cells or water-clear cells are present in some glands, and the nodularity may be visible on gross examination. Oxyphil cells are especially likely to be numerous in cases of chronic renal disease.

Primary chief cell hyperplasia

Approximately 30% of the cases of primary hyperparathyroidism are caused by hyperplasia of the glands, usually of the chief cell type. Partial secretory autonomy is evident. Sometimes, the disorder is familial, and it may occur as part of a multiple endocrine tumor syndrome.[62]

All the glands are enlarged. The lower pair are usually the larger. Total weight may reach 25 gm. Individual glands often appear slightly irregular in outline. They are not adherent to the surrounding tissue. Gland tissue is tan to reddish brown. The cut surface may be smooth or nodular. Microscopically, there are a variable reduction in stromal fat and an increase in cellularity, either diffuse or nodular. Chief cells predominate. Water-clear cells, oxyphil cells, and transitional forms are present in smaller numbers. Nuclei appear normal. Giant forms are rare. Nodules usually are composed of solid masses of chief cells. Irregular microscopic extensions of parathyroid tissue may protrude into the soft tissue adjacent to the glands. It is not possible to separate primary and secondary chief cell hyperplasia on histologic grounds alone.

Although all the parathyroid glands are involved in primary hyperplasia, the process may involve an individual gland incompletely and irregularly. A part of a gland may contain fat and parenchyma that appear normal, thereby resembling the "rim" of normal tissue

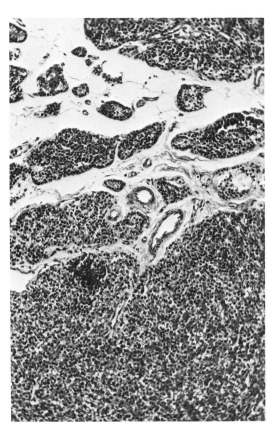

Fig. 35-1 Primary chief cell hyperplasia. Irregular involvement of gland can occur. Several small groups of cells appear to be normal.

outside an adenoma. Also, the hyperplastic cells in primary chief cell hyperplasia form a variety of histologic patterns. Consequently, it is not possible to separate chief cell hyperplasia from adenoma by examining a single gland.[59]

Primary water-clear cell hyperplasia

Primary water-clear cell hyperplasia is an uncommon cause of hyperparathyroidism and may be related to the chief cell type.[44] All the glands are irregularly enlarged, but the upper pair is usually the larger pair. The total weight varies from a few grams to as many as 60 gm. The glands are chocolate brown, not adherent to the surrounding tissue, and their surfaces are irregular with pseudo-podal projections or deep lobulations. Cut surfaces are soft, smooth, and uniform. All of the glands have the same microscopic appearance because they are composed entirely of large water-clear cells. These cells range from 10μ to 40μ in diameter and have nearly uniform, small, dark-staining nuclei about 4μ to 8μ in diameter. Cell patterns include dif-

fuse solid masses, acini with basal orientation of the nuclei, and irregular trabeculae. Nuclear palisading may occur. Giant nuclei may be present in small numbers.

Neoplasms
Parathyroid adenoma

Parathyroid adenoma is the cause of primary hyperparathyroidism in 60% to 70% of patients with the disorder. Two or more adenomas occur in 3% to 6% of all patients with primary hyperparathyroidism. They are more common in the lower pair of glands. Adenomas range in size from less than 100 mg to several hundred grams (rarely), but most weigh only a few grams. A few are palpable on physical examination. There is a rough correlation between the size of the tumor and the degree of hyperfunction. Secretory autonomy is usually present. One or more adenomas may occur as part of a multiple endocrine tumor syndrome, and a variety of thyroid lesions frequently occur in association with adenoma. The tumors are spherical to oval, soft, tan to reddish brown, or occasionally gray, have a smooth capsule, and are usually not adherent to the surrounding tissues. The cut surface may be focally hemorrhagic or cystic, and zones of fibrosis and calcification may be present. Deposits of brown pigment mark the sites of old hemorrhage.

The majority of adenomas are composed of chief cells, either normal or abnormal in appearance, but any cell type can predominate and any single tumor can contain a variety of cell types. Oxyphil cell tumors are often nonfunctional (not always), but with this exception, there is no correlation between the degree of hyperfunction and the cell type. Giant nuclei, bizarre nuclei, and multinucleated cells are fairly common. Mitoses are rare.

The cells may be arranged as simply a solid mass or they may form cords, nests, acini, or follicles resembling thyroid follicles. Nodules of single or mixed patterns may be evident. Commonly one histologic pattern predominates, but in some tumors a variety of patterns is visible.

The remaining tissue of a gland containing an adenoma often forms a "rim" of normal or somewhat atrophic-appearing parathyroid cells outside the capsule of the adenoma. Such tissue usually contains fat and is composed of small chief cells and perhaps some oxyphil cells. When the pathologist finds such a "rim," he can suspect that the altered para-

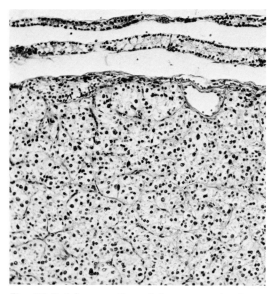

Fig. 35-2 Adenoma. Two delicate strands of remaining glandular tissue above tumor.

thyroid tissue represents an adenoma rather than hyperplasia, but only by locating normal glands elsewhere can the surgeon and pathologist be certain that hyperplasia is not the cause of the hyperparathyroidism.

Carcinoma

Nonfunctional carcinomas are almost impossible to separate from thyroid carcinomas, so that most pathologists require the presence of hyperparathyroidism to make the diagnosis. These rare neoplasms are frequently palpable on physical examination. Parathyroid hyperfunction may be marked. At surgery, carcinoma is nearly always tightly adherent to surrounding tissue and is irregular in shape, but some have resembled typical adenomas. The cut surface is gray, light tan, or brown and is firm, largely as a result of fibrous septa running through the tumor.

Microscopically, the cancer usually consists of solid masses of cells separated by irregular fibrous septa and surrounded by a thick fibrous capsule. The cells may be large chief cells, clear cells, or elongated cells (10μ to 15μ) with eosinophilic to amphophilic cytoplasm and large elongated nuclei. Perivascular palisading is common. Mitotic figures are usually present.

The only certain criterion of malignancy is the presence of metastases, usually in the regional lymph nodes, sometimes in the lungs and abdominal viscera. Local invasion of adjacent soft tissue and the thyroid gland oc-

curs. Recurrence is common, and death is likely. Management of the patient is difficult because of the persistent or recurring hyperparathyroidism.

"Tertiary" hyperparathyroidism

The term "tertiary" hyperparathyroidism describes those rare instances in which long-standing secondary hyperparathyroidism is followed by autonomous hyperparathyroidism. Surgery reveals hyperplasia, adenoma, or carcinoma of the glands, the disorder perhaps having been evoked by the prolonged stimulation of parathyroid tissue. Such cases suggest that parathyroid hyperplasia and neoplasia are closely related and that separation of the various hyperfunctional pathologic processes into categories (hyperplasia, adenoma, carcinoma) may be somewhat artificial.[59, 61]

Hyperparathyroidism with tumors of other organs

A variety of malignant neoplasms have been associated with a syndrome identical to hyperparathyroidism. In some instances, the neoplasms have produced a substance that appears to be parathyroid hormone.[68] In these cases, the parathyroid glands are usually normal. Occasionally, parathyroid hyperplasia apparently has accompanied hormone-secreting tumors. The explanation of this phenomenon is unknown.

Lesions associated with hyperparathyroidism

The hypercalcemia of hyperparathyroidism may result in the deposition of calcium salts (known as metastatic calcification) in a variety of soft tissues. Renal calculi occur in at least half the patients with hyperparathyroidism and often are the reason the patient seeks medical aid. A considerably smaller number of patients have osteoporotic lesions of the skeletal system, the fully developed condition being known as generalized osteitis fibrosa cystica.

Metastatic calcification

The kidneys and blood vessels are the most frequent sites of metastatic calcification, but some deposits, especially in acute hyperparathyroidism, may be found in the lungs, stomach, heart, eyes, and other tissues. Calcium deposition is particularly abundant when there is renal failure with phosphate retention.

In blood vessels, the calcification is mainly in the media and particularly involves elastic

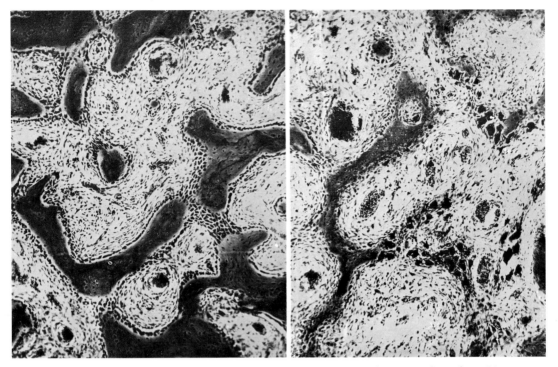

Fig. 35-3 Osteitis fibrosa cystica (Recklinghausen's disease) in hyperparathyroidism. Note irregular arrangement of newly formed bone trabeculae, which exhibit narrow osteoid zones and osteoclastic resorption. Marrow is fibrous and hyperemic. (Courtesy Dr. W. H. Bauer.)

tissue, so that the internal elastic lamella is often prominently calcified. The adjacent intima may be thickened by hyperplasia but usually without calcification. Vascular calcification may be particularly severe in secondary renal hyperparathyroidism in which there is an increased level of blood phosphate. In some patients, ischemic muscle pains in the extremities and even gangrene have resulted.

Generalized osteitis fibrosa cystica

Osteitis fibrosa cystica (Recklinghausen's disease) is characterized by generalized distortion of the skeleton due to lack of sufficient mineralization, with increased osteoclastic resorption, and by replacement of the osseous tissues and marrow spaces by fibrous tissue. In advanced cases, there are giant cell tumors and cysts. Markedly involved bones are soft and are easily deformed or cut. Bone lesions are probably more common with large, active adenomas[46] (see also p. 1721).

The condition is essentially an osteoclastic resorption of bone and its replacement by connective tissue in which there are abortive attempts at new bone formation. When mild, the gross change in the bones is merely a slight porousness and, microscopically, mild generalized osteoporosis and marrow fibrosis. As the condition progresses, there is more loss of osseous tissue, with replacement by connective tissue. Immature and poorly calcified bone develops in the connective tissue. The newly formed bone soon may again undergo resorption. Osteoclasts are abundant. Large fibrous scars develop in the place of the original spongy bone. Brown or giant cell tumors, usually in the jaws or long bones, are colored by blood pigment and consist of multinucleated giant cells in a cellular fibrous stroma. Cysts lined by connective tissue may result from degeneration or hemorrhage but are not always present. Characteristic early roentgenographic changes include subperiosteal resorption of bone, most frequently seen along the margins of the middle phalanges of the fingers. Plasma alkaline phosphatase is increased. Because skeletal collagen is resorbed, urinary hydroxyproline excretion is increased.

Renal lesions

The kidneys may be severely damaged in hyperparathyroidism as a result of the deposition of calcium in the kidneys (nephrocalcinosis) and the formation of renal stones. Excess parathyroid hormone apparently interferes

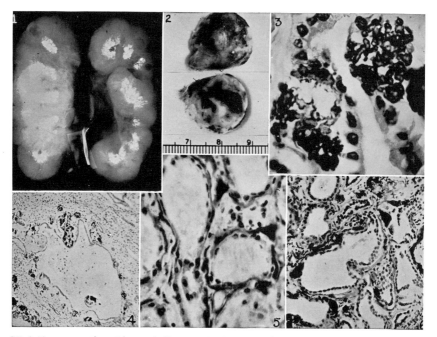

Fig. 35-4 Hyperparathyroid renal disease. **1,** Massive deposits of calcium. **2,** Parathyroid adenoma—external and cut surfaces. Dark area on cut surface is area of hemorrhage (scale in centimeters). **3** to **6,** Interstitial and peritubular calcium deposits in kidneys. (From Anderson, W. A. D.: Endocrinology **24:**372-378, 1939.)

with the ability of the tubules to concentrate urine. In acute hyperparathyroidism, some of the nephrons show calcification of tubular epithelial cells and tubular basement membranes. Calcium casts are formed, at least partly from cellular debris undergoing calcification.

In the milder chronic cases, patchy calcification usually involves cells of the ascending limb of the loop of Henle, the distal convoluted tubule, and the collecting tubule.[49] Casts, usually calcific, are formed partly from desquamated cells and cellular debris and may cause obstruction of the nephron. Some interstitial calcification may occur. Foci of fibrosis with tubular and glomerular atrophy and infiltration by chronic inflammatory cells are common.

In advanced cases fibrosis, inflammation, and nephron destruction are extensive, and calcification of interstitial tissue may be marked. Both atrophy and cystic dilatation of the tubules proximal to obstructing calcific masses may be evident.

Renal calculi are present in 60% or more of cases of hyperparathyroidism and may be the basis for the presenting symptoms. Although hyperparathyroidism is an uncommon cause of renal calculi, investigation for its presence should be made in every patient with renal stones. In some clinics, 10% of individuals with renal stones have hyperparathyroidism. The calculi are predominantly calcium oxalate or calcium phosphate. Kidneys containing stones may have only minor tubular damage, or they may be extensively involved by calcium deposits and the associated parenchymal damage. Hydronephrosis may occur. Pyelonephritis is common in kidneys damaged by stones and by calcinosis.

Renal osteodystrophy and secondary hyperparathyroidism

The osteodystrophy occurring in chronic renal failure is characterized by varying degrees of osteitis fibrosa, osteomalacia, osteoporosis, and osteosclerosis.[78] The clinical and pathologic features in a single patient depend on the pathologic process that predominates during a particular time period. The pathologic processes, in turn, depend on which of the complex metabolic disturbances of uremia are most important in the person affected and how these disturbances are altered by therapeutic measures. Renal lesions of a type in which large amounts of renal parenchyma are lacking or destroyed and those that are stationary or very slowly progressive (renal insufficiency over a prolonged period) may result in these skeletal changes. Hemodialysis and renal transplantation prolong life and thereby have substantially increased the possibility that skeletal disease may develop.

A variety of factors operate to produce skeletal lesions in chronic renal failure. Abnormal metabolism of vitamin D is present and leads to greatly diminished calcium absorption from the intestine and prevents normal calcification of osteoid. Elevation of serum phosphate and the abnormal metabolism of vitamin D impair the bone response to parathyroid hormone. Magnesium depletion may have similar effects. Thus, the reduction in serum calcium causes increased secretion of parathyroid hormone. Acidosis may affect bone directly by using calcium carbonate as a buffer and may interfere with parathyroid function. Metabolic alterations of circulating parathyroid hormone, impaired inactivation of the hormone by the damaged kidney, and a variety of other metabolic abnormalities present in patients with diseased kidneys may affect the bones. The result of these many factors is a tendency for osteomalacia to be more evident in patients with lesser degrees of renal failure. Osteitis fibrosa is usually more prominent in severe renal failure (see also p. 807).

One of the most important complications of the secondary hyperparathyroidism usually present in chronic renal disease is soft tissue calcification. Sites commonly involved are the arteries, heart, kidneys, lungs, stomach, soft tissues around joints, eyes, and skin and subcutaneous tissues. Arterial, myocardial, and renal calcification may have grave clinical effects.

In children, remarkable skeletal deformities and growth disturbances (dwarfism) may result because bone growth is incomplete and the epiphyses are not united. The underlying renal lesion is most commonly a developmental imperfection in the kidneys or urinary tract, such as congenital hypoplasia, congenital polycystic disease, strictures of the ureters, or congenital valves of the urethra. Infection (pyelonephritis) may be added to hydronephrotic atrophy in cases of obstruction in the lower urinary tract and still further decrease the functioning renal parenchyma.

The characteristic changes occurring in the epiphyseal cartilages are probably the result of vitamin D resistance as well as of hyperparathyroidism. The epiphyseal cartilages are greatly increased in bulk but show degenerative changes, defects of calcium deposition, and marked distortions. Stresses and strains cause the cartilage to be bent and twisted, and it may be partially or entirely pushed away from its normal position at the end of the shaft. Extreme deformity often results. The skull may be greatly thickened, and the appearance of the calvaria closely resembles that in Paget's disease of bone.

The kidneys show less calcium deposition than in primary hyperparathyroidism, and renal calculi are less frequent.

OTHER ABNORMALITIES

Parathyroid cysts large enough to be clinically apparent are rare. They may occur within the thyroid gland and the mediastinum as well as in the lower neck near the thyroid gland (p. 1110).

Inflammatory processes in parathyroid tissue are unusual. Sometimes, inflammation in the thyroid gland extends into one or several glands. Rarely, part of the gland tissue is replaced by amyloidosis or by secondary carcinoma, such as carcinomas of the lung and the thyroid gland.

REFERENCES
General; development and structure

1 Castleman, B.: Tumors of parathyroid glands. In Atlas of tumor pathology, Sect. IV, Fasc. 15, Washington, D. C., 1952, Armed Forces Institute of Pathology.
2 Christie, A. C.: J. Clin. Path. **20:**591-602, 1967.
3 Gaillard, P. J., Talmage, R. V., and Budy, A. M.: The parathyroid glands, Chicago, 1965, University of Chicago Press.
4 Gilmour, J. R.: J. Path. Bact. **45:**507-522, 1937.
5 Gilmour, J. R.: J. Path. Bact. **46:**133-149, 1938.
6 Gilmour, J. R.: J. Path. Bact. **48:**187-222, 1939.
7 Gilmour, J. R., and Martin, W. J.: J. Path. Bact. **44:**431-462, 1937.
8 Golden, A., and Canary, J. J.: In Bloodworth, J. M. B., editor: Endocrine pathology, Baltimore, 1968, The Williams & Wilkins Co.
9 Greep, R. O., and Talmage, R. V., editors: The parathyroids, Springfield, Ill., 1961, Charles C Thomas, Publisher.
10 Munger, B. L., and Roth, S. I.: J. Cell. Biol. **16:**379-400, 1963.
11 Roth, S. I., and Munger, B. L.: Virchow Arch. Path. Anat. **335:**389-410, 1962.

Hormones; regulation of calcium metabolism

12 Aurbach, G. D., Potts, J. T., Jr., Chase, L. R., and Melson, G. L.: Ann. Intern. Med. **70:**1243-1265, 1969.
13 Bingham, P. J., Brazell, I. A., and Owen, M.: J. Endocr. **45:**387-400, 1969.
14 Borle, A. B.: Endocrinology **85:**194-199, 1969.
15 Chase, L. R., and Aurbach, G. D.: Science **159:**545-547, 1968.
16 Copp, D. H.: J. Endocr. **43:**137-161, 1969.
17 Epstein, F. H.: Amer. J. Med. **45:**700-714, 1968.
18 Estep, H., Shaw, W. A., Watlington, C., Hobe,

R., Holland, W., and Tucker, St. G.: J. Clin. Endocr. **29**:842-848, 1969.

19 Gudmundsson, T. V., Galante, L., Woodhouse, N. J. Y., Osafo, T. D., Matthews, E. W., MacIntyre, I., Kenny, A. D., and Wiggins, R. C.: Lancet **1**:443-446, 1969.

20 Kyle, L. H.: New Eng. J. Med. **251**:1035-1040, 1954 (milk-alkali syndrome).

21 Raisz, L. G., and Niemann, I.: Endocrinology **85**:446-452, 1969.

22 Selye, H.: Arch. Path. (Chicago) **34**:625-632, 1942.

Pathologic calcification

23 Anderson, W. A. D.: J. Pediat. **14**:375-381, 1939.

24 Anderson, W. A. D.: J. Urol. **44**:29-34, 1940.

25 Barr, D. P.: Physiol. Rev. **12**:593-624, 1932.

26 Lutz, J. F.: Ann. Intern. Med. **14**:1270-1282, 1941 (calcinosis).

27 Mortensen, J. D., and Baggenstoss, A. H.: Amer. J. Clin. Path. **24**:45-63, 1954 (nephrocalcinosis).

28 Mulligan, R. M.: Arch. Path. (Chicago) **43**:177-230, 1947 (metastatic calcification).

29 Parfitt, A. M.: Arch. Intern. Med. (Chicago) **124**:544-556, 1969.

30 Selye, H.: Calciphylaxis, Chicago, 1962, University of Chicago Press.

Hypoparathyroidism; pseudohypoparathyroidism

31 Bronsky, D., Kiamko, R. T., and Waldstein, S. S.: J. Clin. Endocr. **28**:61-65, 1968.

32 Bronsky, D., Kushner, D. S., Dubin, A., and Snapper, I.: Medicine (Balt.) **37**:317-352, 1958.

33 Chase, L. R., Melson, G. L., and Aurbach, G. D.: J. Clin. Invest. **48**:1832-1844, 1969.

34 Drake, T. G., Albright, F., Bauer, W., and Castleman, B.: Ann. Intern. Med. **12**:1751-1765, 1939.

35 Krane, S. M.: J.A.M.A. **178**:472-475, 1961.

36 MacGregor, M. E.: Proc. Roy. Soc. Med. **61**:583-588, 1968.

37 Mann, J. B., Alterman, S., and Hills, A. G.: Ann. Intern. Med. **56**:315-342, 1962.

38 Spinner, M. W., Blizzard, R. M., and Childs, B.: J. Clin. Endocr. **28**:795-804, 1968.

39 Taitz, L. S., Zarate-Salvador, C., and Schwartz, E.: Pediatrics **38**:412-418, 1966.

Hyperparathyroidism

40 Boonstra, C. E., and Jackson, C. E.: Ann. Intern. Med. **63**:468-474, 1965.

41 Castleman, B., and Mallory, T. B.: Amer. J. Path. **11**:1-72, 1935.

42 Cope, O.: Ann. Surg. **114**:706-733, 1941.

43 Dawson, J. W., and Struthers, J. W.: Edinburgh Med. J. **30**:421-564, 1923.

44 Hellström, J., and Ivemark, B. I.: Acta Chir. Scand. suppl. 294, pp. 1-113, 1962.

45 Keating, F. R., Jr.: J.A.M.A. **178**:547-555, 1961.

46 Lloyd, H. M.: Medicine (Balt.) **47**:53-71, 1968.

47 Nicholson, W. F.: Brit. J. Surg. **56**:106-108, 1969 (results of treatment).

48 Pugh, D. G.: Amer. J. Roentgen. **66**:577-586, 1951.

49 Pyrah, L. N., Hodgkinson, A., and Anderson, C. K.: Brit. J. Surg. **53**:245-316, 1966.

50 Rienhoff, W. F., Jr., Rienhoff, W. F., III, Brawley, R. K., and Shelley, W. M.: Ann. Surg. **168**:1061-1074, 1968.

51 Rogers, H. M., Keating, F. R., Jr., Morlock, C. G., and Barker, N. W.: Arch. Intern. Med. (Chicago) **79**:307-321, 1947 (peptic ulcer).

52 Roth, S. I.: Arch. Path. (Chicago) **73**:495-510, 1962.

53 Turchi, J. J., Flandreau, R. H., Forte, A. L., French, G. N., and Ludwig, G. D.: J.A.M.A. **180**:799-804, 1962 (hyperparathyroidism and pancreatitis).

Hyperplasia
Secondary hyperplasia

54 Bernstein, D. S., and Cohen, P.: J. Clin. Endocr. **27**:197-210, 1967 (fluorides).

55 Castleman, B., and Mallory, T. B.: Amer. J. Path. **13**:553-574, 1937 (renal disease).

56 Grimes, B. J., Fisher, B., Finn, F., and Danowski, T. S.: Acta Endocr. (Kobenhavn) **56**:510-520, 1967 (nonosseous, nonparathyroid neoplasms).

Primary hyperplasia

57 Albright, F., Sulkowitch, H. W., and Bloomberg, E.: Arch. Intern. Med. (Chicago) **62**:199-215, 1938.

58 Albright, F., Bloomberg, E., Castleman, B., and Churchill, E. D.: Arch. Intern. Med. (Chicago) **54**:315-329, 1934.

59 Black, W. C., III, and Utley, J. R.: Amer. J. Clin. Path. **49**:761-775, 1968.

60 Cope, O., Keynes, W. M., Roth, S. I., and Castleman, B.: Ann. Surg. **148**:375-388, 1958.

61 Golden, A., Canary, J. J., and Kerwin, D. M.: Amer. J. Med. **38**:562-578, 1965.

62 Steiner, A. L., Goodman, A. D., and Powers, S. R.: Medicine (Balt.) **47**:371-409, 1968 (multiple endocrine tumors).

63 Utley, J. R., and Black, W. C.: Amer. J. Surg. **114**:788-795, 1967.

Neoplasms

64 Barnes, B. A., and Cope, O.: J.A.M.A. **178**:556-559, 1961 (carcinoma).

65 Black, B. K., and Ackerman, L. V.: Cancer **3**:415-444, 1950.

66 Ellis, J. T., and Barr, D. P.: Amer. J. Path. **27**:383-405, 1951 (carcinoma).

67 King, E. S. J., and Wood, B.: J. Path. Bact. **62**:29-35, 1950 (carcinoma).

68 Sherwood, L. M., O'Riordan, J. L. H., Aurbach, G. D., and Potts, J. T., Jr.: J. Clin. Endocr. **27**:140-146, 1967 (nonparathyroid tumors).

69 Sommers, S. C., and Young, T. L.: Amer. J. Path. **28**:673-689, 1952.

70 Woolner, L. B., Keating, F. R., Jr., and Black, B. M.: Cancer **5**:1069-1088, 1952.

Lesions associated with hyperparathyroidism

71 Andersen, D. H., and Schlesinger, E. R.: Amer. J. Dis. Child. **63**:102-125, 1942.

72 Anderson, W. A. D.: Arch. Path. (Chicago) **27**:753-778, 1939.

73 Anderson, W. A. D.: Endocrinology **24**:372-378, 1939.

74 Chown, B., Lee, M., Teal, J., and Currie, R.: J. Path. Bact. **49:**273-290, 1939.
75 Follis, R. H., Jr., and Jackson, D. A.: Bull. Johns Hopkins Hosp. **72:**232-241, 1943 (skeletal changes).
76 Ginzler, A. M., and Jaffe, H. L.: Amer. J. Path. **17:**293-302, 1941.
77 Herbert, F. K., Miller, H. G., and Richardson, G. O.: J. Path. Bact. **53:**161-182, 1941.
78 Kleeman, C. R., Massry, S. G., Coburn, J. W., and Popovtzer, M. M.: Arch. Intern. Med.

(Chicago) **124:**261-268, 1969 (conference on divalent ion metabolism and osteodystrophy in chronic renal failure).
79 Pappenheimer, A. M., and Wilens, S. L.: Amer. J. Path. **11:**73-91, 1935.

Other abnormalities
Cysts

80 Wood, J. W., Johnson, K. G., and Hinds, M. J. A.: Arch. Surg. (Chicago) **92:**785-790, 1966.

Chapter 36

Adrenal glands

Sheldon C. Sommers

STRUCTURE AND FUNCTION

The adrenal glands are glands of mystery and adventure. Before analyzing their pathology, it seems appropriate to mention the aura of romanticism and flamboyance that still clings to their endocrinology. Cannon's homeostasis theory[5] emphasized the adrenal medulla as an emergency source of catecholamines for flight or fight. Selye's general adaptation syndrome[16] popularized adrenocortical reactions after various tissue injuries. Corticosteroids are claimed to participate in most cellular processes. Cortisone and related compounds have been used therapeutically in various diseases of unknown cause as a sort of endocrinologic panacea. Biochemical and functional investigations recently have outdistanced adrenal morphology.

Embryologically, the adrenal medulla is of neural crest ectodermal origin and thus a component of the nervous system. The cortex originates from urogenital ridge mesoderm. Accessory cortical nodules are commonly present in the adrenal capsule. They also are scattered throughout the retroperitoneal space, in the testicular region in 7.5% and beneath the renal capsule in 1.2% of autopsies and less often in the ovaries or broad ligaments. Celiac accessory adrenal glands were found in 32% of autopsies. Chromaffin tissue foci resembling the adrenal medulla and termed paraganglia are peppered throughout the retroperitoneum, forming the prominent infant organ of Zuckerkandl. This organ atrophies and is more difficult to find after puberty.

The human adrenal gland passes through three major developmental phases: fetal, childhood, and adult. The prenatal cortex has an inner fetal zone, similar in location to the X-zone in mice, which disappears within months after birth. Relative to body weight, the adrenal glands are large at birth, weighing 2 gm to 4 gm each, or 8.2 gm ± 3.4 gm together. In anencephalics, the fetal cortical zone atrophies prematurely after the twentieth week of pregnancy, and at birth each adrenal gland weighs only 0.25 gm to 1 gm, with closely packed cortical cells. The changes resemble those after hypophysectomy.

In late childhood, the adrenarche occurs, with increased prepuberal secretion of androgens and related compounds. By then, the adult cortical zonation of glomerulosa, fasciculata, and reticularis has become established. At 11 to 15 years of age, the normal aggregate weight is 8.5 gm in boys and 7.5 gm in girls. Apparently normal adult adrenal glands removed surgically each weigh 4.8 gm ± 0.8 gm in men and 4.1 gm ± 0.8 gm in women. After sudden death, the aggregate adrenal weight is 9.2 gm ± 1.8 gm in the United States. In other autopsies, the normal range is 12.0 gm to 16.0 gm, or 0.21 gm to 0.26 gm per kilogram of body weight. The increase is ascribed to cortical hypertrophy in response to the stress of illness. Crowding of experimental animals leads to adrenocortical hypertrophy and gonadal shrinkage. Comparable effects may occur in human beings, since the combined weight of the adrenal glands at autopsy was 8.78 gm ± 2.43 gm in Jamaican men and 8.22 gm ± 2.18 gm in Jamaican women, compared to 13.82 gm ± 2.80 gm and 12.66 gm ± 2.90 gm in the respective European groups. Most autopsies do not include careful stripping of the periadrenal fat or accurate weighing of the glands and, except for a few series, satisfactory baseline weights are difficult to find.

The flattened right and pyramidal left human adrenal glands each have a head, body, and tail region, with the medulla in the more medial aspect of the head and body.

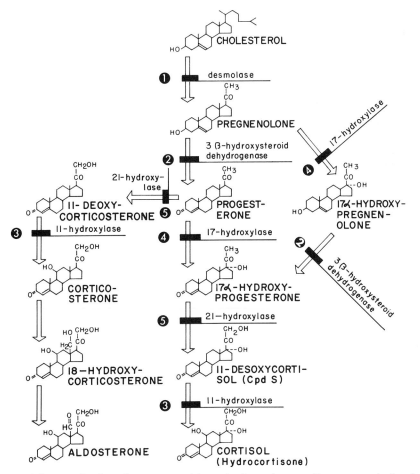

Fig. 36-1 Scheme of adrenal corticosteroid synthetic pathways. Enzymes underlined and numbered correspond to congenital enzymatic deficiencies that block reactions, as discussed in text.

The mid-quartile zona glomerulosa is 6.9% of the volume of the total cortex; zona fasciculata, 69.3%; zona reticularis, 22.7%; medulla, capsule, connective tissue, and vessels make up about 21.5% of the gland volume. The normal cortex measures 1 mm to 2 mm in width, and the total cortical width is significantly related to its volume. The zona fasciculata mid-quartile width of 0.846 mm is statistically significantly correlated with its volume. The human zona glomerulosa is normally discontinuous.

On section, the adrenal cortex is golden yellow with a brown pigmented inner zona reticularis and a gray medulla. In women of menopausal age, the zona reticularis is often prominent. Abundant sudanophilic lipid and cholesterol are present in all three adrenocortical zones. The cells normally appear finely vacuolated in paraffin sections. Zonation may not be obvious histologically, but with experience aided by reticulin stains, the "bishops' crozier" glomerulosa pattern, the linearly arranged fasciculata, and the diagonal network of slightly pigmented reticularis cells can be recognized. The irregularly arranged medullary cells have prominent nuclei and abundant amphophilic cytoplasm. Some vaguely resemble neurons. Some studies have recognized twisted medullary cell cords with basophilic or oncocytic staining. Chromaffinity is a mahogany brown medullary tissue color produced by the oxidant effect of chromate salts or Helly's solution on epinephrine in unfixed tissues.

Electron microscopy demonstrates characteristic platelike mitochondrial cristae in the zona glomerulosa cells, in contrast to tubular mitochondria of zona fasciculata cells. Cortical cells have abundant smooth endoplasmic reticulum like other steroid-secreting cells and a less prominent rough endoplasmic reticulum. Although it contains isolated adrenocortical cells, the adrenal medulla is separated completely from the cortex by a basement membrane. Osmiophilic cytoplasmic catecholamine-storage granules in medullary cells comprise pure epinephrine and norepinephrine types, each surrounded by limiting membranes. The latter have a clear peripheral halo.

Adrenocortical function involves the synthesis and secretion of steroids formed from cholesterol (Fig. 36-1). In the human adult, these include aldosterone, chiefly from the zona glomerulosa, hydrocortisone (cortisol) from the zona fasciculata, and androgens and estrogens predominantly from the zona reticularis. The human fetal cortex responds to both ACTH and chorionic gonadotropin but has relatively little 3β-hydroxysteroid dehydrogenase enzyme activity, which prevents the formation of progesterone and hence of aldosterone and cortisol. Instead, dehydroepiandrosterone and its derivatives are the major steroids secreted, contributing to the placental synthesis of estrogens, particularly estriol.

At birth, the fetal cortical zone degenerates and shrinks and completely involutes within three to twelve months, reducing the aggregate adrenal weight to 5.6-6.3 gm ± 2.0 gm. Failure of the fetal cortex to involute or to develop the 17-hydroxylase, 21-hydroxylase, and 11β-hydroxylase enzymes, which normally occur after the first ten weeks of pregnancy, may result in some instances of congenital adrenal hyperplasia.

In adults, cortisol and total 17-hydroxycorticosteroids have a diurnal secretory cycle with a low point as sleep begins and a peak with daylight and waking. Aside from pituitary control by ACTH and an adrenal growth factor, the cortex has complex interactions with organs such as the kidney and liver and with other endocrine glands, particularly the gonads. In several conditions, both adrenocortical and gonadal abnormalities exist, as in some types of adrenogenital dysgenesis, the Stein-Leventhal syndrome, Morgagni's syndrome, and virilizing and cushingoid states. The juxtaposition of adrenal cortex and medulla suggests interactions comparable to those between the pituitary lobes, but little is known of this in human beings. The adrenal medulla contains predominantly norepinephrine in infants, but thereafter its major hormone is epinephrine.

CONGENITAL ANOMALIES

Absence of both adrenal glands is compatible with life if accessory cortical tissue is present in the retroperitoneum or testes or if sufficient corticosteroids are produced by the brown fat. Aberrant adrenal tissue also may occur in the pancreas or liver. Only one adrenal gland may develop, the two glands may be fused, or there may be bilaterally double adrenal glands. Minor anomalies include adrenohepatic or adrenorenal fusion (commonly with adhesions between the capsules) and true parenchymal union. The fusion usually is unilateral and without functional importance.

Hypoplasia

Hypoplasia of the fetal cortical zone associated with anencephaly has been mentioned, and similar effects occur with prenatal pituitary or nervous system degeneration. Cystic degeneration of the outer cortex is common in premature infants of less than thirty-five weeks gestation. Three types of adrenal hypoplasia are recognized in liveborn infants:

1 Precocious involution of the fetal cortex, which is found in postmaturity or various newborn illnesses. Destructive necrosis and hemorrhage of the fetal cortex are extensive, with infiltrates of neutrophils.

2 Idiopathic hypoplasia, in which the glands weigh only 0.3 gm to 1.8 gm each, with miniature adult type cortices some eight cells thick. Fetal cortex is absent. The affected infants typically develop weight loss, dehydration, hyponatremia, hypoglycemia, and convulsions and die of adrenocortical insufficiency within ten days. One such infant was postmature, and his mother had subnormal urinary estriol levels attributable to a deficiency of fetal adrenal dehydroepiandrosterone precursor. Another was born to a mother who had received cortisone.

3 Cytomegalic adrenocortical hypoplasia, which is rare, usually in males, and evidently involves failure of the fetal cortical zone to involute and a related hypoplasia of the permanent outer cortex. Some instances are familial.

Anaplastic fetal adrenocortical cells are found in 3.5% to 13% of infants at autopsy. Ordinarily, this focal cytomegaly and irregular nuclear hyperchromatism may only represent an atypical involutional change.

Fetal adrenocortical cytomegaly is a characteristic of Beckwith's syndrome, which also includes macroglossia, abnormal umbilicus, somatic gigantism, and severe hypoglycemia. If bilateral adrenocortical cytomegaly is extensive, death may follow in about one month from adrenal insufficiency. One 5-day-old female infant with bilateral adrenal cytomegaly and visceromegaly also had a metastasizing adrenocortical carcinoma of similar appearance. A male adult with cytomegalic adrenocortical hypoplasia suffered from both aldosterone and cortisol deficiencies. Since 20α-hydroxypregnenone was increased, the cytomegalic cells may have been functional; ultrastructural features of steroidogenesis also were found.

Congenital hyperplasia

Congenital adrenal hyperplasia with the adrenogenital syndrome is an uncommon condition believed due to autosomal recessive genes. Its importance lies in the associated anomalies of the external genitalia, the enzyme blocks responsible for the syndrome, and the interrelations of embryonic adrenal and genital tract differentiation thus revealed. The classification of Bongiovanni et al.[22] is useful, since it permits correlation of the individual enzyme deficiencies indicated in Fig. 36-1 with the clinicopathologic alterations.

1 Desmolase deficiency is a rarity associated with lipoid adrenal hyperplasia. The cortical cells lack 17-ketosteroids and contain excessive cholesterol and neutral lipid. Since practically all types of corticosteroid synthesis are blocked, there is no virilization, the blood pressure is low, salt and water loss are common, and death in infancy is frequent. Males usually are hypospadiac and may be regarded as pseudohermaphrodites. Urinary ketosteroids are low.

2 3β-Hydroxysteroid dehydrogenase deficiency is also rare and usually fatal. The affected males are hypospadiac or may possess a vagina. Normal development of the male external genitalia is inhibited since the testis also lacks the enzyme, so that testosterone and related steroids are not produced. Females may be moderately virilized at birth by the weakly androgenic effects of dehydroepiandrosterone and related 5-3β-hydroxysteroid compounds, which comprise almost all the urinary steroids. Ordinarily, low blood pressure, salt loss, hypoadrenal crises, failure to respond to treatment, and death ensue. One survivor had only partially blocked cortisol synthesis, and two others treated with cortisol were hypoglycemic and developed gray or brown skin pigmentation at the ages of 3 months and 6 months, respectively.

3 11-Hydroxylase deficiency is the chief virilizing and hypertensive type of congenital adrenal hyperplasia. The dominant steroid is compound S, urinary 17-ketosteroids are increased, and salt wastage is uncommon. Urinary pregnanetriol is slightly elevated. The progeny of pregnant rats treated with the enzyme inhibitor metyrapone provide an experimental model. Similar clinical and laboratory findings occur in some children with hypertension, adrenal adenoma, malnutrition, or diarrhea. There have been reports of postpubertal girls with polycystic ovaries and some with hypertension who may have incomplete 11-hydroxylase deficiency. Adrenal hyperplasia is not always demonstrated.

4 17-Hydroxylase deficiency is rare. No androgens or estrogens are produced. The urinary 17-ketosteroids are low. Aldosterone and cortisol are deficient. Hypertension is present without salt wastage, since the major steroids produced are deoxycorticosterone and corticosterone. Amenorrhea, incompletely developed secondary sex characteristics, and polycystic ovaries have been found in three seventeen-year old girls. No adrenal tissue was examined. It is uncertain whether the enzyme deficiency is congenital or is associated with adrenal hyperplasia.

5 21-Hydroxylase deficiency accounts for about 90% of all congenital adrenal hyperplasias. It produces the most familiar type of adrenogenital syndrome in infants and children. Virilization in both sexes is moderate or notable. Affected females have clitoral hypertrophy, and labial fusion may simulate a scrotum (Fig. 36-2). Consequently, some individuals have been mistakenly reared as boys. In males, there may be precocious penile enlargement (macrogenitosomia). Both sexes have accelerated somatic growth. The dominant steroid is 17-hydroxyprogesterone, and over twenty urinary steroids that lack C-21 hydroxyl groups are present, with

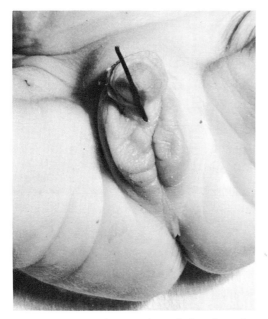

Fig. 36-2 External genitalia of female infant with 21-hydroxylase deficiency and adrenocortical hyperplasia. Appearance typical of female pseudohermaphroditism with adrenogenital syndrome.

androsterone and etiocholanolone predominant among the increased 17-ketosteroids. Pregnanetriol is one urinary 17-hydroxyprogesterone metabolite. The virilizing androgen is testosterone.

A sixth type of enzyme deficiency involves 18-oxidase without cortical hyperplasia.

In embryos, androgens inhibit differentiation of the genital tract along female lines, except in testicular feminization. One consequence is external genitalia of female pseudohermaphroditic appearance. The internal genitalia of embryos and children are less affected by androgens, whereas after puberty luteinized ovarian cysts or testicular Leydig cell hyperplasia may occur. In some cases there is testicular proliferation of accessory adrenocortical cells, but usually the testicular masses are hyperplastic Leydig cells. Female pseudohermaphroditism occasionally follows maternal therapy with progesterone, androgens, or estrogens. Since masculinization is progressive, early diagnosis and continuous cortisone-type steroid therapy are desirable.

In about 30% of patients with 21-hydroxylase deficiency, there are salt loss, a tendency to low blood pressure, sudden collapse with water restriction, and low serum sodium and high potassium levels, as well as hypoglycemia, susceptibility to infections, and brown skin pigmentation. Episodic fever may be attributable to etiocholanolone secretion. Supported by cortisone-type therapy, the individuals may survive to middle age or beyond. Deoxycorticosterone treatment has produced hypertension lasting several months.

Except for desmolase deficiency, the adrenal glands appear similar in all the congenital hyperplasias. The glands are up to five times normal size and may weigh 40 gm to 50 gm each. The cortex is thickened and convoluted, with cells resembling the zona reticularis comprising two-thirds of its total volume (Fig. 36-3). Apparently, the hyperplasia does not represent persistent fetal adrenocortical tissue. In children, the cells generally are not pigmented or stained by fuchsin. The zona fasciculata usually is identifiable microscopically. In adult female pseudohermaphrodites, the hyperplastic zona reticularis is both pigmented and fuchsinophilic. The characteristically increased ACTH that accompanies congenital adrenal hyperplasia has been ascribed to insufficient feedback control by cortisol.

At least three other conditions with adrenal hyperplasia in the newborn infant have been reported. Infants of diabetic mothers may have increased urinary corticoids as part of an edematous, pseudoerythroblastosis syndrome, sometimes with an apparent increase of fetal cortical width. In infants dying of erythroblastosis fetalis or α-thalassemia, the fetal cortex is both thick and excessively vacuolated; the accompanying thymic atrophy suggests adrenal hyperfunction, possibly due to chronic intrauterine hypoxia. Antenatal infection also is reported associated with adrenocortical hyperplasia in the newborn infant.

CHILDHOOD ABNORMALITIES

Hemorrhage. Certain adrenal lesions are more common before puberty, without necessarily being limited to children. Adrenal hemorrhage that destroys both the cortex and medulla may reflect birth trauma, particularly after breech delivery. Waterhouse-Friderichsen syndrome involves bilateral, ordinarily fatal, destructive adrenal hemorrhages, classically associated with meningococcemia. Other gram-negative organisms such as colon bacilli may be responsible, and, less often, diphtheria, varicella, or measles. Gram-negative endotoxin shock, endothelial necrosis, sinusoidal thrombi, and intravascular consumption coagulopathy are implicated in the pathogenesis.

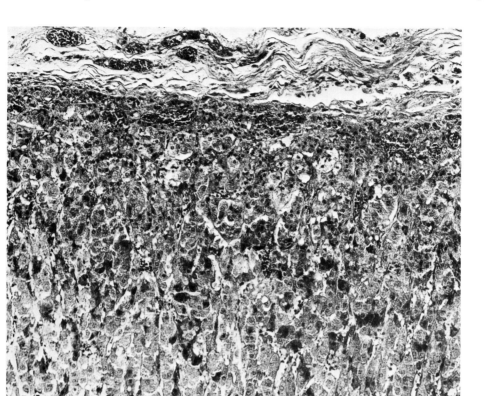

Fig. 36-3 Congenital adrenal hyperplasia associated with female pseudohermaphroditism. Cortical cells irregularly enlarged, with acidophilic granular cytoplasm. (×120.)

Necrosis. Hepatoadrenal necrosis is another usually fatal lesion, especially in premature infants with systemic herpes simplex infection acquired at birth, probably from maternal vaginitis. Both the adrenocortical and hepatic cells are extensively destroyed. Some contain intranuclear Cowdry type A inclusion bodies. Cytomegalic inclusion disease is accompanied by typical, large, acidophil, intranuclear, viral inclusions and cortical necrosis in about one-third of generalized cytomegalovirus infections. A comparable adrenal involvement may occur in adults as a complication of lymphoma, leukemia, or peptic ulcer. Varicella and herpes zoster of the adrenal glands produce medullary intranuclear inclusions.

Granulomas. In about half of the autopsied cases of infantile toxoplasmosis, adrenal granulomas with or without recognizable organisms are found. In generalized histoplasmosis, coccidioidomycosis, and brucellosis, there occur epithelioid, caseous, or partly calcified adrenal granulomas, sometimes extensive enough to cause death from adrenocortical insufficiency. Congenital syphilis may show subcapsular adrenal fibrosis and abundant treponemes. Tuberculous Addison's dis-

ease of children is like the adult condition described below.

Hypoplasia. Adrenocortical cytotoxic hypoplasia, occasionally with persistent cytomegalic cortical cells, characterizes idiopathic Addison's disease of infancy. Histologically, the adrenocortical cells are degenerated, with intermingled lymphocytes and macrophages. Several familial syndromes include childhood Addison's disease, most frequently combined with hypoparathyroidism and candidiasis or pernicious anemia. Adrenocortical insufficiency and death from malnutrition at the age of 4 months or less occur in primary familial xanthomatosis (Wolman's disease). Among various xanthomatous lesions ascribed to inborn lysosomal acid lipase deficiency, the adrenal glands are notably enlarged by cortical foam cells. Adrenal cholesterol, over 90% esterified, is increased twentyfold. There are also adrenocortical necrosis, foreign body reaction to crystallized lipid, and diffuse punctate calcifications that may be radiologically diagnostic. In children, adrenal calcification also follows hemorrhage from birth trauma.

Status thymicolymphaticus. Status thymicolymphaticus is a term applied to adrenocortical functional insufficiency in delicate children who die of ordinarily trivial traumas or viral or other infections. Unusually abundant thymic and other lymphoid tissues are thought to reflect subnormal corticosteroid responses. The adrenal cortex appears cytologically unreactive. The diagnosis is currently unpopular, and the existence of the condition is doubted by many. A comparable condition has been described in certain captive wild animals that died of minor conditions perhaps because of an inadequate adrenocortical reactivity to stress (see also p. 1397).

Cortical insufficiency. Partial adrenocortical insufficiency with selective familial cortisol deficiency in a child was correlated with absence of the zona fasciculata and zona reticularis. Adrenal cortisol unresponsiveness to ACTH, mental retardation, typical facies, dwarfism, and obesity comprise the Prader-Willi syndrome. Familial hypoaldosteronism in infants with 18-oxidase deficiency is accompanied by hyponatremia and hyperkalemia. Urinary corticosterone and related dehydro and tetrahydro compounds are increased. At autopsy, the adrenal glands are not enlarged. Small cells form tubular cords in the peripheral cortex. Functional, sometimes transient, hypoaldosteronism is reported in a few children and young adults but lacks a distinctive lesion.

Cortical hyperfunction. Adrenocortical hyperfunction in children is more often due to adrenal neoplasms than to hyperplasia. Boys may show the "infant Hercules" syndrome of pronounced muscular and somatic development with precocious pseudopuberty, comprised of macrogenitosomia and hirsutism but without testicular tubular or Leydig cell maturation. Girls with either neoplasms or adrenal hyperplasia are more often virilized, with some attributes comparable to Cushing's syndrome in adults. Adrenal medullary hyperplasia has been correlated with hypertension in two children and reported in pancreatic cystic fibrosis.

Neuroblastoma. Neuroblastoma of the medulla is the chief infantile adrenal neoplasm, varying from incidentally found seedlings to massive retroperitoneal tumors. Next to retinoblastoma, this is the most common congenital cancer. The age at diagnosis is less than 1 year in 30% and below 5 years in 80%. Less than 5% of the patients are over 15 years old. Extra-adrenal neuroblastomas arise elsewhere, particularly in the retroperitoneum and posterior mediastinum. When

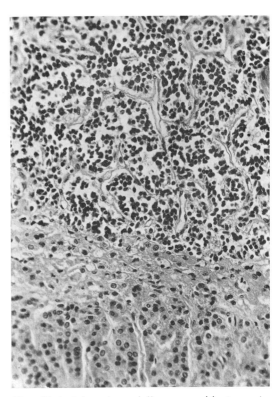

Fig. 36-4 Adrenal medullary neuroblastoma in newborn infant. (×200.)

the primary tumor is small, metastases may first attract attention. Typical profuse osseous metastases, which include the skull and orbit, with resulting exophthalmos, are called the Hutchison type of neuroblastoma. Large hepatic neuroblastomatous metastases constitute the Pepper syndrome.

Adrenal neuroblastomas are grossly or finely nodular, soft, gray-red, and vascular with a peripheral rim of persistent yellow adrenal cortex. Necrosis, hemorrhage, cystic degeneration, and calcification are seen. Microscopically, the viable tumor is composed of small, dark-stained, rounded or unipolar cells, practically without cytoplasm or architecture, arranged among thin-walled sinusoidal vessels (Fig. 36-4). Rosettes with distinctive neuroblastic palisading around spaces resembling primitive neural canals or pseudorosettes similar to those in embryonic sympathetic ganglia distinguish about half of neuroblastomas. Neurites and rosettes are formed in neuroblastoma tissue cultures. Ultrastructurally, most neuroblastomas contain cytoplasmic catecholamine granules, and they occasionally secrete excessive epinephrine.

In related better-differentiated neoplasms classified as ganglioneuroblastomas, foci of

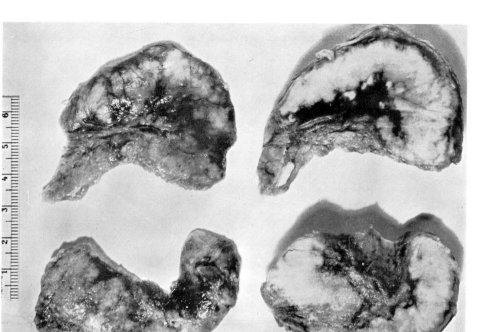

Fig. 36-5 Tuberculosis of adrenal glands in Addison's disease.

immature or mature neurons and nerve fibers are present. Fully differentiated ganglioneuromas are benign. In eleven cases, maturation has been observed from malignant neuroblastoma to benign ganglioneuroma. Sometimes, neuroblastoma and the histologically indistinguishable retinoblastoma regress spontaneously.

HEMORRHAGE AND NECROSIS

Adult adrenal apoplexy involves unilateral or bilateral adrenal hemorrhage, complicating trauma, infections, malignant hypertension, myocardial infarction, toxemia of pregnancy, septic abortion, or anticoagulant therapy. Vascular injury, parenchymal degeneration, venous thrombi, and generalized hemorrhagic or intravascular coagulative states are considered responsible.

Adrenocortical necrosis occurs focally in malaria, tetanus, typhus, Rocky Mountain spotted fever, epidemic hemorrhagic fever, and gram-negative bacterial infections; accompanying acute peptic ulcers; and following abdominal operations. Diffuse bilateral adrenal necrosis and cortical insufficiency are more common in children than in adults but may complicate infected abortion, obstetric shock, and fatal pemphigus vulgaris. Focal necrosis more often follows thromboses of afferent capsular vessels and outer zonal sinusoids, whereas diffuse bilateral adrenocortical necrosis results from long-lasting sinusoidal obstruction and medullary venous thromboses. Combined arterial and venous damage exaggerates both parenchymal necrosis and the subsequent hemorrhage.

INFLAMMATION, ATROPHY, AND ADDISON'S DISEASE

Exudative inflammation is uncommon in the adrenal cortex due to the antiphlogistic effects of corticosteroids. Necrosis exceeds leukocytic infiltration in various viral, mycotic, and bacterial infections that involve the adrenal glands. Granuloma formation is retarded in adrenal tuberculosis, leprosy, coccidioidomycosis, and histoplasmosis, with relatively more organisms and parenchymal destruction and less epithelioid or giant cell reaction and fibrosis than in other tissues. In lesions of extra-adrenal infections, corticoid therapy also reduces granulomas and promotes increased organisms and necrosis.

Foci of lymphocytes and plasma cells localized around adrenal medullary veins usually are associated with comparable infiltrations in the splenic red pulp and surrounding the renal and retroperitoneal veins. These commonly indicate chronic pyelonephritis with retroperitoneal chronic phlebitis rather than intrinsic adrenal disease.

Bilateral destructive adrenocortical tuberculosis is the classic cause of Addison's disease. Weakness, pigmentation of the skin and mucous membranes, hypotension, hypoglycemia, hyponatremia and hyperkalemia, a tendency to dehydration, and adrenal crises with shock following trauma or infections are its salient characteristics. Both adrenal glands are enlarged and largely replaced by caseous granulomas (Fig. 36-5). Forty years ago, 70% of Addison's disease was tuberculous, but idiopathic adrenocortical atrophy now predominates. Amyloidosis accounts for 1% and adrenal replacement by metastatic carcinoma for less than 0.5% of Addison's disease. Lymphoid tissues and pancreatic islets tend toward hyperplasia due to their release from adrenocortical control.

In idiopathic adrenal atrophy, the gland weights are reduced to 1.2 gm to 2.5 gm each and the cortices are narrowed and largely replaced by fibrous tissue (Fig. 36-6). Sometimes, nonspecific granulomas, giant cells, or infiltrates of lymphocytes are present in the cortices and medullae. These lesions comprise so-called cytotoxic atrophy. Periadrenal brown fat may be conspicuous. Familial Addison's

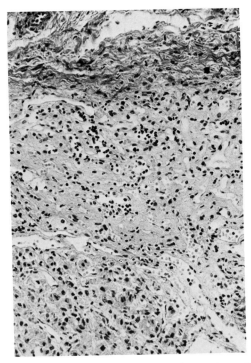

Fig. 36-6 Idiopathic adrenocortical atrophy with Addison's disease. Cortical cells have practically disappeared and stroma is collapsed. Adrenal medulla and central veins can be seen below. (×120.)

disease with atrophic and fibrotic adrenal changes suggests an autosomal recessive transmission.

Combined nontuberculous Addison's disease, hypothyroidism due to chronic thyroiditis, and occasionally hypopituitarism associated with pituitary lymphoid infiltrates constitute Schmidt's syndrome. Circulating antiadrenal mitochondrial and microsomal antibodies are found in the sera of half of the patients with nontuberculous Addison's disease. Diabetes mellitus, chronic hepatitis, gonadal failure, or pernicious anemia sometimes accompany Addison's disease, also suggesting autoimmune reactions. Experimental allergic adrenalitis can be transferred passively by lymphoid cells.

Adrenocortical atrophy secondary to hypophysectomy or pituitary destruction by disease may be extreme. In one adult with panhypopituitarism, the combined weight of the adrenal glands was only 0.8 gm, with cortices ten to twelve cells thick. Giant mitochondria occur posthypophysectomy in the zona fasciculata, reflecting a high progesterone:corticosterone ratio. Long-term cortisone-type therapy for connective tissue diseases, arthritis, or asthma reduces the gland weights by about half, with notable shrinkage of the zona fasciculata and sometimes the zona glomerulosa (Fig. 36-7). In iatrogenic adrenocortical atrophy, the collapsed, condensed cortical stroma may simulate fibrosis. Patients treated with both ACTH and cortisone demonstrate zona fasciculata cytolysis. In wasting diseases like tropical sprue and cirrhosis, comparable adrenocortical atrophy occurs, and it may be uncertain whether hormone therapy or chronic disease is responsible in some instances. Androgen therapy in large amounts has been claimed to produce similar changes in women. Functional adrenocortical insufficiency has been reported after oral contraceptive therapy. An atrophy of the inner zona fasciculata accompanying the aging process, with increased sudanophilic lipid, has been described in men over 50 years of age (see also p. 1428).

DEGENERATIONS AND INFILTRATIONS

As corticosteroids are secreted in acute diseases, the adrenal cortex becomes rapidly depleted of both birefringent and sudanophilic lipid. After six days, the cortical lipid is restored, but in the interval, lipid depletion reflects recent hypersecretion. In chronically ill individuals, adrenal lipid also is frequently depleted. The outer zona fasciculata cells may be reduced in size, producing a lipid depletion reversion pattern. In severe acute trauma, burns, toxemias, and infections like diphtheria, besides the loss of lipid, hyaline protein droplets are found in cortical cells with necrobiosis. The outer zona fasciculata regenerates around the cytolysis, resulting in a hollow cylindrical appearance of the fasciculata cell cords termed Rich's tubular degeneration (Fig. 36-8). Excessive ACTH stimulation is considered responsible for tubular degeneration, while hyaline droplet change has been produced experimentally by methyl androstenediol. Similar hyaline droplets in adrenal medullary cells occur in various chronic diseases. Spironolactone, an aldosterone antagonist, produces laminated sudanophilic myelin-like bodies in the zona glomerulosa cells.

Less specific degenerative changes include adrenal lymphocytic infiltrates near the cortico-medullary junction associated with

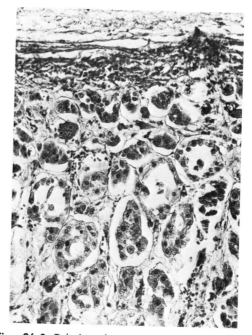

Fig. 36-8 Tubular degeneration resulting from cytolytic degeneration of zona fasciculata with regeneration to form hollow cylinders of cortical cells. (×120.)

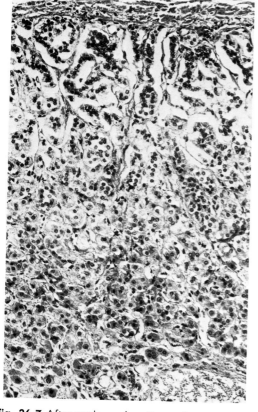

Fig. 36-7 After prolonged cortisone therapy, zona fasciculata cells become shrunken and cortical thickness reduced to 0.5 mm, half the normal width. Zona glomerulosa and zona reticularis unaffected and appear prominent. (×120).

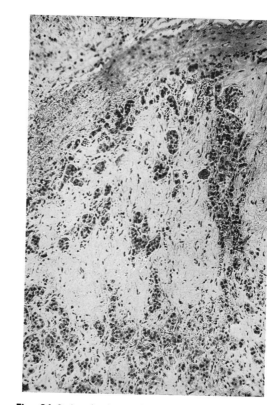

Fig. 36-9 Amyloidosis of adrenal cortex. Capsule at top and adrenocortical cells largely replaced by deposits. (×100.)

fragmented basement membranes. Hyaline fibrotic areas beneath the capsule or in the medulla are commonly secondary to arteriolosclerosis. Relatively little identifiable adrenal medulla may remain. Rarely, there is also medullary calcification and functional insufficiency.

Amyloid is deposited in the zona fasciculata in about 80% of patients with generalized amyloidosis, augmenting the adrenal weights. The zona glomerulosa is involved last, and adrenocortical insufficiency is uncommon (Fig. 36-9). Purely localized adrenal deposits of amyloid have been found in 6% of autopsies. In primary amyloidosis, only the adrenal arteries may be involved.

The zona glomerulosa becomes pigmented in hemosiderosis, and more hemosiderin is deposited here in hemochromatosis.

Fat replaces parts of the adrenal zona fasciculata and zona reticularis occasionally without affecting adrenal weight. A few lymphocytes or hematopoietic foci may be associated with fatty infiltration. The adrenal cortex also is a site of myeloid metaplasia; hematopoiesis is evident in sinusoids of the deep zona fasciculata, compressing the cell cords without significant gland enlargement.

CORTICAL NODULARITY

Approximately half of persons over 50 years of age have nonuniform adrenal cortices with multiple small rounded nodules of zona fasciculata. Regeneration following segmental ischemic adrenocortical atrophy due to local vascular disease accounts for many cortical nodules in older people. The nodular foci may possess more or less lipid than the uninvolved cortex and also differ in histochemical succinic dehydrogenase, esterase, and acid phosphatase reactions. Nodularity is more common with cirrhosis, hypertension, and cancer than with other chronic conditions. Adrenal changes in seasonally breeding wild rabbits suggest that sudden excessive stimulation of the outer cortical zones is responsible for some nodule formation. Adrenocortical nodularity without cortical thickening or increased gland weights does not constitute hyperplasia. Its functional importance is unknown.

HYPERPLASIA, CUSHING'S SYNDROME, AND ADRENAL VIRILISM

Adrenocortical hyperplasia may be either diffuse or nodular (finely or grossly), and it is usually bilateral. Objective and quantitative criteria for the diagnosis include gland weights exceeding the top 5% or above twice the standard deviation from the mean of normal weights and cortices thicker than 2 mm. Usually, hyperplasia involves the zona fasciculata. Exceptions in aldosteronism and adrenal virilism are noted below. Additional less conclusive indications of hyperplasia are irregular extracapsular proliferations of cortical cells, nodules that bulge into the medulla, and cortical cell cuffs around the central veins.

Nonspecific adrenocortical hyperplasia is most common with acromegaly, thyrotoxicosis, hypertension associated with arteriolosclerosis and arteriosclerosis, cancer, and diabetes mellitus. Some cases are unexplained. The adrenal glands of acromegalic patients usually are enlarged and nodular, with exaggerated androgen secretion after ACTH stimulation. Hyperplasia accompanies hyperthyroidism in about 40% of the patients, essential hypertension and arteriosclerosis in 16%, and diabetes mellitus in 3.4%. In both hyperthyroidism and hypertension, increased adrenal weights may be ascribed partly to the frequent terminal complication of congestive heart failure. Adrenocortical hyperplasia is not significantly increased in hypertension, but adrenal nodularity, hyperplasia, and adenomas lumped together are twice as common in hypertensive individuals as in matched normotensive persons. In patients with multiple primary cancers, adrenocortical hyperplasia occurs in 7.5%, compared to 5.2% in those with single cancers. Aside from endocrinologically active neoplasms, cancer sites with relatively frequent nonspecific adrenocortical hyperplasia include the following: endometrium, 19%; prostate, 14%; kidney, 14%; breast, 12%; and large intestine, 9%.

The best understood specific adrenocortical hyperplasia accompanies Cushing's syndrome. As originally described, Cushing's disease is due to an ACTH-secreting basophil pituitary adenoma, but in the much more common *syndrome,* no pituitary tumor is found. The typical patient has a rounded, moon-shaped face, obesity with a "buffalo hump" around the shoulders or a girdle distribution, a plethoric complexion associated with polycythemia, thin skin with easy bruising and abdominal striae, muscle weakness, hypertension, osteoporosis, and a diabetic type of glucose tolerance test. In women, hirsutism, amenorrhea, and mental disturbances are frequent, and acne may be present. Since practically all these changes follow sufficient

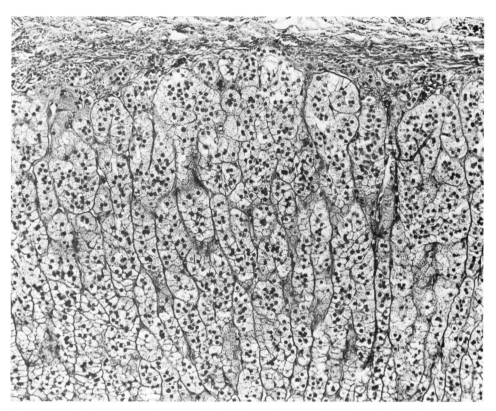

Fig. 36-10 Cushing's syndrome with diffuse adrenocortical hyperplasia. Outer zona fasciculata cells typically enlarged to form club-shaped cords. (×120.)

cortisone or cortisol administration, Cushing's syndrome is attributable to hypercortisolism. Women are affected more frequently than men in a ratio of about 3:1.

In children, Cushing's syndrome is about equally commonly associated with adrenocortical hyperplasia and tumors, but after the age of 10 years, zona fasciculata hyperplasia accounts for approximately 70% of cases. The zona reticularis also may be increased. Cortical adenoma is responsible for about 20% of the cases of adult Cushing's syndrome and adrenocortical carcinoma for 10%. The uninvolved and contralateral cortices are atrophic. Surgically removed glands with diffuse hyperplasia together weigh 14 gm to 26 gm or more in three-quarters of the patients with Cushing's syndrome and 10 gm to 12 gm in one-quarter. The cortices are usually thicker than 2 mm. In equivocal cases, volumetric studies demonstrate zona fasciculata hyperplasia. A distinctive cytologic enlargement and increased cytoplasmic lipid are observed, producing clublike thickenings of the outer zona fasciculata cell cords, with occasional very large cells (Fig. 36-10). The hyperplastic zona fasciculata may compress,

infiltrate, or replace the zona glomerulosa and zona reticularis and penetrate into the medulla. Hyperplasia also includes the zona reticularis in women with virilization, so that in clinical Cushing's syndrome the endocrine hyperfunction is not necessarily restricted to the zona fasciculata and hypercortisolism.

Nodular hyperplasia involves increased adrenal weights and cortices thickened by rounded zona fasciculata nodules, usually 1 mm to 6 mm and occasionally up to 2 cm in diameter. Some individuals are apparently normal endocrinologically. Others have hypertension, edema, and hyperaldosteronism. Grossly, nodular hyperplasia with Cushing's syndrome involves bilateral adrenal hypertrophy up to triple the normal weight and multiple adenomatous nodules that are 1 cm to 5 cm in diameter and yellow, brown, black, or red according to their lipid content and lipochrome or heme pigmentation from hemorrhages. The nodules have variable lipid content and decreased glucose-6-phosphate-dehydrogenase activity (Fig. 36-11). On electron microscopy, the hyperplastic adrenocortical cells possess an abundant smooth endoplasmic reticulum and tubulovesicular

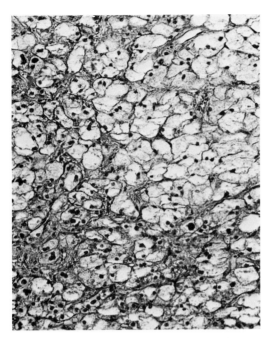

Fig. 36-11 Nodular hyperplasia of zona fasciculata with Cushing's syndrome associated with irregular cellular enlargement and locally increased lipid in adrenocortical cells. (×120.)

mitochondria characteristic of the zona fasciculata.

Nodular adrenocortical dysplasia is an unusual lesion in infants or children with Cushing's syndrome. The glands are not enlarged, and the cortex contains multiple minute nodules up to 2 mm in diameter, notably pigmented by lipochrome and apparently arising from the zona reticularis. The intervening cortical tissue is atrophic. The cortical hyperfunction is unresponsive to ACTH or dexamethasone, unlike the more common ACTH-dependent hyperplasia with Cushing's syndrome.

Cushing's syndrome with bilateral adrenocortical hyperplasia is now usually ascribed to hypothalamic-hypophyseal dysfunction, but some cortical nodules are endocrinologically autonomous. The 11-hydroxycorticosteroid and growth hormone responses to insulin injections are impaired. Compound S and cortisol are both hypersecreted, and if the plasma cortisol level exceeds 55 mg per 100 ml, hypokalemic alkalosis develops. Occasionally, the adrenal glands of patients with Cushing's syndrome secrete largely corticosterone and 11-dehydrocorticosterone (see also p. 1427).

Ectopic ACTH production by nonendocrine tissue tumors is considered responsible for approximately 20% of the cases of Cushing's syndrome. Often, the clinical findings are incomplete or absent, perhaps because the condition has developed rapidly, but hypokalemic alkalosis is a usual finding. Edema, skin pigmentation, and severe diabetes mellitus are more common than in idiopathic Cushing's syndrome. Oat cell carcinoma of the lung is the most frequently associated tumor. Pituitary hyaline basophils are increased, indicating increased circulating cortisone. Other recognized ACTH-secreting tumors include thymic adenocarcinomas, pancreatic islet cell tumors, thyroid medullary carcinomas, and carcinoids of the lung or stomach, among diverse foregut endodermal neoplasms. Neuroblastomas and ovarian, testicular, and other neoplasms also have been implicated.

The adrenal glands in the ectopic ACTH syndrome usually are notably enlarged, two to five times the normal weight. Microscopically, the zona fasciculata cells, particularly near the capsule, are distinctively enlarged, depleted of lipid, and acidophilic (Fig. 36-12). These are effects of maximal ACTH stimulation. Plasma and urine 17-hydroxycorticosteroids and plasma ACTH are increased, and sometimes also compound S and corticosterone. In contrast to typical Cushing's syndrome, dexamethasone suppression fails. Besides ACTH, some neoplasms also produce excessive melanocyte-stimulating hormone, parathyroid hormone, gastrin, glucagon, antidiuretic hormone, norepinephrine, or serotonin. Pancreatic tumors appear the most versatile. Patients with lung carcinomas that do not produce ACTH may secrete excessive 17-hydroxycorticosteroids and cortisone after ACTH administration, as occurs nonspecifically in other severe illnesses.

Iatrogenic adrenocortical hyperplasia has followed prolonged ACTH therapy in leukemic children and in adults with various chronic diseases. Gland weights are nearly doubled. Both the zona fasciculata and zona reticularis are thicker, the individual cells are enlarged, and cholesterol and lipid are reduced. Histochemical reactions for phosphatases, dehydrogenases, and RNA are increased; 11β-hydroxylation is stimulated. The clinical and laboratory findings resemble Cushing's syndrome.

Cushingoid states have some attributes of Cushing's syndrome such as obesity, diabetes mellitus, hirsutism, or hypertension, without a clear-cut correlated hypercortisolism, pituitary and adrenocortical hyperplasia, or neo-

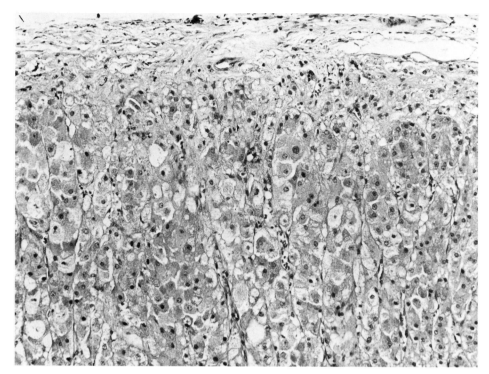

Fig. 36-12 Enlargement and lipid depletion of maximally stimulated outer zona fasciculata cells produced by ectopic ACTH. (×120.)

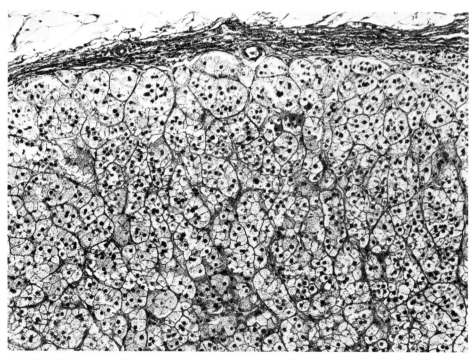

Fig. 36-13 Primary aldosteronism associated with unilateral adrenocortical hyperplasia. Zona glomerulosa cells enlarged and finely granular. (×120.)

plasia. Such conditions include the Morgagni-Stewart-Morel syndrome of obesity and hirsutism with hyperostosis frontalis interna; the Achard-Thiers syndrome of diabetes in bearded women; the "burgeoning women" of Corscaden with obesity, hypertension, arthritis and endometrial hyperplasia or carcinoma; and some instances of the Stein-Leventhal syndrome and Schroeder's "endocrine hypertensive syndrome" with central obesity.

Hyperplasia of the inner zona fasciculata and zona reticularis together characterize adrenal virilism, sometimes called the acquired or adult adrenogenital syndrome. In women, hirsutism, acne, temporal alopecia, squared body contours, deep voice, and clitoral enlargement to some degree frequently accompany Cushing's syndrome. Androgen secretion, particularly dehydroepiandrosterone and 11β-hydroxyandrostenedione, is responsible. Cortisol and corticosterone also are increased. Pure adrenal zona reticularis hyperplasia is unusual. When mild, it may produce only hirsutism. Adrenal hirsutism is estimated to explain about 1% of excessive hair growth in women. Two distinctive characteristics of hyperplastic zona reticularis cells are lipochrome pigment and fuchsinophilia.

Zona glomerulosa hyperplasia, with enlarged lipid-containing cells forming a continuous subcapsular layer at least 100μ wide, is associated with secondary aldosteronism fully developed as a complication of malignant or renovascular hypertension, nephrotic syndrome, cirrhosis with ascites, and other conditions (Fig. 36-13). Nodular hyperplasia of both zonae glomerulosa and fasciculata accompanies cases variously classified as secondary, nontumorous, idiopathic or pseudoprimary aldosteronism. Unilateral nodular hyperplasia is a rare acceptable cause of primary aldosteronism. In sodium restriction the zona glomerulosa ordinarily is increased in thickness with depletion of the cytoplasmic lipid and cholesterol.

NEOPLASMS
Adenoma, primary aldosteronism, and carcinoma

Adrenal cortical adenoma is usually a relatively large, single, rounded mass of yellow-orange adrenocortical tissue, measuring 1 cm to 5 cm in diameter (Fig. 36-14). Larger adenomas up to 12 cm in diameter may show hemorrhages, cystic degeneration, and calcification. The tissue bulges from the cut sur-

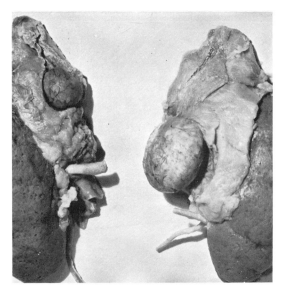

Fig. 36-14 Bilateral cortical adenomas of adrenal glands showing their location in relation to kidneys.

face, indicating compression. Most adenomas are surrounded by a rim of stretched, uninvolved adrenal cortex and have an incomplete fibrous capsule or none. Histologically, adenomas are composed of relatively regular large cells with uniformly abundant lipid, arranged in nodules and cords with a vaguely fasciculate pattern. The margins of contact with uninvolved adrenal cortex are evident, since cells of the latter are zonated, smaller, and contain less lipid. Giant cells with prominent nuclei and cellular polymorphism often present in adrenocortical adenomas are not considered evidence of cancer.

Nodules smaller than 9 mm in diameter sometimes are considered adenomas, but if they are multiple, bilateral, or zonated and lie in the capsule or outside, it is doubtful that they are true adenomas. A genuine adrenocortical adenoma usually is associated with either a normal or atrophic homolateral and contralateral uninvolved gland. When the adrenal cortices are multinodular or hyperplastic, the largest masses represent dominant nodules rather than adenomas.

Adenomas located centrally in the adrenal gland may be difficult to distinguish from pheochromocytomas, and in extra-adrenal sites such as the retroperitoneum or ovary they may be confused with nonchromaffin paragangliomas, Leydig cell tumors, and hypernephroid and other neoplasms. Some differential diagnostic features are given in Table 36-1.

Table 36-1 Differential diagnostic features

Features	Adrenocortical tumor	Pheochromocytoma
Gross appearance	Yellow or orange	Gray, red, or brown
Histology	Cordlike arrangement	Sheets; nests; mosaic or twisted cord pattern
Cytology	Uniform size; squared shapes Cytoplasmic lipid vacuoles; Sudan and cholesterol positive Occasional mitoses	Variable size; polyhedral shapes No lipid vacuoles No mitoses
Chromaffinity	Negative	Positive
Ultrastructure	No catecholamine granules	Catecholamine granules

An adrenal adenoma is found in about 2% of adult autopsies. In the absence of overt endocrine effects and hormonal analyses, these are called "nonfunctional adenomas." Adenomas have been found most commonly in autopsies on elderly, obese, diabetic patients, 30%; women averaging 81 years of age, 29%; hypertensive individuals, 20%; and in almost one-third of patients with the familial multiple endocrine adenomatosis syndrome that also involves the pancreatic islets and the parathyroid, pituitary, and thyroid glands besides peptic ulcerations, gastric mucosal hyperplasia, and colonic villous adenomas.

In children, most adrenal tumors are functional and develop in the first four years of life, with girls being affected about 2.5 times as often as boys. Adrenal tumors commonly become apparent clinically between the ages of 4 and 8 years. In girls, virilization occurs in half the cases, virilization and aspects of Cushing's syndrome occur in one-third, and combined virilizing and feminizing effects occur in 5%. In boys, virilization occurs in two-thirds of the cases and combined virilizing and Cushing's syndrome occurs in one-quarter. Feminizing tumors in children are uncommon. Only a dozen have been reported, half of them carcinomas. Cushing's syndrome occurring under 10 years of age usually is due to an adrenal neoplasm.

About three-quarters of functioning adrenal tumors in children are benign adenomas, 10% of which are bilateral. The remaining quarter are carcinomas. Practically all the carcinomas metastasize and prove fatal. Dehydroepiandrosterone is the chief steroid secreted by virilizing adenomas, and the urinary 17-ketosteroids are increased. Androgens also promote somatic growth and maturation. The testicular tubules and Leydig cells remain undeveloped or there is no menstrual activity, unlike the situation in precocious puberty.

Cortisol hypersecretion typifies Cushing's syndrome. Combined virilization and estrogenization are associated with adrenocortical conversion of dehydroepiandrosterone partly to estradiol.

In adults with Cushing's syndrome, functioning adrenal adenomas characteristically reduce the plasma ACTH, unlike adrenocortical hyperplasia. Hirsutism and acne less commonly accompany adenoma than adrenal carcinoma. Virilizing and feminizing adrenal tumors more often are carcinomas than adenomas. The latter may respond functionally to ACTH and dexamethasone.

Primary aldosteronism is associated with an adrenocortical adenoma in about 90% of cases and with carcinoma, multiple adenomas, and unilateral cortical hyperplasia in the remainder. Fewer than ten authentic cases with adenomas have been reported in children. Before the age of 20 years, most instances of aldosterone hypersecretion have been associated with either bilateral diffuse or nodular cortical hyperplasia. Conn's syndrome (Conn et al.[118]) describes the combination of hypokalemic alkalosis, renal potassium loss, and hypertension which may be cured by removing an aldosterone-secreting adrenal adenoma. Renin is characteristically suppressed, and the renal juxtaglomerular cells are atrophic. Aldosteronomas often are flattened tumors 0.9 cm to 1.5 cm in diameter. They may be impalpable and unidentified until multiple sections of the gland are made. A few are larger, and some have weighed more than 30 gm. Characteristically, they are more orange than yellow, rich in lipid, and histologically resemble other adrenal adenomas, with either a fasciculate or glomerulosal architecture (Fig. 36-15). Biosynthesis of cortisol, corticosterone, and aldosterone is demonstrable. Electron microscopy of seven cases has shown the tumor mito-

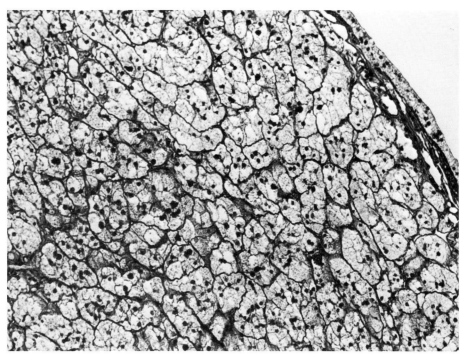

Fig. 36-15 Enlarged lipid-rich cells surrounded by fibrous capsule characterize adrenocortical adenomas, in this instance aldosteronoma. (×120.)

chondria to possess the platelike cristae of zona glomerulosa cells, or tubulovesicular cristae like the zona fasciculata, or a combined "hybrid cell" type. Histochemically, 3-β-hydroxysteroid dehydrogenase activity is reportedly intense.

Hypertension also occurs associated with adenomas which produce corticosterone, desoxycorticosterone, or, more rarely, tetrahydrodeoxycorticosterone. Unlike adenomas, adrenal carcinomas with aldosteronism usually show increased urinary 17-ketosteroids and 17-hydroxycorticosteroids, and biosynthesis in vitro of hydrocortisone, cortisone, and corticosterone also is found. Disturbances in so-called pseudoprimary, nontumorous, or idiopathic aldosteronism may be completely similar to the preoperative clinical and laboratory findings of Conn's syndrome, but the normal-appearing or nodular hyperplastic adrenal glands, if removed, do not benefit the hypertension. Compared to primary aldosteronism, aldosterone hypersecretion and hypokalemia are less notable, and the renal juxtaglomerular cells are not so markedly atrophic. In a few individuals, hyperaldosteronism has been controlled by prednisone therapy or dexamethasone.

Primary aldosteronism without hypokalemia or an aldosteronoma exists but is uncommon

enough to question the diagnosis. The nature of cases with hyperaldosteronism and one or multiple cortical nodules 0.3 cm to 0.8 cm in diameter or bilateral hyperplasia is disputed. Conceivably, they represent transitions from adrenocortical hyperplasia to genuine adenomas. In contrast to other functioning adrenocortical neoplasms, the uninvolved homolateral and the contralateral zona glomerulosa and zona fasciculata in primary aldosteronism have been reported as atrophic, normal, or hyperplastic. In our experience, the uninvolved glomerulosa retains its usual discontinuity and varies within normal limits. Accurate volumetric studies are needed to settle this point. In several cases, aldosteronoma and renal or established essential hypertension were present together, accounting for the failure of adrenalectomy to relieve the hypertension.

Hypoaldosteronism as an isolated adult abnormality is also a puzzling condition. In the first reported case, a large adrenal adenoma containing predominantly compound S was found at autopsy. Other instances have been observed with postoperatively recurrent hypercortisolism, prolonged heparin therapy, or excessive licorice ingestion, or as a functional deficiency with postural hypotension.

Pigmented adrenocortical adenoma, or so-

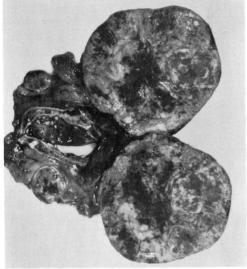

Fig. 36-16 Adrenal carcinoma associated with Cushing's syndrome.

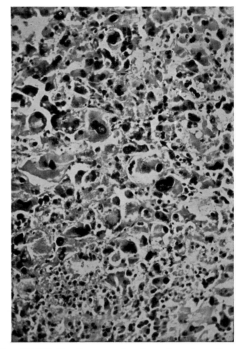

Fig. 36-17 Carcinoma of adrenal cortex. Tumor cells show marked variation in size, shape, and intensity of staining. (×200.)

called black adenoma, is a pathologic curiosity without functional significance. Grossly and microscopically, the cells contain so much brown pigment that they resemble a melanoma, but special stains demonstrate a PAS-positive lipochrome like that of the zona reticularis.

Adrenal carcinomas are predominantly functional. They are distinguished from adenomas by capsular or blood vessel invasion and metastasis. Carcinomas are usually large when first discovered, 7 cm to 20 cm in diameter, and weigh 100 gm to 2400 gm. Hemorrhage, necrosis, and calcification are more common in adrenal carcinomas than in adenomas (Fig. 36-16). Nuclear atypia, large nucleoli, multinucleated cells, mitoses, and compact acidophilic cells are typical of adrenocortical carcinomas, but demonstrable invasion, metastasis, or both are necessary for definite diagnosis (Fig. 36-17). Judged from reported cases, about half of adrenal carcinomas are associated with Cushing's syndrome, 20% with virilization, 4% with these syndromes combined, 12% with feminization, and 4% with aldosteronism and related conditions. Approximately 10% of adrenal carcinomas are nonfunctional. Fever may attract attention to the nonfunctioning type. About twelve large carcinomas have been observed in association with severe hypoglycemia. Most adrenal carcinomas metastasize widely and cause death.

About three-quarters of **feminizing adrenal neoplasms** are carcinomas and one-quarter adenomas. Most develop in men between 20 and 60 years of age, with bilateral gynecomastia, loss of libido, and atrophy of the testes and penis. Obesity, attributes of Cushing's syndrome, and feminine distribution of body hair may be present. Urinary estrogens and usually both 17-ketosteroids and 17-hydroxycorticosteroids are increased, and gonadotropins are decreased. The tumors are not distinguishable histopathologically from other adrenal neoplasms. Estrogen biosynthesis is demonstrable from pregnenolone, progesterone, androstenedione, and testosterone. In women, estrogen-producing adrenal tumors are associated with amenorrhea, hirsutism, and clitoral enlargement. In men with prostatic hypertrophy, the pituitary cytology has suggested ACTH hypersecretion and a mild variant of the adrenogenital syndrome. No feminizing adrenocortical hyperplasia is known in adults.

Feminizing and virilizing adrenal neoplasms that arise in extra-adrenal rests are difficult or impossible to distinguish morphologically from Leydig cell tumors, ovarian lipid cell tumors, Sertoli-type androblastomas, or luteomas of pregnancy. These primary gonadal tumors are ordinarily virilizing and benign, whereas adrenocortical neoplasms that produce sex hormones are predominantly malignant.

Metastatic cancer in the adrenal glands is often bilateral, with tumors commonly less than 2.5 cm in diameter. Initially, the medulla usually is involved. Carcinomas of the lung, particularly of the squamous cell type, form adrenal metastases in one-third of cases. Carcinomas of the breast show metastases in 25% of adrenalectomy specimens and in 30% at autopsy. Carcinomas of the stomach, large intestine, and pancreas frequently metastasize to the adrenal glands. Also, melanomas, renal cell carcinomas, and thyroid carcinomas often spread to the adrenal glands.

Cysts

Aside from rare echinococcal cysts, found in less than 0.5% of patients with echinococcosis, most adrenal cysts are noninflammatory. Pseudocysts lined by fibrous tissue represent residues of remote hematomas or degenerated adenomas. Genuine cysts may be lined by glandular epithelium resembling the adrenal cortex or by endothelium indicating a cavernous lymphangioma or hemangioma. Angiomas may exceed 20 cm in diameter and constitute the largest adrenal cysts. They may have partly calcified walls.

Myelolipoma

Myelolipoma of the adrenal gland is a fatty, gray or red spheroid mass apparently originating in the inner zona fasciculata, usually measuring 0.5 cm to 6 cm in diameter. One such tumor measuring 25 cm in diameter produced pressure symptoms. Histologically, the structure simulates adult hematopoietic bone marrow, with comparable amounts of adipose and myeloid cells (Fig. 36-18). Myelolipomas are not clearly neoplasms and may represent enlarged mesenchymal rests. Sometimes, they accompany obesity or bone marrow failure and may occur also in the intercostal spaces and retroperitoneal or pelvic connective tissue. One woman has been reported with bilateral adrenal tumors composed of brown fat or hibernomas.

Pheochromocytoma and chromaffin paraganglioma

A pheochromocytoma is a medullary adrenal neoplasm that typically secretes epinephrine, norepinephrine, or both. Similar extra-adrenal tumors, conventionally termed chromaffin paragangliomas, may be retroperitoneal, above the aortic bifurcation or

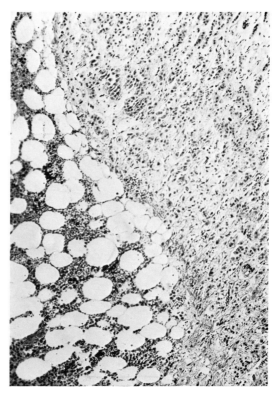

Fig. 36-18 Myelolipoma of adrenal gland. Tissue resembling bone marrow surrounded by adrenal cortex. (×100.)

celiac in location, or attached to the urinary bladder, or within mediastinal, intrathoracic, or intracranial areas. Sporadic pheochromocytomas may be unsuspected and often are found after an elective operation in an individual who develops acute hypertension and subsequent lethal shock under anesthesia. Patients with preoperatively recognized pheochromocytomas have paroxysmal or persistent hypertension, orthostatic hypotension, palpitation, headaches, and flushing or sweating spells in various combinations, with increased urinary vanilmandelic acid and other catecholamine metabolites. About two-thirds have hyperglycemia ascribable to decreased insulin release, and three-quarters are hypermetabolic. Occasionally, diabetes mellitus is cured by removing a pheochromocytoma.

The tumors vary from incidental microscopic findings to masses over 2 kg in weight, but the average weight is 90 gm and the size 5 cm to 6 cm in diameter. Grossly, pheochromocytomas are rounded, gray or red, and circumscribed and are surrounded by stretched adrenal cortex. Hemorrhages, cystic areas, calcification, or a central dense fibrous scar are common (Fig. 36-19). Chromaffin tests on fresh tissue characteristically color pheochro-

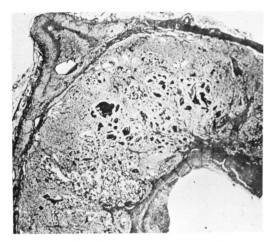

Fig. 36-19 Pheochromocytoma enclosed by adrenal cortex at upper left. Central cystic degeneration and rich sinusoidal vascularity demonstrated. (×8.)

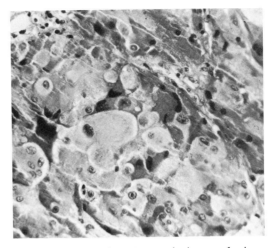

Fig. 36-20 Irregular size and shape of pheochromocytoma cells and nuclei, as well as variable staining of their cytoplasm, are characteristic. Darker colored cells are brown due to the chromaffin reaction. (×350.)

mocytomas dark brown. Occasional tumors containing pure norepinephrine are chromaffin negative; these pheochromocytomas are more common in childhood. Tissue fixed in Helly's or Zenker's fluid demonstrates chromaffinity both grossly and microscopically.

Histologically, pheochromocytomas show notable variability of cell and nuclear size and arrangement. Basic twisted cell cord patterns, basophilic or acidophilic staining, and the presence of fine or coarse intracytoplasmic pigment granules and PAS-stained secretory droplets aid in making the diagnosis (Fig. 36-20). Ultrastructurally identified epinephrine-containing cytoplasmic granules in pheochromocytomas are larger than in the normal medulla. Similar organelles in neuroblastomas and ganglioneuroblastomas explain their occasionally excessive secretion of catecholamines. Catecholamines are stored and secreted from osmiophilic cytoplasmic granules. Differentiation from adrenocortical neoplasms may be difficult microscopically (Table 36-1). Adrenocortical adenoma and pheochromocytoma may occur in the same gland. The periadrenal adipose tissue in cases of pheochromocytoma typically has an excess of brown or hibernating fat.

Whether pheochromocytomas originate from adrenal medullary hyperplasia is uncertain. Homolateral and contralateral hyperplasia of the predominant pheochromocytoma cell type has been reported. In the absence of reliable criteria for identifying hyperplasia of the adrenal medulla, these reports are difficult to evaluate. The association of medullary hyper-

plasia with increased catecholamine excretion has been described in pancreatic cystic fibrosis.

Malignant pheochromocytomas constitute about 6% of all cases. Some are microscopically atypical, more closely resembling neuroblastomas. Others are typical except for gross or microscopic invasion of the periadrenal fat or blood vessels. However, neither gross invasion nor microscopic pleomorphism is a reliable indication of likely recurrence of pheochromocytomas or metastasis. Clinical and pathologic evidence of malignancy often develops years after the original pheochromocytoma was removed, and the metastatic tumor histologically may still appear benign. Multiple benign chromaffin paragangliomas are to be distinguished from malignant pheochromocytoma.

Several syndromes associated with pheochromocytoma include Recklinghausen's neurofibromatosis, Lindau-von Hippel disease and cerebellar hemangioblastoma, Albright's syndrome, multiple mucocutaneous neuromas, and familial multiple endocrine neoplasms that include medullary thyroid carcinoma and hyperparathyroidism due to parathyroid hyperplasia or adenomas. This last combination is also called Sipple's syndrome or multiple endocrine neoplasia type 2 to distinguish it from multiple adenomas of the pituitary gland, parathyroid glands, and pancreatic islets (type 1) and combined papillary thyroid carcinoma and parathyroid adenoma (type 3). Pheochromocytomas are bilateral in about half of the cases of familial pheochro-

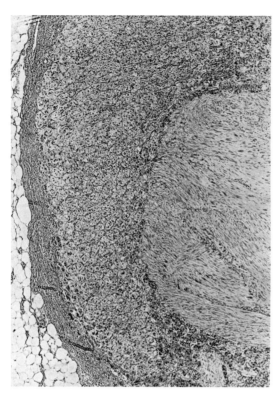

Fig. 36-21 Small neurofibroma of adrenal medulla. (×50.)

mocytoma, compared to 5% of sporadic cases. Autosomal dominant inheritance appears responsible for familial multiple endocrine neoplasia.

Cushing's syndrome caused by a cortisol-secreting pheochromocytoma has been recognized in about twelve cases, including one intrapancreatic chromaffin paraganglioma. Both catecholamines and cortisol were produced by a single tumor.

Renal biopsies from patients with pheochromocytoma show edematous subendothelial changes of the small arteries without arteriolosclerosis, and segmental renal cortical scars are found. The myocardium often shows focal degeneration similar to that produced experimentally with norepinephrine.

Malignant melanoma and other adrenal neoplasms

Primary malignant melanoma in the adrenal gland has been recognized in some twelve cases. Usually, multiple metastases are present elsewhere. The pigment is identified as melanin, and other possible primary sites are excluded. Neural crest melanoblasts are probably the cells of origin.

Other adrenal neoplasms are usually small

benign connective tissue tumors, including neurilemoma, neurofibroma, lipoma, leiomyoma, osteoma, and angioma, as well as mixed mesenchymoma (Fig. 36-21).

REFERENCES
Structure and function

1 Bech, K., Tygstrup, I., and Nerup, J.: Acta Path. Microbiol. Scand. **76:**391-400, 1969 (involution of fetal cortex).
2 Beisel, W. R., and Rapoport, M. I.: New Eng. J. Med. **280:**541-546, 596-604, 1969 (response to infections).
3 Benirschke, K.: Obstet. Gynec. **8:**412-425, 1956 (adrenal in anencephaly).
4 Berry, R. E.: In Pathology annual, vol. 4, (S. C. Sommers, editor), New York, 1969, Appleton-Century-Crofts, pp. 71-88 (normal adrenal glands).
5 Cannon, W. B.: Physiol. Rev. **9:**399-431, 1929 (homeostasis).
5a Christy, N. P., editor: The human adrenal cortex, New York, 1971, Hoeber Medical Division, Harper & Row, Publishers.
6 Dahl, E. V., and Bahn, R. C.: Amer. J. Path. **40:**587-598, 1962 (aberrant testicular adrenal).
7 Dobbie, J. W., and Symington, T.: J. Endocr. **34:**479-489, 1966.
8 Falls, J. L.: Cancer **8:**143-150, 1955 (accessory adrenal in broad ligament).
9 Johannisson, E.: Acta Endocr. (Kobenhavn) **58**(suppl. 130):7-107, 1968 (adrenal development).
10 Lanman, J. T.: Medicine (Balt.) **32:**389-430, 1953 (fetal cortex).
11 LeCompte, P. M.: J. Clin. Endocr. **9:**158-162, 1949 (adrenocortical width).
12 Long, J. A., and Jones, A. L.: Lab. Invest. **17:**355-370, 1967, (fine structure).
13 Mitchell, N., and Angrist, A.: Arch. Path. (Chicago) **35:**46-52, 1943 (adrenal rests in kidney).
14 Orth, D. N., and Island, D. P.: J. Clin. Endocr. **29:**479-486, 1969 (circadian cortisol rhythm).
15 Schulz, D. M., Giordano, D. A., and Schulz, D. H.: Arch. Path. (Chicago) **74:**244-250, 1962 (weights in infants).
16 Selye, H.: J. Clin. Endocr. **6:**117-230, 1946 (adrenal reaction to stress; adaptation syndrome).
17 Stirling, G. A., and Keating, V. J.: Brit. Med. J. **2:**1016-1018, 1958 (weights in Jamaicans).
18 Studzinski, G. P., Hay, D. C. F., and Symington, T.: J. Clin. Endocr. **23:**248-254, 1962 (adrenal weight).
18a Symington, T.: Functional pathology of the adrenal gland, Baltimore, 1969, The Williams & Wilkins Co.
19 Villee, C. A., and Loring, J. M.: J. Clin. Endocr. **25:**307-314, 1965 (newborn adrenal steroids).
19a Villee, D. B.: New Eng. J. Med. **281:**473-484, 533-541, 1969 (fetal adrenal function).

Congenital anomalies

20 Biglieri, E. G., Herron, M. A., and Brust, N.: J. Clin. Invest. **45:**1946-1954, 1966 (17-hydroxylase deficiency).

21 Bolande, R. P.: Amer. J. Path. **34**:137-147, 1958 (adrenal in postmaturity).

22 Bongiovanni, A. M., Eberlein, W. R., Goldman, A. S., and New, M.: Recent Progr. Hormone Res. **23**:375-449, 1967 (congenital adrenocortical hyperplasia).

23 Borit, A., and Kosek, J.: Arch. Path. (Chicago) **88**:58-64, 1969.

24 Clayton, B. E., Edwards, R. W., and Makin, H. L.: J. Endocr. **43**:xivi-xivii, 1969 (other 11-hydroxylase deficiencies).

25 Craig, J. M., and Landing, B. H.: Amer. J. Clin. Path. **21**:940-949, 1951 (adrenal cytomegaly).

26 Dolan, M. F., and Janovski, N. A.: Arch. Path. (Chicago) **86**:22-24, 1968 (adrenohepatic fusion).

27 Ehrlich, E. N., Straus, F. H., II, Hunter, R. L., and Wiest, W. G.: J. Clin. Endocr. **29**:523-538, 1969 (cytomegalic hypoplasia in adult).

28 Gardner, L. I., Sniffen, R. C., Zygmuntowicz, A. S., and Talbot, N. B.: Pediatrics **5**:808-823, 1950 (salt-losing 21-hydroxylase deficiency).

29 Goldman, A. S.: J. Clin. Endocr. **27**:1390-1394, 1967 (experimental 11-hydroxylase inhibition).

30 Kerenyi, N.: Arch. Path. (Chicago) **71**:336-343, 1961 (congenital hypoplasia).

31 Landing, B. H., and Gold, E.: J. Clin. Endocr. **11**:1436-1453, 1951 (adrenogenital syndrome with Leydig cell hyperplasia).

32 Laqueur, G. L., and Harrison, M. B.: Amer. J. Path. **27**:231-245, 1951 (brown fat).

33 Mallin, S. R.: Ann. Intern. Med. **70**:69-75, 1969.

34 Miloslavich, E.: Virchow Arch. Path. Anat. **218**:131-152, 1914.

34a Moncrieff, M. W., Mann, J. R., Goldsmith, A. R., and Chance, G. W.: Postgrad. Med. J. **46**:162-166, 1970 (Beckwith's syndrome).

35 Nellhaus, G.: New Eng. J. Med. **258**:935-938, 1958 (maternal testosterone and masculinization).

36 O'Donohoe, N. V., and Holland, P. D. J.: Arch. Dis. Child. **43**:717-723, 1968 (familial congenital hypoplasia).

37 Oppenheimer, E. H.: Arch. Path. (Chicago) **87**:653-659, 1969 (adrenal in prematurity).

38 Provenzano, R. W.: New Eng. J. Med. **242**:87-89, 1950 (idiopathic hypoplasia).

39 Sherman, F. E., Bass, L. W., and Fetterman, G. H:. Amer. J. Clin. Path. **30**:439-446, 1958 (cytomegaly and carcinoma).

40 Silverman, W. A., editor: Dunham's Premature infants, ed. 3, New York, 1961, Hoeber Medical Division, Harper & Row, Publishers (edema in infants of diabetics).

41 Wiener, M. F., and Dallgaard, S. A.: Arch. Path. (Chicago) **67**:228-233, 1959 (intracranial adrenal).

42 Wilkins, L.: J.A.M.A. **172**:1028-1032, 1960 (maternal progestin and masculinization).

Childhood abnormalities

43 Beckwith, J. B., and Perrin, E. V.: Amer. J. Path. **43**:1089-1104, 1963 (neuroblastoma in situ).

44 Bialestock, D.: Arch. Dis. Child. **36**:465-473, 1961 (hypertension and hyperplastic medulla).

45 Cheatham, W. J., Weller, T. H., Dolan, T. F., Jr., and Dower, J. C.: Amer. J. Path. **32**:1015-1035, 1956 (varicella).

46 Christian, J. J., and Ratcliffe, H. L.: Amer. J. Path. **28**:725-737, 1952 (adrenal hypoplasia and shock in animals).

47 Crocker, A. C., Vawter, G. F., Neuhauser, E. B. D., and Rosowsky, A.: Pediatrics **35**:627-640, 1965 (familial xanthomatosis).

48 Fisher, E. R., and Davis, E.: New Eng. J. Med. **258**:1036-1040, 1958.

48a Guin, G. H., Gilbert, E. F., and Jones, B.: Amer. J. Clin. Path. **51**:126-136, 1969 (neuroblastoma).

49 Horn, R. C., Jr., Koop, C. E., and Kiesewetter, W. B.: Lab. Invest. **5**:106-119, 1956.

50 Kidder, L. A.: Amer. J. Clin. Path. **22**:870-878, 1952 (cytomegalovirus disease).

51 Margaretten, W., Nakai, H., and Landing, B. H.: Amer. J. Dis. Child. **105**:346-351, 1963 (septicemic adrenal hemorrhage).

52 Misugi, K., Misugi, N., and Newton, W. A., Jr.: Arch. Path. (Chicago) **86**:160-170, 1968 (neuroblastoma—ultrastructure).

52a Naeye, R. L., and Blanc, W. A.: New Eng. J. Med. **283**:555-560, 1970 (perinatal infection).

53 Patrizi, G., Middelkamp, J. N., and Reed, C. A.: Amer. J. Clin. Path. **49**:325-341, 1968 (herpes simplex adrenal necrosis).

54 Pearson, G. W.: Brit. Med. J. **1**:1056-1057, 1962 (childhood Addison's disease).

55 Rudd, B. T., Chance, G. W., and Theodoridis, C. G.: Arch. Dis. Child. **44**:244-247, 1969 (Prader-Willi syndrome).

56 Stowens, D.: Arch. Path. (Chicago) **63**:451-459, 1957.

57 Thomison, J. B., and Shapiro, J. L.: Arch. Path. (Chicago) **63**:527-531, 1957.

58 Visser, H. K. A., and Cost, W. S.: Acta Endocr. (Kobenhavn) **47**:589-612, 1964 (18-oxidase deficiency and hypoaldosteronism).

59 Wilkerson, J. A., Van De Water, J. M., and Goepfert, H.: Cancer **20**:1335-1342, 1967 (benign transformation of neuroblastoma).

59a Young, E. P., and Patrick, A. D.: Arch. Dis. Child. **45**:664-668, 1970 (Wolman's disease).

Hemorrhage and necrosis

60 Bove, K. E.: Arch. Path. (Chicago) **80**:418-425, 1965.

61 Fox, B.: Lancet **1**:600-602, 1969.

62 Golden, A.: Amer. J. Clin. Path. **19**:918-928, 1949 (adrenocortical necrosis).

63 Lever, W. F.: Medicine (Balt.) **32**:1-123, 1953 (pemphigus).

64 MacGillivray, I.: Brit. Med. J. **2**:212-216, 1951 (obstetric shock).

65 McKay, D. G.: Disseminated intravascular coagulation, New York, 1965, Hoeber Medical Division, Harper & Row, Publishers, p. 439.

66 Plaut, A.: Amer. J. Path. **31**:93-105, 1955 (adrenal venous thrombi).

67 Sevitt, S.: J. Clin. Path. **8**:185-194, 1955 (post-traumatic apoplexy).

68 Tedeschi, L. G., and Peabody, C. N.: Arch. Path. (Chicago) **73**:6-12, 1962.

Inflammation, atrophy, and Addison's disease

69 Carpenter, C. C. J., Solomon, N., and Silverberg, S. G.: Medicine (Balt.) **43**:153-180, 1964 (Schmidt's syndrome).

70 Das, G., and Becker, M.: J.A.M.A. **207**:2438, 1969 (oral contraceptives and adrenal insufficiency).

71 Frenkel, J. K.: Ann. N. Y. Acad. Sci. **84**:391-439, 1960.

72 Friedman, N. B.: Endocrinology **42**:181-200, 1948.

73 Goudie, R. B., Anderson, J. R., Grav, K. K., and Whyte, W. G.: Lancet **1**:1173-1176, 1966 (adrenal autoantibodies).

74 Guttman, P. H.: Arch. Path. (Chicago) **10**: 742, 895, 1930 (Addison's disease).

75 Heller, E. L., and Camarata, S. J.: Arch. Path. (Chicago) **49**:601-604, 1950 (amyloidosis and Addison's disease).

76 Jantet, G., Crocker, D. W., Shiraki, M., and Moore, F. D.: New Eng. J. Med. **269**:1-7, 1963 (posthypophysectomy atrophy).

77 Kiaer, W., and Norgaard, J. O. R.: Acta Path. Microbiol. Scand. **76**:229-238, 1969 (cytotoxic adrenalitis).

78 Nichols, J., and Delp, M.: J.A.M.A. **185**: 643-646, 1963 (atrophy with hypopituitarism).

79 Sunder, J. H., Bonessi, J. V., Balash, W. R., and Danowski, T. S.: New Eng. J. Med. **272**: 818-824, 1965 (familial Addison's disease).

80 Wuepper, K. D., Wegienka, L. C., and Fudenberg, H. H.: Amer. J. Med. **46**:202-216, 1969.

Degenerations and infiltrations; cortical nodularity

81 Braunstein, H., and Yamaguchi, B. T., Jr.: Amer. J. Path. **44**:113-126, 1964 (nodularity in chronic illness).

82 Currie, A. R., and Symington, T.: In Wolstenholme, G. E. W., and Cameron, M. P., editors: The human adrenal cortex, Boston, 1955, Little, Brown and Co., p. 396 (attempt to correlate histologic changes in anterior hypophysis and adrenal glands in various diseases in man).

82a Dobbie, J. W.: J. Path. **99**:1-18, 1969 (cortical nodules and hyperplasia).

83 Hart, M. N., and Cyrus, A., Jr.: Amer. J. Clin. Path. **49**:387-391, 1968.

84 Jenis, E. H., and Hertzog, R. W.: Arch. Path. (Chicago) **88**:530-539, 1969 (spironolactone effects).

85 Motlik, K., and Janouskova, M.: Virchow Arch. Path. Anat. **336**:427-446, 1963 (experimental hyaline droplet production).

86 Myers, K.: Nature (London) **213**:147-150, 1967 (nodularity in wild rabbits).

87 Ravid, M., Gafni, J., Sohar, E., and Missmahl, H.-P.: J. Clin. Path. **20**:15-20, 1967.

88 Shamma, A. H., Goddard, J. W., and Sommers, S. C.: J. Chronic Dis. **8**:587-598, 1958 (cortical nodularity and hypertension).

89 Stemmerman, M. G., and Auerbach, O.: Arch. Intern. Med. (Chicago) **74**:384-389, 1944 (amyloidosis).

90 Wilbur, O. M., Jr., and Rich, A. R.: Bull. Johns Hopkins Hosp. **93**:321-347, 1953 (tubular degeneration).

Hyperplasia, Cushing's syndrome, and adrenal virilism

91 Ashworth, C. T., and Garvey, R. F.: Amer. J. Path. **34**:1161-1171, 1958.

92 Azzopardi, J. G., and Williams, E. D.: Cancer **22**:274-286, 1968 (ectopic ACTH syndrome).

92a Baer, L., Sommers, S. C., Krakoff, L. R., Newton, M. R., and Laragh, J. H.: Circ. Res. **27** (suppl. 1):203-208, 1970 (pseudoprimary aldosteronism).

93 Beattie, M. K., and Heasman, M. A.: J. Path. Bact. **75**:83-94, 1958 (hypertension).

94 Carr, H. E., Jr., Curtis, G. W., and Thorn, G. W.: Amer. J. Surg. **107**:123-135, 1964 (correlations in Cushing's syndrome and adrenal virilism).

94a Choi, Y., Werk, E. E., and Sholiton, L. J.: Arch. Intern. Med. (Chicago) **125**:1045-1049, 1970 (autonomy of adrenal nodules in Cushing's syndrome).

95 Christy, N. P., and Laragh, J. H.: New Eng. J. Med. **265**:1083-1088, 1961 (hypokalemic alkalosis).

96 Cohen, R. B.: Cancer **19**:552-556, 1966 (histochemistry of Cushing's syndrome—adrenals).

97 Cohen, R. B., Chapman, W. B., and Castleman, B.: Amer. J. Path. **35**:537-561, 1959.

98 Cushing, H.: Bull. Johns Hopkins Hosp. **50**: 137-195, 1932.

98a Granger, P., and Genest, J.: Canad. Med. Ass. J. **103**:34-36, 1970 (adrenal glands in hypertension).

99 Kennedy, J. H., Williams, M. J., and Sommers, S. C.: Ann. Surg. **160**:90-94, 1964 (lung carcinoma and Cushing's syndrome).

100 Landing, B. H., and Feriozi, D.: J. Clin. Endocr. **14**:910-921, 1954 (iatrogenic effects).

101 Lim, N. Y., and Dingman, J. F.: New Eng. J. Med. **271**:1189-1194, 1964 (acromegaly).

102 Meador, C. K., Bowdoin, B., Owen, W. C., Jr., and Farmer, T. A., Jr.: J. Clin. Endocr. **27**:1255-1263, 1967 (nodular dysplasia and Cushing's syndrome).

103 Neville, A. M., and Symington, T.: J. Path. Bact. **93**:19-35, 1967.

104 Nichols, J.: Arch. Path. (Chicago) **62**:419-424, 1956 (low sodium diet).

105 O'Neal, L. W., Kipnis, D. M., Luse, S. A., Lacy, P. E., and Jarett, L.: Cancer **21**:1219-1232, 1968 (ectopic ACTH and other hormones).

106 O'Riordan, J. L. H., Blanshard, G. P., Moxham, A., and Nabarro, J. D. N.: Quart. J. Med. **35**:137-147, 1966.

107 Parker, T. G., and Sommers, S. C.: Arch. Surg. (Chicago) **72**:495-499, 1956 (hyperplasia and cancer).

108 Raker, J. W., Cope, O., and Ackerman, I. P.: Amer. J. Surg. **107**:153-172, 1964.

109 Reidbord, H., and Fisher, E. R.: Arch. Path. (Chicago) **86**:419-426, 1968 (ultrastructure of adrenal in Cushing's syndrome).

110 Ross, E. J., Marshall-Jones, P., and Friedman, M.: Quart. J. Med. **35**:149-192, 1966 (Cushing's syndrome).

111 Rutishauser, E., and Rosner, P.: Virchow Arch. Path. Anat. **337**:175-182, 1963 (pericapsular cortical tissue).

112 Wilens, S. L., and Plair, C. M.: Amer. J.

Path. **41:**225-232, 1962 (hyperplasia and arteriosclerosis).

Neoplasms
Adenomas, primary aldosteronism,
and carcinoma

112a Alterman, S. L., Dominguez, C., Lopez-Gomez, A., and Lieber, A. L.: Cancer **24:**602-609, 1969 (adrenal carcinoma and aldosteronism).

113 Bailey, R. E., Slade, C. I., Lieberman, A. H., and Luetscher, J. A., Jr.: J. Clin. Endocr. **20:** 457-465, 1960 (steroid production of adenomas).

114 Berdjis, C. C.: Oncologia (Basel) **15:**288-311, 1962 (multiple endocrine adenomas).

115 Besser, G. M., and Landon, J.: Brit. Med. J. **4:**552-554, 1968 (tumors with Cushing's syndrome).

116 Birke, G., Franksson, C., Gemzell, C. A., Moberger, G., and Plantin, L. O.: Acta Chir. Scand. **117:**233-246, 1959 (adrenal cortical tumors).

117 Cahill, G. F.: J.A.M.A. **138:**415-425, 1948 (adrenal neoplasms, especially cancer).

118 Conn, J. W., Knopf, R. F., and Nesbit, R. M.: Amer. J. Surg. **107:**159-172, 1964 (primary aldosteronism).

119 Cussen, L. J.: Med. J. Aust. **47**(1):39-41, 1960 (metastases to adrenal).

120 Daly, J. J.: Lancet **2:**710-711, 1956 (adenoma in diabetics).

121 Davis, W. W., Newsome, H. H., Jr., Wright, L. D., Jr., Hammond, W. G., Easton, J., and Bartter, F. C.: Amer. J. Med. **42:**642-647, 1967 (pseudoprimary aldosteronism).

122 De Lima, C. R., Capuano, Y., Ciscato, J. G., Carvalhal, S., and Chiorboli, E.: Obstet. Gynec. **28:**209-212, 1966 (ovarian adrenal rest tumor).

123 Gabrilove, J. L., Sharma, D. C., Wotiz, H. H., and Dorfman, R. I.: Medicine (Balt.) **44:**37-79, 1965 (adrenocortical feminizing tumors).

124 Hudson, J. B., Chobanian, A. V., and Relman, A. S.: New Eng. J. Med. **257:**529-536, 1957 (hypoaldosteronism).

125 Hutter, A. M., Jr., and Kayhoe, D. E.: Amer. J. Med. **41:**572-580, 1966 (adrenocortical carcinoma).

126 Kaplan, N. M.: J. Clin. Invest. **46:**728-734, 1967 (aldosteronoma steroids).

127 Kenny, F. M., Hashida, Y., Askari, H. A., Sieber, W. H., and Fetterman, G. H.: Amer. J. Dis. Child. **115:**445-458, 1968 (virilizing adrenal tumors).

128 Laragh, J. H., Cannon, P. J., and Ames, R. P.: Canad. Med. Ass. J. **90:**248-256, 1964 (secondary aldosteronism).

129 LeCompte, P. M.: Amer. J. Path. **20:**689-707, 1944 (adenoma versus pheochromocytoma).

130 Luders, C. J.: Virchow Arch. Path. Anat. **324:** 123-135, 1953 (pigmented adenoma).

131 Neville, A. M., and Symington, T.: Cancer **19:** 1854-1868, 1966.

132 Reidbord, H., and Fisher, E. R.: Arch. Path. (Chicago) **88:**155-161, 1969 (aldosteronoma ultrastructure).

133 Schteingart, D. E., Oberman, H. A., Friedman, B. A., and Conn, J. W.: Cancer **22:** 1005-1013, 1968 (adenoma versus carcinoma).

134 Sherwin, R. P.: Cancer **12:**861-877, 1959.

135 Silverstein, M. N.: Cancer **23:**142-144, 1969 (hypoglycemia with adrenal tumors).

136 Sommers, S. C., and Terzakis, J. A.: Amer. J. Clin. Path. **54:**303-310, 1970 (aldosteronoma).

137 Spain, D. M., and Weinsaft, P.: Arch. Path. (Chicago) **78:**231-233, 1964 (adenoma in aged women).

138 Walters, W., and Sprague, R. G.: J.A.M.A. **141:**653-656, 1949 (functioning tumors).

139 Wilkins, L.: J. Clin. Endocr. **8:**111-132, 1948 (feminizing tumors).

140 Wood, K. F., Lees, F., and Rosenthal, F. D.: Brit. J. Surg. **45:**41-48, 1957 (nonfunctional adrenal carcinoma).

Cysts; myelolipoma

141 Hodges, F. V., and Ellis, F. R.: Arch. Path. (Chicago) **66:**53-58, 1958.

142 McGregor, A. L.: Acta Med. Scand. suppl. 306, pp. 107-110, 1955 (hibernoma).

143 Mikail, M., and Kirshbaum, A.: J. Urol. **99:** 361-365, 1968.

144 Parsons, L., Jr., and Thompson, J. E.: New Eng. J. Med. **260:**12-15, 1959.

145 Plaut, A.: Amer. J. Path. **34:**487-515, 1958 (myelolipoma).

145a Tulcinsky, D. B., Deutsch, V., and Bubis, J. J.: Brit. J. Surg. **57:**465-467, 1970 (myelolipoma).

Pheochromocytoma; other neoplasms

146 Dick, J. C., Ritchie, G. M., and Thompson, H.: J. Clin. Path. **8:**89-98, 1955 (adrenal melanoma).

147 Edmunds, L. H., Jr.: Ann. Thorac. Surg. **2:** 742-751, 1966 (mediastinal pheochromocytoma).

148 Engelman, K.: Bull. N. Y. Acad. Med. **45:** 851-858, 1969 (associated syndromes).

149 Gifford, R. W., Jr., Kvale, W. F., Maher, F. T., Roth, G. M., and Priestley, J. T.: Proc. Mayo Clin. **39:**281-302, 1964.

150 Ransom, C. L., Landes, R. R., and Gaddy, C. G.: J. Urol. **79:**368-376, 1958 (malignant pheochromocytoma).

151 Rona, G.: Canad. Med. Ass. J. **91:**303-305, 1964 (brown fat changes).

151a Sharp, W. V., and Platt, R. L.: Angiology **22:**141-146, 1971 (pheochromocytoma and Lindau–von Hippel disease).

152 Sherwin, R. P.: Amer. J. Surg. **107:**136-143, 1964.

153 Silva, T. F., and Sommers, S. C.: Amer. J. Med. Sci. **236:**700-704, 1958 (renal changes with pheochromocytoma).

154 Smithwick, R. H., Greer, W. E. R., Robertson, C. W., and Wilkins, R. W.: New Eng. J. Med. **242:**252-257, 1950.

155 Steiner, A. L., Goodman, A. D., and Powers, S. R.: Medicine (Balt.) **47:**371-409, 1968 (familial endocrine neoplasms).

156 Tannenbaum, M.: In Pathology annual, vol. 5 (S. C. Sommers, editor), New York, 1970, Appleton-Century-Crofts, pp. 145-171.

157 Van Vliet, P. D., Burchell, H. B., and Titus, J. L.: New Eng. J. Med. **274:**1102-1108, 1966 (myocardial lesions with pheochromocytoma).

Chapter 37

Female genitalia

Arthur T. Hertig and Hazel Gore

The pathologic anatomy of the female genital system is so intimately interwoven with its embryology, anatomy, endocrinology, and physiology that a chapter on this field in a textbook of general pathology can do no more than give the essentials. Therefore, the student may well wish to consult more extensive texts such as Novak and Woodruff,[18] Netter,[17] Eastman and Hellman,[5] Parkes,[21] Greep,[10] Patten,[33] Papanicolaou,[20] and Zuckerman.[27]

This chapter, arranged by broad subjects rather than by the component parts of the genital system, is essentially the subject matter presented at the Harvard Medical School to the undergraduate students in general pathology and to the postgraduate students in obstetrics and gynecologic pathology. It represents the experience of the senior author in the pathology laboratory of the Boston Lying-in Hospital for thirty years and at the Free Hospital for Women for twenty-five years and in reviewing referred material at Harvard Medical School for the past fourteen years.[12] It is colored by his experience and interest in embryology, clinical obstetrics, and, in general, clinicopathologic correlation.

ANATOMY AND PHYSIOLOGY

The form and function of the various portions of the female genital tract will be reviewed only briefly and to emphasize those features of potential pathologic significance.

Vulva. The vulva consists of the mons veneris, labia majora and labia minora, clitoris, hymen, and vestibule, into which open the urethra, vagina, and minor and major vestibular (Bartholin's) mucus-producing glands. The skin of the mons veneris and external surface of the labia majora is of usual type except for the presence of apocrine sweat glands, which develop at puberty, possess myoepithelium, and are involved in extramammary Paget's disease, hidradenomas, and occasionally hidradenocarcinoma. The inner aspect of the labia majora and all of the labia minora have no hair, less keratinization of the epidermis, and abundant sebaceous glands. The vulva, subject to all the diseases to which the skin is subject elsewhere in the body, is also subject to the specific venereal infections—condyloma acuminatum, lymphopathia venereum, granuloma inguinale, and leukoplakic vulvitis, a precancerous dermatosis. The paraurethral ducts and glands of Skene (homologous to the prostate) and Bartholin's glands (homologous to the bulbourethral glands in the male) are susceptible to and act as reservoirs for gonorrheal infections.

Vagina. The vagina, a collapsed fibromuscular tube, is lined by nonkeratinized stratified squamous epithelium resting upon a thick vascular mucosal stroma surrounded by a double-layered smooth muscle coat that merges into the surrounding endopelvic fascia. The mucosa normally contains no glands although, occasionally, mucus-secreting glands of aberrant cervical or mesonephric origin may be present in the fornices and are potential sources of tumors. Remnants of Gartner's duct (mesonephric) are always present within the wall laterally and may form cysts or undergo neoplasia. The squamous epithelium, under the influence of estrogens, which affect the glycogen content of all but the basal cells, is thick at birth and during pregnancy but thin during childhood, the puerperium, and after the menopause. It probably varies in thickness and histologic pattern during the menstrual cycle. Although the histologic pattern is unsettled, the exfoliative cytologic pattern is well correlated with the various phases of this cycle. Thus, during the early proliferative (postmenstrual) phase, the few but predominant cells are of the precornified type. They gradually become numerous and of cornified type as ovulation approaches. Following ovulation, the numerous individual cells revert to the precornified type with angular folded edges, but later on in the premenstrual phase, these cells are clumped, fragmented, and associated with mucus and polymorphonuclear leukocytes. During childhood, the cells are predominantly basal in type. As pregnancy advances, the numerous precornified cells (often clumped and associated with polymorphonuclear leukocytes) become fewer, smaller, and boat shaped, the so-called "navicular cells." During the puerperium, the cells are predominantly basal, with a few precornified and cornified cells mixed with inflammatory debris. This is similar to the postmenopausal smear, except that the exfoliated cells are all of the basal type and the inflammatory exudate is greater. Knowledge of the normal variation in the vaginal cytology is necessary to interpret the abnormal cells exfoliated from malignant pelvic neoplasms.

Uterus. The nulliparous uterus weighs 40 gm to 50 gm and measures approximately 7.5 cm in length including the cervix, 5 cm in width, and 2.5 cm in thickness at the fundus. The parous uterus weighs 50 gm to 70 gm and is increased in all its dimensions by approximately 1.2 cm. At birth, the cervix is larger than the corpus uteri, but in adults it forms only one-third of the organ. Following the menopause, there is more or less reversal to the infantile form, although the actual size is variable.

At the junction of the cervix and body of the uterus is a short (0.5 cm), ill-defined isthmus that becomes the lower uterine segment during pregnancy. Its mucosa, comparable to the basal endometrium, contains only a few nonmucus-secreting glands in a dense fibroendometrial stroma. Glands and stroma undergo only minimal change during the menstrual cycle and pregnancy. This thin mucosa is confusing in endometrial biopsies or curettage specimens and is transitional between the mucus-secreting endocervix and the typical endometrium lining the flat, triangular-shaped uterine cavity. The latter measures from 3 cm to 3.5 cm in depth and 2.5 cm to 3 cm in width at its base, which lies between the ostia of the fallopian tubes. Therefore, the uterine cavity lies entirely within the corpus, the fundus being above the uterine cavity and between the isthmic regions of the tubes.

Cervix. The cervix is a thick-walled, cylindrical structure composed largely of fibrous tissue. Anatomically, it consists of the portio vaginalis (anatomic portio) and the endocervix. The anatomic portio is that part of the cervix lying external to the external os. Its surface is visualized by the clinician by speculum examination. It includes squamous epithelium and subepithelial stroma and the columnar epithelium and stroma of a clinical erosion or an eversion. The anatomic endocervix lies between the external os and internal os. Histologically, there are three zones, which do not necessarily correspond with anatomic zones. The histologic portio consists of cervical stroma without glands covered by squamous epithelium. The transitional zone, which lies between the histologic portio and endocervix, consists of endocervical stroma and glands (more accurately, crypts[6]) covered by some form of squamous epithelium, often immature. The histologic endocervix consists of endocervical stroma containing glands with surface and glandular columnar epithelium.

In the nullipara, the external os is dimple-like. It may coincide with the squamocolumnar junction but often does not. The endocervical canal is fusiform and flattened anteroposteriorly, the opposing mucosae showing a herringbone pattern of ridges called plicae palmatae, which act as valves. In the multipara, the external os shows more or less lateral or stellate healed lacerations, accompanied by variable degrees of endocervical eversion and erosion. The squamocolumnar junction is now irregular and usually visible from the vagina. The resulting inflammation of the thus-exposed endocervix is accompanied by variable degrees of proliferative repair of squamous and columnar epithelium, the latter usually showing squamous metaplasia (subcylindrical cell hyperplasia) of varying amount and maturity. The mouths of the mucus-secreting endocervical glands in the inflamed area may be blocked by epithelial repair or metaplasia, or both, resulting in nabothian cysts up to 5 cm in diameter.

Histologic changes in the cervical mucosa analogous to those in the endometrium and tube during the menstrual cycle are debatable, although there is no doubt that cervical mucus is more abundant and more permeable to spermatozoa at the time of ovulation. Following the menopause, both types of epithelium become thinner, with virtual cessation of mucin production by the endocervix.

During pregnancy, the increased vascularity, edema, and glandular hyperplasia accompanied by increased mucus secretion result in eversion of the endocervix in the vicinity of the external os. The stage of the immediate gestation and the presence of prior pregnancy will determine the degree and maturity of endocervical subcylindrical cell hyperplasia which, on occasion, may mimic carcinoma in situ but, unlike the latter, tends to involute postpartum. There is probably also a hormonal component in the etiology of such hyperplasia because endocervices in all normal newborn infants show this process, often to a marked degree. A significant number of normal cervices biopsied during pregnancy reveal a pseudodecidual reaction of the subepithelial (usually endocervical) stroma. This reaction is dependent upon estrogen and progesterone stimulation and may be slight or marked, diffuse or patchy, and it may or may not give rise to clinical bleeding. Endometrial glands are not present. Hence, the condition is not endometriosis with superimposed decidual reaction but is related to ectopic endometrial stroma present throughout the genital system, including the retroperitoneal tissue of the tubes, ovaries, and pelvis itself. Its possible relationship to the genesis of endometriosis is discussed elsewhere.

Ovary. In the sexually mature adult, the gonadotropins of the anterior lobe of the pituitary gland and the neuroendocrine control of the hypothalamus regulate the cyclic production of steroid ovarian hormones by the graafian follicle and corpus luteum. Although pure follicle-stimulating hormone (FSH) causes development of follicles to the antrum stage, the addition of luteinizing hormone (LH) is required for full development of the follicle (and presumably ovulation) and for adequate estrogen formation.[8] Further, the follicle is directly stimulated by estrogen, which facilitates the action of FSH and LH and later affects the life of the corpus luteum.

Luteotropic hormone (LTH) is required in addition for adequate progesterone formation in animals, but its role in human physiology is uncertain. Ovulation, with subsequent corpus luteum formation, is required for significant progesterone formation, although on occasion this has been observed with luteinized unruptured follicles.

On occasion, ovulation has been induced in an amenorrheic woman by a combination of human follicle-stimulating hormone and a luteinizing hormone—usually in the form of human chorionic gonadotropin (HCG). Use of materials from other species has involved problems of antibody production. Not only has Gemzell[7] produced ovulation by FSH and HCG, but there also have been successful pregnancies among his patients. More recently, ovulation has been induced by clomiphene citrate, MRL-41, a nonestrogenic compound related to chlorotrianisene, and there have been some subsequent normal pregnancies.[9]

During the classic twenty-eight-day menstrual cycle, the output of steroids is lowest in the first week, and it rises during the second week to a well-defined peak that coincides insofar as may be presently determined with ovulation. Its subsequent fall is accompanied by uterine bleeding in about 5% of patients. There is a subsequent rise usually to a point lower than the "ovulation peak," but this may be ill defined. There is a fall prior to menstruation.

Coincident with the peak of estrogen production, progesterone is elaborated presumably by the corpus luteum.[25] The precise type of cells involved is uncertain. Estrogen and progesterone reach plateau levels during the twentieth to twenty-third days. This coincides with the time during which the ovum is implanting, the endometrium is most edematous, and the corpus luteum is morphologically most active. In the absence of pregnancy and consequent lack of chorionic gonadotropin, degeneration of the corpus luteum ensues. Electron microscopic studies of the active and regressing luteal cell of the corpus luteum of the menstrual cycle and of the corpus luteum of pregnancy have revealed specific patterns that appear related to hormonal production.[1, 2] Estrogen gradually falls, and its urinary excretion begins to rise about the eighth day of the cycle. Blood progesterone, on the other hand, is essentially absent between the onset of menstruation and until the twelfth day, two days prior to ovulation, when blood estrogen reaches its peak.

The general morphologic details of follicle maturation, ovulation, corpus luteum formation, and involution of follicular derivatives may be gained from standard textbooks of histology, but there is still much to be learned. Oogenesis in the human ovary occurs only during fetal life and ceases by the time of birth.[28] It has been shown that germ cells increase steadily from 600,000 two months after fertilization to 6,800,000 in the fifth month, when they have reached a maximum. Thereafter, there is a decline, so that there are about 2,000,000 at birth, but half are atretic. By the seventh year, only 300,000 oocytes persist. Well-developed primordial follicles with granulosa, theca interna, and theca externa layers were previously thought not to come under the influence of the follicle-stimulating hormone until they contained an antrum or cavity within the mass of granulosa cells. Ryan[21a] has stated that pure FSH causes development of the follicle to the antrum stage. Of the several follicles in both ovaries thus stimulated during any one cycle, one ordinarily gains ascendancy, reaches 1.5 cm to 2 cm in diameter as it migrates toward the thinning cortex, and ovulates, probably by a slow process rather than a sudden rupture. The ovum-containing follicular fluid is aspirated by the oviduct, whose fimbriated end is said to be closely approximated to the ovary during ovulation. All other antrum-containing follicles are said to involute after ovulation and before the next cycle begins.

The pathologic aberrations of the normal ovarian cycle result in such important conditions as the following:

1 Failure of ovulation, with resulting sterility, hyperplastic endometrial changes, and one or more cystic follicles or isolated follicle cysts
2 Hemorrhage from recent or old corpus luteum, with or without resulting intraperitoneal hemorrhage
3 Corpus luteum cyst formation, usually associated with pregnancy and resulting in atypical hyperplastic secretory endometrium
4 Varying degrees of persistence of follicular wall elements, with or without luteinization thereof, and with or without associated ovulation, but usually resulting in abnormalities of the menstrual cycle

The ovary in pregnancy may be regarded as pathologic by the uninitiated. It is moderately edematous and always contains foci of pseudodecidua (Fig. 37-53) beneath the germinal epithelium. Such foci occasionally have been mistaken, both grossly and microscopically, for neoplasms. Aside from the obviously enlarged corpus luteum of pregnancy, which is endocrinologically vital to the gestation for about two months, the follicles in varying stages of development and atresia undergo a marked thecal lutein hyperplasia. This reaches its peak of development with hydatidiform mole and choriocarcinoma, the ovaries showing numerous cysts, reaching 3 cm in diameter on occasion, and possessing a thin yellow wall due to the luteinization of the theca interna. Such follicular cysts and cystic follicles involute when the chorionic gonadotropic stimulus is removed.

As the ovary ages, it becomes smaller, firmer, and convoluted, mainly at the expense of the ova, primordial follicles, and cortex. The medulla remains relatively unchanged except for increased prominence of sclerotic vessels. Corpora albicantia persist in the medulla for years postmenopausally. The cortex becomes thin and atrophic and tends to resemble ordinary fibrous tissue except when it undergoes hyperplasia. Minor degrees of the latter are relatively common and probably account for the reappearance of menopausal symptoms during the postmenopausal period. Moderate to marked degrees of hyperplasia (Fig. 37-1) of this presumably estrogenic and probably progesteronic thecal stroma are approximately twice as common in patients with endometrial carcinoma as in comparable control patients of the same age.

Endometrium. The histologic details of the changes that the endometrium undergoes during a classic cycle of twenty-eight days may be found in standard textbooks of histology and gynecologic pathology and in periodicals[3, 19] The cycle is ordinarily described as beginning on the day of onset of menstruation

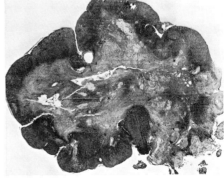

Fig. 37-1 Ovary of 54-year-old postmenopausal patient showing marked cortical stromal hyperplasia resulting in presumed mild estrogenic hormone secretion. Note dense convoluted cervix with infolding of surface epithelium resulting in germinal inclusion cyst formation. (×7.)

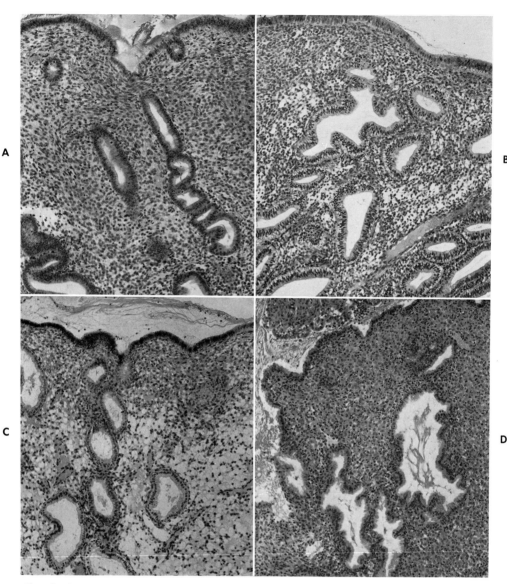

Fig. 37-2 A, Late proliferative endometrium at or about time of ovulation. Tortuous, pseudostratified glands with many mitoses are characteristic. Stroma, without predecidual reaction, may have variable degree of edema. **B,** Sixteen-day secretory endometrium. This early postovulatory endometrium is characterized by tortuous growing glands with irregular vacuolization due to accumulation of glycogen in cytoplasm beneath nuclei. **C,** Twenty-two-day secretory endometrium. Significant features of this stage are massive stromal edema, tortuosity of glands nearing secretory exhaustion, thin-walled blood vessels, and absence of predecidua. This coincides with peak of corpus luteum activity during which time ovum is in process of implanting. **D,** Premenstrual endometrium. This phase is characterized by nearly complete predecidual transformation of stroma, secretory exhaustion of glands which have serrated pattern, and inspissation of secretion. There is also leukocytic infiltration—both polymorphonuclear and monocytic. (×150; from Noyes, R. W., Hertig, A. T., and Rock, J.: Fertil. Steril. **1:**3-25, 1950.)

with the ischemic necrosis of predecidual stroma associated with hemorrhage that undergoes fibrinolysis and accompanied by involution of the remaining secretorily exhausted glands and predecidual stroma. The basal portion of the endometrium is altered little except in pregnancy, although on occasion there may be cyclic glandular response in some foci of the basal part. The middle part waxes and wanes, whereas the upper part is lost during menstruation.

Morphologically, the cycle truly begins

about the seventh day, when the surface epithelium has regenerated from the glands and the latter have involuted to become straight tubular structures with pseudostratified epithelium showing active growth. The stroma is usually edematous, rapidly growing, and of "naked nucleus" type, with wispy cytoplasmic processes joining nuclei of contiguous stromal cells (Fig. 37-2, *A*). The vascular system includes the tips of spiral arterioles, venules, and the intervening capillary bed. From this stage until ovulation (fourteen days ± two days prior to the next expected period), the stroma and glands grow, under the stimulus of a rising estrogen level, until the endometrium reaches a thickness of about 2 mm to 3 mm. It shows markedly tortuous, rapidly growing glands whose cytoplasm is rich in ribonucleic acid and alkaline phosphatase but poor in acid phosphatase, glycogen, and mucopolysaccharides.[16]

About thirty-six hours following ovulation, the first evidence of corpus luteum activity is seen as irregular basal vacuolization of glandular epithelium by the accumulation of glycogen (Fig. 37-2, *B*). During the phase of active secretion, from the seventeenth through the nineteenth day, the segmenting ovum is in the uterine cavity as a free blastocyst that implants on about the twentieth day. Then begins the phase of stromal edema, with continued but declining glandular secretion from the twentieth through the twenty-third day (Fig. 37-2, *C*), during which time the ovum is embedding and the corpus luteum is at its peak of activity. Until the twenty-fourth day, it is impossible to distinguish between pregnant and nonpregnant endometrium unless one finds the ovum, since the corpus luteum is uniformly active during the first nine days of its life whether the patient is pregnant or not. If the patient is not pregnant, the corpus luteum functionally and morphologically involutes, although the predecidual reaction (Fig. 37-2, *D*) in the stroma progresses until menstruation ensues on the twenty-eighth day. If the patient is pregnant, the corpus luteum is functionally and morphologically altered from the twenty-fourth day onward, with associated progestational hyperplasia of the endometrium. This morphologic entity is visible throughout the upper "two-thirds" of the endometrium and consists of:

1 Recrudescence of glandular secretion
2 Accentuation of stromal edema
3 Normal development of predecidual

reaction, beginning about the spiral arterioles and beneath the surface epithelium
4 Increased vascular prominence, with congestion of arterioles, capillaries, and venules[11]

This distinctive picture gradually changes after the first missed menstrual period to become the typical decidua of pregnancy.

Histochemically, secretory or progestational endometrium has increasing acid phosphatase, glycogen, and mucopolysaccharides, with decreasing ribonucleic acid and alkaline phosphatase.

The significant pathologic aberrations of the normal endometrial cycle are as follows:
1 Irregular focal shedding of progestational endometrium, resulting in irregular ripening with resultant bleeding
2 Hyperplasia due to anovulatory ovarian cycles associated with cystic follicles, follicle cysts, or corpus luteum cysts
3 Neoplasia, which is usually the long-delayed aftermath of hyperplasia

It is of interest that neoplastic endometrium has a histochemical pattern comparable to that of secretory endometrium, strongly suggesting that stimulus from both estrogen and progesterone rather than estrogen alone is involved in the genesis of endometrial carcinoma.[16]

EMBRYOLOGY

Knowledge of the embryology of the female genital system is necessary in order to understand its structure and function, as well as its congenital anomalies and tumors. Its development is not only intimately associated with that of the mesonephros, ureter, urinary bladder, rectum, and anus, but also common anlagen participate in the development of the gonads and external genitalia of both sexes. Moreover, two ductal systems develop in every embryo, each system becoming either functional or vestigial, depending upon the sex of the embryo.

A description of the essential phases in the development of the genital organs follows.

Ovary. The indifferent stage of the gonad makes its first appearance as paired thickenings on the ventromedial aspect of the dorsally situated mesonephroi late in the fifth week of development (6.7 mm embryo). Three separate tissues participate in the formation of the gonad:
1 The thickened coelomic epithelium overlying the gonadal ridge

2 The underlying mesenchyma

3 The primordial germ cells

It is generally accepted that the primordial germ cells arise in the early stage of the embryonic disk but are first definitely recognized in the caudal aspect of the yolk sac entoderm of the 3 mm embryo.[36] The germ cells subsequently migrate in and/or are carried passively via the gut epithelium, its mesentery, and the gonadal coelomic epithelium until they reach their ultimate destination in the gonad at the 5 mm stage.[32] This observation has given rise to the erroneous conclusion that the primordial germ cells arose in this so-called "germinal epithelium." The latter is, however, active and thickened and is said by Gillman[29] to give rise to the primary sex cords that result in the granulosa cells of the graafian follicle and the Sertoli cells of the testis. The underlying mesenchyme gives rise to the ovarian theca and the testicular interstitial cells. Judging from tumors arising from gonadal stroma and germinal epithelium, it would seem to us, however, that the gonadal mesenchyme is totipotential for both epithelial and stromal elements of the developing gonad. Such tumors, often producing estrogenic or androgenic steroid hormones or both, show a spectrum of these specific gonadal epithelial and stromal elements, whereas the germinal epithelial tumors form cystomas usually without specific gonadal stroma or steroid hormone production. Admittedly, embryologic facts should not be deduced from oncologic data, but usually a tumor recapitulates some phase in the histogenesis of its parent tissue.

The definitive testis is recognizable at about the 20 mm stage (eighth week of development) by the isolated primordial germ cells lying along the primitive sex cords that gradually evolve into seminiferous tubules, the latter surrounded by interstitial cells. These make their first appearance in the 30 mm stage (ninth week of development) and reach their peak of development at midterm (160 mm), subsequently undergoing involution.

The definitive ovary is recognizable also at about the 20 mm stage by the irregular clusters of sex cords surrounding the isolated primordial germ cells. The sex cord cells, whatever their origin, form primitive granulosa cells that "protect" the primordial ova from the stroma derived from the mesovarial mesenchyme, which invades the medulla and thence the cortex. Such stroma becomes the thecal element of the graafian follicle and

first appears in 100 mm embryos (fourteenth week of development) but is recognized as thecal in nature only when the embryo exceeds 245 mm (twenty-seventh week of development).

Genital ducts. The dorsal paired mesonephric (wolffian) and paramesonephric (müllerian) ducts form the male and female ductal systems, respectively. Both are present during the indifferent stage of sexual differentiation, although the mesonephric system develops first.

The mesonephric duct, succeeding the pronephric duct, which arises during the third week (nine to ten somites), grows caudally to join the allantois (primitive urinary bladder) during the fifth week (7 mm to 8 mm). The metanephric diverticulum, destined to form the ureter and renal pelvis, arises at this time from the mesonephric duct where the latter joins the allantois. In the male, the upper portion of the mesonephric duct, with the few persisting mesonephric tubules opposite the testis, becomes the epididymis and vas deferens. In the female embryo after the tenth week (42 mm to 50 mm stage), the mesonephric tubules and duct begin to undergo atrophy. Remnants persist into adult life, however, as the epoophoron and paraoophoron of the ovarian hilum and mesosalpinx, mesonephric tubules, and ducts in the musculature of the cervix and Gartner's duct rests in the lateral wall of the vagina. Such remnants form simple cysts and also tumors of the mesonephroma group in any of these diverse locations.

The paramesonephric (müllerian) ducts arise early in the seventh week (11 mm stage) lateral and parallel to the mesonephric ducts by an invagination of the coelomic epithelium opposite the cephalic end of the mesonephros. The solid tips burrow caudally through the mesenchyme beneath the coelomic epithelium and cross the mesonephric duct anteriorly at the level of the caudal end of the mesonephros during the eighth week (23 mm stage). By the ninth week (30 mm stage), these paired ducts have fused in the midline and have joined the posterior wall of the urogenital sinus to form the müllerian tubercle. By the eleventh week (56 mm stage), the fusion is complete to form the uterovaginal canal. The unfused paramesonephric ducts form the fallopian tubes, whereas the fused portions form the uterus and a significant portion of the vagina (the upper four-fifths, according to Koff[31]). The lack of agreement as to the extent of müllerian component of the vagina is due to the replacement of the primitive solid epithelium of the müllerian tubercle by that of the urogenital sinus. Patten[33] points out that although the vaginal epithelium may be largely derived from the urogenital sinus, the wall of the vagina is of müllerian origin, and its junction with the vestibule, derived from the urogenital sinus, is marked by the hymen. The possibility has been raised that the epithelia of both vagina and cervix are derived from the urogenital sinus. It has been suggested that this may explain some pathologic changes in the cervix.[6] In the male embryo, after the beginning of the ninth week (30 mm stage), the paramesonephric duct begins to undergo atrophy, presumably because of the growth of the testicular interstitial cells. Remnants of the müllerian ducts persist into adult life only as the appendix testis and the utriculus masculinus of the prostatic urethra.

External genitalia. At the beginning of the eighth week (20 mm), the external genitalia of both sexes are often indistinguishable, since the size and shape of the homologous parts (the genital tubercle, the urogenital sinus opening, genital folds, and genital swellings) are apparently similar. As a result, the majority of embryos of this stage are said to be females, although the gonads are beginning to be histologically separable. During this stage of the phallus period,[34] the male external genitalia are said to be distinguishable from the female by the greater prominence of the urogenital opening in the former. Moreover, the urogenital opening in the male extends the length of the phallus and is more prominent distally, whereas in the female it extends only to the glans and is more prominent proximally.

With continued development in the male, the genital tubercle becomes larger to form the penis, the urethral groove becomes longer and enclosed by the genital folds to form the penile urethra, with coincident separation of the urogenital sinus from the anus, and the genital swellings fuse in the midline to form the scrotum. With continued development in the female, the genital tubercle grows less rapidly, and curves gradually to form the clitoris, the urethra maintains its relationship to the urogenital sinus which widens and deepens to form the vestibule, the genital folds form the labia minora, and the genital swellings become the labia majora. By the end of the tenth week (50 mm), the sex can be correctly determined from the external genitalia, whereas during the eighth week (21 mm to 30 mm) in only 28%, during the ninth week (31 mm to 40 mm) in 36%, and during the tenth week (41 mm to 50 mm) in 90% can the sex be correctly determined.[35]

It is during this critical period when the definitive genital systems are being established in both sexes that congenital anomalies develop.

CONGENITAL ANOMALIES

The several types of congenital anomalies affecting the internal and external genitalia are (1) absence (aplasia or agenesis), (2) hypoplasia (dysgenesis), (3) atresia of tubular or membranous structures, (4) failure of müllerian ducts to fuse in the midline, (5) accessory structures, (6) abnormalities of position, and (7) conditions of intersexuality. Since abnormal gonadal development is often the key to other congenital abnormalities and the abnormalities may involve more than one part of the genital system, the entire subject is discussed briefly as a part of each organ system or region.

Ovary. Absence of the ovary may be unilateral or bilateral. If unilateral, it is almost invariably accompanied by absence of müllerian and wolffian duct derivatives, together with the kidney on that side, presumably as a result of unilateral failure of the urogenital ridge to develop. Even though the ovary is present, unilateral müllerian abnormalities usually are accompanied by ipsilateral ureteral and renal defects, whereas bilateral abnormalities of fusion or complete absence of müllerian structures show less correlation (35%) with renal defects.[48]

Bilateral ovarian agenesis or Turner's syndrome was formerly thought to involve chromosomal females but has now been found to have an XO structure and usually only forty-five chromosomes, although they may be mosaics, XX/XO, or XXX/XO, and rarely XX.[44] The internal and external genitalia with secondary sexual characteristics are of infantile female type, except that the gonad is composed of a minute white fibrous mass or ridge without anatomic evidence of either female or male gonadal elements. This syndrome is associated with congenital anomalies of the skeletal, cardiovascular, and nervous systems—most commonly including short stature (averaging 52 in), web neck, shield-like chest, and cubitus valgus (increased carrying angle). Less commonly, there occur co-arctation of the aorta, hypertension, deafness, mental deficiency, ocular disorders, spina bifida, syndactylism, and malformations of the fingers, toes, and ribs. The gonadotropin level is elevated as in castrated individuals, whereas the 17-ketosteroids are only slightly reduced.

This severe gonadal dysgenesis emphasizes that the embryonic genital ducts are hormonally controlled by their corresponding gonads and that in the absence of an embryonic gonad the müllerian system predominates, presumably because of maternal estrogenic stimulation. Patients with the Klinefelter-Reifenstein-Albright syndrome (sclerosing tubular degeneration of the testis but with interstitial cells), although apparently males with varying degrees of eunuchoidal or female habitus, have an XXY sex chromatin structure and a total of forty-seven chromosomes.[44] A similar condition may occur in chromatin-negative individuals, and this usually is referred to as chromatin-negative Klinefelter's syndrome. Mosaics are common among patients with Klinefelter's syndrome, and a variety of these has been recorded.

True accessory ovaries are rarely seen, may be accompanied by an accessory fallopian tube, are either intraperitoneal or extraperitoneal, and may undergo neoplasia. False accessory ovaries, also uncommon, are merely lobulations of a single organ. Small masses of accessory ovarian tissue may be found in sites occupied by the ovary during its embryonic development and descent, including the hilum, mesovarium, and round and broad ligaments.

Fallopian tubes. Unilateral absence is uncommon and is associated with ureteral and renal abnormalities on the affected side. The rare bilateral absence may be associated with uterine and vaginal agenesis but with normal ovaries attached laterally to the free edge of an "empty" broad ligament, the latter formed by the transverse pelvic septum. More commonly, the ampullar portion of one tube may be absent or rudimentary because of torsion and subsequent ischemic atrophy. Supernumerary tubes with or without ovaries are rare, but duplication of the ampular region (accessory tubes) and accessory tubal ostia are relatively common. Accessory tubes arising anywhere along the course of a tube never communicate with its lumen, but the accessory ostia located near the main ostium always do. Unilateral or bilateral segmental atresia and

persistence of the coiled fetal pattern are other rare anomalies of unknown etiology.

Uterus, vagina, and vulva. The commonest anomaly of the uterus, vagina, and vulva (derived from the fused midline portions of the müllerian ducts caudal to the mesonephroi), is failure of fusion at various levels and to varying degrees. Complete failure of fusion results in two complete genital tracts (uterus duplex separatus), each consisting of ovary, tube, uterus, cervix, and vagina. Pregnancy may occur in either or both uteri. Minimal degrees of fusion failure result in an essentially normal-appearing uterus containing a partial sagittal septum at the fundus (uterus subseptus unicollis). All gradations between complete and minimal failure of fusion occur as follows: (1) uterus septus (two uterine and cervical canals), (2) uterus bicornis unicolli (two horns with one cervix), and (3) uterus duplex bicornis (two horns with two cervices). The asymmetrically developed uterus (uterus unicornis) has a normal ovary, tube, and vagina, but the opposite müllerian and wolffian duct derivatives are absent.

Absence or atresia of the vagina (gynatresia) is said to be due to the failure of the vaginal portions of the müllerian ducts to fuse, followed by disappearance of these primordia. The cause is unknown. The external and the remainder of the internal genitalia are normal. The rare transverse septum is a variant, although a mild degree, of atresia.

Varying degrees of sagittal septation occur in the vagina—from complete duplication associated with uterus duplex separatus to partial septation at the introitus associated with otherwise normal internal genitalia. The complete or partial duplication may be bilaterally equal or unequal, the latter often associated with partial deficiencies of the müllerian duct more proximally and hence associated with anomalies of the urinary system of that side. The anomalous vagina may or may not communicate with the main vagina or the vestibule at the introitus. Associated with such internal duplication there may rarely occur duplication of the external genitalia, including both labia, clitoris, and urethra. Other rare anomalies of the external genitalia include fusion of the labia minora, absence of the mons veneris or clitoris, and common urethral-hymeneal or retrovestibular opening. Rarely, accessory breast tissue (from "milk line") is present in the labia majora and presumably may lactate, undergo cystic change, or develop a malignant tumor. Imperforate hymen, although uncommon, is clinically the most important vulvar anomaly.

Intersexuality. In anomalies of intersexuality, the gonads of an individual may be of one or both sexes, but the ductal and external genital systems show varying degrees of indifferent or heterologous development. The two main types of such ambisexual development with normal chromosomal complement are true hermaphroditism and pseudohermaphroditism.

Barr[37] has shown that, even in true hermaphrodites, examination of the nuclei in skin biopsies will reveal either the female or the male chromatin pattern. Of his nine cases, six were female and three male. Of sixty-four pseudohermaphrodites, the thirty of the female type caused by adrenal hyperplasia all showed the peripheral planoconvex chromatin mass characteristic of the female, and the one female type of nonadrenal origin also showed the female pattern, whereas thirty-three male pseudohermaphrodites all showed the male chromatin pattern. There is some experimental evidence that an excess of the heterologous sex hormone during the sexually indifferent stage of embryonic development may produce pseudohermaphrodites in animals but not in man.[41]

Thompson and Thompson's classification of intersexual states (with a few comments from their text incorporated)[24] follows.

A Intersexual conditions with normal chromosome complement
  1 True hermaphroditism
  2 Pseudohermaphroditism
    a Female
      (1) Adrenogenital syndrome
      (2) Excess of maternal sex hormones
        (a) Endogenous
        (b) Exogenous
      (3) Idiopathic
    b Male
      (1) Testicular feminization
      (2) Idiopathic
B Intersexual conditions with abnormal chromosome complement
  1 Without a Y chromosome
    a Aneuploidy X
      (1) XO—Turner's syndrome (XX/XO; XXX/XO; XX)
      (2) XXX—Superfemale (mental retardation; ? also normal)
      (3) Other
        (a) XXXX—retarded
        (b) XXXXX—retarded
    b Abnormal structure of X
      (1) Deletion
      (2) Isochromosome
      (3) Ring
  2 With a Y chromosome
    a Aneuploidy of X and/or Y
      (1) XXY—Klinefelter's syndrome
      (2) Other
        (a) XXY
        (b) XXXYY } All like Klinefelter's
        (c) XXXXY
    b Abnormal structure of Y
      (1) Small—male or female, but sexually abnormal
      (2) Large—normal male
  3 Mosaics—extreme variability of phenotypes*

True hermaphroditism is the presence in an individual of (1) an ovotestis (both gonadal elements in a single organ) but without other gonadal elements, (2) bilateral ovotestes, (3) an ovotestis in combination with either an ovary or a testis, or (4) an ovary and a testis.[46] In forty cases collected by Weed et al.,[46] four of the patients had the first condition, eleven had the second, fourteen had the third (seven patients with each), and eleven had the fourth condition. Although both types of gonads are represented to some degree or other, usually neither is completely functional. The exception is de Moura's[45] 19-year-old patient with normal male external genitalia who had bled periodically via the urethra for four years and had abdominal cramps in the right side but who was also able to ejaculate motile spermatozoa. At operation, a normal ovary, tube, and uterus were removed from the right side, leaving a normally functioning testis in the left scrotum. The combination of an ovary with müllerian duct on one side and a testis with wolffian duct on the other, the uncommon gynandromorph, is due to local hormonal effect from the embryonic gonad acting on the homologous ductal systems.[41] (It will be recalled that all normal embryos have both müllerian and wolffian ducts on both sides.) Usually, however, the ductal systems of the true hermaphrodite are bilaterally but variably developed, with an infinite variety of combinations of the female and male systems, the müllerian system often being more prominent than the wolffian. The external genitalia occasionally may be male or female but usually are of an indifferent type: enlarged clitoris or small penis showing some degree of hypospadias from failure of the urethral groove to close, bifid scrotum or enlarged labia simulating bifid scrotum, or the female type of urethra opening at the base of the phallus. The mül-

*Slightly modified from Thompson, J. S., and Thompson, M. W.: Genetics in medicine, Philadelphia, 1966, W. B. Saunders Co.

lerian system may open to the outside as a vagina of variable size or may communicate with the urethra. It is impossible to predict on an anatomic basis whether the secondary sexual development at puberty will be male or female.

Pseudohermaphroditism is the presence of a gonad of one sex and, to a variable extent, the internal and external genitalia of the opposite sex. Evans and Riley[38] have reported thirty patients with this condition covering twenty years' experience at the University of Michigan, twelve of the male and eighteen of the female type. The age at which the patient was first seen varied from 1 week to 35 years, but the condition had been long suspected in many of the patients. That it has some genetic basis is suggested by the fact that six of the patients had siblings with comparable defects.

After summarizing reports of 298 cases of hermaphroditism in the literature plus seventy cases of their own, Wilkins et al.[47] classified ambisexual development as follows:

A Female pseudohermaphroditism with congenital adrenal hyperplasia
B Intersexes
   1 True hermaphrodites
   2 Male pseudohermaphroditism
   3 Female pseudohermaphroditism of nonadrenal origin

Congenital adrenal hyperlasia is the commonest variety of female pseudohermaphroditism (168 of the 368 patients).[47] The patients are chromosomal females, possess ovaries, and have a large phallus, with variable labial fusion, but have female genital ducts and show precocious male secondary sexual development at an early age (1 to 4 years). They are characterized clinically by increased excretion of adrenal androgens (2 mg to 5 mg per day of 17-ketosteroids as infants; up to 25 mg to 80 mg per day as adolescents). There also occur the features of excess body growth, accelerated epiphyseal development, progressive hirsutism, acne, and deepening of the voice. The condition is alleviated by cortisone (see also p. 1467).

The true hermaphrodites (forty of the 368 patients[47]) were discussed previously. These develop secondary sex characteristics at puberty in contrast to the patients in Group A.

The male pseudohermaphrodites (151 of the 368 patients[47]) all possess testes, variously located, which do not form spermatozoa but have Sertoli and interstitial cells. It is commonly accepted by gynecologists that these patients usually resemble females, for the apparent females seek their help because of failure to menstruate and to conceive. On the other hand, many of the male pseudohermaphrodites have external genitalia of male type. Indeed, in the group of Wilkins et al.,[47] the external genitalia commonly simulate the male (about two-thirds of cases), may simulate the female (about one-third of cases), but only occasionally are ambiguous (six of the 151 patients). The largest group, simulating the male, have a large-sized to medium-sized phallus with labial fusion to a variable but significant degree, although the internal genitalia may be either male or female. The secondary sexual characteristics of this group are predominantly male, in contrast to those whose internal and external genitalia simulate the female. Kozoll[43] points out that one-third of all male pseudohermaphrodites have inguinal hernias, whereas none of the female pseudohermaphrodites do. Female pseudohermaphrodites of nonadrenal origin (nine of the 368 patients[47]) have a rare form of pseudohermaphroditism, characterized by ovaries, a large phallus, labial fusion, female genital ducts, and secondary female sexual development. Two developed the anomaly in utero during pregnancies complicated by a maternal arrhenoblastoma, an androgen-producing tumor which virilized the mother. It is now known that either estrogen or progesterone administered to the pregnant patient may cause masculinization of the fetus. In a very few instances the cause of female pseudohermaphroditism is obscure.

Wilkins et al.[47] stress that the ambisexual child should be reared on the basis of its sex as determined by its external genitalia rather than its inherent sex, since the attendant sociologic and psychologic factors resulting from such rearing lead to better clinical results than arbitrary decisions based on gonadal or chromosomal sex. Sex is a matter of total personality, not merely genes, gonads, genital system, and endocrines.[39]

PELVIC INFLAMMATORY DISEASE

Pelvic inflammatory disease (Fig. 37-3) is, according to Mohler,[56] a "tissue reaction to some irritant which involves the internal female genitals and their contiguous structures."* It may be considered as a single disease with some organs being more frequently

---

*From Mohler, R. W.: Amer. J. Obstet. Gynec. 57:1077-1086, 1949.

involved than others. The anatomic nature of the female genital tract, by providing a communication between the peritoneal cavity and the outside and because of its physiologic property of adaptability to procreation, is of importance with respect to the natural history of the disease.

Pelvic inflammation is a dynamic process, and the use of qualifying terms such as acute, chronic, or subsiding refers only to facets of the overall condition. Generalized pain of varying intensity limited to the lower abdomen, blood changes indicating reaction to inflammation, and increased erythrocytic sedimentation rate are the usual clinical findings.

A variety of organisms may cause this disease, but the specific forms are of gonorrheal, puerperal, and tuberculous origin. These types differ in their method of spread and their effect on the genital tract.

Gonorrheal type (pelvic inflammation by surface extension)

Gonorrheal inflammation begins from a focus of infection in the lower genital tract, bartholinitis, endocervicitis or urethritis. Not every inflammation of Bartholin's gland is, however, gonococcal. Early there is marked inflammation, followed by blockage of the duct with cyst formation. The cyst, 1 cm to 5 cm in diameter, is lined by a transitional type of epithelium and is surrounded by a variable amount of mucus-secreting glandular tissue.

The infection is transmitted by physical force (e.g., coitus and douche) and extends as an ascending infection along the mucosa. Vulvovaginitis may occur in children but not in adults because of the difference in thickness of the epithelium. An endocervicitis and an endometritis occur in the adult, but the most marked lesion is an endosalpingitis. This results in an acute inflammation of the tubal plicae, with subsequent adherence to form glandlike spaces, healed follicular salpingitis (Fig. 37-4). The infection then extends to the ovary, causing an acute perioophoritis followed by perisalpingitis with relatively little, if any, involvement of the tubal muscle. Usually in the early stages the tube is, grossly,

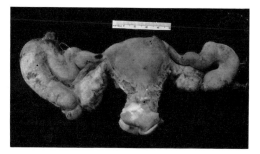

Fig. 37-3 Bilateral pyosalpinx with retort-shaped, sealed tubes, partly adherent to ovaries.

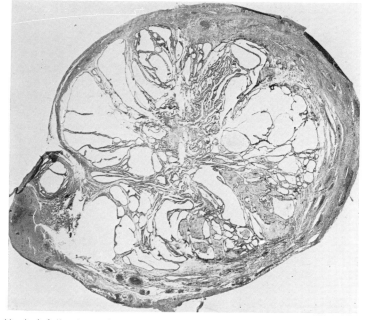

Fig. 37-4 Healed follicular salpingitis with adherence of tubal plicae to form glandlike spaces. This particular case is unusual in that there is an associated tuberculous salpingitis. (×7.)

only slightly reddened and edematous, but with reinfections from the lower genital tract, extensive fibrous adhesions are formed. These often involve the fimbriae with formation of pyosalpinges (Fig. 37-3). Later, there may be development of hydrosalpinges. Further, there may be cystic ovaries due to the periooophoritis, tubo-ovarian abscess, and pelvic abscesses.

Acute gonococcal salpingitis or a flare-up of chronic gonococcal pelvic inflammatory disease rarely, if ever, occurs during a pregnancy.[52]

Treatment and prognosis. Formerly, gonorrheal pelvic inflammation was treated by operation and then by sulfonamides. Now, antibiotics are used, with special effort being made to clear up foci that may cause reinfection. For advanced disease with symptoms, treatment is still surgical.

In very early infection, with treatment the prognosis (both anatomically and physiologically) is said to be good, but in general the prognosis is doubtful, as indicated by an increased incidence of tubal ectopic pregnancy.

Puerperal type (pelvic inflammation by interstitial extension)

The most frequent causative organisms of puerperal pelvic inflammations are the staphylococci and streptococci. Infections with *Escherichia coli, Clostridium welchii,* and the mycoses spread similarly by a break in the continuity of the surface epithelium. Such may happen with dilatation or cauterization of the cervix, curettage of the uterine cavity, induced abortion, or spontaneous interruption of a pregnancy. Usually, this type of pelvic inflammation is associated with pregnancy (puerperal sepsis), and the infection passes via lymphatics or thrombosed venous sinuses and the interstitial tissues of the pelvis to involve the pelvic structures, peritoneum, and bloodstream. Mucosal surfaces are little involved except occasionally by beta-hemolytic streptococcal puerperal infection, which rarely may spread, as does the *Neisseria gonorrhoeae,* via the tubes to the peritoneum. From the usual interstitial extension, there results a pelvic cellulitis, sometimes with abscess formation, together with a perisalpingitis and a periooophoritis.

Treatment and prognosis. Treatment of puerperal pelvic inflammation is by an antibiotic to which the organism is sensitive or by a suitable chemotherapeutic agent.

The prognosis varies with the stage and type of infection.

Tuberculosis

The precise incidence of pelvic tuberculosis is difficult to determine. It varies with the incidence of pulmonary tuberculosis in the community and so differs in various countries. The usual incidence among infertility patients is about 5%. Early endometrial lesions are being seen more frequently because of increased numbers of endometrial biopsies. There is a decrease in the more advanced lesion, the type commonly seen thirty-five years ago.

Most pelvic tuberculosis is diagnosed between the ages of 15 and 40 years, and it is rare after the menopause. Abdominal pain is the commonest symptom, with menstrual abnormalities second. Sterility alone is a prominent complaint, but this varies with the type of clinic in which the patients are seen. Pelvic inflammatory disease occurring in a virgin or defying ordinary treatment is usually tuberculous.

The method of spread to the pelvis is hematogenous. Spread from one pelvic organ to another may be by direct continuity or by hematogenous or lymphatic extension.

Individual organ involvement varies with the series of patients under consideration. Infertility patients with incidentally found endometrial tuberculosis will have an apparently low tubal incidence because often there will not be histologic examination of the tubes.

Gross appearance. The findings in pelvic tuberculosis vary considerably. In early cases, the pelvic organs may appear completely normal. The *tubal lesion* (Fig. 37-4) usually begins in the distal end. There is gradual thickening, and finally the tube is soft although nodular and tortuous. The fimbriated end may or may not be patent. In late stages, the lumen contains caseous material. The peritoneum may be involved, small white tubercles 0.1 cm to 0.2 cm appearing on the surface.

The *endometrium* may be grossly normal or may be caseous. The infection probably spreads directly from the tube to the endometrium, and the myometrium when involved is infected from the endometrium. Involvement of the serous surface always is associated with pelvic peritonitis, probably from spillage from tubes. Cervical lesions may be microscopic only, or there may be gross ulceration. Cervical lesions are probably secondary to endometrial lesions. The uterus is grossly distorted only if there is obstruction to the cervical canal or in the presence of myometrial abscess.

The *ovary* usually is involved only microscopically, probably via lymphatics, but occasionally may be covered by dense adhesions. Careful histologic examination of barely visible adhesions may reveal tubercles. It is probably secondary to tubal involvement, with occasional secondary tubo-ovarian adhesions.

The *vagina* may appear normal or may be nodular and ulcerated. Vaginal involvement is usually secondary to a cervical lesion.

Microscopic appearance. The typical tubercle in pelvic tuberculosis is similar to that described elsewhere (p. 950). In the tube, there is usually an accompanying healed follicular salpingitis (Fig. 37-4), and there is frequently an exuberant epithelial overgrowth, which has sometimes been mistaken for carcinoma. This is accompanied by a variable degree of necrosis.

In early endometrial involvement, the tubercles usually are located superficially and are found in curettings only toward the end of the cycle. Later, they are more extensive and may be necrotic, sometimes with glandular proliferation similar to that in the tube.

The final proof that such a lesion is tuberculous is obtained by culturing the organism from the tissue or, as has been suggested by some authors, from the menstrual discharge. The bacillus also may be demonstrated microscopically.

Complications. Tuberculous peritonitis is a common complication of pelvic tuberculosis. Tubal pregnancy may occur but is rare.

Treatment and prognosis. Formerly, the accepted treatment for pelvic tuberculosis was surgical removal of the diseased organs. Currently, streptomycin, isonicotinic acid hydrazide, and PAS are being used in varying proportions over a long period of time. The prospect of pregnancy in patients with pelvic tuberculosis formerly was negligible, but with modern therapy, the rate is 12% (20% if there are no palpable pelvic masses at the end of therapy). Of the pregnancies, only about one-third proceed to term, one-third abort, and about one-third are tubal ectopic.

Pyometra

Pyometra is pus within the uterine cavity. This is frequently accompanied by a cervical stenosis (although DeVoe and Randall[51] found that 54% of cervical canals were patent, but similar inflammation was present in the cervix whether patent or stenosed). About half the cases of pyometra are associated with a malignant uterine tumor (in order of fre-

quency are untreated cervical cancer, previously irradiated cervical cancer, and endometrial cancer). Benign conditions with which pyometra may be associated are senile atrophy of the genital tract and uterine prolapse. Pyometra also may occur following cauterization or surgery of the cervix. Anaerobic organisms are important, being present alone in 37% of the patients and along with aerobic organisms in an additional 38%. The most prominent symptoms are vaginal discharge, vaginal bleeding, and abdominal pain.

Treatment and prognosis. Treatment of pyometra usually is directed at establishing adequate drainage and treating the underlying lesion.

The presence of pyometra with an untreated malignant tumor of the uterus indicates a poorer prognosis than with the tumor alone. Indeed, in sixty of 208 patients with pyometra complicating malignant uterine disease, pyometra was listed as the primary cause of death.[54]

Vaginitis emphysematosa

In vaginitis emphysematosa,[49, 53] the vagina and cervix are studded with multiple cystic structures, from pinhead size to 2 cm in diameter, lying beneath the surface squamous epithelium, sometimes singly, often in clusters (Fig. 37-5). These are tense and filled with gas that has a high carbon dioxide content.

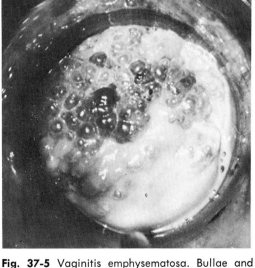

Fig. 37-5 Vaginitis emphysematosa. Bullae and vaginal discharge in upper part of vagina. Photograph taken through cylindrical speculum. (HMS CS-62-321; courtesy Letterman Army Hospital C-2040; from Close, J. M., and Jesurun, H. M.: Obstet. Gynec. **19:**513-516, 1962.)

Microscopically, the surface epithelium may have prominent rete ridges or be hyperkeratotic. Cystic spaces lined by squamous epithelium, giant cells, or nondescript flattened epithelium or a combination of these lie beneath the squamous epithelium, with varying degrees of fibrosis and inflammation. The lesion usually occurs during the reproductive years, is commonly associated with pregnancy, and is of unknown etiology. The current favored theory is that it is a manifestation of microbial vaginitis.

Physiologic salpingitis

Physiologic salpingitis is a nonbacterial acute salpingitis. The tubes are said by Nassberg et al. to be "characterized by a polymorphonuclear leukocyte infiltration, edema of the stroma of the plicae, dilatation of lymphatic vessels of the plicae, leukostasis, and menstrual blood in the tubal lumen."* The condition occurs in about two-thirds of all normal tubes during menstruation.[57] Perhaps it would be observed more often if multiple sections were examined at or soon after menstruation.

Granulomatous salpingitis (nontuberculous)

Granulomatous salpingitis may occur in response to agents other than *Mycobacterium tuberculosis*. They often may be identified by special stains or by physical methods. This

---

*From Nassberg, S., McKay, D. G., and Hertig, A. T.: Amer. J. Obstet. Gynec. 68:130-137, 1954.

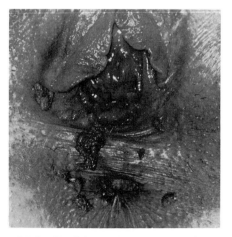

Fig. 37-6 Condylomata acuminata (venereal warts). These multiple papillomas involving perianal region, vulva, vagina, and cervix are of viral origin. Husband of this patient had similar penile lesions.

reaction may be part of a generalized pelvic peritoneal response or occasionally part of a systemic disease. The commonest types are (1) talc granuloma (from a previous abdominal operation), (2) Lipiodol granuloma (or granuloma from any fatty material, e.g., content of a dermoid cyst), (3) fungal granuloma (e.g., actinomycotic), and (4) sarcoidosis.

VULVA
Benign tumors of epithelial origin

Papilloma. Papilloma is an uncommon, usually single, potentially malignant tumor occurring anywhere on the vulva during adult life. Although usually small, it may grow to from 4 cm to 5 cm in diameter. Microscopically, it is composed of papillary processes of squamous epithelium with a scanty central connective tissue core. It should be distinguished from the usually multiple condylomata acuminata (Fig. 37-6).

Endometriosis. Endometriosis of the vulva is not a true neoplasm but may simulate one, both grossly and microscopically. It may arise in two ways: by metaplasia of the pelvic peritoneum accompanying the round ligament or by implantation of viable endometrium following a surgical procedure. Patients with perineal endometriosis usually have a history of trauma. The lesion may reach 1 cm to 2 cm in size and, grossly and microscopically, is similar to endometriosis seen elsewhere.

Hidradenoma. Hidradenoma is a benign tumor of apocrine sweat gland origin, occurring usually in the dermis of the labium majus and only occasionally in the labium minus or the interlabial sulcus. It usually occurs between the ages of 30 and 50 years but has been observed before the age of 20 years (although not before puberty) and in a patient 77 years of age.[73] No lesion has been reported in a black woman.

Hidradenoma is usually a single tumor, measures 0.5 cm to 1.5 cm in diameter, is freely movable and discrete but not encapsulated, and lies beneath the epidermis. Most usually it is an incidental finding, usually diagnosed clinically as a fibroma or wen and producing symptoms only when ulcerating through the skin. When ulcerative, it is red and fungating, mimicking cancer (Fig. 37-7, A). Otherwise, when cut, the tumor may be pale gray, red, or brown.

Microscopically, hidradenoma is well defined from the surrounding tissue (Fig. 37-7, B). The adjacent connective tissue may be

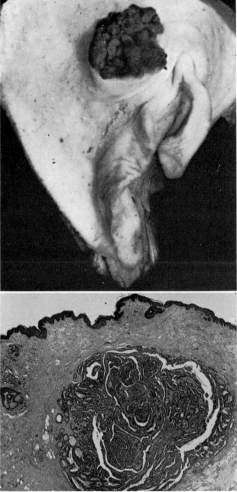

Fig. 37-7 Hidradenoma of vulva. **A,** Tumor rupturing through epidermis (unusual complication) appears as red fungating papillary tumor on right labium majus of otherwise normal vulva. It is to be distinguished from carcinoma. **B,** Fairly well-circumscribed but nonencapsulated tumor lying within dermis. There is slight penetration of surrounding connective tissue, but these tumors are rarely malignant. (×15.)

compressed to form a pseudocapsule, but there is no true capsule. The tumor is composed of multiple gland spaces lined by cuboidal to columnar epithelial cells and a deeper spindle layer, the myoepithelium, with a variable amount of intervening stroma so that the tumor may appear papillomatous or as a solid adenoma. There may be some inflammation or evidence of old hemorrhage. The resemblance to intraductal papillomas of the breast is striking, a fact to be expected

in view of the apocrine origin of both the breast and the vulvar sweat glands from which these tumors arise (see p. 1677).

Malignant tumors of epithelial origin

Carcinoma in situ. The term carcinoma in situ is sometimes used to include several clinicopathologic entities—viz., Bowen's disease, erythroplasia of Queyrat, amelanotic melanoma, and extramammary Paget's disease.[67] Whether these are variants of one or several diseases is unsettled. Indeed, one report claims to show transitions between Bowen's disease and Paget's disease. We believe they are histologically distinct. The tw. better known, Bowen's disease and extramam. mary Paget's disease, are described here.

Bowen's disease. Bowen's disease is an epithelial lesion that may occur anywhere on the skin of middle-aged or elderly patients of either sex, without any predilection for the vulva (p. 1649).

The lesions may be papular or plaquelike, slightly raised above the surface, and reddish brown in color. Early lesions are discrete, but later they coalesce to form large areas with a crusted or dull red, moist surface. Microscopically, the epithelium is markedly thickened—with irregularity in size and shape of cells and numerous mitoses.

Invasive carcinoma may occasionally develop from this lesion, but the disease is not sufficiently common to determine the prognosis statistically.

Extramammary Paget's disease. Extramammary Paget's disease is a rare dermatosis limited to the skin of the axilla and the anogenital region (of either sex). Clinically and pathologically, it resembles Paget's disease of the breast. The lesion is extremely rare but is found more commonly on the labia majora than the labia minora. It has been described in patients from 33 to 84 years of age, predominantly in postmenopausal women (p. 1598).

Grossly, the lesion is red, moist, and sharply demarcated, sometimes with superficial crust formation. The nearby vulva may be swollen and edematous. A firm underlying cancer of variable size may be palpable.

Microscopically, there are typical large clear Paget cells in the epidermis, within or just above the malpighian layer. These cells may coalesce, with resulting loss of the more superficial layers of the squamous epithelium. The underlying carcinoma, when found, is an adenocarcinoma of apocrine sweat gland origin. Finding mucin in the Paget cells has suggested a sweat gland origin for these cells, but this problem has not been settled. Histochemical studies have identified mucin, melanin, and acid and neutral mucopolysaccharides in Paget cells.[85] Except for mucin, these have been demonstrated also in melanoma, Bowen's disease, and erythroplasia of Queyrat. The relatively nonspecific aldehydefuchsin reaction is positive in Paget cells and negative in the others. This has been suggested as an empiric distinguishing feature.[81]

Papillary carcinoma in situ. The term papillary carcinoma in situ has been applied by Clark[75] to a lesion quite distinct clinically from Bowen's disease, although occasionally there may be some overlapping in the histologic pattern. Basically, the lesion is papillary, but it may vary from a granular area, through a papillary lesion grossly similar to and often misdiagnosed as condyloma acuminatum, to a large plaque with a rough papillary surface. In general, the lesion grows slowly in a lateral direction, invading the underlying stroma relatively late, if at all. Histologically, loss of polarity of cells and mitotic activity are prominent.

Melanoma. Melanoma constitutes 2.3% of malignant vulvar neoplasms or 8.3% of melanomas in females. The average age of the patients is about 55 years, but the lesion may appear from youth to old age. The pathogenesis is similar to that of melanomas occurring elsewhere in the body.[69] Pigmented nevi are common on the vulva. Melanomas may have a variable degree of pigmentation, but there is a rare interesting form, the intraepidermal amelanotic melanoma, which simulates Paget's disease. In this form, the lesion is confined to the epidermis. Groups of pale spherical to ovoid cells are present within the epidermis, usually where it joins the underlying dermis. On occasion, it may be impossible for even experienced pathologists to agree that a lesion is amelanotic melanoma or extramammary Paget's disease.

Leukoplakia and kraurosis. White lesions of the vulva, including leukoplakia, kraurosis, and lichen sclerosus et atrophicus, have been described, but there is little agreement regarding their relationship (one to the other) or to their part in the genesis of carcinoma of the vulva. Some consider kraurosis vulvae to be the end stage of leukoplakic vulvitis,[65] whereas others consider them two separate entities.[74, 83, 89]

Leukoplakia is a disease of mucosal or mucocutaneous surfaces or both, with the development of grossly visible thick white plaques. Histologically, there is marked hyperkeratosis in areas in which normally there is only a thin layer of keratin. There is elongation of rete ridges—sometimes uniform, sometimes irregular. Lymphocytes, histiocytes, and plasma cells infiltrate the corium up to the epidermis. There may be hyperkeratosis and thickening (lichenification) of the adjacent true skin.[83]

In kraurosis vulvae, the mucosal surface is paper thin, smooth, shining, and dry. This change merges with the normal skin and usually does not extend beyond the inner aspect of the labia majora. It may be accompanied by varying degrees of narrowing of the introitus or atrophy of the labial structures, but these are strictly atrophic changes and may occur with senile or prematurely senile changes without "kraurosis." Histologically, there is thickening of the stratum corneum, often with atrophy of the remainder of the epithelium. Initially, an area of edema appears in the superficial corium, apparently displacing rather than destroying the elastic tissue fibers.[74] Thin strands of connective tissue pass through this edematous layer, but later a homogeneous, bright pink–staining intercellular substance, presumably collagen, is deposited in the edematous area. Often, an inflammatory zone develops within the dermis immediately below this edematous or scarred area. Focal epithelial hyperplasia and hyperkeratosis (leukoplakia) occasionally may be superimposed on these primary changes within the dermis.

The histologic features of kraurosis vulvae are identical with those of lichen sclerosus et atrophicus. The usual method of differentiation is based upon the presence or absence of extension beyond the vulva. Therefore, those patients with extravulvar cutaneous lesions are considered to have lichen sclerosus et atrophicus. Perhaps these two conditions should be considered as one,[83] the gynecologist seeing one aspect and the dermatologist the other.

Carcinoma of the vulva may follow or be associated with leukoplakic vulvitis (Fig. 37-8) in a significant number of patients. Carcinoma occurring in patients with lichen sclerosus et atrophicus probably arises from superimposed foci of hyperplastic epithelium. There is no evidence that vulvar carcinoma arises from atrophic epithelium, nor has it been shown that leukoplakia will always

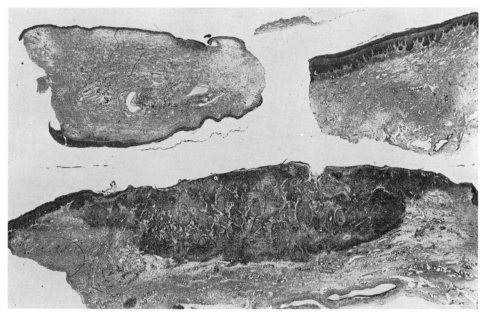

Fig. 37-8 Typical squamous cell carcinoma of vulva apparently associated with leukoplakic vulvitis but not obviously arising therefrom. Hyperkeratotic or leukoplakic lesion at upper right and early squamous cell carcinoma at bottom center. (×12; AFIP 279168-1.)

terminate in cancer if untreated. About 60% of patients with vulvar cancer have leukoplakia elsewhere in the vulva, while of a group of patients with leukoplakia of the vulva, approximately 10% developed squamous cell carcinoma.[89]

Carcinoma of vulva. Carcinoma is the commonest malignant disease of the vulva, ranking third in sites of malignant disease of the female genital tract but constituting only 5% of gynecologic malignant disease and 1% of all cancers. A significant increase in incidence is being observed. Other malignant diseases involving the vulva are malignant melanoma (2%), an occasional adenocarcinoma of Bartholin's gland, and a very rare sarcoma. Carcinoma may occur at any age from the first to the tenth decade, wtih 80% of patients in the postmenopausal years. On rare occasions, it has been diagnosed during pregnancy. Etiologic factors of importance appear to be leukoplakic vulvitis and exposure to certain chemicals in the cotton and cutlery industries.

This lesion is found most commonly on the labium majus, usually on its anterior two-thirds (Fig. 37-9). Clinical staging of tumors is determined by the size of the lesion, either with or without the criteria of palpable lymph nodes. The tumor may be finely papillary or have a granular, ulcerated surface. Usually,

there is adjacent induration due to an accompanying infection. Lymph nodes frequently are involved (50%), but only in late lesions also involving the vagina does the tumor extend to the underlying periosteum, levatores, rectum, urethra, or bladder.

Microscopically, approximately 96% of these tumors are squamous cell carcinomas. They are usually well differentiated, producing pricklelike cells and often with definite pearl formation. These may arise from unicentric or multicentric foci, often (but not always) in a vulva involved by leukoplakic vulvitis.

Basal cell carcinoma constitutes 1.27% to 4% of all vulvar carcinomas, the majority occurring on the labium majus at an average age of 60 years. Two types have been described: a superficial plaque that may persist unchanged for some time and the "rodent ulcer" that begins as a small plaque and later ulcerates. Recently, a microscopic variant, adenocystic basal cell carcinoma, has been described.

Squamous cell carcinoma of the vulva metastasizes most usually via the lymphatics but occasionally via the bloodstream. Indeed, the "kiss" metastasis sometimes observed on the opposite labium is due to lymphatic extension. Vulvar carcinoma spreads first to the superficial inguinal and femoral nodes and

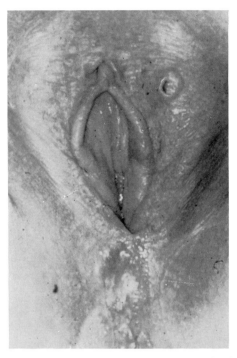

Fig. 37-9 Early squamous cell carcinoma of vulva appearing as small, raised, ulcerated lesion on medial surface of left labium majus. Labium majus is common site of vulvar carcinoma. Leukoplakic vulvitis also present but difficult to see grossly.

then to Cloquet's node, the medial group of the external iliac nodes. It has been said: "The frequency of lymphatic metastasis is to a certain degree an expression of the relative age, histologic type and degree of extension of the primary tumor. This, however, is applicable to a series and has no value to the individual patient."*

In general, the less differentiated the tumor and the younger the patient, the shorter the natural course of the disease. Surgery, (viz., radical vulvectomy and radical lymph node dissection) is the treatment of choice. Radiation has been advocated but is not generally accepted. The absolute cure rate for cancer of the vulva varies from 18.1% to 26.5%.

Hidradenocarcinoma. An extremely rare malignant variant of the hidradenoma recurs after excision and kills by metastasis. Sometimes, there may be difficulty in deciding whether there is invasion at the margin of a hidradenoma because of some irregular scarring resulting in apparent stromal infiltration. Very rarely, hidradenocarcinoma may be

*From Way, S.: Malignant disease of the female genital tract, Philadelphia, 1951, The Blakiston Co.

part of extramammary Paget's disease with involvement of the overlying skin.

Bartholin gland carcinoma. Bartholin gland carcinoma is a rare cancer that probably constitutes less than 1% of vulvar cancers, despite varying reports. The average age is between 49 and 50 years, with an age range from 18 to 91 years. A lesion has been reported in a 25-year-old patient during pregnancy.[76] In its early stage, it is usually a hard, painless nodule deep in the labial fat and may be confused with an inflammatory process. It becomes attached to surrounding tissue, although skin involvement is late and tends to extend deep into fat, muscle, and the pubic bones. The tumor may undergo necrosis, resulting in a fluctuant mass.

The cut surface of the early lesion is firm and pale, whereas the late lesion is loculated, containing stringy mucus separated by a delicate fibrous connective tissue. Microscopically, the Bartholin gland cancers reported have been squamous cell carcinoma (36%), adenocarcinoma (45.7%), carcinoma of various unusual types (8.7%), undifferentiated carcinoma (2.6%), sarcoma (3.5%), and unknown (3.5%).[76] Usually, the adenocarcinoma has a cribriform pattern and only rarely is mucus-secreting. The prognosis is poor, and only about 9% of patients survive five years without disease after treatment. Treatment is surgical, for the tumors are radioresistant.

Benign tumors of connective tissue origin

Benign connective tissue tumors of the vulva are extremely rare, only thirty-four having been seen at the Mayo Clinic in thirty-four years.[88] These varied in diameter from 0.6 cm to 8 cm, except for lipomas, which were up to 17 cm in diameter. The distribution of the tumors was as follows: fibromas, 16; lipomas, 7; hemangiomas, 5; neurofibromas, 2; leiomyomas, 2; ganglioneuroma, 1; and lymphangioma, 1. All were similar to such tumors occurring elsewhere in the body and were histologically benign. None recurred after excision.

Granular cell myoblastoma. Granular cell myoblastoma is a rare tumor of controversial origin and variable malignancy, occurring very rarely in the female genital tract (most usually in the vulva, although sometimes in the vagina and uterus). Most commonly, it is found in the fourth or fifth decade, but it may occur at any age.

The tumor is usually small (less than 4

cm), slow growing, and discrete but not encapsulated.[70] It is firm, with a homogeneous, glistening, pale yellow to grayish white cut surface. Tumors are often superficial, sometimes with ulceration, but may be deeply situated. Microscopically, there are irregularly arranged bundles and sheets of large polyhedral eosinophilic cells with poorly defined margins, eosinophilic cytoplasmic granules, and small dark regular nuclei. Frequently, there is a pseudoepitheliomatous hyperplasia of the overlying squamous epithelium.

Malignant tumors of connective tissue origin

Malignant connective tissue tumors of the vulva are rare, and about 60% occur in the labia majora. Such sarcomas may occur at any age, with the average being 40.5 years—some twenty years younger than that for carcinoma of the vulva. The tumors may vary considerably in size (1 cm to 15 cm) and may be diffuse or discrete. Initially, they lie beneath the skin and then extend and ulcerate through the surface. Usually, the consistency is homogeneous and fleshy but may be soft or firm, and the color varies from white to yellow to red.

The rate of growth of an individual tumor may be variable, remaining stationary for some time and then growing rapidly. Microscopically, it is usually some type of fibrosarcoma but occasionally is a liposarcoma, lymphosarcoma, or rhabdomyosarcoma. The prognosis is poor, and surgery is the usual therapy.

Metastatic tumors

Metastatic tumors may reach the vulva in one of three ways:

1 Via blood vessels, with thrombosis of main vessels and retrograde tumor embolization, as from renal cell carcinoma, ovarian carcinoma and sarcoma, and choriocarcinoma

2 Via lymphatics from other pelvic organs, such as carcinoma of the endometrium, cervix, or vagina

3 By implantation at surgery, a possible but rare event

It is usually possible to distinguish primary and secondary vulvar carcinomas in the early stages, the primary lesion arising from the surface epithelium and the metastatic tumor lying beneath it as a general rule. In later stages, when ulceration has occurred, this distinction may be impossible.

VAGINA
Benign tumors

Papilloma. Papilloma of the vagina is an uncommon single or multiple tumor that may simulate or give rise to carcinoma. It has the usual appearance, both grossly and microscopically, of a papilloma arising from squamous epithelium. It should be distinguished from condyloma acuminatum, which is usually multiple and of viral origin.

Polyp. A polyp is an uncommon vaginal tumor derived from the mucosal stroma and covered by vaginal epithelium. It sometimes contains glandlike structures. It does not appear to have any malignant potential.

Endometriosis. Although not a true neoplasm, endometriosis of the vagina may simulate one. Usually associated with endometriosis elsewhere in the pelvis, it may arise spontaneously or following pelvic surgery. It may occur either in the mucosa or in the muscle of the vagina, in the latter case usually having extended from the pelvic peritoneum to the posterior fornix. A variable overgrowth of muscle may occur, forming adenomyosis or an adenomyoma. Endometriosis in the vagina may undergo cyclic change and, extremely rarely, may give rise to an adenocarcinoma of endometrial type.

Cysts. Two main types of cysts may occur in the vagina. Those arising from remnants of the mesonephros are lined by a cuboidal epithelium, although the cells may become flattened by the cyst contents. Those cysts following surgical procedures are of epidermal inclusion type and are lined by squamous epithelium that is flattened and thinned out to a variable degree. Endometriosis may present as a hemorrhagic cyst. Occasionally, epithelial lining may suggest paramesonephric origin. Vaginitis emphysematosa must be considered when cysts are multiple.

Granulation tissue. Granulation tissue is mentioned with tumors because so often it is mistaken for tumor. It may occur as red nodules in the vault of the vagina following hysterectomy or in the region of a neglected pessary. It may be friable or relatively firm. Microscopically, it is composed of loose connective tissue containing thin-walled blood vessels and is densely infiltrated by plasma cells and some polymorphonuclear leukocytes.

Benign connective tissue tumors. Connective tissue tumors of the vagina are very rare, but the most common type is the leiomyoma. It occurs usually in the fifth decade but may occur in the pregnant patient. Grossly and microscopically, it is similar to these tumors found elsewhere in the female genital tract. It varies from 1.5 cm to 4.5 cm and is usually discrete and easily shelled out but may be diffuse. Other rare benign tumors include fibroma, myoblastic myoma, neurofibroma, and neuroepithelioma.

Benign cystic teratoma (dermoid cyst). Benign cystic teratoma occurs rarely in the vagina[103] and probably arises from a misplaced primordial germ cell that failed to reach its destination during its migration from the yolk sac endoderm. Grossly and microscopically, it is similar to benign cystic teratomas arising in the ovary.

Malignant tumors

Carcinoma in situ. Carcinoma in situ has been reported only rarely. It usually is diagnosed after malignant cells are found in a routine vaginal smear. Koss[15] has observed that carcinoma in situ of the vagina may be found after hysterectomy for cervical carcinoma.

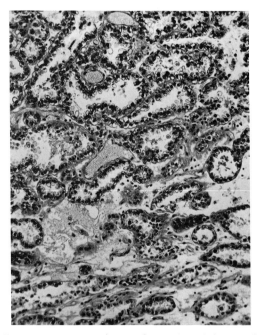

Fig. 37-10 Mesonephroma from vaginal fornix of 21-year-old patient. (This type of tumor may occur anywhere along course of mesonephros and its duct—i.e., ovary, mesovarium, mesosalpinx, cervix, and lateral wall of vagina.) Note characteristic tubules formed by clear "cobblestone" cells. Like all tumors, this type has many variations, although one illustrated is classic. (×100; courtesy St. Luke's Hospital, Bethlehem, Pa.; from Novak, E., Woodruff, J. D., and Novak, E. R.: Amer. J. Obstet. Gynec. **68:**1222-1242, 1954.)

Carcinoma. Primary carcinoma of the vagina is an uncommon disease, constituting about 0.49% of female cancers[61] and 1% of genital cancers.[67] It is usually a disease of postmenopausal women but may occur at any age, with an age range of 24 to 82 years. Whether marital status is relevant is uncertain, for reports are conflicting. Indeed, the only predisposing factor that has been noted is the use of a rubber ring pessary. Whelton and Kottmeier[114] found a wide distribution of lesions, with more in the upper two-thirds posterior and posterolateral areas of the vagina.

Lesions vary from a small nodular tumor (occasionally missed on palpation), to a papillary soft lesion with broad-based stalk (30%), to an ulcerated tumor, usually penetrating, with raised firm borders (over 50%). Usually when first seen, the tumor is larger than 3 cm in diameter.

Microscopically, these carcinomas are of two types: squamous cell carcinoma (89% to 96.7%) and adenocarcinoma (3.3% to 11%). The squamous cell variety is usually of intermediate differentiation (3.9%, grade I; 66%, grade II; 27.2%, grade III; and 2.9%, grade IV). Those rare adenocarcinomas arising from endometriosis resemble endometrial carcinoma. Those from mesonephric tubular and ductal elements resemble mesonephromas, with glandlike spaces lined by flattened cells or large cells with clear cytoplasm (Fig. 37-10).

Growth of carcinoma of the vagina is relatively silent, and the cancer usually is advanced when diagnosed, at least 75% of lesions having already extended or metastasized beyond the vagina. The lymphatics of the upper vagina are carried with the uterine vessels to the obturator and external iliac nodes. The remainder of the vagina is drained by vessels terminating in the internal and external iliac chains of nodes. Lymphatics of the rectovaginal septum may terminate in the nodes of the lateral sacral or promontory groups. Vaginal lymphatics have an indirect connection with the inguinal lymph nodes via anastomoses with lymphatics of the vulva.

The following clinical classification was presented by Whelton and Kottmeier in the hope that there may be more uniform assessment of carcinoma of the vagina.

Stage I

The carcinoma involves 2 cm or less of the vaginal mucosa.

Stage II

A The carcinoma involves more than 2 cm but less than the entire vaginal mucosa in the longitudinal axis.

B The carcinoma infiltrates the paracolpos but does not reach the pelvic wall.

Stage III

A The carcinoma involves the entire vaginal mucosa in the longitudinal axis.

B The carcinomatous infiltration extends to the pelvic wall and is fixed there.

Stage IV

A The carcinoma involves the bladder, urethra, rectum or vulva.

B The carcinoma extends outside the true pelvis, i.e., metastases to the inguinal nodes, to nodes above the pelvic brim or distant metastases.*

Treatment is usually by irradiation. Prognosis is dependent upon the site of the lesion (best in lesions of the upper third of the vagina), the stage of the disease, and the histologic grade of the lesion (the lower the grade, the better the prognosis). Adenocarcinoma has a uniformly poor prognosis. The absolute five-year survival rate is 24% and the ten-year survival 15%. The major causes of death are uremia and cachexia from local pelvic spread of the tumor.

Sarcoma. Fibrosarcomas and their variants tend to occur in adults rather than in children but have been observed from the first through the ninth decades. (Sarcoma botryoides is discussed on p. 1532.) Sarcomas vary in size from 2 cm to 15 cm and may be located anywhere in the vaginal wall. They may be soft or firm, pale gray to pink, homogeneous, and well vascularized, with varying degrees of necrosis and hemorrhage. They may arise from the stroma of the mucosa or the vaginal wall itself. Microscopically, they may be varied, although sarcomas of the myo-, fibro-, myxo-, and angio- types have been described.

These tumors spread locally to kill by uremia and cachexia but may metastasize to the pelvic and retroperitoneal lymph nodes or to distant sites such as lungs, pleura, ribs, and axillary nodes. Treatment is generally unsatisfactory and consists of irradiation or surgery or a combination of both.

Melanoma. Melanoma,[106] the rarest of the malignant vaginal tumors, may occur at almost any age. The reported age range is from 22 to 75 years, with a fairly even scat-

*From Whelton, J., and Kottmeier, H. L.: Acta Obstet. Gynec. Scand. 41:22-40, 1962.

tering. The patients usually present with vaginal bleeding, and there may be one or more lesions. These are similar grossly to melanomas elsewhere in the body, usually more than 1.5 cm in diameter and commonly ulcerated. Usually, the apparently primary lesion is found just within the introitus. Malignant junctional change has been observed at least once, indicating that a vaginal melanoma may be primary, although doubt often has been raised as to whether or not this is so.

Tumors metastatic to vagina. Metastases to the vagina are more common than primary tumors and may occur in several ways:

1 By direct extension, as from the cervix, vulva, bladder, urethra, and rectum

2 By lymphatic permeation or embolization, as from the endometrium, cervix, bladder, or rectum

3 By vascular embolization, as from uterine carcinoma, renal cell carcinoma, ovarian neoplasms, or choriocarcinoma

4 By direct implantation, as from the endometrium or cervix

The commonest secondary tumor of the vagina is from the cervix and occurs in over 70% of patients with cervical carcinoma. Endometrial carcinoma metastasizes to the vagina in 13%. The prognosis is poor even with treatment of both the primary and the metastatic lesion.

CERVIX
Benign conditions

Polyp. Cervical polyps are pedunculated growths from the mucous surface of the cervix. They may arise from the portio vaginalis, the squamocolumnar junction, or the lower endocervix (usually the latter), and they often represent the overgrowth of one of the cervical folds (plicae palmatae). They may be single (88%) or multiple (12%) and may be associated with chronic cervicitis, although this does not seem to be causative.[116] Polyps are found most commonly in parous women in the fifth decade. The incidence is 1.5% of overall admissions to a general hospital and 2.4% of admissions to a gynecologic hospital. (Probably this distribution has changed with the current use of oral contraceptives.)

Cervical polyps vary in size from microscopic to 2 cm or more and are soft in consistency but sometimes shotty (due to nabothian cysts), pink to red in color, and sometimes ulcerated. Microscopically, there is a loose vascular connective tissue, the surface being covered by endocervical epithelium and with occasional cervical glands. The stroma is usually very inflamed. Cervical polyps have a low potential of malignancy, lower indeed than that of the remainder of the cervix.

Papilloma. A papilloma[145] is an epithelial tumor in which the cells cover fingerlike processes or ridges of stroma. Usually these are composed of stratified squamous epithelium with varying degrees of keratinization, covering connective tissue stalks. The various types of neoplasm in the papilloma group are as follows:

1 Cockscomb polyp—polyp occurring during pregnancy on the anatomic portio but probably histologic transitional zone. These are often pleomorphic but regress after delivery.
2 Condyloma acuminatum—probably of inflammatory etiology, usually multiple.
3 True papilloma—usually single, small (0.2 cm to 0.7 cm), and attached at or near the squamocolumnar junction by a broad base. These are potentially malignant, and it is often difficult to determine whether early cancer is present. Microscopically, there is a connective tissue stalk covered by squamous epithelium thrown into papillary folds.

Squamous metaplasia. Small cells have been observed beneath the columnar epithelium of the endocervix. Their origin has been debated, theories ranging from congenital rest to squamous cell ingrowth. These theories are unlikely, and the most acceptable is that they arise from the columnar cells and have the ability to produce squamous cells or more columnar cells. These *subcylindrical cells* may proliferate to form reserve cell

hyperplasia, then begin to differentiate to a squamous pattern, *squamous metaplasia* (Fig. 37-11), and develop into immature squamous epithelium, so-called *leukoparakeratosis*. Rarely, they may become anaplastic or dysplastic, *reserve cell anaplasia,* related to the genesis of carcinoma in situ. Should there be concurrent adenomatous and squamous patterns, there is *adenomatous hyperplasia with squamous metaplasia or squamocolumnar prosoplasia* (Fluhmann).[6]

Leukoplakia. The presence of white patches on the surface of the cervix prior to stain-

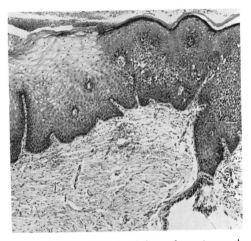

Fig. 37-12 Clinical leukoplakia of cervix, pathologically leukokeratosis (or leukohyperkeratosis since keratin is prominent). Normal squamous epithelium composed of clear glycogen-containing cells is sharply demarcated from cells without glycogen. Above latter is layer of cells containing keratoeleidin granules and layer of keratin. Note epidermidization of gland by presence of squamous epithelium in gland mouth. (×55; AFIP 496589-30102.)

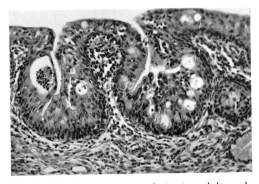

Fig. 37-11 Squamous metaplasia in adult endocervix. Proliferation of cells deep to columnar epithelium resulting in scalloped appearance with remnants of surface mucoid columnar epithelium remaining. (×125; AFIP 320679-23011.)

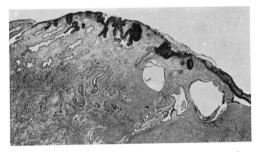

Fig. 37-13 Low-power view of cervix to show location in transitional zone of squamous cell carcinoma in situ, readily distinguished by its deep staining. It extends from region of external os into endocervical canal, filling many glands. (×6; AFIP 573586-53-858; from Hertig, A. T., and Mansell, H.: CA: Bull. Cancer Progr. **6**:196-202, 1956.)

ing with Schiller's iodine is termed leukoplakia. Microscopically, these patches appear
as sharply defined areas with surface hyperkeratosis, the underlying cells lacking glycogen
(Fig. 37-12). This has been termed leukokeratosis (leukohyperkeratosis if exaggerated)
by Schiller.[157]

Squamous cell carcinoma in situ

The presence of morphologically malignant
but noninvasive squamous epithelium along
the surface (or both along the surface and
within the glands) of the cervix but without
stromal invasion constitutes carcinoma in situ
(Fig. 37-13). The true incidence is difficult
to determine, the best estimate being 0.218%.
Age range is from the twenties to the seven-
ties, with most patients being in the thirties.
Since more Papanicolaou smears from teenage girls have been examined, it becomes apparent that this lesion may begin before the
age of 20 years.

In any consideration of cervical lesions, it
must be borne in mind that anatomic and
histologic divisions of the cervix do not always
coincide. The *anatomic portio* extends from
the external os to the vaginal reflexion and
the *anatomic endocervix* from the internal os
to the external os. The *histologic portio* is
composed of fibromuscular stroma covered
by mature squamous epithelium. The *histologic endocervix* consists of endocervical
stroma and glands (tunnels or crypts). When
the endocervical surface is altered in some
way by metaplasia or is covered by a variant
of squamous epithelium, this is termed the
transitional zone. The transitional zone may
be found anatomically within the endocervix
or out on the anatomic portio, and, to
emphasize again, *the histologic and anatomic
portio and endocervix do not necessarily
coincide.*

There are no characteristic gross features
of carcinoma in situ, although experts in the
use of the colposcope claim to be able to
detect the lesion. It usually begins in the
histologic transitional zone where altered surface epithelium overlies former histologic
endocervix. In studies on the cervices of
pregnant and postpartum women, Johnson et
al.[144] have observed that carcinoma in situ
develops through a process of hyperplasia and
anaplasia (dysplasia) of the subcylindrical
(reserve) cells. In a group of forty-eight patients, direct evidence was found in four and
indirect evidence in thirty-seven. In the re-

maining seven patients, there was nothing to
disprove their theory.

Carcinoma in situ may extend into the
anatomic endocervix or out onto the anatomic
portio. Congenital erosion, where the endocervical columnar epithelium extends out onto
the anatomic portio, producing a red cir-
cumoral zone, is a common site. The squamocolumnar junction may be located at varying
points on the portio.[164] Furthermore, the
squamocolumnar junction may no longer be
regular and well defined in the cervix distorted by eversion, laceration, and regenerative epithelial repair associated with the
pregnant, puerperal, or postpartum state.
Occasionally, carcinoma in situ may occur at
the margin or in altered epithelium of a congenital erosion in the virgin patient or in one
who has never been pregnant.

Carcinoma in situ on the anatomic portio
beyond any erosion may be clearly defined by
application of Schiller's solution (1 part
iodine, 2 parts potassium iodide, 300 parts
water) to the cervix cleaned by a mild alkaline solution. Those areas that appear on
initial inspection to be consistent with normal
histologic portio but on application of the
solution fail to stain mahogany brown are
Schiller positive and delineate epithelium that
contains no glycogen. Only a small percentage
(about 5%) of such areas is carcinoma in
situ, the majority being areas of leukoparakeratosis.

There is no way, grossly, to recognize carcinoma in situ involving the endocervical
canal. It is discovered by random biopsy or
endocervical curettage and may be suspected
by the presence of specific cells and cell
clusters in a Papanicolaou smear. The histologic criteria are those of morphologic malignancy in any nonkeratinizing squamous epithelium. There is absence of the normal cellular stratification and polarity, with cellular
pleomorphism, often marked (Fig. 37-14).
Mitotic activity, instead of being confined to
the lower third of the epithelium, may extend
throughout its thickness.

Sometimes, there may be slight surface
stratification (but itself atypical), and this is
probably the in situ form of a pearl-forming
invasive carcinoma.[130] The rare carcinoma in
situ associated with leukoplakia is of this
type. Often at the margin of an invasive carcinoma the epithelium, although not classifiable as carcinoma in situ, is definitely abnormal. The prickle cell layer just above the basal
layer, instead of being two to three cells in

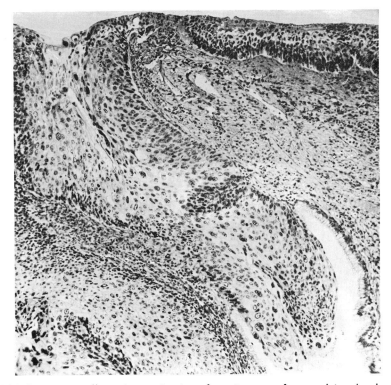

Fig. 37-14 Squamous cell carcinoma in situ of cervix on surface and in gland, growing farther into lumen of gland. (×130; from Hertig, A. T., and Younge, P. A.: Amer. J. Obstet. Gynec. **64**:807-815, 1952.)

thickness, is greatly increased, and the mitoses extend above the lower third. Such is termed *prickle cell hyperplasia* (also called basal cell hyperactivity). Above this is a variable degree of essentially normal surface stratification. Finding prickle cell hyperplasia in a cervical biopsy is an indication for further investigation of that cervix, since it may occur with carcinoma in situ. Its relation to carcinoma in situ, however, is unknown.

Involvement of cervical glands by carcinoma in situ is not considered as invasion but as a change occurring in the glandular epithelium or, occasionally, an extension along the surface of the stroma by the malignant epithelium. It extends into the mouths of glands, destroys the columnar epithelium as it proceeds, and often projects or "prolapses" into the lumen of the gland farther than its line of attachment (Fig. 37-14). It may fill entire glands.

Relationship of carcinoma in situ to carcinoma of cervix. It is extremely difficult to prove that the morphologic entity termed carcinoma in situ inevitably proceeds to invasive carcinoma unless surgically removed or destroyed, because during a biopsy to confirm the diagnosis the lesion may be removed.

Furthermore, in view of present knowledge, once the diagnosis is definitely established, the physician's duty is to treat the patient in some way, attempting to destroy or remove the lesion. Circumstantial evidence that carcinoma in situ is the preinvasive form of squamous cell carcinoma has been accumulated from the following observations:

1 *Comparable prevalence.** Comparable prevalence rates, 0.42% for carcinoma in situ and 0.27% for invasive carcinoma, were found on screening 168,665 patients in Shelby County, Tenn.[125] Upon rescreening 26,005 patients from this group one year later, the incidence of carcinoma in situ was 0.17% and of invasive carcinoma, 0.05%. (There are some discrepancies in varying reports from this study, but all show the same trend.)

2 *Age incidence.* By comparing large groups of patients having carcinoma in situ with those having invasive cancer, it is seen that the in situ lesion usually occurs in people about twelve years younger than does the

*The difference between incidence and prevalence should be noted. Incidence is the number of patients developing a lesion in a given period of time. Prevalence is the number of patients with a lesion in the community at any time.

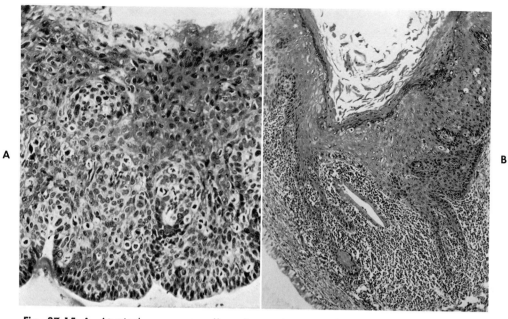

Fig. 37-15 A, Atypical squamous cell carcinoma in situ with cellular pleomorphism and loss of stratification except for surface layers, which are keratinized but have some semblance of stratification. It is probable that this type of carcinoma in situ would develop into well-differentiated squamous cell carcinoma. **B,** "Microcarcinoma" or very early invasive carcinoma of cervix found by making semiserial sections of cervix from which biopsy illustrated in **A** was taken. **(A,** ×150; AFIP 218754-53-9877; **B,** ×75; AFIP 218754-53-9884.)

invasive lesion, although in both there is a wide range. Average age for carcinoma in situ is 38 years and for invasive cancer, 50.1 years.

3 *Racial and ethnic occurrence.*[140] There is a parallel racial occurrence between in situ and invasive lesions. Carcinoma in situ is three and one-half to six times as common in other white women as in Jewish women and invasive carcinoma four to five times as common. Both lesions are about twice as common in black women as in white women. Carcinoma in situ is three times as common and invasive carcinoma seven times as common in Puerto Rican women as in other white women in New York City.

4 *Carcinoma in situ progressing to invasive carcinoma.* In an attempt to determine the progression of carcinoma in situ to invasive carcinoma, two approaches have been used: study of prospective cases and study of retrospective cases.

There are very few prospective cases—viz., those in which a diagnosis of carcinoma in situ has been made, treatment withheld, and the patient allowed to develop invasive carcinoma. This has been done in some countries, and a 22% incidence of invasive carcinoma

has been found after five years by Petersen[155] in Denmark.

Retrospective cases are those in which a diagnosis of invasive carcinoma has been made, and, on investigation of the patient's past history, biopsies have been found containing carcinoma in situ. Unfortunately, it is not possible to be sure in these cases that the invasive carcinoma was not present as a small focus at the time of the original biopsy. In one series, seventeen of twenty-four (71%) prior biopsies showed carcinoma in situ.

5 *Apparent carcinoma in situ showing early invasion.* If carcinoma in situ precedes invasive carcinoma of the cervix, careful study of a large series of cases should indicate the transition between the preinvasive and invasive forms of the disease (Fig. 37-15). From purely practical considerations, it is impossible to make true serial sections or even semiserial sections of every cervix in which carcinoma in situ is diagnosed. In varying series, semiserial sections have been made, with evidence of very early stromal invasion found in from 5% to 23%. In such patients the stromal invasion is so early that these lesions have the same prognosis as the in situ variety.[130]

6 *Diminishing incidence of cervical carci-*

noma (in groups of patients previously studied to detect cervical carcinoma in situ). With mass surveys, such as in Shelby County, Tenn.,[125] there is virtual disappearance of invasive carcinoma from groups of patients screened regularly, with removal from the study group of those with carcinoma in situ. Parallel with the introduction of cancer detection clinics in British Columbia[120] (thought to be screening about half of the female population), there was a 30% reduction in clinically invasive carcinoma in five years.

7 *Invasive carcinoma still showing foci of the in situ pattern.* Again, if carcinoma in situ is the preinvasive form of invasive carcinoma, it would not be surprising to find carcinoma in situ at the margin of a small or early invasive carcinoma (Fig. 37-16). Such proves to be the case, and this phenomenon was first described by Schottlaender and Kermauner[158] in 1912 and frequently is referred to by their names. As the lesion increases in size, it tends to destroy the in situ pattern.

This rather constant association of the carcinoma in situ pattern with early invasive carcinoma of the cervix is the single most important factor in the proper diagnosis and therapy of the preinvasive stage of cervical carcinoma. *Until invasive carcinoma is ruled out by at least a second set of multiple biopsies and a coincidental endocervical curettage, the microscopic diagnosis of carcinoma in situ should mean to both the clinician and pathologist that the patient may well have invasive cervical cancer.* The most popular method of investigation is cold knife conization. To rule out invasive carcinoma, the lines of surgical excision should extend beyond any carcinoma in situ and the specimen should be fixed flat and then cut into multiple labeled blocks so that the entire specimen may be examined.

8 *Light absorption data on carcinoma in situ as compared to invasive carcinoma.* Microscopically, carcinoma in situ looks like carcinoma that has not yet invaded. Foraker[128] has approached this problem photometrically and found that both lesions have similar light absorption data.

9 *Vaginal smear correlation.* Studying only one initial vaginal smear, Graham[135] found malignant cells in 86% to 89% from patients

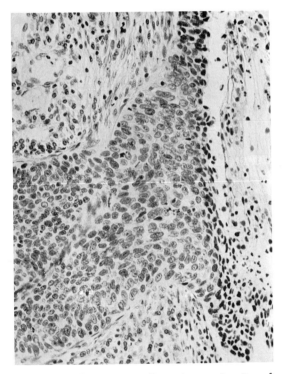

Fig. 37-17 Squamous cell carcinoma in situ of cervix involving surface and extending into and filling endocervical gland. Malignant cells found by Papanicolaou technique are being exfoliated from surface of lesion and appear entangled in overlying mucus. (×320; from Younge, P. A., Hertig, A. T., and Armstrong, D.: Amer. J. Obstet. Gynec. **58:**867-895, 1949.)

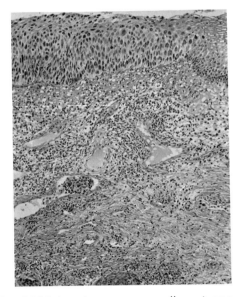

Fig. 37-16 Invasive squamous cell carcinoma of cervix in which in situ pattern is retained on surface at margin of lesion. Surface epithelium on left still retains pattern of carcinoma in situ, but there are nests of invasive carcinoma in underlying connective tissue and within vascular channel. (×60; from Hertig, A. T., and Mansell, H.: CA: Bull. Cancer Progr. **6:**196-202, 1956.)

with carcinoma in situ (Fig. 37-17) and 90% to 96% from patients with invasive carcinoma. Koss[15] has pointed out that the smear pattern may be correlated with the histology. Dyskaryotic cells indicate borderline lesions and a mixture of dyskaryotic and cancer cells suggests carcinoma in situ, whereas cancer cells are the predominant abnormal cells in invasive carcinoma.

Carcinoma in situ of cervix during pregnancy and puerperium. Atypical changes[143] may occur in the squamous epithelium of the cervix during pregnancy, with giant and irregular hyperchromatic nuclei. In such cases, stratification is preserved, together with a normal overall pattern. Such changes must be distinguished from true carcinoma in situ. Indeed, it is thought by some that carcinoma in situ itself may regress after pregnancy, but there is no good proof of this. In a follow-up study of a group of patients by colpomicroscopy through pregnancy and the postpartum period, Richart[156] found that none of the lesions had regressed. Provided invasive carcinoma has been ruled out by careful biopsies, preferably by radial and circumferential biopsies as Johnson and Hertig[143] suggest, carcinoma in situ does not constitute a surgical emergency in pregnancy, so the patient should be followed for some months after the pregnancy has terminated before definite therapy is started. Furthermore, all patients with markedly atypical lesions should be followed into the postpartum period until there is definite evidence of progression or regression. Even those patients whose lesions appear to have regressed should be followed at regular intervals. Those lesions diagnosed by adequate criteria as carcinoma in situ during pregnancy and said to regress postpartum were probably removed completely by the biopsies. In varying series, the incidence of carcinoma in situ during pregnancy varies from 0.35% to 8.4%, the latter seemingly a very high figure.

Clinical management of carcinoma in situ of cervix. The treatment is varied and usually adapted to the individual patient. The commonest method of treatment is complete hysterectomy, with or without conservation of the ovaries, with the line of surgical excision of the vagina controlled by the Schiller test. Those who regard carcinoma in situ as cancer (unqualified) recommend either radiation or Wertheim hysterectomy with radical lymph node dissection. The morbidity and mortality associated with this procedure probably far outweigh any risk of persistence of tumor with a less radical operation. On the other hand, in patients in whom it is of importance to conserve the reproductive function, a shallow cold knife conization may be done, with careful histologic examination to ensure that the lesion has been completely removed. This lesion also has been cured by cauterization and probably on occasion by multiple biopsies, but such therapy is not recommended.

Prediction of complete removal of carcinoma in situ. When submitting a conization specimen, the surgeon should always identify some point (such as 12 o'clock) by a suture. The specimen should be opened at a known point and fixed flat. Parallel blocks should then be made with careful identification and preferably one block to a slide, taking care that the sections include the lines of surgical excision on each block. From a careful examination of endocervical, portio, and deep lines of surgical excision, a calculated estimate may be made of the completeness of removal. Although carcinoma in situ is multifocal, it tends to be so circumferentially rather than in the long axis of the cervix, so that clear lines of excision through histologically normal tissue in all blocks suggest complete removal. A problem exists when there is atypical epithelium at the lines of excision. Therefore, no definite prognostic statement should be made because there is always the possibility that there was sufficient damage to immediately adjacent tissue during the conization procedure to destroy such atypical epithelium, although this should certainly not be presumed.

Carcinoma of cervix uteri

Carcinoma of the cervix is a malignant epithelial neoplasm, most commonly squamous (90% to 95%), sometimes adenocarcinoma (5% to 10%), and rarely adenoacanthoma, although some may be unrecognized. The incidence is 30 per 100,000 females in the United States and has remained constant for about forty years. There are current signs that it is declining. There is a geographic variation in incidence.

Squamous cell carcinoma

Squamous cell carcinoma of the cervix constitutes 11% of all malignant neoplasms in the female. It accounts for 55% to 65% of genital cancer in the female, being second only to breast cancer in frequency. It is less common in Jewish women as compared to

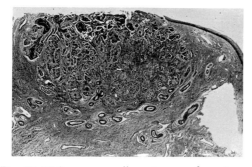

Fig. 37-18 Squamous cell carcinoma of cervix extending into endocervix and deep tissue of cervix but without ulceration of portio epithelium. Position of this small carcinoma indicates that it has most probably arisen within endocervix at squamocolumnar junction. Compare with Fig. 37-13. (×6; AFIP 264079-52094.)

other white patients (1:4),[140] while approximately twice as common in American black women as in white patients. It is at least half as common in the prolapsed cervix as in the normally positioned cervix.[159] The combination of squamous cell carcinoma and prolapse is more common in El Salvador.[124] Squamous cell carcinoma occurs most commonly in patients between 40 and 60 years of age, but it may occur in the twenties and sometimes after the age of 70 years. The average age when diagnosed is 50.1 years.

It usually develops in the region of the squamocolumnar junction (Figs. 37-13 and 37-18) in association with continued inflammation and epithelial regeneration associated with pregnancy and following childbirth. Early marriage or early coitus appears to be an important factor, and divorce, syphilis, and prostitution are more common in these patients. Only rarely do true virgins develop squamous cell carcinoma, and then it is probably in association with inflammation and regeneration at the margin of a congenital erosion.

Gross appearance. The gross appearance of squamous cell carcinoma varies. The apparently benign cervix may harbor tumor that has extended into the endocervix and out into the cervical connective tissue but without ulcerating through the portio epithelium. This is often clinically unsuspected. The smallest lesion visible on the portio is a firm granular area near the external os that bleeds with minimal trauma. More obvious are the three classic types:

1 Excavating type, which results in an irregular, hard ulcer with sloughing base
2 Cauliflower type, which may vary con-

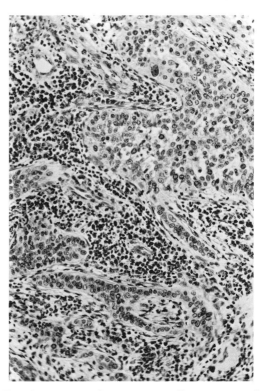

Fig. 37-19 Typical squamous cell carcinoma of cervix has plexiform pattern without keratin formation. (×160; AFIP 264084-1.)

siderably in size and has a coarsely nodular or papillary appearance, often with surface ulceration
3 Flat, infiltrating type (commonest), which may grow out on the cervix without ulcerating the cervical mucosa and may indeed extend the length of the vagina without ulcerating the vaginal mucosa, which is hard and tough and cuts with a gritty consistency, and in which ulceration appears late

Microscopic appearance. Classically, these tumors are nonkeratinizing and belong to the moderately well-differentiated squamous cell carcinomas. They may be classified in a variety of ways. We have used three grades.

Grade I

Numerous epithelial pearls, considerable keratinization with visible intercellular bridges, and less than two mitoses per high-power field (5%)

Grade II

Pearls rare or absent, moderate keratinization, some intercellular bridges, two to four mitoses per high-power field, and moderate pleomorphism of tumor cells (85%) (Fig. 37-19)

Grade III

Absence of pearls, slight keratinization, no intercellular bridges, more than four mitoses per high-power field, and marked cellular pleomorphism (10%)

Criteria for grading cervical carcinoma vary somewhat among students of the subject. Other classifications are those of Broders,[121] Martzloff,[151] and Glucksmann and Spear.[134]

Broders[121] uses four grades, depending on degree of differentiation and divided as follows:

Grade 1—Differentiation ranging from almost 100% to 75%
Grade 2—Differentiation ranging from 75% to 50%
Grade 3—Differentiation ranging from 50% to 25%
Grade 4—Differentiation ranging from 25% to practically 0

Martzloff[151] classifies cervical carcinomas according to the predominant cell as follows:

Spinal cell—Resembling cells of the upper portion of stratum mucosum of normal cervical epithelium (15.5%)
Transitional cell—Representing intermediate variety, corresponding to those cells limited above by spinal cell layer and below by stratum germinativum (66.8%)
Fat spindle cell—Broad spindle cell, resembling more or less the compactly placed basal cells but not true basal cells (12%)
Adenocarcinoma from endocervix—Comprises remaining 5.7%

Glucksmann and Spear classify squamous cell carcinomas as either anaplastic parakeratotic (AP) or anaplastic squamous (AS), constituting 69% and 24.5%, respectively, of cervical cancers. The former are the undifferentiated variety and the latter the more differentiated.

Biology of cervical carcinoma. Staging of cervical carcinoma is a clinical estimation of the extent of the tumor and of the presence or absence of lymph node involvement. That currently used is the modified description tabulated in *Annual Report on the Results of Treatment in Carcinoma of the Uterus and Vagina.*[64]

Stage 0—Intraepithelial (carcinoma in situ)
Stage I—Strictly confined to cervix
Stage II—Infiltrates parametrium but has not reached pelvic wall; involves vagina but not lower third
Stage III—Carcinomatous infiltration has extended into pelvic wall; on rectal examination, infiltration feels firm and nodular; no smooth "cancer-free" space between tumor and pelvic wall; involves lower third of vagina
Stage IV—Involves bladder or rectum or has extended outside true pelvis—i.e., below vaginal inlet, above pelvic brim, distant metastases

Lymph nodes may be divided into a primary group and a secondary group, some nodes of the primary group always being involved before those of the secondary group are involved. The primary group is composed of the parametrial nodes, the paracervical (ureteral) node, and the nodes of the hypogastric, obturator, and external iliac groups. The secondary group includes the sacral, the common iliac, the inguinal, and the aortic (periaortic) nodes.[141]

Radiosensitivity is ably summarized by Ewing when he states: "In general the degree of radiosensitivity runs parallel to the degree of anaplasia of tumor cells, but so many factors enter into clinical malignancy that the parallelism is far from uniform."* It is important to distinguish between radiosensitivity and ultimate curability of a tumor. An anaplastic tumor may be largely destroyed by radiation, but viable cells may remain and continue to grow. The concept of true radiosensitivity (developed by Glucksmann and Spear[134]) is that the resting (potential dividing cells) and the mitotic cells are killed off and that the remaining ones—no longer capable of dividing but still capable of maturing—go on, mature, and thus degenerate.

It is important to determine which tumors are radioresistant so that these may be treated surgically, and this may be assessed on the appearance and apparent viability of surviving tumor cells. To this Gluckmann and Spear[134] add the ability to differentiate while undergoing radiation.

It has been shown that there is a good correlation between clinical stage and five-year survival and also between the degree of radiation response and five-year survival in patients treated by irradiation. In general, 75% of patients with stage I lesions, 50% with stage II, 25% with stage III, and 0% with stage IV are alive and well at five years. The average world figures for all stages is 37.8% alive and well at five years.

Another method for estimation of radiosensitivity of a cervical cancer has been described by Graham[136, 137] from the cytology of the vaginal smear. This sensitivity (RR) is evaluated by the appearance of the *benign* exfoliated vaginal cells after radiation therapy. Furthermore, a prediction of the radiosensitivity may be made in patients with cervical carcinoma prior to irradiation from the appearance of benign exfoliated cells. Changes

---

*From Ewing, J.: Radiology **13**:313-318, 1929.

in these are termed sensitization response (SR).[138] The value of both of these tests has been questioned.[150] From a recent study of the literature, it appears that the RR determination is not being widely used, and there is no evidence that the SR determinations are being utilized other than perhaps by Graham.

The radiosensitivity of cervical cancer metastatic to lymph nodes depends not only upon the sensitivity of the tumor itself but also, of course, upon whether the radiation reaches the nodes in adequate dosage. It is difficult to determine the exact time of onset of cervical cancer, but taking the onset of clinical vaginal bleeding as the starting point (which, of course, it is not), 50% of untreated patients are dead in eleven months and 88% in three years. Bleeding, however, may not invariably be present, 2% of patients with advanced tumors never having bled. Most patients are treated by radium and deep x-ray therapy and only a small proportion (about 3%) by Wertheim hysterectomy and radical lymph node dissection, often with irradiation. Various other radioactive agents are less often employed. Both methods of therapy have fairly similar results in stages I and II in competent hands, and both have their attendant complications.

In general, the principal cause of death is the local extension of the tumor and its effect on the ureters—with subsequent urinary tract obstruction, infection, and uremia. Evidence of ureteral compression and kidney damage is present in 82.8% of untreated patients and 78.6% of treated patients.[123]

Adenocarcinoma

Adenocarcinoma of the cervix[139] is a malignant epithelial neoplasm arising from the endocervical mucosa or glands, situated anywhere from the internal os to the external os, or even beyond in that portion of the endocervix incorporated into the ectocervix as the result of eversion or congenital erosion. Rarely, it may arise from vestigial remnants of wolffian (mesonephric) duct epithelium and is designated as mesonephroma (Fig. 37-10) or mesometanephric carcinoma.

Adenocarcinoma constitutes 4.5% of all malignant cervical neoplasms. Although the average age is about 50 years, it is interesting that cervical cancer occurring in patients under 20 years of age is most likely to be adenocarcinoma. There is an age range from 17 to over 80 years. It is probable that there is an in situ stage of adenocarcinoma of the

cervix,[129] but this has received little attention. There are relatively more unmarried patients with adenocarcinoma of the cervix than with squamous cell carcinoma. The gestational histories of patients with adenocarcinoma are more often similar to those of patients with endometrial carcinoma than to those of patients with squamous cell carcinoma of the cervix.

Atypical changes are sometimes observed in endocervical glands during pregnancy, and the question may be raised whether or not these are related to the genesis of adenocarcinoma. Glucksmann[133] has described an adenoacanthoma of the cervix ("mixed carcinoma"), which is often poorly differentiated. It accounts for 51% of cervical cancers in pregnant women and only 8% of the whole series in his study.

Usually, the tumor appears to have arisen in the anatomic endocervix but obviously may have arisen from glands on the portio or may appear to have arisen diffusely through the cervix. The tumors are most commonly papillary (40%) or ulcerative (34%), but they also may be nodular or polypoid. The type arising in the endocervical canal and growing into the cervical stroma may not produce symptoms until the tumor erodes onto the portio. The diffuse variety may result in marked enlargement and extreme friability of the cervix.

Microscopically, the pattern is extremely varied. The well-differentiated adenocarcinomas may be cervical gland type (Fig. 37-20), gyriform type, papillary type, endometrium-like pattern, or tubal-type pattern. When very well differentiated, these tumors may present a very difficult diagnostic problem.[149] The moderately poorly differentiated type may have a goblet cell pattern or be of signet-ring type. The undifferentiated tumors do not have a significant pattern.[139]

Prognosis seems to be similar to that in squamous cell carcinoma (judging from the literature), but results of treatment in our experience are very poor (18% five-year survival). Radiation response of these tumors is apparently much the same as that of squamous cell carcinoma, although there is no uniform opinion on this subject.

"Pill" cervix

Columnar epithelial proliferation with a resultant small gland adenomatous hyperplasia, together with some varying degrees of squamous metaplasia, has been observed in

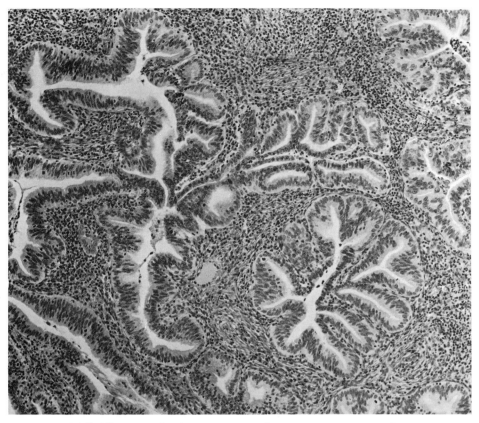

Fig. 37-20 Well-differentiated adenocarcinoma of cervix retaining normal racemose pattern of cervical glands but with irregular piling up of lining cells. (×110.)

some patients taking oral contraceptives.[62, 122, 131, 160] It is often focal and may occur in a preexisting polyp, or its development may result in a polypoid formation. The precise prevalence is difficult to determine because relatively few patients taking the "pill" have had cervical biopsies. It has been observed with the progesterone type of oral contraceptive but what relationship the dosage and length of use have to its development is unknown. At least some patients have developed the pattern after only a few months. Whether prolonged use of oral contraceptives in patients developing this pattern will result in development of neoplastic disease is unknown and is a question for the future.[152] The immediate problem is recognition of this bizarre pattern as one related to the intake of oral contraceptives and one which will regress after their suspension. Furthermore, its differential diagnosis from true adenocarcinoma is most important.

Grossly, the lesion may be polypoid or it may be interpreted as a congenital erosion or an eversion with marked inflammation. Microscopically, there is a proliferation of the columnar epithelium forming small gland spaces, which often are crowded together. The lining epithelium may be flattened, or the cells may be vacuolated. Combined with the squamous metaplasia, this may produce a disturbing tumorlike lesion (Fig. 37-21).

The pattern is an exaggeration of the patterns observed in pregnancy. Also, as in pregnancy, the columnar epithelium of patients taking oral contraceptives is tall with an active mucus-secreting appearance. Also, as in pregnancy, the cervical stroma or the stroma of an endocervical polyp may be edematous. By its very edema the stroma may raise the question of a stromal mesenchymal tumor.

Cervical adenocarcinoma of wolffian (mesonephric) origin

Cervical carcinomas of mesonephric origin are rare[298] but occur at ages ranging from 13 to 71 years. They have no characteristic appearance but usually involve the anterolateral or posterolateral aspect of the cervix, later involving the whole organ. Microscopically, they mimic the mesonephros and range from well-differentiated tubular carcinomas (Fig.

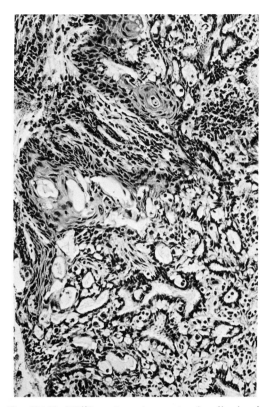

Fig. 37-21 "Pill" pattern in cervix. Small gland adenomatous hyperplasia combined with squamous metaplasia. (×138; HMS CS-66-192; courtesy Dr. J. W. Hamlin and Dr. R. B. Ziegler.)

37-10) to typical clear cell carcinomas of hypernephroid or Grawitz type. Prognosis is probably similar to that of other adenocarcinomas of the cervix.

Sometimes, an adenocarcinoma in a cervical biopsy may have a typical clear cell pattern, but upon examination of the hysterectomy specimen, transitions from an ordinary endocervical gland may be observed. Therefore, the problem of differential diagnosis is not so simple in practice as it appears from written description even when the techniques suggested by McGee et al.[148] are employed. There is another unsolved problem associated with the mesonephric type of carcinoma. The dividing line between very marked, nonneoplastic hyperplasia of mesonephric remnants and early but definite carcinoma may be impossible to draw at this time even when the entire cervix is available for study.

Carcinoma of cervix in pregnancy

About 1% of cervical cancers occur in pregnant women or within four months of delivery, whereas about 0.05% of pregnant patients have the disease.[146] Morphology is similar in the pregnant and the nonpregnant patient, although there are proportionately more adenoacanthomas.[133] Whether pregnancy influences the rate of growth is debated but actually unknown.

True carcinoma should be treated when diagnosed. Competent clinicians differ in their treatment of any individual patient, although theoretically the cancer should be treated unless the pregnancy is at term. The five-year survival rate prior to the middle of the last trimester does not appear to differ from that in the nonpregnant patient, stage for stage, but the apparent cure rates in the last half of the third trimester and in the postpartum period are poor.[146] It is considered unwise to allow such patients to deliver vaginally.

Connective tissue tumors and rare tumors

Leiomyoma of the cervix is said to constitute 0.29% to 15.5% of all leiomyomas of the uterus. Its cause is unknown, but it usually affects multiparas.

Leiomyosarcoma is a rare tumor in the cervix. *Carcinosarcoma* is also an uncommon tumor of the cervix. It is a histologic variant of the malignant mixed müllerian tumor. *Sarcoma botryoides,* a rare tumor of mesenchymal origin, is a variant of the malignant mixed müllerian tumor. It is predominantly a disease of infancy, but it may occur at all ages.

Lymphoma is extremely rare in the cervix, probably as a direct result of the lack of lymphoid tissue in this area. Presumably it arises from the occasional germinal lymphoid follicles found in the cervix.

Hemangioma[132] presents as a wine-colored lesion of the cervix, fading on pressure. The patients usually have a history suggestive of carcinoma. *Hemangioendotheliomas* are said to constitute 0.1% of cervical malignancies and to be radiosensitive.[119]

Ganglioneuroma has been reported by Fingerland and Sikl.[127] This was a tiny polypoid lesion composed largely of Schwann cells with some ganglion cells. *Malignant melanoma* has been reported.

Carcinoma metastatic to cervix. Carcinoma metastatic to the cervix is extremely rare and has been reported from the breast, pancreas, and stomach. There may be cellular infiltration by leukemic cells. The most important feature is the distinction of such tumors from primary carcinoma.[162]

ENDOMYOMETRIUM
Benign conditions of endometrium

Irregular shedding. Irregular shedding[187, 188] of the endometrium is characterized clinically by prolonged and irregular menstruation (bleeding from progestational endometrium), endocrinologically by continued secretion of sodium pregnanediol glucuronide during such bleeding, and pathologically by various degrees of retardation of shedding, involution, and healing of endometrial glands and stroma. In our experience, such endometrium between menstrual periods shows a mosaic pattern composed of areas of variable degrees of maturity and immaturity, especially prominent in the postovulatory period.

"Pill" endometrium. The current common use of oral contraceptives has produced some confusing endometrial patterns. These differ from the classic cycle but beyond that are difficult to classify. Undoubtedly, the pattern varies with the contraceptive agent and with the dosage and with the state of the endometrium at the time such therapy is in-

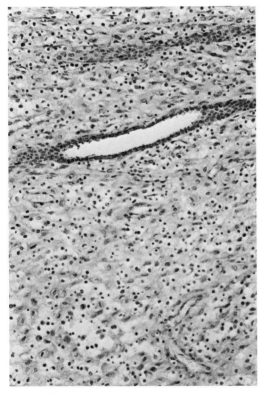

Fig. 37-22 One of numerous patterns seen with oral contraceptive therapy. Gland is small and lined by low epithelium, inactive in appearance, and stroma is of "almost-predecidual" type. (×138; HMS CS-66-205.)

stituted. A common pattern in patients on a combined type of oral contraceptive is that of inactive glands of small lumen lined by low cells—a "dead" appearance—together with a stroma that varies from a definite predecidual pattern (seen with the higher doses previously given) to a rather compact stroma that may suggest predecidua in varying stages of regression (Fig. 37-22). There are usually large thin-walled vessels within the stroma. This pattern is seen when therapy is instituted about the fifth day of the cycle. However, should therapy be started later in the cycle, in a patient with irregular shedding, in a patient recently curetted, or in one recently postpartum or postabortal, there may be a wide spectrum of patterns.

Some contraceptives, when given for a number of successive cycles, may produce vacuolated glandular cells, often a little suggestive of ovulation, but not quite coinciding with the classic picture. Should Enovid be given in large doses for other reasons, there may be a very exuberant stromal development, sometimes so exuberant as to raise the question of neoplastic proliferation because of mitotic activity in the decidua-like stroma.

Polyp. Polypoid growths of the endometrium may be single or multiple and vary from a few millimeters to several centimeters in diameter. They usually appear first in the mid-thirties, while the patient is still menstruating, and may persist after the menopause. They usually arise from the middle or basal third of the endometrium and may or may not be covered by functioning endometrium. The potential of malignancy is similar to that of cystic hyperplasia (about 1%).

Cystic hyperplasia. Cystic hyperplasia of the endometrium is a condition characterized by cystically dilated but active glands lined by a single layer of columnar epithelium or by pseudostratified epithelium (Fig. 37-23, *A*). The stroma is composed of cells with very scanty cytoplasm, but the striking feature is the presence of large, thin-walled stromal sinusoids. It is from these that the bleeding occurs in endometrial hyperplasia. Grossly, the hyperplastic endometrium is soft, pale pink to yellow in color, and variously and irregularly thickened, in a most marked degree forming prominent polypoid areas.

Adenomatous hyperplasia. Probably a later stage of hyperplasia, adenomatous hyperplasia (Hertig's type), shows some glands from which outpouchings are rising and others in which this has already occurred, resulting in

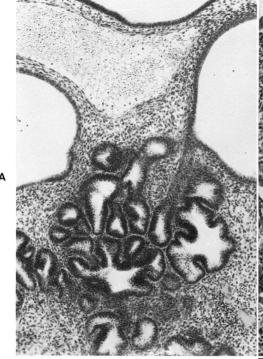

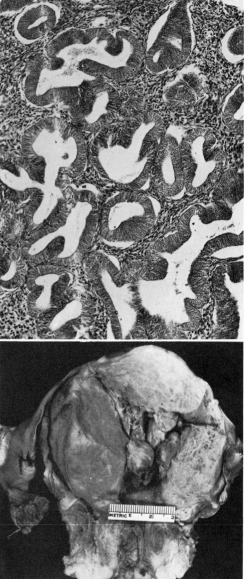

Fig. 37-23 A, Cystic (above) and adenomatous hyperplasia (below) of endometrium, with prominent large thin-walled stromal sinusoid from which bleeding found in this condition occurs, in 22-year-old patient who had been bleeding irregularly and profusely since 17 years of age. **B,** Adenocarcinoma in situ of endometrium from curettage of same patient at 26 years of age. **C,** Adenocarcinoma of endometrium found in uterus of same patient at 30 years of age. Patient died three months after hysterectomy. (**A** and **B,** ×100; from Sommers, S. C., Hertig, A. T., and Bengloff, H.: Cancer **2:**957-963, 1949.)

groupings of multiple small glands lined by cells similar to those in cystic hyperplasia (Fig. 37-23, *A*). The stroma also is similar to that in cystic hyperplasia.

Anaplasia (dysplasia). Anaplasia denotes the dedifferentiation of the cells lining the glands. In the endometrium, this results in pale-staining eosinophilic cells, usually in a single layer but occasionally pseudostratified and usually with only a few mitoses. This pattern has been described as atypical hyperplasia (type II or III) by Campbell and Barter[169] and adenomatous hyperplasia by Gusberg and Kaplan.[178] These lesions may be difficult to differentiate from carcinoma in situ or minimal carcinoma.

Many of the problems in diagnosis of endometrial lesions are related to nomenclature,

and in any institution it should be well established what histologic pattern is meant by each term.

Malignant conditions of endometrium

Carcinoma in situ

Carcinoma in situ of the endometrium has no definite gross appearance, the endometrium showing the features of the hyperplasia in which it is arising. Gusberg and Kaplan[178] apply the term *adenomatous hyperplasia,* which they consider stage 0 carcinoma of the endometrium, to such carcinoma in situ. Microscopically, there are groups of pale glands "back to back," obliterating the intervening stroma, similar to those in actual cancer but without the usual alteration of glandular pattern seen in carcinoma (Fig. 37-23, *B*).

Although carcinoma in situ is found in association with or precedes invasive carcinoma and is morphologically similar to this cancer, it is not identical. It is to be distinguished from typical microscopic adenocarcinoma, which is confined to the endometrium and without evidence of myometrial invasion. Papillary infoldings within glands of carcinoma in situ or small secondary lumina within the gland walls suggest definite adenocarcinoma.

Pedunculated adenomyoma

The finding in curettings of a mixture of normal endometrium and fragments of uterine muscle containing endometrial type glands without any surrounding endometrial stroma suggests a diagnosis of pedunculated adenomyoma. Glands are usually irregular, and squamous elements are common. If the uterus is available, there may be definite superficial myometrial invasion. These lesions persist after curettage and may show myometrial invasion so are best considered as low-grade carcinoma. They usually occur in young patients, often in those with infertility problems.

Carcinoma

Carcinoma arising from the endometrium is usually glandular but sometimes is associated with squamous elements. The reported incidence is about 0.0119% of the female population. This suggests that the disease is only one-third as common as cervical cancer. Reports over the last ten years suggest an increase in endometrial carcinoma, so that its incidence is approaching that of cervical carcinoma. The age range is from the third to the ninth decade, although it has, on rare occasions, been reported before the age of 20 years. The peak incidence is in the sixth decade, but there is another, although much lower, peak in the twenties. Carcinoma of the endometrium is more frequent in spinsters. Married women with this malignant tumor are more likely to have been nulliparous or to have had very few children.

Of general medical and endocrinologic interest is the increased incidence of diabetes mellitus, obesity, breast carcinoma, thyroid disease, and estrogenically hyperactive ovarian lesions in association with endometrial carcinoma, and these also are observed in patients with endometrial hyperplasia.

Etiology. The etiology of carcinoma of the endometrium is unknown, but the clinical, endocrinologic, and pathologic evidence gradually accumulating indicates that it often develops as the result of long-continued, noncyclic stimulation of the endometrium by estrogen (and possibly progesterone), usually of ovarian origin but very rarely artificially administered.[168] It should be noted that the questionably carcinomatous pattern seen in the patient taking such hormones often regresses with the suspension of therapy. Endometrial carcinoma does *not* arise from normal endometrium, but it may arise from abnormal foci within otherwise normal endometrium. This cancer develops through a series of changes that may be generalized or focal in the endometrium. Not all endometria showing these changes ultimately develop endometrial carcinoma. Indeed, very few do. These changes are cystic hyperplasia, adenomatous hyperplasia, anaplasia, and carcinoma in situ. Gradual morphologic transitions have been observed in sequential biopsies on patients who have developed cancer[175] and may be seen in the same endometrial specimen as the cancer.

Prospective studies have indicated that endometrial carcinoma will develop in 2.4% to 3% of premenopausal patients with endometrial hyperplasia and in 12% to 25% of the comparable postmenopausal group.[184] Furthermore, the more atypical or disturbing the hyperplasia, the greater the likelihood that the patient will develop endometrial carcinoma.[169]

Gross appearance. Grossly, there are two types of carcinomas of the endometrium: diffuse and discrete. The diffuse variety may be confined to the endometrium but spread widely through it. It may be polypoid, pale, firm, friable (Fig. 37-23, *C*), and lacking the glistening mucosal surface of cystic hyperplasia. There may be surface ulceration, or the surface may be hemorrhagic or shiny as a result of mucus production. The discrete form may occur anywhere in the uterus (most frequently in the posterior wall) and may be papillary, polypoid, or slightly raised from the surrounding endometrium. Discrete tumors sometimes are localized to the endometrium (17% to 39%), but they usually have invaded the myometrium.

Microscopic appearance. Endometrial carcinoma is basically an adenocarcinoma, which may be well differentiated (Fig. 37-24), moderately well differentiated (Fig. 37-25), or poorly differentiated. In the better-differentiated varieties, glands may vary in size, often having subsidiary gland lumina actually within their walls. Frequently (in as many as

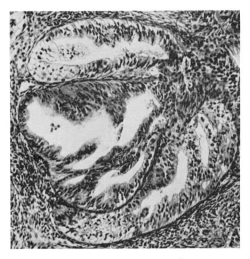

Fig. 37-24 Uncommon secretory adenocarcinoma of endometrium, many cells attempting to recapitulate those of sixteen-day to eighteen-day secretory endometrium. It is of interest that this tumor had already metastasized to ovary, in which there was mature corpus luteum. Question arises as to whether or not this well-differentiated cancer was responding to hormonal action of corpus luteum. (×110.)

20%), there is an accompanying squamous element, such tumors being called adenoacanthomas (Fig. 37-26). In adenoacanthoma, the adenocarcinoma is usually fairly well differentiated but obviously malignant. The squamous element is usually well differentiated and does not necessarily appear malignant histologically but is an integral part of the tumor and takes part in metastases. Rarely, the squamous element may appear histologically to be malignant and may be invading the myometrium.

Secretory carcinoma[175] occasionally may be extremely difficult to diagnose unless there is definite myometrial invasion (Fig. 37-27). Irregular foci of hyperplasia within a secretory endometrium may result in a confusing hyperplastic and hypersecretory pattern, somewhat suggestive of endometrium of pregnancy, best described as *secretory hyperplasia.* Whether or not such foci develop into carcinoma is uncertain, but they may be found in association with definite endometrial adenocarcinoma. We do not know if this curious hyperplastic pattern varies with corpus luteum activity, since we have not seen such a lesion while the remainder of the endometrium was in the proliferative phase.

Foci of secretory activity may be found within the usual endometrial carcinomas, but these pose no diagnostic problem.

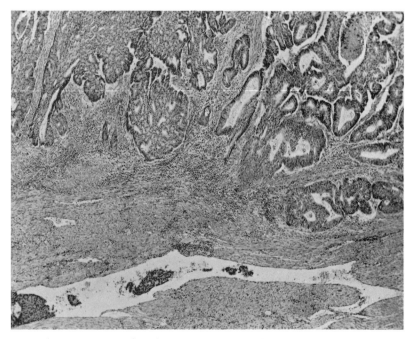

Fig. 37-25 Adenocarcinoma of endometrium, part moderately well differentiated (upper right) and part less well differentiated (upper left), invading myometrium and lymphatic within myometrium. (×46; AFIP 264087-2.)

Clinical staging. Methods of staging[167, 179] endometrial carcinoma vary from the simple and purely clinical method of the Radium-hemmet—operable, technically operable, and inoperable—to complex combinations of clinical evaluation and microscopic findings.

Anatomic spread. Lymphatic spread of endometrial carcinoma is inconstant, and although there are three main channels, there is a rich anastomosis between them. Spread is slower than with cervical carcinoma. Endometrial carcinoma is slow to invade the myometrium but occasionally may penetrate the wall and extend to adjacent intestine or to the broad ligament. Metastases occur to the ovary in about 4% of the patients and often

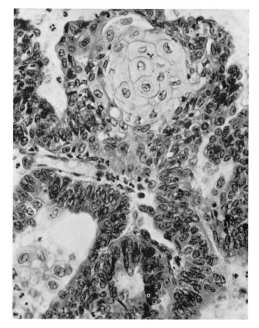

Fig. 37-26 Adenoacanthoma of endometrium. Well-differentiated plaque of squamous cells lies within adenocarcinomatous elements. (×235; AFIP 264048-1.)

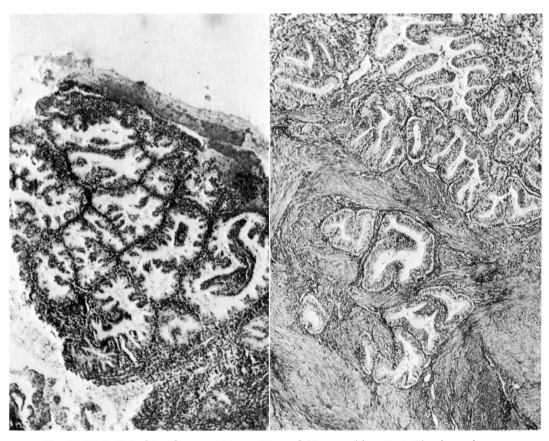

Fig. 37-27 A, Disturbing fragment in curettings of 38-year-old patient. Glands are hypersecretory, with papillary infoldings, but are abnormally crowded. **B,** Invasive secretory carcinoma within myometrium found at hysterectomy six weeks later. (×45; HMS CS-62-2; courtesy Dr. Malcolm L. Barnes; from Gore, H., and Hertig, A. T.: Clin. Obstet. Gynec. **5:**1148-1165, 1962.)

are seen elsewhere in the peritoneum. The commonest distant metastases are in lung and liver.

Current therapy is somewhat varied and may consist of a complete hysterectomy or of preoperative radium with hysterectomy, followed by roentgen therapy. Recently, some patients have been treated by lymph node dissection also. The commonest causes of death are uremia (40%) and pyelonephritis (25%). With modern techniques, the prognosis is good, with five-year survival rates varying from 78% to 94%. The prognosis is related to extent of the tumor and is better if the tumor is well differentiated.

Potent progestational agents that are suppressive rather than curative have been employed for palliation in advanced disease and occasionally for trial therapy of early lesions. Another modern approach is to attempt to produce ovulation, either mechanically through wedge resection of ovaries or biochemically by administration of MER-25 (an analogue of chlorotrianisene) or MRL-141 (clomiphene citrate).[22]

Benign conditions involving myometrium

Adenomyosis uteri. Ectopic nests of endometrium composed of glands and stroma and lying within the myometrium are termed adenomyosis. Usually, it is specified that such nests should be one low-power field beyond the endomyometrial junction. Distribution through the myometrium may be focal or diffuse, with a variable amount of myometrial hypertrophy. The incidence is difficult to determine. In unselected hysterectomies, reports on its incidence vary from 8% to 29%. In uteri removed at autopsy, its incidence was 54%. It never begins before the menarche or after the menopause, but it may manifest itself postmenopausally. The age range is from 27 to 73 years. The symptomatology is variable, the commonest manifestations being menorrhagia, dysmenorrhea, and metrorrhagia. The uterus is usually globoid, slightly enlarged, and often tender.

Of the numerous theories of origin, the most commonly accepted is that of direct invasion of or extension into the myometrium by the endometrium, from its basal portion. Other theories are based mainly on the occurrence of congenital rests or metastatic transmission. A neglected possibility is that it is derived from indifferent stroma lying between muscle bundles. Why any of these happens is unknown.

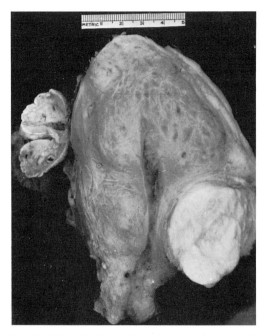

Fig. 37-28 Sagittally sectioned uterus showing diffuse adenomyosis of upper half and typical whorled well-demarcated leiomyoma in lower half.

Grossly, the uterus is usually enlarged and heavier than usual. The enlargement may be focal, but more usually is symmetric. The consistency is firm and, when cut, the myometrium bulges outward with a typical coarse, whorled, fibrous appearance—often with tiny depressed, gray, translucent areas (sometimes hemorrhagic) between the strands of tissue (Fig. 37-28). Microscopically, endometrial glands and stroma lie within the myometrium at a distance equivalent to at least one low-power microscopic field from the endomyometrial junction. These endometrial foci are similar to those of the basal endometrium and hence only rarely undergo cyclic change or hemorrhage. Furthermore, they may undergo all changes seen in endometrium, including hyperplasia, anaplasia, and cancer.[171] Carcinoma is very rare, but sarcoma or carcinosarcoma arising in such an area is even more rare. Another rare finding is a decidual stromal response in adenomyosis during pregnancy, although from examination of uteri removed at the time of therapeutic abortion, it seems that decidual response in adenomyosis may be more common than previously assumed. Oophorectomy is said to cause some regression, but the only definitely curative procedure is surgical removal of the uterus.

Endolymphatic stromal myosis. The pres-

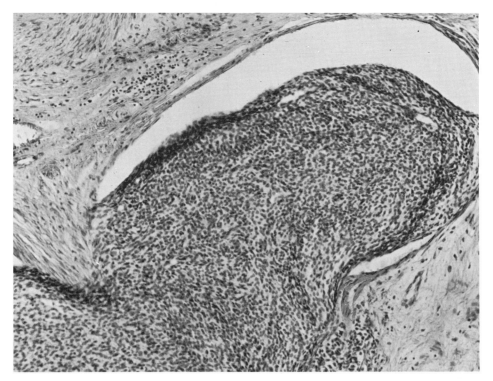

Fig. 37-29 Endolymphatic stromal myosis showing strand of endometrial-type stroma growing into lymphatic. (×130; AFIP 194508.)

ence within the myometrium of strands and masses of a noncollagenous connective tissue, interpreted variously but usually regarded as being of endometrial origin, has been described under many names—most commonly endolymphatic stromal myosis and stromatous endometriosis.[181] This is an extremely rare disease and usually occurs between the ages of 31 and 50 years. There is no constant clinical picture, but most patients have had some abnormal vaginal bleeding. Even the cell of origin is disputed, but the most accepted opinion is that the origin is from endometrial stroma extending into the myometrium (as in adenomyosis) and spreading by lymphatic (Fig. 37-29) or blood vessel permeation or both. Unifocal or multifocal development from tissue already within the myometrium and the possibility that this tumor is a hemangiopericytoma have been suggested. It may occur after the menopause and may continue to grow after castration, thereby differing from adenomyosis and suggesting it is a low-grade sarcoma.

Grossly, the uterus is enlarged usually symmetrically but occasionally focally. The tumor tissue extends through a coarsely meshed myometrium and may appear as yellow or white nodules, usually elastic and rubbery but sometimes pultaceous. Sometimes, it is more finely distributed between the muscle bundles. Microscopically, it is composed of round to oval nuclei with very scanty surrounding cytoplasm, similar in appearance to the endometrial stroma of the proliferative phase. Vascularity is variable within the foci, which may blend with the surrounding myometrium or may be sharply demarcated therefrom.

Its true relation to adenomyosis and to endometrial stromal sarcoma is difficult to determine. It does seem logical, however, that it is part of the broad spectrum of endometrial stromal sarcoma. In the true endolymphatic stromal myosis, the prognosis is fairly good (80% "cure") following surgical removal of all the tumor. The patients who died probably had true endometrial stromal sarcoma. As endolymphatic stromal myosis is so well differentiated, it is not considered to be susceptible to roentgen radiation.

Leiomyoma uteri. Leiomyoma is a well-circumscribed but nonencapsulated benign uterine tumor, composed mainly of muscle but with a variable fibrous connective tissue element (Figs. 37-28 and 37-30). The absolute incidence is difficult to determine,

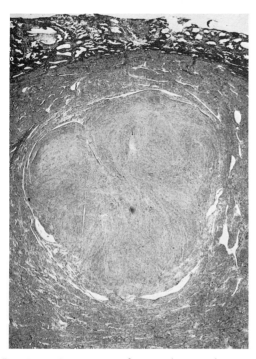

Fig. 37-30 Leiomyoma of uterus lying within myometrium, well demarcated but not encapsulated from surrounding myometrium. (×9¼; AFIP 218754-426.)

varying from 4% to 40% in several reports but most probably occurring in about 25% of women. The tumors are much more common in black than in white patients. Theories of histogenesis are varied, but all are based on some type of connective tissue cell, either immature or mature, within the uterine wall or its blood vessels. Estrogenic stimulation appears in some way to be related to the growth of leiomyomas.

Grossly, leiomyomas may occur anywhere within the uterus, being subserosal (sometimes pedunculated), intramural (Fig. 37-28), or submucosal. They may gradually lose their uterine attachment as they become parasitic on a neighboring organ through fibrinous and, later, fibrous adhesions. Usually, they are multiple but may be single. Leiomyomas are well demarcated from the surrounding muscle, which they may flatten to form a false capsule, but they have no true capsule (Fig. 37-30). Microscopically, the leiomyoma is composed of groups and bundles of smooth muscle fibers in twisted, whorled pattern. Various types of degeneration may occur. Commonest are hyaline and cystic degeneration, less often necrosis (in large tumors) and infection, and occasionally calcification. "Red degeneration"[173] is uncommon, although rela-

tively common in leiomyomas complicating pregnancy. It is due to hemorrhage (with subsequent hemolysis) into an already partially hyalinized leiomyoma. Polycythemia occasionally has been reported in a patient with a large leiomyoma and has been cured by hysterectomy.

Pleomorphism has been observed in some leiomyomas during pregnancy. It may raise a problem in differentiation from leiomyosarcoma although few, if any, mitoses are present. The atypical pattern may well be another manifestation comparable to the Arias-Stella pattern of endometrium and endocervix. Occasional leiomyomas from patients taking oral contraceptives have been edematous and pleomorphic.

Benign metastasizing leiomyoma (intravenous leiomyomatosis). Benign metastasizing leiomyoma is a very rare condition in which a leiomyoma, appearing benign histologically, extends locally via lymphatics or blood vessels and may even produce distant metastases.[200] In such cases, doubt usually is expressed as to whether microscopic sections were adequate. Perhaps a truly malignant area was overlooked, although the "metastases" are as well differentiated as the tumor itself. Harper and Scully[180] consider intravenous leiomyomatosis more common than endolymphatic stromal myosis and believe that it will be found more often if careful search is made. This is not our impression on the basis of our experience. Particular attention should be given to tumors that are cellular or unusually vascular or exhibit vascular thrombosis.

Adenomatoid tumor. Occasional tumors presenting grossly as leiomyomas contain numerous spaces lined by flattened to columnar epithelium, similar to the adenomatoid tumor of the tube. Usually, the muscular component is predominant. Sometimes, the spaces are continuous with the peritoneal surface, suggesting a peritoneal origin. The other distinct possibility is that they are derived from müllerian mesenchyme and are forming a benign "mixed tumor" of the uterus.

Hemangiopericytoma. Hemangiopericytoma is a rare tumor of the uterus and is found also elsewhere in the body. It is composed of nonneoplastic capillary endothelium surrounded by collars of neoplastic capillary pericytes of Zimmerman.[177] These tumors usually have been found in uteri removed for leiomyomas. Hemangiopericytoma is similar, grossly, to the leiomyoma, but is usually less discrete, softer, and more yellow, and it is often mistaken for leiomyosarcoma. Microscopically, there are capillaries, often collapsed and surrounded by a sheath of reticulum that separates them from the collars of spindle-shaped pericytes containing uniform round or oval nuclei but few mitoses. No malignant variant has been reported in the uterus.

Lipoma. Lipoma[174] is a rare tumor of the uterus, composed of adult adipose tissue, often with collagenous and muscular tissue, well demarcated from the surrounding myometrium. Grossly and microscopically, these tumors are similar to lipomas elsewhere in the body, and only one tumor with definite malignant change has been reported.

Malignant tumors of connective tissue origin

Sarcoma is a rare uterine tumor, accounting for 0.07% to 0.15% of gynecologic hospital admissions and comprising 3% or less of all uterine tumors.[195] Highest age incidence is in the fifth decade, with the vast majority occurring after 40 years of age.[194] Malignant connective tissue tumors of the uterus have been classified in many ways. A relatively recent classification is that of Ober, an adaptation of which follows*:

1 Leiomyosarcoma
  a Arising in a leiomyoma
  b Arising diffusely in the uterine wall
2 Mesenchymal sarcoma (malignant mixed müllerian tumor spectrum)
  a Pure homologous (e.g., endometrial stromal sarcoma)
  b Pure heterologous (e.g., rhabdomyosarcoma)
  c Mixed homologous (carcinosarcoma)
  d Mixed heterologous
    (1) Carcinosarcoma (as above with one or more heterologous elements)
    (2) Mixed mesenchymal sarcoma
3 Blood vessel sarcoma (e.g., hemangioendothelioma)
4 Lymphoma
5 Unclassified sarcoma
6 Metastatic sarcoma (not reported)

Indeed, it may well be that the leiomyosarcoma should be included and all tumors grouped as a broad malignant müllerian tumor spectrum.

Leiomyosarcoma

Leiomyosarcomas comprise 50% to 75% of various series of uterine sarcomas. Although it has been suggested that they usually arise in a preexisting leiomyoma, this is doubtful.

*Adapted from Ober, W. B.: Ann. N. Y. Acad. Sci. 75:568-585, 1959.

Only very rarely is there a focus of sarcoma in an otherwise benign leiomyoma. It seems more likely that most of these tumors are malignant at the outset.

Grossly, the tumor may vary from a single nodule to diffuse myometrial involvement. It may extend through the serosal surface to adhere to adjacent structures, or it may project as a polypoid structure into the endometrial cavity. On section, the tumor is of equally varied appearance. It may be indistinguishable from a leiomyoma, although usually some feature will suggest a difference—such as focal loss of the whorled pattern, variation in color, or focal bulging above the level of the cut surface. Usually, such malignant growth arises in the central part of a leiomyoma, but it may arise at the edge and cause early loss of the sharp line of demarcation. The diffuse type of leiomyosarcoma is similarly homogeneous in appearance, varying in color from yellow to pink to gray, and is often hemorrhagic, necrotic, or pultaceous.

Microscopically, leiomyosarcomas are similar to sarcomas in general. The constituent cells are spindle, round, and giant forms. Usually, these are combined in varying proportions, and division of tumors into cell types is impossible. The degree of malignancy cannot always be predicted from the microscopic appearance. That the single most important feature in estimating the prognosis of the patient with leiomyosarcoma is the number of mitoses has been a concept handed down over the past fifty years and only recently questioned. Novak and Woodruff[18] found no survivors after one year if the count were more than ten mitoses per high-power field, using the "worst areas." On the other hand, a low mitosis count does not assure a good prognosis.

Mesenchymal sarcoma

Mesenchymal sarcomas arise in the uterus and are composed of neoplastic stromal elements or an admixture of stromal and epithelial elements. Essentially, mesenchymal tumor is synonymous with that termed malignant mixed müllerian tumor[202] and many other designations. Homologous elements are those direct derivatives of cells usually found in the uterus, whereas heterologous elements are cells or tissues not normally indigenous to the uterus.

Endometrial stromal sarcoma. Endometrial stromal sarcoma is a pale, polypoid, fleshy tu-

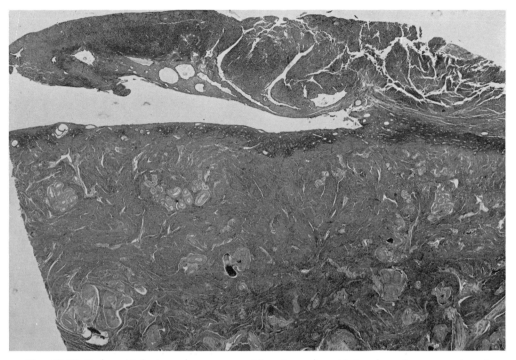

Fig. 37-31 Endometrial stromal sarcoma arising in endometrial polyp. Few normal and cystic endometrial glands surrounded by more normal stroma persist on undersurface of polyp. Endometrium itself is senile. Note thickened myometrial vessels. Same patient as shown in Fig. 37-32. (×8.)

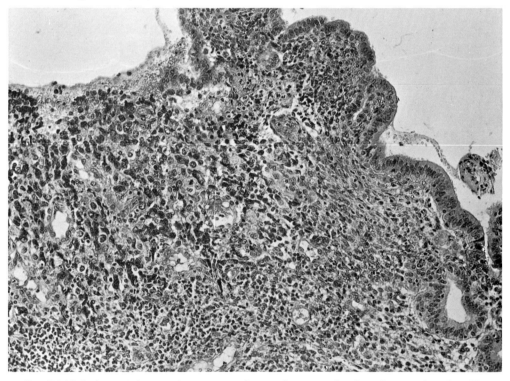

Fig. 37-32 Endometrial stromal sarcoma in biopsy from tip of polyp illustrated in Fig. 37-31. Neoplastic stromal cells (upper left) enlarged, irregular, and pleomorphic, with hyperchromatic nuclei as contrasted to normal stroma (right and below), but glandular cells unaltered. (×250.)

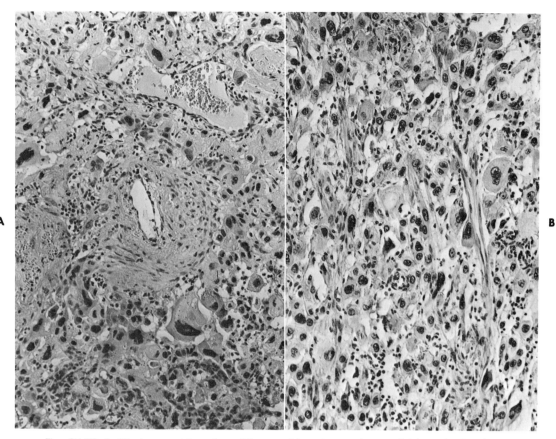

Fig. 37-33 A, Uterine curettings from 23-year-old patient with two children, the last born six months before this specimen taken. Subsequently she had two normal menstrual periods and then intermittent spotting suggesting threatened abortion, but all chorionic gonadotropin determinations were negative. Superficially, this suggested trophoblast but there seemed to be transitions from small to large cells. **B,** Section from 2 cm nodule in hysterectomy specimen of same patient. Tumor cells forming part of walls of small vessels are more suggestive of sarcoma than of trophoblastic neoplasm. (**A** and **B,** Hematoxylin-eosin; ×100; **A,** HMS CS-63-317; **B,** HMS CS-63-317A; **A** and **B,** courtesy Dr. J. A. Mauro and Dr. T. G. Adinolfi.)

mor (Fig. 37-31) usually arising from the uterine fundus. Occasionally, there may be diffuse myometrial invasion without a polypoid tumor. Only rarely is all the endometrium involved. Usually, the tumor is fairly sharply demarcated from more normal endometrium. Microscopically, it is composed of cells that are spindle shaped on longitudinal section and round on cross section. Cytoplasm may be scanty, the cells resembling those of the endometrial stroma in the proliferative phase, or more abundant, so that the constituent cells suggest a resemblance to decidua (Fig. 37-32). There may be giant cells (not to be confused with placental site giant cells or with foreign body giant cells). The higher the mitosis count, as in leiomyosarcomas, the poorer the prognosis.

Malignant mesenchymal lesions mimicking pregnancy. A small group of mesenchymal tumors (Fig. 37-33) from patients giving a history suggestive of pregnancy has been referred to us over the past several years. Although chorionic gonadotropin determinations (when done) have been within normal limits, the lesions have sometimes been labeled atypical choriocarcinoma despite the absence of the usual necrosis. There is often a perivascular tumor arrangement with an overall distribution similar to sarcoma. The vascular pattern is quite distinctive from choriocarcinoma, which develops its own vascular channels by vacuolization of syncytiotrophoblast. Transitions in cell types may be observed. A history of recent pregnancy would not rule out uterine sarcoma, since it is known that pregnancy and uterine sarcoma may be present together.

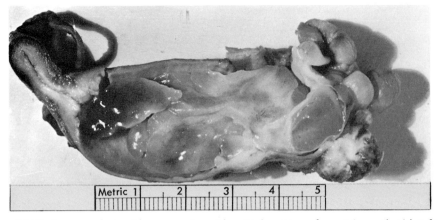

Fig. 37-34 Sarcoma botryoides, seen in midsagittal section, from 16-month-old infant. Tumor, arising from and filling vagina, invaded pelvic tissues, including base of bladder. (Courtesy Dr. S. Farber.)

Spread of uterine sarcoma. Spread of uterine sarcoma is usually by direct extension, frequently by the bloodstream, and only occasionally by lymphatics. The commonest sites of distant metastases are lung and liver.

Treatment and prognosis. Treatment varies, but that commonly employed is total hysterectomy. Whether or not Wertheim hysterectomy should be done is a current problem. Whether radiation is of value in therapy has not yet been definitely established. The prognosis is poor, although somewhat better in patients with sarcomas that seem to arise in a leiomyoma. The five-year survival rate is 20% to 30%.

Malignant mixed müllerian tumor. Malignant mixed müllerian tumor is a useful practical term to include pure heterologous mesenchymal sarcoma and mixed homologous and heterologous mesenchymal sarcomas. These neoplasms arise in the mucosal stroma of the vagina, cervix, and uterus at any time from birth to old age. In children and young people, these tumors are more likely to arise in the vagina (Fig. 37-34) and cervix, whereas in the postmenopausal woman they almost invariably occur in the corpus. Malignant mixed müllerian tumor has been reported rarely in the tube[189] (age range of patients, 5 to 70 years). We have also seen similar tumors of the peritoneum, usually predominantly sarcomatous, apparently arising from stroma similar to müllerian type and lying beneath the peritoneum and also arising primarily in the ovary, presumably from stroma of müllerian potential.

The histogenesis and pathogenesis are unknown, but most widely accepted as the basic

tissue of origin is the müllerian stroma that exists beneath the surface epithelium of the endometrium, cervix, and vagina or that may lie between muscle bundles in the myometrium. Meyer[191] has grouped these tumors on a histogenetic basis into (1) collision tumors formed by the collision of two separate tumors, (2) combination tumors derived from a single cell type, and (3) composition tumors arising from glandular and stromal elements occurring within the one tissue.

Grossly, the tumor is soft, bulky, and polypoid. When occurring in the cervix or vagina, it has the typical appearance of a bunch of grapes. It has a pink to red or purple color and may be small or large, with single or multiple polypoid growths. On section, it is moderately firm, pale, and fibrous. Cartilage is not present in the juvenile form but may be evident, grossly, in the adult form arising in the cervix and endometrium.

When such tumors arise in adults in the cervix or endometrium, they may be diffuse or polypoid. The polypoid appearance apparently is the result of growth into a distensible cavity, since the metastases are diffuse even when the original tumor was markedly polypoid.

Carcinosarcoma (Fig. 37-35) occurring in menopausal patients is polypoid, pedunculated, or sessile, single or multiple, and often sharply demarcated from the myometrium. Externally, it may be coarsely lobulated and smooth or ulcerated. On section, it is soft to firm and occasionally friable and is red to yellow gray in color.

The basic histologic pattern of a malignant mixed müllerian tumor is that of a mesen-

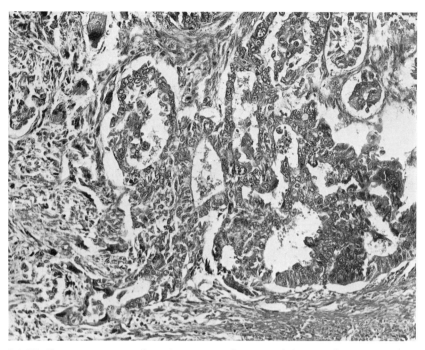

Fig. 37-35 Carcinosarcoma of endometrium showing definite adenocarcinoma (right) within stroma composed of irregular cells, many multinucleated in type. This followed intrauterine radium radiation. (×160.)

chymal sarcoma or myxosarcoma, with or without malignant heterologous elements such as smooth or striated muscle and epithelium. In general, the older the patient, the greater the admixture of heterologous elements and the greater the tendency of such tumors to arise in the cervix and/or endometrium rather than in the vagina and/or cervix. All the heterologous components are assumed to be derived from multipotential stromal cells. It is of interest that carcinosarcoma (Fig. 37-35) has been observed following small doses of uterine radiation. Although patients so treated develop more endometrial carcinoma than the general female population, they develop no more carcinoma than does a similar group of patients (with dysfunctional uterine bleeding) who have not been irradiated. On the other hand, among those cancers occurring in patients who have been irradiated, there is a much higher proportion of carcinosarcoma than in those developing spontaneously.

Pure rhabdomyosarcoma[185] is rare and usually rapidly fatal. Chondrosarcoma and osteosarcoma are even more rare. Mixed sarcomas constitute about 60% of all the mesenchymal tumors.

The juvenile form spreads locally in the pelvis, death resulting from urinary tract and intestinal involvement. The adult form may metastasize, as well as spread locally. Metastases may be found in pelvic, inguinal, retroperitoneal, or mediastinal lymph nodes and in pleura, lungs, pericardium, liver, kidney, and bones. These metastases are usually carcinoma but may be carcinosarcoma or sarcoma, whereas in some patients the metastasis at one site is carcinoma and at another sarcoma.

The prognosis is poor with any type of therapy, the great majority of patients dying in less than two years, although rarely they may survive longer. Treatment of patients with longer survival has usually included radical surgery.

Other sarcomas

Vascular sarcomas are rare.[203] Lymphomas and leukemic infiltration occur in the uterus, but whether or not the uterus is ever the primary site is a difficult problem.

Tumors metastatic to uterus

Uterine metastases may be present as the result of extension or metastasis either from one part of the uterus to another or from other pelvic viscera or by metastasis from distant organs.[170] Cervical carcinoma may extend or, less commonly, metastasize to the endometrium, although extension of endometrial carcinoma to the cervix is more common. The commonest metastatic endometrial tumor is from the ovary (4% of ovarian cancers metastasize to the endometrium), and often it may be impossible to determine in a patient with endometrial and ovarian carcinoma which was primary lesion. Tumors metastatic to the uterus from extrapelvic sites are all carcinomas, the commonest being from the breast and the stomach. This may be related to the frequency of these tumors rather than because of any special predilection for the uterus.

FALLOPIAN TUBE
Benign tumors and tumorlike conditions

Salpingitis isthmica nodosa. Salpingitis isthmica nodosa is a condition of the fallopian tube characterized grossly by one or more nodular thickenings of the isthmus.[211] The exact incidence is difficult to determine but has been reported as 0.8% of autopsied women. It is more common in black patients than in white. The three main theories are that it is congenital, is inflammatory, or is acquired but noninflammatory. Of these, the most convincing is the inflammatory theory.

The lesion is usually bilateral, consisting of single or multiple circumscribed nodules—up to 2.5 cm in diameter and white, yellow, or brown in color, giving the tube a beaded appearance, especially in the isthmic region. Microscopically, it begins as a simple outpocketing of the tubal lumen. Later, glandlike spaces are formed lying within the myosalpinx, with increase in the amount of surrounding muscle. Usually, these spaces are lined by tubal-type epithelium, and their continuity with the tubal lumen has been demonstrated by various techniques. It is analogous to adenomyosis of the uterus.

The lesion itself does not cause symptoms but may be accompanied by symptoms from the associated salpingitis. The commonest complication is sterility, which occurs in about one-half the patients.

Benign cystic teratoma (dermoid cyst). Dermoid cyst of the tube[215] is an extremely rare tumor, most probably arising from a germ cell that lodged in the tubal primordium and thus did not complete its migration to the gonad. Tumors vary from 1 cm to 17 cm in diameter and may weigh as much as 4 lb. Usually, the tumor is unilateral (81%), situated in the right tube (59%), cystic (81%), and grows intraluminally by a pedicle (62%). Microscopically, these tumors resemble dermoids elsewhere in the body, being composed of moderately mature tissues, and may present as struma salpingii.[216]

Hemangioma. Hemangioma is a rare tubal tumor, dark purplish red and mottled in color. It may fill the tubal lumen and consists of dilated, thin-walled blood vessels.

Lymphangioma. Lymphangioma is a rare tumor of the tube that frequently is confused with an adenomatoid tumor of peritoneal origin.

Mesonephroma. Similar to mesonephroma elsewhere in the body, tubal mesonephroma probably arises from mesonephric elements persisting in the broad ligament. It also may be confused with adenomatoid tumor.

Dysgerminoma and granulosa cell tumor. Examples of dysgerminoma and granulosa cell tumor have been described and probably arise from misplaced primordial germ cells and ovarian remnants, respectively.

Endometriosis. Tubal endometriosis is important as a part of generalized pelvic endometriosis or because it may mimic a tumor. It may occur on the serosal surface or in the mucosa of the tube. The etiology of endometriosis of the surface of the tube is probably similar to that in the ovary, whereas in the tubal lumen it probably arises by differentiation of potential endometrial stroma or possibly by heteroplasia of tubal mucosa. On the serosal surface, it consists of irregular red to black nodules, 0.1 cm to 3 cm in diameter, accompanied by a variable amount of scarring. Occurring within the tube, it is soft and hemorrhagic, pouting outward on section.

Microscopically, the lesion is composed of typical endometrial glands and stroma with varying amounts of hemorrhage. Potential endometrial stroma is present in both sites of tubal endometriosis, as shown by the pseudodecidual reaction of pregnancy, which may occur both beneath the serosa and within the connective tissue of the plicae. The cells are large with refractile borders and must be distinguished from metastatic carcinoma.

Adenomatoid tumor. Adenomatoid tumor[219] is a small circumscribed neoplasm confined to the muscular wall of the tube, usually found incidentally and composed of small glandlike spaces lined by cells of mesothelial, endothelial, or even epithelial appearance. There are numerous synonyms for this tumor, indicating theories of origin. Most authors consider that it is of peritoneal origin (and so support the mesothelial theory). The incidence is said to be 0.04%. The age range is from 25 to 86 years, the majority occurring between the ages of 30 and 50 years.

Grossly, these tumors are less than 3 cm in diameter, usually occur immediately beneath the serosa, and are well circumscribed but rarely, if ever, encapsulated. On section, they are homogeneous and white to pinkish gray. Microscopically, the cells vary from flattened endothelium-like elements to a cuboidal or low columnar type, enclosing gland or vessel-like spaces of varying size and shape. Sometimes, the cells may be in solid cords. The cells may be vacuolated, containing mucinlike material. The stroma is fibromuscular, and this appears to be an integral part of the tumor. These tumors have all been incidental findings, so that there is no clinical syndrome. All tubal lesions reported have been benign.

Leiomyoma. Leiomyoma is a very rare tumor in the fallopian tube, usually in the interstitial portion and more commonly on the left side. It varies considerably in size, from very small to 2 kg, and usually is single but may be multiple. It is similar microscopically to leiomyomas elsewhere in the body. It is important to distinguish leiomyoma of the fallopian tube grossly from salpingitis isthmica nodosa, adenomyosis, and adenomatoid tumor.

Lipoma. Lipoma has been found rarely in the tube, usually being removed incidentally during an operation or at postmortem examination.

Malignant tumors
Primary carcinoma

Primary tubal carcinoma is the rarest carcinoma of the female genital tract, constituting 1 in 15,000 to 1 in 20,000 gynecologic admissions, 0.34 to 1.33% of total operations for tubal disease, and 0.16 to 1.11% of genital cancer. Salpingitis is usually present in the tube containing the tumor but not in the other tube. The age range is 18 to 80 years, the majority of patients are between 40 and 65 years, and the average age is 51 to 52 years. Usually, there is a history of diminished fertility in these patients.[213, 217]

Why carcinoma of the tube should be so rare is not understood, but it may be due to the relative stability of the tubal epithelium during the menstrual cycle. Only twice has carcinoma in situ of the tube been reported. Inflammation of the tube does not appear to be etiologically important, because the salpin-

gitis accompanying tubal carcinoma appears to have followed rather than to have preceded it. Tuberculosis likewise does not appear to be important as an etiologic factor.

There is no typical clinical syndrome, commonest symptoms being vaginal discharge and pain. "Hydrops tubae profluens," relief of pain and disappearance of a mass accompanied by profuse vaginal discharge, is more likely to occur with hydrosalpinx and is neither pathognomonic nor a constant finding in tubal carcinoma. Even if this tumor were common, it is unlikely that it would be diagnosed correctly preoperatively because of the nonspecific symptoms and signs. On rare occasions, diagnosis has been suggested by malignant cells in the Papanicolaou smear.

Carcinoma of the tube is usually unilateral, although bilateral in 26% of patients, but without predilection for either side. The appearance depends on the size of the tumor and the patency of the fimbriated end of the tube. If the latter is closed, the tumor may be partially masked by a hydrosalpinx or a pyosalpinx. The tumor itself may vary from 1 cm to 17 cm, may be purple, doughy or firm, granular, gray to yellow, and friable to cheesy in consistency. Usually, it is in the distal third of the tube and may spill into the peritoneal cavity if the ostium is open, but this usually becomes adherent or occluded, so preventing spillage of malignant cells.

It is of importance to distinguish between primary and metastatic tubal carcinoma. In a primary tumor, the main tumor mass should appear grossly to be confined to the tube and to be growing as a papillary endosalpingeal tumor.

Microscopically, in primary tubal carcinoma the epithelium of the endosalpinx is replaced in whole or in part by adenocarcinoma, and the tumor cells are of tubal type. Should the endometrium also contain a focus of carcinoma, its small size, distribution, and histologic characteristics should suggest tubal carcinoma. Tubal carcinomas may be classified in the following three groups[217]:

Grade I

Papillary—a well-differentiated papillary tumor composed of nonciliated columnar cells. The tumor is confined to the mucosa and mitoses are scanty (Fig. 37-36).

Grade II

Papillary-alveolar—less differentiated, with a moderate number of mitoses, but of either papillary or glandular pattern or both

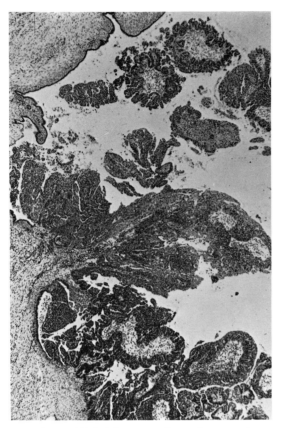

Fig. 37-36 Well-differentiated papillary carcinoma of tube. At left is normal but atrophic tubal mucosa, and tumor appears to arise from it. This feature and absence of tumor elsewhere indicate primary tubal carcinoma. (×40; from Hu, C. Y., Taymor, M. L., and Hertig, A. T.: Amer. J. Obstet. Gynec. **59:**58-67, 1950.)

Grade III

Alveolar-medullary—poorly differentiated, with cells arranged in solid sheets around glandlike spaces, with loss of papillary pattern; frequent mitoses and lymphatic invasion

In any one tumor, there may be marked variation in pattern, but usually the better differentiated the tumor, the better the prognosis.

The usual method of spread is via the lymphatics. The tumor may spread along the tubal mucosa, but usually the fimbriated end of the tube is closed, preventing peritoneal spread. If open, there may be peritoneal implantation, carcinomatosis, ascites, and death. Blood vessel spread accounts for frequent liver involvement. Sometimes, metastases may occur before invasion of the tubal wall. Five-year survival rate (actuarial method) is 34%.

The accepted treatment is total hysterectomy with bilateral salpingo-oophorectomy, followed by deep x-ray therapy. Whether or not this should be accompanied by radical lymph node dissection is uncertain, but probably not.

Sarcoma of fallopian tube

Sarcoma[210] of the fallopian tube is an extremely rare tubal tumor, one-twenty-fifth as common as tubal carcinoma.[222] The age incidence is similar to that for carcinoma. Clinically, there may be discharge or pain, and a pelvic tumor is usually palpable. The tumor has no predilection for either side and is bilateral in one-third of the patients. The tube varies in size from 2 cm to 20 cm, and the contents are usually soft and papillary. Microscopically, there is no constant picture, many types having been described, but the commonest are spindle cell and round cell types. (Malignant mixed müllerian tumor of tube has been mentioned previously.)

Spread may be by direct extension to pelvic tissues or by lymphatic or bloodstream metastases (sometimes to lungs), and occasionally there are secondary growths throughout the peritoneal cavity. Many methods of treatment have been employed, but that currently advocated is total hysterectomy with bilateral salpingo-oophorectomy, followed by deep x-ray irradiation if operation is apparently incomplete. The prognosis is poor.

Carcinoma metastatic to fallopian tube

Metastatic tubal carcinoma is more common than primary tubal carcinoma[213] and occurs in the ratio of 1:650 hospital admissions. The commonest primary sites are the ovary and the endometrium. Tumors metastatic from the ovary are twice as common as those from the endometrium. Most patients with this condition are over 30 years of age and may have generalized metastases or metastases confined to the tube. Clinically, the symptoms are those of the primary tumor, from which the tumor may have spread by lymphatic or bloodstream permeation, direct extension, "implantation," or drop metastasis.

Grossly, these metastatic tumors may be bilateral or unilateral, without predilection for either side. The size of metastases varies widely. Chronic salpingitis is present in about one-third of the tubes. Microscopically, the tumor resembles that of the primary site. The lymphatics of the muscularis and of the mesosalpinx usually are involved. The lymphatics of the endosalpinx and the endosalpinx itself are more rarely involved.

The prognosis is that of the primary tumor. Usually, the prognosis is poor, but some patients with primary endometrial carcinoma remain well for ten years.

OVARY
Nonneoplastic cysts of graafian follicle origin

Cysts may arise at any stage during the evolution or involution of the graafian follicle. Although not of true neoplastic nature, they are included among the ovarian tumors because they may alter the normal physiology, causing abnormal bleeding during sexual maturity or vaginal bleeding in children or young girls. They may occur in association with pregnancy, both normal and abnormal, and cause difficulty in differential diagnosis. Furthermore, they may twist or rupture.

When the product of the graafian follicle shall be considered cystic is a problem. It is fairly generally accepted that the normal developing follicle does not exceed 1.5 cm in diameter before rupturing. Follicles larger than that but less than 2.5 cm in diameter are termed cystic follicles, and those 2.5 cm and over, follicular cysts. Similarly, a corpus luteum over 2.5 cm is considered a corpus luteum cyst.

Cystic structures derived from unruptured follicle. Follicular cysts may be single or multiple and lie within or distort the ovarian cortex. They contain fluid that may be clear and colorless or straw colored or sometimes hemorrhagic. The wall may be white and glistening or hemorrhagic, and sometimes it is yellow because of variable degrees of luteinization of theca. If multiple, cystic follicular derivatives tend to be small and of fairly uniform size, 0.3 cm to 0.5 cm in diameter.

Microscopically, in cystic follicles an oocyte undergoing atresia may be seen. Usually, there is some degree of granulosa cell degeneration, although in some cystic follicles there may be continued granulosa cell activity as evidenced by mitoses. Theca is present in variable amounts and with variable degrees of activity. Occasionally in postmenopausal women, a *luteinized unruptured follicle* may be found. In this, the theca may be luteinized, and the endometrium may show atypical but suggestive secretory changes and be associated with some atypical endometrial bleeding.

In pregnancy, the remaining follicles may respond physiologically to the chorionic gonadotropin produced by the placenta, with resulting luteinization of the theca interna. This

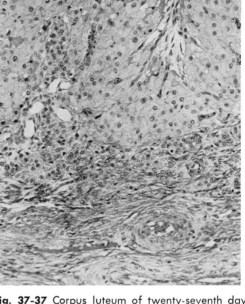

Fig. 37-37 Corpus luteum of twenty-seventh day of menstrual cycle (i.e., a thirteen-day corpus luteum). Convoluted pattern with thecal cells at margin, some being caught up in convolutions of masses of large, pale, luteinized granulosa cells. (×125.)

is most marked with choriocarcinoma and with hydatidiform mole when the ovaries may be enlarged and polycystic.[62] Such luteinized follicles usually involute within six weeks after complete removal of a hydatidiform mole and may do so after removal of a choriocarcinoma if no metastases exist, although they may recur when there is recurrence of the choriocarcinoma. Similar polycystic ovaries with luteinization also have been described in pregnant patients with Rh sensitization, with multiple pregnancy, and occasionally with apparently normal pregnancy. Sometimes, the cysts are not prominent, but there may be sheets of luteinized cells in the ovary. This seems to be a spectrum phenomenon, hyperreactio luteinalis, of which the so-called luteoma of pregnancy is a part.

Cystic structures derived from normally ruptured follicle. The corpus luteum (Fig. 37-37), being derived from a cystic structure, is always potentially cystic. Usually, the cavity rapidly fills with a gray to red coagulum that becomes organized and so contracts.[25] Why some corpora lutea become cystic is not definitely established, although some authors believe it is due to massive hemorrhage into the central portion. They may reach up to 11 cm in diameter, although such a large size is unusual. Grossly, the difference between a cystic corpus luteum and a corpus luteum cyst is of degree only, due mainly to the size of the cyst cavity. The lining is usually smooth without evidence of gross hemorrhage, and the cavity compresses, flattens, and distorts the surrounding corpus luteum. The functioning tissue changes from gray to yellow to yellow-orange color and finally to white, when it becomes a corpus albicans.

Microscopically, all elements of the corpus luteum are present—viz., central coagulum, organizing fibrous tissue, granulosa lutein, and theca lutein cells.

Stein-Leventhal syndrome. The Stein-Leventhal syndrome[230] is characterized clinically by secondary amenorrhea, sterility, and hirsutism, and pathologically by bilateral polycystic ovaries, occurring in the second and third decades. Currently, there is discussion whether the Stein-Leventhal syndrome should include patients clinically similar but with small ovaries. Further, attention recently has been drawn to the possibility that this syndrome represents a multiglandular disturbance. Occasionally, pregnancy has occurred before the onset of the syndrome. The ovaries are enlarged and white, and on section there is a thick fibrous surface surrounding a stroma containing multiple cystic follicles. Often, there is hyperplasia of the theca interna cells with luteinization. Corpora lutea and corpora albicantia are absent because of failure of ovulation. The endometrium is usually proliferative and sometimes slightly hyperplastic but occasionally shows slight secretory changes, presumably due to thecal hyperplasia. Although it was originally claimed that these patients never develop cancer, adenocarcinoma has been reported in these patients—37% of the group studied by Jackson and Dockerty.[229] On the other hand, all young women with endometrial carcinoma do not have Stein-Leventhal syndrome.

Treatment in the past has been wedge resection or some form of disruption of the surface of the ovary. Currently, this is considered to be the last, not the first, therapeutic approach.[14] Cortisone or prednisone are considered the best initial therapy if thyroid and pituitary function are normal. There has been increased emphasis in recent years on the in-duction of ovulation by biochemical techniques, notably clomiphene.

Classification of ovarian tumors

The ovary is a complex structure from an embryologic, anatomic, and functional standpoint, so it is little wonder that its tumors often are difficult to understand. Many different classifications have been suggested—based upon hormonal activity, anatomy, the simple gross or the microscopic benignancy or malignancy of the lesion, or on a histogenetic basis. The latter seems to be the most logical approach. For this reason a simple classification has been developed that is a modification of a system previously proposed. This includes only the true tumors of the ovary and omits those follicular derivatives that may be mistaken for a neoplasm. It must, however, be remembered that such nonneoplastic swellings may occur, and they should be considered in a differential diagnosis.

1 Gonadal stromal tumors
  a Granulosa–theca cell tumor
  b Arrhenoblastoma
  c Gynandroblastoma
2 Germ cell tumors
  a Undifferentiated (pure germ cell type)
    (1) Dysgerminoma
  b Extraembryonic
    (1) Nongestational choriocarcinoma
    (2) Endodermal sinus tumor (Teilum)
  c Embryonic
    (1) Benign cystic teratoma (and struma ovarii)
    (2) Solid well-differentiated teratoma
    (3) Malignant teratoma
    (4) Teratocarcinoma
  d Various admixtures of types
1 and 2 Mixed gonadal stromal and germ cell tumors
  a Gonadoblastoma
3 Cystomas (tumors of "germinal" epithelial origin)
  a Serous cystadenoma and cystadenocarcinoma
  b Mucinous cystadenoma and cystadenocarcinoma
  c Endometrial cystoma—benign and malignant
  d Cystadenofibroma—benign and malignant
4 Congenital rest tumors
  a Adrenal rest tumor
  b Mesometanephric rest tumor
  c Brenner tumor
  d Hilar cell tumor
5 Nonintrinsic connective tissue tumors
6 Metastatic tumors

Gonadal stromal tumors

Granulosa–theca cell tumor. The granulosa–theca cell tumor (feminizing mesenchymal tumor) of the ovary is composed of the different elements of the graafian follicle wall in varying proportions and stages of activity, maturity, and regression. The term thus includes a wide spectrum of tumors ranging from the almost pure granulosa cell tumor, with few thecal elements, to the mixed granulosa–theca cell tumor, to the apparently pure thecoma, and it includes varying degrees of luteinization of any of these elements, the most marked degree constituting a luteoma. These tumors arise from cortical stromal elements, but whether directly or from cells surviving in a follicle undergoing atresia, or by both methods, is not definitely established. They constitute 3.6% to 9% of ovarian tumors and may occur at any age, although 60% to 70% occur in the postmenopausal period.

Of interest are the conditions frequently accompanying these tumors, possibly related to their hormone production. The steroid hormonally active cell, both in these tumors and in the normal follicle, has been thought to be the thecal cell, but this has not been definitely established. Endometrial carcinoma is found in 11% to 15% of patients with these tumors, whereas if patients over 50 years of age only are considered, this incidence is 24% to 27%.[234, 239] Furthermore, a high incidence of leiomyomas, chronic cystic mastitis, and breast carcinoma has been reported. Ascites and hydrothorax may accompany a feminizing mesenchymal tumor but also may be due to metastatic growth or may occur with a completely benign thecoma or fibroma, probably on the basis of circulatory disturbance (Meigs' syndrome). The commonest clinical symptom is uterine bleeding due to endometrial hyperplasia or active endometrium, and this may have been present for from two to ten years.

Grossly, these tumors are usually unilateral, with approximately equal distribution on either side, only 12% to 17.5% being bilateral. They vary in size from 0.4 cm to 40 cm in diameter, with no correlation between the age of the patient, the size of the tumor, or the duration of the symptoms. The surface is usually smooth and may be lobulated, and only rarely are there adhesions. The appearance and consistency of the cut surface depend on the relative proportions of the constituent elements, and the color depends upon the degree of luteinization. Granulosa cell elements give a soft consistency, and thecal cell elements are tough and fibrous. Luteinization imparts varying degrees of yellow color to the tumor. There may be cystic areas, hemorrhage, and necrosis. In predominantly theca

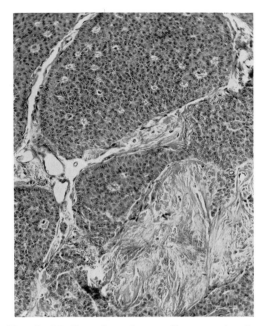

Fig. 37-38 Granulosa-theca cell tumor showing both epithelial and stromal elements. Granulosa cells arranged in folliculoid pattern. There is collagenization of thecal stroma which is analogous to hyalinization of theca externa in formation of atretic follicle and corpus albicans. (×120; AFIP 264079-4.)

cell tumors, there may be edema or calcification.

The microscopic pattern is extremely varied, for the two constituent cells may occur in any proportion (Fig. 37-38). Granulosa cells are uniform in size with poorly defined cytoplasmic margins. The cytoplasm is eosinophilic and slightly granular with large round to oval, evenly staining nuclei. Theca cells are elongated with ovoid nuclei and resemble plump fibroblasts. Differentiation from these may be difficult. Furthermore, deciding whether or not some cells are of granulosa or theca type may be difficult. Silver stains are of value because of the pattern of the reticulum network, which surrounds groups of granulosa cells and does not penetrate such groups to surround an individual cell. On the other hand, each theca cell is surrounded by reticulum. Many arrangements of granulosa cells are described, the commonest being folliculoid, trabeculoid, cylindroid, and sarcomatoid. The theca cells are arranged in interlacing whorls, sheets, or bundles, and often scattered throughout are short tufts, bands, or nests of collagen. Luteinization may occur in any of the elements with increase in pale cytoplasm, which may be vacuolated and better defined.

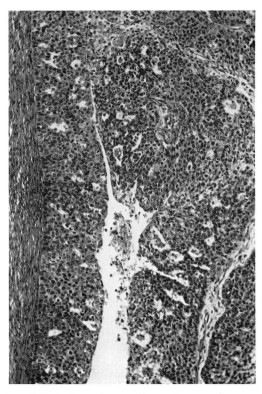

Fig. 37-39 Granulosa cell carcinoma of ovary with retention of granulosa cell pattern but with numerous mitoses and some cellular pleomorphism. (×100; AFIP 218754-53-4536.)

These resemble the luteinized cells of all elements of the normally developing follicle.

Histologically, there is a definite entity recognizable as granulosa cell carcinoma (Fig. 37-39), with variation in size of granulosa cells and many mitoses but a benign-appearing theca, but such tumors are rare. More often, a granulosa cell carcinoma may be suspected, but it may be impossible to differentiate it from a relatively poorly differentiated serous cystadenocarcinoma. The presence of a thecal stroma is of no assistance in the diagnosis, because there may be an ovarian cortical stromal response (histologically mimicking a thecal stroma) with almost any type of primary or metastatic ovarian carcinoma. A certain number of apparently benign granulosa cell tumors, however, behave as malignant tumors and may recur late, even up to twenty-seven years after removal of the primary tumor. Histologically, there is no way to recognize the potential recurrence of such apparently benign tumors. Recurrence is usually in older patients and is said to occur in 20% to 30% of predominantly granulosa cell tumors. Theca cell tumors are almost invariably benign. Only extremely rare malignant tumors have been reported, and some of these appear to be sarcomas without any identifying features. The spread of granulosa cell tumors when malignant—similar to that of any other ovarian cancer—is first and most strikingly to the peritoneum, next and less often to the retroperitoneal lymph nodes, and finally, infrequently, to distant sites.

"Luteoma" of pregnancy. A luteinized granulosa–theca cell tumor has been observed on several occasions quite incidentally at cesarean section. Grossly, these lesions vary from multiple small nodules up to 1.5 cm in diameter. Of nine cases in our files, six patients had a cesarean section for a viable infant, one an abortion, one a tubal pregnancy, and one, a choriocarcinoma. Malinak and Miller[238] have reported reoperating two months after luteoma was found in one ovary at cesarean section and finding ill-defined yellow areas in the other ovary composed of regressing luteinized cells (Fig. 37-40). This suggests that the "luteoma" of pregnancy is either a hormonally dependent "tumor" or a massive hyperplasia in the hyperreactio luteinalis spectrum (p. 1538). We have seen regression in another patient in material from a second operation.

Since the corpus luteum of pregnancy has been observed with luteomas, it seems most likely that they arose directly from ovarian cortical stroma or immature follicles. Usually, they have no obvious hormonal effect because of pregnancy. With the rare masculinizing type, there may be a hirsute masculinized mother and a temporarily masculinized female infant.

Microscopically, the cell pattern mimics that of the corpus luteum of pregnancy but does not have its distinctive architecture, and the cells are larger than in the normal corpus luteum of pregnancy. There are usually large, pale, luteinized granulosa cells, often with peripherally vacuolated margins, and darker cells that we have previously labeled "k" cells of thecal origin, but their function and indeed their origin are not understood.

Arrhenoblastoma. Arrhenoblastoma, or Sertoli–Leydig cell tumor, is a mesenchymal tumor that recapitulates varying aspects of the embryonic testis and may cause clinical defeminization and masculinization. It is a rare tumor. Only about 240 have been recorded in the world literature. Arrhenoblastomas have been reported in patients from 9 to 78 years of age, but most usually occur in the

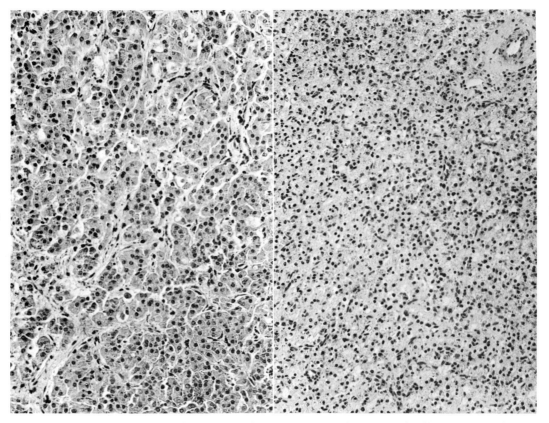

Fig. 37-40 A, Pregnancy "luteoma" with typical large pale luteinized cells. Section is of one of multiple brown-red nodules in ovary removed at cesarean section. Female infant was temporarily masculinized. **B,** Section from ill-defined yellow area in other ovary, removed two months post partum. These cells seem similar to those of "luteoma," albeit undergoing regressive changes. (**A** and **B,** Hematoxylin-eosin; ×100; **A,** CS-64-182; **B,** CS-64-182A; **A** and **B,** courtesy Dr. L. R. Malinak and Dr. G. V. Miller.)

late twenties and early thirties. They usually appear in previously normal women. Indeed, in a study of twenty-nine arrhenoblastomas and their hosts, O'Hern and Neubecker[245] observed that all were positive for nuclear sex chromatin.

Because these tumors occur in young women, arrhenoblastomas may precede, complicate, or follow pregnancy. A functioning arrhenoblastoma, however, will inhibit ovulation so that pregnancy will not occur. Any hormonal activity of such a tumor associated with pregnancy must have arisen after gestation was established. (This rare complication of pregnancy may cause the female embryo to become a pseudohermaphrodite if the virilization occurs sufficiently early in gestation.) Manifestations of defeminization in these women include falling hair, atrophy of the other ovary, atrophy of the breasts, and amenorrhea. These manifestations are followed by masculinization—viz., hirsutism, hy-

pertrophy of the clitoris, and hypertrophy of the larynx, with male voice. With removal of the tumor, there is return to normal except for structural changes (such as hypertrophy of the larynx and clitoris), but signs of masculinity return with recurrence of the growth.

Interest has been focused on the hormonal production by these tumors. Morris and Scully[231] have observed that virilized women with arrhenoblastomas usually have a urinary 17-ketosteroid excretion within the normal range or just beyond; rarely is it high. Therefore, it has been postulated that testosterone, which is potent and need not be present in large quantities, may well be the virilizing hormone.

There are numerous theories of origin, the most logical being that it arises from ovarian cortical stroma, an origin similar to that of the feminizing mesenchymal tumor. For this reason, it is often difficult to decide histologically to which group the less differentiated

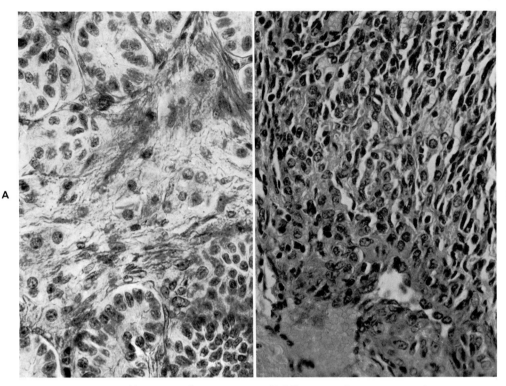

Fig. 37-41 Arrhenoblastoma of ovary. **A,** Well-differentiated type. No virilization, possibly because of microscopic size of tumor. Tubules within mesenchymal stroma and also interstitial cells containing crystalloids of Reinke. **B,** Sarcomatoid type, containing pale, polyhedral interstitial or Leydig cells. Virilization disappeared postoperatively. (**A,** ×400; FHWS-54-899; ×400; **B,** ×315; AFIP 264047-3.)

tumors belong or if, indeed, the tumor is a *gynandroblastoma* containing elements of both feminizing and masculinizing stroma.

The gross appearance is not pathognomonic. The arrhenoblastoma varies in size from microscopic to 28 cm in diameter. It is usually unilateral (5% are bilateral). The surface is usually smooth, but there may be adhesions. On section, the tumor is white to gray with a suggestion of yellow. Small tumors are solid and fibrous. Larger tumors may be soft with hemorrhage and necrosis. They may contain cysts but without papillary projections.

Microscopically, there are three types:

1 A well-differentiated tumor (Fig. 37-41, *A*) with prominent and distinct tubules and suggestive or definite interstitial cells

2 An intermediate type with abortive tubule formation with prominent interstitial cells

3 A sarcomatoid type (Fig. 37-41, *B*) whose sarcoma-like stroma may show variable degrees of differentiation and which may or may not contain typical interstitial cells

Tubules, when they occur, are lined by a low columnar epithelium. Interstitial cells are large, with eosinophilic and sometimes pigmented cytoplasm, similar in appearance to those in the cryptorchid testis. These tumors are usually benign, with a good prognosis after simple removal of the ovary, but about 20% are malignant. Some authors believe this is pessimistic because of the inclusion of some carcinomas.

Gynandroblastoma. The gynandroblastoma is a rare tumor occurring in patients with simultaneous androgenic and estrogenic manifestations.[248] It appears likely that it is a tumor of indifferent gonadal mesenchyme still possessing a bisexual potential which it expresses in both its epithelium and its stroma. The patients usually are virilized to a varying degree—often over a long period of time, with variable amounts of endometrial hyperplasia leading to uterine bleeding. Age range is from 24 to 59 years.

Grossly, the tumors are unremarkable, measure from 1 cm to 20 cm in diameter, and may be solid or partly cystic. The tumor may be predominantly granulosa–theca cell type with significant admixtures and transitions to arrhenoblastoma or vice versa. The main histologic pattern may not correspond with the clinical hormonal pattern. The gynandroblastomas we have seen have not been morphologically malignant, but it must be presumed that such a variant is possible.

Gonadal stromal response to other ovarian tumors. Primary ovarian tumors, not usually hormonally active (Brenner tumor, cystadenofibroma), and metastatic ovarian lesions may sometimes be estrogenic, very rarely androgenic. The integral stroma of the primary tumor or the ovarian stromal response to a primary or metastatic ovarian lesion morphologically may resemble ovarian cortical stroma, often with clear cells variously described as thecomatosis or thecosis. An apparent estrogenic effect has been demonstrated by high cornification index in the vaginal smear and occasional endometrial hyperplasia. On rare occasions, the response has been androgenic.

Germ cell tumors

Dysgerminoma. Dysgerminoma is an epithelial tumor of typical large vesicular cells, indistinguishable morphologically and histochemically from the primordial germ cells of the sexually indifferent embryonic gonad, arranged in lobules or strands separated by a variable amount of connective tissue stroma infiltrated by lymphocytes and histologically similar to the seminoma testis. These tumors constitute about 4% to 5% of malignant ovarian tumors and 1% of all ovarian tumors. The age range is from 2 to 76 years, the tumors most commonly occurring between the ages of 11 and 30 years. The dysgerminoma arises from primordial germ cells at a point in development prior to differentiation into male and female types. These germ cells, first recognizable in the 3 mm embryo, have migrated from the yolk sac of the embryo via the gut mesentery to the genitourinary ridge.

The dysgerminoma occurs more frequently (50%) on the right than on the left (35%) and is sometimes (15%) bilateral. It varies in size from 2 cm to a size filling the abdominal cavity. The tumor may be encapsulated, and the surface may be smooth or irregular. On section, it is rubbery to soft in consistency and yellow to pinkish gray in color.

Microscopically, the cells are large, arranged in groups and cords separated by fibrous stroma, and infiltrated by a varying number of lymphocytes. It is not possible to predict the degree of malignancy from the histologic picture. Giant cell reaction within the tumor is not uncommon and was formerly confused with tuberculosis. A tuberculoid reaction to a lipid in the lung in these patients has occasionally been misdiagnosed as pulmonary "tuberculosis."[257]

Dysgerminoma may occur with a benign cystic teratoma, either as a relatively small focus in the benign cystic teratoma, or the dysgerminoma may be the main tumor and contain a cyst lined by stratified squamous epithelium. Dysgerminoma also may occur with a nongestational choriocarcinoma or with an endodermal sinus tumor as a component part of a teratocarcinoma or malignant teratoma. Occasionally, a positive Aschheim-Zondek test may be obtained, and this is due to the coexistence of a choriocarcinoma. Dysgerminoma may complicate pregnancy, not because of any specific predisposition but because pregnancy and dysgerminoma both occur in young women.

Treatment depends upon tumor extent, as does prognosis. If unilateral and confined within one ovary, most patients will be cured by salpingo-oophorectomy. On the other hand, those bilateral lesions and those unilateral tumors extending beyond the limits of the ovary have a poor prognosis even with radical surgery. The tumors are radiosensitive and occasionaly appear to be radiocurable. The five-year survival rate is 27%.[256]

Nongestational choriocarcinoma. Choriocarcinoma is a rare primary ovarian tumor composed of syncytiotrophoblastic and cytotrophoblastic elements. Only before the age of puberty is it possible to state that a pure choriocarcinoma is of primary teratogenic origin.[260] We have seen a choriocarcinoma of the ovary that at first appeared to be pure so was thought to be gestational, but its nongestational origin was established when a band of dysgerminoma was identified at its margin in one section. After puberty, choriocarcinoma of the ovary is more likely to have followed a pregnancy either primarily ovarian related to an ovarian pregnancy or secondarily ovarian related to a choriocarcinoma arising from an intrauterine or tubal pregnancy.

Grossly, choriocarcinomas of the ovary may measure up to 16 cm in diameter. The surface may be smooth or be coarse and nodular with a thin capsule, and the tumor may have already ruptured. On section, hemorrhage is prominent, and often there is necrosis. Microscopically, these tumors have the typical appearance of a choriocarcinoma—viz., interlacing strands of syncytiotrophoblast and groups of cytotrophoblastic cells. Other elements may be present in the same tumor,[258] most commonly foci of dysgerminoma.[259] This tumor probably originates from a primordial germ cell. (The primordial trophoblast is the first definitive tissue to differentiate in the fertilized ovum.) The tumor produces chorionic gonadotropin and will give a positive pregnancy test. Treatment is similar to that of any ovarian cancer. Methotrexate therapy has been unsuccessful with teratomatous choriocarcinoma. The prognosis is poor.

Endodermal sinus tumor (Teilum[264]). Endodermal sinus tumor, also described as Schiller's mesonephroma ovarii, is considered by Teilum to recapitulate stages in the phylogenetic development of extraembryonic structures such as allantois and yolk sac. These tumors have sometimes been described as embryonal carcinoma of the ovary, but the latter very often contain a variety of germ cell tumor patterns. Endodermal sinus tumors usually occur in the first three decades, and Huntington et al.[261] have pointed out that there are similar patterns in male and female children.

Grossly, the tumors vary in size from several centimeters to 25 cm or more, but usually they are about 15 cm in diameter. Usually, the surface is smooth, but there may be extension of the tumor. The cut surface is soft and friable and is variable in color. It may be cystic with foci of necrosis.

Microscopically, the characteristic feature is a "glomerulus-like" unit, with a central thin-walled vessel surrounded by loose connective tissue with a covering of cuboidal or columnar cells seeming to project into a cavity lined by endothelial cells. Otherwise, the tumor is composed of loose mesenchymal tissue of stellate cells, tending to form a system of communicating cavities and channels.

In a series of these tumors in young children, Huntington et al.[261] found that four of six patients with testicular tumor were well for more than four years. One of two patients with ovarian tumor was well over ten years, and both children with retroperitoneal tumor were dead. The usual recommended therapy is total hysterectomy and bilateral salpingo-oophorectomy, with or without postoperative radiation. The tumors do not seem to be sensitive to radiation. Although this is a malignant tumor, provided the neoplasm is apparently confined to one ovary, it may be worthwhile to remove only the tube and ovary on that side. The prognosis is very poor with any type of therapy, but perhaps with this more conservative approach an occasional normal child may survive.

We know of one patient in whom the Teilum tumor and its metastases regressed in response to Mithramycin therapy but recurred when therapy was suspended because of toxicity. The patient died before any type of maintenance dosage could be established.

Benign cystic teratoma. Benign cystic teratoma ("dermoid cyst") of the ovary is composed of any combination of well-differentiated ectodermal, mesodermal, and endodermal elements.[267, 269] The incidence of benign cystic teratomas among all ovarian neoplasms is about 25%. The majority occur during the reproductive life of the patient, but there is no relation between the age of the patient and the size of the tumor. The distribution of these tumors along the line of migration of the germ cells, most commonly in the gonad or the midline, suggests that they arise parthenogenetically from a primordial germ cell. This possibility is supported by finding segmenting ova in the ovary.

Most investigators agree that teratomatous tumors in the female have a female sex chromatin pattern. The true picture in male teratomatous tumors, however, is not clear. Theiss et al.[272] found all seminomas were of male nuclear sex, but in a review of the literature Matz[268] found half of the teratomas in males have a male chromatin pattern and half a female chromatin pattern with a small group of mosaics. With more consistent observations, some light may be shed on the genesis of teratomas. Identification of sex chromatin in very malignant tumors is considered generally unreliable.

Benign cystic teratomas have been found to be bilateral in 8% to 40%, the remainder being fairly equally distributed on both sides. Usually, the tumor is less than 10 cm but may vary from less than 1 cm to 30 to 40 cm in diameter. It is usually round, with a smooth surface, but there may be dense surface adhesions if there has been any leakage of contents. Usually, the tumor is fluctuant at body temperature, but the contents become more lardaceous when allowed to stand at room temperature. Usually, the cyst is unilocular but occasionally may be multilocular, and it is usually lined by "skin." There may be one or more solid areas containing one or more grossly evident fetal structures or organs, such as bone, cartilage, teeth, or, rarely, an eye. These elevations are covered by skin from which may be growing long hairs. The contents may be thick and greasy or thin and serous and may contain strands of hair.

Microscopically, ectodermal derivatives may be found in 100%, mesodermal in 92%, and endodermal in 72% of these tumors.[267] Stratified squamous epithelium and its derivatives (hair follicles and sebaceous glands) are the most commonly found structures and contribute to the formation of the cyst contents (Fig. 37-42). Other structures frequently seen are brain, nerve, teeth, bone, smooth muscle, and respiratory tract epithelium.

Treatment for the completely benign cystic teratoma is removal of the tumor and careful inspection of the other ovary. On rare occasions, the tumor may be dissected out. The prognosis is excellent.

Malignant change occasionally occurs in one of the elements of an otherwise benign cystic teratoma (0.5% to 5% of tumors). Usually, this is a squamous cell carcinoma,[270] but it may be a carcinoid, a thyroid carcinoma, a sarcoma, or even a malignant melanoma. The prognosis in such patients is poor.

Struma ovarii. A benign cystic teratoma, struma ovarii is composed entirely of thyroid tissue, or, if mixed, the thyroid element is by far the most prominent feature. Small amounts of thyroid tissue are common in the benign cystic teratoma and do not constitute struma ovarii. This is a very rare tumor. Although 240 examples of this tumor had been reported up to 1961,[273] it is doubtful that all of these met the strict criteria for struma ovarii.

Age range of patients is 6 to 74 years, with most patients in the reproductive age group. Tumors range in size from 0.6 cm upward, usually being 6 cm to 8 cm in diameter. Usually, the struma ovarii is unilateral, with a smooth surface and occasionally with adhesions. On section, there may be amber thyroid tissue, or it may be dull and red if colloid is absent. Microscopically, the tissue is identical with the thyroid gland and is composed of multiple follicles of varying size, lined with cuboidal or flattened cells and containing colloid material retracting from the lining and frequently vacuolated at the margins, or the tumor pattern may resemble any of the abnormal histologic patterns of the thyroid gland. About 12% of these tumors are functioning,[274] and in some patients there is very definite relief of hyperthyroidism after oophorectomy. The treatment and prognosis are similar to those for benign cystic teratoma.

Occasionally, struma ovarii may be malignant, but it is more usual for carcinoma to arise in a focus of thyroid in a benign cystic teratoma. There may be blood vessel invasion. Such tumors may implant locally, spread by lymphatics to form nodules in the liver, or spread via the bloodstream, resulting in metastases in bone.

Solid well-differentiated teratoma. Solid well-differentiated teratoma is a solid tumor, usually over 15 cm in diameter, with smooth surface and white to yellow or hemorrhagic cut surface often with numerous small cysts. Histologically, all the elements are well differentiated, although some mitotic activity may be observed.[275] These tumors tend to recur and may implant on the peritoneum. Peterson[276] studied a group of such tumors and found those most likely to recur contained glial tissue.

This tumor seems to be part of a spectrum representing the well-differentiated end, with the malignant teratoma at the undifferentiated end. Attempts have been made to correlate degree of differentiation with prognosis, but series of patients are small.[277]

Malignant teratoma. Malignant teratoma[282] has been described as a "compact, solid, rapidly growing neoplasm composed of tissues which are frequently wholly undifferentiated, corresponding to various stages of fetal development and revealing only isolated tend-

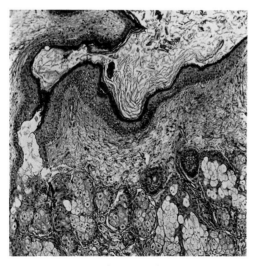

Fig. 37-42 Lining of typical benign cystic teratoma (dermoid cyst) of ovary. Squamous epithelium has prominent sebaceous glands and above it is abundant keratinized debris. (×75; AFIP 510588-07023.)

ency to more completely developed organlike formation."* It occurs most frequently in children and young women.

These tumors constitute 0.015% of ovarian tumors and less than 1% of teratomatous growths. The most commonly accepted origin is the development from a primitive unfertilized ovum.

Malignant teratoma is usually unilateral, more or less maintaining the shape of the ovary. Often, there are adhesions, and in about one-third there is either direct extension or metastasis to other abdominal organs. Microscopically, there is a wide variation of elements usually in varying degrees of differentiation and often reminiscent of developing embryonic tissue. There is often an undifferentiated stroma with nests of cells suggesting neural crest. Foci of better-differentiated tissue may suggest sarcoma or carcinoma. Epithelial structures may resemble embryonic or fetal glandular structures. Islands of elastic or hyaline cartilage, bone, lymphoid tissue, and smooth or striated muscle may be seen. Skin is rare.

Sometimes, there is overgrowth or exclusive growth of epithelial elements, with the formation of an undifferentiated carcinoma, usually with large irregular cells unlike those of müllerian carcinoma or any other recognizable type from any part of the body. Such tumors are termed *teratocarcinoma*.

Malignant teratomas are treated surgically by removal of the uterus, cervix, both tubes, and both ovaries, followed by deep roentgen radiation. The prognosis is poor, with only about 5% five-year cure rate in the first fifty-four patients reported in the literature. More recently, in a group of seventeen patients, most of whom were treated often by unilateral salpingo-oophorectomy, seven are living and well five months to more than eight years later.[278] All who survived were treated by unilateral salpingo-oophorectomy. In those patients whose tumor is composed mainly of a loose pleomorphic stromal tissue, sometimes with papillary or acinar structures (perhaps a Teilum tumor pattern), often termed *embryonal carcinoma*,[281] the prognosis is worse. If the tumor is apparently confined to one ovary, it may be advisable to remove only that tube and ovary. Should the tumor be biologically very malignant, it probably has already spread. If not, the patient may have been cured.

*From Curtis, A. H.: Surg. Gynec. Obstet. **81**:504-506, 1948.

Germ cell tumors of mixed patterns. Various combinations of patterns have been observed. Almost every theoretical combination has been reported.

Gonadoblastoma.[283-285] It seems most convenient to place gonadoblastoma with the germ cell tumors, although it recapitulates the whole embryonic gonad since it contains germ cells, Sertoli-granulosa cells, and Leydig-theca cells. Patients in whom these tumors have been found have primary amenorrhea and lack sexual development. Features may be eunuchoidal. Turner's syndrome may be present, and the patients are masculinized. Patients have a male sex chromatin pattern, 46/XY (four patients), or sex chromosome mosaicism, XO/XY.

Grossly, the tumor is similar to a dysgerminoma. Often, there is disseminated calcification. Microscopically, the tumor contains germ cells, which may be in nests with lymphoid stroma with an outer rim of Sertoli-

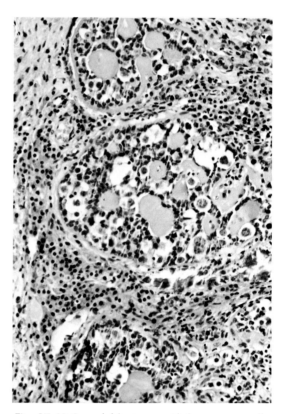

Fig. 37-43 Gonadoblastoma with large germ cells surrounded by Sertoli-granulosa cells and separated by diffuse growth of Leydig-theca cells. Note hyaline deposits with surrounding Sertoli-granulosa rim. (×160; material courtesy Dr. J. Teter, Warsaw, Poland; photograph courtesy Dr. R. E. Scully; from Scully, R. E.: In Grady, H. G., and Smith, H. C., Jr., editors: The ovary; copyrighted by The Williams & Wilkins Co.)

granulosa cells, or the Sertoli-granulosa cells may be arranged around individual cells or may surround spaces containing eosinophilic material (Fig. 37-43). The stroma may be "cellular" or may contain large polyhedral cells of Leydig-theca type.

This tumor has been called gonocytoma III by Teter. In his classification gonocytoma I corresponds with dysgerminoma. Gonocytoma II consists of germ cells and Sertoli-granulosa cells. This occurs in girls and boys, and the sex chromatin pattern corresponds with the external sexual characteristics. Sexual development is normal or precocious, somatic development is normal, and the tumors have estrogenic activity. Teter also mentions a gonocytoma IV, which is a pure dysgerminoma associated with clinical virilization. There is an overgrowth of Leydig (or hilar) cells adjacent to the tumor or in the opposite ovary.

The malignant potential of the gonadoblastoma has not been established. In one malignant gonadoblastoma, there were other malignant teratomatous elements that may well have accounted for the malignant course.

Cystomas (tumors of "germinal" epithelial origin)

The surface epithelium of the ovary is flattened to cuboidal in type and is modified pelvic peritoneum derived from the coelomic epithelium covering the urogenital ridge in the embryo. The term germinal is applied to this because earlier anatomists thought the primordial ova were derived therefrom—a theory now discarded. The surface epithelium is, however, embryonically related to the part of the coelomic epithelium that infolds to form the müllerian duct. The müllerian potential harbored in this epithelium is seen in the three types of cystomas derived therefrom: (1) the serous, recapitulating the tubal epithelium; (2) the mucinous, the cervical epithelium; and (3) the endometrial, the endometrium, by association with the underlying potential or actual endometrial stroma.[289]

In some texts, benign and malignant tumors are sharply separated, but it seems rather that each type of cystoma exhibits a spectrum extending from the definitely benign to the obviously malignant.

An attempt to establish an international classification was made by the Cancer Committee of the International Federation of Gynecology and Obstetrics in Stockholm in 1961. It was considered advisable to introduce an intermediate group for borderline tumors be-

cause the prognosis for these (85% to 90% five-year survival, however treated) is much better than for ovarian carcinoma in general. In this group of tumors, there were papillary processes, irregular piling up of epithelium, and nuclear pleomorphism but no demonstrable evidence of tumor infiltration (previously, these were called low-grade carcinomas). The following classification was therefore suggested (unpublished data).

1 Serous cystomas
  a Serous cystadenoma, benign
  b Proliferating serous cystadenoma without stromal invasion (possibly malignant) (type specimen shown in Fig. 37-46)
  c Serous cystadenocarcinoma, all grades
2 Mucinous cystomas
  a Mucinous cystadenoma, benign
  b Proliferating mucinous cystadenoma without stromal invasion (possibly malignant)
  c Mucinous cystadenocarcinoma, all grades
3 Endometrioid tumors
  a ? Is endometriosis a true tumor, or should this correspond with benign endometrioma? (at present undecided)
  b Proliferating endometrioid cystadenoma without stromal invasion (possibly malignant)
  c Endometrioid adenocarcinoma, all grades
4 Undifferentiated carcinoma (cell type unknown)

Serous cystadenoma and cystadenocarcinoma. Serous cystadenoma is a cystic neoplasm containing from one to many locules. It is derived from the germinal epithelium (Fig. 37-44) and resembles the mucosa of the fallopian tube (Fig. 37-45). It is one of the commoner ovarian tumors, constituting 29.1% of ovarian neoplasms (23.5% of all benign tumors and 60.3% of all malignant tumors).[225] The benign tumors are commonest from ages 20 to 50 and the malignant from 30 to 60 years.

There may be wide variations in gross appearance from the benign to the malignant. In the benign tumors, the surface of the ovary is smooth, and the cysts are lined by a smooth glistening mucosa. The presence of papillae is always a suspicious feature, and carcinoma must be considered, but the tumor may belong to the borderline group (Fig. 37-46). If the papillae have extended through to the surface of the ovary, even the more benign tumors may recur at a later time as a result of the seeding of the peritoneum by these processes. The latter may remain dormant for a variable length of time and then grow, perhaps into a less-differentiated tumor. In some cysts, the whole lining may be papillary, or there may be nodules of solid tumor. The latter type is obviously malignant and the former most probably malignant.

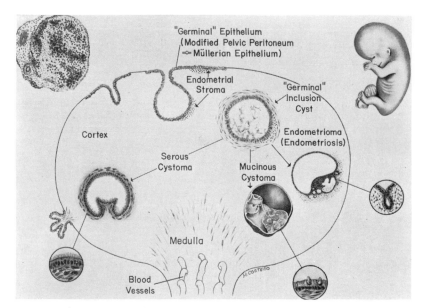

Fig. 37-44 Semidiagrammatic drawing of ovary to illustrate origin and types of cystomas derived from "germinal" epithelium. Note papillary growth on surface and various types of cystic tumors derived from infolding of this type of epithelium. Embryonic ovary and müllerian duct (top left) is drawn from 35 mm embryo (top right) and illustrates embryonic similarity of müllerian duct to germinal epithelium. The three types of cystomas (and their malignant counterparts) derived from "germinal" inclusion cysts are serous, endometrial, and mucinous—all recapitulating müllerian system, to which germinal epithelium is embryologically very closely related. Low-power and high-power drawings are from actual specimens. (From Hertig, A. T., and Gore, H. M.: Rocky Mountain Med. J. **55**:47-50, 1958.)

Papillary processes may actually arise from the surface germinal epithelium of the ovary, and these may behave in a manner similar to those previously described. In any one tumor, there may be extreme variations, from the completely benign to the obviously malignant. The benign tumor is most usually cystic, occasionally with solid connective tissue masses (as in the cystadenofibroma), whereas the malignant tumor is usually semisolid (cystic with solid areas of 2 cm or more). The benign serous cystoma tends to be unilateral and 5 cm to 10 cm in diameter, whereas the malignant serous cystadenocarcinoma tends rather to be bilateral and over 15 cm in diameter.

Microscopically, the epithelial cells may be cuboidal and similar to those of the germinal epithelium, or they may be of tubal ciliated type. In the benign tumors, the cysts usually are lined by a single layer of cells, and any papillae that may be present are likewise covered by a single layer of regular cells. Once these cells become even slightly pleomorphic, irregularly arranged, or piled up upon one another, forming papillary processes of the epithelium itself, the tumor is probably in the borderline group. The solid areas are composed of adenocarcinoma, sometimes fairly well differentiated, with definite papillary and acinar arrangement. The less-differentiated tumors are composed of solid masses of irregular cells with very little pattern. Concentrically rounded psammoma bodies, apparently a product of the interaction of pelvic peritoneum and underlying stroma, may occur in any of these tumors, and in the poorly differentiated carcinoma they may be the only means of identifying its germinal epithelial origin.

Intermediate histologic malignancy is most common, but relative frequency of grades is as follows: grade I, 27%; grade II, 39%; and grade III, 34%. In a study by Santesson,[290] benign tumors constituted 7%, borderline 37%, and malignant 56%.

Histologically benign tumors do not spread unless there are surface papillary foci from which papillae have been swept off to lodge on the pelvic or abdominal peritoneum, to be followed by slow or rapid growth or to remain dormant for many years and then to grow. For this reason, it may sometimes be difficult to determine whether a given tumor is benign or malignant. Histologic grading is considered by some to be related to the tendency to me-

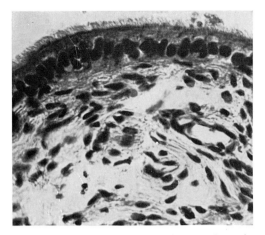

Fig. 37-45 Ciliated serous epithelium from benign serous cystadenoma of ovary. Note resemblance to tubal epithelium. (×100.)

tastasize and also to the five-year survival rate.

Once metastases occur, they are found in descending frequency in the pelvis, abdomen, and uterus. Of patients with ovarian carcinoma, over half already have metastases when first seen. Serous tumors tend to spread directly to the pelvic and abdominal peritoneum and to grow as surface implantations. In addition, they metastasize to aortic, mediastinal, and supraclavicular nodes and, later, to lungs and liver. The frequency of bilateral involvement (up to 20% of benign, 32% of malignant, and 50% of undifferentiated malignant tumors) is probably best explained by histogenesis rather than metastasis, since one would expect more uterine involvement if metastasis were the explanation. Furthermore, there may be additional primary foci elsewhere in the peritoneum. The treatment of choice for the malignant tumors is total hysterectomy and bilateral salpingo-oophorectomy, followed by roentgen irradiation. It is impossible to evaluate accurately the value of roentgen irradiation because of the absence of comparable control series. Nor has it been possible to evaluate radioactive gold or chemotherapy for the same reason.

Mucinous cystadenoma and cystadenocarcinoma. Mucinous cystadenoma is another cystic neoplasm containing from one to many locules, although usually many, derived from the germinal epithelium and resembling cervical epithelium. These tumors constitute 21% of all ovarian tumors and 24.5% of benign ovarian tumors.[225] The malignant variety is very rare (3.1% of all ovarian tumors). The benign form is commonest in the age group 20 to 50 years and the malignant form be-

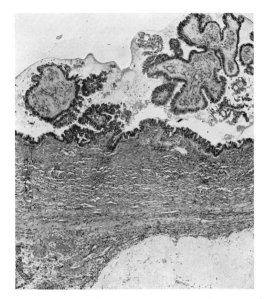

Fig. 37-46 Proliferating serous cystadenoma of ovary without invasion (possibly malignant). Its resemblance to tubal mucosa accounts for synonym endosalpingioma. Epithelium is pleomorphic and is itself beginning to form small papillary epithelial processes. Fibrous mass (below right) is corpus albicans. (×46; AFIP 264082-1.)

tween the ages of 40 and 60 years. There are multiple theories of origin. The two currently supported theories are (1) origin from germinal epithelium (which we think the most usual) and (2) origin as a monophyletic teratoma.[18]

Mucinous cystadenoma is potentially the largest ovarian neoplasm. It varies from 1 cm to 50 cm in greatest diameter and may weigh over sixty-six pounds. It tends to be unilateral, but 4.8% are bilateral in the benign form and 23.4% in the malignant group. Hemorrhagic infarction may occur because of the twisting of the pedicle in a benign tumor but is less likely in a malignant tumor when adherent to adjacent structures. The serosal surface is smooth and pink to gray in color, with the number of locules determining the shape of the tumor. Cross section reveals numerous cysts of varying size, some large and others small, giving a spongelike appearance. The fluid is usually stringy and mucinous. In benign tumors, the lining of the locules is smooth and glistening, with tall cells containing mucoid cytoplasm and basal nuclei (Figs. 37-47 to 37-49). Truly solid or friable areas and papillary processes indicate malignancy. Solid fibrous Brenner tumors or benign cystic teratomas (dermoids) may occur coincidentally. Because of the latter association, the origin of the mucinous cystoma as a monophyletic teratoma is considered the most probable in such a situation.

We have recently seen an atypical mucinous cystadenoma, superficially suggesting adenocarcinoma but, on further examination, bearing a striking resemblance to the "pill" pattern of the cervix. It was learned that the patient had been taking an oral contraceptive.

The malignant mucinous cystadenocarcinomas are more likely to be large and bilateral, to rupture spontaneously, and to be adherent to surrounding pelvic tissues. Microscopically, there is cellular pleomorphism, with the other usual features of cancer (Fig. 37-49). There may be gross evidence of metastatic serosal growth of the tumor either as similar mucinous adenocarcinoma or in the form of gelatinous myxoma peritonei. Often, the malignant cells may be overshadowed by the mucus they produce in this inevitably fatal complication. Whether myxoma peritonei may be associated with a benign tumor is a debatable point.

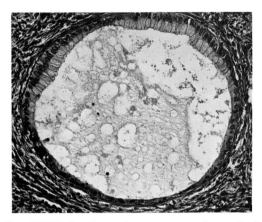

Fig. 37-47 Small ovarian cystoma of germinal epithelial derivation, lined partly by tall mucinous epithelium with pale mucoid cytoplasm containing basal nuclei and partly by undifferentiated cuboidal cells. (×75.)

Endometrial cystoma—benign and malignant. Ovarian endometrial cystomas are composed of functioning endometrial stroma and glands (necessary for "cystoma") within the ovary (see endometriosis). Grossly, they may vary from microscopic size to 10 cm or 15 cm in diameter. Early lesions are usually multiple, but later they may coalesce, forming the typical "chocolate cyst" containing dark brown, altered blood. The lining of the cyst

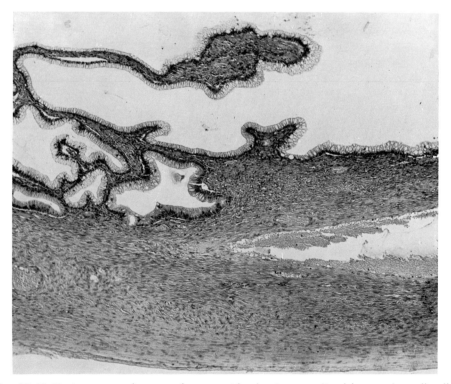

Fig. 37-48 Mucinous cystadenoma of ovary with gland spaces lined by regular tall cells containing pale mucoid cytoplasm. Note resemblance to endocervical mucosa. (×70; AFIP 316189-23112.)

in the early stages may be pink and soft, but in later stages it is brown and shaggy. The rare malignant forms are 2.7 cm to 16 cm in diameter, and the cyst wall may give rise to papillary processes and may contain solid areas.

Microscopically, these tumors are similar to endometriosis elsewhere. Here also, the longer the endometrium has functioned with resulting distortion of the cyst lining, the more difficult it is to establish the endometrial nature of the lesion. This is epitomized in the aphorism that the better the endometriosis is histologically, the poorer is the clinical evidence therefor, and vice versa. Many perfect examples of endometriosis are discovered as incidental findings in surgically removed pelvic organs. Malignant tumors arising in such lesions may have an adenocarcinomatous or an adenoacanthomatous pattern,[292] as in the endometrium itself. Rarely does the stroma become sarcomatous. Even more rare is the carcinosarcoma arising in ovarian endometriosis.

Cystadenofibroma—benign and malignant. Cystadenofibroma[291] is a fibroepithelial tumor of the ovary in which the epithelial component is derived from the germinal epithelium and the connective tissue from the cortical stroma of the ovary. This is a variant of the cystoma, usually of serous type. The dense stroma often is its most conspicuous feature. Small tumors are probably relatively common, but the large typical unilateral fibrous tumor with multiple cysts is extremely rare. Over 90% of these tumors are found after the age of 40 years.

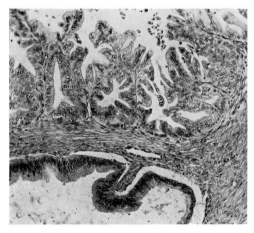

Fig. 37-49 Mucinous cystadenocarcinoma of ovary composed of typical cells with pale mucoid cytoplasm. In lower part of field is mucinous gland lined by irregular but better-differentiated cells. (×110; AFIP 264081-1.)

Grossly, the tumor may be apparently solid, with multiple small cysts, or it may be composed mainly of a large cyst with a small amount of more solid tumor on one side. It varies in size from 0.4 cm to 15 cm in diameter. Papillary processes may occur on the surface or in the lining of the cysts.

Microscopically, the cysts usually are lined by epithelium similar to that of the serous cystoma. Sometimes, the epithelium is mucinous, and we have seen one tumor with mucinous epithelium accompanied by squamous metaplasia. These cysts also may be foci of endometriosis. Furthermore, within one tumor, there may be varying combinations of all three. An occasional cystadenoma has a clear cell epithelial element, and whether this is truly a wolffian type or some germinal epithelial variation has not yet been determined. Stromal component may be white fibrous type or dense cortical stroma, or it may histologically resemble a thecoma, even with luteinization. This is not surprising, since occasionally these cystadenofibromas are associated with an estrogenic effect.

Rarely do these tumors undergo malignant change. However, when this change occurs, it involves the epithelial element. Occasionally, an apparently benign tumor may behave in malignant fashion, usually to the extent of a single omental metastasis.

Carcinosarcoma. Sarcoma, carcinosarcoma, and malignant mixed müllerian tumor in the ovary have been described, and their genesis is probably related to the potential endometrial stroma lying beneath the germinal epithelium.

Congenital rest tumors

Congenital rest tumors are a varied group of tumors for which origin from an embryonic structure is postulated. All of these tumors are rare—not of great practical importance but interesting from the point of histogenesis and histology.

Adrenal rest tumor. Adrenal rest tumors[294] are rare masculinizing ovarian tumors that grossly and histologically resemble the cortical tissues of the adrenal gland. Some poorly differentiated and unusual ovarian carcinomas suggest adrenal cortical carcinoma. It is entirely possible that such a diagnosis is not being made more often because it has not been considered. The adrenal rest tumor occurs in patients ranging in age from 6 to 71 years. It usually is unilateral and varies in size from microscopic to 30 cm in diameter but generally is small (42% less than 5 cm). It usually is encapsulated, lobulated, solid, rubbery, and yellow. Microscopically, it is composed of cords, nests, and strands of polyhedral, lipid-containing cells and is practically indistinguishable from glomerulosa and fasciculata of adrenal cortex. Clinically, all reported patients have had some features of masculinization. Malignant variants constitute 21%. Taylor and Norris[295] consider that an artificial division is made in separating adrenal-like tumors, hilus cell tumors, and stromal luteomas. They group them together as lipid cell tumors.

Mesometanephric rest tumor. Mesonephroma is an uncommon malignant ovarian tumor that morphologically recapitulates the mesonephros. Similar tumors may arise anywhere along the course of the mesonephros, and so present as vaginal, cervical, parovarian, ovarian, or retroperitoneal tumors[298] (Fig. 37-10). This tumor is rare and is found in patients ranging in age from 8 months to 69 years. Some of the young patients may well have had a teratoma. Indeed, there is considerable confusion with Teilum's endodermal sinus tumor. The mesonephroma is of medium to large size, usually about 15 cm in diameter, and may have a smooth surface or one roughened by adhesions. On section, it is soft with cystic areas. Microscopically, the tumor has a tubular pattern formed by flattened or cuboidal cells with oval nuclei and scanty clear cytoplasm.

The clear cell or Grawitz type carcinoma of the ovary or metanephroma belongs to this general group. Clear cells are arranged in sheets and tubules similar to the clear cell carcinoma of the kidney, and there is a similar tendency to extend into blood vessels. Clinically, this is similar to any other malignant ovarian tumor[298] and should be treated as such. When apparently confined to the ovary, the mortality rate is 50%. With spread beyond, it approaches 100%.

Brenner tumor. The Brenner tumor is composed of two elements—a dense, fibrous, usually nonhormone-producing stroma (but sometimes apparently estrogenic) surrounding nests of transitional or urinary tractlike epithelium. The incidence is 1.5% to 2% of all ovarian tumors. It occurs in patients ranging in age from 6 to 81 years, the great majority occurring between 41 and 70 years of age. About 20% of the tumors are associated with mucinous cystomas.[301] Proposed theories of genesis are (1) germinal epithelial or pelvic

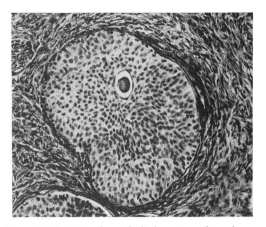

Fig. 37-50 Typical epithelial nest within dense, hormonally inactive fibrous stroma characterizes Brenner tumor. Small cavity contains shrunken inspissated material. (×140; AFIP 305334-1-4-2.)

peritoneal origin, (2) rete ovarii origin, (3) teratomatous origin, (4) ovarian stromal origin, (5) Brenner's original concept of origin from a graafian follicle, and (6) Walthard cell rests in the cortex of the ovary.

Brenner tumors are usually unilateral (8% bilateral), and they vary in size from microscopic to 30 cm in diameter, with one-third less than 1 cm. They may be solid or cystic, with small cysts appearing even in the solid tumors.

Microscopically, there are two essential components: the dense abundant stroma and typical epithelial nests composed of "compact, polyhedral, squamouslike epithelial cells" (Fig. 37-50). These cells are ovoid with an oval nucleus in which there is a characteristic longitudinal groove. The epithelial nests sometimes become cystic. The stromal cells usually are elongated with spindle-shaped dark nuclei, sometimes with hyalinization or calcification. This may resemble stroma of hilar or medullary origin. Sometimes, the stroma is similar to ovarian cortical stroma and sometimes resembles a thecoma.

In Tighe's series[301] of thirty-seven patients (assuming those without endometrial biopsies were normal), there were six with endometrial carcinoma, suggesting that at least 23% of Brenner tumors are hormonally active. Very rare malignant Brenner tumors have been reported. Histologically, the malignant variants have a transitional cell carcinoma pattern resembling a low-grade carcinoma of the bladder.

Hilar cell tumor. Hilar cell tumor[302] is extremely rare and is composed of those cells normally present in the hilum of the ovary.[304,

[306] It usually is associated with nonmyelinated nerves and is indistinguishable, microscopically, from the interstitial cells of Leydig in the normal testis or in an arrhenoblastoma. The age range in reported cases is from 39 to 86 years—usually 46 to 54 years. Usually, the tumor is unilateral, although occasionally it may be bilateral. When small, it is located in the hilar region, is clearly demarcated, is homogeneous, fleshy or soft and friable, and yellow to brown in color, with some mottling, and it is occasionally hemorrhagic.

Microscopically, the cells may be elongated, oval, or polygonal and have eosinophilic cytoplasm. They contain lipochrome pigment and occasionally crystalloids microchemically indistinguishable from the albuminoid Reinke crystalloids in the interstitial cells of the testis. These are relatively large bar-shaped eosinophilic bodies that may lie within the limits of the cell or may distort it. The nucleus is vesicular and contains one to three nucleoli.

These tumors usually are associated with masculinization, although there has been an occasional report of a hilar cell tumor that was apparently estrogenic. That some of these tumors were luteomas seems possible. Only when there are definite Reinke crystalloids is there no doubt about the diagnosis. Most patients have normal or slightly raised ketosteroid excretion. To date, no acceptable malignant hilar cell tumor has been reported.

Nonintrinsic connective tissue tumors

Fibroma. Fibroma is a connective tissue tumor of the ovary composed of fibroblasts and a varying amount of collagen. It constitutes about 1.7% to 5% of all surgically removed ovarian tumors and occurs most usually in middle-aged to elderly women. There is no typical clinical picture, but there is ascites in about one-third of the patients in whom the tumor is larger than 6 cm in diameter. It is bilateral in about 10%, and rarely there are multiple tumors in one ovary.[307] The ovary may be completely or partially replaced. The tumor is well defined, tough, and fibrous, with a whorled pattern. It may be gritty or stony hard as a result of calcification, or it may be red from infarction.

Microscopically, the tumor is composed of thin, spindle-shaped cells arranged in bundles, giving the tissue a fasciculated appearance. It may be difficult to distinguish from thecoma. The origin of cells is not absolutely determined, but it is suggested that they are from one of the following: (1) ovarian cortical connective tissue, (2) connective tissue of the capsule of the ovary, or (3) connective tissue of blood vessel, medulla, hilum, or corpus albicans.

Treatment is simple removal of the tumor, and prognosis is excellent.

Fibrosarcoma. Fibrosarcoma, the malignant variant of the fibroma, is extremely rare, comprising less than 1% of the fibromas of the ovary. Usually, it is unilateral, grayish white, firm, and nodular or lobulated, altogether grossly indistinguishable from the fibroma. The center is often soft and necrotic. It may grow to 40 cm in diameter.

The microscopic pattern varies from a cellular fibroma to a very pleomorphic sarcoma with prominent vascularity.

Accepted treatment is total hysterectomy with bilateral salpingo-oophorectomy followed by irradiation, usually with good results in the low-grade type. The prognosis is poor with more anaplastic tumors, due to local pelvic recurrence and vascular metastases.

Lymphoma. Lymphoma of the ovary, including both primary and metastatic lesions, has been reported in patients from 18 months to 73 years of age. In no patients were there adequate data to be certain the lesion was primary. Most died in fewer than five years (of thirty-five patients, one was living at sixteen years, one died at six years without disease, and one was living at one year). Tumors are bilateral in 43% of the patients and usually are grossly nodular, and brainlike, varying from gray to reddish gray. More than half the tumors are more than 15 cm in diameter. Of thirty-five tumors, fourteen were lymphocytic lymphoma, ten were lymphoblastoma, ten were reticulum cell lymphoma, and one was giant follicular lymphoma.

Metastatic tumors to ovary

The term Krukenberg tumor[311] often is used synonymously with tumor metastatic to the ovary. Since there is no general agreement as to what constitutes a Krukenberg tumor, perhaps this term should be avoided. The most usual concept of this tumor is bilateral bulky ovarian metastases that fail to distort the shape of the ovary. Such tumors often are mucoid in consistency and microscopically contain "signet-ring" cells and an active connective tissue response to such cells. This usually represents a metastasis from a gastrointestinal cancer. They may be accompanied by estrogenic or androgenic phenomena.

The incidence of tumors metastatic to the

ovary[310] is 5% to 20% of malignant ovarian tumors. They tend to occur in a slightly younger age group (22 to 60 years of age; average, 42 to 48 years) than does primary ovarian cancer. By far the commonest primary site is the stomach and then the intestine, with the uterus and the breast not nearly so common.

Grossly, these metastases may be unilateral, although far more frequently they are bilateral. They vary considerably in size, from those found microscopically in an atrophic ovary to masses 24 cm in diameter. On section, they may be firm, soft, mucoid, or myxomatous and may be white, gray, red, or mottled.

Microscopically, metastatic tumors may mimic primary ovarian tumors, be difficult to distinguish from the normal ovary, or be obviously metastatic. They may be composed of large rounded or polyhedral cells, or clear cells with mucoid cystoplasm, or typical "signet-ring" cells in which mucus compresses the nucleus against the side of the cell. Cells may be scattered individually in the stroma or be arranged in strands or acini. The stroma is of fibrous type, varying from a dense to a loose areolar arrangement and is sometimes apparently estrogenic. Rare examples of an androgenic effect have been reported. They may

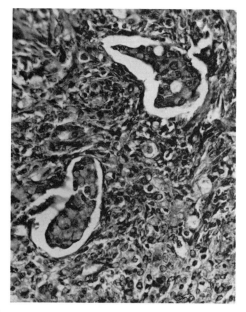

Fig. 37-51 Carcinoma metastatic to ovary with plugs of tumor cells lying within lymphatics. Many cells are of signet-ring type with nucleus compressed against one side of cell. Note sarcomatoid appearance of stroma. (×115; Ovarian Tumor Registry 1395.)

mimic several primary tumors (such as arrhenoblastoma, hilar cell tumor, and mesometanephroma) and sometimes may be difficult to distinguish from simple thecomatosis.

The method of spread varies but may occur by one of the following methods[312]:

1 Spread by peritoneal sedimentation
2 Spread by lymphatic channels, which must include the theory of retrograde spread (Fig. 37-51)
3 Extension by continuity
4 Spread by the bloodstream

Treatment is palliative and the prognosis that of the primary tumor with metastases. Whether or not there is a primary "Krukenberg" tumor with "signet-ring" cells and sarcomatoid stroma is debatable.

Ovarian cancer complicating pregnancy

Ovarian cancer and pregnancy may occur together, since 39%[225] of ovarian cancer occurs in the premenopausal period. The incidence of ovarian tumors in pregnancy is 1:900 pregnancies and of malignant tumors, 1:18,000 pregnancies. Dermoid cysts are the commonest tumors, constituting 20% to 60% of varying series, and benign nonneoplastic cysts (e.g., corpus luteum cyst) are the most common cause of ovarian enlargement.

Data concerning the type and distribution of malignant tumors in pregnancy are given in Table 37-1.

Treatment of these tumors is similar to that in the nonpregnant patient but is complicated by social factors. The prognosis in the treated patient is similar to that for the nonpregnant treated patient.

Endometriosis

Endometriosis is the presence of functioning endometrium located in ectopic sites throughout the genital organs, usually beneath the

Table 37-1 Type and distribution of malignant tumors in pregnancy

Recorded pathology	Cases	%
Dysgerminoma	14	20
Krukenberg tumor	10	14
Carcinoma	9	13
Papillary cystadenocarcinoma	7	10
Adenocarcinoma	6	8.5
Sarcoma	6	8.5
Arrhenoblastoma	4	6
Granulosa cell tumor	14	20
(Granulosa cell carcinoma)	(2)	(3)
	70	100

pelvic peritoneum and most commonly in the ovaries (Fig. 37-52). True or indirect endometriosis is to be distinguished from direct endometriosis. The latter involves the uterine wall, is often associated with some muscular response, and is properly termed adenomyosis.

Genesis. There have been four main concepts[317] of origin of endometriosis:

1 *Embryonic rests, müllerian (Russell) or wolffian (Recklinghausen).* This embryonic rest theory is not entirely supported by modern observation. Nevertheless, the universally present endometrial type of stroma beneath the pelvic peritoneum, and from which we believe endometriosis develops, is, in a very real sense, a congenital rest.

2 *Transtubal transport of endometrial fragments in menstrual blood with subsequent implantation of these fragments on pelvic peritoneum.*[320, 321, 323] The implantation theory presupposes that the endometrium that may reach the peritoneal cavity by reflux bleeding during menstruation will be viable, a fact substantiated by tissue culture.[319] Endometriosis has been produced experimentally in the

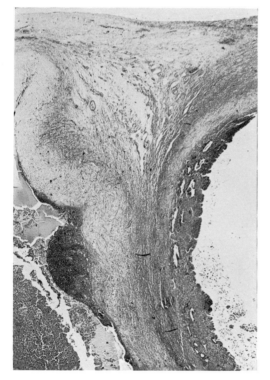

Fig. 37-52 Endometriosis of ovary. On right, cyst is lined by well-preserved secretory endometrium, but on left, there has been prior breakdown and bleeding ("menstruation") so that only scanty endometrial tissue is recognizable. (×20; AFIP 218754-52-514.)

monkey by surgically diverting the menstrual flow into the peritoneal cavity.[323] Such endometriosis may have been due to fragments displaced by surgery or fragments shed during menstruation, or indeed may have arisen from the inflammatory or inductive effect of menstrual blood itself on the pelvic peritoneum and its focal endometrial stroma. Implantation is no doubt the mechanism of the genesis of postoperative endometriosis, as in the laparotomy wound, the episiotomy scar, the portio of the cervix after cauterization, or Bartholin's gland after incision and drainage.

3 *Coelomic metaplasia.* The coelomic metaplasia theory[18] is supported by the known müllerian potential of the coelomic mesothelium and the universal presence of the endometrial-type stroma in a distribution comparable to that of endometriosis. That such endometrial stroma is universally present is shown by the gray-yellow, raised, congested patches of pseudodecidua seen immediately beneath the pelvic peritoneum during pregnancy[322, 325] and most frequently involving the ovary (Fig. 37-53). It is possible that the irritating factors inherent in the menstrual blood produce and further act upon an organizing pelvic peritonitis, incorporating potential endometrial epithelium and actual endometrial stroma. In support of this theory, it is of importance to note that endometriosis of the pelvis lies beneath the pelvic peritoneum rather than as a discrete area on the surface. Endometriosis of the vulva at the insertion of the round ligament is best explained by this concept.

4 *Lymphatic or vascular metastatic origin.* The lymphatic or vascular metastatic origin of endometriosis has been suggested by the finding of endometrial-type glands with or without endometrial stroma in lymph nodes, pleura, vulva, kidney, and skin. We have not seen endometrial stroma in such areas within lymph nodes and have not seen good morphologic evidence that this mechanism could explain early endometriosis either as well as, or to the exclusion of, the coelomic epithelium-endometrial stroma metaplasia concept. Indeed, these are probably peritoneal inclusions and do not represent metastases.

Prevalence and distribution. The prevalence of endometriosis in various clinics is 21.8% to 32%, with an age range of 20 to 63 years, most cases occurring in the fourth and fifth decades. It occurs most commonly in the ovary and then in the uterosacral ligaments and the rectovaginal septum.

Pathologic changes. Endometriosis varies

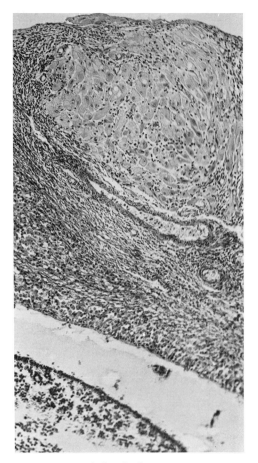

Fig. 37-53 Pseudodecidual reaction occurring in ovary beneath germinal epithelium and above tunica albuginea. Multiple foci of this type are found in ovaries of all pregnant patients, although they do not have endometriosis. It occasionally occurs near corpus luteum or in senescent ovary showing cortical stromal hyperplasia. Note prominent luteinized theca interna of atretic follicle below. (×100; AFIP 294919-17074.)

from tiny congested nodules (of microscopic size) to large hemorrhagic areas beneath the pelvic peritoneum or large cysts in the ovary containing so-called "chocolate" material. There may be a varying number of surface fibrous tags and varying amounts of subserosal fibrosis, with puckering of the surrounding tissue. Cysts in the ovary may be multiple at first but later single. The lining may be thin and sometimes granular or thick and velvety, depending on the condition of the endometrium. The nature of the lining depends on the menstrual phase, the duration of the process, the amount of bleeding, and the reaction to such bleeding.

The stroma is the functional element in endometriosis, so that a diagnosis may be made on the presence of this element alone. Frequently, both endometrial stroma and epithelium are present, often with glands. There is a variable amount of old to recent focal stromal hemorrhage. When the hemorrhage is more extensive, it often has destroyed the architecture of the endometrium, which is replaced by aggregations of hemosiderin-laden macrophages. The endometrium may have responded to cyclic hormonal stimulation and thus have the pattern of any phase of the menstrual cycle (Fig. 37-52). Occasionally, there may be cystic and adenomatous hyperplasia of the endometriosis. Indeed, malignant change may occur in one or both elements, more commonly in the glandular element. It is postulated that primary carcinosarcoma of the ovary or malignant mixed müllerian tumor of the ovary arises from such endometriosis or from stroma of endometrial potential.

In pregnancy, the endometrial stroma of endometriosis may respond to hormonal stimulation by forming true decidua (i.e., glands plus stroma). Endometriosis in pregnancy is to be distinguished from pseudodecidual reaction (Fig. 37-53) in that the former is functioning ectopic endometrium, whatever its origin, whereas the latter is in the nature of a truly congenital rest of pure endometrial stroma. Such stroma is always present beneath the pelvic peritoneum and is particularly observable during pregnancy and probably plays a significant role in the pathogenesis of endometriosis.

Currently, therapy is often by steroid substances.[14, 318]

PLACENTA, AMNION, AND UMBILICAL CORD
Development[12, 338]

Placenta. Significant stages in the formation of the placenta are as follows:

1 Implantation of the six-day to seven-day blastocyst, with formation of solid trophoblast from its wall at the point of contact with the endometrium (Fig. 37-54, *A*).

2 Gradual peripheral orientation of the syncytiotrophoblast in which vacuoles appear and then coalesce to form the intervillous space; central orientation of the cytotrophoblast, which proliferates as isolated masses, forerunners of the primordial villi; these occur from the ninth to thirteenth day of development (Fig. 37-54, *B*).

3 Conversion of the cytotrophoblastic masses

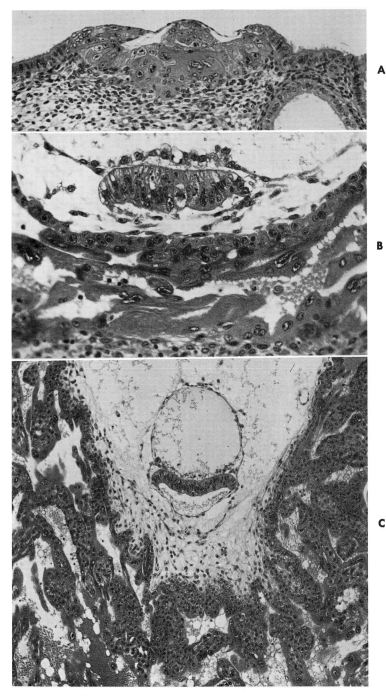

Fig. 37-54 A, Human 7½-day ovum superficially implanted for thirty-six hours on edematous twenty-two-day secretory endometrium. Note solid trophoblast, derived from blastocyst wall at its contact with endometrium and composed of pale cytotrophoblast and darker syncytiotrophoblast. **B,** Human 12½-day ovum showing embryonic disc (above) and adjacent trophoblast in contact (below) with predecidual stroma of twenty-six-day secretory endometrium. Note inner cytotrophoblast beginning to form primordial chorionic villi and outer syncytiotrophoblast whose lacunar spaces contain maternal blood, beginning of uteroplacental circulation. **C,** Human 14-day ovum showing embryo (upper center) surrounded by early chorion frondosum. Note simple unbranched primordial villi composed largely of central cytotrophoblastic core, beginning to form mesenchymal core and surrounded by syncytium which lines intervillous space. (**A,** ×150; **B,** ×250; **C,** ×100; **A** and **C,** courtesy Department of Embryology, Carnegie Institution of Washington, Carnegie No. 7801; from Heuser, C. H., Rock, J., and Hertig, A. T.: Contrib. Embryol. **31:**85-100, 1945; **B,** courtesy Department of Embryology, Carnegie Institution of Washington, Carnegie No. 7700; from Hertig, A. T., and Rock, J.: Contrib. Embryol. **29:**127-156, 1941.)

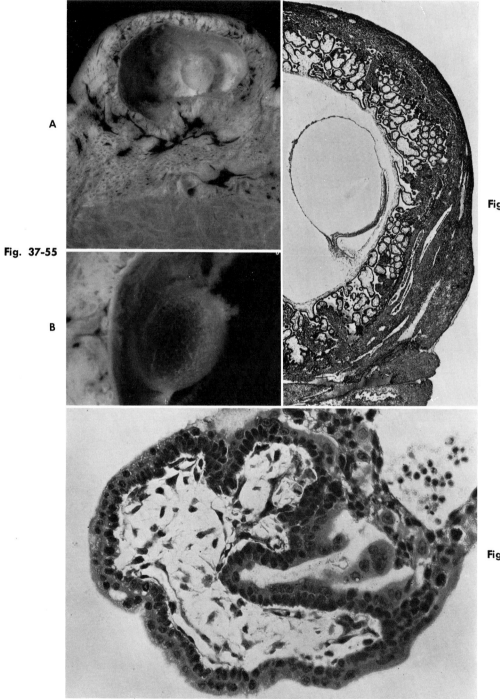

A

B

Fig. 37-55

Fig. 37-56

Fig. 37-57

Figs. 37-55 to **37-57** For legends see opposite page.

covered by syncytiotrophoblast to primordial villi from the fourteenth through the seventeenth day (Figs. 37-54, *C*, and 37-57).

4 Branching of primordial villi from the eighteenth day on through the first trimester. Each primordial villus with its derivatives constitutes a cotyledon of the mature placenta (Figs. 37-55 and 37-56).

5 Gradual enlargement of the entire ovum from the twentieth day to the twentieth week, resulting in (1) obliteration of the entire uterine cavity by fusion of decidua capsularis and decidua vera, (2) progressive thinning of the abembryonic chorion to become the chorion laeve, (3) progressive growth of the amnion, with gradual obliteration of the chorionic cavity by fusion of chorionic and amniotic fibrous tissue, and (4) progressive growth of the chorion frondosum, forming eight to fifteen cotyledons, constituting the placenta (Figs. 37-58 and 37-59).

Amnion. Significant phases in the formation of the amnion are as follows:

1 Its in situ delamination from the adjacent cytotrophoblast of the implanting ovum during the seventh to ninth day of development

2 Resulting formation of a veil-like membrane over and attached to the periphery of the circular concave germ disc during the ninth to the thirteenth day of development (Fig. 37-54, *B*)

3 Gradual transformation of this membrane to amniotic epithelium during the fourteenth to twenty-fifth day of development (Fig. 37-54, *C*)

4 Simultaneous accumulation of a second mesoblastic layer

5 Progressive distention of the amniotic cavity, growth of the embryo, and its "prolapse" into the amniotic cavity

6 Gradual obliteration of the chorionic cavity by fusion of connective tissue of amnion and chorion

Umbilical cord. Significant stages in the formation of the umbilical cord are as follows:

1 Its origin as a mass of chorionically derived mesoblast at the caudal end of the embryonic disc when the latter develops its longitudinal axis during the fourteenth to sixteenth day (Fig. 37-56)

2 Gradual shifting of the caudally located body stalk to a more ventrally situated umbilical cord as the embryo grows caudally

3 Gradual "prolapse" of the embryo accompanied by its cord into the amniotic cavity and simultaneous covering of the cord by amniotic epithelium

Spontaneous abortion

Spontaneous abortion[351] is synonymous with miscarriage and is defined as the premature termination of a medically nonviable pregnancy of less than 27 to 28 weeks of age. The legal age of viability is considerably less, however, and averages about 20 weeks.

The incidence of spontaneous abortion is approximately 12% as determined from a single large private practice but probably is closer to 20%, since many abortions pass unrecognized.[335] About one-half of all miscarriages occur from the tenth to the thirteenth week, irrespective of the apparent etiology. As a general rule, the more defective the fertilized ovum, the earlier the miscarriage occurs—the majority before the end of the first

Fig. 37-55 Gross and microscopic aspects of chorionic, embryonic, and body stalk development at 19 days developmental age (33 days menstrual age). **A,** Ovisac and implantation site bisected to show embryo, chorionic cavity, and chorionic villi around entire circumference. Thin *decidua capsularis* above, *decidua vera* laterally, and *decidua basalis* below, but above myometrium. For gross details of embryo viewed at right angles, see **B. B,** Embryo showing yolk sac with blood islands (right), curved germ disk (left), and crescent-shaped amniotic cavity between chorionic membrane (extreme left) and body stalk (below). For microscopic details (in mirror image), see Fig. 37-56. (**A,** ×4; Carnegie No. 8671, seq. 2; **B,** ×12; Carnegie No. 8671, seq. 6.)

Fig. 37-56 Midsagittal section of embryo, body stalk, and adjacent chorion, latter representing one-half of chorion and including both *chorion laeve* (top) and *chorion frondosum* (bottom). (Carnegie No. 8671, sect. 10-4-2.)

Fig. 37-57 Detail of chorionic villus from pregnancy comparable to that shown in Figs. 37-55 and 37-56. Note immature stroma containing developing blood vessels. Trophoblast consists of outer syncytium and inner Langhans' epithelium. Between streamers of solid trophoblast (upper right) are maternal blood cells within intervillous space. (×300; courtesy Department of Embryology, Carnegie Institution of Washington, Carnegie No. 5960, sect. 5-2-1; from Hertig, A. T.: Contrib. Embryol. **25:**37-82, 1935.)

Fig. 37-58

Fig. 37-59

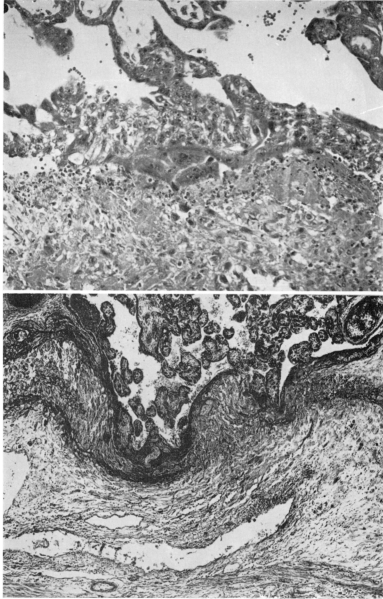

Fig. 37-58 Primordial chorionic villus from normal human ovum of about 18 days. This villus, comparable to that shown in Fig. 37-57, is continuous with cytotrophoblast of cell column and placental floor, latter contiguous with underlying decidua basalis. Note remnants of peripheral syncytiotrophoblast, which is giving rise to giant cells of placental site. (×150; AFIP 218754-548.)

Fig. 37-59 Implantation site from 7-month normal pregnancy. Essential features are floor of placenta, composed of cytotrophoblast to which chorionic villi (above) are attached, and adherent endometrium below. Rohr's fibrinoid layer plainly visible at upper left (within trophoblast) and Nitabuch's at lower left (between trophoblast and decidua). As term approaches, these two layers fuse and tend to become one, comparable to what is seen in middle of illustration. (×50; from Irving, F. C., and Hertig, A. T.: Surg. Gynec. Obstet. **64**:178-200, 1937.)

trimester. Middle-trimester abortions are rare, most defective or poorly implanted ova having already been aborted, whereas the third-trimester complications of premature labor or rupture of the membranes or both, with or without intrauterine fetal death, have not yet begun to appear.

The most frequent causes of spontaneous abortion appear to be absence of the embryo, its early death with resorption, severe abnormality of the embryo, or later death of the embryo. Less commonly, the conceptus has focally or diffusely defective trophoblast (placental tissue) or is abnormally implanted.

Maternal factors include criminal abortion, uterine abnormalities, and febrile and inflammatory diseases. Trauma is frequently (1.3%) mentioned as a cause. Its true incidence is only about 0.1%, the actual cause of the abortion usually having been present sometime prior to the trauma. In about one-quarter of all abortions, there is no apparent cause, and these are the ones that theoretically might be prevented.

The decidua associated with spontaneous abortion uniformly shows thrombosis of blood vessels, focal necrosis with polymorphonuclear and mononuclear leukocytic infiltration, and focal or diffuse recent interstitial hemorrhage. The histologic picture, analogous endocrinologically and pathologically to a delayed menstruation, is the result of the gradual withdrawal of the steroid hormonal "support" of the decidua by the syncytiotrophoblast and/or corpus luteum. (It is necessary for the corpus luteum to function under stimulation of chorionic gonadotropin from the cytotrophoblast for the first eight to ten weeks, when analogous functions are assumed by the trophoblast.)

Szulman[363] has studied the chromosomal constitution of abortuses. While findings were normal in fifteen therapeutic abortuses, sixteen of twenty-five spontaneous abortuses had abnormal karyotypes, including triploidy known to be lethal in higher vertebrates. Kerr and Rashad[344] found one mongoloid 47 XY trisomy G among fifteen induced abortuses. Five of fifteen first-trimester spontaneous abortuses had chromosomal anomalies, especially associated with an empty chorionic sac, whereas only one of twenty second-trimester abortuses had an abnormal chromosomal pattern.

Considering the gross type of abortus, Singh and Carr[358] found that 6% of anatomically normal specimens and 48.4% of abnormal specimens have a chromosomal anomaly.

It is of interest that of 327 abortuses analyzed for sex chromatin, 127 had an XX pattern, 135 an XY pattern, and twenty an XO pattern.[344]

Hydatidiform mole

An uncommon (1 in 2,000 in the United States) complication of pregnancy, hydatidiform mole, is characterized by the progressive swelling of the stroma of the chorionic villi, associated with disappearance of the fetal vascular system and accompanied by a variable amount of trophoblastic proliferation.[334]

The common pathogenic factor in such swelling is absence or early death of the embryo during the first three or four weeks of development, with consequent disappearance of fetal vessels. The process of swelling is due to functional trophoblast on villi deprived of a functional fetal circulation. Hydatidiform swelling, which is, therefore, *not* a degeneration, occurs in three principal situations:

1 The chorionic villi of the majority of "blighted" ova, which constitute about one-half of all spontaneous abortions or nearly 5% of *all* pregnancies

2 Focally throughout otherwise normally developing placentas whose fetuses are alive and whose chorionic circulation functions *except* in those focal areas; appears to be related to a villous vascular anomaly and is a cause of some mid-trimester abortions

3 The margin of normally developing placentas where the chorionic villi are alive but the fetal circulation is becoming embarrassed by the development of the chorion laeve

A true hydatidiform mole is a temporarily missed abortion of a "blighted" ovum whose microscopic hydatid swelling has become macroscopic during the additional eight weeks it has been retained in utero, but whose trophoblast was probably abnormal from the beginning. Correlated with these anatomic changes, there may be excessive size of the uterus (although 25% of uteri are expected size, 25% smaller), bleeding from the uterus via the vagina due to disruption of the normally closed intervillous space, excessive though variable rise in chorionic gonadotropin titer,[329] and frequent bilateral ovarian enlargement, up to 15 cm. Even when there is no gross enlargement, microscopic cysts of follicular origin with prominent luteinized theca interna and sheets of theca lutein cells may be observed. This pattern has been observed most usually with hydatidiform mole and choriocarcinoma but rarely may be associated with a clinically normal pregnancy.[357] These enlarged ovaries return to normal size after complete removal of the trophoblast, and there is no indication for their surgical removal. Failure to involute is an indication of persisting trophoblastic tissue.

As a consequence of the trophoblastic activity, there may be (1) invasion of the uterine wall by one or more hydatidiform molar villi, (2) malignant neoplasia of the trophoblast, resulting in choriocarcinoma, or (3) rarely, "metastasis" of intact hydatidiform villi to the parametrium, local pelvic structures, lungs, or elsewhere in the body.

Grossly, the vesicles of a hydatidiform mole are characteristically discrete, rounded, translucent, and variable in size from bare visibility up to 10 mm in diameter (Figs. 37-60 and 37-61). They may or may not still possess threadlike attachment to the villus from which they arose and of which they are merely a ballooned-up grapelike branch. Foci of trophoblastic proliferation are grossly visible under low diameters of magnification as opaque areas.

The spontaneously expelled or operatively removed hydatidiform mole is usually bulky and may total up to 3 liters, although sometimes its volume is small. The grapelike villi are embedded in variable amounts of old and recent blood clot. The chorionic sac, usually empty (Fig. 37-60) or containing a small defective, macerated embryo (Fig. 37-61) can be identified unless the sac has been traumatically ruptured.

Microscopically, the hydatidiform villus shows striking variation in the degree of trophoblastic proliferation (Figs. 37-62 and 37-64, A). The cytotrophoblast may be present as an orderly Langhans' epithelium, but more often it has proliferated as irregular masses whose pleomorphism and mitotic activity vary from specimen to specimen and from area to

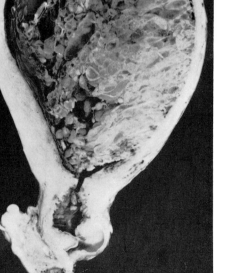

Fig. 37-60 Midsagittal section of typical molar uterus approaching term size, although of only about 20 weeks' gestational age. Uterine cavity is greatly distended but small oval, centrally located chorionic sac may still be identified. (Courtesy Dr. H. Sheehan and AFIP.)

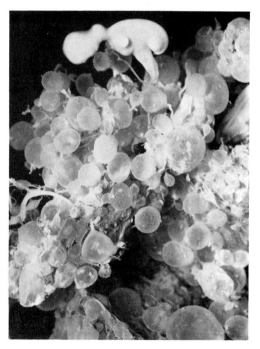

Fig. 37-61 Grapelike vesicles of varying size constituting hydatidiform mole. Stunted, macerated fetus of approximately 6 weeks' menstrual age was within intact chorionic sac (not shown here) when mole was delivered at hysterectomy. This is unusual, chorionic sac usually being empty. (×2; Carnegie No. 8723, seq. 1; from Hertig, A. T.: In Meigs, J. V., and Sturgis, S. H., editors: Progress in gynecology, vol. II, Grune & Stratton, Inc.; by permission.)

area within the same specimen. The syncytiotrophoblast also varies in appearance, from
the regular layer covering Langhans' epithelium to an irregularly festooned mass containing lacunae (Fig. 37-62) representing the
primitive intervillous space. Primitive syncytiotrophoblast also may be mixed with primitive cytotrophoblast, and indeed the cells may
be so pleomorphic and anaplastic that it is
difficult to distinguish cell types.[337]

The avascular fibrous tissue of the villus
forms a layer adjacent to the trophoblast and
so lines the fluid-filled cavity of the villus.
This fluid is analogous to that of the early normal chorion.

The amount of trophoblastic proliferation
and its degree of undifferentiation are, in general, proportional to the tendency of the
hydatidiform mole to become locally invasive
(chorioadenoma destruens) or to become

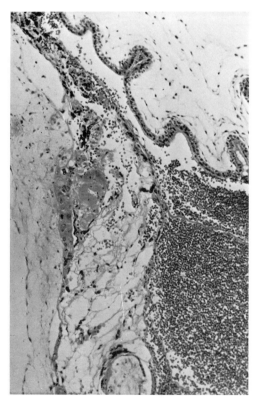

Fig. 37-62 Group II mole (probably benign). Despite benign appearance, patient developed clinically invasive mole (chorioadenoma destruens)
five weeks after evacuation of mole. These portions of two villi show normal double-layered
trophoblast on upper right and pleomorphism of
Langhans' epithelium and vacuolization of syncytiotrophoblast on other villus. (×110; from
Hertig, A. T., and Sheldon, W. H.: Amer. J.
Obstet. Gynec. **53:**1-36, 1947.)

truly neoplastic (choriocarcinoma). This has
been shown by one of us (A.T.H.), who
found that in grouping moles based on the
hyperplasia and anaplasia of the trophoblast,
the higher the group, the more likely was the
patient to develop a chorioma.[337] Nevertheless, it is impossible from microscopic examination of the individual mole to predict the
ultimate clinical outcome. Curettings are more
important, although not absolutely diagnostic
in evaluating potential malignancy, for they
represent the trophoblast actually in juxtaposition to the endometrium. Moreover, the
most *malignant-appearing* trophoblast of a
hydatidiform mole does not accurately resemble the choriocarcinoma that may arise from
it (Fig. 37-64).

The diagnosis of retained or intramyome-
trial trophoblast (either invasive mole or choriocarcinoma) may be suspected on the basis
of subinvolution of the uterus, with continued
bleeding per vaginam and failure of the chorionic gonadotropin to return to normal or to
have fallen almost to normal by four weeks.

The definite diagnosis of invasive mole may
be made only by finding invasive molar villi
within the myometrium (Fig. 37-63). The
definite diagnosis of choriocarcinoma (following a mole or, indeed, any type of pregnancy)
depends upon the finding of typical plexiform
masses of pure immature neoplastic cytotrophoblast and syncytiotrophoblast in curettings,
mixed with necrotic blood clot, within the
myometrium or in a metastatic site[331] (Fig.
37-64, *B*).

Primary hydatidiform mole has been described as occurring in the fallopian tube.
Such lesions are usually blighted ova with
grossly evident hydatidiform swelling of the
villi. It is possible that a true mole could
occur, but the limiting factor is probably the
wall of the tube, which would be likely to
rupture before a true mole had developed.
Kika and Matuda[345] have described a specimen that approaches a true hydatidiform
mole but is probably of transitional type.[335]

Chorionepithelioma
(chorioma)

Chorionepithelioma is a term introduced in
1895 by Marchand and applied to a malignant tumor of trophoblast, usually fatal. This
has been applied loosely to several conditions,
with resulting confusion.[337]

Syncytial endometritis. Syncytial endometritis or atypical chorionepithelioma is merely
an exaggeration of the normal penetration

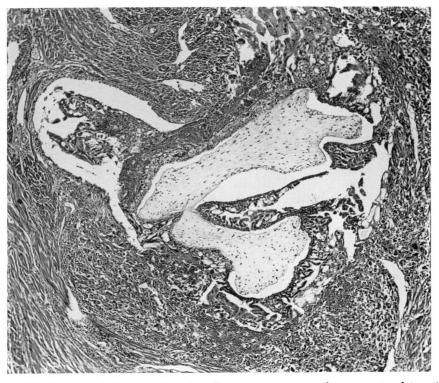

Fig. 37-63 Single hydatidiform villus invading myometrium, pathognomonic of invasive mole. (×48; AFIP No. 298593-2.)

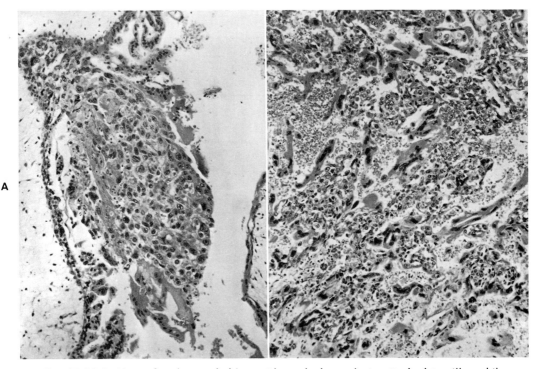

Fig. 37-64 A, Mass of molar trophoblast with marked anaplasia attached to villus while remainder of trophoblast is not unusually active. Although mole gave rise to chorio-carcinoma, this trophoblast does not resemble that of tumor shown in **B. B,** Renal metas-tasis of typical choriocarcinoma occurring in patient whose original mole is shown in **A.** Patient died sixteen months following delivery of hydatidiform mole. (×110; courtesy Rhode Island Hospital, Providence; AFIP 218754-562 and 218754-563.)

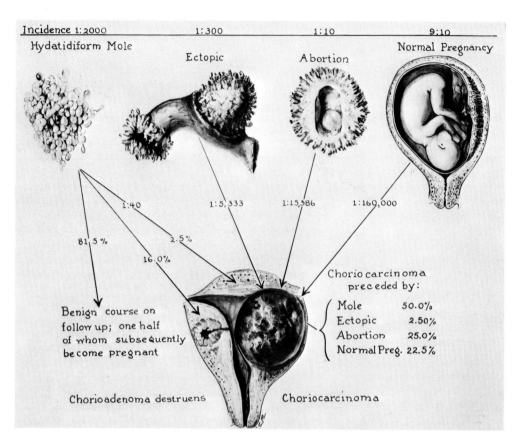

Incidence 1:2000   1:300   1:10   9:10

Hydatidiform Mole   Ectopic   Abortion   Normal Pregnancy

1:40   1:5,333   1:15,386   1:160,000

81.5%   2.5%

16.0%

Benign course on follow up; one half of whom subsequently become pregnant

Choriocarcinoma preceded by:

Mole   50.0%
Ectopic   2.50%
Abortion   25.0%
Normal Preg. 22.5%

Chorioadenoma destruens   Choriocarcinoma

Fig. 37-65 Schematic representation of relationship between various types of pregnancy and chorioadenoma destruens and choriocarcinoma. (Adapted from Hertig, A. T.: In Meigs, J. V., and Sturgis, S. H., editors: Progress in gynecology, vol. II, Grune & Stratton, Inc.; by permission.)

and invasion of decidua and myometrium beneath the placental site by multinucleated giant cells of trophoblastic origin. It is neither a true inflammation nor a neoplasm and has never been conclusively demonstrated to have become clinically malignant.

"Chorionepithelioma in situ." "Chorionepithelioma in situ" is a debatable lesion that is characterized by the presence of small foci of apparently neoplastic chorionic epithelium within decidua, its vessels, or small cavities apparently created by the trophoblast. It is cured by curettage.

Invasive mole. Invasive mole or chorioadenoma destruens (Fig. 37-63) is a locally invasive nonneoplastic variant of the hydatidiform mole and is associated with or follows only that condition. It is theoretically possible that the invasive mole may follow the focal true mole in an otherwise normal placenta.[335] It occurs in about 16% of molar pregnancies. It begins initially as a single villus that invades, is swept into, or lodges within one of the numerous large veins of the placental site.

It usually becomes clinically evident four to twelve weeks following passage of the mole.

Grossly, the lesion is characterized by one or occasionally several discrete or coalescing hemorrhagic areas of variable size within the myometrium. The average one varies from 5 mm to 15 mm in diameter. The lesion may be solid, as a result of laminated blood clot, or cavitated if such hemorrhage has failed to clot or has secondarily sloughed out. The lesion is due to one or more intact hydatidiform chorionic villi, which may be demonstrated microscopically in the depths of the lesion. It usually runs a benign course, but the molar villi may penetrate the serosa, with resultant hemorrhage or sepsis. Rarely, it may give rise to metastases in the pelvic structures, the lung, the spinal cord, or the brain with hemorrhage. These *may* involute, but chemotherapy is advisable. It is usually uncertain whether these metastases are metastatic mole or choriocarcinoma, but therapy is the same for both.

Choriocarcinoma. Choriocarcinoma may be associated with or follow any type of pregnancy but is relatively more common following molar gestations (Fig. 37-65). It occurs in approximately 1 in 40,000 consecutive pregnancies. The interval between the primary pregnancy and clinical evidence of choriocarcinoma may be from days to years but is usually about four to six months. Coincidental or early tendency to vascular metastasis is biologically characteristic of the disease. It largely explains why uteri are so often negative even though metastases subsequently develop, why prophylactic postmolar hysterectomy usually fails to cure the disease, and why hysterectomy, once the disease has developed, also usually fails to prevent a fatal outcome.

The choriocarcinoma, when present in the uterus, tends to be located in the corpus, usually in the upper half, although the uterus may be devoid of tumor even though the metastases are present elsewhere. Primary gestational choriocarcinoma may occur in the tube, in the ovary, and in the cervix. The lesion may vary from a few millimeters to 10 cm in diameter. It is always hemorrhagic and may present as a large fungating lesion in the uterine cavity, with variable involvement of the myometrium, or it may be almost completely within the myometrium and require careful serial blocking of the uterus to discover its location. The cut surface reveals soft to firm hemorrhagic areas with variable degrees of cavitation. The tumor is usually irregular in outline and may or may not be circumscribed, but it is never encapsulated.

Microscopically, there may be a relatively large amount of hemorrhage and a proportionately small amount of tumor, which is located mainly at the periphery of the lesion. Vascular permeation and/or metastases are seen at the periphery of the tumor. The trophoblast itself varies somewhat from tumor to tumor, but in general forms the typical plexiform pattern of cytotrophoblast covered by syncytiotrophoblast characteristic of the developing trophoblast of the eleven-day to thirteen-day ovum. (Compare Figs. 37-54, *C,* and 37-58 with Fig. 37-64, *B*). The cytotrophoblast shows variable degrees of pleomorphism and rates of growth, although usually the cells are uniform and only moderately rapidly growing. The syncytiotrophoblast, although variably pleomorphic, never grows by mitosis. Modern studies indicate it is derived from cytotrophoblast.[364]

Metastases via the vascular system most commonly are found in the lung (60%), vagina (40%), brain (17%), liver (16%), and kidney (13%). Such metastases, like the parent tumor, are composed largely of blood clot, with the tumor located mainly at the periphery. Not all hemorrhagic vaginal nodules are choriocarcinoma. Benign deported trophoblast may cause local hemorrhage. Such a lesion may involute merely after incision. We have seen these benign vaginal nodules only with hydatidiform mole and choriocarcinoma but believe they could occur with a normal intrauterine pregnancy.

One of the most curious biologic characteristics of choriocarcinomatous metastases is their occasional disappearance following removal of the primary uterine tumor. Upon this biologic principle, not understood but presumably related to the ability of residual trophoblast in lungs and myometrium to regress following normal pregnancy, depends the modern therapeutic approach to choriocarcinoma. Current evidence indicates the value of chemotherapy (usually methotrexate), *under the supervision of a chemotherapist experienced* in the management of patients with choriocarcinoma. It usually is considered preferable not to remove the uterus unless satisfactory remission of the disease is not obtained with adequate chemotherapy. The entire problem of the therapy of trophoblastic disease is complicated and should be undertaken only by those having considerable experience and adequate laboratory facilities.[339, 340, 353] Patients are being cured and subsequently having normal pregnancies.

Although the prognosis for choriocarcinoma has generally been poor, a 15% five-year survival was observed without metastases and a 6% five-year survival with metastases before the introduction of chemotherapy. With methotrexate, the five-year survival rate approached 50% in the earlier groups of patients[339] but currently approaches 80%.[326]

If the disease is fatal, death usually occurs within the first year. Death is due to multiple metastases that usually kill by their numbers and location (in the brain or the lungs) but occasionally may kill be uncontrollable hemorrhage (in the brain, the vagina, or an abdominal viscus).

Examination of placenta

For accurate evaluation of the placenta, adequate clinical data should be available. Significant gross features should be noted and recorded, including careful examination of membranes, the maternal, fetal, and cut surfaces of the placenta, and the umbilical cord.

Placental blocks for histologic study should be prepared from the margin, including the membranes, the central portion, and the cord, leaving normal surfaces intact and preserving important anatomic relationships.[328] Special studies may include histochemical techniques.[348]

Abnormalities of placental development

The two important factors influencing placental development are (1) the quality of the primitive trophoblast and (2) its degree of maternal blood supply. Factors influencing the trophoblast are site and depth of implantation.

Anomalies of shape. Anomalies of shape include the following:

1 Placenta bipartita, tripartita, multipartita
2 Placenta duplex (two small and equal-appearing, although separated, placentas vascularly united directly to the umbilical cord)
3 Placenta succenturiata (caused by development of one or more primordial villi of the abembryonic chorion)

Placenta extrachorialis. The term placenta extrachorialis includes placenta circumvallata and placenta circummarginata. In these conditions, the transition from membranous to villous chorion occurs at a variable distance from the edge of the placenta rather than at its usual site, the placental edge. It may be partial or involve the entire circumference. In 18% of placentas, there was placenta extrachorialis.[355] The marginate pattern is about ten times as common as the circumvallate, but they may occur together. The gross pattern varies from a thin fibrous ring to a broad regular or irregular zone of extrachorionic placental tissue.

Microscopically, the yellow rim is composed of decidua, either capsularis and basalis fused or basalis alone. The yellow color is due to necrosis and fibrin deposition within this devitalized decidua lying between the chorion laeve and chorion frondosum.

This anomaly[341] is probably due to a small blastocyst and/or its relatively shallow implantation, although there is not general agreement on this.

Placenta membranacea. Placenta membranacea is essentially an anomaly due to deep implantation, the placenta continuing to cover the whole or most of the chorionic sac, as it continues to obtain nourishment from the surrounding endometrium.

Placenta accreta. Placenta accreta is an abnormal adherence of the placenta to the myometrium and is due to focal or diffuse lack of decidua basalis between the placental trophoblast and myometrium. Rarely, it may be due to deep implantation, but more usually it is due to defective decidua at the site of implantation. Thin endometrium may be due to trauma from previous curettage, destruction by infection, or deficient regeneration, or it may be physiologic when near the tubal ostia and in the lower uterine segment. Complete placenta accreta is uncommon, partial is more common, and focal relatively common (10% of manually removed placentas). Placental polyp is a variant of focal placenta accreta where placental site vessels have failed to involute. These polyps are composed microscopically of "ghost villi" and necrotic or degenerating trophoblast enmeshed in laminated blood clot of varying ages.

Placenta increta and placenta percreta. Placenta increta and placenta percreta are variants of placenta accreta. In placenta increta, the trophoblast penetrates deeply into the myometrium, whereas in placenta percreta, the trophoblast penetrates the entire uterine wall with subsequent rupture of the uterus.

Twin placenta.[328] Dichorionic twin placentas show varying degrees of fusion or approximation but seldom anastomosis of the fetal vascular systems. In contrast, monochorionic twin placentas appear as a single, large, irregular placenta with two cords and variable anastomosis of the fetal vascular system. The two amniotic sacs are usually present and form the partition between the two amniotic cavities. Rarely, the two fetuses are within a single amniotic cavity (monoamniotic twins). Placentas of multiple pregnancy other than twins show varying degrees and combinations of monochorionic and dichorionic twinning. Monochorionic twin placentas are always uniovular, whereas dichorionic twin placentas may be uniovular or binovular.

Degenerations of placenta

Degenerations of the placenta include a number of pathologic processes whose common denominators are the aging of the placental trophoblast and the vascular changes of the uteroplacental circulation, with their sequelae. The latter may be on a physiologic or a pathologic basis.

Fibrinoid degeneration. Fibrinoid degeneration of the cytotrophoblast accompanies and increases with the normal aging of the placenta, first appearing as homogeneous, fibrin-containing material between the individual cells during the fourth month.

Cystic degeneration. Cystic degeneration may occur in the cytotrophoblast.

Calcification. Calcification occurs in areas of fibrinoid and cystic degeneration of the cytotrophoblast and appears as a fine lacelike pattern, opaque yellow in color, and of gritty consistency, usually on the maternal surface.

Infarction. Infarction is due to interference with maternal circulation to, through, or from the placenta (but *never* to loss of fetal circulation). The appearance depends upon the location of the maternal vascular obstruction. Whether infarction of the placenta causes harm to the fetus depends on many factors, including the cause of the underlying infarction, the speed at which it occurs, and the extent to which the placenta has been infarcted.

Ischemic infarction. Ischemic infarction is associated with occlusion of spiral arteriolar sinusoids. Such infarcts are continuous with the maternal surface, are sharply circumscribed, and vary from a few millimeters to an entire cotyledon. Microscopically, the villi are in varying stages of necrosis. There is no intervillous fibrin deposition except secondarily at the periphery, which is in contact with normally flowing maternal blood. These ischemic infarcts are relatively frequent but not always associated with the hypertensive albuminuric toxemia of pregnancy, either with or without previous essential hypertension chronic glomerulonephritis, or pyelonephritis.

Placental lesions in toxemia of pregnancy

The essential placental lesion in toxemia[333] is a premature appearance of and an increase in the amount of degeneration in the syncytium during the last trimester.[365, 366] This process begins first in the regularly spaced nuclei (excluding those forming "knots"), ultimately resulting in their disappearance and leaving the cytoplasm as a thin hyalinized nonnucleated surface covering the villus. Normally at term this process involves only 10% to 40% of terminal functional villous branches, whereas in the eclamptic placenta it varies from 90% to 100%. The more severe the toxemia, the greater the placental involvement.[359, 360] Furthermore, the change tends to be greater in those cases complicated by a previous essential hypertension.

Inflammation of placenta

Acute chorionitis. The commonest cause of acute chorionitis is pyogenic bacteria from the vagina or cervix gaining access to the membranes following premature spontaneous or operative rupture of the membranes. It may occur during prolonged labor whether the membranes are ruptured or not. Grossly, the placenta and membranes are not characteristic, but, microscopically, there is marked diffuse polymorphonuclear leukocytic infiltration of amniotic and chorionic membranes, with or without visible bacteria but often with an associated angiitis and occasionally with thromboses. There may be extension of the inflammatory process to the placental tissue beneath the chorionic plate. Acute diffuse placental inflammation usually is associated with maternal septicemia or traumatic instrumentation of the uterine cavity. The infant may be infected either through its vascular system from the chorion or through its respiratory system from infected amniotic sac contents.[346]

Tuberculosis. In active maternal tuberculosis, the placenta is only occasionally involved and then via the hematogenous route.[354] The infant may contract tuberculosis in utero, and on such occasions tuberculous involvement of the placenta has usually been demonstrated. Placental tuberculosis indicates a probable fetal involvement of about 60%.[368]

Grossly, the lesions may occur as small yellow or large caseous foci, but in miliary tuberculosis[332] they are of pinhead size. Microscopically, there may be decidual involvement, with caseation but without typical tubercle formation. Most common is intervillous involvement, with tubercle formation. Intravillous tubercles are less common, while intravascular and chorioamniotic lesions are extremely rare.[367]

Syphilis. In the syphilitic pregnant patient, the grossly involved placenta has been described as large and boggy, with a pale yellow maternal surface showing large greasy friable cotyledons and, microscopically, enlarged, crowded, fibrous, avascular, and club-shaped villi. Modern investigation, however, indicates that the placenta of the pregnant syphilitic woman has no pathognomonic gross appearance. It varies with the degree of maturity of the placenta and also with the degree of involvement. McCord said: "Formerly I believed that there was a definite histological appearance of the placenta that was a constant pattern for syphilis but I no longer think that is true. I still believe, however, that in a placenta, in or about term, where there is a definite crowding of the villi, absence of the blood vessels, and an increase of stroma cells, the condition is usually syphilitic. The more premature the placenta the greater the difficulty one encounters in making a diagnosis of placental syphilis."* Absolute diagnosis of syphilis in a placenta depends upon identification of spirochetes in tissue from the cord and placenta or in scrapings from umbilical vein walls.

In untreated or inadequately treated pregnant patients with a strongly positive Wassermann reaction, the placenta is more likely to be definitely or probably involved if the infant is stillborn or dies in the hospital (21% of infants dying; 2.4% of infants surviving).[347] Moreover, of syphilitic infants dying of or with the disease, the placenta is definitely or probably diagnostic of the disease in about one-half of the cases. This lack of correlation epitomizes the difficulty in the objective diagnosis of the syphilitic placenta. It has been suggested by many German authors, recently Hörman,[342] that the spirochete passes through the placenta to involve the fetus and that placental change is secondary.

Viral infections. Viruses that affect the placenta of the fetus or both[42] are those of German measles[40, 362] (rubella), measles[330] (rubeola), chickenpox (varicella), smallpox (variola), mumps (epidemic parotitis), anterior poliomyelitis, and viral pneumonia. The fetus may contract all of these except rubella, in which case congenital anomalies of the fetal lens, ears, or heart often result from maternal infections during the second, third, and fourth months, respectively.[362] Stigmata of viral infections have not been reported in such placentas, but we have seen typical intranuclear inclusions in the syncytium of the placenta of a five-month fetus contracting smallpox in utero.

Toxoplasmosis. Toxoplasmosis is transmitted from the mother to the fetus via the placenta. Microscopically, the villi show pseudocysts containing organisms but without evidence of surrounding inflammation.[327]

Malaria. The maternal blood in the intervillous space in malarial patients contains parasites during an acute attack. The placental structure is unaltered so that fetal involvement is rare, although it may occur.[369]

---

*From McCord, J. R.: Amer. J. Obstet. Gynec. **28:** 743-750, 1934.

Chorioangioma

Chorioangioma is the commonest true tumor of the placenta if accepted as a hemangioma—as it is by most authors. There is overgrowth of fetal blood vessels, connective tissue, and trophoblast so that it has been considered by some to be a hamartoma.

This tumor varies from microscopic size to 8 cm to 10 cm in diameter. It may occur as a single tumor or as multiple tumors. The chorioangioma is well circumscribed, firm, and red. The cut surface is plum colored with fine bleeding points.

Microscopically, the tumor has a well-differentiated capillary pattern of benign endothelium embedded in fibrous tissue. The trophoblast merely surrounds the tumor, which is actually a distorted villus. This is the only placental tissue that depends for its viability upon continuity of fetal vessels. No clinical significance has been noted by the senior author in his experience.

ECTOPIC PREGNANCY

An ectopic pregnancy[373] is one that has implanted anywhere outside the limits of the endometrial cavity. The blastocyst implants when it is sufficiently developed, usually at about 6 days of age, irrespective of where it should happen to be. The fact that the tube is the commonest site of ectopic pregnancy is probably due to a physiologic or mechanical slowing down of the rate of progress of the ovum through the tube or to a delay in its entry into the tube. Development proceeds as in the endometrial cavity except that the trophoblast and chorionic villi extend into the tubal muscle rather than into a mass of decidua, often resulting in perforation of the tube. According to Beacham et al.,[370] of 1,805 ectopic pregnancies coming to operation, 74% had ruptured, 12% had been aborted into the abdomen, and 14% had not yet ruptured. The current death rate is 0.25%. About 10% of patients have had a prior ectopic pregnancy.

Often, the tube is the site of healed follicular salpingitis (Fig. 37-4) (usually of gonorrheal origin), sometimes salpingitis isthmica nodosa, and very rarely tuberculous salpingitis. There may be varying degrees of pseudo-decidual reaction in the tubal plicae, although it must be remembered that this had not been present at the time of implantation. A variable degree of acute inflammation may be present. If slight rupture or slow leakage of blood has occurred, there may be extensive peritoneal organization suggesting endometriosis.

No doubt the endometrium undergoes changes of early pregnancy, but when the pregnancy dies or is dislodged, there is a variable amount of endometrial bleeding and breakdown analogous to menstruation or spontaneous abortion. Of endometria examined at the time of diagnosis or removal of a tubal ectopic pregnancy, only 19% show the decidual reaction of pregnancy.[372] The remainder represent varying stages of the cycle and have undoubtedly regenerated following death of the pregnancy (regenerating, 5%; proliferative, 30%), or there may have been subsequent ovulation (secretory, 39%).

Rarely, a fertilized ovum may develop within the ovary.[371] It is not certain whether this is an ovum that did not escape from the follicle, a primary ovarian implantation, or a secondary implantation following tubal abortion. The pathognomonic feature is trophoblast attached to undoubted ovarian tissue.

In recent years there have been numerous reports of cervical and abdominal pregnancies, either primary or secondary.

There may be twin ectopic pregnancies either in the same tube or in opposite tubes, or there may be coincident intrauterine and extrauterine pregnancies.

REFERENCES

Anatomy and physiology

1 Adams, E. C., and Hertig, A. T.: J. Cell Biol. **41:**696-715, 1969 (corpus luteum of menstruation).

2 Adams, E. C., and Hertig, A. T.: J. Cell Biol. **41:**716-735, 1969 (corpus luteum of pregnancy).

3 Bartelmetz, G. W.: Amer. J. Anat. **98:**69-95, 1956 (endometrium).

4 Carey, H. M.: In Carey, H. M., editor: Human reproductive physiology, New York, 1963, Pergamon Press, Inc., chap. 3 (biosynthesis of sex hormones).

5 Eastman, N. J., and Hellman, L. M.: Williams' Obstetrics, ed. 14, New York, 1971, Appleton-Century-Crofts.

6 Fluhmann, C. F.: The cervix and its diseases, Philadelphia, 1961, W. B. Saunders Co.

7 Gemzell, C. A.: In Villee, C. A., editor: Control of ovulation, New York, 1961, Pergamon Press, Inc. (induction of ovulation in human by human pituitary gonadotropin).

8 Grady, H. G., and Smith, D. E., editors: The ovary, Baltimore, 1963, The Williams & Wilkins Co.

9 Greenblatt, R. B., Roy, S., Mahesh, V. B., Barfield, W. E., and Jungck, E. C.: Amer. J. Obstet. Gynec. **84:**900-912, 1962 (induction of ovulation).

10 Greep, R. O.: Histology, ed. 2, New York, 1966, The Blakiston Co.

11 Hertig, A. T.: Lab. Invest. **13:**1153-1191, 1964 (gestational hyperplasia of endometrium).

12 Hertig, A. T.: Human trophoblast, Springfield, Ill., 1968, Charles C Thomas, Publisher.

13 Hisaw, F. L.: Physiol. Rev. **27:**95-119, 1947 (graafian follicle and ovulation).

14 Kistner, R. W.: Gynecology; principles and practice, ed. 2, Chicago, 1971, Year Book Medical Publishers, Inc.

15 Koss, L. G.: Diagnostic cytology, and its histopathologic bases, ed. 2, Philadelphia, 1968, J. B. Lippincott Co.

16 McKay, D. G., Hertig, A. T., Bardawil, W. A., and Velardo, J. T.: Obstet. Gynec. **8:**22-39, 140-156, 1956 (histochemistry of endometrium).

17 Netter, F. H.: The Ciba collection of medical illustrations, vol. 2, Summit, N. J., 1954, Ciba Pharmaceutical Co. (reproductive system).

18 Novak, E. R., and Woodruff, J. D.: Gynecologic and obstetric pathology; with clinical and endocrine relations, ed. 6, Philadelphia, 1967, W. B. Saunders Co.

19 Noyes, R. W., Hertig, A. T., and Rock, J.: Fertil. Steril. **1:**3-25, 1950 (dating endometrial biopsy).

20 Papanicolaou, G. N.: Atlas of exfoliative cytology, Cambridge, Mass., 1954, Harvard University Press.

21 Parkes, A. E.: Marshall's Physiology of reproduction, vol. 2, London, 1952, Longmans, Green & Co. Ltd.

21a Ryan, K. J.: In Grady, H. G., and Smith, D. E., editors: The ovary, Baltimore, 1963, The Williams & Wilkins Co.

22 Smith, O. W., Smith, G. V., and Kistner, R. W.: J.A.M.A. **184:**878-886, 1963 (MER-25 and clomiphene).

23 Smout, C. F. V., Jacoby, F., and Lillie, E. W.: Gynaecological and obstetrical anatomy and functional histology, ed. 4, Baltimore, 1969, The Williams & Wilkins Co.

24 Thompson, J. S., and Thompson, M. W.: Genetics in medicine, Philadelphia, 1966, W. B. Saunders Co.

25 White, R. F., Hertig, A. T., Rock, J., and Adams, E. C.: Carnegie Institution of Washington Pub. No. 592, Contrib. Embryol. **34:**55-74, 1951 (corpus luteum of pregnancy).

26 Woll, E., Hertig, A. T., Smith, G. V., and Johnson, L. C.: Amer. J. Obstet. Gynec. **56:**617-633, 1948 (ovary in endometrial carcinoma).

27 Zuckerman, S., editor: The ovary, vols. 1 and 2, New York, 1962, Academic Press, Inc.

Embryology

28 Baker, T. G.: Proc. Roy. Soc. [Biol.] **158:**417-433, 1963 (quantitative and cytologic study of germ cells).

29 Gillman, J.: Carnegie Institution of Washington Pub. No. 575, Contrib. Embryol. **32:**81-131, 1948 (development of gonads and histogenesis of ovarian tumors).

30 Hertig, A. T., Rock, J., Adams, E. C., and Mulligan, W. J.: Carnegie Institution of Washington Pub. No. 603, Contrib. Embryol. **35:**199-220, 1954 (ovum).

31 Koff, A. K.: Carnegie Institution of Wash-

ington Pub. No. 443, Contrib. Embryol. **24:** 59-90, 1933 (vagina).

32 McKay, D. G., Hertig, A. T., Adams, E. C., and Danziger, S.: Anat. Rec. **117:**201-219, 1953 (germ cells of human embryos).

33 Patten, B. M.: Human embryology, ed. 3, New York, 1968, The Blakiston Co.

34 Spaulding, M. H.: Carnegie Institution of Washington Pub. No. 276, Contrib. Embryol. **13:**67-88, 1921 (external genitalia).

35 Wilson, K. M.: Carnegie Institution of Washington Pub. No. 363, Contrib. Embryol. **18:** 23-30, 1926 (external genitalia and sex glands).

36 Witschi, E.: Carnegie Institution of Washington Pub. No. 575, Contrib. Embryol. **32:**67-80, 1948 (germ cells of human embryos).

Congenital anomalies

37 Barr, M. L.: Anat. Rec. **121:**387, 1955 (chromosomal sex).

38 Evans, T. N., and Riley, G. M.: Obstet. Gynec. **2:**363-378, 1953 (pseudohermaphroditism).

39 Foss, G. L.: Brit. Med. J. **2:**1907-1909, 1960 (intersex states).

40 Gray, M. J.: Obstet. Gynec. **23:**526-527, 1964 (rubella soon after conception).

41 Grumbach, M. M.: Van Wyk, J. J., and Wilkins, L.: J. Clin. Endocr. **15:**1161-1193, 1955 (chromosomal sex).

42 Kaye, B. M., and Reaney, B. V.: Obstet. Gynec. **19:**618-622, 1962 (virus disease in pregnancy).

43 Kozoll, D. D.: Arch. Surg. (Chicago) **45:**578-595, 1942 (pseudohermaphroditism).

44 Lennon, B.: In Harrison, C. V., editor: Recent advances in pathology, ed. 7, Boston, 1960, Little, Brown and Co. (nuclear sexing).

45 de Moura, A. C., and Basto, L. P.: J. Urol. **56:**725-730, 1946 (hermaphroditism).

46 Weed, J. C., Segaloff, A. B., Weiner, W. B., and Douglas, J. W.: J. Clin. Endocr. **7:**741-748, 1947 (hermaphroditism).

47 Wilkins, L., Grumbach, M. M., Van Wyk, J. J., and Shepard, T. H.: Pediatrics **16:**287-300, 1955 (hermaphroditism).

48 Woolf, R. B., and Allen, W. M.: Obstet. Gynec. **2:**236-265, 1953.

Pelvic inflammatory disease

49 Close, J. M., and Jesurun, H. M.: Obstet. Gynec. **19:**513-516, 1962 (emphysematous vaginitis).

50 Crossen, R. J.: Diseases of women, ed. 10, St. Louis, 1953, The C. V. Mosby Co., chap. 9, pp. 595-632 (pelvic inflammation).

51 DeVoe, R. W., and Randall, L. M.: Amer. J. Obstet. Gynec. **58:**784-789, 1949 (pyometra).

52 Friedman, S., and Bobrow, M. L.: Obstet. Gynec. **14:**417-425, 1959 (pelvic inflammatory disease in pregnancy).

53 Gardner, H. L., and Fernet, P.: Amer. J. Obstet. Gynec. **88:**680-694, 1964 (vaginitis emphysematosa).

54 Henriksen, E.: Amer. J. Obstet. Gynec. **72:** 884-895, 1956 (pyometra and malignant lesions).

55 Malkani, P. K., and Rajani, C. K.: Obstet. Gynec. **14:**600-611, 1959 (pelvic tuberculosis).

56 Mohler, R. W.: Amer. J. Obstet. Gynec. **57:** 1077-1086, 1949 (classification).

57 Nassberg, S., McKay, D. G., and Hertig, A. T.: Amer. J. Obstet. Gynec. **67:**130-137, 1954 (physiologic salpingitis).

58 Snaith, L. M., and Barns, T.: Lancet **1:**712-716, 1962 (pelvic tuberculosis).

59 Sutherland, A. M.: Amer. J. Obstet. Gynec. **79:**486-497, 1960 (genital tuberculosis).

Tumors
General

60 Corscaden, J.: Gynecologic cancer, ed. 3, Baltimore, 1962, The Williams & Wilkins Co.

61 Harnett, W. L.: A survey of cancer in London, London, 1952, British Empire Cancer Campaign.

62 Hertig, A. T., and Gore, H.: In Atlas of tumor pathology, Sect. IX, Fasc. 33, Washington, D. C., 1956, 1960, 1961, and 1968, Armed Forces Institute of Pathology (tumors of female sex organs; hydatidiform mole and choriocarcinoma; vulva, vagina and uterus, and supplement; tube and ovary).

63 Kottmeier, H. L.: Carcinoma of the female genitalia, The Abraham Flexner Lectures, Series 11, Baltimore, 1953, The Williams & Wilkins Co.

64 Kottmeier, H. L., editor: Annual report on the results of treatment in carcinoma of the uterus and vagina, vol. 13, Stockholm, 1964, P. A. Norstedt, & Söner.

65 Meigs, J. V.: Tumors of the female pelvic organs, New York, 1934, The Macmillan Co.

66 Way, S.: Malignant disease of the female genital tract, Philadelphia, 1951, The Blakiston Co.

67 Willis, R. A.: Pathology of tumours, ed. 3, London, 1960, Butterworth & Co. (Publishers) Ltd.

Vulva

68 Abell, M. R.: Amer. J. Obstet. Gynec. **86:** 470-482, 1963 (adenocystic basal cell carcinoma).

69 Allen, A. C.: The skin, St. Louis, 1954, The C. V. Mosby Co., chap. 24.

70 Birch, H. W., and Sondag, D. R.: Obstet. Gynec. **18:**443-453, 1961 (granular cell myoblastoma).

71 Boutselis, J. G., Ullery, J. C., and Teteris, N. J.: Obstet. Gynec. **22:**713-724, 1963 (carcinoma).

72 Burdick, C. O., and Warner, P. O.: Obstet. Gynec. **23:**396-400, 1964 (simultaneous Bowen's and Paget's diseases).

73 Chung, J. T., and Greene, R. R.: Amer. J. Obstet. Gynec. **75:**310-318, 1958 (hidradenoma).

74 Clark, W. H., Jr.: Bull. Tulane Univ. Med. Fac. **16:**123-128, 1957 (leukoplakia and kraurosis).

75 Clark, W. H., Jr.: Personal communication, 1960.

76 Dennis, E. J., III, Hester, L. L., Jr., and Wilson, L. A.: Obstet. Gynec. **6:**291-296, 1955 (Bartholin gland carcinoma).

77 Drake, J. A., and Whitfield, A.: Brit. J. Derm. **41**:177-187, 1929 (Paget's disease).

78 Eichner, E.: Obstet. Gynec. **21**:608-613, 1963 (adenoid cystic carcinoma of Bartholin's gland).

79 Embrey, M. P.: J. Obstet. Gynaec. Brit. Comm. **68**:503-504, 1961 (carcinoma complicating condylomata acuminata).

80 Finn, J. L., and McFadden, J. P.: Amer. J. Obstet. Gynec. **67**:181-183, 1954 (carcinoma of Bartholin's gland).

81 Helwig, E. B., and Graham, J. H.: Cancer **16**: 387-403, 1963 (Paget's disease).

82 Henry, S. A.: Ann. Roy. Coll. Surg. Eng. **7**: 425-454, 1950 (relation of cancer to occupation).

83 Hyman, A. B., and Falk, H. C.: Obstet. Gynec. **12**:407-413, 1958 ("leukoplakia").

84 Janovski, N. A., and Ames, S.: Obstet. Gynec. **22**:697-708, 1963 (lichen sclerosus et atrophicus).

85 Janovski, N. A., Marshall, D., and Taki, I.: Amer. J. Obstet. Gynec. **84**:523-536, 1962 (histochemistry).

86 Jeffcoate, T. N. A., and Woodcock, A. S.: Brit. Med. J. **2**:127-134, 1961 (premalignant lesions).

87 Kehrer, E.: In Viet-Stocckel, Handbuch der Gynäkologie, vol. 5, ed. 3, Munich, 1929, J. F. Bergmann, Part I, pp. 1-696.

88 Lovelady, S. B., McDonald, J. R., and Waugh, J. M.: Amer. J. Obstet. Gynec. **42**:309-313, 1941 (benign tumors).

89 McAdams, A. J., Jr., and Kistner, R. W.: Cancer **11**:740-757, 1958 (leukoplakia and carcinoma).

90 Merrill, J. A., and Ross, N. L.: Cancer **14**: 13-20, 1961 (cancer).

91 Pick, L.: Virchow Arch. Path. Anat. **175**: 312-364, 1904 (hidradenoma).

92 Prince, L. N., and Abrams, J.: Amer. J. Obstet. Gynec. **73**:890-893, 1957 (endometriosis of perineum).

93 Taki, I., and Janovski, N. A.: Obstet. Gynec. **18**:385-402, 1961 (histochemistry of Paget's disease).

94 Taussig, F. J.: Amer. J. Obstet. Gynec. **33**: 1017-1026, 1937 (sarcoma).

95 Taussig, F. J.: Surg. Clin. N. Amer. **18**:1309-1314, 1938 (metastatic tumors).

96 Way, S.: Ann. Roy. Coll. Surg. Eng. **3**:187-209, 1948 (lymphatic drainage).

97 Wilson, J. M.: Arch. Surg. (Chicago) **43**:101-112, 1941 (basal cell carcinoma).

98 Woodruff, J. D., and Richardson, E. H., Jr.: Obstet. Gynec. **10**:10-16, 1957 (malignant Paget's disease).

Vagina

99 Bennett, H. G., Jr., and Ehrlich, M. M.: Amer. J. Obstet. Gynec. **42**:314-320, 1941 (myoma).

100 Diehl, W. K., and Haught, J. S.: Amer. J. Obstet. Gynec. **52**:302-310, 1946 (sarcoma).

101 Evans, D. M. D., and Hughes, H.: J. Obstet. Gynaec. Brit. Comm. **68**:247-253, 1961 (cysts).

102 Ferguson, J. H., and Maclure, J. G. Amer. J. Obstet. Gynec. **87**:326-336, 1963 (intra-epithelial carcinoma).

103 Johnson, H. W.: Canad. Med. Ass. J. **41**:386, 1939 (dermoid cyst).

104 Livingstone, R. G.: Primary carcinoma of the vagina, Springfield, Ill., 1950, Charles C Thomas, Publisher.

105 Martzloff, K. H., and Manlove, C. H.: Surg. Gynec. Obstet. **88**:145-154, 1949 (metastases).

106 Mullaney, J.: J. Path. Bact. **81**:473-480, 1961 (melanoma).

107 Quan, A., and Birnbaum, S.: Obstet. Gynec. **18**:360-362, 1961 (leiomyoma).

108 Reich, W. J., Nechtow, M. J., and Abrams, R.: Amer. J. Obst. Gynec. **56**:1192-1194, 1948 (endometriosis).

109 Samuels, B., Bradburn, D. M., and Johnson, C. G.: Amer. J. Obstet. Gynec. **82**:393-396, 1961 (carcinoma in situ).

110 Schonberg, L. A., Oliver, R., Burks, N., and Derieux, G. H.: Obstet. Gynec. **22**:234-236, 1963.

111 Schram, M.: Obstet. Gynec. **12**:195-198, 1958 (leiomyosarcoma).

112 Strachan, G. I.: J. Obstet. Gynaec. Brit. Emp. **46**:711-720, 1939 (vaginal implantations from uterine carcinoma).

113 Tracy, S. E.: Amer. J. Obstet. Gynec. **19**:279-285, 1930 (sarcoma).

114 Whelton, J., and Kottmeier, H. L.: Acta Obstet. Gynec. Scand. **41**:22-40, 1962 (carcinoma).

115 Whitehouse, W. L., and Porteous, C. R.: J. Obstet. Gynaec. Brit. Comm. **69**:481-485, 1962 (carcinoma).

Cervix

116 Aaro, L. A., Jacobson, L. J., and Soule, E. H.: Obstet. Gynec. **21**:659-665, 1963 (polyps).

117 Abell, M. R.: Amer. J. Clin. Path. **36**:248-255, 1961 (primary melanoblastoma).

118 Bergsjø, P.: Acta Obstet. Gynec. Scand. **42**: 85-92, 1963 (adenocarcinoma).

119 Bowing, H. H., Fricke, R. E., and McClellan, J. T.: Amer. J. Roentgen. **57**:653-658, 1947 (hemangioendothelioma).

120 Boyes, D. A., Fidler, H. K., and Lock, D. R.: Brit. Med. J. **1**:203-205, 1962 (carcinoma reduced by cancer clinics).

121 Broders, A. C.: Minn. Med. **8**:726-730, 1925 (grading of carcinoma).

122 Candy, J., and Abell, M. R.: J.A.M.A. **203**: 323-326, 1968 ("pill" cervix).

123 DeAlvarez, R. R.: Amer. J. Obstet. Gynec. **54**:91-96, 1947 (causes of death in cancer of cervix).

124 Diaz-Bazan, N.: Obstet. Gynec. **23**:281-288, 1964 (cervical carcinoma and procidentia).

125 Dunn, J. E.: Amer. J. Public Health **48**:861-873, 1958 (Memphis-Shelby County investigations).

126 Ewing, J.: Radiology **13**:313-318, 1929 (radiosensitivity).

127 Fingerland, A., and Šikl, H.: J. Path. Bact. **47**:631-634, 1938 (ganglioneuroma).

128 Foraker, A. G.: Arch. Path. (Chicago) **53**: 250-256, 1952 (light-absorption data in cancer).

129 Friedell, G. H., and McKay, D. G.: Cancer **6**:887-897, 1953 (adenocarcinoma in situ).

130 Friedell, G. H., Hertig, A. T., and Younge, P. A.: Arch. Path. (Chicago) **66**:494-503,

1958 (early stromal invasion in carcinoma in situ).

131 Gall, S. A., Bourgeois, C. H., and Maguire, R.: J.A.M.A. **207**:2243-2247, 1969 ("pill" cervix).

132 Gerbie, A. B., Hirsch, M. R., and Greene, R. R.: Obstet. Gynec. **69**:499-507, 1955 (vascular tumors).

133 Glucksmann, A.: Cancer **10**:831-837, 1957 ("mixed carcinoma").

134 Glucksmann, A., and Spear, F. G.: Brit. J. Radiol. **18**:313-322, 1945 (radiation effect on carcinoma).

135 Graham, J. B., Sotto, L. S. J., and Paloucek, F. P.: Carcinoma of the cervix, Philadelphia, 1962, W. B. Saunders Co.

136 Graham, R. M.: Surg. Gynec. Obstet. **84**: 153-165, 1947 (cellular changes in radiation response).

137 Graham, R. M.: Surg. Gynec. Obstet. **84**:166-173, 1947 (prognostic significance of radiation response).

138 Graham, R. M., and Graham, J. B.: Cancer **6**:215-223, 1953 (sensitization response).

139 Gusberg, S. A., and Corscaden, J. A.: Cancer **4**:1066-1072, 1951 (adenocarcinoma).

140 Haenszel, W., and Hillhouse, M.: J. Nat. Cancer Inst. **22**:1157-1181, 1959 (uterine cancer morbidity—racial groups).

141 Henriksen, E.: Amer. J. Obstet. Gynec. **58**: 924-942, 1949 (lymphatic spread of carcinoma).

142 Hertig, A. T., and Gore, H.: Amer. J. Roentgen. **87**:48-55, 1962 (radiosensitivity and histopathology).

143 Johnson, L. D., and Hertig, A. T.: J. Iowa Med. Soc. **48**:283-293, 1958 (carcinoma in situ, especially in pregnancy).

144 Johnson, L. D., Easterday, C. L., Gore, H., and Hertig, A. T.: Cancer **17**:213-229, 1964 (histogenesis of carcinoma in situ).

145 Kistner, R. W., and Hertig, A. T.: Obstet. Gynec. **6**:147-161, 1955 (papillomas).

146 Kistner, R. W., Gorbach, A. C., and Smith, G. V.: Obstet. Gynec. **9**:554-560, 1957 (cancer in pregnancy).

147 Koss, L. G., Stewart, F., Foote, F. W., Jordan, M. J., Bader, G. M., and Day, E.: Cancer **16**: 1160-1211, 1963 (prospective study of in situ lesions).

148 McGee, C. T., Cromer, D. W., and Greene, R. R.: Amer. J. Obstet. Gynec. **84**:358-366, 1962 (differentiation between mesonephric and endocervical adenocarcinoma).

149 McKelvey, J. L., and Goodlin, R. R.: Cancer **16**:549-557, 1963 (adenoma malignum).

150 McLennan, M. T., and McLennan, C. E.: Obstet. Gynec. **24**:161-168, 1964 (appraisal of radiation response).

151 Martzloff, K. H.: Bull. Johns Hopkins Hosp. **34**:141-149, 1923 (carcinoma).

152 Melamed, M. R., Koss, L. G., Flehinger, B. J., Kelisky, R. P., and Dubrow, H.: Brit. Med. J. **3**:195-200, 1969 (relation of "pill" to carcinoma in situ).

153 Newman, H. F., and Northup, J. D.: Amer. J. Obstet. Gynec. **84**:1816-1819, 1962 (mucosal polyps).

154 Ostergard, D. R., and Morton, D. G.: Amer.

J. Obstet. Gynec. **99**:1006-1015, 1967 (multiple malignancies).

155 Petersen, O.: Amer. J. Obstet. Gynec. **72**: 1063-1071, 1956 (spontaneous course of precancerous conditions).

156 Richart, R. M.: Amer. J. Obstet. Gynec. **87**: 474-477, 1963 (neoplasia in pregnancy).

157 Schiller, W.: Amer. J. Obstet. Gynec. **35**:17-38, 1938 (leukoplakia).

158 Schottlaender, J., and Kermauner, F.: Zur Kenntnis des Uteruskarzinoms, Berlin, 1912, S. Karger.

159 Stone, B. H., and Mansell, H.: Obstet. Gynec. **5**:198-200, 1955 (procidentia).

160 Taylor, H. B., Irey, N. S., and Norris, H. J.: J.A.M.A. **202**:637-639, 1967 ("pill" cervix).

161 Twombly, G. H., and Di Palma, S.: Amer. J. Roentgen. **65**:691-697, 1951 (spread of cancer).

162 Wallach, J. B., and Edberg, S.: Amer. J. Obstet. Gynec. **77**:990-995, 1959 (metastatic carcinoma).

163 Warren, S.: Arch. Path. (Chicago) **12**:783-786, 1931 (grading of carcinoma of cervix).

164 Younge, P. A.: Obstet. Gynec. **10**:469-481, 1957 (cancer).

Endomyometrium

165 Andrews, W. C.: Obstet. Gynec. Survey **16**: 747-767, 1961 (estrogens and endometrial carcinoma).

166 Boutselis, J. G., and Ullery, J. C.: Obstet. Gynec. **20**:23-35, 1962 (sarcoma).

167 Boutselis, J. G., Bair, J. R., Vorys, N., and Ullery, J. C.: Amer. J. Obstet. Gynec. **85**: 994-1001, 1963 (carcinoma).

168 Bromberg, Y. M., Liban, E., and Laufer, A.: Obstet. Gynec. **14**:221-226, 1959 (carcinoma after estrogen administration).

169 Campbell, P. E., and Barter, R. A.: J. Obstet. Gynaec. Brit. Comm. **68**:668-672, 1961 (atypical hyperplasia and its significance).

170 Charache, H.: Amer. J. Surg. **53**:152-157, 1941 (metastatic carcinoma).

171 Colman, H. I., and Rosenthal, A. H.: Obstet. Gynec. **14**:342-348, 1959 (carcinoma in adenomyosis).

172 Emge, L. A.: Amer. J. Obstet. Gynec. **83**: 1541-1563, 1962 (adenomyosis).

173 Faulkner, R. L.: Amer. J. Obstet. Gynec. **53**: 474-482, 1947 (degeneration of myomas).

174 Gonzalez Angulo, A., and Kaufman, R. H.: Obstet. Gynec. **19**:494-498, 1962 (lipomatous tumor).

175 Gore, H., and Hertig, A. T.: Clin. Obstet. Gynec. **5**:1148-1165, 1962 (premalignant lesions).

176 Grant, E. C. G.: J. Obstet. Gynaec. Brit. Comm. **74**:908-918, 1967 ("pill" endometrium).

177 Greene, R. R., and Gerbie, A. B.: Obstet. Gynec. **3**:150-159, 1954 (hemangiopericytoma).

178 Gusberg, S. B., and Kaplan, A. L.: Amer. J. Obstet. Gynec. **87**:662-678, 1963 (cancer precursors).

179 Gusberg, S. B., and Yannopoulos, D.: Amer. J. Obstet. Gynec. **88**:157-162, 1964 (corpus cancer).

180 Harper, R. S., and Scully, R. E.: Obstet.

Gynec. **18:**519-529, 1961 (intravenous leiomyomatosis).

181 Hunter, W. C.: Amer. J. Obstet. Gynec. **83:** 1564-1573, 1962 (stromal endometriosis).

182 Idelson, M. G., and Davids, A. M.: Obstet. Gynec. **21:**78-85, 1963 (metastasis of leiomyoma).

183 Kistner, R. W.: Clin. Obstet. Gynec. **5:**1166-1180, 1962 (hormonal therapy).

184 Kucera, F.: Zbl. Gynaek. **79:**347-350, 1957 (histogenesis of carcinoma).

185 Kulka, E. W., and Douglas, G. W.: Cancer **5:**727-736, 1952 (rhabdomyosarcoma).

186 McBride, J. M.: J. Obstet. Gynaec. Brit. Emp. **66:**288-296, 1959 (premenopausal hyperplasia and carcinoma).

187 McKelvey, J. L., and Samuels, L. T.: Amer. J. Obstet. Gynec. **53:**627-636, 1947 (irregular shedding).

188 McLennan, C. E.: Amer. J. Obstet. Gynec. **64:**988-998, 1952 (irregular shedding).

189 McQueeney, A. J., Carswell, B. L., and Sheehan, W. J.: Obstet. Gynec. **23:**338-343, 1964 (malignant mixed müllerian tumor in tube).

190 Marshall, J. F., and Morris, D. S.: Ann. Surg. **149:**126-134, 1959 (intravenous leiomyomatosis).

191 Meyer, R.: Zbl. Allg. Path. **30:**291-296, 1919-1920.

192 Meyer, R.: Z. Geburtsh. Gynaek. **85:**440-466, 1923.

193 Meyer, R.: In Henke, F., and Lubarsch, O., editors: Handbuch der speziellen pathologischen Anatomie und Histologie, vol. 7, Berlin, 1930, Julius Springer (Uterussarkome).

194 Novak, E., and Anderson, D. F.: Amer. J. Obstet. Gynec. **34:**740-761, 1937 (sarcoma).

195 Ober, W. B.: Ann. N. Y. Acad. Sci. **75:**568-585, 1959 (sarcoma).

196 Ober, W. B., and Tovell, H. M. M.: Amer. J. Obstet. Gynec. **77:**246-268, 1959 (mesenchymal sarcoma).

197 Ober, W. B., and Tovell, H. M. M.: Bull. Sloane Hosp. Women **5:**65-76, 1959 (malignant lymphoma).

198 Rothman, D., and Rennard, M.: Obstet. Gynec. **21:**102-105, 1963 (myoma-erythrocytosis syndrome).

199 Sandberg, E. C., and Cohn, F.: Amer. J. Obstet. Gynec. **84:**1457-1465, 1962 (adenomyosis in pregnancy).

200 Steiner, P. E.: Amer. J. Path. **15:**89-110, 1939 (metastasizing fibroleiomyoma).

201 Stemmermann, G. N.: Amer. J. Obstet. Gynec. **82:**1261-1266, 1961 (carcinoma metastatic to uterus).

202 Sternberg, W. H., Clark, W. H., and Smith, R. C.: Cancer **7:**704-724, 1954 (malignant mixed müllerian tumor).

203 Stout, A. P.: In Atlas of tumor pathology, Sect. II, Fasc. 5, Washington, D. C., 1953, Armed Forces Institute of Pathology (tumors of soft tissues).

204 Twombly, G. H., Scheiner, S., and Levitz, M.: Amer. J. Obstet. Gynec. **82:**424-427, 1961 (endometrial cancer, obesity, and estrogenic excretion).

205 Vellios, F., Stander, R. W., and Huber, C. P.: Amer. J. Clin. Path. **39:**496-505, 1963.

206 Weingold, A. B., and Boltuch, S. M.: Amer.

J. Obstet. Gynec. **82:**1267-1272, 1961 (extragenital metastases to uterus).

207 Weisbrot, I. M., and Janovski, N. A.: Amer. J. Clin. Path. **39:**273-283, 1963 (endometrial stromal sarcoma).

208 Williams, T. J., and Woodruff, J. D.: Obstet. Gynec. Survey **17:**1-18, 1962 (malignant mixed müllerian tumor).

Fallopian tube

209 Aaron, J. B.: Amer. J. Obstet. Gynec. **42:** 1080-1086, 1941 (dermoid cyst).

210 Abrams, J., Kazal, H. L., and Hobbs, R. E.: Amer. J. Obstet. Gynec. **75:**180-182, 1958 (sarcoma).

211 Benjamin, C. L., and Beaver, D. C.: Amer. J. Clin. Path. **21:**212-222, 1951 (salpingitis isthmica nodosa).

212 Dede, J. A., and Janovski, N. A.: Obstet. Gynec. **22:**461-467, 1963 (lipoma).

213 Finn, W. F., and Javert, C. T.: Cancer **2:**803-814, 1949 (primary and metastatic cancer).

214 Green, T. H., Jr., and Scully, R. E.: Clin. Obstet. Gynec. **5:**886-906, 1961 (tumors).

215 Grimes, H. G., and Kornmesser, J. G.: Obstet. Gynec. **16:**85-88, 1960 (benign cystic teratoma).

216 Henriksen, E.: Obstet. Gynec. **5:**833-835, 1955 (struma salpingii).

217 Hu, C. Y., Taymor, M. L., and Hertig, A. T.: Amer. J. Obstet. Gynec. **59:**58-67, 1950 (carcinoma).

218 Hurlbutt, F. R., and Nelson, H. B.: Obstet. Gynec. **21:**730-736, 1963 (carcinoma).

219 Ragins, A. B., and Crane, R. D.: Amer. J. Path. **24:**933-945, 1948 (adenomatoid tumor).

220 Roberts, C. L., and Marshall, H. K.: Amer. J. Obstet. Gynec. **82:**364-366, 1961 (fibromyoma).

221 Ryan, G. M.: Amer. J. Obstet. Gynec. **84:** 198, 1962 (carcinoma in situ).

222 Scheffey, L. C., Lang, W. R., and Nugent, F. B.: Amer. J. Obstet. Gynec. **52:**904-916, 1946 (sarcoma).

223 Schenck, S. B., and Mackles, A.: Amer. J. Obstet. Gynec. **81:**782-783, 1961 (positive Pap smear).

224 Sedlis, A.: Obstet. Gynec. Survey **16:**209-226, 1961 (carcinoma).

Ovary
General

225 Allan, M. S., and Hertig, A. T.: Amer. J. Obstet. Gynec. **58:**640-653, 1949 (carcinoma).

226 Benedict, P. H., Cohen, R. B., Cope, O., and Scully, R. E.: Fertil. Steril. **13:**380-395, 1962 (Stein-Leventhal syndrome—ovary and adrenal).

227 Girouard, D. P., Barclay, D. L., and Collins, C. G.: Obstet. Gynec. **23:**513-525, 1964.

228 Grady, H. G., and Smith, H. C., Jr., editors: The ovary, Baltimore, 1963, The Williams & Wilkins Co.

229 Jackson, R. L., and Dockerty, M. B.: Amer. J. Obstet. Gynec. **73:**161-173, 1957 (Stein-Leventhal syndrome and endometrial carcinoma).

230 Leventhal, M. L.: Amer. J. Obstet. Gynec. **76:** 825-838, 1958 (Stein-Leventhal syndrome).

231 Morris, J. M., and Scully, R. E.: Endocrine

pathology of the ovary, St. Louis, 1958, The C. V. Mosby Co.

232 Munnell, E. W., and Taylor, H. C., Jr.: Amer. J. Obstet. Gynec. **58:**943-959, 1949 (carcinoma).

233 Taymor, M. L., and Barnard, R.: Fertil. Steril. **13:**501-512, 1962 (luteinizing hormone excretion).

Gonadal stromal tumors
Granulosa–theca cell tumors

234 Banner, E. A., and Dockerty, M. B.: Surg. Gynec. Obstet. **81:**234-242, 1945 (theca cell tumors).

235 Greene, R. R., Holzwarth, D., and Roddick, J. W., Jr.: Amer. J. Obstet. Gynec. **88:**1001-1011, 1964 ("luteomas" of pregnancy).

236 Hughesdon, P. E.: J. Obstet. Gynaec. Brit. Emp. **65:**540-552, 1958 (origin).

237 McKay, D. G., Hertig, A. T., and Hickey, W. F.: Obstet. Gynec. **1:**125-136, 1953 (histogenesis).

238 Malinak, L. R., and Miller, G. V.: Amer. J. Obstet. Gynec. **91:**251-259, 1965 ("luteoma" of pregnancy).

239 Mansell, H., and Hertig, A. T.: Obstet. Gynec. **6:**385-394, 1955 (endometrial carcinoma).

240 Meigs, J. V., and Cass, J. W.: Amer. J. Obstet. Gynec. **33:**249-267, 1937 (fibroma).

241 Scully, R. E.: Cancer **17:**769-778, 1964 (luteoma).

242 Sjöstedt, S., and Wahlén, T.: Acta Obstet. Gynec. Scand. **40**(suppl. 6):1-26, 1961 (prognosis).

243 Traut, H. F., and Marchetti, A. A.: Surg. Gynec. Obstet. **70:**632-642, 1940.

Arrhenoblastoma

244 Hughesdon, P. E., and Fraser, L. T.: Acta Obstet. Gynec. Scand. **32**(suppl. 4):1-78, 1953.

245 O'Hern, T. M., and Neubecker, R. D.: Obstet. Gynec. **19:**758-770, 1962.

246 Pedowitz, P., and O'Brien, F. B.: Obstet. Gynec. **16:**62-77, 1960.

247 Savard, K., Gut, M., Dorfman, R. I., Gabrilove, J. L., and Soffer, L. J.: J. Clin. Endocr. **21:**165-174, 1961 (androgen production).

Gynandroblastoma

248 Emig, O. R., Hertig, A. T., and Rowe, F. J.: Obstet. Gynec. **13:**135-151, 1959.

249 Hartford, W. K., and Russell, H. T.: Obstet. Gynec. **22:**648-653, 1963 (vaginal cytology).

250 Neubecker, R. D., and Breen, S. L.: Amer. J. Clin. Path. **38:**60-69, 1962.

Gonadal stromal response to other ovarian tumors

251 Hughesdon, P. E.: J. Obstet. Gynaec. Brit. Emp. **65:**702-709, 1958.

252 Scully, R. E., and Richardson, G. S.: Cancer **14:**827-840, 1961.

253 Woodruff, J. D., Williams, T. J., and Goldberg, B.: Amer. J. Obstet. Gynec. **87:**679-698, 1963.

Germ cell tumors
Dysgerminoma ovarii

254 Hughesdon, P. E.: J. Obstet. Gynaec. Brit. Emp. **66:**566-576, 1959 (origin).

255 Mueller, C. W., Topkins, P., and Lapp, W. A.: Amer. J. Obstet. Gynec. **60:**153-159, 1950.

256 Pedowitz, P., Felmus, L. B., and Grayzel, D. M.: Amer. J. Obstet. Gynec. **70:**1284-1297, 1955.

257 Weintraub, L. R., Rosenblatt, P., and Brandman, L.: Amer. J. Obstet. Gynec. **61:**1167-1170, 1951 (tuberculoid reaction).

Primary choriocarcinoma

258 Dixon, F. J., and Moore, R. A.: In Atlas of tumor pathology, Sect. VIII, Fascs. 31 and 32, Washington, D. C., 1952, Armed Forces Institute of Pathology.

259 Neigus, I.: Amer. J. Obstet. Gynec. **69:**838-847, 1955.

260 Oliver, H. M., and Horne, E. O.: New Eng. J. Med. **239:**14-16, 1948.

Endodermal sinus tumor (Teilum)

261 Huntington, R. W., Jr., Morgenstern, N. L., Sargent, J. A., Giem, R. N., Richards, A., and Hanford, K. C.: Cancer **16:**34-47, 1963 (in young children).

262 Neubecker, R. D., and Breen, J. L.: Cancer **15:**546-556, 1962.

263 Santesson, L., and Marrubini, G.: Acta Obstet. Gynec. Scand. **36:**399-419, 1957.

264 Teilum, G.: Cancer **12:**1092-1105, 1959 (in ovary and testis).

Benign cystic teratoma

265 Afonso, J. F., Martin, G. M., Nisco, F. S., and de Alvarez, R. R.: Amer. J. Obstet. Gynec. **84:**667-676, 1962 (melanogenic ovarian tumors).

266 Kelley, R. R., and Scully, R. E.: Cancer **14:**989-1000, 1961 (cancer in dermoid cysts).

267 Marcial-Rojas, R. A., and Medina, R.: Arch. Path. (Chicago) **66:**577-589, 1958.

268 Matz, M. H.: Obstet. Gynec. Survey **16:**591-605, 1961.

269 Peterson, W. F., Prevost, E. C., Edmunds, F. T., Hundley, J. M., Jr., and Morris, F. K.: Amer. J. Obstet. Gynec. **70:**368-382, 1955 (benign cystic teratoma).

270 Peterson, W. F., Prevost, E. C., Edmunds, F. T., Hundley, J. M., Jr., and Morris, F. K.: Amer. J. Obstet. Gynec. **71:**173-189, 1956 (epidermoid carcinoma in benign cystic teratoma).

271 Shettles, L. B.: Nature (London) **178:**1131, 1956 (intrafollicular cleavage of ovum).

272 Theiss, E. A., Ashley, D. J. B., and Mostofi, F. K.: Cancer **13:**323-327, 1960 (nuclear sex).

Struma ovarii

273 Marcus, C. C., and Marcus, S. L.: Amer. J. Obstet. Gynec. **81:**752-762, 1961.

274 Smith, F. G.: Arch. Surg. (Chicago) **53:**603-626, 1946.

Solid well-differentiated teratoma

275 Benirschke, K., Easterday, C., and Abramson, D.: Obstet. Gynec. **15:**512-521, 1960.

276 Peterson, W. F.: Amer. J. Obstet. Gynec. **72:**1094-1102, 1956.

277 Thurlbeck, W. M., and Scully, R. E.: Cancer **13:**804-811, 1960.

Malignant teratoma

278 Breen, J. L., and Neubecker, R. D.: Obstet.
Gynec. **21**:669-681, 1963.
279 Curtis, A. H.: Surg. Gynec. Obstet. **81**:504-
506, 1948.
280 Murray, R. C., and Hofmeister, F. J.: Obstet.
Gynec. **18**:474-479, 1961.
281 Neubecker, R. D., and Breen, J. L.: Cancer
15:546-556, 1962 (embryonal carcinoma).
282 Novak, E. R.: Amer. J. Obstet. Gynec. **56**:
300-310, 1948.

Gonadoblastoma

283 Teter, J.: Amer. J. Obstet. Gynec. **84**:722-
730, 1962.
284 Teter, J.: Acta Path. Microbiol. Scand. **58**:
306-320, 1963.
285 Teter, J., Philip, J., Wecewicz, G., and Po-
tocki, J.: Acta Endocr. (Kobenhavn) **46**:1-11,
1964.

**Cystomas (tumors of "germinal" epithelial
origin)**

286 Campbell, J. S., Magner, D., and Fournier,
P.: Cancer **14**:817-826, 1961 (adenoacanthoma
of ovary and uterus).
287 Cariker, M., and Dockerty, M. B.: Cancer
7:302-310, 1954 (cystadenocarcinoma).
288 Corner, G. W., Jr., Hu, C. Y., and Hertig,
A. T.: Amer. J. Obstet. Gynec. **59**:760-774,
1950 (carcinoma arising in endometriosis).
289 Hertig, A. T., and Gore, H. M.: Rocky Mountain Med. J. **55**:47-50, 1958 (classification).
290 Santesson, L.: In The morphologic precursors
of cancer, Proceedings of International Conference, University of Perugia, Italy, 1961, p.
699 (histopathologic evaluation of malignancy).
291 Scott, R. B.: Amer. J. Obstet. Gynec. **43**:733-
751, 1942 (cystadenofibroma).
292 Thompson, J. D.: Obstet. Gynec. **9**:403-416,
1957 (adenoacanthoma).
293 Woodruff, J. D., Bie, L. S., and Sherman,
R. J.: Obstet. Gynec. **16**:699-712, 1960
(mucinous tumors).

Congenital rest tumors
Adrenal rest tumor

294 Pedowitz, P., and Pomerance, W.: Obstet.
Gynec. **19**:183-194, 1962.
295 Taylor, H. B., and Norris, H. J.: Cancer **20**:
1953-1962, 1967 (lipid cell tumor).

Mesometanephric rest tumor

296 Janovski, N. A., and Weir, J. H.: Obstet.
Gynec. **19**:57-63, 1962 (histologic and histochemical).
297 Lee, R. A., Dockerty, M. B., Wilson, R. B.,
and Symmonds, R. E.: Amer. J. Obstet.
Gynec. **84**:677-681, 1962.
298 Novak, E., Woodruff, J. D., and Novak, E. R.:
Amer. J. Obstet. Gynec. **68**:1222-1242, 1954.
299 Novak, E. R., and Woodruff, J. D.: Amer. J.
Obstet. Gynec. **77**:632-644, 1959.

Brenner tumor

300 Idelson, M. G.: Obstet. Gynec. Survey **18**:246-
267, 1963 (malignancy, histogenesis, and
estrogen production).

301 Tighe, J. R.: J. Obstet. Gynaec. Brit. Comm.
68:292-296, 1961.

Hilar cell tumor

302 Boivin, Y., and Richart, R. M.: Cancer **18**:
231-240, 1965 (hilus cell tumor).
303 Goodwin, J. W., Ehrmann, R. L., and Leavitt,
T., Jr.: Obstet. Gynec. **19**:467-470, 1962.
304 Merrill, J. A.: Amer. J. Obstet. Gynec. **78**:
1258-1271, 1959 (hilus cells).
305 Novak, E. R., and Mattingly, R. F.: Obstet.
Gynec. **15**:425-432, 1960.
306 Sternberg, W. H.: Amer. J. Path. **25**:493-521,
1949.

Nonintrinsic connective tissue tumors
Fibroma

307 Dockerty, M. B., and Masson, J. C.: Amer.
J. Obstet. Gynec. **47**:741-752, 1944.

Lymphoma

308 Collins, J., and Piper, P. G.: Obstet. Gynec.
20:686-689, 1962.
309 Woodruff, J. D., Noli Castillo, R. D., and
Novak, E. R.: Amer. J. Obstet. Gynec. **85**:
912-918, 1963.

Metastatic tumors to ovary

310 Jarcho, J.: Amer. J. Surg. **41**:538-564, 1938
(Krukenberg tumor).
311 Krukenberg, F.: Arch. Gynaek. **50**:287-321,
1896 (fibrosarcoma ovarii mucocellulare).
312 Leffel, J. M., Masson, J. C., and Dockerty,
M. B.: Ann. Surg. **115**:102-113, 1942.
313 Woodruff, J. D., and Novak, E. R.: Obstet.
Gynec. **15**:351-360, 1960 (Krukenberg).

Ovarian cancer complicating pregnancy

314 Falk, H. C., and Bunkin, I. A.: Amer. J.
Obstet. Gynec. **54**:82-87, 1947.
315 Gustafson, G. W., Gardiner, S. H., and Stout,
F. E.: Amer. J. Obstet. Gynec. **67**:1210-1223,
1954.
316 Hamilton, H. G., and Higgins, R. S.: Int.
Abst. Surg. **89**:525-531, 1949.

Endometriosis

317 Gardner, G. H., Greene, R. R., and Ranney,
B.: Obstet. Gynec. **1**:615-637, 1953 (histogenesis).
318 Kistner, R. W.: Clin. Pharmacol. Ther. **1**:525-
537, 1960 (treatment).
319 Markee, J. E.: Carnegie Institution of Washington Pub. No. 518, Contrib. Embryol. **28**:
221-308, 1940 (menstruation in endometrial
implants).
320 Sampson, J. A.: Arch. Surg. (Chicago) **10**:1-
72, 1925 (endometrial carcinoma of ovary).
321 Scott, R. B., and Te Linde, R. W.: Obstet.
Gynec. **4**:502-510, 1954 (clinical endometriosis).
322 Tedeschi, L. G., and Botta, G. C.: Amer. J.
Obstet. Gynec. **84**:631-637, 1962 (appendiceal
decidual reaction).
323 Te Linde, R. W., and Scott, R. B.: Amer. J.
Obstet. Gynec. **60**:1147-1173, 1950 (experimental).
324 Weller, C. V.: Amer. J. Path. **11**:281-286,
1935 (of umbilicus).

325 Weller, C. V.: Amer. J. Path. **11**:287-290, 1935 (ectopic decidual reaction).

Placenta, amnion, and umbilical cord

326 Bagshawe, K. D.: Choriocarcinoma; the clinical biology of the trophoblast and its tumours, Baltimore, 1969, The Williams & Wilkins Co.
327 Beckett, R. S., and Flynn, F. J.: New Eng. J. Med. **249**:345-350, 1953 (toxoplasmosis).
328 Benirschke, K.: Obstet. Gynec. **18**:309-333, 334-337, 1961 (placenta and twin placenta).
329 Delfs, E.: Obstet. Gynec. **9**:1-24, 1957 (quantitative chorionic gonadotropin).
330 Dyer, I.: Southern Med. J. **33**:601-604, 1940 (measles complicating pregnancy).
331 Gore, H., and Hertig, A. T.: Clin. Obstet. Gynec. **10**:269-289, 1967 (problems in diagnosis of trophoblast).
332 Helmer, M.: Brit. Med. J. **2**:1341, 1952 (miliary tuberculosis).
333 Hertig, A. T.: Clinics **4**:602-614, 1945 (toxemias of pregnancy).
334 Hertig, A. T., and Edmonds, H. W.: Arch. Path. (Chicago) **30**:260-291, 1940 (hydatidiform mole).
335 Hertig, A. T., and Gore, H:. In Davis, C. H., and Carter, B., editors: Gynecology and obstetrics, Hagerstown, Md., 1959 and 1965, W. F. Prior Co., (diseases of ovum).
336 Hertig, A. T., and Gore, H.: In Nealon, T. F., Jr., editor: Management of the patient with cancer, Philadelphia, 1965, W. B. Saunders Co., (trophoblastic lesions).
337 Hertig, A. T., and Sheldon, W. H.: Amer. J. Obstet. Gynec. **53**:1-36, 1947 (grouping of hydatidiform mole).
338 Hertig, A. T., Rock, J., and Adams, E. C.: Amer. J. Anat. **98**:435-493, 1956 (human ova).
339 Hertz, R., Lewis, J., Jr., and Lipsett, M. B.: Amer. J. Obstet. Gynec. **82**:631-640, 1961 (chemotherapy of choriocarcinoma; follow-up data on patients—personal communication from J. Lewis).
340 Hertz, R., Ross, G. T., and Lipsett, M. B.: Amer. J. Obstet. Gynec. **86**:808-814, 1963 (chemotherapy of nonmetastatic trophoblastic disease).
341 Hobbs, J. E., and Price, C. N.: Amer. J. Obstet. Gynec. **39**:39-44, 1940 (placenta circumvallata).
342 Hörmann, G.: Arch. Gynaek. **184**:481-521, 1954 (placenta and syphilis).
343 Jacobson, F. J., and Enzer, N.: Amer. J. Obstet. Gynec. **78**:868-875, 1959 ("benign" molar metastasis to lung).
344 Kerr, M., and Rashad, M. N.: Amer. J. Obstet. Gynec. **94**:322-339, 1966 (chromosomes in abortions).
345 Kika, K., and Matuda, I.: Obstet. Gynec. **9**: 224-227, 1957 (primary tubal hydatidiform mole).
346 Kobak, A. J.: Amer. J. Obstet. Gynec. **19**:299-316, 1930 (fetal bacteremia).
347 McCord, J. R.: Amer. J. Obstet. Gynec. **28**: 743-750, 1934 (syphilis).
348 McKay, D. G., Hertig, A. T., Adams, E. C., and Richardson, M. V.: Obstet. Gynec. **12**:1-36, 1958 (histochemistry).

349 McKay, D. G., Robey, C. C., Hertig, A. T., and Richardson, M. V.: Obstet. Gynec. **69**: 722-734, 1955 (fluid of hydatidiform moles).
350 McKay, D. G., Robey, C. C., Hertig, A. T., and Richardson, M. V.: Obstet. Gynec. **69**: 735-741, 1955 (chorionic and amniotic fluid).
351 MacMahon, B., Hertig, A. T., and Ingalls, T.: Obstet. Gynec. **4**:477-483, 1954 (abortion).
352 Montgomery, T. L.: Amer. J. Obstet. Gynec. **31**:253-267, 1936 (fibrosis).
353 Ross, G. T., Goldstein, D. P., Hertz, R., Lipsett, M. B., and Odell, W. D.: Amer. J. Obstet. Gynec. **93**:223-229, 1965 (treatment of metastatic trophoblastic disease).
354 Schaefer, G.: Amer. J. Obstet. Gynec. **38**: 1066-1067, 1939 (tuberculosis).
355 Scott, J. S.: J. Obstet. Gynaec. Brit. Emp. **67**:904-918, 1960 (placenta extrachorialis).
356 Sexton, L. I., Hertig, A. T., Reid, D. E., Kellogg, F. S., and Patterson, W. S.: Amer. J. Obstet. Gynec. **59**:13-24, 1950 (premature separation).
357 Shettles, L. B.: Obstet. Gynec. **21**:339-342, 1963 (theca lutein cysts in pregnancy).
358 Singh, R. P., and Carr, D. H.: Obstet. Gynec. **29**:806-818, 1967 (chromosomes and anatomic findings in abortions).
359 Smith, O. W., and Smith, G. V. S.: Amer. J. Obstet. Gynec. **33**:365-379, 1937 (pregnancy toxemia).
360 Sommers, S. C., Lawley, T. B., and Hertig, A. T.: Amer. J. Obstet. Gynec. **58**:1010-1013, 1949 (placenta in pregnancy treated by stilbestrol).
361 Stein, I. F.: Amer. J. Obstet. Gynec. **38**:1068-1070, 1939 (tubal pregnancy with tuberculous salpingitis).
362 Swan, C., Tostevin, A. L., and Black, G. H. B.: Med. J. Aust. **2**:889-908, 1946 (rubella).
363 Szulman, A. E.: New Eng. J. Med. **272**:811-818, 1965 (chromosomal aberrations in abortion).
364 Tao, T. W.: Thesis, Harvard University, Cambridge, Mass., 1962 (organ culture of trophoblast).
365 Tenney, B., Jr.: Amer. J. Obstet. Gynec. **31**: 1024-1028, 1936 (syncytial degeneration).
366 Tenney, B. Jr., and Parker, F., Jr.: Amer. J. Obstet. Gynec. **39**:1000-1005, 1940 (toxemia of pregnancy).
367 Warthin, A. S.: J. Infect. Dis. **4**:347-368, 1907 (tuberculosis).
368 Whitman, R. C., and Greene, L. W.: Arch. Intern. Med. (Chicago) **29**:261-273, 1922 (tuberculosis).
369 Wickramasuriya, G. A. W.: J. Obstet. Gynaec. Brit. Emp. **42**:816-834, 1935 (malaria).

Ectopic pregnancy

370 Beacham, W. D., Webster, H. D., and Beacham, D. W.: Amer. J. Obstet. Gynec. **72**: 830-834, 1956.
371 Bercovici, B., Pfau, A., and Liban, E.: Obstet. Gynec. **12**:596-600, 1958 (primary ovarian pregnancy).
372 Romney, S. L., Hertig, A. T., and Reid, D. E.: Surg. Gynec. Obstet. **91**:605-611, 1950.
373 Schiffer, M. A.: Amer. J. Obstet. Gynec. **86**: 264-270, 1963.

Chapter 38

Breast

Joseph F. Kuzma

DEVELOPMENT AND STRUCTURE

General anatomy. The adult female breast is a modified compound alveolar secretory gland derived from the skin. It is composed of approximately twenty irregular lobes radiating from the central nipple area. Each lobe has an excretory duct with a local dilatation of the duct beneath the nipple known as the sinus lactiferous. The ducts do not anastomose, although two or more may have a common opening at the nipple. Multiple duct branchings (lobes) ending in clusters of epithelial cells (lobules) constitute the parenchyma. Large ducts at the nipple are lined by stratified squamous epithelium that gradually merges with the columnar cells of the smaller ducts. The peripheral portions have low columnar cells, frequently of two layers, that blend into the cuboid cells of the lobules. Just within the basement membrane, fibrillar elongated cells derived from epithelium (myoepithelial cells) may be seen.[6]

The stroma immediately supporting the lobules of the breast is known as the intralobular connective tissue, which is continuous with the periductal tissue. The periductal and intralobular tissue varies with the functional state and may be considered as a part of the "parenchyma." It is loose reticular or myxomatous in appearance and is sharply defined from the more dense interlobar substance. Except during pregnancy and lactation, the bulk of the breast is made up of connective tissue and fat.

Embryology. As in all mammals, the human breast develops in a primitive epidermal thickening known as the milk line, which extends bilaterally on the ventral surface between the upper and lower limb attachments. In the human embryo, the milk line appears at about the sixth week. This primitive line then gradually atrophies, but at the ninth week the site of the permanent mammae can be recog-

nized by the persistence of the epithelial thickening (primitive nipple buds). By the sixth month of development, some fifteen to twenty solid epithelial cords extend into the corium from the basal layer of the primitive nipple. By the ninth month, these branching cords have developed a lumen and may have two or three layers of cells.

Neonatal mammary gland. At birth, the breast consists of moderately branched, extremely dilated ducts containing pinkish secretion material. The breasts of both sexes show similar change. The influence of the maternal hormones promotes epithelial proliferation so that the terminal portions of the ducts have columnar epithelium with secretory buds. Whatever secretion is developed is derived from the duct epithelium, since the phase of lobular development has not yet been accomplished. The periductal tissue is quite vascular at this time. Approximately two weeks after birth, the columnar cells recede in height, become vacuolated, and are cast off. The adjacent connective tissue then fills the areas occupied by the dilated ducts. In 60% of infants, clinical examination reveals enlargement, induration, and congestion. These findings may be confused with true inflammation, which is much less common.

Mammary gland of adolescence. Before the onset of menstruation, there is a gradual development, with physical enlargement of the breast. This generally takes place over a period of three to five years. Enlargement in the mass of the breast is brought about by proliferation of all its components. Proliferation of periductal stroma keeps pace with growth of the ducts. The intervening connective tissue increases in proportion. The ducts themselves elongate and divide. Their terminal branches, where growth is greatest, dilate and form bunches of cystlike structures.

Microscopically, at this time the dilated

ducts show proliferation of the epithelium in the form of pseudostratification and clump formation. Such clumps are particularly prominent about the ends of the smaller branched ducts and indicate the sites of future acinar development. As the growth proceeds, the solid clumps of cells (of ductules) undergo central autolysis and thereby become epithelium-lined channels. However, not all portions of the breast develop simultaneously or to the same degree. Elaboration of estrogenic hormone by the ovary is responsible for this phase of development.[3]

Mammary gland of sexual maturity. Influence of the sexual cycle upon the breast was described by Rosenburg[11] in 1922 and later substantiated by Ingleby.[25] The cellular activity of the breast is somewhat parallel to that of the endometrium. During the phase of menstruation, breast epithelium shows shrinkage of the duct branches, with desquamation and atrophy of the epithelial cells. The cells that remain are relatively small, low columnar, and have deeply staining nuclei. They are very closely associated with the more deeply situated undifferentiated basal cells. In the relatively dense periductal connective tissue, small round cells may be prominent. Several days after cessation of menstruation, the proliferative phase becomes evident. This is characterized by expansion of the duct system, increase in the size and number of the epithelial cells, and development of a soft, edematous, pale-staining, relatively acellular periductal connective tissue. Shortly thereafter, the multiple branchings of the ducts continue, under the influence of luteal hormone, to the point of definable lobule formations of crowded epithelial cells. However, this is not uniform.

The premenstrual hyperplasia of columnar cells is accompanied by an abortive "secretory" activity. Patients attest to moderate volume changes and sensations of fullness, heaviness, or tenderness in the premenstrual period. The relationship between the periductal tissue and the epithelium is, therefore, converse. During the epithelial proliferation phase, the surrounding periductal tissue softens, develops a mucoid character, and becomes considerably decreased in bulk. When secretion takes place into the ducts, the distention may further obscure the periductal connective tissue. With the advent of epithelial involution, the connective tissue proliferates and replaces the area occupied by the large duct or lobule. At this time, it is moderately cellular. Cyclic changes are not seen in amenorrhea associated with castration or chronic illness such as tuberculosis or diabetes.

Mammary gland in pregnancy and lactation. In pregnancy, the earliest external change detected in the mammary gland is the moderate increase in firmness of the breast, associated with enlargement of the superficial veins, and the gradually developing pigmentation of the areola and nipple. The first three months of pregnancy are characterized by cellular proliferation. This is particularly marked at the blind ends of the branched ducts and in the sites of lobular development. As the epithelial tissue becomes more and more prominent, the periductal tissue softens and has a less intense staining character. Eventually, the lobular proliferation is characterized by forms of acini with their acinar ducts accompanied by a delicate vascular connective tissue bed. It has been pointed out that the centralmost parts of breast beneath the nipple develop blind duct pouches that may act as reservoirs.[9]

At term, superficial epithelial cells of the breast have differentiated into fat-containing (colostrum) cells. Such cells are shed in variable amounts and constitute what is known as the initial secretion of the breast (colostrum). Shortly after delivery, the basal cells lining the dilated acini become the secretory epithelium, with pale cytoplasm and various globules (Fig. 38-1). This lactation cytologic change is accompanied by immense increase in the secretory lobules. Acinar differentiation and secretory function are promoted by luteal hormones, pregnancy placental hormones, and the lactogenic stimulus of the pituitary gland. Quite remarkable mammotropic and lactational effects have been observed in young patients of both sexes treated with high doses of certain tranquilizing drugs.[8, 10]

In the phase of involution following lactation, the collapse of the dilated secretory lobules and ducts may be followed by failure of adequate connective tissue growth, producing thereby a breast of a flattened contour and flabby consistency. The irregularity of involution, the persistence of dilated ducts, and the periductal and perilobular lymphocytic infiltration may constitute chronic cystic mastitis. However, it is generally accepted that mastodynia disappears and cystic disease of the breast improves after lactation. This may be due to luteal hormone influence.

Tumor formations are adversely influenced by pregnancy and lactation. Fibroadenomas grow rapidly and may increase remarkably.

Carcinoma of the breast in pregnancy is a high-grade malignancy with a very poor prognosis.[5] *Mammary infarcts* during pregnancy may be indistinguishable, by clinical criteria, from malignancy,[7] whereas histologically it may not be clear whether such ischemic accidents occur in focal gravid hypertrophy or other lesions such as fibroadenoma.

Senile breast. After menopause, the striking change in the breast is the atrophy of the acini and lobules, with gradual epithelial involution progressing toward the nipple from the periphery. The involution is frequently irregular and quite commonly accompanied by dilated ducts lined by small, deeply stained epithelial cells. Eventually, the stroma also decreases in bulk, by nature of sclerosis and loss of cellularity. Dilatation of atrophic ducts along with retention of acellular debris, *duct ectasia,* is a common finding in this age group. Significant inflammatory changes about the

ducts induced by the retained "secretions" is called *periductal mastitis.*

CONGENITAL ANOMALIES

The commonest anomaly of breast development is the growth of supernumerary breast parts. Frequently, this is merely the presence of accessory nipples (polythelia) along the milk line.[13] In the white population, the greater number of these are said to appear below the normal breast and are somewhat more common in the male than in the female.

More important from the clinical standpoint is the presence of accessory breast tissue (polymastia) in the axilla. Frequently, this is not associated with the presence of a nipple and areola and may not be recognized until painful swelling and tenderness develop with the advent of pregnancy. Likewise, the possibility of development of cancer in an axillary ectopic breast is ever present.

Amastia results from the disappearance of the entire mammary line, including the usually defined bud of epithelial proliferation in the thoracic area.

HYPERTROPHY

Hypertrophy of one or both breasts may take place at any time and is brought about by abnormal hormonal relationships. Before puberty, hypertrophy is usually bilateral and is frequently the physical evidence of estrogen-

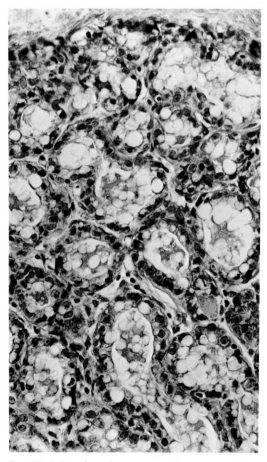

Fig. 38-1 Developed acini actively secreting (lactation) in lobule of breast at term pregnancy. (×320.)

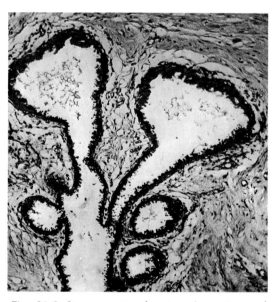

Fig. 38-2 Gynecomastia showing elongation and abortive budding of ducts, which are surrounded by loose periductal stroma in which lymphocytes are evident.

producing tumors. These include granulosa cell tumors of the ovary, chorioepithelioma of the ovary, adrenal gland (cortical cell) tumors, and pituitary tumors. Such changes are reversible, as evidenced by regression of the breast size following extirpation of the hormone-producing tumors.

At the time of adolescence or shortly thereafter, irreversible hypertrophy of one or both breasts may take place (virginal hypertrophy). The breast may become extremely pendulous, the veins enlarged, and the nipple drawn into the pendulous mass. Prominent histologic change is the increase of the fibrous tissue and the attempted lobular formation. According to Geschickter,[3] such an increase in the size of the breast rests in its inherent abnormal sensitivity to estrogenic hormones. Sensitivity may not be bilaterally the same.

In both the precocious hypertrophy and the true virginal hypertrophy, the estrogenic activity is evidenced by duct epithelial hyperplasia and hypertrophy accompanied by irregular, meager secretory activity. The development of acini depends upon luteal hormones and pituitary influence rather than on estrogens. The finding of follicular cysts of the ovary or a fibroadenoma in such a breast has been noted.

Gynecomastia (hypertrophy of male breast)[14]

The development and growth of the male breast parallels that of the female up to the time of adolescence. Abnormal enlargement of the breast may take place at any period of life, most frequently in boyhood and in senility. Usually, only one breast is involved, with no appreciable difference of incidence in respect to the left or right. In the majority, the enlargement is evident as a buttonlike swelling beneath the areola. In unusual circumstances, the breast enlarges and assumes proportions similar to that of the virginal female breast. The condition is best expressed in the words of Karsner:

"Gynecomastia is an enlargement of the mammary gland or glands of males due to proliferation of connective tissue, dense in the general stroma and often loosely arranged in periductal regions, together with variable degrees of multiplication, elongation, or branching of ducts, or of all three, without formation of true acini, accompanied by periductal or more widespread infiltration of lymphocytes, plasma cells, large mononuclear cells, and occasionally eosinophils, or neutrophilic polymorphonuclear cells, or both; secretion is frequently present in ducts, may be discharged spontaneously or manually expressed, but rarely if ever is it true colostrum or milk. This definition excludes pseudogynecomastia, due to the deposition of fat in the

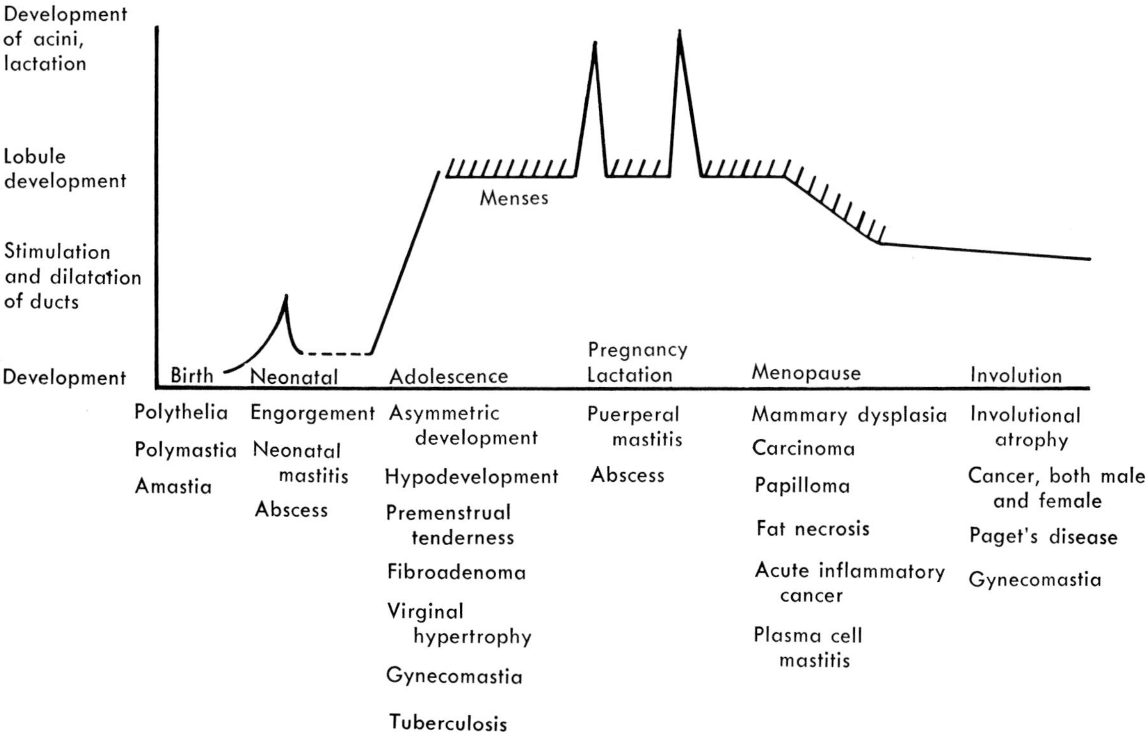

Fig. 38-3 Diseases of breast according to life stage.

mammary regions, as well as suppurative or other essentially inflammatory processes, granulomatous lesions, and neoplasms, either benign or malignant"* (Fig. 38-2).

Gynecomastia is many times more common than carcinoma of the male breast. There is no relationship between carcinoma and gynecomastia. Enlargement of shape and form of the male breast approaching the proportions of the conventional female breast can be produced by the administration of synthetic estrogens, whereas lactational secretion and enlargement occasionally are induced by high doses of tranquilizers.[8, 10] Hormonal imbalance, with actual or relative increase of estrogenic hormones or end-organ sensitivity, is the practical consideration for the etiology of gynecomastia.[16] True gynecomastia does not appear in eunuchs, although it is found in association with certain hypogonadal syndromes (i.e., Klinefelter and Reifenstein) and with testicular atrophy following mumps orchitis, trauma, or simple involution (androgenic decline) of later years.

In starvation and in cirrhosis of the liver, the failure of proper "deestrogenation" also may be associated with hypertrophy of the male breast. A number of hormone-producing tumors have been recorded in a causative association with gynecomastia—viz., choriocarcinomas of the testis or other sites, Leydig or Sertoli cell tumors, pituitary adenomas, and adrenocortical cell tumors. Although there is doubt that injury is a causative factor, it cannot be denied that it may provoke a more rapid increase in growth.

INFLAMMATIONS
Acute mastitis

Acute bacterial mastitis most often occurs in primiparas during the first few weeks of nursing. The causative agent (generally *Staphylococcus aureus* and less commonly streptococcus) invades the breast through fissures of the nipples and the exposed lymphatics or by way of the milk ducts. Breast engorgement following irregularity of nursing incident to cracked nipples enhances the possibility of bacterial invasion.

The painful, swollen, indurated, reddened, and hot breast may be exquisitely tender. Changes are either diffuse or focal. With the advent of suppuration, localization and softening become apparent. Abscesses have classic

---

*From Karsner, H. T.: Amer. J. Path. **22:**235-315, 1946.

locations (viz., subareolar, parenchymal, or stromal and retromammary).

Early cases of puerperal mastitis can easily be confused with acute inflammatory carcinoma, or vice versa. In the later stages, repair and fixation to the skin may likewise be erroneously interpreted. The axillary nodes frequently are enlarged and generally are tender. Gross findings of suppuration or abscess formation and microscopic changes of acute inflammation are in no way peculiar in this organ. Rarely, however, a late-appearing subacute or a relapsing puerperal mastitis may closely resemble plasma cell mastitis or tuberculosis.

Plasma cell mastitis

The uncommon entity known as plasma cell mastitis (pseudotuberculosis) occurs after pregnancy (multiple) in women about 40 years of age. A history of difficult nursing (inverted nipples, cracked nipples, death of infant) is elicited in 50% of the cases.[18] Stasis and inspissation of secretions initiate this inflammatory disease. It is chemical in nature rather than bacterial and actually constitutes a type of foreign body reaction as evidenced by eosinophils, foam cells, giant cells, colostrum cells, and fatty acid crystals.

The lesion is one of induration beneath a quadrant of the areola associated with a lump formation and distortion of the nipple. It may be accompanied by pain and tenderness of variable degree or by a cloudy discharge from the nipple. At times, it is multicentric in origin. The ducts may be palpably thickened and the axillary nodes enlarged. The diseased area presents a level cut surface of grayish mottled character punctuated by distorted ducts, expressed secretions, and minute areas of necrosis.

Microscopic appearance at times is very similar to tuberculosis. Epithelioid cells and giant cells may be clustered in a tubercle-like arrangement. However, polymorphonuclear cells are quite common, and foam cells are prominent. The most characteristic findings are the absence of caseation, the absence of tubercle bacilli, and the predominance of plasma cells (Fig. 38-4). The grouping of giant cells and foam cells about lipid crystals is a prominent feature and may resemble fat necrosis.

Variable amounts of connective tissue in the phase of regeneration and repair increase the hardness of the area and cause retraction of the nipple. Clinically and grossly, therefore,

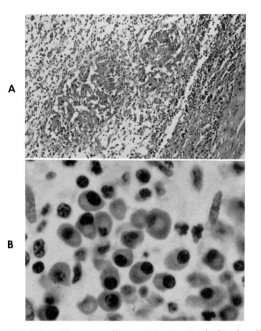

Fig. 38-4 Plasma cell mastitis. **A,** Epithelioid cell tubercles at periphery of lesion. **B,** Cellular complement. (**A,** ×100; **B,** ×750.)

there may be striking resemblance to mammary carcinoma. However, the poorly defined diffuse induration, without chalk streaks or cicatrization but with minute cysts of fatty material, makes possible the differential diagnosis of plasma cell mastitis from carcinoma in most cases.

Chronic mastitis

Chronic mastitis, with the exception of the chronic puerperal mastitis, is a granulomatous inflammation. In most instances, it is secondary to a systemic disease, such as tuberculosis, blastomycosis, actinomycosis, or syphilis.

Fat necrosis

A peculiar and unusual breast "tumor" is occasionally encountered in fat, pendulous breasts following "injury." A history of physical violence to the breast, however, is elicited in less than one-half of the women with this condition. Indeed, fat necrosis may be associated with a suppurative disease of the breast, with carcinoma, with ischemia produced by pressure, and with "biopsy" breast surgery.[22] Symptoms may be present for months or years.

Clinical characteristics of a hard, somewhat fixed lump in the absence of discoloration of the skin easily may be misinterpreted as that of a malignant tumor. In the early stages, the lesion appears as a well-defined, firm, solid,

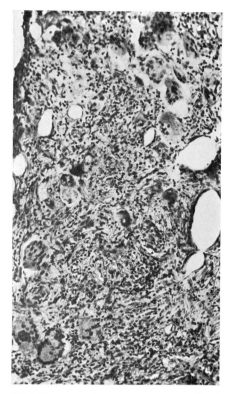

Fig. 38-5 Fat necrosis. Lesion is rather old, showing numerous multinucleated giant cells, spaces occupied by lipids, moderate fibrosis, and numerous small round cells.

homogeneous, lardaceous substance. As necrosis progresses, it may change to a light yellow, orange, brown, or brownish red color, depending upon presence or absence of hemorrhage. Cyst formation, hemorrhage, calcification, stellate scarring, and fixation are almost constant in the old lesion.

Histologic architecture of acute inflammation in the adipose tissue may be more striking than "fat necrosis." Polymorphonuclear cells, plasma cells, lymphocytes, and monocytes are constant. The monocytes may be of epithelioid or foam type but generally form foreign body giant cells. Early stages of the disease present opaque fat cells (fat saponification), and later there is found true necrosis with the presence of cholesterol crystals (sharp, angular clefts) and calcification (Fig. 38-5).

MAMMARY DYSPLASIA

Under the heading mammary dysplasia one must present a historically heterogeneous, challenging group of conditions composed of lesions fundamentally so similar that it becomes advantageous (if not imperative) to consider them under a single, descriptive, defining term. The many points of similarity in development, clinical expression, and histology greatly outweight those of dissimilarity. It has taken the period from Brodie in 1846 and Reclus in 1883 up to our time to evolve the present-day concept of a single disease in various forms—maladie cystique (Reclus), mastopathia cystica (Aschoff), fibrocystic disease, cystic hyperplasia, chronic cystic mastitis, or Schimmelbusch's disease, mazoplasia, cystiphorous desquamative epithelial hyperplasia (Cheatle, Cutler), fibroadenomatosis cystica (Semb), and mammary dysplasia (Geschickter). Present feeling is that the confusing nomenclature had birth in the arbitrarily selected criteria of lesions without cognizance of one essential disorder in somewhat different qualitative and quantitative phases.

Mammary dysplasia is essentially an abnormal interplay of parenchyma and stroma, developed and expressed by failure of reciprocal proliferation and involution (i.e., anatomic consequences of abnormal physiology). The paramount change centers about the breast lobule of sexual maturity. The condition, therefore, is not very active in postmenopausal life, nor is it a disease of the male breast. It is, moreover, neither inflammatory nor neoplastic, and the irrevocable term of chronic cystic mastitis is not generic. Anatomic changes of this condition are the reflection of ovarian hormonal imbalance (viz., corpus luteum deficiency with relative or absolute hyperestrinism) acting upon the susceptible breast over a long period of time.[26, 30] In the few cases investigated, pregnanediol levels were found to be lower than normal (11.6 mg per premenstrual cycle as compared with a normal of 30 mg).[3, 29]

Basically, the condition consists of lumpiness and cysts of the mammary gland. It is found in women chiefly in the last decade of reproductive life but, although developing in this period, it may not have prominent symptoms or be recognized until after the menopause. It commonly is bilateral and associated with premenstrual pain. The upper outer quadrant of the breast is chiefly involved. The hormonal irregularity also is evident in sterility or irregular menstruation. Failure of pregnancy and lactation or disturbances attending these physiologic processes predispose to mammary dysplasia, whereas normal pregnancy and lactation are the best therapies. Many cases apparently subside spontaneously.

Writers frequently refer to the relation of

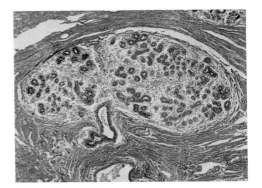

Fig. 38-6 Normal lobule. Mature, well-developed lobule with sharp distinction between lobular parenchymal connective tissue and that of general stroma. (×40.)

chronic cystic mastitis to mammary carcinoma. Warren[36] found mammary carcinoma four and one-half times more frequently in a group with chronic cystic mastitis, irrespective of age, than in the normal population. An autopsy study of the adult human breast is reported by Sandison,[32] who noted incidence of lobular adenosis, sclerosing adenosis, epithelial hyperplasias, and sundry associated changes. Special reference is made to proliferative epithelial changes. Others also place importance upon epithelial hyperplasia as a finding having a significant frequency relationship to subsequent cancer of the breast.[34, 61] A discussion of estrogen as an important factor in breast cancer, as well as in chronic cystic mastitis, is provided by Womack.[37]

On the basis of histologic interplay (in the lobule) between epithelium, myoepithelium, lobular connective tissue, stromal connective tissue, and inflammatory cells, mammary dysplasia may be multiform (Table 38-1).

Pronounced mixtures of these occur frequently in a single lesion (Fig. 38-7).[3, 30]

Mazoplasia (mastodynia, early phase with minimal change)

Gross appearance. In mazoplasia, the mammary gland is involved by a periodic swelling and diffuse granularity of the affected area. One-fourth of the patients may develop adenosis. Cutting is somewhat difficult and a section so made presents a white, poorly demarcated, dense, irregular, stiff, and tough substance marked by minute pinkish dots of the parenchyma.

Microscopic appearance. The essential change in mazoplasia is a moderate thickening and increase of the lobular stroma and its fusion with the general connective tissue.

Table 38-1 Forms of mammary dysplasia

	Mazoplasia (least change)	Adenosis	Cystic mastitis (greatest change)
Epithelium	Normal?	Hyperplastic	Atrophic or "apocrine" change
Stroma	Slightly increased	Intralobular increase	Sclerotic
Lobules	Slightly irregular	Large; irregular; very cellular	Atrophic; irregular; cystic
Cysts	Microscopic	Variable	Large; macroscopic
Area	Diffuse area involved	Periphery of breast	Midzone
Inflammation	None	Generally little	Prominent

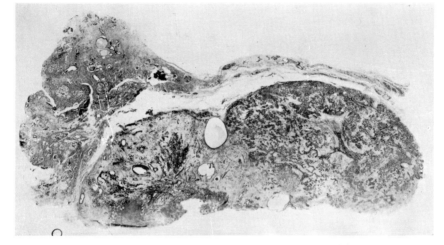

Fig. 38-7 Single encapsulated nodule showing various patterns of breast disease within one lesion—cystic disease, adenosis, adenoma, intracanalicular fibroadenoma, and extensive lobular carcinoma.

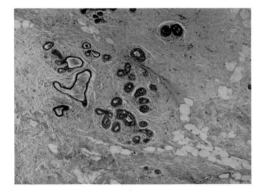

Fig. 38-8 Mazoplasia. Loss of distinction between lobular and stromal connective tissue and cystic dilatation of ductule. (×45.)

Microscopically, the ducts are dilated, and the lobules are variable in size and irregular in outline. The epithelium may be nearly normal or multilayered, secretory, or vacuolated, flat, or desquamating—more commonly all phases may be encountered in the perusal of large sections. However, the deviations from normal are usually not very pronounced (Fig. 38-8).

Adenosis

Gross appearance. In adenosis, the breast is rather small and fibrous in character. It has an easily palpable, exaggerated parenchyma with sharp peripheral boundaries. The nodularity to palpation, which is quite characteristic, is mostly peripheral. The gland cuts with difficulty. Involved areas resemble mazoplasia but have three differences:

1 Minute pinhead-sized to pea-sized clear cysts
2 Small, rubbery-hard, finely granular, speckled, shotlike areas containing yellowish, grumous plugs closely associated with the cysts
3 Irregular clustering of enlarged tan-pink lobules forming a discrete area of increased consistency

Microscopic appearance. Diffuse fibrosis with loss of distinction between intralobular and periductal connective tissue and the general stroma is characteristic of adenosis. Many ductules are dilated and contain clear or cloudy fluid. The epithelium is usually hyperplastic and lines the proliferating ductules with several layers of cells—at times forming minute papillomas or "spilling" out of its confines to cause considerable disorganization of the lobules (Fig. 38-9). Separation and disorganization of the lobules by advanced intralobular fibrosis accompanied by epithelial proliferation resembling glandular growth and invasion has been termed *sclerosing adenoma-*

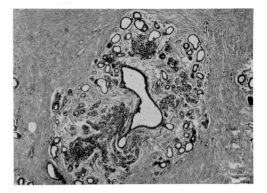

Fig. 38-9 Adenosis. Lobule with early cyst formation and "spilling" out of epithelial cells into lobular stroma. (×40.)

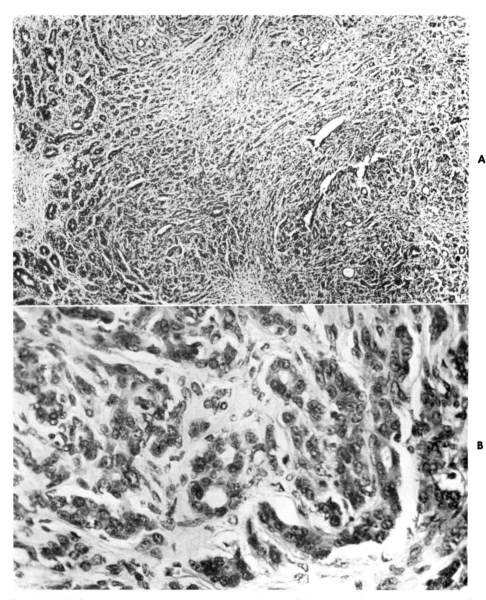

Fig. 38-10 Sclerosing adenomatosis. **A,** Four lobules of breast represented in pattern of delicate filigree architecture. **B,** High-power magnification of central portion of one lobule. Admixture of fibrous stroma with disorganized glands closely mimics pattern of infiltrating adenocarcinoma.

tosis or fibrosing adenoma (Fig. 38-10). Such a lobule presents a filigree pattern and frequently is associated with myoepithelial hyperplasia. Although the lesion is benign, its histologic appearance may easily be misinterpreted as cancer.[35]

Cystic disease

Gross appearance. In cystic disease, the breast is likely to be a little more fatty than in mazoplasia and adenosis. It presents a round, smooth, tense, movable mass averaging 3 cm to 4 cm in diameter, which transilluminates and may be fluctuant. The area is closer to the center of the breast than is adenosis. Sections show an exaggerated pattern of adenosis. Cysts are variable, multiple, and large and protrude into the stromal fat. They are somewhat translucent, causing the light brownish contents to appear bluish through the cyst wall (blue dome cyst). The shotty areas are also larger, harder, and more yellowish. On pressure in some cases, abundant pasty material can be expressed in the form of ribbons.

Microscopic appearance. In cystic disease, the irregular lobules are small, acini are few, and ductules are dilated and filled with amorphous granular material. Larger cysts have atrophic, flattened, or absent epithelium accompanied by a very dense, sclerotic, outlining stroma. Epithelial involution is the keynote, to which, however, there are two exceptions:

1 The occasionally persistent focus of hyperplasia or papilloma formation
2 The hyperplasia of apocrine-like glands

This latter finding is a prominent feature, although similar glands may be found in many otherwise normal breasts or be associated with fibroadenoma, papilloma, or sclerosing adenomatosis. The glands are variable and large. The lining acidophilic epithelium is very tall and commonly presents plump papillary projections. Nuclei are nearly basilar in position and are round and light-staining. Knobby free margins of the tall cells are characteristic. Lymphocytic or mononuclear infiltrations around ducts, smaller cysts, and in the lobules are both prominent and constant. In some instances, myoepithelial proliferation adds to the epithelial hyperplasia (Fig. 38-11). Epithelial hyperplasia in cystic disease may be considerable in some instances and occasionally is associated with the presence of cancer in the same area, in an adjacent site, or even in the opposite breast.

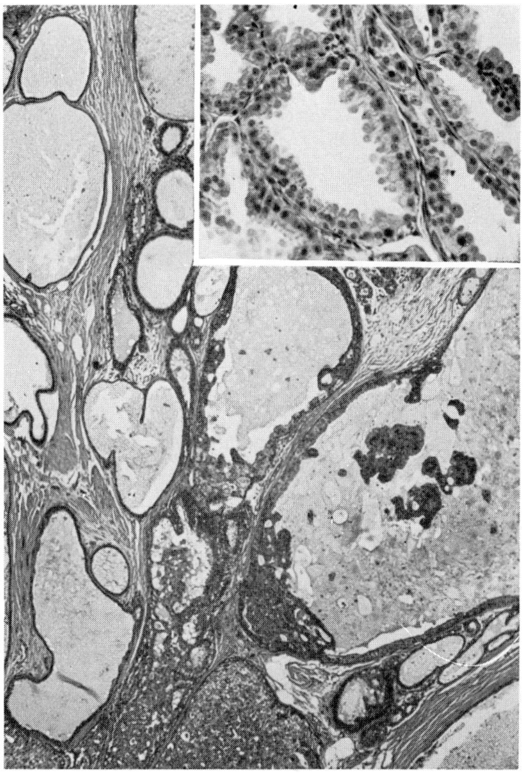

Chemical analysis of fluid aspirated from

Fig. 38-11 Chronic cystic mastitis with atrophy, intracystic epithelial proliferation, and duct carcinoma. Inset shows high magnification of apocrine type of epithelium. (×40.)

cystic disease of the breast reveals that potassium, nonprotein nitrogen, and cholesterol are considerably higher than in the blood, while sodium, chlorides, glucose, and total protein are lower. The sum of potassium and sodium is roughly about 200 mEq, and potassium is frequently very high (i.e., 140 mEq). The pH of the fluid is 7.1 to 7.4. There is no correlation with age of patient or duration of cyst.[28]

Miscellaneous cystic disorders

Galactocele. A galactocele or milk cyst develops in young females during lactation. The contents are truly milky or inspissated. It develops presumably because of duct obstruction. The cyst wall may show areas of necrosis, round cell infiltration, and condensation of the adjacent stroma. It is a rare occurrence.

Dilated ducts. Dilated ducts or ductule ectasia occurs at or after the menopause and consists of visible or palpable dilated ducts filled with a puttylike material beneath the nipple. Ducts show desquamating secretory epithelium with lymphocytes and monocytes in the duct walls. The inflammatory reaction

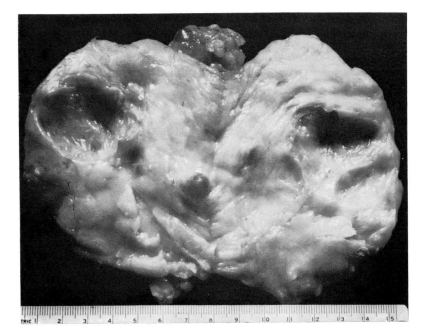

Fig. 38-12 Cystic disease of breast. Larger cyst is bisected and shows glistening smooth lining. In center is smaller bulging cyst.

is in response to chemical irritation of decomposition. The condition is the result of irregular proliferation and secretion in women 50 years of age or over.

Ductule ectasia and *periductal mastitis* have certain common features and may, in fact, express slightly different dimensions of the same basic disorder—postmenopausal atrophy, stasis, and inflammation. Plasma cell mastitis appears earlier in life. Nonetheless, some authors hold that it is ductule ectasia-periductal mastitis, albeit florid.

Summary

Errors of hormonal interplay and breast tissue responsiveness eventuate in clinical abnormalities of anatomy—benign lumps and masses—collectively referred to as mammary dysplasia. Inclusions of adenoma, fibroadenoma, etc., which have similar pathogenesis, would be reasonable. However, because these are local circumscribed manifestations of proliferation, they are traditionally classified under *tumors*.

TUMORS
Benign tumors
Fibroadenoma

Fibroadenoma is a slowly growing, estrogen-induced, benign tumor occurring in females, most often before the age of 30 years.[39, 42] It begins as mammary dysplasia

with an overgrowth of young myxomatous intralobular connective tissue and variable epithelial proliferations. Often, it is associated with other forms of dysplasia such as adenosis and cyst formation. The reason why a focal area should be affected by hormonal imbalance (hyperestrinism or hypersensitivity to estrin) has not been explained. Menopause usually results in cessation of the growth of the tumor, while pregnancy and lactation cause it to grow readily.[41]

The condition is usually solitary but occasionally multiple, bilateral, or recurring. The skin overlying the tumor and the axillary nodes shows no change. The tumor is movable, solid, rubbery in consistency, and smooth or lobulated. Its average size is about 3.5 cm. It does not transilluminate.

The gross appearance of fibroadenoma is distinctly different from that of any other mammary tumor. Its encapsulation, partial or complete, and its rubbery consistency allow sectioning only if the tumor is firmly held, or else it will slip and roll away from the knife. A sharp distinct edge outlines the decidedly elevated, flat, or slightly convex cut (or sectioned) surface. Firmer lesions are grayish white. Softer ones are pink. Either form, however, is grossly homogeneous. The surface made by section may present a fine granularity or a delicately fissured geographic pattern. Old lesions are hyalinized and may be

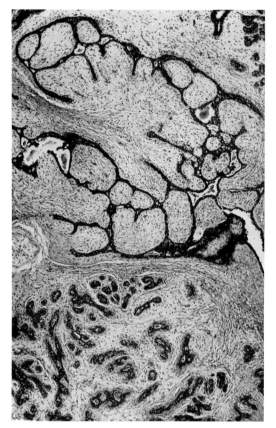

Fig. 38-13 Fibroadenoma showing intracanalicular formation at top, and pericanalicular arrangement in lobule at bottom.

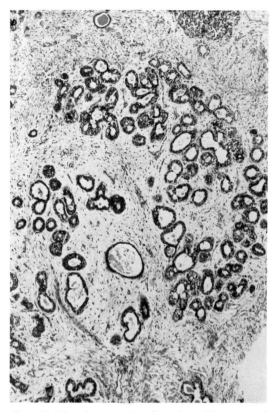

Fig. 38-14 Adenoma. Combined proliferation of young lobular connective tissue and epithelium. (×40.)

calcified. Three histologic variations are acceptable, depending probably upon the rate of growth of the connective tissue rather than on its origin.[42] Names applied (intracanalicular fibroadenoma, pericanalicular fibroadenoma, and adenoma) are based on the predominance of either connective tissue or glands and their relationships, for no fibroadenoma is a pure histologic type.

Intracanalicular fibroadenoma (intracanalicular myxoma). In intracanalicular fibroadenoma, the connective tissue is active and proliferating. Large polypoid masses growing into the parenchymal channels, thereby becoming covered by epithelium, produce a mosaic of distorted myxomatous discs. The epithelium is intimately applied to these projections and is continuous with that of the duct. It is atrophic at points of physical contact and heaped up or multilayered in dilated segments of the elongated tortuous ductules. Huge formations of this type, 10 cm or greater in diameter, are known as *giant intracanalicular myxoma* or *cystosarcoma phyllodes* (see sarcoma, p. 1602).

Pericanalicular fibroadenoma. Pericanalicular fibroadenoma has a denser stroma than intracanalicular fibroadenoma. Both epithelium and stroma in proliferation make up the tumor. The ductules and lobules are hyperplastic and distorted by connective tissue growth. More typical, however, are sweeping, encircling bands of dense connective tissue about the ductules and glands.

Adenoma. Adenoma differs from intracanalicular and pericanalicular fibroadenomas in its remarkable epithelial proliferation of mature, irregular, closely packed glands outlined by tall, partly secreting epithelium. It may be so cellular as to recall the histology of adenocarcinoma. However, there are usually a neighboring connective tissue hyperplasia and lobular distortion or a close resemblance to fetal breast tissue ("fetal adenoma") (Fig. 38-14).

Papilloma

Intraductal or intracystic papillomas occur predominantly in parous women at or shortly before the menopause. The papilloma appears

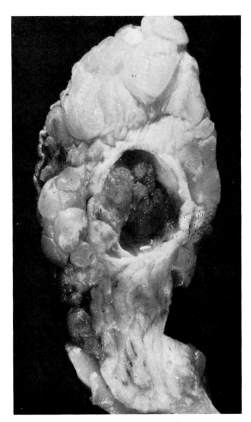

Fig. 38-15 Intracystic papilloma.

as a firm, granular, raspberry-like nodule, filling a duct or forming a small nipplelike projection on the wall of a cyst beneath the areola (Fig. 38-15). Larger lesions have a delicately fissured surface of villous or arborescent character. A cloudy sanguineous fluid fills the cyst or duct and accounts for the spontaneous or induced bleeding from the nipple in more than one-half of the cases. Papillomas are commonly multiple.

The microscopic structure of papillomas is a complex arrangement of fibrovascular stalks bearing epithelial surfaces. A lesser number is delicately villous, with a single layer or two of epithelial cells, uniform in size and polarity. Others with broad connective tissue stalks tend to irregularly aggregate clusters of epithelial and myoepithelial cells between the stalks. In smaller ducts, a similar lesion called *papillomatosis* is essentially an epithelial/myoepithelial syncytium with little supporting fibrovascular tissue (Fig. 38-16.)

The biologic behavior of highly cellular lesions having epithelial bridging or perforated sheets of cells (cribriform) is difficult to assess. The potential for development of malignancy has been both affirmed and denied. Cytologic characteristics and evidence of invasion remain the most important criteria. I share the opinion that some papillomas become malig-

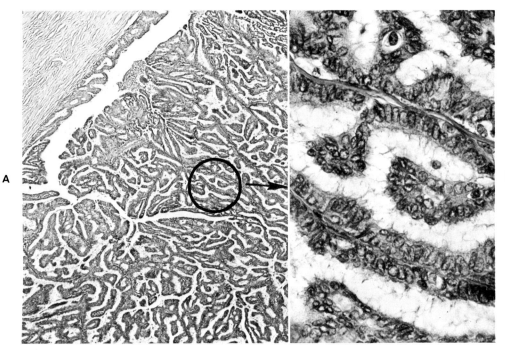

Fig. 38-16 Papilloma. **A,** Arborescent pattern of delicate papillary formations in a large papilloma. **B,** Enlargement of encircled area.

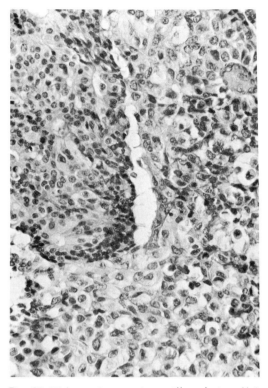

Fig. 38-17 Large intracystic papillary lesion. Uniform cellular pattern of benign lesion depicted at upper left, while remainder is cytologically malignant and histologically infiltrating. Presumed that all of lesion was benign in character at one time. (×320.)

nant, a fact likely to be confused by our tendency to reverse our original diagnoses. Fig. 38-17 is essentially a lesion of uniform cytology in cribriform pattern, which most pathologists diagnose as benign, replaced in part by cells of malignant cytologic characteristics and demonstrable aggressiveness. The relationship of intraductal papillary proliferations to subsequent carcinoma in the same or opposite breast is discussed in several reports.[43, 48, 61]

Adenoma of nipple

A somewhat distinct lesion of papillomatosis, adenosis, fibromyxoid stroma, and spurious infiltration occurs in or beneath the nipple (Fig. 38-18). It has considerable resemblance to the variegated patterns of canine mammary tumors. It is benign although misinterpreted as malignant much too often. This lesion is described under the heading *subareolar duct papillomatosis* in the *Atlas of tumor pathology.*[47]

Malignant tumors

Incidence. Mammary carcinoma may affect either breast, accessory breast tissue, or the male gland. Incidence of carcinoma of the breast is nearly twice the rate of malignancy found at any other site, in either male or fe-

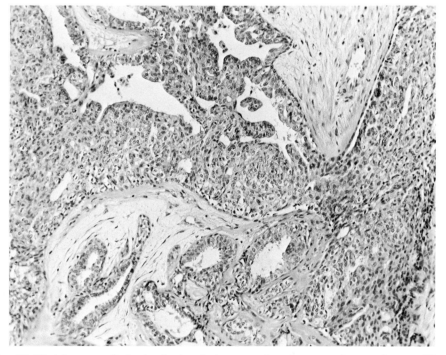

Fig. 38-18 Adenoma of nipple. Benign lesion too often interpreted as malignant. Histologically, it is mixture of papillomatosis and adenosis, but cells with benign cytologic features should be most helpful in making correct diagnosis. (×125.)

male.[61] Risk of breast cancer for the American female is presently stated to be 1 : 16[66] and rate of incidence is increasing in women under 55 years of age.[62] Most cancers are discovered shortly before, during, or just after the menopause. The older the patient, the more probable it is that a single lump in the breast is a carcinoma.

Predisposition. It appears that breasts which have not achieved full anatomic and physiologic potential (prolonged lactation) or have certain benign lesions are more prone to develop cancer.[37, 100] Breast cancer occurs more commonly in single women, infertile married women, and late-married women, suggesting that unopposed estrogen activity during a long reproduction life-span is the most significant factor. Mammary cancer in cows is almost nonexistent.[92, 93] Ovarian cortical hyperplasia has been reported in postmenopausal women with breast cancer, and cancer of the male breast has developed following estrogen therapy for prostate cancer. Breast cancer reportedly does not develop after prepubertal castration.

The role of heredity in the development of cancer is not understood, although a number of recorded instances show development of breast cancer in siblings and successive generations. The risk is two to three times greater in women with familial history of breast cancer than in the general population. Identification of high-risk breast cancer groups is the subject of a recent report.[63] The experimental work in reference to heredity and to the "milk factor" is not directly applicable to human beings.

The part played by trauma in the development of mammary tumors is negligible. This is borne out by the infrequency of breast carcinoma compared to the frequency of injury and the lack of relationship between the size of the tumor and the time factor following injury. Most tumors are much too large when noticed to have been initiated by a dated physical violence. However, it must be conceded that degeneration and hemorrhage may occur in a tumor as a result of injury and that its rate of growth may be accelerated.

Etiology. The cause of mammary cancer is not completely known. The highly specialized biologically active mammary tissue under the influences of hormones (especially estrogen) undergoes periodic hyperplasia and involution. Imbalances lead to mammary dysplasia or to accentuated repair and hyperplasia that eventually cross the threshold of neoplasia.

This is more than speculation, since estrogens act principally upon the ducts and ductules from which most carcinomas arise. Geschickter states: "All of the estrogens of sufficient potency for clinical use will produce mammary cancer in the rat regardless of chemical composition or physiologic potency. . . ."*

Unusual proliferative histologic patterns in the cervix and breast have been attributed to the "pill," but at the present time contraceptive pills are neither indicted nor absolved in the increasing incidence of breast cancer in women roughly at menopause or younger.[60, 71, 76, 97] More precise information of target tissue response in relation to formation/excretion and administration of estrogens (estriol, estradiol, and estrone) is necessary to answer any questions regarding the use of contraceptive pills and potential breast cancer. On the other hand, estrogens by mouth, implantation, and inunction apparently have induced breast cancers in transsexual individuals.[95] Cancer of the male breast also is reported in patients with cancer of prostate treated by synthetic estrogens over a long period of time.[64] Some, however, interpret this as metastasis from the prostate, not primary breast cancer.[54] An acceptable case is reported.[83]

A survey of multiple primary cancers in females strongly suggests a positive incidence interrelationship among cancers of the breast, genital organs, and gastrointestinal tract.[89]

Pathologic anatomy. Malignant tumors arise most frequently in the upper outer quadrant of the breast. The central area is next in frequency and then the upper inner quadrant, followed by the lower inner quadrant.[3] The lesions arising far out in the periphery of the breast metastasize to regional nodes earlier than those arising in the central portion, but lesions of the inner quadrants have a less favorable prognosis because of mediastinal metastasis. In the elderly individual, cancer is likely to be of a hard fibrous character. In the small atrophic breast, duct carcinoma of comedo variety is seen. In the atrophic but fatty breast, early metastasis may arise from a very small focus of carcinoma. Young women, particularly with pregnancy, are likely to have a highly anaplastic, rapidly growing malignancy.

The classic example of carcinoma of the breast is a single, hard, poorly movable, nonelastic, easily cut nodule. Sections have a dry,

*From Geschickter, C. F.: Diseases of the breast, ed. 2, Philadelphia, 1945, J. B. Lippincott Co.

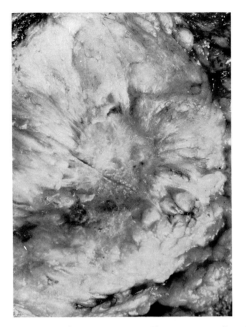

Fig. 38-19 Adenocarcinoma. Classic example of so-called scirrhous adenocarcinoma with a depressed infiltrating flat mass showing chalk streaks.

gritty, opaque surface marked by radiating, translucent lines of connective tissue accompanied by small yellowish or opaque grayish dots and streaks. The central portion of the tumor is slightly concave, and the margins extend into the stroma, between which the fat lobules may protrude above the level of the tumor. Therefore, the border may be scalloped. The concave surface, the chalky streaks, the pouting fat tissue, and the blending of the tumor with the stroma in a radiating fashion are the paramount characteristics (Fig. 38-19).

The lesion may be firm enough to grate on cutting, and if one cuts thin slices of the tumor, these maintain an extremely sharp edge and a level surface. The tissue appears extremely turgid and is not elastic or flexible. The infiltration of the connective tissue produces a contraction of the dermal papillae and of Cooper's ligaments, thereby developing the "orange peel" appearance of the skin. Periductal invasion causes retraction of the nipple (Fig. 38-20). Intimate fixation to breast stroma and sometimes to the underlying fascia makes the tumor limited in movement. Such cancers are "scirrhous" or carcinomas with "productive fibrosis." Other gross types include the medullary opaque white or pink soft tumors, frequently with hemorrhage and necrosis; mucoid or gelatinous; papillary

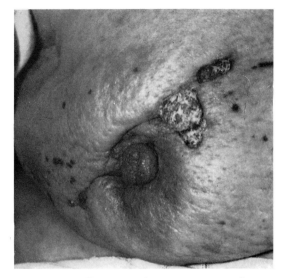

Fig. 38-20 Infiltrating adenocarcinoma producing retraction of nipple, marked dimpling of skin, and invasion of skin surface.

and soft; circumscribed; intracystic; and comedo (Fig. 16-17).

More than 90% of the malignant mammary gland tumors arise from the epithelium of the duct system, either the large or the small channels. Acinar carcinomas and sarcomas comprise the remainder. Basic features of adenocarcinoma may be found in virtually any mammary carcinoma, although one or another modification of histologic architecture may predominate, and several varieties may occur in one tumor.

Prognosis. According to one report, average duration of life from onset of symptoms for untreated breast cancer is 3.3 years, and only 18% survive five years.[4] In treated patients without positive axillary nodes, five-year survival is approximately 80%. For those with disease in axillary nodes, it is about 50%.

Single events and combinations thereof that portend poor prognosis include the following[62a]:

1 Primary tumor greater than 4 cm in diameter
2 Involvement of nipple by tumor (axillary nodes generally positive in such cases)
3 Edema and thickening of skin
4 High grade of malignancy (the young and pregnant female)
5 Enlarged, deep, or fixed axillary nodes
6 Internal mammary node involvement
7 Absence of plasma cell reactions in duct carcinomas
8 Predetermined biologic factors

The latter, according to MacDonald,[79] explain why 55% of breast cancer patients are not controlled by any means, 25% depend upon treatment for control, and 20% do well without treatment (Fig. 16-8). For survival figures related to specific histologic types, see the *Atlas of tumor pathology*.[47] It must be recognized that the foregoing figures relate to clinical cancers of the breast detected largely by the patient herself. Continuing missionary work is required for the discovery and treatment of the disease in a preclinical presymptomatic phase. As Shimkin stated, ". . . the overwhelming single determinant of prognosis is the stage of the disease at initial definitive treatment."*

Clinical orientation. Cancer of the breast is the leading neoplasm in the female. Each year, 65,000 new cases are discovered, while 25,000 patients die of the disease. The challenge is to discover the more than 300,000 potential breast cancer victims in the next five years in a population of more than 36,000,000 women 40 years of age or older.[88] Curability of breast cancer, although dependent upon many factors, resides largely in the premise that dissemination (incurability) of the disease is a function of duration and size of the lesion when first discovered. Even the smallest clinically detected lesion has had several years of existence in a preclinical phase. Nonetheless, more than three-fourths of all breast cancers are discovered by the patient when the average size is 5 cm, and the disease is local in less than one-half. Annual physical examinations by physicians interested in breast cancer will find cancer in about 1 in 700 examinations, but three out of four of these women will have disease localized to the breast. Mammography will detect three preclinical lesions (average size, 1 cm) per 1,000 examinations when the disease is only local in 80%. Evidence suggests that mammography picks up lesions several years earlier than clinical examination.[82] Mammography has limited accuracy in small atrophic breast and in women under 40 years of age and always must be considered complementary to clinical examination.[94] Overall false negative evaluation is about 15%. Xerography, thermography, and ultrasonics all have utility, although not precisely quantitated at this time. A schedule of repeated periodic clinical examinations with mammography is presently advised.[73]

What is the fate of women with biopsy-

benign proliferations of the breast? Identification of cytohistologic transitions of a benign proliferative disorder into a clinically aggressive lesion is observed only infrequently. This fact, however, should not deny a greater risk of breast cancer in women with benign lesions, not by virtue of the benign process but rather by nature of the breast tissue whose capacity for cellular proliferation is already established.[43, 56, 75, 86] By analogy, familial-hereditary factors that increase risk of breast cancer are not identified histologically.

One single fact bears irrefutably upon the incidence of breast cancer—it is the history of cancer in one breast. If we agree on any one point, this is it. The incidence of contralateral breast cancer is many times greater than in the general female population, and particularly so for those under 50 years of age.[66] Incidence rate for contralateral breast cancer is stated as 1% per year. Biopsy of the clinically negative breast at the time of mastectomy for cancer is positive for cancer in about 15%. Bilateral synchronous cancers (contralateral not infiltrating) are approximately 10%.[99]

In premenopausal women, breast cancer is likely to be estrogen "dependent," and any procedure for decreasing the estrogen titer may be beneficial to the patient. Postmenopausal women are different. Their skeletal metastasis may be significantly improved by estrogen therapy.[74] It has been reported that differences in steroid metabolism/excretion are demonstrable in breast cancer patients.[58]

Radical surgery for breast cancer, with its severe disruption of the lymphatics, at times is responsible for severe and persistent edema of the upper extremity. In rare instances, a lymphangiosarcoma arises in the skin and soft tissues of such an arm[93] (Fig. 38-21 and p. 1668).

Clinical stage classification. A clinical stage classification of cancer of the breast has been developed by the American Joint Committee on Cancer Staging and End Results Reporting.[52]

Biopsy. Biopsy should be "excisional"—total skillful removal of the tumor whenever possible. "Incisional" biopsy is permissible for very large lesions. Needle aspiration biopsy provides satisfactory documentation for infiltrating lesions, clearly benign conditions, and cysts. Spontaneous breast secretions are subject to the "Pap smear" technique of diagnosis, but there is understandable reluctance to manipulation of the breast or its tumor for

---

*From Shimkin, M. B.: In discussion of Cutler, S. J., and Connelly, R. R.: Cancer 23:767-774, 1969.

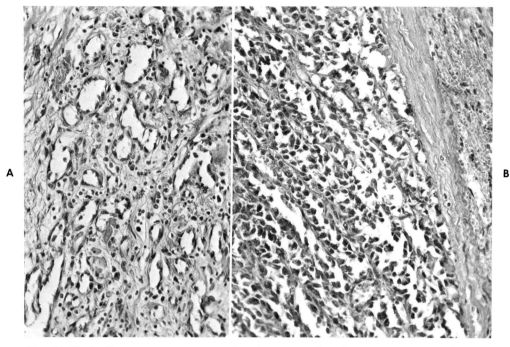

Fig. 38-21 A, Chronic postmastectomy lymph stasis or lymphangiectasis. **B,** Lymphangio-sarcoma (same case).

the purpose of producing exfoliation or "secretion" for cytodiagnosis. The degree of risk in transferring cancer cells and inoculating the lymphovascular system by any of the procedures just mentioned is yet to be assessed.

Metastasis. The principal route of metastasis is lymphatic, notably to the axilla, since the majority of lesions are found in the upper outer quadrant of the breast. Of the general group of carcinomas at the time of operation, 47% have axillary metastasis.[55] In instances of bilateral simultaneous mammary cancers, 71% have axillary involvement. The lesions that are diagnosed as grade IV are associated with 84% axillary metastasis.[50] Other lymphatic routes involve the lower cervical chain, the supraclavicular and infraclavicular lymph nodes, and the intercostal, retrosternal, and mediastinal routes, particularly from the medial and lower quadrants of the breast. There is also an epigastric pathway that may lead directly to the mediastinal or abdominal nodes.

Intramammary secondary foci are not too uncommon, and extension across the midline to the opposite breast occurs occasionally. The skin may be involved by way of the periductal lymphatics, lymphatics of Cooper's ligament, or by direct continuity. Multiple nodular cutaneous metastasis of the chest wall is known

as cancer *en cuirasse*. Visceral metastases are most prominent in the lungs and pleura, occurring in over one-half of the patients. The liver, bone, brain, adrenal gland, and spleen follow in order of frequency. Dissemination of tumor cells to the spine and brain may be explained by vertebral vascular communications that favor retrograde spread.[101] It is peculiar that both cutaneous and osseous metastases are very unusual distal to the elbows and knees. Symptomatic (bleeding) gastrointestinal metastases of breast cancers appear to be related to adrenal steroid therapy.[53, 72]

Classification of mammary cancer

Mammary tumors may be classified according to gross characteristics (scirrhous, colloid, medullary), histologic characteristic (adenocarcinoma, carcinoma simplex, sarcoma), histogenesis (duct, lobule, acini), or activity (infiltrating, noninfiltrating). It is obvious, therefore, that a classification can readily become both confusing and unwieldy. Terms denoting histology are based on the predominant architecture and not on purity of the lesion. It should be noted, therefore, that many patterns may be seen in any one carcinoma (Fig. 38-22). A working classification may well combine the various features that make a tu-

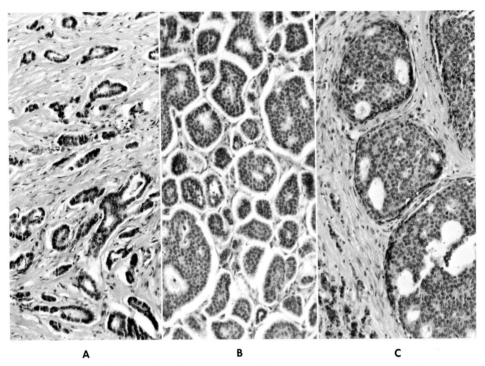

A   B   C

Fig. 38-22 Three different histologic patterns of breast cancer present in single primary lesion, 2.5 cm in width. Adenocarcinoma with fibrosis, **A,** carcinoma simplex, **B,** and duct carcinoma with invasion, **C,** are represented.

mor histologically, clinically, or otherwise distinct. The following orientation scheme, to which benign tumors have been added, is modified from Foote and Stewart:*

Benign

1 Epithelial
  a Papillomas
2 Mixed epithelial and mesodermal
  a Fibroadenoma
    (1) Intracanalicular
    (2) Pericanalicular
    (3) Adenoma
3 Mesodermal—breast tumors only by geography and in no way distinctive in mammary gland (viz., lipoma, angioma, fibroma, myoma)

Malignant

1 Mammary ducts
  a Noninfiltrating tumors
    (1) Papillary carcinoma
    (2) Comedocarcinoma or duct carcinoma
  b Infiltrating tumors (adenocarcinoma)
    (1) Paget's disease
    (2) Papillary carcinoma
    (3) Comedocarcinoma
    (4) Adenocarcinoma with productive fibrosis (scirrhous, simplex)
    (5) Medulla carcinoma
    (6) Mucinous carcinoma

*Modified from Foote, F. W., Jr., and Stewart, F. W.: Surgery **19:**74-99, 1946.

2 Mammary lobules
  a Noninfiltrating—"in situ"
  b Infiltrating—lobular adenocarcinoma
3 Epithelial or mesodermal origins such as tumors of skin, skin appendages, and supporting tissues of breast; same as found elsewhere in body—dermoid cyst, sweat gland tumors, basal or squamous cell carcinoma of skin, liposarcoma, etc.

Adenocarcinoma

Apparently three-fourths of mammary carcinomas are associated with desmoplasia and generally have been called scirrhous carcinoma. The average age of occurrence is about 50 years, duration of symptoms ordinarily is less than a year, and the lesion averages 2 cm to 3 cm in diameter. Almost two-thirds of the patients have axillary gland metastasis at the time of removal. The classic signs of mammary cancer generally refer to this particular form.

The histologic hallmark is productive fibrosis and hyalinization in the tumor. Cancer cells in very small clusters and in single rows occupy the irregular cleft spaces between collagen bundles (Fig. 38-23). Large groups of cancers with isolated tubular formations have been designated as "carcinoma simplex." Others are chiefly glandular. Periductal and perivascular infiltrations are common.

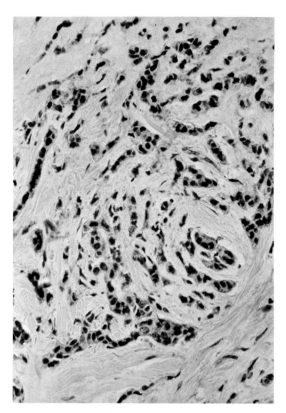

Fig. 38-23 Scirrhous carcinoma. Note dense stroma with narrow columns of tumor cells.

Medullary carcinoma

Approximately 5% to 10% of the malignant tumors belong to the group called medullary carcinoma. This tumor is characterized by a deeply situated, midzonal, circumscribed, movable mass. The skin may be stretched over the bulging mass, but it does not show dimpling and is generally free of ulceration. The gross lesion appears as a soft, partially cystic or hemorrhagic, bulky, somewhat opaque white tumor. It frequently resembles lymphoid tissue or has encephaloid characteristics. It is generally spherical and in two-thirds of the cases is larger than 5 cm in diameter. Such a tumor generally grows slowly but may rapidly enlarge because of hemorrhage or necrosis. Prognosis is better than in adenocarcinoma.

The microscopic picture is that of a highly cellular tumor composed of large, oval or polygonal cells with slightly basophilic cytoplasm and vesicular nuclei with prominent nucleoli. The pattern may be large broad sheets or wide roughly parallel bands of tumor cells. At times, only the periphery of the tumor is viable, the remainder having been converted to a cyst by autolysis and hemorrhage. Usually, a generous lymphocyte infiltration accompanies the epithelial cells and forms an important histologic characteristic.

Circumscribed (but infiltrating) cancer is a name given to medullary carcinomas which are grossly sharply demarcated and histologically rich in plasma cells.

Comedocarcinoma

This tumor, comprising somewhat less than 10% of the mammary carcinomas, is so named from the physical characteristics of plugs of pasty material expressed from the surface of the tumor. It is a slowly growing tumor that may have a course extending over years. It averages 5 cm in diameter, is rather soft, and in only 15% of the cases has involved axillary nodes. Three-fourths of the patients survive a five-year period, with radical mastectomy. A central location of the tumor is associated with cloudy nipple discharge in approximately one-third of the cases. Skin ulceration and retraction of the nipple are very late findings. It occurs particularly in women after the menopause and is more frequently associated with chronic cystic mastitis than other carcinomas.[3] It arises from the small or intermediate ducts, and in its growth the ducts of a given portion of the breast become filled with plugs of tumor cells. The tumor is usually somewhat circumscribed, quite firm in consistency, and grayish in color. It has an infiltrating gross appearance, but it is not so hard as the scirrhous carcinoma. The tumor areas present grayish dots, from which ribbonlike plugs of yellowish gray pasty material or solid tumor plugs are extruded upon pressure.

Microscopic characteristics are those of many cores of highly cellular epithelial tissue, generally containing a central granular amorphous eosinophilic necrosis. The larger the area, the more prominent the necrosis. The pattern frequently follows that of the duct system. Occasionally, there is liquefaction of some of the cells in the epithelial layer, giving an appearance of accessory acinar formation. Such, however, are not vascularized. The cells are generally small and dark and have dense nuclei. Cells nearer the center may be larger and less intensely stained. Hyperchromatism, mitoses, and loss of polarity are quite prominent. In its invasion, it very commonly mimics other histologic patterns such as gland formation, papillary structures, and productive fibrosis. Occasionally, the cellular

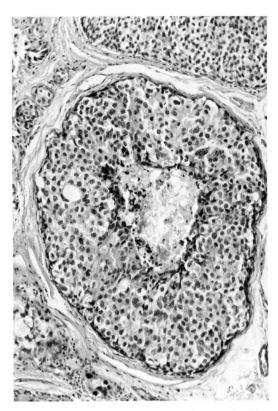

Fig. 38-24 Comedocarcinoma. Large ductlike structure has central debris and uniform small cells.

growth is confined to the duct system. It is then known as a noninfiltrating variety and is adequately treated by simple mastectomy.[93] However, one must be certain of the absence of infiltration (Fig. 38-24).

Duct carcinoma

Duct carcinoma is quite similar to comedocarcinoma, but it ordinarily lacks the central necrosis of the tumor cell discs. It is more rapid in its progress, with a brief period of symptoms, and is more commonly associated with pain or discharge from the nipple and involvement of axillary nodes.[3] It arises from the central ducts.

The microscopic picture is that of a profuse growth of the duct epithelium, forming large clear cells with large nuclei, prominent nucleoli, and frequent mitoses. Minute papillary-like projections and accessory acinar formation are more prominent than in comedocarcinoma. Pleomorphism is noteworthy. In some instances, clear areas within the tumor-filled ducts are evident, but eosinophilic necrosis is not striking in the typical case. Both comedocarcinoma and duct carcinoma are of

ductal origin, and both are noninfiltrating intraductal proliferations for an indefinite period of time (very good prognosis) prior to demonstrable infiltration and aggression.

Paget's disease

Paget's disease is a chronic eczematoid thelitis associated with a central duct carcinoma. It has a course of long duration that begins with subjective symptoms of burning, itching, or soreness of the nipple, followed by physical findings of hyperemia and enlargement. This change extends to the areola and is accompanied by fissuring, weeping or oozing, crust formation, and eventually ulceration and destruction of the nipple. Occasionally, the nipple changes are preceded by a definable lump in the breast. Paget's disease comprises less than 5% of mammary carcinomas and occurs in an older age group of women than the usual carcinoma. Approximately one-third of the patients have axillary node metastasis, but if the lesion is limited to the nipple, prognosis is very good. Gross examination of the tissue beneath the nipple area shows dilated thick ducts containing grumous pasty material. Some ducts also may be identified as being filled with cell masses, fixed and indurated. The periductal infiltration produces a fairly well-defined tumor not different from that previously described, although it may be very small.

The nipple and cutaneous manifestations of the disease are characterized by the presence of very large, pale, vacuolated cells (Paget cells) in the rete pegs of the epithelium. These may show large hyperchromatic nuclei and mitoses. The epidermis, therefore, has a "moth-eaten" histologic appearance (Figs. 38-25 and 38-26). Question still exists whether Paget cells represent an epidermoid carcinoma of the nipple arising in situ, whether they represent an intraepithelial metastasis from the constantly present underlying duct carcinoma, or whether they are just "peculiar cells" found in some cases of duct carcinoma.[1, 69, 81, 85] It is probably correct that Paget's disease is not a primary tumor of the squamous epithelium of the nipple, since in its metastasis it does not have epidermoid characteristics. There is some evidence of intraepithelial spread of the duct cancer cells. However, not infrequent confusion with superficial melanoma, chiefly in extramammary sites, and confusion vice versa, suggests needed rethinking regarding the possible role of melanocytes in Paget's disease.[84]

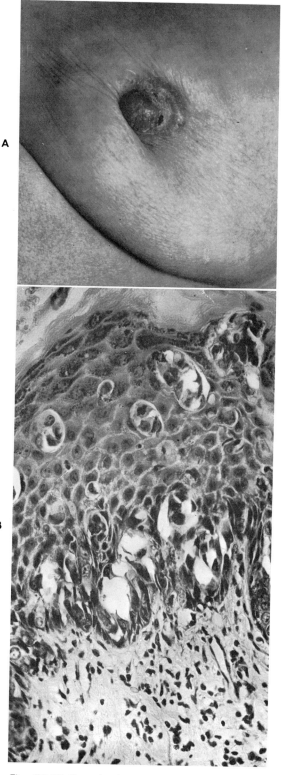

Papillary adenocarcinoma

A centrally located tumor, papillary adenocarcinoma grows slowly and frequently is 5 cm or more in diameter. It occurs mainly in the 35-year to 40-year age group. It is commonly associated with discharge from the nipple and the presence of a large, soft, bulky nodule. With central hemorrhage or cyst formation, it may be fluctuant. In the late stages, it loses its movable characteristics and ulcerates through the skin. Axillary node involvement is quite late and not prominent. The microscopic architecture is papillary in type, showing a communicating dendritic pattern. The cells are variable, in some instances forming large sheets and in other instances forming single cell layers. Lymphoid cells about the borders are not unusual. Histologic invasion is evident at the attachment of the papillary mass and is characterized by cells of mod-

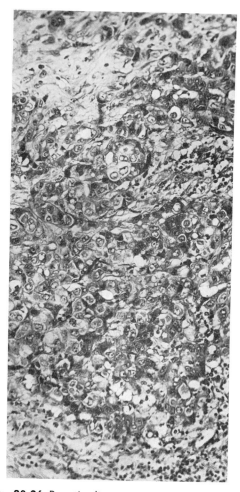

Fig. 38-25 Paget's disease of nipple. **A,** Nipple is retracted, and surrounding its base there is scaling dermatitis associated with thickening and induration of periphery of areola. **B,** Epithelium shows surface hyperkeratosis and very marked disorganization of its basal portions, numerous vacuoles, and many large extremely pale cells. Note mitotic figure.

Fig. 38-26 Paget's disease metastasis to axillary lymph node. Cells are large and clear, maintaining histologic features of nipple skin changes.

erate hyperchromatism, lack of polarity, and frequent mitoses. Invasion is the best evidence of malignancy. Other histologic and cytologic criteria many times fail to accurately differentiate papilloma from papillary carcinoma.

Mucinous carcinoma

Mucinous carcinoma is an adenocarcinoma also known by the name of colloid or gelatinous carcinoma. It is not a common lesion. It grows rather slowly and is associated with late metastasis and lack of nipple retraction.

Grossly, the tumor is fairly well demarcated but not encapsulated. It produces a spherical mass of moderately firm character, with a translucent, moist, gelatinous or slimy surface marked by a delicately interlacing pattern of more solid, opaque tissue. Its gross characteristics frequently closely resemble those of mixed tumor of the parotid gland. On cutting, strings of mucoid material may adhere to the knife. It is very slippery, and small particles of mucoid material can easily be removed from the tumor by scraping. The

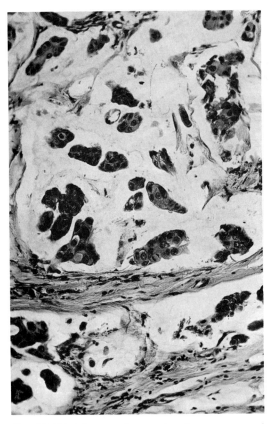

Fig. 38-27 Adenocarcinoma showing compressed clusters of tumor cells with abundant extracellular mucinous material.

bulging droplets of slimy material are most pronounced after formalin fixation.

The typical microscopic picture is that of a multilocular cystlike formation. The spaces contain a light grayish blue–staining amorphous material. At some point around the periphery of these spaces, small clusters of deeply stained epithelial cells may be evident (Fig. 38-27). They generally are poor in detail, apparently because of mechanical pressure. Between such cystic spaces, the breast stroma and parenchyma may be infiltrated by columns and nests of deeply stained epithelial cells. These have round solid nuclei, eccentrically placed. The cytoplasm contains a single small or large vacuole. "Signet-ring" forms are produced by large amounts of intracellular mucoid substance. When the predominant picture consists of large mucoid spaces with few cells, the tumor is usually slow in its growth and metastasizes very late. However, the presence of cellular areas in which the cells are of "signet-ring" type (intracellular mucus) always makes such tumors unpredictable.

Infrequently, mucinous carcinoma presents as an ill-defined tumor with nondestructive extensive infiltrations by large granular cells with small round nuclei. Resemblance to granular cell myoblastoma (a benign tumor of the breast) may be striking (Fig. 38-28). Multiple blocks should be examined to identify malignant nuclear features, cytoplasmic vacuoles, single rows of hyperplastic cells, and proliferative epithelial abnormalities.

Acute inflammatory carcinoma

Acute inflammatory carcinoma is a condition occurring in the obese pendulous breasts of young women, especially during lactation (50%). It comprises 1% of mammary carcinomas and is a special tumor only by virtue of clinical findings. It very closely resembles an acute inflammation of the breast and has been called erysipeloid carcinoma or carcinomatous mastitis. It generally is associated with outstanding signs and symptoms of inflammation—both local and generalized. It is sudden in onset, showing a rapidly developing discoloration and induration of the breast. It develops an intense reddish purple hue that may extend onto the chest wall or to the opposite breast. The skin is hot and dry and frequently shows a diffuse scaling. It has a particularly indurated feel. The crusted nipple generally is retracted so as to be barely visible. Frequently, the breast substance pre-

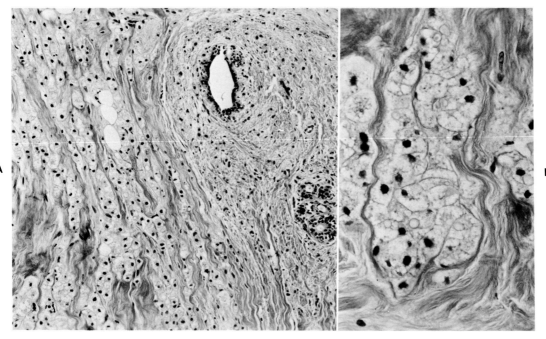

Fig. 38-28 Unusual histologic pattern of infiltrating and metastasizing mucinous carcinoma masquerading as "granular cell myoblastoma." (**A,** ×160; **B,** ×390.)

sents no definable tumor but a diffuse brawny induration. On gross examination of such a breast, a very thick edematous skin and breast stroma are readily identified. In many instances, the fat and stroma are poorly demarcated and there is diffuse induration of all structures. In rare instances, a large, centrally situated, poorly defined mass can be identified, and this generally has the characteristics of an infiltrating adenocarcinoma. Histologic characteristics are not specific, but infiltration of the subepidermal lymphatics and vessels is the identifying feature. This apparently represents retrograde lymphatic metastasis from blockage of the deeply situated lymph channels.[76] Similar minute clusters of neoplastic cells infiltrate throughout the breast substance. One-half of the patients develop widespread skin metastasis, and more than three-fourths of the patients have axillary metastasis when seen.

Lobular carcinoma

Carcinoma originating in ductules of the histoanatomic units called lobules and distending its ductules without invasion is known as *in situ lobular carcinoma*. Multicentric independent foci of disease and bilaterality are additional characteristics. In situ lobular carcinoma frequently is demonstrable in breasts removed for clinical cancer, in the contralateral breast on biopsy, and in bi-opsied benign lesions.[66, 77] It is a presymptomatic, preclinical microscopic cancer not suspected or identified by gross examination of breast tissue. Diagnosis is histologic—viz., epithelial filling and distention of ductules by a single type cell population, uniform in size, shape, and round dark nuclei in a constant repetitive pattern. Simple excision of the lesion is inadequate (Fig. 38-29). Presently, we interpret other patterns of ductular proliferations (nondistending multiform cells irregularly spaced) as less than cancer, and record them as "atypical epithelial proliferation," "duct adenosis," "papillomatosis," "suspicious ductular hyperplasia," etc. A system of quantitation of histologic features predicting biologic behavior of some lesions has been proposed.[56] Another decade or two will pass before we properly and affirmatively associate the "atypicalities" with evolution of in situ lobular carcinoma. More than twenty-five years have been invested in gaining convincing facts for the general acceptance of "lobular in situ carcinoma" as a stage of clinical carcinoma.

Infiltrating and metastasizing lobular carcinomas comprise approximately 10% of all breast cancers and derive from in situ lobular forms.[82] Transitions between the two patterns are clear. Infiltration of fibrous and fatty stroma is by relatively small uniform cells,

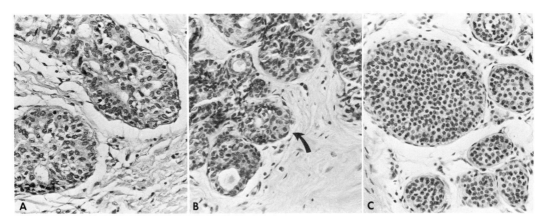

Fig. 38-29 Examples of lobular epithelial proliferations. **A** and **B**, Benign. **C**, Malignant—lobular in situ carcinoma. **A**, Terminal ductular atypical proliferation. **B**, Atypical lobular hyperplasia. Compare cytology at end of arrow with **C**. **C**, In situ lobular carcinoma. Single type cell population with uniform dispersion in distended ductules. The specimen shown in **B** suggests positive relationship between atypical lobular hyperplasia and lobular carcinoma in situ by cluster of carcinoma in situ kind of cells. What does specimen shown in **A** mean in high-risk women? In postmenopausal women? (**A** to **C**, ×320.)

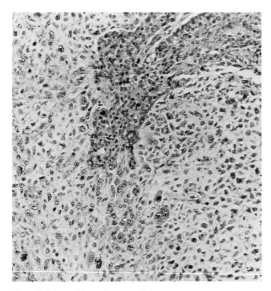

Fig. 38-30 Chondromucoid sarcomatous metaplasia in carcinoma of breast. Darker epithelial component blends with sarcomatous features just below midfield.

chiefly single or in rows, as beads on a string, reminiscent of scirrhous adenocarcinoma. Gross specimen characteristics of increased density and turgor may be ill-defined.

Rare tumors

Histologic patterns of rarely encountered epithelial tumors include squamous cell carcinoma, adenoid cystic carcinoma, sweat gland type carcinoma, and carcinoma showing mesenchymal metaplasia, chondromatous or osseous (Figs. 38-30 and 38-31).

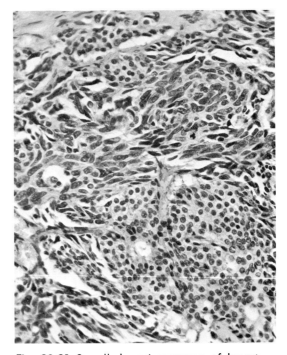

Fig. 38-31 So-called carcinosarcoma of breast—infiltrating carcinoma of breast having histologic features of sarcoma.

Sarcoma

The specialized mesenchyma of the breast, along with epithelium, has the capacity to form tumors—i.e., fibroadenoma or giant myxofibroadenoma. Lobulations and cystic formations in very large tumors of this type are emphasized by the designation "*cystosarcoma phyllodes,*" although a very small number

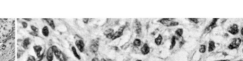
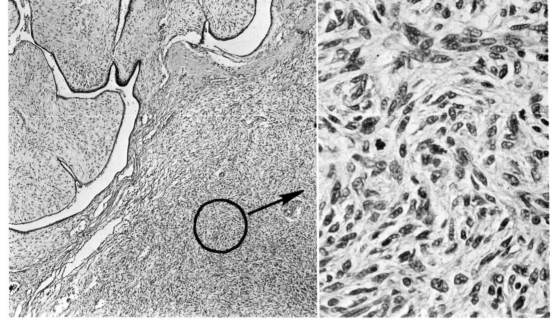

Fig. 38-32 A, Cystosarcoma phyllodes, malignant form showing cellular atypical stroma. **B,** Enlargement of area in circle.

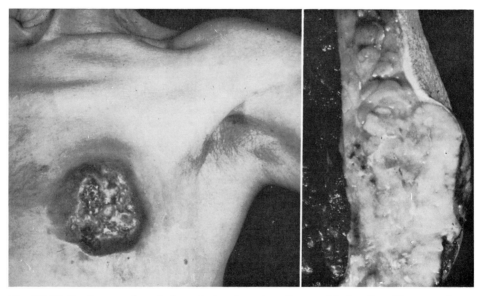

Fig. 38-33 Carcinoma of male breast showing ulceration and induration. Gross specimen reveals attachment to pectoral muscle and invasion of skin.

actually are malignant. The lesion may be very large, yet not infiltrative. Few are frankly malignant, metastasizing (to lungs rather than axillary nodes) as fibrosarcomas, liposarcomas, or mixtures including muscle tissue. To avoid errors, it is preferred to add "benign" or "malignant" to the diagnosis of cystosarcoma phyllodes (Fig. 38-32).

Other sarcomas not in context with fibroadenoma or epithelial participation are by and large much more malignant: liposarcoma, fibrosarcoma, leiomyosarcoma, soft parts osteogenic sarcoma, and angiosarcoma. The latter may appear deceptively innocent. Hodgkin's disease, reticulum cell sarcoma, lymphosarcoma, and malignant fibrohistiocytic proliferations in the breast are seldom local disease only. Granular cell myoblastoma may be a "tumor of the breast."

Cancer of male breast

Cancer of the male breast (Fig. 38-33), although infrequent, presents clinical and pathologic findings quite similar to those of cancer of the female breast. The report of Treves and Holleb presents an unusually rich experience with this disease[98] (see also discussion of gynecomastia, p. 1581).

REFERENCES
General

1 Cutler, M.: Tumors of the breast, Philadelphia, 1962, J. B. Lippincott Co.
2 Ewing, J.: Neoplastic diseases, Philadelphia, 1940, W. B. Saunders Co.
3 Geschickter, C. F.: Diseases of the breast, ed. 2, Philadelphia, 1945, J. B. Lippincott Co.

Development and structure

4 Bloom, H. J. G., editor: Symposium on the prognosis of malignant tumors of the breast, New York, 1962, Hafner Publishing Co., Inc.
5 Bunker, M. L., and Peters, M. V.: Amer. J. Obstet. Gynec. 85:312-321, 1963.
6 Eggeling, H. V.: In von Molloendorff, W., editor: Handbuch der mikroskopischen Anatomie des Menschens, Berlin, 1927, Julius Springer (die Milchdruse).
7 Hasson, J., and Pope, C. H.: Surgery 49:313-316, 1962.
8 Khazan, N., Primo, C., Danon, A., Assael, M., Sulman, F. G., and Winnik, H. Z.: Arch. Int. Pharmacodyn. 136:291-305, 1962.
9 Koeneke, I. A.: Amer. J. Obstet. Gynec. 27:584-592, 1934.
10 Robinson, B.: Med. J. Aust. 2:239-241, 1957.
11 Rosenburg, A.: Frankfurt. Z. Path. 27:466-506, 1922.
12 Schultz, A.: In Henke, F., and Lubarsch, O.: Handbuch der speziellen pathologischen Anatomie und Histologie, Berlin, 1933, Julius Springer (pathologische Anatomie der Brustdruse).
13 Weinshel, L. R., and Demakopoulos, N.: Amer. J. Surg. 60:76-80, 1943.

Hypertrophy
Gynecomastia

14 Greenblatt, R. B., and Perez-Ballester, B.: Med. Asp. Hum. Sex. 3:52-63, 1969.
15 Karsner, H. T.: Amer. J. Path. 22:235-315, 1946.
16 Treves, N.: Cancer 11:1083-1102, 1958.

Inflammations
Plasma cell mastitis

17 Adair, F. E.: Arch. Surg. (Chicago) 26:735-749, 1933.
18 Cromar, C. D. L., and Dockerty, M. B.: Proc. Staff Meet. Mayo Clin. 16:775-783, 1941.

Chronic mastitis
Tuberculosis

19 Webster, C. S.: Amer. J. Surg. 45:557-562, 1939.

Syphilis

20 Stokes, J. H.: Modern clinical syphilology, ed. 2, Philadelphia, 1934, W. B. Saunders Co., p. 1301.

Fat necrosis

21 Adair, F. E., and Munzer, J. T.: Amer. J. Surg. 74:117-128, 1947.
22 Menville, J. G.: Amer. J. Cancer 24:797-806, 1935.

Mammary dysplasia

23 Bloodgood, J. C.: Arch. Surg. (Chicago) 3:445, 1921.
24 Bloodgood, J. C.: J.A.M.A. 93:1056-1059, 1929.
25 Ingleby, H.: Arch. Path. (Chicago) 33:573-588, 1942.
26 Kier, L. C., Hickey, R. C., Keettel, W. C., and Womack, N. A.: Trans. Southern Surg. Ass. 73:229-232, 1951.
27 Kuzma, J. F.: Amer. J. Path. 19:473-489, 1943.
28 Kuzma, J. F.: Unpublished data, 1960.
29 Lewis, D., and Geschickter, C. F.: Amer. J. Surg. 24:280-304, 1934.
30 Nathanson, I. T.: Surgery 16:108-140, 1944.
31 Ochsner, A.: Postgrad. Med. 33:133-138, 1963.
32 Sandison, A. T.: An autopsy study of the adult human breast, 1961, National Cancer Institute Monograph No. 8, United States Public Health Service.
33 Semb, C.: Acta Chir. Scand. 64(suppl. 10):1-484, 1928.
34 Swerdlow, M., and Humphrey, L. J.: Arch. Surg. (Chicago) 87:457-460, 1963.
35 Urban, J. A., and Adair, F. E.: Cancer 2:625-634, 1949.
36 Warren, S.: Surgery 19:32-39, 1946.
37 Womack, N. A.: Amer. Surg. 24:618-629, 1958.

Tumors
Benign tumors
Fibroadenoma

38 Cooper, W. G., Jr., and Ackerman, L. V.: Surg. Gynec. Obstet. 77:279-283, 1943.
39 Geschickter, C. F., Lewis, D. D., and Hartman, C. G.: Amer. J. Cancer 21:828-859, 1934.
40 Ingleby, H.: Arch. Path. (Chicago) 14:21-41, 1932.
41 Moran, C. S.: Arch. Surg. (Chicago) 31:688-708, 1935.
42 Oliver, R. L., and Major, R. C.: Amer. J. Cancer 21:1-85, 1934.

Papilloma

43 Davis, J. B.: Progr. Clin. Cancer 3:221-224, 1967 (cystic disease of breast: relationship to mammary cancer).
44 Gray, H. K., and Wood, G. A.: Arch. Surg. (Chicago) 42:203-208, 1941.

45 Hart, D.: Arch. Surg. (Chicago) **14:**793-835, 1927.
46 Kraus, F. T., and Neubecker, R. D.: Cancer **15:**444-455, 1962.
47 McDivitt, R. W., Stewart, F. W., and Berg, J. W.: Tumors of the breast. In Atlas of tumor pathology, Series 2, Fasc. 2, Washington, D. C., 1968, Armed Forces Institute of Pathology, p. 12.
48 McLaughlin, C. W., Jr., Schenken, J. R., and Tamisiea, J. X.: Ann. Surg. **153:**735-744, 1961.
49 Saphir, O., and Parker, M. L.: Amer. J. Path. **16:**189-210, 1940.

Malignant tumors

50 Adair, F. E.: New York J. Med. **59:**2149-2153, 1959.
51 Adair, F. E., and Herrmann, J. B.: Surgery **19:**55-73, 1946 (sarcoma).
52 American Joint Committee on Cancer Staging and End Results Reporting: Clinical staging system for cancer of the breast, 1962.
53 Asch, M. J., Wiedel, P. D., and Habif, D. V.: Arch. Surg. (Chicago) **96:**840-843, 1968.
54 Benson, W. R.: Cancer **10:**1235-1245, 1957.
55 Berkson, J., Harrington, S. W., Clagett, O. T., Kirklin, J. W., Dockerty, M. B., and McDonald; J. R.: Proc. Staff Meet. Mayo Clin. **32:**645-670, 1957.
56 Black, M. M., and Chabon, A. B.: In Pathology annual, vol. 4 (S. C. Sommers, editor), New York, 1969, Appleton-Century-Crofts, p. 185-210.
57 Bloodgood, J. C.: Amer. J. Cancer **22:**842-853, 1934.
58 Bulbrook, R. D., Hayward, J. L., Spicer, C. C., and Thomas, B. S.: Lancet **2:**1238-1240, 1962.
59 Cheatle, G. L., and Cutler, M.: Arch. Surg. (Chicago) **20:**569-590, 1930.
60 Cole, P., and MacMahon, B.: Lancet **1:**604-606, 1969.
61 Copeland, M. M.: Amer. Surg. **29:**304-316, 1963.
62 Cutler, S. J., and Connelly, R. R.: Cancer **23:** 767-771, 1969.
62a Denoix, P., and Rouquette, C., editors: Symposium on the prognosis of malignant tumours of the breast, New York, 1963, Pitman Publishing Corp.
63 Dunn, J. E., Jr.: Cancer **23:**775-780, 1969.
64 Edelman, S.: J. Mount Sinai Hosp. N. Y. **34:** 578-586, 1967.
65 Egan, R. L.: Amer. J. Roentgen. **88:**1095-1101, 1962.
66 Ferber, B., Handy, V. H., Gerhardt, P. R., and Soloman, M.: Cancer in New York State, exclusive of New York City, 1941-1960: a review of incidence, mortality, probability, and survivorship, Albany, N. Y., 1962, New York State Department of Health, Bureau of Cancer Control.
67 Foot, N. C.: Arch. Path. (Chicago) **33:**905-916, 1942.
68 Foote, F. W., Jr., and Stewart, F. W.: Amer. J. Path. **17:**491-496, 1941.
69 Foote, F. W., Jr., and Stewart, F. W.: Surgery **19:**74-99, 1946.
70 Fox, S. L.: Ann. Surg. **100:**401-421, 1934 (sarcoma).

71 Goldenberg, V.E., Wiegenstein, L., and Mottet, N. K.: Amer. J. Clin. Path. **49:**52-59, 1968.
72 Hartmann, W. H., and Sherlock, P.: Cancer **14:**426-431, 1961.
73 Hayward, J. L.: Proc. Roy. Soc. Med. **59:** 1204-1208, 1966.
74 Jessiman, A. G., and Moore, F. D.: New Eng. J. Med. **254:**846-853, 900-906, 947-952, 1956.
75 Leis, H. P., Jr., and Bowers, W. F.: Western J. Surg. Obstet. Gynec. **72:**171-176, 1964.
76 Lemon, H. M.: Cancer **23:**781-790, 1969.
77 Lewison, E. F.: Milit. Med. **129:**115-123, 1964.
78 MacCarty, W. C.: Proc. Staff Meet Mayo Clin. **12:**817-822, 1937.
79 MacDonald, I. G.: Surg. Gynec. Obst. **92:** 443-452, 1951.
80 Massopust, L. C.: Surg. Gynec. Obstet. **86:** 54-58, 1948 (infrared photography).
81 Muir, R.: J. Path. Bact. **49:**299-312, 1939.
82 Newman, W.: Ann. Surg. **164:**305-314, 1966.
83 O'Grady, W. P., and McDivitt, R. W.: Arch. Path. (Chicago) **88:**162-165, 1969.
84 Orr, J. W., and Parish, D. J.: J. Path. Bact. **84:**201-208, 1962.
85 Paget, J.: St. Barth. Hosp. Rep. **10:**87-89, 1874.
86 Potter, J. F., Slimbaugh, W. P., and Woodward, S. C.: Ann. Surg. **167:**829-838, 1968.
87 Rogers, H., and Flo, S.: New Eng. J. Med. **226:**841-844, 1942 (sarcoma).
88 Ross, W. L.: Cancer **23:**762-766, 1969.
89 Schoenberg, B. S., Greenberg, R. A., and Eisenberg, H.: J. Nat. Cancer Inst. **43:**15-32, 1969.
90 Shimkin, M. B.: In discussion of Cutler, S. J., and Connelly, R. R.: Cancer **23:**767-774, 1969.
91 Sommers, S. C., and Teloh, H. A.: Arch. Path. (Chicago) **53:**160-166, 1952.
92 Stewart, F. W.: In Atlas of tumor pathology, Sect. IX, Fasc. 34, Washington, D. C., 1950, Armed Forces Institute of Pathology (tumors of breast).
93 Stewart, F. W., and Treves, N.: Cancer **1:**64-81, 1948.
94 Strax, P., Venet, L., Shapiro, S., and Gross, S.: Cancer **20:**2184-2188, 1967.
95 Symmers, W. S.: Brit. Med. J. **2:**83-85, 1968.
96 Taylor, G. W., and Meltzer, A.: Amer. J. Cancer **33:**33-49, 1938.
97 Taylor, H. B., Irey, N. S., and Norris, H. J.: J.A.M.A. **202:**637-639, 1967.
98 Treves, N., and Holleb, A. I.: Cancer **8:**1239-1250, 1955.
99 Urban, J. A.: Cancer **20:**1867-1870, 1967.
100 Wynder, E. L., Bross, I. J., and Hirayama, T.: Cancer **13:**559-601, 1960.

Metastasis

101 Batson, O. V.: Ann. Surg. **112:**138-149, 1940.
102 Dorn, H. F., and Cutler, S. J.: Morbidity from cancer in the United States, Public Health Monograph No. 29, Washington, D. C., 1955, Government Printing Office.
103 Saphir, O., and Parker, M. L.: Arch. Surg. (Chicago) **42:**1003-1018, 1941.
104 Warren, S., and Witham, E. N.: Surg. Gynec. Obstet. **57:**81-85, 1933.

Chapter 39

Skin

Arthur C. Allen

There is a sizable group of dermatoses that has significant morphologic individuality. In many instances, the distinguishing features are so clear cut that a diagnosis may be offered on examination merely of the histologic slide. In other cases, a small range of diagnoses may be suggested by the section. In the remainder, the microscopic changes give no diagnostic help in the absence of a clinical history. Although the size of the last group will obviously be determined by the experience of the examiner, the percentage of cases that falls into it can be made sufficiently low as to merit the lagging interest of the general pathologist. One of the major difficulties in the learning of dermatopathology is that the changes usually are not of the "all-or-none" or *qualitatively* distinct variety but are often a matter of weighted *quantitative* differences. The proper judgment of these differences depends on a knowledge of the normal histologic range of the structures of the skin, as well as on an ability to add up and interpret a whole series of aberrations in these structures.

Obviously, only a small segment of cutaneous pathology can be included in this chapter. Accordingly, it would seem to underscore the applicability of dermatopathology best if some of the many lesions diagnosable by histologic characteristics alone were given preference over those less easily recognizable. For the latter, the reader may refer to the general references.[1-6]

STRUCTURE OF NORMAL SKIN

The skin normally varies in color, elasticity, thickness, blood supply, and texture depending on anatomic location, age, state of nutrition, endocrinologic status, and race of the individual. With the unaided eye, fine (Blaschko's) ridges are noted over the skin generally, and coarse folds, allowing for movement, are present, particularly over the joints.

Between the ridges are *sulci of Heidenhain.* The ridges are further marked by delicate, crisscross, triangular or polygonal lines. In recent years, there has been considerable interest in the science of *dermatoglyphics,* which deals with the interpretation of detailed patterns of sulci, furrows, and ridges of the palms. Dermatoglyphic abnormalities have been observed in patients with rubella, psoriasis, neurofibromatosis, anonychia, a variety of chromosomal abnormalities, and in some disorders otherwise unassociated with cutaneous manifestations.[7]

The ostia of sweat glands, the pores, open onto the ridges. The hair, of course, varies, too, in texture, length, density, contour, and color depending on age, race, sex, etc. The smooth, hairless skin, or the skin with fine vellus hairs, is known as *glabrous* skin. The epidermis varies over most of the body from 0.07 mm to 0.12 mm and from 0.8 mm to 1.4 mm or more on the palms and soles. The cutis has a corresponding range of thickness. The junction of the cutis and the subcutis or subcuticular fat is usually indistinct, except in certain regions such as the forehead, ear, perineum, and scrotum.

Fig. 39-1 represents a diagram of normal skin. It is of diagnostic use to bear in mind that the skin varies in different parts of the body. For example, sebaceous glands are particularly prominent about the face, especially in the region of the nose, so that diagnoses of hyperplasia or adenoma of sebaceous glands should take this feature into account. The epidermis is normally thin and the rete ridges relatively inconspicuous over the tibia, the breasts, and the flexor surfaces of forearms. This variant should not, therefore, be mistaken for atrophy. Similarly, the dermis over the lower legs, for example, is normally much less thick than it is in many other portions of the body, so that, again, the possibil-

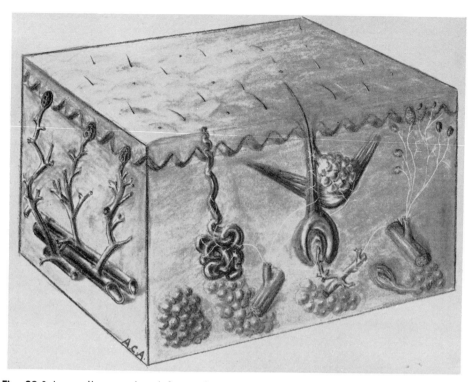

Fig. 39-1 In smaller panel at left are shown arteries, veins, and lymphatic vessels, along with their plexuses within papillae. In reality, plexuses of all three types of vessels overlap in same regions. In larger front panel are included appendages, nerves, and subcutaneous fat. Tubular sweat gland on left reaches surface through duct that, in its course through epidermis, maintains its own epithelial lining. Ductal ostium or sweat pore is independent of hair follicle. In center is pilosebaceous apparatus comprising hair follicle, sebaceous glands, and arrectores pilorum. Nerves and vessels supplying critical papillae are shown at deep portion of follicle. Sebaceous gland is intimately linked to hair follicle, into which its duct empties directly. Arrectores pilorum not only stiffen hair shaft but, as may be surmised from position illustrated, also help, by contraction, to expel contents of sebaceous gland and to constrict superficial vessels. On right are shown nerves and nerve endings—corpuscles of Merkel-Ranvier, Meissner, Ruffini, Krause, and Pacini. Nerve fibers entwined about appendages are also illustrated. (From Allen, A. C.: The skin, Grune & Stratton, Inc.; by permission.)

ity of confusion with atrophy exists. The elastic tissue of the dermis shows such a large range in its quantity, as well as in the degree of fraying and splintering of the fibers, even in normal tissues, that considerable caution should be used in concluding that abnormalities of elastic tissue are present. Finally, the normally thick stratum corneum of the sole of the foot may prompt the diagnosis of keratoderma. These are a few of the examples of the variation in cutaneous histology, an accurate evaluation of which is clearly essential for an appraisal of some of the qualitatively similar pathologic changes.

Epidermis

The epidermis is composed of the following layers:

1 Basal cell layer (stratum germinativum)

2 Prickle cell layers (stratum spinosum, rete muscosum, rete malpighii)
3 Granular layers (stratum granulosum)
4 Stratum lucidum
5 Cornified layer (stratum corneum)

The basal cell layer is one cell thick and forms the junction between epidermis and dermis. The nuclei are relatively hyperchromatic, arranged perpendicular to the epidermal "basement membrane," and normally contain a few mitoses as evidence of the activity of a layer that serves in part as the progenitor of the remainder of the epidermis. Interspersed in the basal layer are cells with a clear zone separating and often compressing most of the cytoplasm and nucleus away from the cell wall (the so-called "cellule claire"). The cytoplasm may or may not contain melanin, but these cells are likely to be dopa-positive and, accordingly, are melanocytes. Not all melanocytes of the basal layer are "clear cells." Ultrastructurally, the melanocytes contain melanosomes but are thought by most observers to contain few or no desmosomes or tonofilaments. As a matter of fact, such structures may be noted, albeit often reduced in number, not only in many melanocytes but, more vividly and meaningfully, also in the marginal cells of melanocarcinomas in situ (Fig. 39-46). The fairly universal insistence that keratinocytes lack lysosomes has contributed to the circular reasoning that melanocytes are *ipso facto* nonkeratinocytes inasmuch as they contain these organelles. A directly contrary observation has recently clearly indicated that keratinocytes are characterized by *Odland bodies,* which are membrane-coating granules, keratinosomes, or lysosomes.[112] For a long time it has been accepted, on debatable evidence, that melanocytes are really nerve endings that migrated from the neural crest, became incorporated in the epidermis, and later constituted the source of some pigmented nevi. In our opinion, the process of conversion of basal cells and keratinocytes into melanocytes normally takes place continuously and may be retarded (as in vitiligo) or accelerated (as in sunburn). Actually, as would be anticipated, the numbers of dopa-reactive epidermal melanocytes have been found to be increased following irradiation with ultraviolet light, although contrary results previously had been reported.[82] In other words, the activation of basal cells and keratinocytes into melanocytes varies in speed and extent with different age groups, races, and stimuli. However, it would be misleading to fail to acknowledge that the concept of neurogenesis of melanocytes, nevi, and melanocarcinomas is the popular one at the moment.

The emphasis on cytochemical, functional, and ultrastructural differences, such as differences in organelles or content of enzymes and hormones, as a basis for differences in histogenesis seems to be somewhat overdrawn. The hiatus in this kind of histogenetic logic is that comparable, informative cellular situations are overlooked. For example, no one doubts the common genesis of the intestinal argentaffin and its accompanying mucosal epithelial cell, or the various cells of the gastric mucosa, or the ACTH-secreting cell of the oat cell carcinoma and the nonhormonal bronchial epithelium. Moreover, the presence of an enzyme (e.g., dopa oxidase) in one cell and its absence in an adjacent basal cell or keratinocyte does not prove a difference in histogenesis between the melanocyte and the other epidermal cells any more than the presence of serotonin in the argentaffin cells of intestinal glands establishes an embryogenesis different from that of the adjacent mucous or Paneth cell of the mucosa.

There appears to be as much validity to a concept of dual genesis for epidermal melanocytes and keratinocytes on the basis of difference in organelles as there is for concluding, for example, that Paneth, goblet, and enterochromaffin cells of a duodenal crypt represent three separate histogenetic lines. It is no surprise that recent ultrastructural studies have confirmed the histogenetic unity of these intestinal cells—i.e., their derivation from a common less differentiated cell.[101]

There has been a revival of interest in the nature of the controverted intraepidermal, aurophilic **Langerhans' cell.** To some, it is a worn-out ("effete") melanocyte with a debatable capacity to manufacture or even to phagocytose melanin. To others, it is a form of intraepidermal neural element with a spectrum of "neural enzymes," including ATPase and leucine aminopeptidase. To still others, it is a histiocyte that has wandered into the epidermis and is identical with the histiocytes of "histiocytosis X." Ultrastructurally, it was forcefully emphasized that this cell possessed a specific racquet-shaped organelle but, as was to be expected, similar organelles have been observed in other organs such as the thymus gland. More recently, it has been admitted, in a refreshing reversal of opinion, that Langerhans' cells are not related to melanocytes, that they are not derived from the neural crest, and that "the whole question of their nature, derivation, and function must be regarded as wide open again."* This, one hundred years after the description of these epidermal cells by Langerhans! It will come as no surprise that, to the author, this cell has always appeared to be a modulated keratinocyte which, like other keratinocytes, has a variable content of enzymes, pigment, and organelles depending on its functional stage.[2] Obviously, these features are conditioned by genetics and the response to stimuli at a given time.

The prickle cells are several layers thick, the number varying in different parts of the body. The cells are joined by cytoplasmic

*From Breathnach, A. S., Silvers, W. K., Smith, J., and Heyner, S.: J. Invest. Derm. **50:**147-160, 1968; copyrighted by The Williams & Wilkins Co.

bridges (spines, prickles, desmosomes), which serve as the most easily recognizable identification of such cells, both in squamous cell neoplasms and in metaplastic processes. The intracellular cytoplasmic *tonofilaments* generally are regarded as the precursors of keratin. Glycogen is usually present. The generally accepted absence of lysosomes in keratinocytes recently has been disputed, thereby narrowing the supposed differences between keratinocytes and melanocytes.[37]

The *stratum granulosum* averages about two layers thick and is composed of cells with blue, round cytoplasmic granules of keratohyalin. The chemical nature of the keratohyaline granules remains essentially obscure. Although superficially resembling nuclear material, they are Feulgen negative and PAS negative and contain no protein-bound sulfhydryl groups. They appear as electron-dense bodies and apparently contain tonofilaments. The granules are also osmophilic, are digested with elastase, and are presumed to be closely related histogenetically to keratin. The stratum lucidum, which is practically confined to the palms and soles, is a clear, homogeneous, acidophilic, anuclear, thin layer of "eleidin."

The *stratum corneum,* also normally without nuclei, is made up of various thicknesses of keratin. The stratum corneum, particularly its lower half, is important as the barrier in regulating the transfer of water through the skin. Fat globules may be present in the two uppermost layers.

PAS-positive, diastase-resistant mucopolysaccharides are present in the epidermis and are presumed to play a role in binding or cementing the epidermal cells together. Since keratinization normally takes place in the upper layers of epidermis, the acid mucopolysaccharides are presumably degraded, allowing the keratin to be discarded as invisible flakes. With incomplete degradation of the mucopolysaccharides, visible coherent, parakeratotic scales occur, as in psoriasis.[88]

The elaboration of adequate lipoprotein with a particular species of sterol ester is apparently necessary for normal keratinization. Compounds that inhibit cholesterol synthesis, for example, may lead to disordered ichthyotic keratinization.[113] The obvious mucus-producing capacity of epidermis is manifested in some epidermal carcinomas and in *follicular mucinosis.* There is convincing histologic evidence to indicate that a true epidermal basement membrane, equivalent, for example, to the one surrounding glands, does not exist. Basement membranes in other locations, such as those about sweat glands, renal tubules, etc., are argyrophilic. No such continuous epidermal basement membrane is demonstrable with silver stains, although an illusion of one occasionally is created by argyrophilic granules of melanin aligned in the basal layer. On the other hand, stains with the periodic acid–Schiff reagent do reveal what appear to be interrupted segments of a basement membrane. This simulation is caused by the presence of polysaccharides that have been irregularly concentrated by the varying densities of the subepidermal collagen, especially with edema of the upper cutis. In this connection, one other fact should be mentioned again. Basal cells do have "intercellular" bridges (desmosomes) that bind them to the overlying cells of the stratum spinosum and, in their upper portions, to each other. To the corium they are attached by semidesmosomes to an ultrastructurally visible membrane called an *"adepidermal lamina,"* visible only electronmicroscopically and not equivalent to the argyrophilic structures readily detectable even in routine stains, as mentioned.

Dermis

The dermis or corium is divided into the superficial pars papillaris and the deeper pars reticularis. The papillae of the dermis alternate with projections of epidermis called *rete ridges.* The length of the papillae, the thickness of the overlying epidermal plate, the vascularity, the edema, and the direction and consistency of the collagenous fibers of the papillae are all of diagnostic value. In the papillary portion, the fibers of collagen tend to run vertically. In the deeper part, the fibers are rather loosely dispersed in a horizontal direction. Accuracy in evaluating changes in the consistency, tinctorial qualities, and cellularity of the collagen and elastic tissue of the dermis furnishes the basis for many diagnoses. With electron microscopy, elastic fibers show a fibrillar structure within an otherwise almost homogeneous matrix in which dense elements are embedded but in which the characteristic periodicity of collagen is lacking.[26]

The cutaneous *appendages* include the sweat glands, sebaceous glands, hair follicles, arrectores pilorum, and nails. The sweat glands are coiled glands of two varieties: eccrine and apocrine.

The *eccrine* glands are universally distributed in the skin and are made up of several coils of tubular glands lying deep in the dermis. These glands empty their secretion into tubules traversing the dermis and epidermis, opening into the fine ridges of the skin as pores. The coils are lined by two principal layers of cells: (1) the more superficial, basophilic, *dark,* granular mucopolysaccharide-containing cells and (2) the more basilar, acidophilic *clear* or chief cells. There may be some interdigitation between these cells. A flattened third type of cell, the myoepithelial or "basket" cell, is interposed between these secretory cells and the basement membrane. A large battery of enzymes is detectable in the eccrine glands, including oxidases, dehydrogenases, phosphorylases, alkaline phosphatase, and glucuronidases. Their presence has been utilized in defining certain of the neoplasms of sweat glands. The ducts are lined also by two layers of epithelial cells, but the myoepithelium is absent. The inner lining of the ducts of sweat glands is keratinized in their course through the epidermis, and, indeed, some of the neoplasms of sweat glands show evidence of squamous cell metaplasia. In any case, the inner hyaline membrane of the ducts often serves as a clue to the genesis of these neoplasms.

The *apocrine glands* occur in the axilla, groin, nipple, umbilicus, anus, and genital region. The apocrine glands are easily recognized by their large lumens, prominence of secretory cytoplasmic granules, and rows of myoepithelial cells longitudinally oriented below the cuboidal or columnar secretory cells. The periglandular basement membrane is especially conspicuous. Light yellow, sudanophilic granules, as well as granules of hemosiderin and a minimum of glycogen, are commonly present. Mucin normally is present within the lumen and cells of apocrine glands and is PAS positive and diastase resistant. Desmosomes, similar to those of keratinocytes, have been noted.[43] The ultrastructural observation of canaliculi, particularly, suggests that an eccrine type as well as an apocrine (i.e., apically erosive) type of secretion occurs.[25] Secretory activity varies with the menstrual cycle. The ducts of the apocrine glands usually open in close relationship to the hair follicles but may reach the surface independently, as do the eccrine glands.

The *sebaceous* or *holocrine glands* are racemose structures that serve mainly as appendages to the hair follicles to which they are attached. Each alveolus is rimmed by a basement membrane surrounding one or two layers of squamous cells, internal to which are the characteristic sebaceous cells with small round nuclei and abundant, finely latticed, fatty cytoplasm. The sebaceous cells are pushed toward the duct, wherein they finally rupture and release their fatty contents in the hair follicle. Modifications of sebaceous glands occur in the eyelids and ears, in the areolae of the nipple, and in the male and female genitalia (glandulae odoriferae). In these regions, they are unconnected with hairs or hair follicles. The amount of sebum secreted is about the same in the adolescent boy and girl, shows no appreciable change in the aging female, and decreases in the aging male. Ectopic sebaceous glands may be found in the salivary glands and in the glans penis. Such ectopic glands of the corona penis are often referred to as Tyson's glands. Actually, Tyson appears to have described a beaded rim of fibroepithelial pearly nodules about the corona.

The *hair* consists of a shaft which, at its lower end, enlarges into a bulb. The bulb embraces an invaginating dermal papilla, through which the hair receives its blood supply. The intracutaneous portion of the hair shaft and the bulb are enclosed in a hair follicle. The hair shaft is made up of a cuticle, a sheath, and a more or less pigmented cortex and medulla, the latter being absent in lanugo hairs.

The *arrectores pilorum* are bands of smooth muscle originating in or near the papillary layer of the dermis and inserting at several points into the outer layer of adjacent hair follicles just above their papillae. The direction of the muscle is at an angle to the hairs so that their contraction ("goose flesh") causes the hairs to be erected. At the same time, the superficial vessels are constricted to avoid cooling, and sebaceous secretion is expelled by the pressure of the contracting arrectores pilorum. However, there is some disagreement as to this last function.

The *blood* and *lymphatic vessels* of the skin are arranged in plexuses. The arterial vessels are derived from the subcutaneous arteries, which give off plexuses to the papillary layer, as well as to the reticular layer and the various appendages. It has been suggested that the selective localization of infiltrate to various components of the dermis is related to the pattern of these plexuses. In the skin of certain regions of the body, particularly the fingers, there are, normally, arteriovenous shunts or *glomera* that serve to regulate blood flow and surface temperature. The glomus is composed of an afferent arteriole, a shunt called the Sucquet-Hoyer canal, and an efferent vein. The canal is lined by layers of rounded glomus cells that have a contractile function. The veins also form plexuses in the papillary, subpapillary, and deep reticular layers, as well as about the appendages.

The lymphatic plexuses are localized principally in the papillae and at the junction of dermis and subcutaneous tissue. The deeper lymphatic vessels have valves.

The *nerves* of the skin are preponderantly medullated. A few are nonmedullated and lead to the blood vessels, smooth muscles, epidermis, hair follicles, and glands. The specialized nerve endings include the corpuscles of *Vater-Pacini*, which are found in the deep layers of the skin and subcutaneous tissue, in the mucous membranes, and in the conjunctiva and cornea. These structures are particularly numerous in the skin of the nipple and external genital organs. Other nerve endings are the *Meissner corpuscles* of the papillae of the skin of palms, soles, and tips of fingers and toes, the end bulbs of *Krause,* which are smaller than but structurally similar to the Meissner corpuscles and are found in the external genitalia, the elongated, dermal corpuscles of *Ruffini*, and the intraepidermal disclike, tactile *Merkel-Ranvier* corpuscles, which are identified with silver stains and are present in the epidermis and external root sheath of hairs. The endings are presumably receptors for touch (Merkel-Ranvier and Meissner corpuscles), pressure (pacinian corpuscles), heat (corpuscles of Ruffini), and cold (end bulbs of Krause).

DEFINITIONS
Clinical terms

macule circumscribed flat area of altered coloration of skin; evanescent or permanent; varies in size from pinhead to several centimeters, in color from red (erythema), brown (ephelis), and the various colors of blood pigment (petechiae and ecchymoses) to white (vitiligo), and in shape from circular, polygonal, linear to the polymorphous varieties of erythema multiforme.

papule circumscribed elevated area; varies in size from pinhead to about 5 mm, in surface contour from flat, conical, pointed circular to umbilicated, in color from red, yellow, white to violaceous, and in shape of base from round to more or less polygonal (e.g., papules of lichen planus and psoriasis); the papule, as well as the macule, may provoke pruritus, burning sensation, anesthesia, and pain or may cause no symptoms; both macules and papules may be overlain by scales.

nodule an enlarged papule varying in size from about 0.5 cm to 2 cm, usually deep-seated, involving the lower dermis and subcutaneous fat (e.g., the nodules of rheumatoid arthritis and leprosy).

vesicle circumscribed, single or grouped elevations of the epidermis, beneath which are collections containing serum, plasma, or blood; surface may be flat, globoid, or umbilicated (e.g., smallpox and eczema).

pustule vesicle containing pus predominantly (e.g., impetigo).

bulla (bleb) similar to vesicle, except that the bullae are larger, varying from 0.5 cm to more than 8 cm (e.g., pemphigus).

scale loosened, imperfectly cornified, parakeratotic superficial layer of skin which is shed as fine, branny, dirty white, yellowish keratinous dust or large pearly white flakes; distribution may be focal or universal and usually is associated with inflammation of the skin (e.g., psoriasis and exfoliative dermatitis) but need not be (as in ichthyosis).

crust residue of dried serum, blood, pus, and epithelial, keratinous, and bacterial debris; crusts vary in color from yellow to green to dark brown, depending on the admixture of the different ingredients, and in consistency from a thin superficial and watery (as in impetigo) to a thick, bulky and loosely or firmly attached covering of a rupioid syphiloderm; crusts follow the oozing of serum, blood, or pus in a disrupted, eroded, or ulcerated epidermis (as in eczema, impetigo, smallpox, abrasions, and other conditions).

excoriation (erosion) superficial erosion and ulceration produced mechanically, usually by the fingernails in scratching pruritic skin or in picking at various lesions (as in "neurotic excoriations").

fissure (rhagade) linear, often crusted, tender, painful defect in continuity of the skin, occurring usually at mucocutaneous junctions at sites where there is normally considerable elasticity of the skin (e.g., about the anus, mouth, fingers, palms, and soles) and also in certain diseases (e.g., syphilis, nonspecific anal fissures, keratoderma, intertrigo, and eczema).

ulcer defect of the skin, deeper than an erosion or excoriation, extending at least into the dermis; the edges may be ragged, punched out in appearance, undermined or everted; the floor may be glazed or granular, puriform or hemorrhagic, and shallow or deep; the outline of an ulcer may be circular, serpiginous, crescentic, ovoid, or irregular; ulcers may be painless or exquisitely sensitive; they heal generally by concentric scarring and epithelization (e.g., tropical, diphtheritic, and varicose ulcers).

lichenification thickening of the skin with exaggeration of its normal markings so that the striae form a crisscross pattern; follows chronic irritation of pruritic skin.

comedo keratinous plug, sometimes admixed with bacteria and inflammatory cells, within ducts of sebaceous glands; characteristic of acne.

Histologic terms

acanthosis thickening through hyperplasia of the rete malpighii; may exist without hyperkeratosis (Fig. 39-15).

hyperkeratosis thickening of the keratinized layer, the stratum corneum; generally is associated with a prominent stratum granulosum (Fig. 39-33).

parakeratosis persistence of nuclei in the stratum corneum, signifying the presence clinically of a loosely adherent scale (e.g., dandruff); characterized by the absence or marked diminution of the stratum granulosum, except in the stage of healing (Fig. 39-15); with fluorescence microscopy (with acridine orange, rhodamine B, and thioflavine S), hyperkeratosis is reflected by orthrochromasia and brilliance and parakeratosis by dullness and metachromatic color changes.

spongiosis intercellular edema of the epidermis which, when marked, progresses to vesiculation (e.g., eczema).

acantholysis separation of individual cells from the stratum spinosum, with loss of prickles and consequent isolation within the fluid of a vesicle (e.g., pemphigus).

ballooning degeneration one of the diagnostic morphologic phenomena leading to vesiculation in viral diseases; characterized by the isolation of a cell from its neighbors, especially in the lower layers of the epidermis, the withdrawing of its prickles following intracytoplasmic edema and vacuolization, and the amitotic division of its nucleus so as to form a multinucleated giant cell (e.g., variola, but, particularly, herpes and varicella).

reticular colliquation a characteristic of the cutaneous vesicles due to viruses, as in ballooning degeneration; the cytoplasm of several cells becomes edematous, granular, coalescent, and partially disintegrated; the residual cytoplasm forms reticulated septa that separate multiloculated intraepidermal collections of fluid or vesicles; the nuclei become small, pyknotic, or completely karyorrhectic.

dyskeratosis abnormality of development or distinctive alteration of epidermal cells; two types are distinguished: (1) benign dyskeratosis—e.g., the molluscum bodies of molluscum contagiosum, represented by swollen brightly eosinophilic cells, mostly of the stratum granulosum, containing virus elementary bodies, or the *corps ronds* and *grains* of the stratum granulosum and stratum corneum, respectively, as noted in Darier's disease; in molluscum contagiosum, the dyskeratosis is owing to a virus; (2) malignant dyskeratosis—anaplastic changes such as hyperchromatism, changes in polarity, increase in mitotic figures, and enlargement of nuclei and nucleoli so as to signify potential or actual development of carcinoma (Fig. 39-35).

pseudoepitheliomatous hyperplasia marked acanthosis with extensive downgrowth of rete ridges such as may occur at the periphery of an ulcer, in bromodermas, and following insect bites; occasionally, the exuberant epidermal hyperplasia is mistaken for carcinoma as in so-called molluscum sebaceum or keratoacanthoma (Fig. 39-52).

liquefaction degeneration obliteration of the line of demarcation of epidermis and dermis by edema of the basal cells and subepidermal dermis, as well as by the presence of inflammatory cells at this junction (e.g., lichen planus and lupus erythematosus) (Fig. 39-11).

Eponyms

Eponyms are a part of the literature of the diseases of any organ and are especially common in dermatologic parlance. There are obvious disadvantages to the use of an eponym instead of an objective descriptive name for a disease entity. On the other hand, to honor a pioneering observer by attaching his or her name to a symptom complex adds a degree of historical warmth and color that may compensate for the loss of immediate definition. Only a small fraction of the many existing eponyms are herein included. The generally familiar or the uncommonly used eponyms have been omitted.

Albright's syndrome polyostotic fibrous dysplasia, cutaneous pigmentation (café-au-lait), and precocious puberty.

Bazin's disease erythema induratum.

Behçet's triple symptom complex iritis, with ulcers of mouth and genitalia.

Bockhart's impetigo superficial staphylococcic folliculitis.

Brooke's tumor trichoepithelioma; epithelioma adenoides cysticum.

Buschke's disease scleredema adultorum.

Carrión's disease verruga peruana; Oroya fever.

Chediak-Higashi syndrome oculocutaneous albinism, photophobia, anemia, infections, and characteristic leukocytic granules.

Darier-Roussy sarcoid subcutaneous sarcoid.

Degos' disease malignant atrophic papulosis; papular mucinosis.

Duhring's disease dermatitis herpetiformis.

Ehlers-Danlos syndrome hyperelastosis cutis, dermatorrhexis, and laxity of joints.

Fordyce's disease heterotopic sebaceous glands of mucous membranes of lips and oral cavity.

Fox-Fordyce disease chronic, pruritic papular eruption of axilla, groin, and genitalia.

Gardner's syndrome familial polyposis of the large intestine, with adenocarcinoma, osteomas of skull and long bones, and epidermal cysts and neurofibromas of skin.

Gougerot-Blum disease pigmented purpuric lichenoid dermatitis, principally of lower extremities.

Habermann's disease pityriasis lichenoides et varioliforma acuta.

Hailey-Hailey disease chronic benign familial pemphigus (so-called bullous Darier's disease).

Hallopeau's acrodermatitis acrodermatitis continua; dermatitis repens.

Hutchinson's syndrome a triad of stigmata of congenital syphilis—interstitial keratitis, peg-shaped, notched incisor teeth, and nerve deafness.

Kast's syndrome association of cutaneous hemangiomas with chondromas or dyschondroplasia.

Letterer-Siwe disease malignant, usually nonlipid histiocytosis or "reticulosis" of skin and viscera of infants and occasionally of older children ("histiocytosis X").

Lewandowsky's disease rosacea-like tuberculid.

Maffucci's syndrome cutaneous hemangiomas associated with dyschondroplasia and "spider" hands.

Majocchi's disease purpura annularis telangiectodes with characteristic vascular changes in the skin.

Moeller's glossitis chronic superficial excoriations of tongue.

Pautrier-Woringer syndrome dermatopathic lymphadenopathy.

Peutz-Jehgers syndrome oral melanosis associated with intestinal polyposis.

Prader-Willi syndrome lipodystrophic diabetes, acanthosis nigricans, obesity, sexual infantilism, muscular hypotonia, and short stature.

Pringle's adenoma sebaceum associated with tuberous sclerosis.

Reiter's syndrome nonspecific urethritis, arthritis, conjunctivitis, and often dermatitis identical with keratoderma blennorrhagicum.

Rendu-Osler-Weber syndrome hereditary hemorrhagic telangiectasia.

Riehl's melanosis melanosis of oral mucous membranes.

Romberg's disease progressive atrophy of face along distribution of fifth cranial nerve.

Schamberg's disease progressive pigmentary purpuric dermatosis of lower extremities.

Senear-Usher syndrome pemphigus erythematodes.

Sjögren's syndrome keratoconjunctivitis sicca, xerostomia, rhinitis and laryngitis sicca, alopecia, and sclerodermatous changes.

Spiegler-Fendt sarcoid benign dense lymphocytic nodularity of skin clinically resembling sarcoid and histologically easily confused with lymphosarcoma or leukemia cutis.

Stevens-Johnson syndrome severe form of erythema multiforme characterized by fever, severe malaise, and erosions of mucous membranes, conjunctivae, and genitalia.

Sturge-Weber syndrome nevus flammeus (hemangioma), contralateral hemiparesis, epilepsy, mental retardation, and cerebral calcification.

Sutton's disease periadenitis mucosa necrotica recurrens; chronic aphthous stomatitis.

Vogt-Kóyanagi syndrome bilateral uveitis, premature alopecia and graying of the hair, dysacousia, and symmetric vitiligo, especially of the extremities.

Weber syndrome hypertrophy of a limb due to congenital hemangiectasia.

Weber-Christian syndrome relapsing, febrile, nodular panniculitis.

Werner's syndrome scleroderma, poikiloderma, bilateral cataracts, pluriglandular dysfunction, and premature graying of hair.

CUTANEOUS-VISCERAL DISEASE

The cutaneous reflection of visceral disease is finally coming to be accorded the significance it has long merited. It is relevant to note that because of the increasing awareness of the importance of the association of visceral with cutaneous diseases, graduate students of dermatology are requesting more sophisticated training in internal medicine, as recent surveys emphasize. A simple listing of some of the cutaneous manifestations of visceral lesions, many of which have become apparent within the past decade, will underscore this vital relationship:

1 Pigmentations
  a Acanthosis nigricans of adults ("malignant" type)—commonly associated with visceral adenocarcinoma
  b Acanthosis nigricans (juvenile)—occasionally associated with congenital lipodystrophy and insulin-resistant diabetes or with Rud's syndrome (tetany, epilepsy, anemia, and mental retardation; also with ichthyosis hystrix)
  c Peutz-Jehgers syndrome—focal mucosal and cutaneous pigmentation with gastrointestinal polyps and, rarely, with carcinomas
  d Hemochromatosis—with pigmentary cirrhosis of liver and diabetes mellitus
  e Addison's disease
  f Incontinentia pigmenti—with neurologic and cardiac abnormalities
  g Ochronosis—with cardiac disease
  h Phenylketonuria—with neurologic manifestations
  i Pellagra
  j Café-au-lait spots—with Recklinghausen's disease and fibrous dysplasia
  k Chediak-Higashi syndrome—with specific leukocytic inclusions, semialbinism, etc.

2 Miscellaneous nonbullous dermatoses
  a Lupus erythematosus—with nephritis, carditis, and hypersplenism
  b Dermatomyositis in adults—with visceral cancer
  c Ichthyosis in adults—with lymphomas
  d Alopecia mucinosa—with mycosis fungoides
  e Erythema annulare (gyratum)—with rheumatic fever and cancer
  f Pyoderma gangrenosum—with ulcerative colitis
  g Sarcoidosis and other granulomatous diseases—with visceral involvement

3 Vesiculobullous lesions
  a Zoster—with malignant lymphomas (occasionally, dermatitis herpetiformis, pemphigoid, and erythema multiforme bullosum are associated with visceral cancers)
  b Acrodermatitis enteropathica
  c Bullous lesions—with porphyrias
  d Dermatitis herpetiformis—with intestinal disease (spruelike)
  e Toxic epidermal necrolysis—several instances associated with malignant lymphomas

4 Urticaria
  a Urticaria pigmentosum—with involvement of bones, liver, spleen, and lymph nodes
  b Urticaria—with amyloidosis, nerve deafness, and renal disease

5 Diseases of collagen and elastic tissue
  a Scleroderma—with renal, cardiac, and gastrointestinal lesions
  b Pseudoxanthoma elasticum—with ocular and cardiac lesions
  c Ehlers-Danlos syndrome—increased serum hexosamine; involvement of vessels, heart, and gastrointestinal tract
  d Cutis laxa
  e Necrobiosis lipoidica diabeticorum—with diabetes mellitus

f Circumscribed myxedema—with exophthalmic goiter

g Amyloidosis (primary and secondary)—with myeloma (primary amyloidosis), chronic infections (secondary amyloidosis), etc.

6 Vascular diseases

a Angiokeratoma of Fabry—with renal and vascular lesions

b Allergic granulomatosis—with visceral angiitis

c Degos' syndrome—thromboangiitis of skin and intestines

d Blue, rubber-bleb nevus—with intestinal angiomas

e Neurocutaneous-vascular syndromes
  (1) Sturge-Weber syndrome—cutaneous angiomatosis, epilepsy, etc.
  (2) Ataxia-telangiectasia
  (3) Rendu-Osler-Weber syndrome—with arteriovenous fistulas of lung, brain, etc.

7 Metabolic disorders

a Xanthomatoses—with diabetes mellitus, von Gierke's disease, biliary cirrhosis, lipid nephrosis, and essential familial hypercholesterolemia

b Lipidoses with cutaneous infiltration—reticulohistiocytic granulomas (lipid dermatoarthritis); lipid proteinosis; gangliosidoses and other sphingolipidoses (Fabry's, Tay-Sachs, Gaucher's etc.)

c Mucopolysaccharidoses—e.g., Hurler's syndrome

d Dysproteinemias—including Waldenström's macroglobulinemia (with malignant lymphomas), cryoglobulinemias (with cutaneous infarcts), and multiple myeloma (with cutaneous infiltration)

8 Cutaneous tumors

a Arsenical lesions (keratoses, Bowen's disease, etc.)—with visceral cancers in limited percentage

b Kaposi's sarcoma—with malignant lymphomas

c Sebaceous adenomas—with tuberous sclerosis

d Basal cell nevus syndrome and other neurocutaneous syndromes

DERMATOSES

In order to set up what may possibly be a more workable and more orderly classification of the varieties of dermatoses than seems currently to exist for pathologists, the diseases of the skin have been divided primarily into histologic categories. While some overlapping of criteria is present, it is hoped that the basis for the classification is, in general, sufficiently defined to be of practical value. The diseases discussed are not only those that the pathologist is most likely to encounter but also those that, with minor exceptions, are diagnosable on histologic changes alone.

Diseases principally of epidermis

Hyperplasias

Darier's disease. Clinically, Darier's disease (keratosis follicularis; psorospermosis) is recognized by the development early of small,

uniform, firm, reddish brown, greasy keratinous papules that subsequently become coalescent, papillomatous, and crusted and acquire an offensive odor. The lesions tend to be located about the face and neck and spread to the chest, limbs, and loins. The palms and nails may be involved, as may the oral mucosa. The disease occurs principally in the second and third decades.

The histologic picture is so distinctive as to be pathognomonic and consists of the following:

1 Focal, truncated masses of keratin, usually partially parakeratinized, especially near the surface, may be located over the ostia of hair follicles or over the interfollicular epidermis. For this reason, the term *keratosis follicularis* is inaccurate.

2 *Corps ronds*, or dyskeratotic cells, practically limited to the stratum granulosum, contain nuclei that are rounded and encircled by a clear cytoplasmic halo. The keratohyaline granules that characterize the cells of the stratum granulosum are usually absent in the *corps ronds*.

3 The "grains" are cells basically similar to the *corps ronds* but occur in the lower portion of the overlying keratinous masses and consist of cells with perinuclear spaces in the parakeratotic foci. Desmosomes tend to disappear from the dyskeratotic cells of Darier's disease, apparently after redistribution of the tonofilaments.[24]

4 The suprabasilar cleavage of the epidermis at the junction of the basal layer and the lowermost layer of the stratum spinosum forms a lacuna or small vesicle with a papillary base (Fig. 39-2). In addition, there may be a nondescript hyperemia and perivascular infiltrate of mononuclear cells in the upper corium.

The lesions that may offer some difficulty in differentiation are the isolated keratosis follicularis and benign chronic familial pemphigus (bullous Darier's disease). Verrucal or isolated keratosis follicularis, originally recorded in 1948 in the first edition of this text and elsewhere in the same year, is histologically similar to Darier's disease, although the lesions of the latter appear more regular, smaller, and often multiple even in the same section.[10] This verrucal lesion is likely to be single and has a predilection for the scalp. We (and others) have seen an identical histologic picture in the wall of the epidermal inclusion or pilosebaceous cysts. Accordingly, it

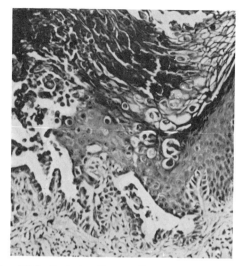

Fig. 39-2 Darier's disease (keratosis follicularis) showing suprabasilar cleavage, corps ronds, grains, and marked parakeratosis. (Hematoxylin-eosin.)

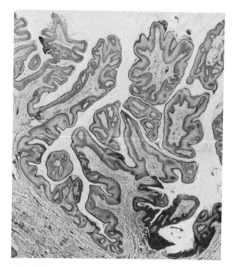

Fig. 39-3 Acanthosis nigricans with melanin pigmentation of basal layer. (Hematoxylin-eosin.)

now seems likely that so-called "isolated Darier's disease" or "warty dyskeratoma," which we originally thought was congenital, is derived from banal epidermal inclusion or pilosebaceous cysts or possibly occasionally from comedones. The relationship of this entity to the genodermatosis of Darier's disease is merely the minor histologic resemblance.

The benign chronic familial pemphigus shows prominence of the suprabasilar cleavage but lacks an appreciable keratinous mass. *Corps ronds* and grains (Fig. 39-2) are relatively inconspicuous. *Verruca vulgaris, porokeratosus Mibelli, keratosis pilaris,* and *lichen spinulosus* offer some differential difficulties histologically by virtue of the presence of focal keratinous masses or projections, but the other criteria of Darier's disease are absent in these lesions. Also to be distinguished from Darier's disease are hypertrophic lichen planus, pityriasis rubra pilaris, phrynoderma, keratosis follicularis contagiosa of children (Brooke), and Kyrle's disease. The latter (known, too, as hyperkeratosis follicularis et parafollicularis in cutem peneterans) does not appear to occur in children and is unrelated to trauma. An association with hepatic disease and altered carbohydrate metabolism has been suggested. This interesting genodermatosis is characterized by a partially parakeratotic plug protruding from the trough of invaginated epidermis, or follicle, with a moderate lymphocytic and histiocytic dermal reaction, at times with foreign body reaction to the penetrating keratin. This reaction is absent in elastosis perfor-

ans serpiginosa and basophilic perforating collagenosis.

Acanthosis nigricans. Acanthosis nigricans appears as patches of gray-black, warty masses with a predilection for the axilla, groin, submammary region, elbows, knees, and, occasionally, oral mucous membranes. Two types are recognized: juvenile and adult. The distinction is based on age rather than any difference in appearance of the lesions.

The juvenile type, unlike the adult form, is not associated with cancer, although, in some instances, it may accompany lipodystrophies and mental retardation.[29] The adult type is prone to be associated with visceral cancer—in about 50% of the patients, particularly in those beyond the fourth decade.[29] In about 65% of the patients, the associated cancer is a gastric adenocarcinoma. Adenocarcinomas of other viscera, such as lung and infrequently uterus, may be found. Occasionally, the acanthosis nigricans may appear to antedate the visceral cancer. The association of acanthosis nigricans and abdominal cancer in elderly people is a very real (if poorly understood) phenomenon and may be dependent in some instances on the encroachment on the sympathetic nerve chain by the cancer. Dermatomyositis, erythema nodosum, zoster, symmetric palmar and plantar erythema, exfoliative dermatitis, and Bowen's disease are some of the other dermatoses that may reflect the presence of visceral cancer.

The histologic picture of acanthosis nigricans is that of a papillary hyperkeratosis, in most areas disproportionately greater than the underlying acanthosis. The epidermis is thrown into folds by its excessive lateral growth and in sections often appears reticulated where rete ridges have joined. The basal layer is densely pigmented with fine argyrophilic melanin granules (Fig. 39-3), and a few chromatophores lie in the upper corium. This folding of a hyperkeratotic epidermis in which the basal layer is diffusely darkened as an almost solid line of melanin is characteristic of acanthosis nigricans. There is no anaplasia of the epidermis even in those cases accompanied by abdominal neoplasms. Oral florid papillomatosis may be associated with acanthosis nigricans. The lesions histologically simulated by acanthosis nigricans are xeroderma pigmentosum, various forms of verrucae, including seborrheic keratosis (pigmented papilloma), the pseudoacanthosis nigricans associated with obesity, and, because of the basal pigmentation, Addison's disease and nevus unius lateris.

Molluscum contagiosum. Molluscum contagiosum is a mildly contagious autoinoculable disease of the skin, caused by a virus and characterized by pinhead-sized to pea-sized waxy, firm, buttonlike, often pruritic papules occurring on the face, trunk, and genital regions particularly and on the feet rarely. The lesions develop slowly over a period of weeks and may remain indefinitely without therapy. The disease appears especially in children and may occur in epidemic proportions in institutions. Molluscum contagiosum may occur in deceptively giant forms and apparently may be transmitted venerally.[65]

The histologic picture should be immediately recognizable. The connective tissue papillae between the lobules are compressed or altogether obliterated, so that the inwardly projecting lobules appear as a bulbous downgrowth. This lobulation of the epidermis is almost as suggestive of the diagnosis as is the pathognomonic feature, the molluscum bodies, and may serve to help differentiate this lesion from verrucae, particularly when the molluscum bodies happen to be inconspicuous. The molluscum bodies are clustered cells, principally of the stratum granulosum but also of the stratum spinosum, which are enlarged, as are virus-infected cells generally, and contain homogeneously smooth, brightly eosinophilic cytoplasm. The nucleus is inconspicuously flattened to one side of the cell, and keratohyaline granules tend to disappear. The cytoplasm, when studied with vital stains, appears actually to contain many elementary bodies

(Lipschütz) embedded in a mucoid matrix. These dyskeratotic cells are enclosed in an eosinophilic, keratin-like membrane that resembles the dense cell membranes of plants. The molluscum bodies have been confused with the brightly eosinophilic cells of the stratum granulosum that are often prominent in verruca vulgaris. The virus seen electron microscopically measures 300 mμ × 200 mμ × 100 mμ, is characteristically brick shaped, and contains a dumbbell-shaped nucleoid. The virus replicates in the cytoplasm rather than nucleus.[64] Specific fluorescence staining of the inclusion bodies with tagged antibodies of serum from infected human beings and rabbits has been demonstrated.[33]

Vesicles

The vesicles of various diseases may closely simulate each other clinically. Inasmuch as the prognostication, even as to fatality, may depend on the exact diagnosis, it is clearly important that the diagnostic histologic features be definitely evaluated. In general, three types of vesicles occur: (1) eczematous, (2) cleavage (e.g., dermatitis herpetiformis, pemphigus, epidermolysis bullosa, impetigo, and burns), and (3) viral (e.g., smallpox, chickenpox, and herpes).

Eczema. Eczema, which is derived from a verb meaning "to boil out," is in most instances the cutaneous response of a skin sensitive to an allergen. The response may begin as an erythema and evolve through the papular, vesicular, pustular, and exfoliative stages. Some cases of eczema remain in one of the phases (e.g., eczema rubrum, eczema squamosum, eczema papulosum), but in most instances, the disease passes through the stage of vesiculation. From the histologic point of view, the vesicle of eczema, whatever the etiology, is basically the same whether the allergen is an external irritant, ingested food, or the product of superficial fungi, as in the epidermophytid. Moreover, the histologic picture of the eczematous vesicle differs sharply from that of pemphigus, dermatitis herpetiformis and the viral lesions of smallpox, chickenpox, and herpes.

The vesicle of eczema begins as foci of spongiosis in the rete malpighii. The intercellular edema progresses so as to form microvesicles that coalesce with adjacent vesicles similarly formed. The walls of such vesicles are the compressed epidermal cells that usually are arranged as septa in the large blisters. Histologic changes of this sort occur also in the vesicles of pompholyx, dyshidrosis, acro-dermatitis perstans, and other eruptions of unknown etiology that are localized principally to the hands, as well as in the vesicles of pustular bacterids. The latter are usually sterile pustules of the palms and soles and are assumed to be provoked by allergic reactions to bacterial products.

Cleavage vesicles. Some years ago, we applied the term "cleavage" to those vesicles formed by the separation or "cleavage" of the epidermis or dermis through a single horizontal plane.[10] The cleavage may occur at any level of the epidermis and, occasionally, may split the upper dermis. The precise level of cleavage usually embodies a key diagnostic clue. The following discussion is of representative types of cleavage vesicles.

The lesions of *dermatitis herpetiformis (Duhring's disease)* are symmetrically distributed in groups in the scapular regions, on the buttocks, or on the extremities. The lesions may be erythematous macules or papules, but in most cases they are characterized by vesicles that may vary from those detectable only microscopically to large bullae. The disease may be accompanied by mild constitutional symptoms and signs. Itching, burning, and pricking sensations almost always are present. The disease is characterized by spontaneous remissions and relapses. The etiology is unknown. The iodide sensitivity test is no longer regarded as specific for dermatitis herpetiformis. The lesions respond remarkably in most instances to penicillin and sulfapyridine but usually do not react satisfactorily to other sulfonamides. The patients must be kept on maintenance doses of these chemotherapeutic agents, failing which the eruption reappears.

A juvenile form of dermatitis herpetiformis has been described which differs symptomatically from the adult form. The latter tends to be more chronic, is associated with pruritus, is polymorphic, leaves scarring and pigmentation, and responds more consistently to dapsone and sulfapyridine.[36]

The microscopic features of the vesicle of dermatitis herpetiformis consist of a collection of serum, fibrin, and a few neutrophilic and eosinophilic leukocytes that have cleaved and lifted the entire epidermis from the corium. The epidermis itself shows no other constant change. Of diagnostic importance is the change in the dermal base of the vesicle— i.e., particularly, the flattened papillae that are edematous and infiltrated with cells of the same type that are found in the vesicle itself. The absence of eosinophilic leukocytes by no means precludes the diagnosis of dermatitis herpetiformis, although those cells often are noted in considerable numbers. Occasionally, eosinophils, both within the fluid of the vesicle and in the underlying dermis, occur in pemphigus, particularly in *pemphigus vegetans.*

The fully developed lesion of dermatitis herpetiformis is rarely a diagnostic problem, but frequently a very early or, at least, a very small lesion is biopsied at a stage prior to appreciable vesiculation. The principal clue in these is the occurrence of small clusters of leukocytes, immediately subepidermal and associated with a suggestion of edema and leukocytic reaction in a small bit of the underlying dermis (Fig. 39-4). The accurate diagnosis of this particular vesicle is of critical importance because of the possibility of confusion with the fatal disease pemphigus. As mentioned, the presence of eosinophilic leukocytes in the infiltrate is of appreciable aid in the diagnosis of dermatitis herpetiformis, but their presence is not so constant as is usually stated. Often, the vesicles of the varieties of pemphigus and of epidermolysis bullosa are bland in the sense that they provoke little or no dermal reaction—in contradistinction to those of dermatitis herpetiformis. However, there are sufficient exceptions to this rule so that the mere presence of inflammatory reaction does not preclude the possibility of pemphigus, although in epidermolysis bullosa such

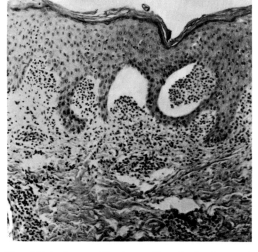

Fig. 39-4 Dermatitis herpetiformis in its early stage showing cleavage of epidermis from dermis by collections of leukocytes. (Hematoxylin-eosin.)

reaction is usually due to trauma or secondary infection and is rarely an intrinsic part of the disease. Furthermore, some of the vesicles of epidermolysis bullosa occur not at the suprabasilar level or at the junction of the epidermis and dermis but between the stratum corneum and stratum granulosum or at some level of the rete malpighii. Similarly, the vesicle of impetigo contagiosum is formed between the stratum corneum and rete malpighii and, consequently, is easily distinguished from that of dermatitis herpetiformis. In addition, there is generally considerably more purulent exudate within the lesion of impetigo contagiosum. The vesicles of the viral lesions, (i.e., smallpox, chickenpox, and herpes simplex, and herpes zoster) are easily recognized by their distinctive inclusion bodies, reticular colliquation, and ballooning degeneration (see definitions, p. 1611).

Pemphigus refers to a group of diseases, commonly fatal and characterized by bullous lesions. The cause is unknown. The disease involves both sexes equally, mainly between 40 and 70 years of age, and most frequently begins in the mucous membranes of the mouth or in the skin of the trunk. Rarely, pemphigus vulgaris is observed in children.[54] Pemphigus is fatal in somewhat over 50% of the patients. The several varieties include pemphigus vulgaris, pemphigus foliaceus, and pemphigus vegetans. These forms are entities primarily on the basis of the acuteness of the disease or the type of lesions accompanying the vesicles—e.g., the foul-smelling scales of pemphigus foliaceus and the fungoid papillomatous masses of pemphigus vegetans. Pemphigus erythematodes (Senear-Usher syndrome) previously was regarded as a separate entity with a good prognosis. It is now believed that this condition is actually a variant of pemphigus in which the erythematous stage may be prolonged. The incidence of pemphigus vulgaris is about four times that of all the other varieties combined. Bullae are observed at some time in the course of pemphigus foliaceus and vegetans. The group name is applied also to benign chronic familial pemphigus (Hailey-Hailey disease), but there is reason to believe that this disease is quite distinct from the usually fatal varieties of pemphigus. The actual cause of death in uncomplicated pemphigus is not clear, although the loss of proteins and electrolytes in the bullous fluid is probably a significant factor. The prognosis for patients with pemphigus is better if the disease develops before the age of 40 years and is treated with steroids early in its course.

The histologic picture of the cutaneous lesion of pemphigus is as follows:

1 The typical vesicle or bulla consists of a collection of serous fluid, most often at the suprabasilar layer of the epidermis, but occasionally the split is in the midst of the rete malpighii or at the dermal-epidermal junction. As a rule, there is little or no reaction in the dermis, although, as stated previously, there are many exceptions in which the upper dermis or submucosa is crowded with polymorphonuclear leukocytes admixed with the various mononuclear cells (i.e., lymphocytes, plasma cells, and histiocytes). Such a vesicle or bulla characterizes *pemphigus vulgaris* but may be a part of the picture of other varieties of pemphigus (Fig. 39-5). In addition, rounded epidermal cells, loosened by "acantholysis" (Tzanck cells) frequently are found in the vesicles of pemphigus, but, as stated, they are not pathognomonic of this disease. These acantholytic cells may be recognized in smears of vesicles stained with hematoxylin and eosin and may be distinguished from cells of viral vesicles, for example. They are characterized by the disintegration of desmosomes and the separation, disorganization, and loss of tonofilaments, a sequence of events accompanying acantholysis not only in other dermatoses but also in some epidermal neoplasms, particularly melanocarcinomas. The

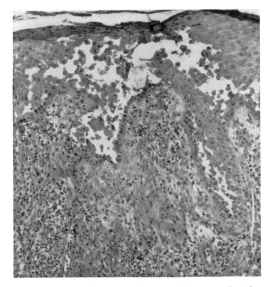

Fig. 39-5 Pemphigus vulgaris with suprabasilar cleavage and isolated clusters of epidermal cells within vesicle. These are acantholytic cells of Tzanck. (Hematoxylin-eosin.)

vulnerability of the desmosomes is regarded as the principal pathogenetic basis of pemphigus, a concept reinforced by immunofluorescence demonstration of the fixation of autoantibodies at these intercellular sites. As indicated, autoimmune antibodies may be demonstrated by fluorescence in the intercellular spaces of the epidermis of patients with pemphigus vulgaris. In bullous pemphigoid, the antibodies are localized to the position of the basement membrane.

The histologic differentiation of pemphigus vulgaris from "bullous pemphigoid" is often not so clear cut as was implied when the latter term was coined. The early mucosal involvement, the relative lack of inflammation, the abundance of acantholysis, and the suprabasilar (versus epidermal-dermal) cleavage, are features more indicative of pemphigus. *Benign mucosal* pemphigoid may involve the conjunctiva, oronasal cavity, larynx, esophagus, and genitalia. The histology is like that of bullous pemphigoid except for the occurrence of cicatrization as a consequence of the submucosal inflammatory reaction. It is probable that pemphigoid is a variant of *erythema multiforme bullosum,* as is the *Stevens-Johnson syndrome.* Pemphigoid may, on occasion, be associated with visceral cancer[72] (Fig. 39-6).

Painful, tender, acute *toxic epidermal necrolysis,* with rapid onset and recovery or rapid demise, is a newly emphasized entry resembling glabrous pemphigoid or pemphigus and thought to be due to drug, viral, or bacterial sensitivity. The offending drugs include barbiturates, sulfonamides, penicillin, phenylbutazone, hydantoins, salicylates, antihistamines, and others. Histologically, the cleavage may be at one of several levels: dermal-epidermal as in erythema multiforme bullosum, suprabasilar as in pemphigus, or within the upper rete malpighii. Scattered foci of necrosis of keratinocytes may be present, and some of these may appear in the vesicles as acantholytic cells. Few or no inflammatory changes occur within the dermis unless secondarily infected, thereby closely simulating erythema multiforme bullosum. Several instances have been associated with malignant lymphomas.

The association of systemic lupus erythematosus with bullous pemphigoid and with pemphigus erythematodes has reinforced the concept of the simultaneous presence of multiple autoimmune diseases. The suggestive evidence is not only clinical and histologic but also immunologic in the form of fluorescent antibodies in the basement membrane zone (for pemphigoid) and intercellular antibodies (for pemphigus).[55]

Bullae also may result following the use of anticoagulants.[83] These bullae are subepidermal and histologically simulate erythema multiforme.

2 In *pemphigus vegetans,* in addition to the bulla just described, there is an associated diagnostic lesion consisting of marked acanthosis with prominent prolongation of the rete ridges, between which are brilliantly dense collections of eosinophilic leukocytes. The eosinophils may migrate into the epidermis, which may become ulcerated and be the seat of intraepidermal microabscesses. The ulcerations, the intraepidermal abscesses, and the extensive acanthosis with winding reticulated ridges may simulate a bromoderma or the reaction to deep fungal infections such as coccidioidomycosis.

3 In *pemphigus foliaceus,* the typical bulla often is immediately adjacent to a unique acanthosis. Often, the fluid accumulates between layers of the upper rete malpighii. If the accumulation of fluid is minimal, the cleavage may be sufficient to separate the uppermost portion of the epidermis by crude pressure of the thumb on the skin of the patient (Nikolsky's sign). The ridges are rounded and formed in congeries so that in a single section they may appear isolated in the

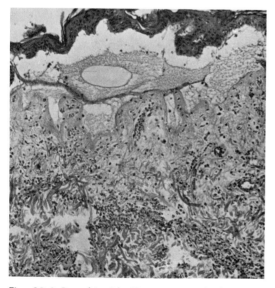

Fig. 39-6 Pemphigoid. Cleavage vesicle between epidermis and dermis with relatively sparse dermal reaction. Tzanck cells are absent. (Hematoxylin-eosin.)

deep dermis, as in an early squamous cell carcinoma. This type of acanthosis resembles most the epidermal proliferation often seen overlying myoblastomas. The epidermal proliferation usually is accompanied by a polymorphous cellular infiltrate of neutrophilic leukocytes and mononuclear cells. Tzanck cells are present in both pemphigus foliaceus and pemphigus vegetans, and in lesser numbers, in Hailey-Hailey disease and other vesicular dermatoses.

Epidermolysis bullosa occurs soon after birth (congenital) or may first appear in the second or third decade (so-called acquired type). There are two varieties of epidermolysis bullosa: simple and dystrophic. In the simple type, the lesions occur, after slight trauma, on any portion of the body and regress, leaving merely temporary pigmentation but no permanent changes. The dystrophic type is characterized by lesions of the extremities, provoked by minimal trauma and associated with pigmentation, milia (epidermal cysts), atrophy, destruction of nails, cicatrizations, and syndactylism.

Both the simple and dystrophic types may be congenital or acquired. The histology is that of a pressure vesicle with cleavage often at the junction of the stratum corneum and stratum granulosum or between the epidermis and dermis, especially in the dystrophic type (Fig. 39-7). The inflammatory reaction

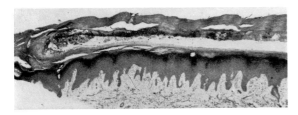

Fig. 39-7 Epidermolysis bullosa. Cleavage vesicle in stratum corneum, unlike deeper, dystrophic form. (Hematoxylin-eosin.)

within both the vesicle and the underlying dermis is mild except in regions, such as the feet, that are easily traumatized and infected. The small epidermal inclusions lie in the dermis beneath or at the margins of the vesicles. A congenital disturbance of the dermal elastic tissue is said to occur in the dystrophic type. The evidence for this is not satisfactory. However, necrosis of upper dermal collagen and elastic tissue may occur in the dystrophic form and may result in severe contractures of the extremities with bony absorption. Involvement of the conjunctiva, oral mucosa, and esophagus may develop, heralding a poor prognosis. The epidermal inclusion cysts are particularly prone to appear in the dystrophic form and reflect, in part, the dermal isolation of portions of sweat ducts and rete ridges that subsequently form the cysts. The relative lack of inflammatory cellular response within and beneath the vesicles is of diagnostic usefulness in differentiating them from other vesicles with cleavages at corresponding sites. The bullae of dystrophic epidermolysis bullosa have been attributed to the specifically higher local production of collagenase in contrast with pemphigus vulgaris and bullous pemphigoid.[31] A picture simulating epidermolysis bullosa may follow the administration of penicillamine.

Subcorneal pustular dermatosis is considered to be a special vesicular entity. The lesions, which tend to affect particularly middle-aged women, appear as minute gyrate or annular groups of erythematous, superficial vesiculopustules localized chiefly to the intertriginous areas about the breasts, axillae, and groins. The lesions respond to sulfapyridine, as do those of Duhring's disease.

Histologically, the changes consist of cleavage vesicles and pustules located immediately beneath the stratum corneum, as the name indicates. Eosinophils are not a part of the picture, although occasionally acantholytic cells may be present. The exudate is usually

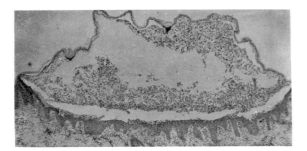

Fig. 39-8 Impetigo contagiosum. Superficial cleavage vesicle with purulent exudate. (Hematoxylin-eosin; AFIP 99848.)

sterile—unlike that of impetigo contagiosa, which the lesion otherwise resembles histologically.

Viral vesicles. Smallpox (variola), chickenpox (varicella), alastrim, vaccinia (cowpox), herpangina, herpes simplex, and herpes zoster (shingles) are described in Chapter 11. In contrast to the ease with which most of the exanthemas are differentiable clinically is the difficulty or impossibility of differentiating the vesicles histologically. Nevertheless, there are certain features common to each of these vesicles that at least permit the recognition of each, histologically, as a vesicle produced by a virus. These features include (1) *reticular colliquation* by which the epidermis becomes transformed into multiple locules bounded by a reticulum of drawn-out, stringy, cytoplasmic septa and (2) *ballooning degeneration,* the formation of multinucleated giant cells in the lower layers of the rete malpighii.

It is stated that in the vesicle of smallpox, reticular colliquation proceeds at a faster pace, particularly at the periphery of the lesion, than does ballooning degeneration, and thereby accounts for the umbilication of this vesicle. In smallpox, Guarnieri bodies are found as eosinophilic, varying-sized, round, cytoplasmic inclusions—especially in those cells that are at the base of the vesicle, including those undergoing ballooning degeneration. In addition, eosinophilic intranuclear inclusions with margination of the nuclear chromatin are common in these cells. In the vesicles of herpes, these intranuclear inclusions are referred to as "zoster bodies of Lipschütz," although they are morphologically similar to the intranuclear inclusions of the other viral vesicles.

The scarring that follows some of these vesicles (e.g., those of zoster and occasionally of smallpox) is an index of the prior inflammatory destruction of the upper corium. As a rule, edema and infiltrate of inflammatory cells are present in the upper dermis of most vesicles of the various viral diseases. The residual scarring, however, appears to reflect the greater intensity and destructiveness of the process. The virus of zoster appears capable of producing the clinical picture of varicella in susceptible individuals. It is suggested that steroids increase this susceptibility.

Relatively recently, a new entity referred to as "*herpangina*" has been described. It is a benign, febrile, self-limited disease of viral etiology, affecting children chiefly and characterized by a sudden onset of grayish white, papulovesicular, oral or pharyngeal lesions with a surrounding red areola. Histologic studies of the vesicles are not available, but one would anticipate that they would resemble the vesicles of herpes.

Another controverted disease that now appears clearly virogenic is *Kaposi's varicelliform eruption*. This disease is really either disseminated herpes simplex or generalized vaccinia, often inoculated in skin made receptive by a preceding dermatosis such as eczema or atopic dermatitis. The rapid diagnosis of viral vesicles is expedited by the use of smears of the vesicular contents. This cytodiagnostic method is particularly useful with the viral vesicles as opposed to other types in which excessive dependence may be placed on acantholytic cells. It is hypothesized that the virus of varicella-zoster remains latent in sensory ganglia after a preceding varicella and hematogenous dissemination of the virus occurs with subsequent activation.[46]

Superficial mycoses. Superficial mycoses are included in this section because of their involvement of epidermis principally. The mycoses are separated into the superficial type (ringworm, tinea corporis, and favus) and the deep type (blastomycosis, coccidioidomycosis, actinomycosis, etc.). Superficial mycoses are divided, according to the region affected, into tinea capitis, barbae, corporis, cruris, and pedis or epidermophytosis. Several kinds of fungi may be responsible for the same clinical type of lesion. On the other hand, the form and chronicity of ringworm may vary considerably with the causative fungus. For example, *Trichophyton* infection of the feet presents as a dry, scaly dermatosis, whereas that due to *Epidermophyton* appears vesicular and moist. It has therefore been suggested that the etiology, as well as the anatomic region, be indicated in the name—e.g., tinea corporis trichophytica. However, usage sanctions the retention of additional names for varieties of ringworm infection that have distinguishing features of pattern, color, severity, or chronicity of lesions—such as favus, kerion (ringworm of scalp complicated by abscesses), tinea imbricata, tinea versicolor, and others.

Botryomycosis is merely a bacterial infection histologically confused with actinomycosis because of the eosinophilic radiate or asteroid formation about the colonies of bacteria. The etiologic agent is usually a staphylococcus, but streptococci and proteus organisms also may produce this pattern. Gram stains on histologic sections facilitate the diagnosis.

The fungus may be observed in wet smears of scrapings soaked in sodium or potassium hydroxide, or they may be cultured on special media, such as Sabouraud's agar. However, with the exceptions of tinea versicolor and favus, it is rare to observe the fungus in a routine paraffin section of a lesion of ringworm. Generally, the histologic picture comprises merely the presence of scales or vesicles along with subepidermal hyperemia and slight perivascular cuffing by mononuclear cells. In tinea versicolor, the spores and hyphae of *Microsporon furfur* are usually abundant and confined to the stratum corneum. In favus, the large scutula, or matted scales, contain myriads of the fungus.

The vesicle of ringworm, no matter where the lesion is located, is an eczematous vesicle, usually multiloculated, and the morphologic result of excessive spongiosis. This type of vesicle is the picture of the dermatophytid or allergic manifestation of the fungal infection. The dermatophytids are sterile of fungi and are caused by the cutaneous reaction to the products of fungi transported probably through the blood or lymph. For example, the dermatophytids following ringworm of the feet often occur on the hands. It has been suggested that sensitizing antibiotic therapy with preparations from fungi such as penicillin may be responsible in some measure for the dermatophytids following superficial mycoses. The deep mycoses are described in Chapter 12.

Scabies. Another lesion of the epidermis that is often recognizable in a fortunate histologic section is caused by *Acarus scabiei*. The disease is characterized by the occurrence of intensely pruritic papules, vesicles, pustules, and excoriations usually located in relation to the burrow, cuniculus, or gallery dug by the mite of the *Acarus* into the epidermis. These lesions tend to occur in the webs of the fingers, on the wrists, in the genital regions, and beneath the breast. The disease is contagious and, in most instances, is transmitted by direct bodily contact with an infected individual. The diagnosis may be made clinically by picking the female mite out of the burrow and identifying it with the low-power lens of the microscope.

Histologically, none of the lesions of scabies is diagnostic except the burrow with the tenant mite. However, the mite often may not be included in the section, but the presence of ova or fecal material of the *Acarus* within the burrow or merely the presence of the gallery itself is strongly presumptive evidence of scabies. The burrow is a superficial epidermal defect extending obliquely through the thickened stratum corneum, which serves as a roof to shelter the *Acarus*.

A form of scabies may be transmitted to man by mites that infest dogs, cats, birds, and monkeys. So-called *Norwegian scabies* appears to be merely a more fulminant form of ordinary scabies.

The *Demodex folliculorum,* the acarid commonly found within the keratinous follicular plugs of comedones, has generally been regarded as an innocuous infestation. More recently, the innocuous nature of infestation with *Demodex folliculorum* has been questioned. Blepharitis, for example, has been attributed to this arthropod.

Diseases affecting both epidermis and dermis

In this discussion are included those histologic entities to which changes in both the epidermis and the dermis jointly contribute to the morphologic diagnosis.

Lupus erythematosus

Lupus erythematosus occurs in two principal forms: acute and chronic or discoid.

Discoid lupus erythematosus. The discoid variety is fortunately the more common and manifests itself by stationary or slowly progressive coalescent macules or plaques covered irregularly with fine, whitish or yellowish, greasy scales and associated with focal gray patches of atrophy and keratotic plugging of follicles. The lesions usually are well defined (hence, discoid) and show a predilection for the malar areas and bridge of the nose distributed in the shape of a butterfly. The process is not limited to this area but may occur also on other parts of the face, the scalp, the neck, extremities, and elsewhere. In any location, the lesions are aggravated by exposure to sunlight or other forms of irradiation. The lesions may regress completely, but usually there is residual, rather typical superficial scarring with pigmentation or leukoderma and alopecia. Acute changes also may be superimposed on the discoid lesions. Carcinomatous transformations (squamous cell) may occur in the chronic process, probably for nonspecific reasons similar to those that obtain in some other forms of chronic cicatrizing ulcerations. The lesions respond remarkably well to antimalarial drugs.

The histologic features of the discoid variety

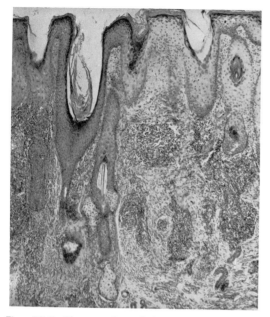

Fig. 39-9 Chronic discoid lupus erythematosus with alternating acanthosis and atrophy, liquefaction degeneration, keratinous plugs in follicles, superficial telangiectases, and dense collections of dermal lymphocytes. (Hematoxylin-eosin; from Allen, A. C.: Arch. Derm. Syph. [Chicago] **57:**19-56, 1948.)

of lupus erythematosus are easily recognizable in most cases. They include the following:

1 Alternating acanthosis and atrophy of the epidermis, with the process infrequently progressing to squamous cell carcinoma

2 Liquefaction degeneration of the basal layer

3 Hyperemia or telangiectasis and edema of the papillary and subpapillary layer of the dermis

4 Dense collections of mononucelar cells, principally lymphocytes, in the upper and midportions of the dermis, most concentrated about the appendages, often with atrophy and consequent alopecia (Fig. 39-9)

5 Focal depigmentation of the basal layer along with clusters of melanophages secondary to the subepidermal inflammation

6 As we have long ago noted, a PAS-positive, fragmented, pseudobasement membrane produced by the concentration of polysaccharides in the edematous dermis immediately beneath the epidermis

Basophilic "degeneration" of collagen in the upper dermis is a completely unreliable criterion of chronic lupus erythematosus, inasmuch as it is found normally in the skin of the malar regions, especially in the older age

groups of patients. Changes in vessels, other than telangiectasis, are not part of the picture of discoid lupus erythematosus. The lesions of *rosacea* may occasionally offer differential diagnostic difficulty because of the presence of keratotic plugs and erythema. The epidermal changes and mid-dermal masses of lymphocytes favor lupus erythematosus. Occasionally, the collections of lymphocytes extend into the underlying panniculus *(lupus erythematosus profundus)* and may be mistaken for Weber-Christian disease. Similar dense masses of lymphocytes in the dermis may be confused with a malignant lymphoma, the benign dermal lymphocytosis of Jessner, or the potpourri of lesions labeled Spiegler-Fendt sarcoid.

Acute lupus erythematosus. The acute (or "subacute") lupus erythematosus may occur as a focal, transient reaction to sunlight or may be part of the spontaneous fatal systemization of the disease. These acute lesions may be superimposed on the chronic process or may affect previously uninvolved skin. The chronic lesion is assumed to be complicated by the disseminated form in the rarest instances. However, while this may be the impression clinically, the histologic data belie this impression somewhat. It is estimated that in only 1% of the patients does discoid lupus erythematosus evolve into the systemic form.[81] Moreover, the presence of antinuclear antibodies in many patients wtih chronic lupus erythematosus suggests to some observers an immunologic relationship to the systemic disease. Antinuclear antibodies as demonstrated by fluorescence microscopy are found in patients with systemic lupus erythematosus as well as in patients with other so-called autoimmune diseases. What is of special interest is that such antibodies are present in about half of the cases of chronic discoid lupus erythematosus.[76] These antibodies appear to be absent in eruptions due to light sensitivity.

In the acute cases, the skin becomes reddened, edematous, and sometimes purpuric, with patchy macules that may coalesce into an erysipeloid, somewhat mottled malar flush. On the hands, the lesions may be erythematous or purpuric and macular or papular. Elsewhere, they may take other forms such as vesicles, bullae, scaling macules, and telangiectases. When the acute process complicates the discoid lesion, fresh superficial or even moderately deep ulcerations may occur, in addition to the other changes mentioned, particularly at the advancing periphery of the old lesion. As stated, the acute cutaneous phenomena may be a localized reaction to sunlight without systemic complications. In the disseminated variety, which occurs particularly but by no means exclusively in young women, the constitutional signs and symptoms include fever, thrombopenia, leukopenia, excessive gamma globulinemia, splenomegaly, arthralgias, valvular disease (Libman-Sacks disease), anorexia, vomiting, diarrhea, dysphagia, abdominal pain, and lymphadenitis. The principal causes of death are renal insufficiency, bacterial endocarditis, cardiac failure, pulmonary tuberculosis, sepsis, or pneumonia (see also pp. 499 and 1320).

As with the discoid variety, the etiology of the disseminated type is obscure, although— because of clinical and laboratory features (reaction to sunlight, occasional porphyrinuria, and antinuclear antibodies) and histologic changes (fibrinoid degeneration of collagen and focal necrosis of lymph nodes)— the underlying pathogenesis has been attributed by some investigators to an unexplained allergic or autoimmune mechanism. However, the overwhelming selection of females is difficult to reconcile with such a universal phenomenon as allergy, unless, perhaps, the allergen is a product of a sex-linked haptene. Similarly, the recent finding of viruslike inclusions in the tissues of patients with systemic lupus erythematosus is difficult to reconcile with the predominance of this disorder among women if the inclusions are considered etiologic.

The acute histologic changes in the skin are recognized in an exaggeration of the liquefaction degeneration of the basal layer of the epidermis with eosinophilic swelling of the cytoplasm of the basal cells, edema of the papillary and subpapillary layers, necrobiosis with karyorrhexis and nuclear distortion of inflammatory cells in the upper dermis, telangiectasis, and, occasionally, fibrinoid degeneration of foci of collagen in this region, as well as of the walls of some of the arterioles. The latter change is inconstant and is surely not responsible for the other cutaneous alterations. Circulating antibodies have been demonstrated at the dermal-epidermal junction by immunofluorescence studies. Characteristic histologic changes occur in other organs in the disseminated disease. These include the following:

1 Atypical verrucous endocarditis (Libman-Sacks disease) recognizable by the hematoxylin bodies of Gross (coalescent nuclear debris analogous to the phenomenon of the LE cell naturally showing a positive Feulgen reaction for nucleic acids) and the extensive fibrinoid swelling of the cardiac valves, especially in the often-overlooked pockets of the posterior mitral leaflet (p. 647 and Fig. 18-37)

2 Striking fibrinoid alteration of the interstitial collagen of the myocardium that may, but need not, be mistaken for Aschoff bodies

3 Concentric dense rings of collagen, apparently thickened reticulum, about the central splenic arterioles (Figs. 31-22 and 31-23)

4 Focal fibrinoid swelling of the walls of glomerular capillaries ("wire loops")

With the exception of the splenic lesion, these changes are practically pathognomonic of disseminated lupus erythematosus and occur rarely in such presumably closely related diseases as scleroderma and dermatomyositis. The splenic changes apparently do occur infrequently in minimal form in other diseases. The glomerular alterations may be so widespread as to cause renal insufficiency and a clinical picture of glomerulonephritis in about one-third of the patients, often with the nephrotic syndrome. The atypical verrucous endocarditis offers an optimal nidus for the implantation and growth of bacteria so that

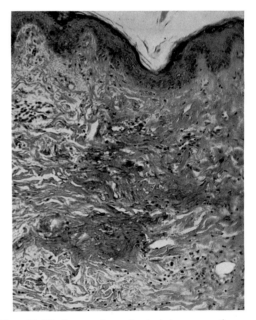

Fig. 39-10 Acute disseminated lupus erythematosus with fibrinoid necrosis of dermal collagen, an uncommon finding in skin in this disorder. (Hematoxylin-eosin.)

bacterial endocarditis is a common terminating event in this disease (Figs. 39-10 and 39-11).

Undoubtedly, one of the most provocative discoveries in the field of cutaneous-visceral integration of the last few decades has been the phenomenon of the LE cell. Cytologically, the phenomnon is manifested typically by a rosette of neutrophilic leukocytes about a mononuclear cell (apparently a lymphocyte) or, less typically, by a neutrophilic leukocyte with a cytoplasmic vacuole or a cytoplasmic inclusion of a nuclear fragment. Often, there is excessive clumping of platelets. The essence of this phenomenon resides in the gamma globulin of the serum of patients with disseminated lupus erythematosus and may be observed not only with cells of the patient's marrow but with cells of the peripheral blood. It also may be observed with normal cells (human or animal) after mixture with the patient's serum. Similar cells are noted in a cantharides-induced blister in the skin of individuals with disseminated lupus erythematosus. It is of interest, but by now not surprising, to record the dramatic remissions initiated by cortisone and ACTH in profoundly ill patients. With this improvement, the number of

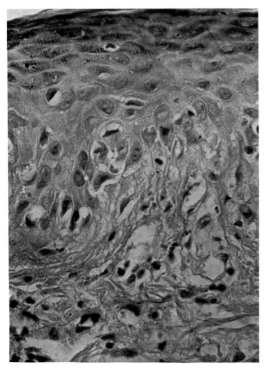

Fig. 39-11 Acute disseminated lupus erythematosus with marked liquefaction degeneration at epidermal-dermal junction. (Hematoxylin-eosin.)

LE cells diminishes and may completely disappear. Some instances of a positive LE phenomenon have been recorded in multiple myeloma, leukemia, Hodgkin's disease, rheumatoid arthritis, viral hepatitis, acquired hemolytic anemia, and reactions to drugs (phenylbutazone and hydralazine) and in association with infection or contamination of serum with *Aspergillus niger* or *Trichophyton gypseum*. It is of interest that the LE cell does not occur in scleroderma and dermatomyositis, which, together with disseminated lupus erythematosus, have been gratuitously linked as diffuse vascular or diffuse collagen disease—notwithstanding this and other discrepancies. Moreover, there is adequate reason to conclude that no one of these diseases is either a diffuse vascular disease or a generalized disease of collagen. Review of the histology of even a small number of autopsies in such cases quickly reveals that the involvement of vessels or collagen is, as a rule, neither diffuse nor itself responsible for the clinical picture, with the exception of scleroderma.

Dermatomyositis

Dermatomyositis has been discussed in the chapter on hypersensitivity diseases (p. 502). It will suffice to state here that although the purplish red, finely scaly edematous rash located principally about the upper face is fairly diagnostic, the histologic picture of the skin is not. It consists chiefly of spotty parakeratosis, some liquefaction degeneration at the epidermal-dermal junction, and edema of the upper dermis. However, the vacuolar sarcolysis, coagulation necrosis, and acute inflammatory changes in the swollen muscle fibers may be strongly suggestive. As stated, the search for vascular alterations is generally fruitless (Fig. 39-12).

The pathogenetic and etiologic spectra of myositides are expanding rapidly and form an intriguing chapter dealing with viruses, unresolved relationship to visceral cancer, lesions of the thymus, etc. It appears evident that some of the confusion related to dermatomyositis is that a variety of myositic disorders as well as systemic lupus erythematosus and scleroderma are mistakenly considered to be dermatomyositis. The presence of dermal mucin in a specimen with no specific pattern is stated to be suggestive of dermatomyositis.[52]

Psoriasis

Psoriasis is characterized by reddish brown papules, covered with silvery white micaceous

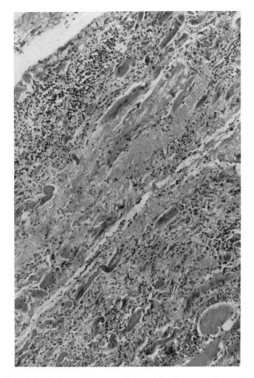

Fig. 39-12 Dermatomyositis with dense inflammatory cells interspersed among atrophic muscle fibers. (Hematoxylin-eosin.)

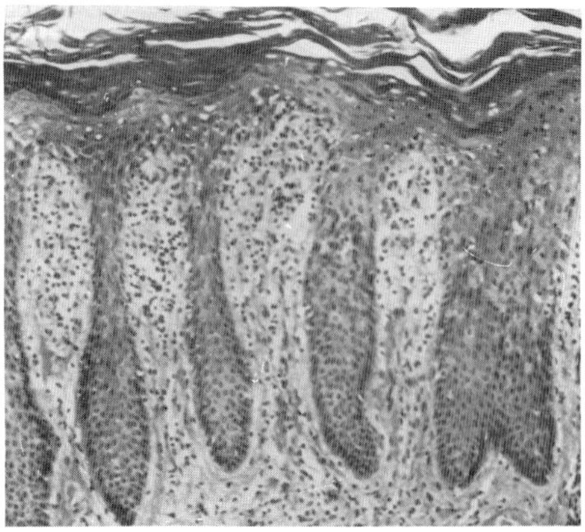

Fig. 39-13 Psoriasis with conspicuous parakeratosis, elongated, clubbed rete ridges, thinned suprapapillary epidermis, and rigid vessels in papillae. (Hematoxylin-eosin.)

scales with a predilection for symmetric distribution on the extremities, especially on the knees and elbows. Lesions may occur also on the scalp, upper back, face, and genitalia and over the sacrum. The nails often are involved and become thickened, dirty white, irregularly laminated, rigid, and brittle. The disease is notoriously chronic although remissions may occur spontaneously and after certain therapy, as following exposure to x-rays or to ultraviolet ray therapy.

Occasionally, a widespread erythroderma or exfoliative dermatitis may complicate psoriasis, either spontaneously or, more particularly, after vigorous therapy. Another complication of psoriasis is arthritis, occurring usually in association with the generalized erythroderma. Occasionally, the arthritis is deforming and persistently ankylotic, as in rheumatoid arthritis.

The use of various qualifying terms such as psoriasis punctata, psoriasis guttata, psoriasis rupioides, psoriasis follicularis, psoriasis nummularis, and others reflects simply the predominant pattern of the lesions.

The histologic features of psoriasis (Fig. 39-13) are as follows:

1 Acanthosis with regular downgrowth of the rete ridges to about the same dermal level

2 Rounded test tube–shaped tips of the rete ridges

3 Prolongation of the papillae, frequently with single vessels (venules) extending the length of the papillae as if rigid rather than tortuous

4 Thin epidermal plates over the elongated papillae, which offer so little covering for the dilated vessels of the papillae that bleeding occurs when a scale is lifted (Auspitz's sign)

5 Prominent parakeratosis, usually extending the length of the lesion rather than focally

6 Absence or sparsity of stratum granulosum

7 Microabscesses (of Munro) in the upper rete malpighii

In addition, there is an absence of spongiosis, as a rule, except in the immediate vicinity of the epidermal microabscesses. Intracellular edema in the rete malpighii is common. The papillae are infiltrated chiefly with lymphocytes and histiocytes. In lesions that are in the early stage of development, some of these features, such as the rounding of the ridges and the elongation of the papillae with thin epidermal plates, may be absent. Furthermore, as in other dermatoses, recent therapy, trauma, or secondary infection obviously will modify the pattern. However, in patients in whom there has been a superimposed exfoliative dermatitis, the basic histologic picture of the psoriatic lesion tends to persist and thereby may help differentation from the exfoliative stage of *mycosis fungoides,* a problem

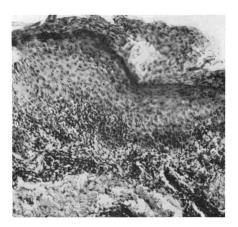

Fig. 39-14 Parapsoriasis with spotty parakeratosis, acanthosis, transepidermal migration of inflammatory cells, and infiltrate immediately subepidermal. (Hematoxylin-eosin.)

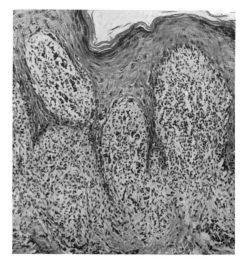

Fig. 39-15 Lichen planus with hyperkeratosis, acanthosis, pointed rete ridges, liquefaction degeneration, and dense subepidermal inflammatory zone. (Hematoxylin-eosin.)

that occasionally arises (Fig. 39-51). Neurodermatitis may simulate psoriasis so closely as to be histologically indistinguishable. As a rule, however, the psoriasiform features listed previously are irregular or less developed in neurodermatitis or individual changes are altogether lacking.

Parapsoriasis. Parapsoriasis—notwithstanding the name—is not otherwise related to psoriasis. The disease is characterized by erythematous macules covered with fine scales and distributed on the trunk and extremities. The lesions are extremely resistant to therapy.

The histologic changes of parapsoriasis are said to be quite nonspecific and to simulate psoriasis, seborrheic dermatitis, lichen planus, a macular syphiloderm, or the early stage of mycosis fungoides. Although the changes may simulate these other diseases, the specific diagnosis of parapsoriasis may be made with considerable assurance in many cases on the basis of the histologic changes alone. These changes include the spotty, thin areas of parakeratosis, slight to moderate acanthosis, vertical arrangement with some hyperchromatism of the basal layer along with slight liquefaction degeneration and, perhaps most revealing, the localization of inflammatory cells, mostly mononuclear, in the immediately subepidermal zone. The infiltrate hugs the epidermis tightly, and characteristically some of the inflammatory cells are located in the epidermis in their transepidermal migration (Fig. 39-14). The absence or sparsity of plasma cells and of endarteritis helps to eliminate syphilis as a possibility. The presence of parakeratosis and a minimal stratum granulosum, as well as the shape of the ridges, easily

distinguish parapsoriasis from lichen planus. One of the serious errors of histologic diagnosis is mislabeling as parapsoriasis (en plaque) the early stage of mycosis fungoides. This error is made both clinically and histologically.

Lichen planus

Lichen planus is generally easily recognized clinically by the irregular, violaceous, glistening, flat-topped, pruritic papules, covered with a thin, horny, adherent film and distributed symmetrically, particularly along the flexor aspects of the wrists, forearms, and legs. The usual form of lichen planus tends to resolve spontaneously after a year or so.

On careful examination, minute whitish points and lines (Wickham's striae) are seen on the surface of the papules. The disease is chronic, may last from months to years, and is rarely associated with constitutional reaction except in some of the hyperacute cases. The principal varieties include lichen planus, lichen planus hypertrophicus, and lichen planus atrophicus. During World War II, many soldiers who had received Atabrine for suppressing malaria developed cutaneous lesions that simulated lichen planus, more especially lichen planus hypertrophicus. However, Atabrine dermatitis differed from lichen planus in its localization (face, scalp, and nails), in its greater severity, in its common association with eczematous and exfoliative dermatitis, and in its response following removal of the patient from tropical climates and withdrawal of the drug. Also associated with Atabrine dermatitis were occasional severe or fatal systemic reactions, including aplastic anemia, hepatitis, and necrotizing nephrosis.[2]

The histology of lichen planus is strikingly characteristic and comprises:

1 Hyperkeratosis
2 Prominence of the stratum granulosum
3 Acanthosis, with elongated, saw-toothed rete ridges
4 Liquefaction degeneration of the basal layer
5 A mononuclear infiltrate consisting mostly of lymphocytes and histiocytes, sharply limited to the papillary and subpapillary layers of the dermis (Fig. 39-15)

In the atrophic form the ridges are flattened and the dermal infiltrate is sparse and replaced by an increased density of collagen containing somewhat thickened arterioles. Those lesions of Atabrine dermatitis that clinically resemble lichen planus carry that similarity into the histologic picture.

Keratoderma blennorrhagicum

Infrequently, perhaps in about 1 in 5,000 cases, there develops an ugly eruption following the contraction of gonorrheal urethritis. This eruption is called keratoderma blenorrhagicum or gonorrheal keratosis and is associated with a nonsuppurative migrating arthritis and gonorrheal urethritis that persist in spite of chemotherapy. The cutaneous lesions appear several weeks following the urethritis, do not contain gonococci, according to most observers, and clear only after disappearance of the urethritis. The lesions of the skin are identical with those of *Reiter's syndrome,* which is associated with a presumed "nonspecific" urethritis, conjunctivitis, and nonsuppurative arthritis. In both the keratoderma and Reiter's syndrome, evolution of the disease is essentially similar. In both, the arthritis clears, as a rule, without residual damage to the joints. In the few cases tested, the complement fixation test for gonorrhea was negative in Reiter's syndrome. More recently, the pleuropneumonia or "L" organisms have been considered responsible for Reiter's syndrome.

The histologic features of keratoderma blennorrhagicum are as follows:

1 Prominent parakeratosis with excessive loosening of the scales so that they may be difficult to include in the histologic sections
2 Acanthosis with elongation and rounding

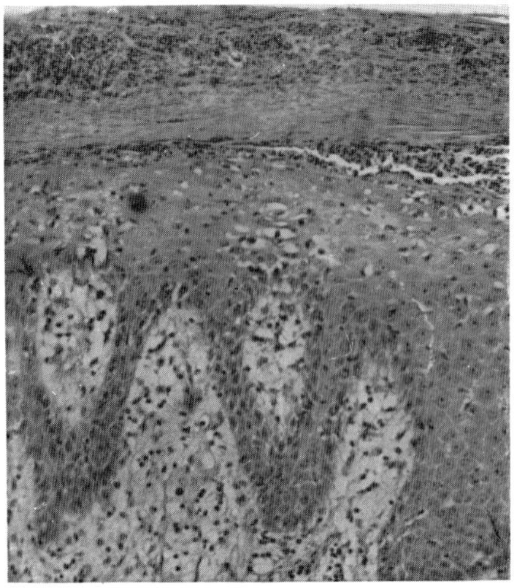

Fig. 39-16 Keratoderma blennorrhagicum with prominent parakeratosis and acanthosis, clubbed rete ridges, and diffusely scattered leukocytes. (Hematoxylin-eosin.)

of the ends of the rete ridges, very much as in psoriasis, so that pustular psoriasis may be a difficult differential diagnostic problem
3 Elongation of the papillae but generally not as strikingly as in psoriasis because the overlying epidermal plate usually is not so thinned as in the latter disease
4 Numerous polymorphonuclear leukocytes, particularly in the upper rete malpighii and in the scales

The leukocytes tend not to be clustered densely into epidermal abscesses, but rather they are scattered more or less evenly and tend to occur in lacunae. The infiltration of the vascular papillae is principally of lymphocytes and histiocytes (Fig. 39-16). No gonococci are demonstrable by bacterial stains, although they are said to have been cultured in a few instances. Moreover, notwithstanding the abundance of polymorphonuclear leukocytes, the commonplace staphylococci are so few in these lesions that often they, too, are not demonstrable even with special bacterial stains. It has been presumed that the development of the cutaneous lesions several weeks after the urethritis, the usual absence of gonococci in the lesions, the intractability of the lesions to local therapy, their spontaneous resolution after the urethritis has been cleared, and the distribution of the skin lesions in the pattern of epidermophytids all suggest an allergic basis for the eruption. It is, of course, well known, but occasionally forgotten, that the histologic response to allergy may consist of vesicles and polymorphonuclear exudation in addition to the more generally recognized reactions of eosinophilia, plasmocytosis, and fibrinoid degeneration of collagen.

Diseases principally of dermis
Urticaria pigmentosa

Urticaria pigmentosa is a chronic disease of the skin that begins usually in the first year of life but may start shortly after puberty or in later adult life, selecting particularly males of light complexion. In a significant number of patients with urticaria pigmentosa there is a history of asthma or hay fever. The eruption, characteristically, is made up of oval, 0.5 cm to 2.5 cm, pigmented, yellowish-to-reddish brown, macular, papular, and even nodular lesions occurring on the back especially but also on the face, scalp, palms, and soles. Infrequently, a patient will have merely a solitary nodule of urticaria pigmentosa. Solitary mastocytomas generally are detected by the first month of life and comprise about 10% to 15% of all instances of cutaneous mastocytosis. The disseminated cutaneous form usually develops by the next few months. About 25% of cases appear late in teenage or adult life, between the ages of 15 and 40 years, occurring equally in males and females.

Occasionally, the eruptions may be sufficiently yellow to simulate xanthomatosis. The lesions are often intensely pruritic and, when irritated, become reddened, swollen, and urticarial—i.e., they show evidence of dermographism. They may persist for years and, in many instances, disappear spontaneously. In those patients in whom the lesions of urticaria pigmentosa appear in childhood and are confined to the skin, the likelihood of spontaneous resolution during adolescence is great. In those in whom the lesions first appear in adolescence or later, the possibility of their persistence and systemization is considerable.

Systemic involvement (bones, liver, lymph nodes, spleen etc.) occurs in about 10% of patients, mostly in adults, and about one-third of these develop the equivalent of a mast cell leukemia. Uncommonly, a solitary nodule or mastocytoma is followed by dissemination to the viscera or to the remainder of the skin. Such dissemination is said not to occur if the nodule remains solitary for approximately two months.[22]

The histologic picture of urticaria pigmentosa is distinctive. In the more striking examples, the upper one-half to two-thirds of the dermis is replaced by a compact zone

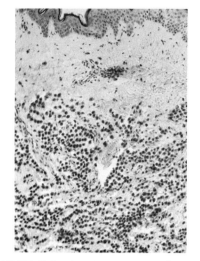

Fig. 39-17 Urticaria pigmentosa with superficial edema of cutis and extensive numbers of mast cells in remainder of dermis. (Hematoxylin-eosin.)

of mast cells that obscure the dermal landmarks (Fig. 39-17). The mast cells should be recognized in sections stained with the routine hematoxylin and eosin, notwithstanding their simulation of ordinary histiocytes and of plasma cells. Frequently, under high magnification, even with this routine stain, the cytoplasmic granules of mast cells may be discerned. These granules are, of course, more clearly demonstrable in metachromatic stains, such as Giemsa's or toluidine blue. The granules are presumed to contain histamine, heparin, and possibly serotonin. In some cases, mast cells are present in smaller numbers and are dispersed as clumps of ten to twenty cells about the mid-dermal vessels. In these instances, nice judgment may be required to differentiate the presence of mast cells in normal and abnormal numbers. In addition to the mast cells, there often are subepidermal edema (urticaria), chromatophores containing melanin in the upper dermis, and eosinophilic leukocytes scattered among the mast cells. Melanosis of the basal layer of the epidermis also may be present. The full-blown picture of urticaria pigmentosa closely resembles the so-called mastocytoma of dogs. Systemic foci of infiltrations of mast cells are found also in the viscera—e.g., in the spleen, liver, and lymph nodes. Routine histologic sections of urticaria pigmentosa are commonly mistaken for leukemia, nevi, malignant melanomas, and Letterer-Siwe disease. Resignation to the teaching that mast cells cannot be detected or strongly suspected with stains of hematoxylin and eosin is, in large part, responsible for these serious errors. Collections of mast cells may produce lytic and diffuse sclerotic lesions of bones as well as hepatosplenomegaly. As indicated, other organs may be involved.

Simple urticaria may be caused in a variety of ways: by drugs, allergenic foods, infections (melioidosis), ultraviolet irradiation *(urticaria solare),* and, fairly commonly, emotional disturbances. Urticaria solare follows immediately after exposure to light of sufficient intensity and of proper wavelength, usually in the violet or blue part of the spectrum.

Erysipelas

Erysipelas is described in the chapter on bacterial diseases (p. 286).

Acute febrile neutrophilic dermatosis

Acute febrile neutrophilic dermatosis might be mentioned here. This entity refers to a relapsing erysipeloid cellulitis of unknown etiology, occurring preponderantly in women, described by Sweet in 1964.[98] The face is commonly involved.

Diseases of collagen

Keloid. A keloid is a hypertrophic cutaneous scar that develops as a reaction to burns of various sorts, incisions, insect bites, vaccinations, and other stimuli. Ulcerated keloids are prone to undergo carcinomatous transformation of the epidermis after a long interval, particularly those due to burns or associated with chronic sinuses, as in osteomyelitis. The dermal portion of a keloid is not more likely to become sarcomatous than the dermis elsewhere. Rarely, a keloid resolves spontaneously.

The histologic features of a keloid include thick, homogeneously eosinophilic bands of collagen admixed with thin collagenous fibers and large active fibroblasts. The sweat glands, sebaceous glands, follicles, and arrectores pilorum are atrophic, destroyed, or displaced by the scar. The epidermis may be atrophic or only slightly altered by fusion and irregular pattern of the ridges. The ordinary scar of the skin is more cellular than a keloid and is composed of uniformly thinner collagenous fibers. In both instances, elastic tissue is diminished or absent. The keloidal reaction of hypertrophic collagenous bundles and large fibroblasts is characteristic of dermatitis papillaris capillitii (keloidal acne), which

occurs particularly in the nuchal region and, with the associated extensive plasmocellular reaction, represents a type of response to folliculitis.

Balanitis xerotica obliterans. Balanitis xerotica obliterans constitutes another disease of collagen that appears clinically as whitish, firm, coalescent papules or a sclerotic plaque of the glans penis and foreskin and occurs, often, following circumcision. The disease is of some importance because the process tends to extend to the urethral meatus, causing stenosis of the orifice. The lesion is to be differentiated clinically from erythroplasia of Queyrat and circumscribed scleroderma. There is likelihood that balanitis xerotica obliterans is a form of lichen sclerosus et atrophicus, which tends to occur on the vulva.

The histologic picture consists of:

1 Atrophic epidermis or epithelium with loss of rete ridges

2 Striking homogenization of the collagen affecting about one-third of the upper dermis

3 A more or less dense zone of lymphocytes and histiocytes beneath the homogenized collagen (Fig. 39-18)

The small arteries and arterioles of the upper and middle dermis may show evidence of endarteritis obliterans, but this process is sufficiently inconstant as not to warrant the use of the qualification "obliterans" in the name of the disease. Furthermore, on the basis of other cutaneous atrophy, there is considerable reason to believe that the vascular change does not initiate the collagenous

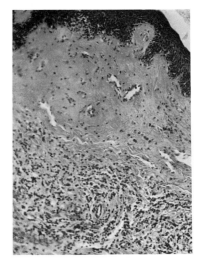

Fig. 39-18 Balanitis xerotica obliterans with homogenization of subepidermal collagen over zone of inflammatory cells. (Hematoxylin-eosin.)

change but perhaps is an incidental secondary reaction as in other kinds of chronic inflammations (e.g., chronic gastric ulcer).

In lichen sclerosus et atrophicus, the initial change is a subepidermal edema that subsequently progresses to the characteristically homogenized densely sclerotic collagen in which the elastic fibers are diminished because of their displacement downward. The edema may be so great as to cause actual vesiculation at the epidermal-dermal junction.

Acrodermatitis chronica atrophicans. Acrodermatitis chronica atrophicans presents the basic qualitative histologic features of balanitis xerotica obliterans—i.e., atrophy of the epidermis and a subepidermal homogenized zone of collagen beneath which is a dense zone of mononuclear cells (Fig. 39-19). The major difference lies in the constantly wider zones of homogenization and cellular reaction in balanitis xerotica obliterans. In addition, the epidermis is hyperkeratotic. There are loss of dermal elastic tissue and atrophy of appendages in acrodermatitis chronica atrophicans.

Clinically, however, there is no resemblance between the two diseases. Acrodermatitis chronica atrophicans begins as erythematous, slightly edematous macules that later become wrinkled, atrophic, and sclerodermatoid. As the prefix *acro-* indicates, the disease tends to select the extremities, particularly the hands and feet and the extensor surfaces of the elbows and knees.

The condition occurs predominantly in

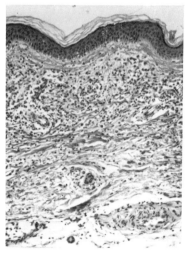

Fig. 39-19 Acrodermatitis chronica atrophicans with thin zone of hyalinized subepidermal collagen and deeper layer of inflammatory cells. (Hematoxylin-eosin.)

middle-aged women. It has been reported that individuals with this disease are prone to develop epidermoid carcinomas of the skin. However, thus far the statistical documentation lacks conviction, just as it does for the corresponding complication in psoriasis, in the absence of arsenical or x-ray therapy.

Granuloma annulare. Granuloma annulare is a chronic eruption made up of papules or nodules grouped in a ringed or circinate arrangement with a tendency to occur on the dorsa of the fingers and hands and on the elbows, neck, feet, ankles, and buttocks, particularly of children and young adults. The lesions can be palpated intracutaneously rather than subcutaneously, as can the rheumatic nodules.

The etiology of the disease is unknown. Because of the histology, a rheumatic basis for the disease comes to mind but here, too, clinical evidence is lacking. Allergy is a probable factor. We have seen two cases associated with disseminated allergic granulomatous arteritis. The histologic picture of granuloma annulare has been observed also as a reaction to the *Culicoides furans,* a biting gnat.

Histologically, granuloma annulare is characterized by an intradermal oval or circular focus of fibrinoid degeneration of collagen. These necrotic foci of dermal collagen really suggest infarcts, although corresponding occlusion of adjacent vessels is not regularly noted. About such a focus there are palisaded rows of epithelioid cells or histiocytes, some of which may be vacuolated by fat (Fig. 39-20). It is the combination of fibrinoid alteration of collagen and palisaded histiocytes that suggests a possible rheumatic etiology. In fact, the histologic features of granuloma annulare are identical with those of the rheumatic nodule—the only difference being the location of the latter in the subcutaneous tissue, adjacent to or within synovial membranes. Certainly, the histologic picture is not that of tuberculosis, although the characteristic fibrinoid degeneration of the collagen of granuloma annulare and the rheumatic nodule has been mistaken for the caseation of tuberculosis, a simulation that usually can be detected easily. There may be considerable difficulty, however, in recognizing early or small lesions of granuloma annulare in which the only clue may be a minimal smudgy fibrinoid swelling of collagen with clumps of a few histiocytes, some vacuolated and others partially palisaded. These minute lesions may be confused with xan-

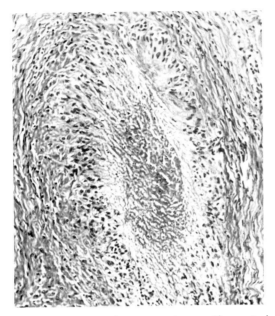

Fig. 39-20 Granuloma annulare with central fibrinoid necrosis of dermal collagen surrounded by palisaded epithelioid histiocytes. (Hematoxylin-eosin; from Allen, A. C.: Arch. Derm. Syph. [Chicago] **57**:19-56, 1948.)

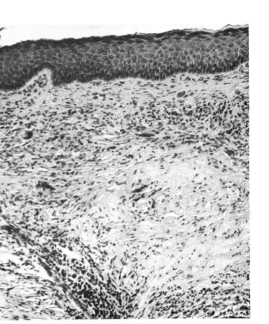

Fig. 39-21 Necrobiosis lipoidica diabeticorum with irregularly homogenized, degenerated dermal collagen and tuberculoid granulomas at periphery. (Hematoxylin-eosin.)

thoses, necrobiosis lipoidica diabeticorum, or leprosy. Of course, Aschoff bodies are absent in granuloma annulare, as they are in the subcutaneous rheumatic nodule. They are confined to the heart.

Necrobiosis lipoidica diabeticorum. Necrobiosis lipoidica diabeticorum is a disease characterized by oval, circular, firm, sharply defined plaques with yellowish centers and violaceous peripheries, occurring predominantly on the legs but found also on the forearms, palms, soles, neck, and face. The centers of the lesions are prone to ulcerate. Trauma, often inconspicuous, may initiate the lesions. In about 50% to 80% of the patients, the disease is associated with diabetes. In about 10%, the lesions precede the onset of diabetes. In the remainder, diabetes does not develop. Obviously, the recognition of necrobiosis lipoidica diabeticorum can be of remarkably prophetic importance.

Clinically, the disease must be differentiated from other such focal diseases of collagen as granuloma annulare, amyloidosis, morphea, and lipidproteinosis, as well as the granulomas of sarcoid and erythema induratum, which tend, also, to occur on the extremities. The diabetic state in some instances of necrobiosis lipoidica diabeticorum may be missed with the standard glucose tolerance test and dis-

covered with the cortisone glucose tolerance test.[70]

The basic histologic change of necrobiosis diabeticorum consists of ischemic-like degeneration of collagen, occurring in irregular patches, especially in the upper dermis. In well-developed foci, the altered collagen is swollen and somewhat granular, with loss of fibrils and with a diminution in nuclei of fibrocytes. At the periphery of the collagenous alteration are small collections of histiocytes often arranged about Langhans' giant cells and simulating sarcoid or tuberculosis (Fig. 39-21). This giant cell reaction occasionally may involve the walls of veins to produce a giant cell phlebitis reminiscent of the reaction in temporal arteritis. Vacuoles may be present in the cytoplasm of the giant cells and histiocytes, but fat is found infrequently within the cells of these lesions, although extracellular fat is detectable about the altered collagen.

Scleroderma. There are two basic varieties of scleroderma, the differentiation of which is of great importance prognostically: (1) morphea or circumscribed scleroderma and (2) diffuse scleroderma.

Circumscribed scleroderma occurs as well-delimited, round or oval plaques with whitish, yellowish, or ivory-colored centers and violaceous peripheries. Occasionally, the plaques

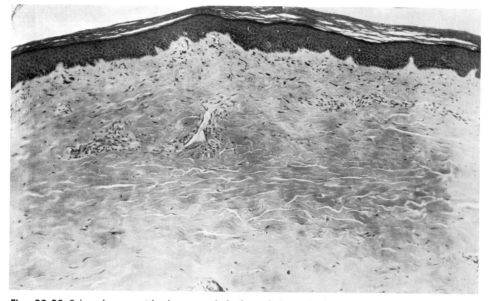

Fig. 39-22 Scleroderma with dense and thickened dermal fibers, atrophy of appendages and epidermis, and melanin pigmentation of basal layer. (Hematoxylin-eosin.)

correspond in distribution to the innervation of a cutaneous nerve, so that a trophic origin has been suggested. Degeneration and regeneration of dermal nerves are said to occur with characteristic patterns in scleroderma and acrosclerosis. *Morphea guttata* or *white-spot disease* is a modification of circumscribed scleroderma characterized by varying-sized chalk white patches on the chest and neck. Rarely does circumscribed scleroderma progress into the often fatal diffuse scleroderma. Usually, the lesions clear, with a barely noticeable thin atrophic area as a residuum. *Linear scleroderma* of an extremity may be associated with melorheostosis or linear hyperostosis of the underlying bone.

Diffuse scleroderma, which affects women twice as often as men, begins insidiously—usually as edema of the hands, other parts of the extremities, or neck—and extends inexorably on to sclerosis that stiffens, binds, and limits the mobility of the affected part. Ulcerations may occur over bony prominence. Calcareous cutaneous deposits and pigmentation, the latter of such a degree as to simulate Addison's disease, are frequent. The normal cutaneous lines become obliterated. Diminution in sweating, hyperesthesias, and pruritus may occur. Sclerosis limited to the hands in association with the vasospastic symptoms of Raynaud's disease is called acrosclerosis or sclerodactylia. In actuality, this symptom complex presents a phase of diffuse sclero-

derma, although the progress to the fatal disease is not invariable (see pp. 503 and 745).

Systemic sclerosis refers to diffuse scleroderma with visceral involvement. Dense fibrosis may affect the myocardium and the esophagus and other portions of the gastrointestinal tract. The lungs may be affected with cystic fibrosis, particularly at the bases. Renal vessels may present the histologic picture of accelerated nephrosclerosis, and, if widespread, will indeed be associated with malignant hypertension. The glomeruli may show conspicuous diffuse membranous glomerulonephritis. The cardiac fibrosis or the cystic pulmonary changes may lead to myocardial failure.

The histologic sections of morphea cannot be differentiated from those of diffuse scleroderma. The principal changes involve the collagenous fibers, which become hypertrophied through edema and then atrophy. The atrophic fibers are no longer loosely disposed as in the normal dermis but are compressed into dense, compact, collagenous masses, with diminution of fibrocytic nuclei and obliteration of spaces between collagenous bundles so that the thickness of the dermis is visibly decreased (Fig. 39-22). Inflammatory reaction may be absent or, in the early stages, abundant, particularly as focal collections of mononuclear cells disposed about appendages. The appendages (hair, sweat glands, and sebaceous glands) are atrophic. Elastic fibers may be diminished or distorted, but they represent the least informative alteration and are unduly emphasized in the literature. The epidermis may be normal, but usually it is atrophic, with flattened rete ridges and a hyperpigmented basal layer. Subepidermal melanin-containing chromatophores may be increased. In conjunction with the collagenous atrophy, small arteries and arterioles may become secondarily sclerotic. Calcific or even ossified foci (osteoma cutis) may replace the altered collagen of the dermis and subcutaneous septa. The deposits of calcium may be so extensive as to camouflage the primary diagnosis and be dismissed as "calcinosis." Superficial dermal telangiectasia is common, possibly as a consequence of sclerosis of deeper vessels.

Atrophic myositis may accompany the cutaneous lesions, although uncommonly to the degree found in *dermatomyositis* or *poikilodermatomyositis,* in which the inflammatory reaction in the skeletal muscles may be extreme, despite the usual nondescript subepidermal edema and focal liquefaction degeneration in the latter diseases. Here, again, it is emphasized that neither *diffuse* vascular nor *diffuse* visceral collagenous changes occur in dermatomyositis or poikilodermatomyositis any more than they do in the vast majority of cases of diffuse lupus erythematosus or even systemic sclerosis.

In view of the association between sclerosis of skin and lung (systemic sclerosis, burns, healed infarcts, etc.) on the one hand and carcinoma on the other, it may be anticipated that carcinoma of the skin would be a complication of diffuse scleroderma. This latter association is rare and may, perhaps, be a reflection of the duration of the sclerosis.

Scleredema. Scleredema (Buschke's disease) is to be distinguished from scleroderma. Although the entity is commonly known as *scleredema adultorum,* it does involve children in an appreciable percentage of cases.

Scleredema is usually a self-limited disease characterized by a tough, nonpitting, uniform edema of the head and neck, producing a masklike expression and restricted motion that simulates scleroderma. The periphery of the process is sharply palpable. The disease generally runs its course in from several months to a year and a half, leaving no residuum. Recurrences have been recorded.

The lesion differs from scleroderma in the absence of pigmentation, the rarity of involvement of the hands and feet, and complete resolution with rarest exceptions. The usually self-limited scleredema of Buschke is distin-

guished from the long-lasting, often extensive scleredema associated with diabetes mellitus.

The histologic picture of scleredema is that of striking edema and hypertrophy of tight collagenous bundles so that, despite the compactness of the bundles, the thickness of the dermis is distinctly increased over normal. The epidermis, vessels, elastic tissue, and muscle show no changes. The changes of *sclerema neonatorum* are altogether different from scleredema or scleroderma and consist of the precipitation of fatty acid crystals and foreign body reaction in the subcutaneous fat, possibly due to a deficiency of olein in the fat, with consequent raising of its melting point. The localized, nodular sclerema, which some believe may result from birth trauma, is a self-limited disorder. The diffuse form, which may involve also visceral (e.g., periadrenal and perirenal) fat, is a fatal disease. Scleredema and scleroderma are to be differentiated also from *myxedema* of either the circumscribed or the diffuse type. In *myxedema,* unlike either scleredema or scleroderma, there are focal granularity, irregular vacuolization, and looseness of the collagen bundles due to the presence therein of interfibrillary fluid and nonsulfated acid mucopolysaccharides (as demonstrated with alcian blue and colloidal iron). It is stated that the heart and voluntary muscles (e.g., tongue) also may be affected.

The epidermis tends to be hyperkeratotic. Circumscribed myxedema occurs in association with hyperthyroidism and has been associated with clubbing of the nails.

Lipid proteinosis. Lipid proteinosis *(hyalinosis cutis et mucosae)* is another remarkable disease affecting dermal collagen and its vessels. The disease generally manifests itself in infancy and is characterized by verrucous yellowish plaques, especially on the hands, feet, elbows, and face. The lesions may involve also the mouth and larynx. In the latter location, the woody consistency of the lesions may cause a stenosis severe enough to require tracheotomy. Persistant hoarseness is a common symptom. Disturbances in phospholipids are inconstant. A familial tendency toward diabetes mellitus is occasionally present. It does not now appear that the entity is a primary lipidosis but rather that the lipid is normal in composition incidental to other tissue changes, especially those of collagen. One form of lipid proteinosis is light sensitive and occurs with erythropoietic porphyria.

The histologic features of lipid proteinosis are a hyperkeratotic and acanthotic epidermis

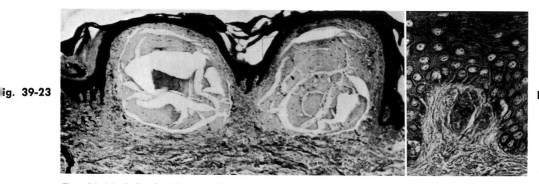

Fig. 39-24

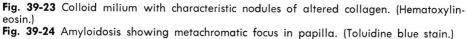

Fig. 39-23 Colloid milium with characteristic nodules of altered collagen. (Hematoxylin-eosin.)

Fig. 39-24 Amyloidosis showing metachromatic focus in papilla. (Toluidine blue stain.)

overlying eosinophilic homogenized collagen in the upper dermis. The walls of arterioles and small arteries of this region are thickened. A fat stain reveals dense sudanophilic deposits in and about their walls, as well as in the stroma. No foam cells are present such as are found in *Fabry's disease (angiokeratoma corporis diffusum)*. The serum lipids are normal, as a rule. It is stated that the fat is combined with the protein of the collagen and therefore resists ordinary fat solvents. This property was not borne out in two cases personally observed. As might be expected, the hyalinized collagen is PAS positive and diastase resistant and stains metachromatically with toluidine blue. Accordingly, the entity has been designated a "lipoglycoproteinosis."

Amyloidosis. Amyloidosis may be confined to the skin, or the cutaneous lesions may represent part of a systemic process. The eruption is characterized by pruritus and brownish papules, nodules, or plaques, occurring particularly on the legs. Histologically, there are focal areas of bland homogenization of dense collagen, occasionally scattered in the dermis but often located as subepidermal round masses (lichen amyloidosis) which stain metachromatically with the ordinary stains for amyloid.

The subepidermal nodules of amyloidosis *(lichen amyloidosis)* tend to be restricted to the skin. The nodular, para-articular masses of amyloid, along with amyloidotic macroglossia, are likely to be a manifestation of primary amyloidosis (para-amyloidosis) and to be associated with myeloma or related plasmocytosis and globulinemias. The cutaneous manifestations of amyloidosis secondary to leprosy, tuberculosis, rheumatoid arthritis, Hodgkin's disease, chronic suppuration, etc. may be detectable only microscopically. The amyloid of primary amyloidosis tends to resist metachromatic stains in contrast with amyloid of secondary amyloidosis. Rarely, epidermolysis bullosa may overlay secondary amyloidosis of the skin.[71]

The histologic picture of lichen amyloidosis may closely simulate *colloid milium*, in which, too, there is a homogeneous alteration, with swelling into nodular masses of the subepidermal collagen (Fig. 39-23). However, the collagen of colloid milium does not stain metachromatically, and, in addition, the fibers in this disease appear looser, more edematous, and more friable than do those of amyloidosis (Fig. 39-24).

Clinically, colloid milium appears as small translucent papules from 1 mm to 5 mm in diameter, occurring commonly on the exposed areas, particularly the face, of fair-skinned individuals, more commonly men.

Circumscribed myxedema. Circumscribed or localized myxedema occurs in association with exophthalmic Graves' disease. It appears as a fairly demarcated nonpitting, solidly edematous, usually bilateral plaque of the pretibial region, at times extending to the dorsa of the feet.

Persistently elevated serum levels of "long-acting" thyroid stimulator (LATS) are the rule in patients with pretibial myxedema. In some instances, LATS has been detected in homogenates of tissue from the affected areas in concentrations significantly higher than in unaffected tissue. It is hypothesized that LATS acts as a specific antibody which, when fixed in tissue, elicits the characteristic local edematous reaction[60] (see also p. 1436).

Histologically, abundant basophilic mucin is found separating and fragmenting dermal collagenous bundles, without inflammatory reaction other than an occasional increase of mast cells. The diffuse myxedema of hypothyroidism is characterized by swelling of the collagenous bundles by interfibrillary mucin, which, in some instances, is demonstrable with alcian or toluidine blue. There is less disruption of the collagenous bundles in diffuse myxedema than in circumscribed myxedema of hyperthyroidism. These lesions are to be distinguished from the nonendocrinogenic subepidermal mucinous papules of *lichen myxedematosis* or *papular mucinosis*.

Mucinous cysts

Mucinous dermal cysts, often loosely referred to as "synovial cysts" or "myxoid cysts," are seen as single, smooth, and firm 5 mm to 6 mm nodules at the bases of distal phalanges. The overlying epidermis is likely to be slightly thinned but not otherwise significantly altered. The cyst contains a mucinous, clear material quite like that of synovial cysts, and the similarity extends to the histologic structure. The mucin is PAS negative but contains large amounts of hyaluronic acid as reflected in the positive alcian blue stain.[53] There is no communication of these cysts with bursae or joint cavities.

Microscopically, the cyst is found to be unilocular or multilocular and to be derived from a simple liquefaction of the dermal collagen so that no mesothelial or endothelial lining is present. Such a lining may be simulated by compressed fibrocytes of the dermal collagenous fibers. Essentially, this picture is analogous to that found in what are also loosely called synovial cysts of tendons or ganglions. These, too, do not represent cysts of expanded synovial walls with mesothelial lining but, rather, foci of mucinous degeneration of collagen of tendon or synovia. The mucinous dermal cyst may become obliterated by fibrosis and calcification.

Diseases of elastic tissue

Although alterations in elastic tissue, especially diminution and fraying, occur in many dermatoses, there are several principal, primary disorders of elastic tissue: (1) cutis hyperelastica (Ehlers-Danlos syndrome), (2) pseudoxanthoma elasticum, (3) senile elastosis, (4) elastoma dorsi, (5) elastosis perforans serpiginosa, and (6) dermatolysis (cutis laxa).

Cutis hyperelastica. Cutis hyperelastica (Ehlers-Danlos syndrome) is a familial disease characterized by hyperelastic velvety skin ("rubber skin") associated with hyperlaxity and hyperextensibility of the joints and the

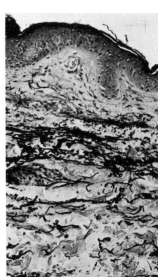

Fig. 39-25 Hyperelastosis cutis. (Weigert-van Gieson.)

tendency of the skin to bleed, tear, and scar following slight trauma. The disorder may be associated with skeletal deformities, including arachnodactyly, blue sclerae (as in *Löbstein's syndrome*), dilatation of viscera (trachea, esophagus, and colon), pulmonary blebs, dissecting aneurysms, etc.

Histologically, abundant compact masses of elastic fibers throughout the dermis are demonstrable by Weigert's stain for elastic tissue (Fig. 39-25). The suggestion that the increase in elastic fibers is illusionary rather than real is not borne out by personal observations. There appears to be no qualitative alteration in these or in the collagenous fibers. The tendency for calcification, as observed in elastica fibers in pseudoxanthoma elasticum and in degenerative arterial diseases, is not apparent in the elastic fibers of Ehlers-Danlos syndrome. Edema of the superficial dermis, with disruption of the normal wavy pattern of the dermal collagenous fibers, may be observed. On the other hand, calcification within the panniculus may be present.

Pseudoxanthoma elasticum. Pseudoxanthoma elasticum is another hereditary disease in which yellowish papules and plaques symmetrically distributed are found in abnormally lax skin of the neck, axilla, groin, and cubital and popliteal spaces. Other parts of the body are less frequently involved.

In histologic sections, the elastic fibers are easily detectable, even in routine preparations stained with hematoxylin and eosin, as masses of basophilic, curved, small, partially calcified,

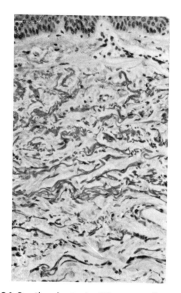

Fig. 39-26 Senile elastosis. (Hematoxylin-eosin.)

fragmented curlicues, with a tendency toward concentration near the mid-dermis. Occasionally, there are associated disheveled, foreign body type of granulomas. In about 50% of the patients with pseudoxanthoma elasticum there occur ophthalmoscopically visible "angioid streaks" in the retina that are said to be similar to the dermal changes histologically and are attributed to cracking of Bruch's elastic membrane of the choroid. The histologic evidence, however, is limited.

Pseudoxanthoma elasticum may be associated with changes in the cardiovascular system, including arterial aneurysms and calcification and degeneration of elastic tissue of arteries. Other congenital cardiovascular, gastrointestinal, and genitourinary defects may occur with the syndrome. Rarely, this syndrome is associated with cutis hyperelastica and with osteitis deformans.

Senile elastosis. Senile elastosis is the term used to describe the loss of elasticity of the skin of elderly people, as noted particularly on the face and the dorsum of the hands (i.e., the exposed portions of the body). This condition is found associated also with epidermal neoplasms, discoid lupus erythematosus, radiodermatitis, and other diseases. In microscopic sections, the change is represented by a subpapillary zone of basophilic alteration of swollen elastic fibers.

This form of elastosis may or may not be associated with atrophy of the epidermis and appendages (Fig. 39-26). It is of interest that, notwithstanding the increase in elastic tissue,

such skin is characterized by a loss of elasticity as if the physical properties of these fibers had been altered or as if collagenous fibers had acquired the staining properties of elastic tissue.

Elastofibroma dorsi. Elastofibroma dorsi refers to an apparently reactive fibrouslike tumefaction localized preponderantly to the scapula but occurring also near the ischial tuberosity and greater trochanter. The surprising histolgic finding is the presence of numerous clusters of thick and fragmented elastic fibers, readily recognizable by their eosinophilia even in sections stained with hematoxylin and eosin. Although these fibers lack the periodicity of collagen and are digested with elastase, there are reasons to suggest origin from denatured collagen. These fibers, which do not contain fat or calcium, exhibit differences from those of the elastic laminae of arteries, elastotic degeneration of the skin, and pseudoxanthoma elasticum.[99]

Elastofibroma dorsi is to be distinguished from the familial fibromas or "collagenomas" recently described in which no change in the elastic tissue was noted.[42]

Elastosis perforans serpiginosa. Another lesion involving elastic tissue is called elastosis perforans serpiginosa. It is characterized by groups of arciform or circinate, erythematous, acuminate, keratotic papules, usually on the face and neck.

The histology is made diagnostic by the compact packets of curled, frayed, thickened basophilic elastic fibers over which the epidermis is acanthotic and hyperkeratotic. The papule or plug is owing chiefly to the penetration and extrusion through the epidermis of masses of elastic fibers. Lymphocytes and foreign body type of giant cells surround the lesion. The pattern simulates that of Kyrle's disease (hyperkeratosis follicularis in cutem penetrans), in which the extruded plugs are keratinous rather than elastic tissue.

Specific granulomas

Of the specific granulomas of the skin, the following should be mentioned: those due to tuberculosis, sarcoidosis, berylliosis, leprosy, brucellosis, leishmaniasis, syphilis, and granuloma inguinale, granulomas due to atypical acid-fast bacilli, and those due to deep fungi, such as sporotrichosis, blastomycosis, coccidioidomycosis, and histoplasmosis.

Tuberculosis cutis. Tuberculosis cutis may assume a large variety of clinical forms of which lupus vulgaris, scrofuloderma, tuberculosis cutis verrucosa, miliary cutaneous tuberculosis, and many kinds of tuberculids are a few examples. While differing prognostic implications usually make the precise diagnosis of tuberculosis of significance, the important service the pathologist is expected to render is to name the overall tuberculous process. In this, the problem is complicated by the difficulty with which the sparse tubercle bacilli are demonstrable in paraffin sections of the skin, so that the tubercle is usually the chief basis for the diagnosis. Unfortunately, many agents other than tubercle bacilli are capable of producing tubercles. Moreover, the tubercle often is incompletely formed, and reliance is then placed on such suggestions as epithelioid cells clustered or palisaded in the vicinity or in a matrix of caseated tissue, with or without giant cells. The cutaneous reaction of leishmaniasis, as well as of histoplasmosis and other fungi, is often tuberculoid, but the detection of the respective organisms in histiocytes and giant cells establishes the diagnosis.

Of increasing interest are the cutaneous granulomas produced by "atypical" acid-fast bacilli or, more accurately, bacilli that, although acid-fast, are basically different in drug sensitivity as well as in cultural and pathogenetic respects from the *Mycobacterium tuberculosis*. Runyon's classification of these strains into four groups—photochromogens (e.g., *Mycobacterium balnei*), scotochromogens, Battey strain, and "rapid growers"—is a workable one. Not all of the granulomas produced by these organisms have a tuberculoid structure histologically. Some appear quite nonspecific.[59]

Sarcoidosis. The histologic diagnosis of *Boeck's sarcoid* is made on the finding of dermal hyperplastic tubercles, with or without giant cells and Schaumann's or asteroid bodies but in the absence of caseation. Usually, the tubercules are surrounded by dense bands of collagen stroma. No tubercle bacilli are detectable. The term *Darier-Roussy sarcoid* is reserved for an essentially similar histologic process occurring in the deep dermis and subcutaneous fat, thereby resembling erythema induratum. Confusion arises from the simulation of the tuberculous process by the tissue reaction in the tuberculoid form of leprosy, in the syphilitic gumma, and by the tissue response in blastomycosis, coccidioidomycosis, leishmaniasis, and sporotrichosis. Moreover, in some instances of sarcoid, a form of fibrinoid degeneration simulating caseation may occur (p. 939).

Sarcoidosis responds well to cortisone. A diagnostic test for sarcoidosis, called the *Kveim test*, consists of injecting intradermally a brei of tissue known to be involved with Boeck's sarcoid and observing the delayed clinical and histologic reaction to the injection several weeks later.

Berylliosis and brucellosis. The granulomas of berylliosis (usually acquired by inoculation of the beryllium phosphors from broken fluorescent lamps) and those of *brucellosis* may be histologically indistinguishable from those of sarcoidosis or tuberculosis. Silca granulomas are distinguished by the presence of birefringent silica crystals within giant cells. Zirconium in stick deodorants may also cause giant cell granulomas. The *Brucella* organisms may be recovered from culture or after animal inoculation of the diseased tissue.

Other granulomas. The remainder of the granulomatous lesions, including those of leprosy, syphilis and other venereal diseases, the deep mycoses and parasitic infestation, etc., are discussed in other chapters.

PIGMENTATIONS

The abnormalities of cutaneous pigmentation may be considered under two principal categories: metallic and nonmetallic.

Metallic abnormalities of cutaneous pigmentation

The exogenous pigmentations are chiefly those due to metals introduced into the body in a variety of ways, including ingestion, parenteral administration, inunction, and intradermal injection. In general, the metallic pigmentations provoke at least an increased deposition of melanin in the basal layer and in dermal chromatophores. The brown **arsenic pigmentation** due to the ingestion of, particularly, trivalent arsenicals (in Fowler's solution, sodium cacodylate, or arsenic trioxide) often is associated with keratosis of the palms and soles. Histologically, there are relative hyperkeratosis with atrophy of the remainder of the epidermis, hyperchromatism, and a tendency toward palisading of the basal cells and increased melanin deposits in these cells as well as in the chromatophores of the upper dermis, which usually is edematous.

Argyria, in which the skin is discolored bluish gray, may follow the ingestion of silver nitrate, formerly used in the treatment of peptic ulcers, or the application of this drug as well as colloidal silver compounds (Argyrol and Neo-Silvol) to mucous membranes. The

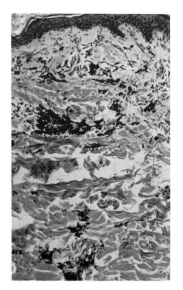

Fig. 39-27 Tattoo with irregular deposits of black-appearing pigment. (Hematoxylin-eosin.)

pigmentation is particularly marked in those areas of the skin exposed to light. The black granules of silver are noted especially in the argyrophilic basement membrane of the sweat glands but also in the connective tissue about sebaceous glands and hair follicles and just beneath the epidermis.

Chrysiasis, due to the parenteral use of gold preparations, as in the treatment of chronic lupus erythematosus, causes an ash-gray or mauve pigmentation characterized histologically by irregular, large granules located chiefly in chromatophores and in the walls of blood vessels. A somewhat similar histologic picture is caused by pigmentation due to **bismuth** and **mercury.**

In **tattoos,** the pigmentation is the result of the deposition of various metallic and vegetable pigments (e.g., cinnabar or red mercuric sulfide) both within chromatophores and extracellularly in irregularly large clumps sometimes surrounded by foreign body reaction (Fig. 39-27). Discoid lupus erythematosus may selectively involve the red areas of tattoos (mercuric sulfide) and spare the blue. Similarly, individuals sensitive to mercury may show allergic reactions in the red portions. Conversely, syphilitic lesions may spare these mercury-impregnated red components of tattoos.

Nonmetallic abnormalities of cutaneous pigmentation

The nonmetallic abnormalities of cutaneous pigmentation include those due to hemo-chromatosis, Addison's disease, pellagra, Peutz-Jeghers syndrome, acanthosis nigricans, chloasma, melanosis of Riehl, ephelides (freckles), sunburn, purpuras, tinea versicolor, and pinta. Several of these entities illustrate once again the cutaneous reflection of visceral disease.

In **hemochromatosis** (bronze diabetes), hemosiderin and, less noticeably, hemofuscin are deposited as brownish granules in melanophores principally and diagnostically about sweat glands. In addition, there is increased melanin in the epidermis and adjacent chromatophores. This cutaneous lesion is commonly associated with deposits of the pigments in the pancreas, liver, and lymph nodes and the development of diabetes mellitus and cirrhosis of the liver.

In **Addison's disease,** there is an excessive deposit of melanin in the basal layer of the epidermis and in underlying melanophores. A similar histologic picture is found in the ordinary freckle (ephelis), sunburn, and chloasma (the latter especially during pregnancy).

Melanosis of Riehl, often associated with malnutrition, is characterized by brown macular discolorations of the face, neck, and, occasionally, hands. Histologically, there is irregular pigmentation by melanin of the basal layer and chromatophores, in addition to telangiectasis, varying degrees of hyperkeratosis, liquefaction degeneration of the basal layer, and partial obliteration of the rete ridges. A similar picture is seen in tar melanosis, the occupational dermatosis probably concerned with photosensitization.

The **Peutz-Jeghers syndrome** consists of melanosis of the lips, oral mucosa, and digits in patients with gastrointestinal polyposis.

Increased pigmentation of the skin follows a variety of cutaneous purpuras: **purpura annularis telangiectodes** (Majocchi's disease), **Schamberg's disease,** and **pigmented purpuric lichenoid dermatitis** of Gougerot and Blum. Each of these disorders occurs selectively on the lower extremities. The pigment in these cases is hemosiderin, which is deposited in chromatophores in the upper dermis. **Angioma serpiginosum,** which is also rather loosely included in the category of cutaneous purpuras, is really an inflammatory telangiectasia and usually shows little or no hemosiderin. In all of these "purpuras," which are unassociated with systemic disorders, there are inflammatory cells (principally lymphocytes and histiocytes) localized in the upper dermis, especially about arterioles and capillaries, which may have swollen and prominent endothelium.

This latter finding is particularly true of Majocchi's disease. There is some question as to whether or not these conditions are actually different phases of the same basic vascular disease. Occasionally, these purpuric lesions, particularly those of *Majocchi's disease,* may be confused histologically with the vascular changes of **periarteritis nodosa** or bacterial and rickettsial arteritis. The changes of **thrombophlebitis migrans** and of **thrombo-angiitis obliterans** are discussed elsewhere (p. 746).

Of great interest is another truly diffuse vascular disease characterized by thromobocytopenia, purpura, a usually fulminant, fatal course (although rare protracted cases have occurred), and a specific histologic picture of fibrinoid necrosis and plateletlike *verrucal* thickening of the walls of dilated arterioles and capillaries. In the past, the disease has been called generalized platelet thrombosis or some variant of this term. However, the histogenesis of the entire lesion from the vascular walls would seem to make the designation **thrombocytopenic verrucal angionecrosis** more appropriate as was long ago suggested.[1] These cases are rarely diagnosed clinically. Inasmuch as the vascular necrosis occurs in the skin as well as the viscera, a skin or muscle biopsy is called for in obscure instances of thrombocytopenic purpura. There is strongly suggestive clinical and histologic evidence of a factor of hypersensitivity in this primarily diffuse vascular disease. Accordingly, we should attribute the thrombocytopenia to an allergic response rather than to depletion by so-called generalized thrombosis, which, as already indicated, and despite certain immunofluorescence studies, does not occur, as previously indicated.[1]

Achromia should be mentioned among the abnormalities of cutaneous pigmentation. The congenital absence of pigment is referred to as partial or complete albinism or leukoderma. **Vitiligo** or acquired leukoderma is usually of unknown etiology. The depigmented patches may be rimmed by hyperpigmented borders and the histologic sections reveal the depigmented and hyperpigmented basal layers in the respective portions. Vitiliginous areas may occur also in any lesion in which there are considerable liquefaction degeneration of the basal layer and encroachment onto this layer by inflammatory cells. *Pinta* and *lichen planus* are cases in point. In both, the melanin is extracted from the basal layer, phagocytized by chromatophores, and carried away to regional lymph nodes. Vitiliginous patches occur in patients with tinea versicolor, partly because the areas affected by the fungus prevent absorption of ultraviolet irradiation and partly because the fungus itself actively causes a degree of depigmentation. In skin that has been planed for scars of acne, there is a tendency for the unabraded skin to become hyperpigmented and for the abraded epidermis to regenerate with less pigmentation than the original.

DISEASES OF APPENDAGES

Limitations of space permit no more than the briefest mention of the nonneoplastic diseases of the cutaneous appendages.

Sweat glands

The disorders of the sweat glands include hyperhidrosis, congenital or acquired hypohidrosis, miliaria (prickly heat and tropical or thermogenic hypohidrosis with plugging of the sweat ducts by hydropic edematous epithelium), bromhidrosis (fetid sweat), chromhidrosis (colored sweat), hidradenitis suppurativa of the apocrine glands, and Fox-Fordyce disease (pruritic papular chronic adenitis of the sweat glands of the axillae, nipples, and pubic and perineal regions).

Sebaceous glands

The diseases of the sebaceous glands include varieties of seborrhea, hyposteatosis or diminished secretion, comedones, acne in its several forms, and rhinophyma.

Hair

The *abnormal conditions of the hair* are many. Hypertrichosis, the alopecias of the cicatricial types (pseudopelade, folliculitis decalvans, and chronic lupus erythematosus of the scalp) and the noncicatricial types (alopecia areata, ordinary male baldness, fungal infections, etc.), fragile hairs (fragilitas crinium), trichorrhexis nodosa, pili torti (twisted hairs), fungal infections such as piedra and trichomycosis nodosa, and trichostasis spinulosa (multiple lanugo hairs in a single follicle) constitute a few of the problems.

One of the more interesting disorders of hair follicles is called *alopecia mucinosa* or follicular mucinosis. It is characterized histologically initially by intracellular and subsequently extracellular mucin within the hair sheaths, perifollicular inflammatory cells, and loss of hair shafts. The mucin stains with alcian blue and is PAS negative. The significant fact concerning this lesion is that in individuals over 40 years of age it represents strongly presumptive evidence of the early stage of mycosis fungoides.

Nails

The diseases of the nails are of particular interest not only for the involvement of the nails themselves but for the accessory information they reflect on systemic disorders. *Beau's lines* are transverse furrows in the nail that date periods of severe acute illnesses or of inflammations near the nail folds, leading to the arrest of function of the matrix.

The discoloration and the thickening of the nail due to psoriasis, eczema, or fungi, the spoon nails (*koilonychia*) associated with trauma, eczema, and the Plummer-Vinson syndrome, the brittleness (onychorrhexis) following the use of certain chemicals or in vitamin A deficiency, the loss of nails (onycholysis) after trauma or systemic diseases such as hypothyroidism, and the whitening of nails (leukonychia) represent some of the changes that affect the nails.

PANNICULITIS

Several diseases of the subcutaneous fat simulate each other closely histologically but have different prognostic and etiologic implications: (1) erythema induratum (Bazin's disease), (2) nodular, nonsuppurative, febrile, relapsing panniculitis (Weber-Christian disease), (3) erythema nodosum, (4) nodular vasculitis, and (5) erythema pernio (chilblain).

Erythema induratum. Erythema induratum appears as chronic, recurring, often ulcerated, bluish red nodosities (of the calves of the legs, particularly). The lesions generally are found in patients with frank tuberculosis elsewhere. Histologically, tubercles, as a rule of an incomplete or atypical variety, are found in the subcutaneous fat. Caseation may or may not be present. Fat necrosis and fat atrophy associated with nonspecific inflammation of the fibrous septa, fat, and lower dermis are present. Endarterial and endophlebitis inflammation and proliferation are seen commonly. Tubercle bacilli are rarely found in these lesions, although positive results have been reported from guinea pig inoculation of the tissue.

Subacute nodular migratory panniculitis. Subacute nodular migratory panniculitis, which may follow acute infections such as tonsillitis, appears similar to erythema induratum histologically.

Nodular, nonsuppurative, febrile, relapsing panniculitis (Weber-Christian disease). Nodular, nonsuppurative, febrile, relapsing, panniculitis is observed preponderantly in women and is characterized by bluish discoloration of the skin over firm subcutaneous nodules on the extremities and trunk, usually associated with otherwise unexplained fever. Isolated cases have responded to chemotherapy (sulfapyridine and penicillin). Fatalities have occurred in several cases, but autopsy findings were not especially enlightening except for the steatitis in the pretracheal, mediastinal, and retroperitoneal regions. The recently recorded instances of "mesenteric panniculitis" appear unrelated.

In sections of what are regarded as typical cases, the fat itself is infiltrated chiefly with lymphocytes and histiocytes, but the septa are relatively spared. So-called "wücher" atrophy of fat (replacement of atrophied fat by fat-laden histiocytes), foreign body giant cell reaction, and endophlebitis and endarteritis are also present. However, the septa, although relatively spared, often are infiltrated and edematous. Therefore, the involvement of the septa cannot be used as a criterion for excluding the possibility of Weber-Christian disease, although if they are free, the evidence is considerable that the panniculitis belongs to this category.

Although "nonsuppurative" is included in the name of the entity, the fact is that sterile abscesses occasionally are noted along with cystic liquefaction necrosis and focal calcification. It has been suggested that Weber-Christian disease is of diverse etiology and in some instances is owing to pancreatitis.[40]

Erythema nodosum. Erythema nodosum occurs clinically as tender, pale red to livid blue nodules, principally on the anterior aspect of the lower extremities. These lesions, unlike those of erythema induratum, do not ulcerate, are transient, lasting only for several weeks on an average, and are not necessarily associated with a tuberculous process elsewhere. The disease may be one manifestation of a variety of unrelated infections, including coccidioidomycosis, leprosy, syphilis, viral diseases (e.g., measles, cat-scratch fever), and ringworm, or it may follow lymphomas, the ingestion of drugs, or the administration of a vaccine.

The histologic picture of erythema nodosum is much like that of erythema induratum with the addition that there is a greater tendency in erythema nodosum for nonspecific inflammation of the middle and lower dermis, which is practically spared in erythema induratum.

Nodular vasculitis. Nodular vasculitis occurs chiefly in older women and refers to the often recurrent nodosities that are more painful, are of shorter duration, and have less tendency to ulcerate than the lesions of erythema induratum.

The histologic picture of nodular vasculitis is the same as that of Bazin's disease.

Erythema pernio. Erythema pernio occurs usually on the hands and feet as tender, red, pruritic macules provoked by cold.

The histologic picture may closely simulate that of erythema induratum, as may the lesions produced in response to cold allergy.

Miscellaneous forms. Miscellaneous forms of panniculitis include those secondary to trauma, insulin injections, pancreatitis, allergic reactions (including those following insect bites), angiitis, cryoglobulinemia, and sclerosing lipogranulomas.

VASCULAR DISORDERS

There is a broad spectrum of vascular disorders in which the skin plays a prominent clinical and, at times, diagnostic, role. A few of these are mentioned in Chapter 20. Additional ones, with probable or clear-cut vascular involvement, include the cutaneous lesions of rheumatic fever, subacute bacterial endocarditis, typhus fevers, and other infections, Degos' syndrome, allergenic vasculitides, necrobiosis lipoidica diabeticorum, the vascular changes of diabetes mellitus and hypertension, granuloma annulare, rheumatoid granuloma, Mucha-Habermann's disease, the purpuric dermatoses, and others.

A form of superficial, subcutaneous thrombophlebitis known as **Mondor's disease** is characterized clinically by a linear, cordlike induration with an overlying cutaneous groove extending usually from the axilla toward the nipple. The lesion may be mistaken for a neoplasm clinically.

XANTHOSES

The xanthoses may be simply classified as follows:

1 Normolipemic
  A Juvenile xanthoma
  B Xanthoma disseminatum
2 Hyperlipemic
  A Xanthoma diabeticorum

  B Xanthoma tuberosum multiplex
  C Xanthoma eruptiva (in association with lipid nephrosis, von Gierke's disease, diabetes mellitus, biliary cirrhosis, hypothyroidism, idiopathic hyperlipemia)
  D Xanthelasma (± 50% with hyperlipemia)
  E Xanthoma planum (± 50% with hyperlipemia) (in association with biliary cirrhosis, diabetes mellitus, myeloma and other dysproteinemias)

Other dermatoses characterized by the presence of lipid include lipid proteinosis, angiokeratoma of Fabry, necrobiosis lipoidica diabeticorum, lipid dermatoarthritis (reticulohistiocytoma), Hand-Schüller-Christian disease, Niemann-Pick disease, and Gaucher's disease. These are described elsewhere in this book.

Many of the lesions included in this classification are often classified with neoplasms. Actually, none is really a neoplasm in the usual sense of neoplasia. Most are obviously a reflection of disordered metabolism of lipids or lipoproteins, but it would constitute no major contribution to hasten to discard the term xanthoma. The differentiation of these various xanthoses is often important from the prognostic and therapeutic viewpoints, although in many instances the distinction cannot be made on the basis of histology alone. Moreover, several of these types of lesions often are combined in the same patient.

Juvenile xanthoma

Juvenile xanthomas usually appear during the first two years of life. Occasionally, they may develop during adolescence. The lesions are yellow, several millimeters to centimeters in diameter, solitary or distributed in the skin over most of the body. The head is the predilected site. The extensor aspects of the extremities are also prominently involved. Extracutaneous lesions may occur in the eye, tongue, vulva, lungs, and visceral fat. The serum lipids are normal. In general, the disorder runs a benign course and the nodules tend to disappear in from one to three years, particularly near puberty. The rare presence of these lesions in visceral fat and serous membranes does not preclude survival and is not to be mistaken for a form of malignant histiocytosis.

Histologically, the nodules are characterized by packed lipid histiocytes interspersed with eosinophilic leukocytes, scattered lymphocytes, and numerous well-formed rosettes of histiocytes (Touton giant cells) (Fig. 39-28). Applying granuloma to this one form of xanthosis adds little clarification.

What needs to be explained is the mechanism by which dermal histiocytes of normolipinic individuals become laden with lipid.

Xanthoma disseminatum

Xanthoma disseminatum refers to an uncommon type of xanthomatosis which is nonfamilial and rarely is associated with hypercholesterolemia or diabetes mellitus. The lesions appear as fine papules, nodules, or plaques with a predilection for the flexor surfaces of extremities. Mucous membranes (mouth, pharynx, glottis, and trachea), as well as the sclera and brain, including the hypothalamus and pituitary gland, may be involved. The involvement of the latter may lead to diabetes insipidus.

The histology of xanthoma disseminatum is essentially similar to that of the xanthomas associated with hyperlipidemia. The dermis is occupied by rows or clumps of sudanophilic birefringent lipid with few or no giant cells, varying amounts of fibrosis, and scattered lymphocytes. Extracellular cholesterolosis may be conspicuous.

Xanthoma diabeticorum

The lesions of xanthoma diabeticorum appear as small, yellow to brown, discrete or confluent eruptive papules resembling those of xanthoma disseminatum but located predominantly on the extensor, rather than flexor, aspects of the extremities and on the palms and soles. Other distinctive features include the suddenness of involution and evolution of the lesions, the marked pruritus, and the association with diabetes mellitus and marked lipemia, both usually of a severe degree. The lesions tend to respond to the therapy for diabetes mellitus.

Although blood cholesterol levels as high as 1,300 mg% have been reported in patients with xanthomatosis, it is now coming to be appreciated that factors other than hyperlipemia are concerned with the deposition of fat in blood vessels as well as skin. These factors include the size of fat molecules and the ratio of the concentrations of the various lipids to each other, with consequent abnormality of emulsifying conditions.

Xanthoma tuberosum multiplex and xanthoma eruptiva

Xanthoma tuberosum multiplex refers to a familial disorder with essential hypercholesterolemia and characterized by oval, circular, or irregularly shaped discrete and coalescent

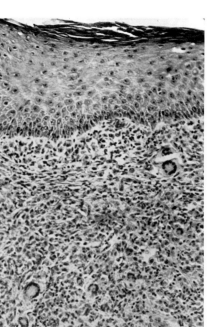

Fig. 39-28 Xanthoma tuberosum with numerous lipid histiocytes, some of which are congregated as Touton giant cells. (Hematoxylin-eosin.)

plaques, nodules, or bosselated tuberosities, some pedunculated. These occur predominantly on the extensor surfaces of the extremities, particularly the elbows, knees, and heels. The palms and soles also may be affected along with tendon sheaths. These tuberous xanthomas, associated with hyper-β-lipoproteinemia, characteristically are localized to sites of pressure or trauma, presumably owing to increased vascular permeability to the lipids that subsequently saturate macrophages. If this is indeed the mechanism, it is not clear why there is, as a rule, no concomitant hemosiderosis. The lesions, which tend to develop slowly and to remain stationary for many years, are among the commonest form of xanthomas (Fig. 39-28).

Xanthoma tuberosum occurs also in patients with essential or idiopathic hypertriglyceridemia. Such patients may, in addition, develop *eruptive xanthomas*. These small, papular lesions of **xanthoma eruptiva** occur in association with the secondary hypercholesterolemia or hyperphospholipidemia of biliary obstruction, lipid nephrosis, von Gierke's disease, and myxedema or following the lactescent hypertriglyceridemia of idiopathic (primary)

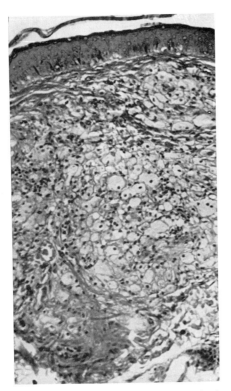

Fig. 39-29 Xanthelasma of eyelid with lipid-filled histiocytes. (Hematoxylin-eosin.)

hyperlipemia. Xanthoma tuberosum and xanthelasma may also appear in patients with idiopathic hyperlipemia. The red-rimmed, pink, eruptive xanthomas in patients with severe diabetes with hypertriglyceridemia tend to respond to antidiabetic therapy.

Xanthelasma

Xanthelasma, the commonest form of cutaneous xanthosis, appears as a flat or slightly and irregularly raised and outlined, yellow to brown, soft, oblong papule or plaque in the upper eyelid, usually near the inner canthus. It may occur alone or in association with any of the other forms of xanthomas, with or without elevation of serum lipids. Hypercholesterolemia was found in 33% of men and 40% of women with xanthelasma palpebrum. Hyperlipemia occurred in 58% of men and 60% of women.[74]

The histologic picture is essentially that of bland, pure clusters of lipid-laden foam cells with a minimum or absence of desmoplasia, giant cells, or inflammatory cells (Fig. 39-29).

Xanthoma planum

Xanthoma planum represents the least common form of xanthosis and, in essence, is the morphologic (gross and histologic) equivalent of xanthelasma distributed chiefly on the scalp, neck, and folds of the extremities as well as in old scars. Its association with multiple myeloma and other dysproteinemias has been recently emphasized.[34]

RETICULOHISTIOCYTOMA (RETICULOHISTIOCYTIC GRANULOMA)

The entity reticulohistiocytoma, which was so named in 1948, produces remarkable lesions, the extent and nature of which are still being investigated.[8, 10] Because of the association with arthritis, it has more recently been designated *lipid dermatoarthritis*.[8] Originally, this condition was thought to be limited to the skin and was regarded as a form of ganglioneuroma because of the superficial simulation of ganglion cells by the histiocytes.

Clinically, the disease is characterized by cutaneous papules and nodules (rarely solitary) and, often, by an associated disabling polyarthritis. The nodules may resemble xanthomas, and, indeed xanthelasma is present in about one-fourth of the patients.

Histologically, the cutaneous lesions are characterized by histiocytes with abundant basophilic cytoplasm intermingled with lymphocytes and occasionally scattered eosinophilic leukocytes (Fig. 39-30). The infiltrate tends to be confined to the upper dermis, with resulting moderate atrophy of the overlying epidermis. The cytoplasm of the histiocytes reacts positively with Sudan black B and PAS stains and is presumed to contain a glycolipid.

"ATYPICAL FIBROXANTHOMA"

There has been considerable interest in the past few years in an ulceronodular lesion of the exposed skin (chiefly the ears and cheeks) of elderly people. The lesion has been called "atypical fibroxanthoma" and resembles an anaplastic sarcoma with spindle cells and multinucleated giant cells, as well as bizarre cells with single, large hyperchromatic nuclei, mitoses often abnormal (tripolar), and some intracellular lipid. The striking feature is the disparity between the histologic anaplasia and the benign course, as thus far recorded. Some of these are undoubtedly nonpigmented spindle cell melanocarcinomas. It should be recalled that fat may be present in melanocarcinomas.[1]

NEOPLASMS OF SKIN

The following classification of neoplasms of the skin is based on the segregation of cutane-

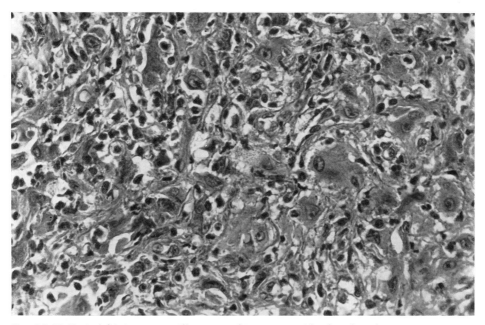

Fig. 39-30 Reticulohistiocytoma, illustrating histiocytes with abundant homogeneous cytoplasm loosely admixed with few lymphocytes and eosinophilic leukocytes. (Hematoxylin-eosin; from Allen, A. C.: The skin, Grune & Stratton, Inc.; by permission.)

ous neoplasms with respect to their location and/or histogenesis from epidermis, dermis proper, and appendages. In the ensuing discussion, several of the lesions are taken out of the order of the outline for purposes of clarity of presentation.

Epidermis

A Benign
  1 Verruca (including vulgaris, digitata, filiformis, plantaris, and juvenilis)
  2 Seborrheic keratosis
  3 Condyloma acuminatum
  4 Keratoacanthoma
  5 Junctional nevus
B Precancerous
  1 Senile keratosis
  2 Leukoplakia
  3 Xeroderma pigmentosum
  4 Bowen's disease
  5 Erythroplasia of Queyrat
C Malignant
  1 Basal cell carcinoma
  2 Squamous cell carcinoma
  3 Melanocarcinoma (malignant melanoma), including melanotic freckle of Hutchinson
  4 Paget's disease

Dermis

A Nevus
  1 Intradermal nevus (common mole)
  2 Compound nevus (dermis and epidermis)
  3 Juvenile melanoma (dermis and epidermis)
  4 Blue nevus (Jadassohn-Tièche)
B Tumors of vessels
  1 Lymphangioma
  2 Hemangioma

  3 Angiokeratoma (dermis and epidermis)
  4 Glomus tumor
  5 Hemangiopericytoma
  6 Kaposi's iliopathic hemorrhagic sarcoma
  7 Postmastectomy lymphangiosarcoma
  8 Sclerosing hemangioma (dermatofibroma lenticulare)
  9 Dermatofibrosarcoma protuberans
  10 Angiosarcoma
C Fibroma and fibrosarcoma
D Neurofibroma and neurofibrosarcoma
E Tumors of muscle
  1 Leiomyoma (arrectores pilorum)
  2 Angiomyoma
  3 Myoblastoma (genesis?)
F Osteoma
G Xanthomas (discussed in previous section)
H Lymphomas and allied diseases
I Metastatic neoplasms

Appendages

A Sweat glands
  1 Adenoma or epithelioma
    (a) Ductal
    (b) Glandular
  2 Carcinoma
B Sebaceous glands
  1 Adenoma
  2 Carcinoma
C Hair follicles
  1 Brooke's tumor—trichoepithelioma or epithelioma adenoides cysticum
D Miscellaneous cysts
  1 Dermoid
  2 Epidermoid
  3 Pilosebaceous
  4 Calcifying epithelioma

Benign lesions of epidermis
Verruca (wart)

The verrucae or warts represent thickenings or projections of epidermis to which are traditionally, if inconsistently, applied one of several adjectives in accordance with the shape, location, or other clinical feature of the lesion: verruca vulgaris, verruca plantaris, verruca digitata, verruca filiformis, verruca plana juvenilis, and verruca senilis.

The **verruca vulgaris** is the papillary wart common in children and found especially on the fingers, palms, and forearms. They occur singly or in groups. There is some question as to whether or not these tumors merit inclusion under "neoplasms," inasmuch as they may disappear spontaneously or, as in some reported cases, under psychotherapy, including placebos. The possibility that these lesions are due to viruses is still strongly considered and fortified by evidence from electron microscopy of viral particles.

Histologically, the verruca vulgaris is characterized by a papillary acanthosis surmounted by friable keratotic material. The cells of the stratum granulosum are often acidophilic and vacuolated (Fig. 39-31). The basophilic intranuclear inclusions of the verrucae are related to the viral particles rather than the osmophilic intranuclear eosinophilic material, which is related to keratin. A loose infiltration of various mononuclear cells may be present in the papillae. Carcinomatous transformation of these lesions must occur rarely, if ever, although occasionally a verrucal form of senile keratosis or a squamous

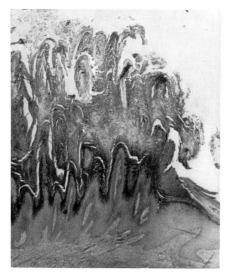

Fig. 39-31 Verruca vulgaris. (Hematoxylin-eosin.)

cell carcinoma with a prominent papillary hyperkeratotic surface is erroneously regarded as having arisen from a verruca vulgaris.

Oral florid papillomatosis comprises benign condylomatoid verrucal masses covering large portions of the buccal mucosa. These presumably are of viral origin.

An oral and genital lesion histologically similar to condyloma occurs with the entity called *dyskeratosis congenita,* which may be associated with a variety of ectodermal and mesodermal changes, including hyperpigmentation of the skin, reticulated poikilodermatous changes, dystrophic nails, deforming atrophic arthritic changes, dental dystrophies, cardiovascular changes, testicular atrophy, and hypersplenism.

The **verruca digitata** occurs chiefly on the scalp, face, and neck. It is distinguished from verruca vulgaris principally because the digitated lesion is made up of long fronds that may be separated down to the base of the lesion.

The **verruca filiformis,** which occurs chiefly on the eyelid, is merely a single slender projection of skin, composed of a core of connective tissue representing the elongated dermal papilla covered by epidermis showing little acanthosis and hyperkeratosis. In this respect, these verrucae differ from the verruca vulgaris.

The **verruca plantaris** clinically simulates a callosity of the sole of the foot. The two are distinguished by the observance in the plantar wart of the soft papillary verrucal acanthosis after the hyperkeratotic portion has been removed. In the callus, stripping of the horny material leaves the flat epidermis.

The **verruca plana juvenilis** is generally a smooth, relatively flat wart that is prone to occur on the dorsum of the hands of adolescents. It may closely simulate the lesions of epidermodysplasia verruciformis, although the latter differ in their distribution and in their occurrence in an older age group.

Histologically, the verruca plana is characterized by acanthosis and hyperkeratosis. The acanthosis is relatively greater than in the callosity. Without knowledge of the clinical picture, verruca plana may be confused microscopically with various keratodermas, although the vacuolization of the cells of the stratum granulosum may be of differential help.

The "hard nevus of Unna" is essentially a verruca plana. *Acrokeratosis verruciformis* is the name applied to other verrucal lesions, hereditary in character and occurring symmetrically on the hands and feet. These lesions histologically tend to lack the loose basketweave appearance present in the upper layers of the warts of epidermodysplasia verruciformis.

The *seborrheic keratosis* is labeled also *verruca senilis* or *pigmented papilloma*. The term verruca senilis is not well chosen, for the reason that the lesions often appear in young people and acanthosis is the feature of note. Seborrheic keratosis is used by the dermatologists and emphasizes the greasy feeling to the touch imparted by the abundant fatty keratinous nests within the lesion. These lesions occur particularly on the trunk and forehead and are usually dark brown, elevated, and sharply delimited.

The histologic picture is that of abruptly thickened epidermis that encloses nests of laminated keratin resulting from focal, irregular maturation of epidermis partially inverted within the core of the lesion. In places, the central pearls are incompletely developed and present large mature squamous cells without the keratinous nests. The surrounding cells are usually focally pigmented with fine brown granules of melanin and superficially resemble basal cells. However, close examination often reveals residual intercellular bridges that help identify them as squamous cells, notwithstanding statements to the contrary. Many of these *epithelial cells are dopa positive*. In our judgment, the pigment is produced by the tumor cells (i.e., the keratinocytes). Others assume

that the pigment is inoculated into the tumor cells by nonneoplastic melanocytes carried along with the tumor. This same judgment applies to the condylomatous, so-called "melanoacanthoma." Rare cases of malignant transformation of the seborrheic keratosis have been recorded.[15] These have included basal cell carcinomas and malignant melanomas.[2, 15]

A lesion that has many of the cellular characteristics of the verruca pigmentosum is the so-called "inverted papilloma," which grows downward rather than outward from the epidermal surface. The "inverted papilloma" often is associated with an inflammatory reaction of mononuclear cells at its base, very much as are the senile keratoses (Fig. 39-32). The lesion referred to as "eccrine porothelioma" or "acrosyringoma" closely resembles the earliest stage of seborrheic keratosis. The *Degos* or *clear cell acanthoma* also is reminiscent of an initial stage in the development of seborrheic keratosis. Glycogen is present in the clear cells.

Keratoacanthoma

The problem of pseudoepitheliomatous hyperplasia is directly related to the histologically difficult subject of so-called *"self-healing squamous cell carcinomas,"* also more or less equivalently labeled *molluscum sebaceum* and *molluscum pseudocarcinomatosum*. Most commonly, these occur in elderly males, although even adolescents may be affected, especially if there has been contact with oils. The lesions appear as single or multiple nodules that are smooth except for the characteristic umbilication of the central keratin. The nodules often regress spontaneously in about two months, leaving little or no scar. Recurrences have been recorded.

Histologically, as already implied, the nodules are not really carcinomas but, rather, coalescent comedones or keratinous masses with prominent pseudoepitheliomatous hyperplasia at their bases (see Fig. 39-37). Giant keratoacanthomas may become incredibly large, particularly on the face, and may recur after incomplete excision. The well-differentiated, keratoacanthomatous pattern in the rapid recurrence supports the original diagnosis, although considerable self-confidence may be required to maintain it. An important clue is the absence of significant atypia in the epidermis at the margins of the keratoacanthomas.

Notwithstanding the occasional recurrences following incomplete removal, these lesions

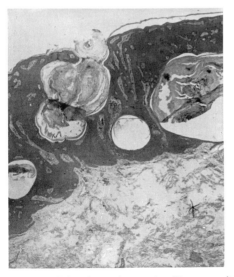

Fig. 39-32 Seborrheic keratosis. (Hematoxylin-eosin.)

are benign. On the other hand, the attention that has been focused on keratoacanthomas has perforce led to misdiagnosis of squamous cell carcinomas as keratoacanthomas. An analogous problem exists in the erroneous diagnosis of melanocarcinomas as juvenile melanomas. As might have been anticipated, an impressive number of instances of carcinomas are being erroneously diagnosed keratoacanthomas.[49]

A variety of the lesion has been designated "generalized eruptive keratoacanthoma." These may be so numerous as to cover most of the body and involve even the oral mucosa.[108]

Precancerous lesions

The precancerous lesions of the skin include senile keratosis, Bowen's disease, erythroplasia of Queyrat, and the *active* junctional nevus. Each of these entities is characterized by atypia or "dyskeratosis" of cells that, importantly, is confined to the limits of the epidermis. To such lesions the term "carcinoma in situ" is often applied. "Precancerous" as applied to these lesions connotes, in a crude measure, the relatively high degree of probability with which they are likely to undergo malignant degeneration rather than the inevitability of such a complication. *Kraurosis vulvae,* a term which has become unpopular in recent years, had been used diversely either in place of vulval lichen sclerosis et atrophicus, on the one hand, or as equivalent to epidermoid carcinoma in situ, on the other.

Senile keratosis

The senile keratoses are irregular brownish patches of epidermis roughened by horny scales, occurring characteristically on the dorsa of the hands of aged people. Histologically similar lesions may follow irradiation and exposure to arsenic or to the elements of the weather. They may be single or several, or they may occur in great numbers over many parts of the body.

Microscopically, they are characterized chiefly by dyskeratosis of the cells of the basal layer and adjacent layers of the rete malpighii. These cells show hyperchromatism, loss of polarity, increased numbers of mitotic figures, and irregularity of size and shape of nuclei. Hyperkeratosis and parakeratosis of varying degrees are responsible for the roughened surface. Inflammatory cells, principally mononuclear, are present in the subepidermal tissue. These cells often encroach onto the epidermis so as to obscure the integrity of the

"basement membrane" and occasionally prompt the premature and erroneous impression of infiltrating carcinoma. The cutaneous horn in many instances represents a senile keratosis with an accumulation of keratinous material in the form of a projecting spur. The same type of horny projection may be superimposed also on verrucae.

Leukoplakia

Leukoplakia is a term that merits some discussion of its usage. As applied clinically, or grossly, it refers to whitish patches of mucosa that encompass not only cancerous or "precancerous" foci, but also those benign patches of mucosa thickened and whitened by mycoses, lichen planus, reaction to dentures, smoking, etc. Nevertheless, to many surgeons and pathologists (probably to most of them), leukoplakia connotes a carcinoma in situ or a lesion morphologically approaching an intraepithelial carcinoma. The difficulty is that the diagnosis often is rendered as merely "leukoplakia" when the pathologist is not certain in his or her own mind that there is or is not sufficient atypia to warrant a designation of leukokeratosis or of carcinoma in situ. This is very much the situation with lesions of the cervix, when the diagnosis is hedged with such terms as "basal cell hyperplasia" or "dyskaryosis"—to the bewilderment of the clinician. Surely, there are instances in which the pathologist may not be certain of the malignant potential of such a "whitish patch," but it would appear more informative if this uncertainty were indicated rather than concealed euphemistically.

Xeroderma pigmentosum

Xeroderma pigmentosum is a potentially cancerous familial disease of the skin, usually first manifested early in childhood. It is characterized clinically by areas of atrophy, as well as isolated and coalescent scaly patches of keratosis showing varying amounts of pigmentation. A hyper-α-2-globulinemia has been found consistently in patients with xeroderma pigmentosum, and it has been hypothesized that this abnormality is related to ceruloplasmin.

Histologically, the changes in xeroderma pigmentosum are those of irregular atrophy, acanthosis, and hyperkeratosis, with excessive deposits of melanin in the basal layer and lowermost layers of the stratum spinosum, as well as in chromatophores in the upper dermis (Fig. 39-33). Xeroderma pigmentosum

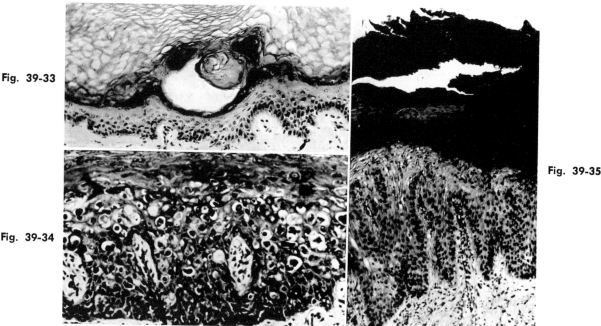

Fig. 39-33 Fig. 39-34 Fig. 39-35

Fig. 39-33 Xeroderma pigmentosum showing hyperkeratosis, epidermal atrophy, and pigmentation. (Hematoxylin-eosin; AFIP 97125.)
Fig. 39-34 Bowen's disease with diffuse cellular atypia. (Hematoxylin-eosin.)
Fig. 39-35 Leukoplakia with marked parakeratosis, acanthosis, some basilar atypia, and subepithelial inflammation. (Hematoxylin-eosin.)

may be complicated by junctional nevi, basal cell or squamous cell carcinomas, and melanocarcinomas.

Bowen's disease

Bowen's disease occurs as irregular, scaly, slowly progressive, usually brownish patches on the trunk, buttocks, and extremities. It is estimated that approximately one-third of patients develop evidence of visceral cancer within six to ten years after the initial diagnosis of Bowen's disease.[75]

Microscopically, the principal feature of the lesions is the presence of isolated dyskeratotic cells scattered haphazardly in all layers of the epidermis (Fig. 39-34). These cells often have large, hyperchromatic single or double nuclei surrounded by cytoplasmic halos. Mitotic figures are numerous in these altered cells. Hyperkeratosis or parakeratosis may be marked. The acanthosis is usually uniform, but irregular thickening may be present (Fig. 39-35).

Electron microscopic study of the dyskeratotic cells discloses displaced cytoplasmic fascicular aggregations of tonofilaments and separation of the desmosomal-tonofilament attachments.[90] This desmosomal-tonofilament dissociation would be anticipated not only

from the acantholytic appearance of Bowen's cells as seen under light microscopy, but also from the ultrastructural studies of acantholytic cells in other lesions such as Darier's disease, pemphigus vulgaris, etc.[24] In our judgment, as previously stated, a basically similar retraction of tonofilaments and loss of desmosomes occur in the conversion of keratinocytes to neval and melanocarcinomatous cells.

Erythroplasia of Queyrat

Erythroplasia of Queyrat is the precancerous lesion occurring principally on the glans penis but also on the vulva and on mucous membranes of the mouth. In addition, the acanthotic thickening associated with erythroplasia is often characterized by long rete ridges that are psoriasiform or attached to each other in a reticulated pattern. A cytologic pattern somewhat similar to that of Bowen's disease occurs in the nipple and adjacent areas of the female breast in **Paget's disease**. However, unlike the lesions just described, Paget's disease is associated with carcinoma of the underlying mammary ducts. As indicated elsewhere, we find the evidence for the conclusion that so-called extramammary Paget's disease is associated with underlying adenocarcinoma of apocrine or eccrine glands somewhat less than convincing.[2] In our judgment, the vast majority of such lesions are pagetoid melanocarcinomas. The small group of remaining lesions includes epidermoid carcinomas and metastatic mucin-producing carcinomas, principally from the bowel and occasionally from other organs such as the ovaries.

The much emphasized presence of mucopolysaccharides within epidermal cells hardly precludes the possibility that they are keratinocytes. Among several kinds of evidence is the clear fact that under the influence of an excess of vitamin A, keratinocytes are modulated into mucus-secreting cells.[50]

Malignant lesions of epidermis

The malignant lesions of the epidermis include basal cell carcinoma, squamous cell carcinoma, Paget's disease, and melanocarcinoma.

Basal cell carcinoma

The term "carcinoma" is preferred to "epithelioma" in connection with the basal cell tumors that belong to the general group of rodent ulcers. If left untreated, these neoplasms will progress, erode, and infiltrate neighboring bone and cartilage in a manner that would seem to merit the designation "cancer" despite the infrequency of metastasis. Actually, over fifty instances of metastasizing basal cell carcinomas have been recorded.[27] The term epithelioma might best be reserved for the form of basal cell proliferation that does not show these invasive characteristics—i.e., the trichoepithelioma, otherwise known as epithelioma adenoides cysticum or Brooke's tumor (p. 1679).

Basal cell carcinomas occur predominantly in blond, fair-skinned people in the region of the face bounded by the hairline, ears, and upper lip. A tumor of the skin of the tip of the nose, however, is more likely to be a squamous carcinoma provided it is not a keratoacanthoma. Basal cell tumors are not confined to the face, but may, in small numbers, occur in the skin of any part of the body, although there is a tendency to desmoplasia in those located away from the face. Squamous cell carcinomas of the anal canal, which are aggressive, particularly if they are located above the anal verge, may appear deceptively similar to basal cell carcinomas. Indeed, some of these are labeled "basaloid"—to the surgeon's confusion.

The basal cell carcinoma begins as a smooth, slightly elevated papule that may be scaly at first but tends soon to ulcerate centrally as the lesion spreads peripherally beneath the epidermis. Characteristically, the ulcer is rimmed by a waxy, smooth, firm, rolled border representing the intact epidermis, which is wrapped over but not yet invaded by the underlying and undermining neoplastic nests. If neglected, the tumor may advance to a grotesque erosion of large portions of the soft tissue, as well as the cartilage and bone of the face (Fig. 11-20). Early treatment by irradiation, excision, or the various other means of local destruction is usually adequate. The advantage of treatment of neoplasms by excision is that it then becomes possible to know by histologic examination not only the precise type of tumor present, but also whether or not the excised tumor is bounded by normal tissue.

Histologically, although there is considerable variability to the pattern of the basal cell carcinomas, there are sufficient characteristics in common so as to make them recognizable with relative ease. They are made up of nests of closely packed cells of uniform size and oval shape, with dark nuclei separated by a small amount of spineless cytoplasm. The nests often are rimmed by a single layer of similar cells arranged, however, in a neat radial pattern and strongly reminiscent of the more or less vertically arranged basal cells forming the lowermost layer of the normal epidermis or of the hair shafts. Mitotic figures are usually fairly common. Such nests may be observed arising not only from the basal portion of the epidermis, but also from the corresponding layer of the hair shaft or from both sources in the same tumor. The presence in these tumors of cells of the same type as those that line both the epidermis and the hair follicle would appear to account for the origin of these neoplasms from either of these structures. This is by no means equivalent to maintaining that embryonic rests of hair matrix, in one or another phase of its development, are the source of basal cell carcinomas. The basal cells of *adult* epidermis do have a limited range of reaction to *carcinogenic* stimulation. One major form such a reaction takes is to produce hair matrixes in the disheveled manner of a basal cell carcinoma, just as in response to *normal* growth stimuli the basal cells produce the orderly components of hair. In other words, when carcinogenic agents such as arsenic or x-irradiation produce basal cell carcinomas, they do so not by activating embryonic rests of hair follicles but by provoking neoplastic change in previously normally situated *adult* basal cells. The origin of basal cell carcinomas from any part of the mature pilary complex is demonstrable also in the skin of rats to which anthramine and methylcholanthrene have been applied.

The histology of basal cell carcinomas may vary in the following ways:

1 By the presence of edematous stroma rimmed by neoplastic cells to form the *alveolar or cystic* type
2 By excessive, dense, hyalinized stroma between nests of basal cells to give the *morphea* type
3 By the presence of foci of squamous cells or pearls, occasionally calcified, in the centers of nests of basal cells

This last modification has been called *basosquamous cell* (transitional or metatypical cell) *carcinoma*. It is stated that the keratin produced by basal cell carcinomas differs from that produced by squamous cell carcinomas in the histochemically demonstrable presence of cystine ("hair follicle keratin") in the basal cell cancers.[45] There is, in addition, the *comedo* type of basal cell carcinoma in which the cores of the masses of basal cells are necrotic.

In terms of prognosis, it has yet to be shown with any degree of credibility that there is any significant difference in these types. This matter is emphasized because of the general belief to the contrary. In particular, it is commonly stated that a basal cell carcinoma with areas of squamous cells represents a tumor with a more precarious prognosis than the ordinary basal cell carcinoma. This concept is based on the assumption that the squamous element of the neoplasm is prone to metastasize. This impression has no basis in fact. It is much more reasonable and in accord with their behavior to regard such areas of keratinized squamous cells simply as evidence of maturation of the central portion of the collection of basal cells rather than as an indication of dedifferentiation. On the other hand, it is true that infrequently there is observed in the same histologic field evidence of a true squamous cell carcinoma alongside a basal cell carcinoma. Such a squamous cell carcinoma would, of course, not be expected to behave as innocently as the squamous portions of a basosquamous carcinoma. Occasionally, some spindle cell areas of squamous cell carcinoma superficially resemble basal cell nests, and a misinterpretation of this resemblance is in some cases responsible for the notion that basosquamous cell carcinomas have a greater tendency to metastasize than do the pure basal cell cancers. If the tumor is to be irradiated, the therapist may be interested to know of the amount and character of the stroma and may want to modify the dosage accordingly. However, in actual practice, radiotherapists usually do not feel the need to vary the dosage with the histologic character of the basal cell carcinoma, inasmuch as a sufficiently destructive dose is used to take care of such variations.

Superficial epitheliomatosis, or multicentric basal cell carcinoma, is a special variety of the basal cell tumors. These lesions occur predominantly on the trunk either as dry and scaly or moist and eczematous, slowly enlarging plaques. Histologically, the lesions are small basal cell carcinomas arising from multiple foci in the basal layers of epidermis. The lesion is differentiated from the Jadassohn type of intraepidermal basal cell carcinoma, in which the neoplastic cells appear to be growing upward toward the surface from the basal cell layer instead of into the dermis. In the superficial lesions, as well as in other cutaneous "carcinomas in situ," arsenic should be suspected as a possible etiologic factor (Fig. 39-36).

The so-called "premalignant fibroepithelial tumor" is really part of the spectrum of variants of basal cell carcinomas and hardly merits such segregation.

In situ and, infrequently, superficially invasive basal cell carcinomas may complicate sclerosing angiomas.[41] The existence of these fairly innocuous lesions has been disputed, but in our judgment they are indistinguishable from "superficial epitheliomatosis" and we believe would be so diagnosed if seen without the underlying angioma.

Basal cell nevus syndrome

Basal cell carcinomas, along with a variety of adnexal hamartomas, may occur as a congenital hereditary phenomenon known as the basal cell nevus syndrome. These lesions may vary from several on the face to hundreds on the trunk and extremities. The associated lesions or symptom complexes may include pseudohypoparathyroidism, ovarian fibromas, mesenteric cysts, dental cysts, bifid ribs, spina bifida, hypertelorism, broad nasal root, bridging of the sella turcica, calcification of the falx cerebri, and agenesis of the corpus callosum. Occasionally, granulomatous or ulcerative colitis may be present.

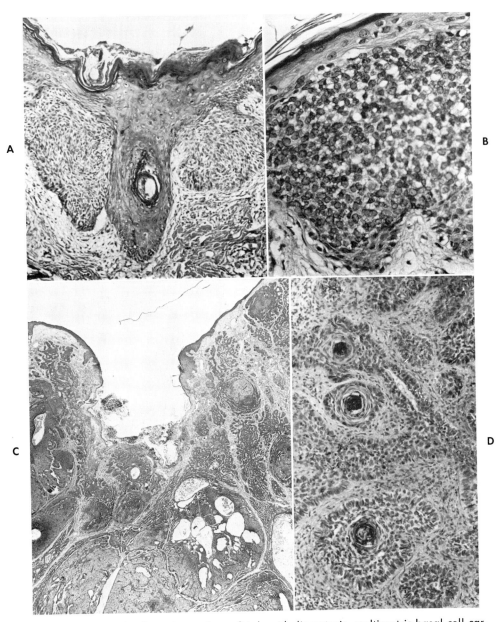

Fig. 39-36 A, Basal cell carcinoma (superficial epitheliomatosis, multicentric basal cell carcinoma). **B,** Intraepidermal basal cell carcinoma (Jadassohn type). **C,** Basal cell carcinoma with central ulceration, smooth borders (clinically waxy), and variegated picture of neoplasm. **D,** Basal cell carcinoma, so-called metatypical or basosquamous cell carcinoma, with central mature, squamous nests. (**A** to **D,** Hematoxylin-eosin.)

Squamous cell carcinoma

The squamous cell carcinoma may occur in the skin of any part of the body, but there is a predilection for the exposed areas, particularly the face and hands. Certain sources of chronic irritation definitely predispose to squamous cell carcinoma. These include pipe smoking, particularly clay pipes, irritation to the scrotum as incurred by chimney sweeps, the exposure to arsenic, tar, and carcinogenic oils that soak the clothes and abdomen of the mule spinner, the constant contact of the abdomen with the small charcoal heaters causing the so-called kangri cancers observed in the Kashmir regions, the exposure of susceptible blond skins to actinic rays and other elements of the weather, the unexplained cancerous irritant that is present in old scars as from burns or osteomyelitis, the vague irritant of syphilitic leukoplakia, and a variety of others.

The sources of the arsenic include that used therapeutically (Fowler's solution, arsphenamine, etc.), orchard sprays, and contaminated water from artesian wells (e.g., of Taiwan). In the latter instance, the cutaneous manifestations may be endemic and include a broad spectrum comprising benign-appearing keratoses, keratoses with fronds or ridges of early basal cell carcinoma, multicentric in situ and invasive basal cell carcinomas, Bowen's disease in its many variations, epidermoid carcinomas, and combinations of any of these lesions.[114] Scars following vaccination may be complicated infrequently by basal cell carcinomas, squamous cell carcinomas, and melanocarcinomas. The basal and squamous cell carcinomas tend to occur in individuals with the type of skin vulnerable to damage from exposure to ultraviolet light.[85] However, in most instances of squamous cell carcinoma, the source of irritation or stimulation is not apparent.

Clinically, the lesion begins as a superficially scaly, slightly indurated area that bleeds, crusts, and resists casual therapy. With growth, the surface becomes ulcerated or hornified and the base indurated. The ulceration may extend to a deforming depth. The sectioned surface is granular and is grayish white flecked with yellow. Usually, the limits of the neoplasm may be determined even by gross inspection of the cut surface.

Microscopically, these carcinomas are characterized by irregular nests of epidermal cells that have infiltrated the dermis for varying depths. The nests of a squamous cell carcinoma may include cells representing any layer of the epidermis from the basal layer to the stratum corneum. In well-differentiated lesions, the intercellular spines and the central keratinous nests, or the "epithelial pearls," easily identify the origin of the tumor from squamous epithelium. In highly anaplastic lesions, these elements may be altogether lacking. Indeed, the anaplasia may be so extreme in occasional squamous cell carcinomas that they may be almost indistinguishable from spindle cell sarcomas. These spindle cell *carcinomas* almost always follow irradiation and are controlled with difficulty. They are not to be confused with the unimportant, focal areas of spindle cells occurring in many basal cell carcinomas or with the spindle cell melanocarcinomas. Another variety characterized by

intercellular edema, particularly affecting the central cells of the neoplastic nests that are rimmed by basilar cells is occasionally mistaken for sebaceous or sweat gland carcinomas or even adamantinomas.

Often of greater practical importance than determining the precise type of carcinoma is the decision as to whether or not an isolated nest of cells represents actual carcinomatous invasion or is merely an obliquely cut rete ridge in an area of *pseudoepitheliomatous hyperplasia*. In some instances, the decision may be most difficult to make. However, the cells of a ridge in hyperplastic epidermis are quite differentiated and tend to resemble very closely the cells of the neighboring, obviously benign ridges and epidermis. The neighboring ridges—elongated, curved, and yet attached to the epidermis and cut perpendicularly—help to indicate that the isolated nest of cells actually represents an obliquely cut ridge rather than cancer. Another problem arises when abundant subepidermal inflammatory cells are present, some of which may have migrated across the "basement membrane" and lower epidermis, thereby obscuring the integrity of or even actually interrupting the "basement membrane." Since disruption of the basement membrane is one of the standard (if unreliable) criteria for provoking at least the suspicion of carcinoma, it becomes of some limited importance to judge, particularly by the anaplasia of the epidermal cells involved, whether or not the disruption is owing merely to inflammation or to early cancer (Figs. 39-37 and 39-38).

The squamous cell carcinomas of the skin are, as a rule, not so anaplastic as the corresponding lesions of mucous membranes such as the lip or uterine cervix. Accordingly, metastases are considerably more common following squamous cell carcinoma of the mucous membranes than of the skin. While this difference is the rule, there are conspicuous exceptions. One of the most anaplastic squamous cell carcinomas of our experience occurred in a scar following a burn of the skin of the leg. The tumor metastasized widely to the viscera.

Effects of ionizing radiation on skin

Ionizing radiation is used therapeutically for a great variety of inflammatory diseases, including acne, psoriasis, eczema, and plantar warts. Such treatment is usually at least temporarily effective for the dermatosis, but se-

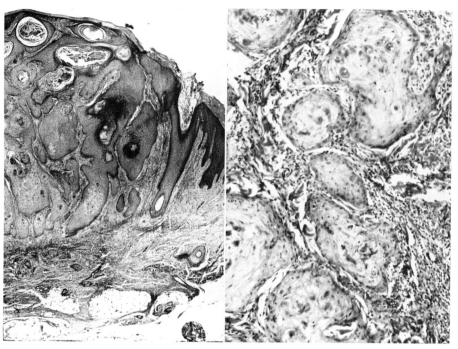

Fig. 39-37 Keratoacanthoma simulating squamous cell carcinoma. (Hematoxylin-eosin.)
Fig. 39-38 Deep margin of keratoacanthoma easily mistaken for squamous cell carcinoma.
(Hematoxylin-eosin.)

quelae in the form of acute and chronic radiodermatitis occur often enough to warrant serious concern. It is estimated that carcinomas complicate approximately 20% of instances of chronic radiodermatitis. This complication may occur over a wide span of years, from three or four to more than fifty, with a median of from twelve to eighteen years. Because of the great time interval between the induction of therapy and the onset of complications, the frequency of such complications may be underestimated by therapists.

The usual type of cutaneous cancer following radiotherapy is the squamous cell carcinoma, but basal cell carcinomas also may occur, particularly in areas about the face where such tumors are prone to arise "spontaneously." As previously mentioned, spindle cell carcinomas are an especially anaplastic variety of squamous cell cancers produced by irradiation (see Fig. 16-29).

Pigmented nevi

The term *nevus* is used by dermatologists to refer to any congenital blemish. Therefore, they refer not only to pigmented nevi but also to vascular nevi, sebaceous gland nevi, sweat gland nevi, and others. However, to others,

"nevus" denotes a neoplasm derived from pigmented or, at least, dopa-positive cells. We have classified these nevi and their malignant counterparts as follows*:

A Benign
  1 Junctional nevus (Fig. 39-39)
  2 Intradermal nevus (Figs. 39-40 and 39-41)
  3 Compound nevus (including halo nevus) (Fig. 39-42)
  4 Juvenile melanoma (Fig. 39-43)
  5 Blue nevus—cellular blue nevus (Figs. 39-44 and 39-45)
B Malignant
  1 Melanocarcinoma (Figs. 39-45 and 39-46)
    (a) Superficial (including melanotic freckle of Hutchinson)
    (b) Deep
  2 Malignant blue nevus

Junctional nevus

The junctional nevus, also known as dermoepidermal or marginal nevus, is of concern because it is a direct forerunner of the melanocarcinoma. Happily, this malignant transformation of junctional nevi occurs relatively infrequently.

The uncomplicated junctional nevus ap-

---

*Slightly modified from Allen, A. C.: Cancer 2:28-56, 1949, and Allen, A. C., and Spitz, S.: Cancer 6:1-45, 1953.

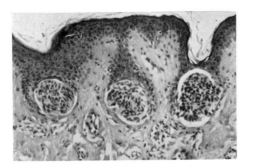

Fig. 39-39 Junctional nevus. (Hematoxylin-eosin; from Allen, A. C.: Cancer **2**:28-56, 1949.)

pears as a flat, smooth, generally hairless, light-brown to dark-brown mole. The lesions may be single or multiple. Their smooth appearance may be altered by their combination with an underlying intradermal nevus (compound). *Unfortunately, it is not always possible to diagnose them accurately clinically.* However, it may be assumed that pigmented moles on the ventral surface of the hands and the feet and on the genitalia are usually junctional nevi or, at least, have a junctional component in the form of a compound nevus.

Histologically, the junctional nevus is easily recognized by the clusters of enlarged, rounded, loosened cells of the basal and adjacent prickle cells of the epidermis. In addition, these cells lose their prickles and cohesion with neighboring cells, and many become powdered with fine granules of melanin. This acantholysis is reflected ultrastructurally in the partial to complete loss of desmosomes and tonofilaments, although residua of these structures are readily noted at the periphery of the "junctional" or acantholytic focus. If mitotic figures are present and the nuclei show any noteworthy anaplasia, the lesion may be assumed to have been on the verge of melanocarcinomatous transformation. Accordingly, depending on the extent of the atypia, these lesions are designated *"active junctional nevi"* or *"melanocarcinomas in situ."* The process may be diffuse along a strip of epidermis or it may be focal, with normal or skipped areas of epidermis intervening between involved portions. In the latter case, judgment as to the adequacy of normal margin bordering the lesion must be made with caution, inasmuch as the section may be removed through one of the intervening, unaltered areas (Fig. 39-39).

It is generally believed that the cells of the junctional nevus are derived from specialized nerve endings intercalated in the basal layer as clear cells. These cells are regarded by most observers as similar to or indentical with Merkel-Ranvier corpuscles. However, it seems that such a restricted view disregards the occurrence of cells of the junctional nevus (many dopa positive) not only in a continuous row in the basal layer, but also as isolated cells high in the prickle cell layers, the stratum granulosum, and even well into the stratum corneum. This phenomenon we believe to occur not by proliferation of neurogenic cells within the epidermis, as many believe, but, rather, by the alteration *in situ* of the preexisting epidermal cells, as a few formerly thought (Fig. 39-46).

It has long ago been clearly shown that the dendrites, which to many seem automatically to connote neurogenesis, may be entirely absent in many of these cells. Unlike truly neurogenic dendritic cells of neurons, which are attached to axon fibers for the transmission of impulses, or, for that matter, unlike true cutaneous nerve endings such as Meissner's or pacinian corpuscles, such fibers are found rarely (if unequivocally ever) leading to or from dendritic melanoblasts. On the other hand, the axon fibers of neurons of Meissner's or pacinian corpuscles are demonstrable with relative ease and constancy by silver preparations. Actually, when the dendrites of melanocytes are seen with silver stains, they are made evident *not because of an intrinsic argyrophilia* such as is possessed by cells of true neurons *but because of the argyrophilia of the contained granules of melanin.* The supranuclear localization of pigment within the prickle cells is, in itself, indicative of an *in situ* origin rather than by "a nipped-off" dendrite belonging to a neighboring cell or by the diffusion of tyrosinase from a clear cell. In the latter instances, it would be expected that the granules of pigment would be diffusely deposited or engulfed as in melanophores or histiocytes.

The detection of cholinesterase in nevi has been used as supporting evidence of the neurogenesis of nevi. As Mishima and Schaub state, cholinesterase has an "infinity of localizations in various nonneural tissues,"* so conclusions as to the origin of neval cells based principally on the presence of this enzyme are obviously unjustified. It is, of course, a brilliantly established fact that the pigment of skin, hair, and

*From Mishima, Y., and Schaub, F. F., Jr.: J. Invest. Derm. **41**:243-245, 1963; copyrighted by The Williams & Wilkins Co.

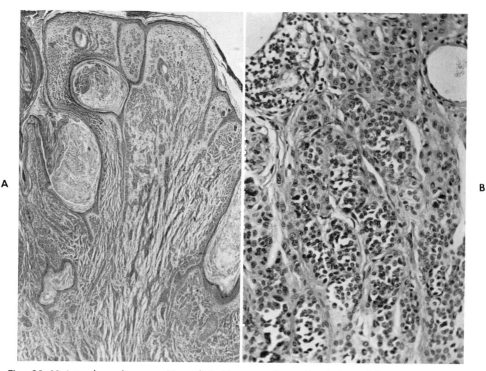

Fig. 39-40 Intradermal nevus. (**A** and **B**, Hematoxylin-eosin; **A** from Allen, A. C.: Cancer 2:28-56, 1949.)

feathers may be controlled by the transposition of the embryonic cells of the neural crest. That neural *control* of many varieties of pigmentation exists is obvious. However, to conclude from this that the cells of the neural crest are incorporated in the epidermis as melanocytes is to fail, in effect, to distinguish the artist from his pigments.

The addition of these facts, supplemented by evidence from the direct examination of many junctional nevi and melanocarcinomas, indicates that basal cells principally, but also prickle cells or keratinocytes, may become converted to melanocytes and that the junctional nevi are derived from these cells. As we have often suggested and apparently ineffectively illustrated, an objective study of the peripheral, intraepidermal portions of junctional nevi or melanocarcinomas in situ clearly discloses the transition of keratinocytes into these lesions[1, 2, 12] (Fig. 39-46).

Intradermal nevus

The intradermal nevus, or common mole, is the ordinary pigmented spot which few people are altogether spared. The mole may be flat or raised, with or without hairs, papillary and keratotic. Intradermal nevi may be present at birth or may develop in later years.

They tend to become more prominent at the time of puberty.

Histologically, the tumor is composed of nests and cords of cells with round, moderately chromatic nuclei surrounded by an even, easily seen rim of cytoplasm. Melanin pigment, when present, usually is limited to the superficial cells in the upper dermis. Similarly, the cells in the upper part of the lesion are more likely to be dopa positive than are the deeper ones.* Mitotic figures are seen rarely in these nevi in adults. Occasionally, hyperchromatism and enlargement of nuclei are simulated by mere agglutination of neval cells. The neval cells characteristically trail off into the depths of the dermis, and rarely into the

---

*The dopa-positive cells are melanoblasts (or melanocytes). There is no convincing evidence to indicate that the tyrosinase reaction is practically or even theoretically of use in differentiating the active junctional nevus from a superficial melanocarcinoma as others have suggested.

Melanophores are merely phagocytes that engulf and transport melanin. Melanophores are dopa negative. A pigmented neval cell or melanoblast may be dopa negative because its enzyme has been completely utilized at a given time or has never been developed. The cells of a nonpigmented (amelanotic) melanoma may be dopa positive. However, not all cells of a pigmented or nonpigmented melanocarcinoma are necessarily dopa positive.

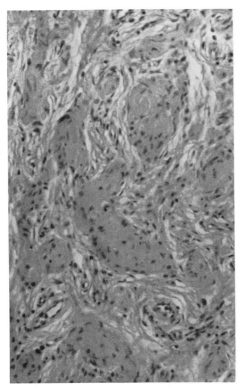

Fig. 39-41 So-called "lames foliacées," which are really no more than foci of collagenization about neval cells. Unlike Meissner corpuscles, which they resemble, even ultrastructurally, these structures become more prominent with increasing age and are practically absent in children. (Hematoxylin-eosin; from Allen, A. C.: Cancer **2:** 28-56, 1949.)

subcutis, without sharp limitation. The overlying epidermis usually is thinned and may be flat or papillary, with or without hyperkeratosis (Figs. 39-40 and 39-41).

There is impressive histologic basis for the conclusion that the ordinary intradermal mole that is *not* overlain by a junctional nevus rarely becomes malignant. We have seen one such instance involving the scalp of a child.

The origin of the cells of the common mole is still unsettled. The possibilities include the following: (1) epidermal cells, (2) specialized "nerve endings" similar to Merkel-Ranvier corpuscles, and (3) dermal nerves. Those who subscribe to the epidermal origin of the intradermal nevus assume, as Unna did, that the altered epidermal cells drop off ("abtropfung") and migrate into the dermis. Those who believe in the neurogenesis of pigmented nevi suggest that the neval cells arise from dermal nerves or their sheaths, as well as from the intraepidermal nerve endings or cells that

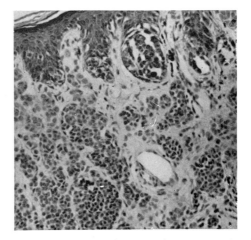

Fig. 39-42 Compound nevus showing junctional and intradermal components. (Hematoxylin-eosin.)

migrated from the neural crest. The frequency with which intradermal nevi are associated with loosened nests of epidermal cells that appear about to drop off (junctional changes) makes the epidermal origin of the common mole (as well as the junctional nevus) the likeliest possibility. This frequent association of the junctional change with the intradermal nevus can hardly be fortuitous, inasmuch as the change is rarely seen with blue nevi and yet is infrequently absent in the moles of children, normally diminishing in frequency and prominence after puberty.

Compound nevus

In about 98% of the intradermal nevi occurring prior to puberty and in about 12% of nevi of adults, there is an associated junctional change[12] (Fig. 39-42). For lesions with this combination of features, the term "compound nevus" was suggested by us many years ago.[12] It recently has been stated that silver stains are of appreciable help in distinguishing compound nevi from malignant melanomas. This, unfortunately, is not correct.

Clinically, as stated, there is no way to be certain as to whether or not an intradermal nevus is compounded with a junctional nevus. This fact emphasizes the importance of histologic examination of all excised nevi. As is indicated in the discussion of melanocarcinomas, the compound nevus has the capacity for undergoing malignant transformation by virtue of its junctional component. This conversion takes place relatively infrequently. The possibility exists that an intradermal nevus may, on occasion, develop overlying junctional change.

Juvenile melanoma

Juvenile melanoma is the name applied to a special form of compound nevus occurring predominantly in children. In the past, these lesions were considered to be histologically malignant but clinically benign. In other words, if the patient was prepubertal, these moles were arbitrarily labeled benign.

It was not until the basic histologic definition of these was first published in 1948 by the late Dr. Sophie Spitz that the morphologic distinction between the juvenile melanomas and true melanocarcinomas began to become evident[94] (Fig. 39-43). It is now reasonably apparent that this much-needed definition has served in a most practical way to clarify portions of a gravely confused problem.

Briefly, the distinguishing features of the juvenile melanomas are those of the compound nevi, with the addition of myogenous-appearing, occasionally spindled, single and multinucleated giant cells with abundant basophilic cytoplasm, often loosely dispersed in an edematous upper cutis. According to Wells and Farthing,[105] cholinesterases are absent in juvenile melanomas, although a contrary finding was noted by Winkelmann.[107] We have found no basis for believing that the juvenile

melanoma, which, as indicated, is really a special form of compound nevus, is any more likely to become malignant than is the ordinary compound nevus.

With increasing experience, it has become possible to recognize the juvenile melanomas for what they are on the interpretation of the histologic picture alone. On this basis, the scope of the significance of the juvenile melanoma has been extended by our discovery that this lesion may be found in adults, preponderantly in the second, third, and fourth decades but occasionally in older patients.[15] The practical importance of this observation is obvious when it is realized that, previously, benign juvenile melanomas were treated as cancers.

Frequently, it is possible to estimate the approximate ages of individuals from certain histologic features of their nevi. These features include the quality of the junctional changes (often abundant and yet qualitatively torpid-looking in children), the compact cellularity of the intradermal component of the nevi in children, the increasing prominence, because of collagenization, of the "lâmes foliacées" with increasing age and their virtual absence in children, and the elements of the juvenile melanoma as outlined previously. The juvenile melanomas undergo involutional fibrosis, as do other types of nevi[13, 14] (Fig. 39-41).

Currently, there is unfortunately an increasing tendency to submit for histologic examination the shaved top of a pigmented lesion. Such a superficial biopsy not only complicates the problems of histologic diagnosis and the determination of cleared margins, but also leads to local recurrences of incompletely removed lesions. These local recurrences may be treacherously difficult to diagnose correctly.

Tragically, radical operations have been performed under the mistaken impression that the juvenile melanoma was malignant, just as they have for keratoacanthoma. A tabulation of some of the misdiagnoses has been recently recorded.[89]

There has been a good deal of objection to our use of "juvenile melanoma" (rather than "spindle cell nevus," for example) for a lesion that is benign and occurs occasionally in adults. Actually, we have always used the term in a descriptive, histologic sense, much as the terms embryonal rhabdomyosarcoma, fetal adenoma of the thyroid gland, infantile fibrolipoma, juvenile nasopharyngeal angiofibroma, and juvenile carcinoma of the breast

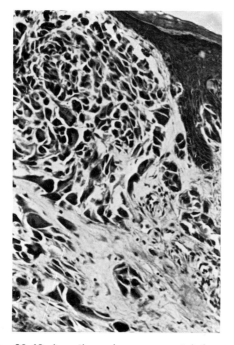

Fig. 39-43 Juvenile melanoma, special form of compound nevus simulating melanocarcinoma. (Hematoxylin-eosin; from Spitz, S.: Amer. J. Path. **24:**591-609, 1948.)

are used. These terms are applied to tumors of adults by the very ones who rather inconsistently object to the corresponding designation "juvenile" in this instance.

Furthermore, the embryonal rhabdomyosarcoma, for example, was originally believed to be confined to infants, children, and teenagers but are now known to occur even in the seventh decade of life.[93] Further, just as with some of these other tumors, the juvenile melanoma occurs in youngsters with an overwhelming preponderance, and our discovery of its presence in adults in 1953 is merely a dividend of the application of the histologic criteria for the diagnosis of this lesion as first enunciated by Spitz in 1948.[94] Finally, while it is true that "melanoma" generally carries with it a malignant connotation, the hard fact is that many malignant melanomas, particularly those of the spindle cell variety or those with prominent giant cells, are being mislabeled juvenile melanoma or spindle cell nevus. Accordingly, the use of "juvenile melanoma" serves the important practical purpose of viewing with added caution the acceptance of a given evaluation of a lesion so diagnosed. Sometimes, it seems to have been forgotten that, after all, it was not many years ago that no one claimed to be able to distinguish the juvenile melanoma from the malignant mela-

noma, and, in a great many laboratories, this problem has obviously been far from resolved.

Blue nevus

The blue or Jadassohn-Tièche nevus appears as a flat or slightly elevated blue or bluish black lesion, occurring particularly on the trunk and extremities and often mistaken clinically for a malignant melanoma. It is structurally essentially the same as the *Mongolian spot* or the nevus of Ota. The former is found in the sacral region in the last half of embryonic life or the first year of infancy, disappearing thereafter. The nevus of Ota occurs in the eye and on the skin of the face.

Histologically, these nevi are composed of interlacing fasciculi of spindle cells with long cytoplasmic processes and oval fibrocytoid nuclei. The cells are usually much more loosely disposed than those of the blue nevus. If the pigment were not present, the histologic picture of the blue nevus would resemble that of a dermal neurofibroma, and, indeed, it is possible that the basic morphogenesis of the two is similar. However, many of the cells of the blue nevus and the Mongolian spot are dopa positive. Abundant melanin pigment may obliterate the details of most of the cells of the blue nevus. In addition, the neoplastic cells are interspersed with numerous pigment-laden

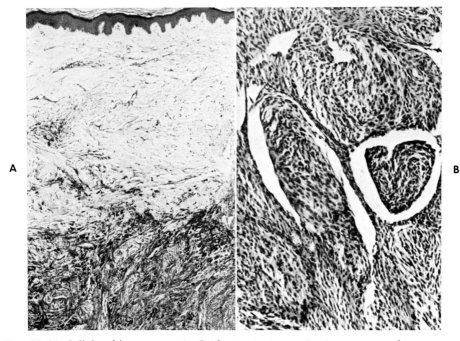

Fig. 39-44 Cellular blue nevus. **A,** Epidermis is intact. **B,** Appearance of invasion of lymphatics is an illusion characteristic of this lesion and is secondary to artifactual shrinkage. (**A** and **B,** Hematoxylin-eosin; from Allen, A. C.: Cancer **2:**28-56, 1949.)

chromatophores. Usually, the neval cells lie deep in the dermis, or occasionally they are directly apposed to the epidermis. The color of the nevus is, of course, dependent not only on the amount of pigment present, but also on the distance of the lesion from the epidermis. Infrequently, the blue nevus is combined with the ordinary intradermal nevus (common mole) and with the junctional nevus.

There is a striking variant of the blue nevus that is frequently incorrectly diagnosed as melanosarcoma. Some years ago, we termed this lesion *cellular blue nevus*.[12] It occurs in about 50% of cases in the skin of the buttocks and the dorsum of the hands or feet. The epidermis is unchanged. The cells of this tumor show no significant anaplasia, and mitotic figures almost always are absent. Fused nuclei often simulate the hyperchromasia of activity. One of the features that characterize the lesion is the cross sections of fasciculi surrounded by clear zones, giving the illusion that the whorls are metastases in lymphatics when they actually represent artifactitious shrinkage and cleavage of the fasciculi (Fig. 39-44). The melanosomes of the cellular blue nevus are stated to have a distinctive ultrastructure.[87]

Blue nevi undergo malignant change with consoling rarity. We have seen somewhat over forty examples of malignant blue nevi. While it appears obvious that the diagnosis of sarcomatous transformation of a blue nevus is often made unjustifiably, it is incorrect to assume, as some do, that such cancers do not occur.

■   ■   ■

Several eponyms continue to be applied to pigmented lesions that, unfortunately, are still poorly defined histologically. Among these are Hutchinson's lentigo or freckle and melanoma of Dubreuilh.

Senile lentigo

The senile lentigo is a common lesion occurring on exposed surfaces in approximately one-third of individuals past middle age. It is characterized histologically by hyperkeratosis and parakeratosis and fringelike elongation of the hyperpigmented rete ridges, often showing an increase in basilar "clear cells" or minimal junctional change.

Melanotic freckle of Hutchinson

Much attention has been given recently to essentially restatements of information concerning the melanotic freckle of Hutchinson, also known as *la mélanose circonscrite précancéreuse de Dubreuilh, senile* or *malignant freckle, precancerous* or *acquired melanosis, premalignant lentigo,* and *lentigo maligna.* Actually, this lesion is characteristically a relatively slow-growing lesion of the face, generally of elderly patients, which evolves from epidermal melanosis to a junctional nevus with varying degrees of activity and, finally, if the patient lives long enough, to a superficial and then deep melanocarcinoma. As we have long ago documented, the melanocarcinomas of the face, especially those of women, tend to be associated with a better prognosis than those of most other regions of the body.[15] Their histogenesis, however, is no different from any other junctional nevus or from the melanocarcinoma derived therefrom, although there are forcefully unequivocal statements to the contrary.

Recently, an inherited entity referred to as the *"multiple lentigines syndrome"* has been described and is stated to include cardiac and ocular defects, deafness, genital anomalies, and retardation of growth.[39]

Halo nevi

Halo nevi (leukoderma acquisitum centrifugum, Sutton's nevus) refers to the progressive centripetal extension of a zone of depigmentation about a nevus. The depigmentation appears to be provoked by subepidermal inflammation. Similar rings of depigmentation may occur about small melanocarcinomas.

A broad spectrum of hypotheses ranging from antigen-antibody reaction to neurotropic disturbance has been suggested to explain the local vitiligo or leukoderma. The most reasonable is that the depigmentation is secondary to the underlying inflammatory reaction similar to the depigmentation that may follow lichen planus.

Melanocarcinoma

The melanocarcinoma *(malignant melanoma)* of the skin ranks with the choriocarcinoma for the widespread metastases to which it gives rise. As previously indicated, we have classified the malignant melanomas as follows*:

1 Melanocarcinomas (from junctional nevus or compound nevus [or juvenile melanoma])
    (a) Superficial
    (b) Deep
2 Malignant blue nevus

*From Allen, A. C., and Spitz, S.: Cancer **6:**1-45, 1953.

Clinically, the malignant melanoma is preceded usually by a flat, hairless mole, pigmented light to dark brown. When such a mole, which may have appeared the same for years, begins to darken, it probably has already undergone at least local malignant transformation. The changes of ulceration, increase in size, and bleeding lend a serious increment to the prognosis.

A mole that is hairy, elevated, and papillary is uncommonly the site of cancer, although the insurance is by no means absolute—for the histologic reasons to be explained. In some instances, the neoplasm appears to arise de novo, especially on the scrotum, palms, and soles. In these regions, the common (intradermal) mole rarely occurs, but the small, flat, often unnoticed, frecklelike junctional or compound nevus frequently is present. Because the lesions of the soles and genitalia are likely to have a junctional component, tend to escape inspection, and are located in areas that appear to have a proportionately higher incidence of malignant melanomas than other anatomic sites, it would seem reasonable to have such nevi removed electively from these sites when feasible.

In many instances, the benign deeply pigmented blue nevus is mistaken for a developing malignant melanoma. As stated, metastasizing melanomas are uncommon prior to the age of puberty, although we have recorded a number of such cases. In each of these instances, the histologic picture could be distinguished from that of the juvenile melanomas but not from the melanocarcinomas of adults.[15]

Melanocarcinomas in black persons. Melanomas are said also to be uncommon in blacks, a phenomenon that has been considered analogous to the frequency of the melanoma in white or gray horses in contrast to the incidence in darkly pigmented ones. However, the statistics on this matter are not always clearly presented, usually for the reason that the ratio of the white to the black population in the particular institution is not taken into account. In a study in which this ratio was properly considered the relative incidence in the white group was about four times that in the black. In another study, the ratio was even lower. In the South African black, a large percentage of the melanomas occur on the feet, a fact that has been attributed to the trauma undergone by the bare feet. Moreover, the chronic irritation of a shoe, belt, or shoulder strap or the stimulation of an electrocoagulating current used in excisional ther-

apy has been vigorously blamed, with inadequate documentation, for the change of a mole into a malignant melanoma.

Histology and histogenesis. There is considerable variation in the cellular pattern of the melanocarcinomas. The primary lesion may simulate a squamous cell carcinoma, a spindle or basal cell carcinoma, an adenocarcinoma, a neurofibrosarcoma, or other neoplasms. The usual melanocarcinoma is composed of cells arranged as compact masses with some cords and alveoli. The cells are likely to be more or less uniform in size and shape. The nuclei of the primary lesion commonly do not exhibit the classic evidence of anaplasia. Mitotic figures may not be numerous, despite the aggressiveness of the neoplasm. Often, the nuclei are vacuolated and contain large acidophilic nucleoli resembling inclusion bodies, sometimes containing melanin. Melanin pigment may be present or absent without prognostic influence. In the neoplastic cells, the pigment tends to be of a uniform, fine granularity, whereas in the chromatophores, the pigment granules are likely to be more irregular in size and shape.

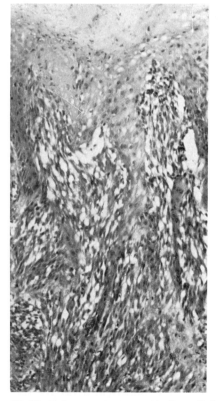

Fig. 39-45 Melanocarcinoma, spindle cell form, showing origin from epidermis. Often confused with juvenile melanomas. (Hematoxylin-eosin; from Allen, A. C.: Cancer **2:**28-56, 1949.)

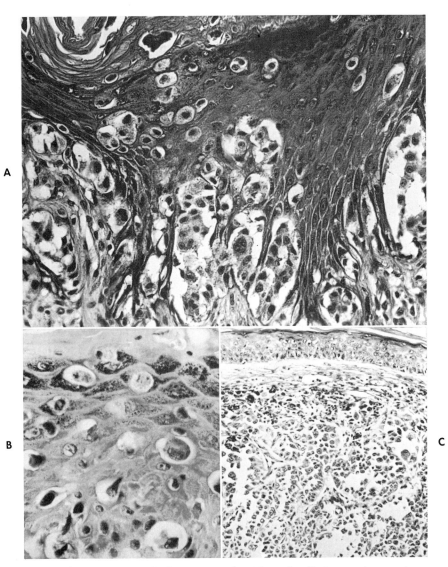

Fig. 39-46 Melanocarcinoma. **A,** Conversion of epidermal cells into melanocarcinomatous cells. **B,** In situ transformation of epidermal cells into melanocarcinomatous cells. **C,** Metastatic melanocarcinoma to skin showing overlying intact epidermis—criterion for primary versus metastatic melanocarcinoma. (**A** to **C,** Hematoxylin-eosin; from Allen, A. C.: Cancer **2:**28-56, 1949.)

One of the most helpful histologic aids in diagnosis is the active junctional change overlying and continuous with the dermal portion of the cancer. The cells of the rete ridges may be so loosened as to be incorporated in the dermal neoplasm, with consequent partial dissolution of the ridges. Isolated, spherical, haloed cells, often powdered with fine melanin granules, may be found as far up as the stratum corneum. Such intraepithelial cells are, in our opinion, the source of practically all melanocarcinomas of the skin and mucous membranes (blue nevi excepted). These cancerous cells are not related to Langhans'

cells or Merkel-Ranvier corpuscles but actually seem to have been, originally, cells derived from various layers of the epidermis. Nor is it true, as some believe, that these cells within the epidermis are metastatic from the underlying tumor within the dermis. Evidence for the autochthonous epidermal origin is found not only in the occurrence of such cells within the epidermis alone in early junctional nevi or superficial malignant melanomas but also in their absence in the epidermis overlying a snugly apposed dermal metastasis of a melanoma (Figs. 39-45 and 39-46), a criterion that distinguishes the primary from the

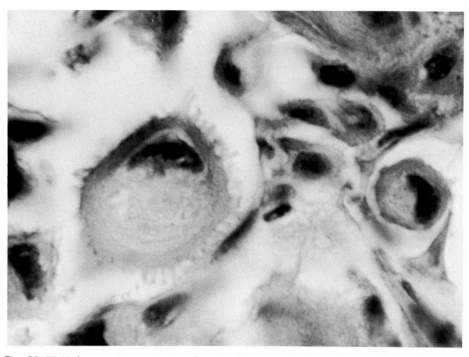

Fig. 39-47 Melanocarcinoma in situ showing histogenesis of neoplasm cells from keratino-cytes. Residue of identifying "prickles" and atypical neoplastic nuclei are evident. (Hema-toxylin-eosin; ×1000.)

metastatic melanocarcinoma (Fig. 39-47). If melanocytes indeed migrate to the epidermis from the neural crest, what is their source when the epidermis is ulcerated? It is not enough to state merely that they simply regenerate, because left unexplained is the mechanism of their distribution to approximately every tenth cell of the basal layer. Such a pattern of distribution would seem to require origin from a preexisting adjacent basal cell.

Active junctional nevus. It is now apparent that when a malignant melanoma appears to be superimposed onto a benign intradermal nevus, there was originally present a clinically obvious or latent junctional nevus that itself was the source of the malignant melanoma. Routine studies of the epidermis of the primary melanocarcinomas of skin (and mucous membranes, including conjunctiva) demonstrate this junctional change. In other words, the melanocarcinoma arising in the skin would actually seem to be a peculiarly virulent variant of an epidermogenic carcinoma, a view originally expressed decades ago by Unna in 1893.[102] Why the malignant melanoma behaves usually more aggressively than other epidermal carcinomas is not yet known. Occasionally, it becomes a problem to decide

if a given lesion is still in the stage of junctional nevus or whether it has become a melanocarcinoma in situ. The histologic diagnosis of a *superficial melanocarcinoma* must, in the last analysis, depend upon finding evidence of invasion of the dermis by the cells of the *active junctional nevus.*

Actually, all junctional nevi, by definition, exhibit a kind of activity or dynamics in the form of varying stages of acantholysis of the intraepidermal cells. However, with this reservation, we have in the past applied the term "active junctional nevus" to the one with nuclear atypia, mitotic figures, and often with large, pagetoid cells scattered singly or in clumps to various levels of the epidermis. Such a lesion is equivalent to "melanocarcinoma in situ." The presence of such an active junctional nevus should lead to a painstaking search for dermal invasion with the help of multiple sections. The histologic criteria for the distinction of a superficial melanocarcinoma—from an active junctional nevus on the one hand and a deep melanocarcinoma on the other—are essentially similar to those used for distinguishing a superficial squamous cell carcinoma from leukoplakia and from a deeply infiltrating carcinoma. Incidentally, the marked degree of pseudoepitheliomatous hyperplasia so commonly associated with melanocarcinomas is largely responsible for mistaking these neoplasms for squamous cell carcinomas. Such epithelial hyperplasia constitutes, in this instance, an additional increment of evidence in favor of the epithelial genesis of melanocarcinomas.[15] It should be emphasized that the concept of the epithelial origin of nevi of the skin and mucous membranes, including the conjunctiva, in no way precludes a neuroectodermal origin of the melanomas of the choroid and uveal tract.

Prognosis. The prognosis of melanocarcinomas, while always serious, is not quite so hopeless as generally believed. The following are factors in the prognosis[15]:

1 Superficial melanocarcinomas. The survival rate in patients with superficial melanocarcinomas is about 75%, as opposed to from 10% to 39% (depending on age and sex) in those with deep melanocarcinomas.

2 Sex. The overall prognosis is considerably better for women, exclusive of those with melanocarcinomas of the mucous membranes.

3 Location. The skin of the head and neck region appears to be the most favorable site.

4 Regional node metastasis. Of course, regional node metastasis is an ominous prognostic portent, but such metastasis does not preclude survival.

5 Five-year survivals. Survival for five years is not necessarily tantamount to cure. Approximately 13% of patients died of metastases five years or more after the diagnosis was made or after the initial therapy.

6 Adequate statistical evidence is lacking that pregnancy is a detrimental factor in the activation of junctional nevi or acceleration of growth of melanocarcinomas. On the other hand, well-documented examples of *spontaneous regression* of malignant melanomas following pregnancy have been recorded.[102] Documented disappearance of metastases from melanocarcinoma has been noted following the transfusion of blood from a donor whose malignant melanoma had undergone spontaneous regression.[97]

7 Local recurrences are usually the result either of failure to remove the junctional change at the margins of the tumor or of reactivation of junctional change at or near the margin of excision. Patients with a melanocarcinoma appear to have a *systemic diathesis for activation* of junctional nevi, which in a considerable percentage of cases (3.5%) leads to multiple primary melanocarcinomas.

8 Such histologic features as the content of melanin and the absence of appreciable polymorphism or mitotic figures are not significantly contributory in the evaluation of the prognosis.

9 Prophylaxis. In view of the fact that moles in certain locations are generally junctional or compound nevi, it would seem wise, prophylactically, to remove, when feasible, isolated nevi of the soles and genitalia if they are larger than 0.5 cm in diameter.

10 Melanocarcinomas of the mucous membranes of the oronasopharynx, larynx, bronchus, esophagus, gallbladder, genitalia, including cervix, and anorectal region are almost uniformly fatal. Undoubtedly, some of the contributory reasons for their grave prognosis is the delay in detection and in accurate histologic diagnosis, the frequent injudicious therapy, the difficulties in adequate operative removal, and possibly such extraneous factors as chronic infection and repeated trauma. In approximately 15% of 337 patients, the tumors arose in these various mucous membranes (exclusive of the conjunctiva). The ulceration of the junctional change and the absence of appreciable amounts of pigment in about 50% of the melanomas of mucous membranes increase the difficulties of histologic diagnosis.

Tumors of vessels
Lymphangioma

The number of histologic and clinical variants, as well as the difficulty in distinguishing neoplasia of lymphatic vessels from ectasias, anomalies, and proliferations due to stasis, has led to the application of needlessly confusing names. The same situation exists with respect to the angiomas, but in both instances it has existed so long that scrapping of terminology at this point would add to the confusion.

The **lymphangioma simplex** is a soft, compressible, grayish pink nodule. The nodules are often multiple and grouped irregularly. Although the skin of the genitalia is the common site for these tumors, they are found also on the lips and tongue and may be associated with a macroglossia or macrocheilia. They are composed of varying-sized, endothelium-lined, thin-walled vessels, either empty or containing lymph with occasional leukocytes. Some of the channels may contain a few red blood cells. There is an abundant proliferation of endothelial cells in a proportion of the tumors, to which the designation **lymphangioma tuberosum multiplex** or **lymphangioendothelioma** has been applied.

Lymphangioma cutis circumscriptum occurs in the skin of the face, chest, or extremities in the form of a single tumor or of multiple, projecting, somewhat papillary, verrucose nodules. They may resemble opalescent vesicles, and there may be an associated telangiectasis. Histologically, they are composed of dilated lymphatic vessels in the upper dermis and are so closely linked to the epidermis as to appear incorporated in it. The overlying epidermis may be irregularly atrophied and acanthotic as well as hyperkeratotic in a papillary manner so as to simulate the angiokeratomas (see also p. 764).

The **lymphangioma cavernosum** may be small and circumscribed, or it may extend diffusely over an extensive area, causing macrodactylia, for example. Histologically, the lymphatic channels are markedly dilated and may extend into fat and muscle, as do the so-called infiltrating angiomas. The unencapsulated extensions are in neither instance evidence of malignant transformation, but they do complicate local removal.

The **lymphangioma cysticum coli** or **hygroma** is a congenital lesion that arises usually in the neck and submaxillary regions and is histologically similar to the lymphangioma cavernosum in both structure and extension. The hygroma may ramify widely upward to the parotid area, downward as far as the mediastinum, and inward to lie precariously close to the trachea and adjacent structures. The lymphangioma cysticum may occur also in the region of the sacrum (pp. 764 and 1110).

It may be impossible histologically to differentiate neoplasms or dysontogenetic tumors of lymphatic vessels from the focal and occasionally nodular lymphangiectasis that follows stasis due to scarring of skin or inflammatory reactions within lymph nodes. The differentiation may be dependent on a complete clinical picture. Often, there is an associated telangiectasia that may complicate the interpretation, as may the accidental presence of a few red blood cells in the lymphatics. The overall impression of these tumors of the lymphatic vessels is that they represent ectasias, either congenital or acquired, secondary to atresias, and are occasionally concomitantly associated with venous dilatation. Certainly, the occurrence of multiple benign tumors of lymphatic vessels in an irregular group does not suggest multicentric neoplasia as much as simple ectasias due either to faulty intrinsic development of the vessels or to errors in development of related structures such as lymph nodes, with resultant changes in lymphodynamics.

Hemangioma

The problems of the pathogenesis and terminology of tumors of blood vessels are even more complicated than those of lymphangiomas. Theoretically, a true hemangioma is to be differentiated from a simple dilatation of blood vessels by its independence from the adjacent normal circulatory channels. A hemangioma enlarges, therefore, by growth of its own elements rather than by incorporation of nearby vessels. In practice, however, these criteria are seldom applied, and accordingly many ectasias, hyperemias, and hyperplasias are included as neoplasias. The hemangiomas may be classified simply as capillary, cavernous, or mixed (p. 762).

The **capillary angioma** corresponds clinically to the familiar "port-wine" stain common on the face and neck, but it exists also as simple small "vascular nevi" or birthmarks. In infants, such angiomas may be composed of compact masses of endothelial cells in which the capillary lumina are obscured in many areas. These proliferations often extend from the dermis into the subcutaneous tissue. The extension of the lesion beyond the dermis and its rich cellularity may provoke the erroneous diagnosis of angiosarcoma.[95] However, such angiomatous formations are usually sufficiently characteristic as to make possible the diagnosis of benign *infantile angioma* on the basis of histologic appearance alone. The capillary angioma may be confused histologically also with granuloma pyogenicum, particularly if the former is ulcerated and inflamed, as the latter usually is. The granuloma pyogenicum, however, is characteristically polypoid, generally has been present for no longer than one to three months, and bleeds easily and repeatedly. The histology of the granuloma pyogenicum is identical with the so-called "pregnancy tumor" that occurs in the oral mucosa during the period of gestation. Thrombocytopenia may be associated with giant vascular tumors. The remission of the thrombocytopenia following removal of the hemangioma suggests that the tumor may occasionally serve as a reservoir for the platelets.

The *sclerosing hemangioma* appears to be a special variety of capillary angioma, although few dermatologists subscribe to this interpretation. They prefer to regard the lesion as a dermatofibroma lenticulare, histiocytoma, or

merely subepidermal fibrosis. The lesions occur chiefly on the extremities and present
clinically as single, firm, and slightly elevated
intracutaneous nodules, averaging several millimeters to a centimeter in diameter. Their
sectioned surface is smooth and yellow.

Histologically, more or less of the dermis is
replaced by spindle cells, arranged generally
in tight curlicues, although in some areas these
cells appear to enclose tiny spaces suggestive
of the lumina of capillaries. In a few cases,
the lumina are so large and numerous as to
make the vascular nature of this lesion obvious. Usually, the cells are vacuolated by lipid,
and in some cases the fat content is the most
striking feature. Dark brown granules of
hemosiderin are often present in many of the
cells. At times, the iron pigment may be so
abundant that some observers, confusing the
pigment with melanin, have succumbed to the
serious error of labeling the lesion a malignant
melanoma. The overlying epidermis may be
normal, atrophied, moderately acanthotic, or
the site of a superimposed basal cell carcinoma.[41] In some instances, a sharply delimited
subepidermal zone of the dermis is spared. A
similar free zone is seen in the dermal neurofibroma, although perhaps not so frequently
(Fig. 39-48). The sclerosing hemangioma may
sometimes be justifiably confused with the
neurofibroma when, as not infrequently occurs, the deeper portion of the lesion is composed of fasciculi of spindle cells such as
characterize the neurofibroma.

Occasionally, a fibrotic tumor resembling
the sclerosing hemangioma, particularly of
the trunk, recurs locally with formation of
satellite nodules. Usually, such tumors originally extended into the subcutaneous fat and
were removed incompletely. These tumors,
called *dermatofibrosarcoma protuberans,* give
rise to distant metastases in the rarest instances.

The **cavernous hemangiomas** are histologically similar to the cavernous lymphangiomas
except for the presence of blood in the congeries of vessels. The vessels may ramify progressively in the subcutaneous fat, fascia, and
intermuscular septa. The extensions may be
so wide and inaccessible as to make surgical
removal an exceedingly difficult procedure.
The term infiltrating angioma is more aptly
applied to such tumors than is angiosarcoma.

Clinically, the cavernous hemangiomas present on the skin surface as purple, single,
globular or multilobular tumors or as the flat
or slightly elevated "strawberry" nevus of in-

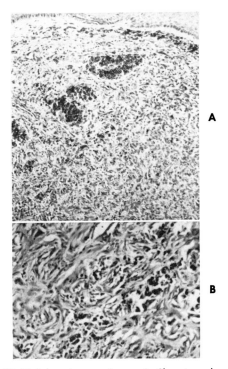

Fig. 39-48 Sclerosing angioma. **A,** Showing abundant hemosiderin. **B,** Vascular nature evident.
(**A** and **B,** Hematoxylin-eosin.)

fants. The angiomas may be multiple and may
cause, or at least be associated with, enlargement and distortion of an area of the body
in the vicinity of the tumors. The distortion
from edema and hypertrophy of an arm
(*Weber syndrome,* 1907) may be so great as
to require amputation because of the sheer
weight of the extremity.

Other syndromes associated with anomalies
of blood vessels include the Sturge-Weber syndrome (nevus flammeus of the face, cerebral
angiomatosis, hemiplegia, and mental retardation), Maffucci's syndrome (angiomas with
dyschondroplasia), and heredofamilial angiomatosis *(Rendu-Osler-Weber disease).* Cutaneous angiomas also may be part of the complex of *multiple congenital angiomas* found
in the viscera, particularly in the cerebellum
and retina, and known as *Hippel's disease.*
The *"blue rubber-bleb nevus"* appears to be
a form of venous hamartoma involving both
skin and gastrointestinal tract. It is characterized by pain, sweating, and a sensation of
dermal "herniation."[86]

The *angiokeratoma* or telangiectatic wart
represents a variety of cavernous hemangioma
that is structurally similar to the lymphangioma cutis circumscriptum. The dilated blood
channels are located high in the papillae and

are so intimately associated with the epidermis as to appear actually within it in many places. The overlying epidermis is usually papillary, acanthotic, and hyperkeratotic. Clinically, the lesions are dark purplish red, firm, the size of a pinhead or split pea, and located in the scrotum, ears, fingers, and toes. The lesions often are associated with some circulatory disturbance such as might follow chilblains and varicosities. This type that tends to occur on the extensor surface of the extremities is known as the *Mibelli* type of angiokeratoma as opposed to *Fordyce's* type without associated pernio. The *angiokeratoma of Fabry* may be associated with lesions of viscera, particularly the kidneys and vessels, with characteristic foam cells. Patients with angiokeratoma of Fabry may excrete increased amounts of the glycoproteins ceramide trihexoside and dihexoside. Examination of the urine for these glycoproteins may aid in the detection of the disorder in members of the families of patients.[77]

Spider "angiomas," which are really small telangiectases, possibly with arteriovenous shunts, occur with chronic hepatic damage as in Laennec's cirrhosis, as well as in pregnancy. They are thought to be an effect of excess of estrogenic hormones.

The term hemangioendothelioma is rather gratuitously and hedgingly applied to hemangiomas in which there is a relative prominence of endothelial cells with or without atypia. The implication in its use is that the neoplasm shows greater activity and therefore presents more likelihood of local recurrence than the ordinary hemangioma. The evidence for this presumption is questionable. A similar situation exists with respect to the use of "lymphangioendothelioma." Unfortunately, the name "hemangioendothelioma," rather than angiosarcoma, is sometimes applied to the frankly malignant tumor.

Angiosarcoma

Primary solitary angiosarcoma of the skin, exclusive of Kaposi's hemorrhagic sarcoma, is rare. However, several cases have been recorded in which visceral metastases have occurred. The metastases tend to be more cellular and anaplastic than the original growth. Others have been reported as malignant vascular tumors of skin under the title hemangioendothelioma, but in most instances evidence of origin from dermis, as well as of the cancerous characteristics, is not convincingly presented. Knowledge of the

rarity of such tumors is of practical importance because of its tempering effect on the tendency to call sarcomatous those nonmetastasizing angiomas with abundant endothelial cells or those that have infiltrated into the subcutaneous fat and beyond into the muscles. The Kaposi sarcoma, on the other hand, represents a process of vastly different significance.

Kaposi's idiopathic hemorrhagic sarcoma

Kaposi's sarcoma begins as reddish to purplish brown, discrete or grouped, painful, tender nodules varying from 1 mm to 2 mm in size to about 1 cm. They occur particularly on the hands and feet, although they may start in the skin of any part of the body. The incidence is about ten times as great in men as in women, and the disease is seen especially in elderly patients, although it has been described in children. The surface of the nodules may be telangiectatic, but often it is verrucose. Local purpura and bullae may be associated with the lesions. Lymphatic blockage with elephantiasis of the extremities is common and is reminiscent of the edema associated with postmastectomy lymphangiosarcoma. The course of the disease is slow, the nodules often involuting, with resultant atrophic scarring and pigmentation. The condition may last from one to fully twenty-five years, although the average duration is from five to ten years. The disease is found chiefly in Italian and Jewish people.

The lesions may involve extensive areas of the skin and nearly every organ of the body. The gastrointestinal tract, mesenteric nodes, liver, and lungs are the most common sites, although even the osseous and central nervous systems may be affected. The question is unsettled as to whether these lesions are truly metastases or actually multicentric foci of a neoplasm. The intestinal lesions of Kaposi's sarcoma, unlike most other metastatic lesions, have a predilection for the inner coats rather than the serosa. In this location, the tumors give rise to profuse hemorrhage. This difference in location in the intestinal tract between the Kaposi sarcoma and other metastatic tumors is a bit of evidence in favor of the multicentric origin of the former. Visceral tumors histologically identical with Kaposi's sarcoma have been found infrequently without cutaneous involvement. Patients with Kaposi's sarcoma die of hemorrhage from an intestinal lesion, intercurrent infection, extensive visceral involvement, or complicating malignant lymphomas.

Kaposi's sarcoma is a form of angiosarcoma that is so varied histologically as frequently to cause difficulty in the interpretation of a given slide. In one phase, perhaps the earliest, the picture is that of a simple hemangioma or of foci of hyperemic, nonspecific granulation tissue characterized by clusters of capillaries placed closely together, with or without a sprinkling of mononuclear cells and histiocytes containing hemosiderin in the intervening and often edematous stroma. At this stage, the endothelial cells may be quite regular, without mitotic figures or other evidence of anaplasia. The important histologic clue is the disposition of these vascular foci not only near the epidermis, *but also isolated about appendages in the deeper layers of the dermis.* The presence of such vascular foci at a distance from the surface of the skin is suspiciously unlike the ordinary pattern of the response of skin to inflammation. In more advanced lesions, there occurs proliferation of spindle cells and fibroblasts in association with scattered lymphocytes and histiocytes. The cells appear to form abortive capillaries, and in the actively growing lesions these cells are large and hyperchromatic and contain mitotic figures. In the later stages, there is a tendency toward focal necrosis of the neoplastic tissue and subsequent fibrosis. These variegated pictures may be observed not only at different stages of the disease but often within a single lesion.

Relation of Kaposi's sarcoma to malignant lymphomas. There is an increasing number of reports in the literature of the simultaneous occurrence of Kaposi's sarcoma with one or another of the malignant lymphomas, including Hodgkin's disease, lymphatic leukemia, lymphosarcoma, and mycosis fungoides. For both statistical and histologic reasons, the latter comprising evidence of transition of the two processes within the same lesion, the association is not considered coincidental.

Postmastectomy lymphangiosarcoma

In 1948, an entity described as lymphangiosarcoma was recorded[96] as a complication of postmastectomy lymphedema of the upper extremity. The lymphangiosarcoma in the skin of the edematous arm developed six to twenty-four years after the mastectomy, the lymphedema having existed during the entire latent period. In one instance, the tumor of the breast was benign. There was no relation-ship between the use of radiation and the development of the lymphangiosarcoma.

Histologically, the sarcoma has a range of variation quite equal to that of Kaposi's sarcoma, and indeed in many sections one cannot be certain that the neoplastic elements are lymphatic vessels rather than blood sinuses. The tumor is capable of metastasizing. Rare instances of lymphangiosarcoma as a complication of the lymphedema of filariasis have been recorded. The mechanism of cancerogenesis in the cases of lymphedema is obscure (see Fig. 38-21).

Glomus tumor

In the corium of the skin of the fingertips, particularly in the nail beds, around the joints of the extremities, and over the scapulae and coccyx, there are normally arteriovenous shunts or glomera. These are composed of an afferent artery, the Sucquet-Hoyer canal or shunt, and an efferent vein. The artery is surrounded by several layers of small, spherical, uniform glomus cells that superficially resemble the cells of the intradermal nevus and that are presumed to control the flow of blood by their contractility. Nonmedullated nerves and bundles of smooth muscle are intimately associated with the shunt. Tumors of this structure are called glomangiomas, angiomyoneuromas, glomus tumors, or neuromyoarterial aneurysms. They are most common in the nail bed but occur elsewhere on the extremities and trunk and even deep to the skin in muscles and joints, as well as in viscera. No instance of tumor occurring in the coccygeal glomus has been observed.

Glomus tumors appear as purplish red spots several millimeters in diameter, which are often clinically diagnosable by a characteristically lancinating pain, remarkably severe in view of the small size of the tumors. Not all glomangiomas, however, are associated with this characteristic symptom which occasionally is simulated by dermal angiomyomas.

Histologically, the glomus tumors range from compact masses of uniform glomus cells with few vascular channels to cavernous skeins of vessels cuffed by these cells. The vessels of the tumors tend to be small, especially in the nail bed. The identifying features are the several rows of peritheliomatously arranged glomus cells in which mitotic figures are rare or absent. These cells may be so numerous as to obliterate vascular lumina and to resemble a basal cell tumor or a variety of sweat gland adenoma. Nonmedullated nerves usually are discerned, but there appears to be no apparent relationship between the pain and the number or location of these nerves. Occasionally, glomus tumors are called simply hemangiomas or glomangioid tumors because of the presence of only two or three perivascular rows of glomus cells. However, such tumors have been observed with the typical symptomatology of glomangiomas. Ultrastructural studies reveal masses of cytoplasmic fibers suggestive of a transition from smooth muscle cells.[100, 103]

Tumors of muscle

Two varieties of tumors of dermal muscle are described: leiomyoma (arising from arrectores pilorum) and angiomyoma. What are called "granular cell myoblastomas" are lesions that were thought to have been myogenic.

Leiomyoma cutis

The leiomyoma cutis occurs singly or in groups of as many as dozens of firm and usually pea-sized nodules, which are often tender and painful. Histologically, they are composed of interlacing sheets of smooth muscle that may resemble a haphazard compact collection of arrectores pilorum (Fig. 39-49). Infrequently, the nuclei are large, irregular in size and shape, and hyperchromatic so as to merit the term *leiomyosarcoma cutis* or *dermatomyosarcoma*. However, these lesions rarely metastasize.

Angiomyoma

The angiomyoma presents as a small nondescript nodule that, microscopically, is made up of circular masses of smooth muscle strongly reminiscent of the media of arteries. The residual arterial lumen is discernible in the core of many of the masses of muscle. These lesions remain benign. Occasionally, they may be found in the subcutaneous fat or even more deeply in the fascia or intermuscular septa of the extremities. As stated, they may cause the sharp pain generally associated with glomangiomas.

Myoblastoma

The "granular cell myoblastoma" is found as a nodule in the skin of various parts of the body, as well as on the mucous membranes, particularly of the tongue and isolated sites such as the larynx, thyroid gland, breast, gallbladder, esophagus, stomach, appendix, pituitary gland, and uvea.

Histologically, the tumors are composed of nests and alveoli of large cells with small, centrally placed nuclei in cytoplasm loosely stippled with eosinophilic granules, occasionally replaced by polyhedral crystalloids. These PAS-positive granules appear to contain lipoprotein or glycolipid and ultrastructurally appear amorphous, vesicular, vacuolar, or particulate.[17] The cells closely resemble those of a xanthoma, but fat stains are negative. On close examination, it is observed that the cytoplasm is not actually vacuolated, as are lipid histiocytes. The loose dispersion of granules that simulate vacuoles has been thought to represent embryonic fibrils of striated muscle cells. Such a hypothesis is open to question, inasmuch as these tumors are present in the corium and other sites where striated muscle does not occur. The same objection may be leveled at the hypothesis that these cells represent degenerated adult striated fibers, although in sites where striated muscle is normally present, such as the tongue, this kind of transition occasionally is suggested. In our opinion, the evidence for the neurogenesis is not considered adequate. The concept of a fibroblastic origin has been advanced and appears far more

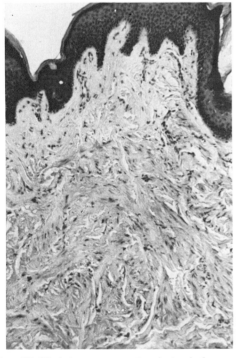

Fig. 39-49 Leiomyoma cutis derived from arrectores pilorum. (Hematoxylin-eosin.)

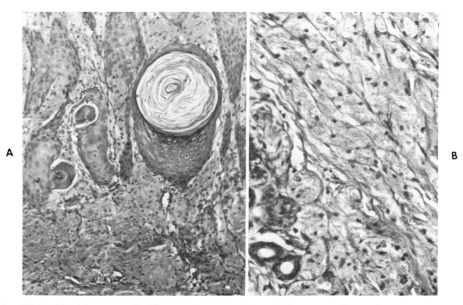

Fig. 39-50 Myoblastoma. **A,** Characteristic pseudoepitheliomatous hyperplasia. **B,** Granular cytoplasm and uniform small nuclei. (**A** and **B,** Hematoxylin-eosin.)

convincing. In any event, whether or not these tumors are proved eventually to be fibroblastic, it is clear that they are easily recognizable histologic entities that rarely, if ever, metastasize.

Some of the so-called malignant granular cell myoblastomas are, in reality, unrelated rhabdomyosarcomas in which a few of the cells happen to be granular. One of the remarkable and distinctive features of many of the myoblastomas is the characteristic epithelial or epidermal acanthosis that overlies the lesion. This feature is not present in association with frank cutaneous leiomyomas. As a rule, dermal neoplasms leave the epidermis essentially unaltered or cause its atrophy through compression. The myoblastomas, on the other hand, appear to provoke a degree of acanthosis that may simulate squamous cell carcinoma. It is as if some epidermal irritant were present in the cells of the myoblastoma (Fig. 39-50). An analogous epidermal proliferation overlies many of the sclerosing angiomas, as previously mentioned.

Fibroma

Cutaneous fibroma. The diagnosis of cutaneous fibroma is usually found on careful review to include dermatofibroma lenticulare or sclerosing hemangioma, neurofibroma, leiomyoma, keloids, and other scars. This confusion does not apply to the pedunculated soft lipofibromas (fibroma molle) in which the fibrous component closely simulates the normal dermal collagen. Undoubtedly, some of the spindle-shaped squamous cell carcinomas and melanocarcinomas have been mistaken for fibrosarcomas and "atypical fibroxanthomas" of the skin.

Neurofibroma

Neurofibroma may occur in the skin as a single tumor or as multiple nodules. In the latter condition, the entity is classified as neurofibromatosis or Recklinghausen's disease and may be associated with café-au-lait pigmented spots and neurofibromas of the sympathetic system, as well as of motor and sensory nerve trunks. The tumors of the skin may be so numerous as to cover almost the entire body from scalp to feet.

The histogenesis of the tumors is complex. The axis-cylinders, as well as the nerve sheaths (neurolemma) and endoneurium, participate to a varying extent, so that the histologic picture may be altered accordingly. The tumor derived predominantly from nerve sheaths (neurolemmoma) tends to manifest more obvious palisading of cells (Antoni A structure), degenerating, edematous microcystic foci (Antoni B), and hyaline Verocay bodies. Occasionally, the neurolemmoma presents marked central necrosis and such excessive telangiectasis is to be mistaken for an angioma. An examination of the periphery of these degenerated tumors usually reveals the telltale palisading of the neurolemmoma. A small percentage of the cutaneous neurofibromas show sufficient hyperchromatism and irregularity in size and shape of nuclei as to suggest sarcomatous degeneration. However, here, too, metastases from these neoplasms of the skin are rare, although local recurrence is fairly frequent. On the other hand, malignant changes in the visceral neurofibromas are common and may take the form of extensive, fatal, local infiltrations or metastases (p. 570). The benign neurolemmoma (schwannoma) undergoes malignant change with extreme rarity. However, malignant neurolemmomas occur, but these are presumed not to have developed from a benign neurolemmoma but to have been malignant from the start. These, too, are uncommon.

Osteoma

Osteoma cutis, an example merely of heterotopic bone, represents a metaplastic change of dermal collagen rather than true neoplasia. The lesion occurs as small nodules, as a rule, in scleroderma or syphilis, in association with acne or intradermal nevi, with hyperparathyroidism, and following trauma or after cystotomies—because of the osteogenic potentialities of urinary tract epithelium or without apparent reason.

The histologic picture may include fat and even marrow cells in addition to the bony trabeculae. In recent years, the phenomenon of *"cutaneous calciphylaxis"* has been emphasized by Selye. This phenomenon is characterized by the production of large cutaneous plaques in rats pretreated with oral dihydrotachysterol and challenged by the subcutaneous infiltration of ferric dextran. The phenomenon is inhibited by topical stress in the form of local trauma, the application of formalin, croton oil, or other irritants, and the use of agents (e.g., polymyxin) that cause degranulation of mast cells and the liberation of histamine.

Lymphomas and allied diseases

The lymphomas and allied diseases of the skin include mycosis fungoides, Hodgkin's disease, lymphosarcoma, and leukemia.

Mycosis fungoides

Mycosis fungoides (also known as granuloma fungoides—both names inaccurately chosen) is a fatal disease, primarily and principally of the skin, that is characterized clinically by three stages: (1) premycotic, (2) infiltrative, and (3) stage of fungoid tumefaction.

The premycotic stage is characterized by eczematoid, severely pruritic, erythrodermic, scaly, well-defined patches or by a generalized erythroderma. The eruption in this phase may simulate eczema, psoriasis, parapsoriasis, seborrheic dermatitis, or a nonspecific exfoliative dermatitis. This stage may persist for months or years and may be impossible to diagnose with assurance either clinically or microscopically. In the second or infiltrative stage, firm, slightly elevated, bluish-red plaques arise—both in the previously involved and the uninvolved areas. Partial or incomplete loss of hair from the scalp and other regions may occur. The last or fungoid stage follows the infiltrative period by several months.

The tumors vary in diameter up to about 10 cm or larger and are prone to ulcerate. In each of the stages, spontaneous remissions may be noted, but these are temporary. Of interest in this respect is the regression—albeit temporary—of cutaneous lesions of mycosis fungoides following reactions of delayed hypersensitivity provoked directly in the lesions.[84] The diagnosis in the few reported instances of cure must be questioned. In some cases, the preliminary two stages do not develop. This form is called mycosis fungoides d'emblée. True instances of mycosis fungoides d'emblée must be exceedingly rare. Undoubtedly, most of the recorded cases are, in reality, examples of Hodgkin's disease, reticulum cell sarcoma, or leukemia. *Sézary's disease or reticulosis* is, in our judgment, a variant of mycosis fungoides.

The histologic picture of the first or premycotic stage is usually not diagnostic and may resemble one of the many conditions simulated clinically. However, even in this phase of the disease, there is a tendency for the infiltrate to be confined as a zone in the upper dermis and for the epidermis to appear psoriasiform. Occasionally, large, single or binucleated hyperchromatic cells are observed, as well as a rare infiltrative cell in mitosis, affording a clue. In the subsequent stages, the infiltrate, still selecting the upper dermis principally, becomes dense and polymorphous. In this variegated infiltrate, the presence of eosinophilic leukocytes and cells that simulate the Sternberg-Reed cell of Hodgkin's disease and often an abundance of small and large (Marschalko) plasma cells constitute the evidence for mycosis fungoides.

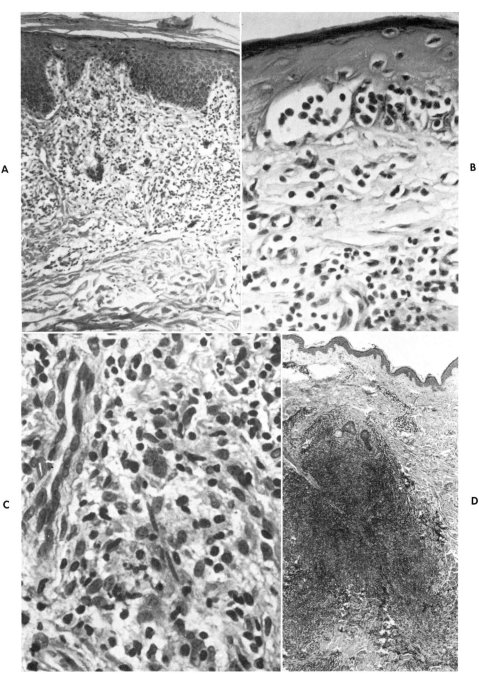

Fig. 39-51 A, Mycosis fungoides in so-called premycotic stage. **B,** Mycosis fungoides illustrating Pautrier "microabscesses," consisting of infiltrate extending from dermis into epidermis. **C,** Mycosis fungoides in tumor stage. **D,** Lymphosarcoma of skin showing density of infiltration without relationship to epidermis as exists in mycosis fungoides. (**A** to **D,** Hematoxylin-eosin.)

In addition, there is a tendency toward scattered clumping of cells of the infiltrate. The epidermis tends to be moderately acanthotic and acanthotic with focal spongiosis and small intraepidermal "microabscesses of Darier-

Pautrier." These "microabscesses" are actually foci of tumor cells that have extended into the epidermis. Their absence does not preclude the diagnosis (Fig. 39-51, *A* and *B*). The quality of the infiltrate may be indistinguishable from that of Hodgkin's disease. The cutaneous infiltrate of Hodgkin's disease tends to be irregularly distributed in parts of the dermis.

Potentially, the most revealing and yet most disputed morphologic clues to the nature of mycosis fungoides are the findings at autopsy. It generally is stated that mycosis fungoides invariably or almost always terminates with the visceral involvement by Hodgkin's disease, lymphosarcoma in its various forms, or leukemia. This has not been true in our experience. We have found visceral involvement by overt malignant lymphoma in about 15% of cases. The peripheral lymph nodes often are enlarged because of their drainage of pigment, etc. from the infiltrated skin. Such nodes—now called "dermatopathic lymphadenopathy"—show partial obliteration of their architecture by reticulum cell hyperplasia, deposits of melanin and fat, and—what is an especially common and presumptive clue in mycosis fungoides—viz., numerous plasma cells. Similar plasma cells are generally in the bone marrow and spleen, and occasionally even contain Russell bodies. These nonspecifically altered lymph nodes of Pautrier and Woringer[73] may easily be mistaken for those of Hodgkin's disease. In this country, they were first adequately described again by Hurwitt[47] in 1942.

It appears reasonable to conclude:

1 That although the cutaneous tumefactions of mycosis fungoides may closely simulate or be indistinguishable from Hodgkin's disease or reticulum cell sarcoma, the *viscera are commonly spared*

2 That mycosis fungoides in the early stages prior to tumefaction is usually diagnosable by the integrated histologic changes in the epidermis and dermis

3 That the plasma cell is one of the chief components of the infiltrate of the skin and viscera and the reasons for its presence should be investigated from the points of view particularly of altered blood proteins and reactions to allergens

Hodgkin's disease; lymphosarcoma; leukemia

The criteria for the histologic recognition in the skin of Hodgkin's disease, lymphosarcoma, and the various leukemias are the same as those used for the visceral lesions. Additional clues are offered by the almost constant denseness of the infiltrate, immediately noted with low-power magnification,

and the selectivity of the infiltrate for the upper dermis in some instances of leukemia (Fig. 39-51, *D*). An important deceptive feature of the lymphomas is the occurrence also of quite *nonspecific cutaneous reactions* in which neoplastic cells are absent. These reactions may take the clinical form of toxic erythema, excoriated pruritic exfoliative erythroderma, generalized pigmentation, urticaria, and zoster. Severe nonspecific cutaneous reactions lead to the changes in the regional lymph nodes, dermatopathic lymphadenopathy, which may become so enlarged as to be clinically indistinguishable from lymphomas. Undoubtedly one of the most difficult neoplasms to evaluate from a biopsy specimen of skin is Letterer-Siwe disease of infancy or the related malignant histiocytoses of childhood—i.e, the so-called reticuloendothelioses, histiocytosis X, or lipid and nonlipid histiocytoses. The crux of the problem is the decision as to whether or not the cutaneous lesion indicates visceral involvement and a fatal prognosis or merely a local histiocytosis or variant of xanthomatosis. In the briefest terms, it may be stated that, in general, the degree of anaplasia and the compactness of the infiltrate of the monocytoid cells in the upper dermis are of great importance in suggesting the grave nature of the disease. However, remarkable disparities have been noted by Spitz.[95]

Another source of clinical and histologic confusion is the entity known as *Spiegler-Fendt sarcoid,* which is characterized by grouped, local or disseminated, bright red nodules. The histologic diagnosis is based principally on the finding of mature lymphocytes, as well as reticulum cells either scattered or as germinal centers of follicles. Anaplasia of the infiltrate or histologic evidence of appreciable activity is lacking. It is obvious that differentiation of this lesion from lymphosarcoma must, at times, require a great nicety of judgment. Indeed, some of the cases originally but erroneously considered to be Spiegler-Fendt sarcoid have been recorded as having terminated in lymphosarcoma. Further confusion results from the use of the term *"benign lymphocytoma,"* which is popular in dermatologic literature. This lesion, which may be single or multiple, resembles Boeck's sarcoid, leukemic infiltration, or discoid lupus erythematosus clinically. Histologically, it consists essentially of dense masses of mature lymphocytes that may be arranged in follicles with germinal centers. As would be anticipated, the lesions are highly radiosensitive.

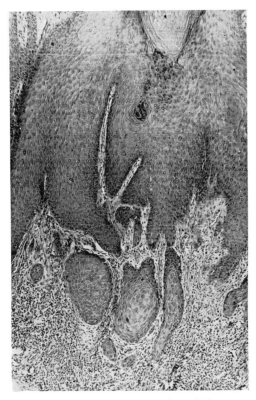

Fig. 39-52 Tick bite with pseudoepitheliomatous hyperplasia simulating squamous cell carcinoma. (Hematoxylin-eosin; from Allen, A. C.: Amer. J. Path. **24**:367-387, 1948; AFIP 95767.)

Still another lesion commonly mistaken for one of the lymphomas is that produced by the bites of insects and ticks. The reaction usually consists of eosinophilic leukocytes, histiocytes, plasma cells, and reticulum cells, the latter occasionally binucleated and even in mitosis. In some lesions, there are also prominent lymphoid follicles with germinal centers. Many patients with such an innocuous reaction have been given the grave diagnosis of Hodgkin's disease, mycosis fungoides, or lymphosarcoma. Part of the reason for the error is that it is not generally appreciated that the reaction to arthopods may persist for many months. The presence of only a single lesion is suggestive evidence, in doubtful cases, of an insect bite. On the other hand, an isolated lesion may occur also in the neoplastic conditions. Incidentally, another deceptive reaction to the venom of insects and ticks is the pseudoepitheliomatous hyperplasias which may be mistaken for squamous cell carcinoma[11] (Fig. 39-52).

Eosinophilic granulomas and *Jessner's lymphocytosis* of the skin of the face also may be erroneously misinterpreted as forms of ma-lignant lymphomas. *"Lethal midline granuloma"* refers to a fulminant, destructive ulceration of the nose and paranasal tissues probably due to either *Wegener's granulomatosis* or one of the malignant lymphomas. The abundant necrosis, along with secondary vascular involvement, commonly obscures the precise histologic diagnosis.

Metastatic neoplasms

Cancerous metastases reach the skin by direct invasion or through the lymphatics or blood vessels. The most common metastases include those from carcinomas of the breast, uterus, lung, gastrointestinal tract, pancreas, thyroid gland, and prostate gland, in addition to those from melanocarcinomas, epidermoid carcinomas and lymphomas, and sarcomas of bone, muscle and fascia.

There is generally little difficulty in recognizing the metastatic character of a tumor in the skin except, of course, in the case of the lymphomas and in Kaposi's sarcoma. In both of these instances, the possibility of autochthonous multicentric origin is to be considered. Plasma cell myeloma occasionally involves skin. A nodule of malignant melanoma usually may be recognized as metastatic by the presence of an overlying intact epidermis showing no evidence of junctional change. Occasionally, a metastatic focus of adenocarcinoma is mistaken for a primary cutaneous carcinoma of sweat gland origin, or extramammary Paget's disease.

Tumors of dermal appendages

Following is a classification of benign tumors of the sweat apparatus:

Ductal (syringal)

A Eccrine
 1 Inverted, papillary syringoma ("eccrine poroma," intraepidermal and/or dermal)
 2 Lobular syringoma ("eccrine spiradenoma")
 3 Lobular hyalinized syringoma ("cylindroma")
 4 Diffuse syringoma

B Apocrine
 1 Syringocystadenoma papilliferum

Glandular

 1 Eccrine cystadenoma
  (a) With chondral metaplasia
 2 Apocrine cystoma or cystadenoma
 3 Hamartomas

Sweat glands

There is obviously an abundance of histologic variants of tumors of sweat gland or

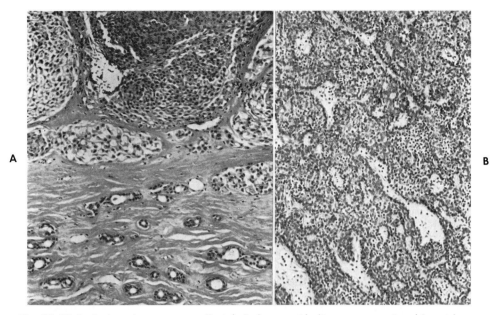

Fig. 39-53 A, Syringadenoma—usually labeled myoepithelioma on questionable evidence. **B,** Lobular syringadenoma (so-called "eccrine spiradenoma"). (**A** and **B,** Hematoxylin-eosin.)

duct origin. As a result, a great number of terms have arisen that often are used ambiguously and applied inconsistently. It would seem that no practical purpose would be denied if all the neoplasms of sweat glands were labeled simply as solid or cystic syringadenoma or syringocarcinoma. However, the range of histologic variation is so great as to lead not infrequently to serious diagnostic errors—such as the mistaking of a sweat gland adenoma for a basal or a squamous cell carcinoma, malignant melanoma, or even synovioma. It may be worthwhile, therefore, at least to mention and illustrate the various sweat gland tumors. Despite their histologic variations, in almost all instances there are foci of cells that indicate their source by their resemblance to sweat glands or ducts. In many instances of the solid syringadenoma, the hard, smooth, hyalinized, collagenous stroma is a clue to the nature of the tumor. In others, large cells with abundant acidophilic cytoplasm—cells that some observers (on insecure evidence) believe to be myoepithelial—suggest origin from sweat ducts (Fig. 39-53). In a considerable number of the cystic syringadenomas, the stratified epithelium frequently is papillated, and the individual cells are vacuolated with glycogen (Fig. 39-54, *D*).

The inverted papillary syringoma (eccrine poroma), which was first segregated by Pinkus et al.,[80] occurs as a single, slightly raised or pedunculated tumor predominantly on the soles, insteps, and palms. The lesion extends downward into the dermis from the stratum corneum as papillary, reticulated bands of compact, uniform, rarely pigmented, nonkeratinizing, phosphorylase-positive cells suggestive of origin from the sweat duct. Often, there is a fairly sharp demarcation from the adjacent epidermis. A similar lesion, comprised apparently of thickened, winding masses of ductal origin, may be confined to the dermis. The so-called clear cell hidroadenoma—the lesion that was once labeled "myoepithelioma"—is probably a partially cystic variant of the papillary syringoma in which abundant glycogen is present in the proliferating ductal cells. It might be anticipated that the underlying sweat glands would be dilated as a consequence of these presumably obstructive lesions. We have, in fact, seen a single instance of grossly visible cyst formation in the sweat glands subtending this type of syringoma. We have not observed or read of other instances of such glandular dilatation.

The terms *"eccrine poroepithelioma"* and *"acrospiroma"* also have been applied to what are believed to be intraepidermal proliferations of sweat duct origin of patterns somewhat different from the syringoma. It is apparent that seborrheic keratoses and even melanocarcinomas in situ are being included in this category.

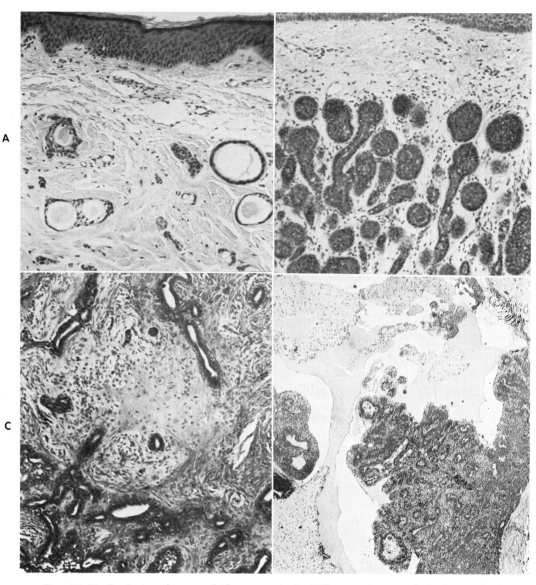

Fig. 39-54 A, Syringadenoma (hidrocystoma). **B,** Diffuse syringoma (spiradenoma). **C,** Syringadenoma with chondral metaplasia ("mixed" tumor) such as occurs in salivary and lacrimal glands. **D,** Syringocystadenoma. (**A** to **D,** Hematoxylin-eosin.)

The **lobular syringoma** ("eccrine spiradenoma") presents usually as a solitary firm nodule which is occasionally painful, as emphasized by Kersting and Helwig.[57] A photomicrograph of this lesion was included in the first edition of this text (1948) as an example of a sweat gland adenoma. The tumor is characteristically lobulated and composed of compact acini with predominant proliferation of the outer darker, lymphocytoid-appearing epithelial cells as distinct from the lighter, larger inner cells that often lie beneath a residual cuticle-like structure. The origin of these tu-

mors from the sweat duct is vividly demonstrable in the early or incompletely developed lesion.

A variant of the lobular syringoma is characterized by conspicuous, *hyalinized* bands of collagen surrounding and intertwining among the lobules and its cells (Fig. 39-55). This lesion ("**turban tumor**" "**cylindroma**") tends to be multiple and may be so extensive as to cover the scalp. Both types of lobular syringoma remain benign.

The "**diffuse syringoma**" usually occurs as multiple, small, soft yellowish papules on the

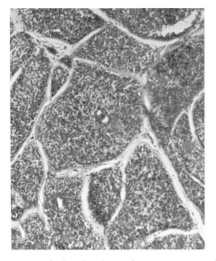

Fig. 39-55 Lobular hyalinized syringoma (turban tumor). (Hematoxylin-eosin.)

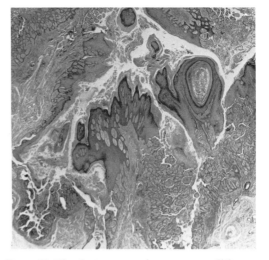

Fig. 39-56 Syringocystadenoma papilliferum. (Hematoxylin-eosin.)

chest, back, and face. The overlying epidermis is intact or may appear glistening. Histologically, the lesion is composed of minute cysts scattered through the upper dermis (hence, "diffuse" versus "lobular" syringoma). The cysts are noted to be dilated sweat ducts containing inspissated secretion and, occasionally, keratin and characterized by epithelial spurs coming off the outer walls.

The **syringocystadenoma papilliferum** tends to occur as a solitary lesion of the scalp or forehead in patients of all ages. The overlying epidermis may be smooth or ulcerated. The histologic picture is easily recognizable by the cystic, papillary lesion projecting onto the surface from the upper dermis (Fig. 39-56). The papillary components are lined by two layers of cells, a deeper layer of small cuboidal cells and an outer layer of tall columnar cells. The luminal secretion of the latter at times is mistaken for cilia, and such tumors in the cervical region have been mistaken for odd branchiogenic fistulas. Frequently, the lining is altered focally by squamous cell metaplasia that extends into underlying sweat ducts and glands. There is often considerable surrounding inflammatory reaction and a common association with hamartomas of sebaceous glands, piliary structures, and small basal cell carcinomas.

The term *"hidradenoma papilliferum"* is applied to the corresponding tumor of the labia majora or adjacent region which also simulates the papilloma of the subareolar mammary ducts.

The eccrine and apocrine **cystadenomas** oc-

cur on the face as solitary small translucent nodules and are easily identified by their lining epithelium. Some of these are regarded as retention cysts and are called "hidrocystomas." Chondral metaplasia may occur in eccrine or apocrine cystadenomas. As we indicated some thirty years ago, the genesis of such cartilage is epithelial, as it is in corresponding tumors of the salivary, lacrimal, and mammary glands.[9]

Cystic syringoadenoma. The clear cell, solid, or partially cystic syringoadenoma or hidradenoma (unsupportably labeled "myoepithelioma") tends to be single, with a predilection for middle-aged and older women, and to occur in any region of the body. The tumors are likely to be sharply delimited and usually occur in the dermis but occasionally extend to the subcutis. In some instances, the lesions are in direct contact with the epidermis often thickened by pseudoepitheliomatous hyperplasia. The tumor cells are arranged in solid or cystic masses, the latter lined by stratified or papillary epithelium of characteristically clear, grossly vacuolated large polyhedral cells. These cells contain abundant glycogen.

In some instances, there are tubular lumens lined by cuboidal cells and scattered through the lesion. Portions of the walls of the cysts may be lined by double layers of cuboidal cells which, too, suggest their origin from sweat glands. These tumors contain abundant phosphorylase, esterases, and respiratory enzymes characteristic of tissue derived from sweat glands.[111] The stroma commonly is focally homogenized and, as we have long emphasized, is in itself suggestive of the syringo-adenomatous nature of these tumors.

Syringocarcinoma. There is a tendency to diagnose sweat gland adenomas as malignant not because of anaplasia of the cells but because of the irregular ramification of nests of cells into adjacent dermis. On the other hand, some of the basal and squamous cell carcinomas characterized by small, discrete nests of cells are mistaken for sweat gland tumors—as are adenocarcinomas metastatic to skin, as well as melanocarcinomas. As a rule, the uncommon sweat gland carcinomas are of a low grade of virulence, as are carcinomas of appendages generally. There have been notable exceptions.

■ ■ ■

The diagnosis of tumors of the sweat ducts or glands is usually made without difficulty with the light microscope. Electronmicroscopic and histochemical studies offer supplementary information. However, electronmicroscopic and histochemical criteria that appear of decisive differential use in the recognition of normal structures of the sweat apparatus are apparently not always applicable to neoplasms. The widely prevalent notion that the validity of conclusions parallels the magnification needs reexamination. In general, amylophorylase, branching enzyme, succinic dehydrogenase, and leucine aminopeptidase are regarded as indicative of eccrine ducts and glands, whereas acid phosphatase and β-glucuronidase are stated to be characteristic of apocrine glands. And yet, the lobular hyalinized syringoma ("cylindroma"), for example, which is clearly of eccrine origin, has been found by some investigators histochemically to suggest apocrine as opposed to eccrine origin.

Sebaceous glands

Adenomas of sebaceous glands occur as small yellowish papules principally on and beside the nose, cheeks, and forehead. In many cases of multiple adenomas, there are associated verrucae, neurofibromas, subungual fibrosis, and shagreen patches. The "shagreen" patches of tuberous sclerosis are nodules or elevated masses of skin produced by the proliferation and sclerosis of dermal collagen. This sclerosis may easily be mistaken histologically for scleroderma. The overlying epidermis may be normal or acanthotically reticulated. In some cases, the patients develop tuberous sclerosis of the cerebral cortex and present the triad of sebaceous adenoma, mental deficiency, and epilepsy (p. 1787). These patients also may have visceral tumors, such as renal angiolipomas. Poliosis, café-au-lait spots, fibroepithelial tags, and hemangiomas also may be associated with this entity.

The histologic picture is that of an overgrowth of sebaceous glands without apparent linkage to the hair apparatus. Often, it is difficult to be sure that the process is not simple hyperplasia rather than neoplasia. There is another histologic form of sebaceous adenoma, characterized by a proliferation of the basal cells lining the sebaceous glands interspersed with isolated sebaceous cells. Rarely, a metastasizing sebaceous gland carcinoma develops in which at least a few scattered sebaceous cells help to identify the source (Figs. 39-57 and 39-58).

Nevus sebaceus of Jadassohn. The term "nevus sebaceus" of Jadassohn is applied to hamartomatous or dysembryogenetic papular or nodular tumefactions of sebaceous glands or the pilosebaceous apparatus. Such malformations may be associated with other ectodermal or mesodermal malformations. Over-

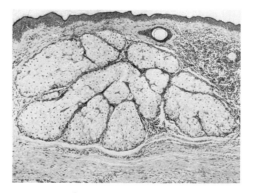

Fig. 39-57 Sebaceous gland adenoma. (Hematoxylin-eosin; AFIP 97228.)

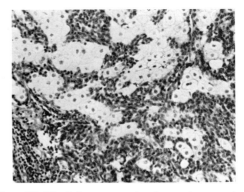

Fig. 39-58 Sebaceous gland carcinoma—low grade. (Hematoxylin-eosin.)

lying or adjacent verrucal epidermal hyperplasia, a variety of sweat or lacrimal gland adenomas, focal alopecia, dermoids, dermal lipomas, angiomas, or basal cell carcinomas may accompany the lesion. Occasionally, it may be combined with ocular and cerebral lesions, with mental retardation and convulsions, as a form of *neurocutaneous* syndrome.

Hair follicles

There is a divergence of opinion as to the types of neoplasms that may arise from hair follicles. Many observers believe that basal cell carcinomas are derived from *embryonic* hair follicles. However, as previously stated, the histologic evidence favors the view that basal cell carcinomas arise from the mature basal cells wherever they lie—at the base of the epidermis, at the periphery of sebaceous glands, or in the outermost layer of the hair follicles. However, the tumor that probably does arise from hair follicles is known synonymously as *trichoepithelioma, Brooke's tumor,* or *epithelioma adenoides cysticum* (Fig. 39-59). Some observers believe that the origin of this tumor from sweat or sebaceous glands is a possibility. The lesion tends to be familial and appears as multiple smooth nodules on the face and chest.

Histologically, unlike most basal cell carcinomas, the tumor is overlain by intact epidermis. The lesion is made up of varying-sized units of cysts filled with keratin and lined with stratified squamous epithelium, from which nests of basal cells proliferate. The trichoepithelioma is benign, unlike the basal cell "epithelioma."

Cysts

The **dermoid cyst** is a congenital cutaneous inclusion occurring usually in the skin of the forehead, especially in the supraorbital region or midline. **Epidermoid cysts** also may be congenital and familial, particularly *steatocystoma multiplex,* but commonly they are the result of trauma (including insect bites) or inflammatory downgrowth, with separation and eventual isolation and encystment of a fragment of epidermis. As we have previously indicated, "sebaceous cyst" is the term loosely applied to cysts that are, in actuality, derived from the entire pilary or pilosebaceous apparatus rather than from the sebaceous gland alone.[2] These keratinous cysts are lined by ordinary stratified squamous epithelium with, rarely, some residual sebaceous cells in one segment of the lining. Usually, the sebaceous cells have been obliterated in the mature cyst. Accordingly, we have labeled them *pilosebaceous cysts,* although pilary cysts might be even more appropriate. This disparity has been recognized by others, particularly Kligman.[58]

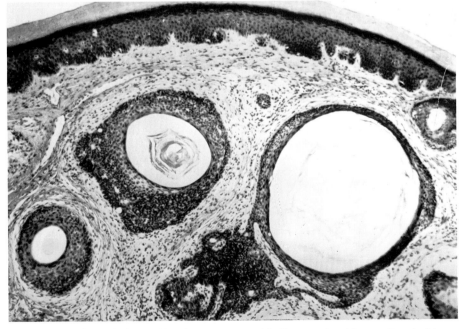

Fig. 39-59 Trichoepithelioma (Brooke's tumor; epithelioma adenoides cysticum). (Hematoxylin-eosin.)

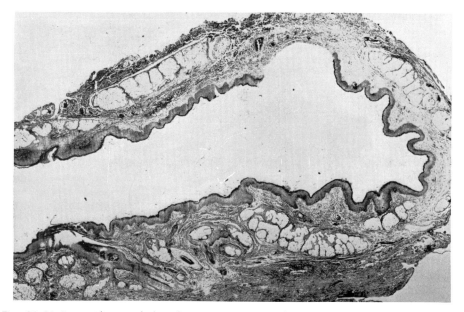

Fig. 39-60 Dermoid cyst of skin showing numerous sebaceous glands and hair follicles. (Hematoxylin-eosin.)

Grossly, the dermoid cannot be differentiated from pilosebaceous and epidermoid cysts. Histologically, the wall of the cyst is actually skin with all of its appendages, often with a prominence of sebaceous glands (Fig. 39-60). The epidermoid and sebaceous cysts differ from the dermoid cysts in that the former lack the appendages and their walls are made up of stratified squamous epidermis surrounded by fibrous tissue. As a rule, it is impossible to distinguish the epidermoid from the pilosebaceous cyst. Infrequently, evidence of the relation of the cyst to a contiguous sebaceous gland may persist. The criteria that have been set up for the differentiation are unreliable. The epithelium of both tends to be nonpigmented.

The contents of each of the cysts are predominantly a beige-colored, greasy keratin, representing in reality the stratum corneum, which in these instances cannot be shed but accumulates in the epidermal enclosures. There is also much fat within the laminated keratin, which either may not be demonstrable in routine sections or may be seen as cholesterin slits. In the dermoid cysts, hairs may be included. Occasionally, the lining epithelium may proliferate as papillary buds, either externally or inward toward the lumen of the cyst. Because of the irregularity of these proliferations and perhaps because of their superficial resemblance to the carcinomas of epidermis, there is a tendency to classify these hyperplasias or benign proliferations as cancer—a tendency not warranted by their behavior.

The *calcifying epithelioma* is an exaggeration of this process of proliferation, which frequently is misinterpreted as cancer. Histologically, this lesion is usually a sharply circumscribed mass of disheveled fragments of epithelium, many of which are necrotic and often partially calcified. The epithelial cells have a basaloid character, although it is likely that they are predominantly of prickle cell origin. This pattern has suggested to some observers an attempt of cells with the ever-invoked "pluripotentiality" to form abortive hair and so has been labeled "pilomatrixoma"—about as felicitous etymologically as it is conceptually. It is more likely that the process represents a form of hyperplasia, as stated, and, further, that this pattern is, in reality, simulation of hair matrix that may occur also in nonpilary sites of proliferation of stratified squamous cells. A foreign body reaction associated with cholesterin deposits is common, as are calcification and even extensive ossification of the stroma. From the observation of early and transitional stages in the development of these lesions, it appears that they arise from the proliferation of the lining of epidermal and pilosebaceous cysts and, infrequently, even of cysts of sweat glands.

Actual cancerous transformation of the lining of cysts is an infrequent occurrence. The incidence of 1% to 6% quoted in the literature is probably high. A figure of about 0.5% would appear to be more representative. On the other hand, squamous cell carcinoma complicating epidermal inclusion cysts of sheep is common.

REFERENCES

General

1 Allen, A. C.: The skin; a clinicopathologic treatise, St. Louis, 1954, The C. V. Mosby Co.
2 Allen, A. C.: The skin; a clinicopathologic treatise, ed. 2, New York, 1967, Grune & Stratton, Inc.
3 Lever, W. F.: Histopathology of the skin, ed. 4, Philadelphia, 1967, J. B. Lippincott Co.
4 Montagna, W.: The structure and function of skin, ed. 2, New York, 1962, Academic Press, Inc.
5 Montgomery, H.: Dermatopathology, vols. I and II, Philadelphia, 1967, Hoeber Medical Division, Harper & Row, Publishers.
6 Rook, A., Wilkinson, D. S., and Ebling, F. J. G.: Textbook of dermatology, vols. I and II, Oxford, 1968, Blackwell Scientific Publications.

Specific

7 Achs, R., Harper, R. G., and Siegel, M.: New Eng. J. Med. **274**:141-150, 1966 (dermatoglyphics).
8 Albert, J., Bruce, W., Allen, A. C., and Blank, H.: Amer. J. Med. **28**:661-667, 1960 (reticulohistiocytomas).
9 Allen, A. C.: Arch. Path. (Chicago) **29**:589-624, 1940 (origin of cartilage in mixed tumors).
10 Allen, A. C.: Arch. Derm. Syph. (Chicago) **57**:19-56, 1948 (survey of cutaneous diseases, World War II).
11 Allen, A. C.: Amer. J. Path. **24**:367-387, 1948 (insect bites).
12 Allen, A. C.: Cancer **2**:28-56, 1949 (nevi and malignant melanomas).
13 Allen, A. C.: Surg. Gynec. Obstet. **104**:753-754, 1957 (juvenile melanomas).
14 Allen, A. C.: Ann. N. Y. Acad. Sci. **100**:29-48, 1963 (juvenile melanomas).
15 Allen, A. C., and Spitz, S.: Cancer **6**:1-45, 1953 (nevi and malignant melanomas).
16 Allen, A. C., and Spitz, S.: Arch. Derm. Syph. (Chicago) **69**:150-171, 1954 (histogenesis of pigmented nevi).
17 Aparicio, S. R., and Lumsden, C. E.: J. Path. **97**:339-355, 1969 (granular cell myoblastoma).
18 Bailey, G., Rosenbaum, J. M., and Anderson, B.: J.A.M.A. **191**:979-982, 1965 (toxic epidermal necrolysis).
19 Blank, H., and Roth, F. J., Jr.: Arch. Derm. (Chicago) **79**:259-266, 1959 (griseofulvin therapy).
20 Breathnach, A. S., and Wyllie, L. M.: J. Invest. Derm. **45**:401-403, 1965.
21 Breathnach, A. S., Silvers, W. K., Smith, J., and Heyner, S.: J. Invest. Derm. **50**:147-160, 1968 (Langerhans' cells).

22 Caplan, R. M.: Arch. Derm. (Chicago) **87**:146-157, 1963 (urticaria pigmentosum).
23 Carne, H. R., Lloyd, L. C., and Carter, H. B.: J. Path. Bact. **86**:305-315, 1963 (carcinoma in cysts of skin).
24 Caulfield, J. B., and Wilgram, G. F.: J. Invest. Derm. **41**:57-65, 1963 (ultrastructure of acantholysis).
25 Charles, A.: J. Anat. **93**:226-232, 1959 (apocrine glands).
26 Charles, A.: Brit. J. Derm. **73**:57-60, 1961 (ultrastructure of elastic fibers).
27 Coleta, D. F., Haentze, F. E., and Thomas, C. C.: Cancer **22**:879-884, 1968 (metastasizing basal cell carcinomas).
28 Curth, H. O.: Arch. Derm. Syph. (Chicago) **66**:761-762, 1952 (Behçet's syndrome).
29 Curth, H. O., Hilberg, A. W., and Machacek, G. F.: Cancer **15**:364-382, 1962 (acanthosis nigricans).
30 Dubois, E. L., and Martel, S.: Ann. Intern. Med. **44**:482-496, 1956 (systemic manifestations of discoid lupus erythematosus).
31 Eisen, A. Z.: J. Invest. Derm. **52**:449-453, 1969 (collagenase in epidermolysis bullosa).
32 Emmerson, R. W.: Brit. J. Derm. **81**:395-413, 1969 (follicular mucinosis).
33 Epstein, W. L., Senecal, I., Krasnobrod, H., and Massing, A. M.: J. Invest. Derm. **40**:51-59, 1963 (viral inclusions).
34 Feiwel, M.: Brit. J. Derm. **80**:719-729, 1968 (xanthomas and dysproteinemias).
35 Fell, H. B.: In Montagna, W., and Lobutz, W. C., Jr., editors: The epidermis, New York, 1964, Academic Press, Inc., chap. IV.
36 Ganpule, M.: Brit. J. Derm. **79**:221-228, 1967 (juvenile dermatitis herpetiformis).
37 Gazzolo, L., and Prunieras, M.: J. Invest. Derm. **51**:186-189, 1968 (lysosomes and keratinocytes).
38 Goodman, R. M., Smith, E. W., Paton, D., Bergman, R. A., Siegel, C. L., Ottesen, O. E., Shelley, W. M., Pusch, A. L., and McKusick, V. A.: Medicine (Balt.) **42**:297-334, 1963 (pseudoxanthoma elasticum).
39 Gorlin, R. J., Anderson, R. C., and Blaw, M.: Amer. J. Dis. Child. **117**:652-662, 1969 (multiple lentigines syndrome).
40 Graciansky, P. de: Brit. J. Derm. **79**:278-283, 1967 (panniculitis).
41 Halpryn, H. J., and Allen, A. C.: Arch. Derm. (Chicago) **80**:160-166, 1959 (epidermal changes overlying sclerosing angiomas).
42 Henderson, R., Wheeler, C. E., Jr., and Abele, D. C.: Arch. Derm. (Chicago) **98**:23-27, 1968 ("collagenoma").
43 Hibbs, R. G.: J. Invest. Derm. **38**:77-84, 1962 (apocrine glands).
44 Hirsch, J. G., Cohn, Z. A., Morse, S. I., Schaedler, R. W., Siltzbach, L. E., Ellis, J. T., and Chase, M. W.: New Eng. J. Med. **265**:827-830, 1961 (Kveim test).
45 Holmes, E. J.: Amer. J. Clin. Path. **52**:86, 1969 (abstract—presented at Interim Meeting, Feb., 1969).
46 Hope-Simpson, R. E.: Proc. Roy. Soc. Med. **58**:9-20, 1965 (pathogenesis of zoster).
47 Hurwitt, E.: J. Invest. Derm. **5**:197-204, 1942 (dermatopathic lymphadenopathy).

48 Hyman, A. B., and Dreizin, D. M.: Dermatologica (Basel) **127**:309-316, 1963 ("isolated Darier's disease").

49 Jackson, I. T.: Lancet **1**:490-492, 1969 (misdiagnosed keratoacanthomas).

50 Jackson, S. F., and Fell, H. B.: Develop. Biol. **7**:394-419, 1963 (mucus-producing keratinocytes).

51 Järvi, O. H., Saxén, A. E., Hopsu-Havu, V. K., Wartiovaara, J. J., and Vaissalo, V. T.: Cancer **23**:42-63, 1969 (elastofibroma).

52 Janis, J. F., and Winkelmann, R. K.: Arch. Derm. (Chicago) **97**:640-650, 1968 (dermatomyositis).

53 Johnson, W. C., and Helwig, E. B.: Arch. Derm. (Chicago) **93**:13-20, 1966 (mucinous cysts).

54 Jordon, R. E., Ihrig, J. J., and Perry, H. O.: Arch. Derm. (Chicago) **99**:176-179, 1969 (childhood pemphigus vulgaris).

55 Jordon, R. E., Muller, S. A., Hale, W. L., and Beutner, E. H.: Arch. Derm. (Chicago) **99**:17-25, 1969 (systemic lupus erythematosus and pemphigoid).

56 Kempson, R. L., and McGavran, M. H.: Cancer **17**:1463-1471, 1964 (atypical fibroxanthomas).

57 Kersting, D. W., and Helwig, E. B.: Arch. Derm. (Chicago) **73**:199-227, 1956 (eccrine spiradenoma).

58 Kligman, A. M.: Arch. Derm. (Chicago) **89**:253-256, 1964 ("sebaceous cysts").

59 Knox, J. M., Gever, S. G., Freeman, R. G., and Whitcomb, F.: Arch. Derm. (Chicago) **84**:386-391, 1961 (atypical acid fast bacilli).

60 Kriss, J. P., Pleshakov, V., and Chien, J. R.: J. Clin. Endocr. **241**:1005-1028, 1964 (LATS and pretibial myxedema).

61 Kroe, D. J., and Pitcock, J. A.: Amer. J. Clin. Path. **51**:487-492, 1969.

62 Laksmipathi, T., and Hunt, K. M.: Brit. J. Derm. **79**:267-270, 1967 (metastasizing basal cell carcinoma).

63 Lever, W. F.: Pemphigus and pemphigoid, Springfield, Ill., 1965, Charles C Thomas, Publisher.

64 Lutzner, M. A.: Arch. Derm. (Chicago) **87**:436-444, 1963.

65 Lynch, P. J., and Minkin, W.: Arch. Derm. (Chicago) **98**:141-143, 1968.

66 Mehregan, A. H.: Arch. Derm. (Chicago) **90**:274-279, 1964 (apocrine cystadenoma).

67 Mehregan, A. H.: Arch. Derm. (Chicago) **97**:381-393, 1968 (perforating elastosis).

68 Mehregan, A. H., and Pinkus, H.: Arch. Derm. (Chicago) **91**:574-588, 1965 (organoid nevi).

69 Mishima, Y., and Schaub, F. F., Jr.: J. Invest. Derm. **41**:243-245, 1963 (cholinesterase in junction nevus).

70 Muller, S. A., and Winkelmann, R. K.: J.A.M.A. **195**:433-436, 1966 (necrobiosis lipoidica diabeticorum).

71 Muller, S. A., Sams, W. M., Jr., and Dobson, R. L.: Arch. Derm. (Chicago) **99**:739-747, 1969 (epidermolysis bullosa and amyloidosis).

72 Parsons, R. L., and Savin, J. A.: Brit. J. Cancer **22**:669-672, 1969 (pemphigoid and cancer).

73 Pautrier, L. M., and Woringer, F.: Bull. Soc. Franc. Derm. Syph. **39**:947-955, 1932 (dermatopathic lymphadenopathy).

74 Pedace, F. J., and Winkelmann, R. K.: J.A.M.A. **193**:893-894, 1965 (xanthelasma).

75 Peterka, E. S., Lynch, F. W., and Goltz, R. W.: Arch. Derm. (Chicago) **84**:623-629, 1961 (Bowen's disease and visceral cancer).

76 Peterson, W. C., Jr., and Gokcen, M.: Arch. Derm. (Chicago) **86**:783-787, 1962 (antinuclear factors in chronic lupus erythematosus).

77 Philippart, M., Sarlieve, L., and Manacorda, A.: Pediatrics **43**:201-206, 1969 (Fabry's disease).

78 Pinkus, H.: Arch. Derm. (Chicago) **76**:419-426, 1957 (alopecia mucinosa).

79 Pinkus, H.: Arch. Derm. (Chicago) **91**:24-37, 1965 (fibroepithelial tumors).

80 Pinkus, H., Rogin, J. R., and Goldman, P.: Arch. Derm. (Chicago) **74**:511-521, 1956 (eccrine poroma).

81 Polák, L., and Turk, J. L.: J. Invest. Derm. **52**:219-232, 1969 (immunology of dermatoses).

82 Quevedo, W. C., Jr., Szabó, G., and Virks, J.: J. Invest. Derm. **52**:287-290, 1969 (UV irradiation and melanocytes).

83 Rapp, Y., Miller, S. P., and Schwartz, A. R.: Arch. Derm. (Chicago) **99**:161-169, 1969 (bullae due to anticoagulants).

84 Ratner, A. C., Waldorf, D. S., and Van Scott, E. J.: Cancer **21**:83-88, 1968 (hypersensitivity in mycosis fungoides).

85 Reed, W. B., and Wilson-Jones, E.: Arch. Derm. (Chicago) **98**:132-135, 1968 (carcinomas and vaccination scars).

86 Rice, J. S., and Fischer, D. S.: Arch. Derm. (Chicago) **86**:503-511, 1962 (blue rubber–bleb nevus).

87 Rodriguez, H. A., and Ackerman, L. V.: Cancer **21**:393-405, 1968 (cellular blue nevus; ultrastructure).

88 Roe, D. A., Flesch, P., and Esoda, E. C.: Arch. Derm. (Chicago) **84**:213-218, 1961 (epidermal mucopolysaccharides).

89 Saksela, E., and Rintala, A.: Cancer **22**:1308-1314, 1968 (juvenile melanoma).

90 Seiji, M., and Mizuno, F.: Arch Derm. (Chicago) **99**:3-16, 1969 (ultrastructure of Bowen's disease).

91 Selye, H.: Calciphylaxis, Chicago, 1962, University of Chicago Press.

92 Shrank, A. B., and Doniach, D.: Arch. Derm. (Chicago) **87**:677-685, 1963 (serum autoantibody pattern in chronic lupus erythematosus).

93 Soule, E. H., Gertz, M., and Henderson, E. D.: Cancer **23**:1336-1346, 1969 (embryonal rhabdomyosarcoma in older age groups).

94 Spitz, S.: Amer. J. Path. **24**:591-609, 1948 (juvenile melanomas).

95 Spitz, S.: J. Amer. Med. Wom. Ass. **6**:209-219, 1951 (clinicohistologic disparities of tumors).

96 Stewart, F. W., and Treves, N.: Cancer **1**:64-81, 1948 (postmastectomy lymphangiosarcoma).

97 Sumner, W. C., and Foraker, A. G.: Cancer **13**:79-81, 1960 (spontaneous regression of melanocarcinomas).

98 Sweet, R. D.: Brit. J. Derm. **76**:349-356, 1964 (neutrophilic dermatosis).

99 Tighe, J. R., Clark, A. E., and Turvey, D. J.: J. Clin. Path. **21**:463-469, 1968 (elastofibroma dorsi).

100 Toker, C.: Cancer **23**:487-492, 1969 (ultrastructure of glomangioma).

101 Troughton, W. D., and Trier, J. S.: J. Cell Biol. **41**:251-268, 1969 (derivation of Paneth's cells).

102 Unna, P.: Berl. Klin. Wschr. **30**:14-16, 1893 (epithelial origin of melanocarcinomas).

103 Venkatachalam, M. A., and Greally, J. G.: Cancer **23**:1176-1184, 1969 (ultrastructure of glomus cells).

104 Waisman, M.: Arch. Derm. (Chicago) **86**:525-529, 1962 (botryomycosis).

105 Wells, G. C., and Farthing, G. J.: Brit. J. Derm. **78**:380-387, 1966 (cholinesterase in juvenile melanomas).

106 Winkelmann, R. K.: Nerve endings in normal and pathologic skin, Springfield, Ill., 1960, Charles C Thomas, Publisher.

107 Winkelmann, R. K.: Cancer **14**:1001-1004, 1961 (cholinesterases).

108 Winkelmann, R. K., and Brown, J.: Arch. Derm. (Chicago) **97**:615-623, 1968 (eruptive keratoacanthomas).

109 Winkelmann, R. K., and McLeod, W. A.: Arch. Derm. (Chicago) **94**:50-55, 1966 (dermal syringoma).

110 Winkelmann, R. K., and Sams, W. M., Jr.: Cancer **23**:406-415, 1969 (elastofibroma).

111 Winkelmann, R. K., and Wolff, K.: Arch. Derm. (Chicago) **97**:651-661, 1968 (hidradenomas).

112 Wolff, K., and Holubar, K.: Arch. Klin Exp. Derm. **231**:1-19, 1967 (keratinosomes).

113 Yardley, H. J.: Brit. J. Derm. **81**(suppl. 2):29-38, 1969 (sterols and keratinization)

114 Yeh, S., How, S. W., and Lin, C. S.: Cancer **21**:312-339, 1968 (arsenic cancers).

115 Zimmer, J. G., McAllister, B. M., and Demis, D. J.: J. Invest. Derm. **44**:33-37, 1965 (mucopolysaccharides in mast cells).

Bones

Granville A. Bennett

For convenience in presentation, the disorders of the skeletal system are treated separately in two parts: bones (Chapter 40) and joints (Chapter 41). It is to be remembered that the term *bone* may be used to designate either a particular kind of mineralized mesenchymal tissue (osseous tissue) or one of the individual units of the skeleton (e.g., humerus or tibia). The joints or articulations are those skeletal structures, comprised, in varying proportions, of cartilage, fibrous connective tissue, and synovia that unite two or more bones to form a functioning part of the skeleton (Fig. 40-1). Although many pathologic states affect both bones and joints in a given region,

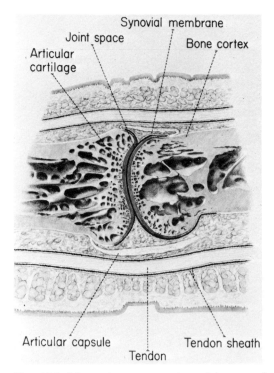

Fig. 40-1 Schematic representation of bone and joint structures.

it is necessary to consider separately each anatomic unit and to describe the alterations that primarily or predominately affect it (see also Chapter 41).

Osseous or bony tissues are susceptible to most, if not all, of the deleterious agents and unfavorable circumstances that affect the soft tissues of the body. Thus, bone reacts to physical and chemical injuries, to nutritional, metabolic, and endocrine disturbances, and to circumstances that are related to environment and heredity. In addition, the cellular components that are incorporated in osseous tissue give rise to a variety of neoplasms.

In its reaction to adverse conditions, bone often behaves quite differently from the other tissues and organs of the body. Such differences are attributable, in most instances, either to the peculiar mechanisms that are responsible for bone development and growth or to the special anatomic and physiologic characteristics of this interesting tissue. It is necessary, therefore, that the known facts related to the embryology, anatomy, and physiology of bone be kept in mind in the study of all skeletal lesions.

NORMAL OSSEOUS TISSUE

Bone is to be regarded as a highly specialized form of connective tissue. Developmentally, it emerges from primitive connective tissues—either by direct transformation of undifferentiated mesenchyme into bone (membranous bone formation) or by the more complicated process of ossification of cartilage (endochondral bone formation). Irrespective of its mode of formation, bone, when fully developed, differs from ordinary connective tissue in several important details. It is relatively cell poor, and such cells as are present are either widely separated from one another and segregated in lacunar spaces as osteocytes, or they are distributed as a single layer of cells upon the bone surfaces, where they form a continuous envelope surrounding all bony structures. The latter cells, depending on their position, constitute either the periosteal or the endosteal layer.

In their resting state, the endosteal and periosteal cells resemble unstimulated fibroblasts. They are elongated and flattened in shape and contain small, darkly staining, rod-shaped or oval nuclei. There can be little doubt that this cell layer plays an important role in the exchange of metabolites between the vascular system and the more distant osteocytes enclosed within the lacunar spaces in the adjacent bony tissue (Fig. 40-2). This function is made possible by the intercommunicating channels (canaliculi) that range between the bone surfaces and the lacunar spaces that enclose the segregated osteocytes

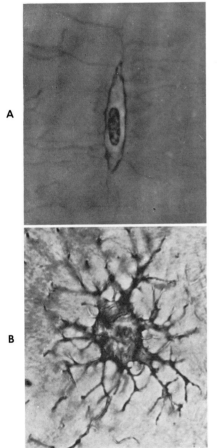

Fig. 40-2 A, Osteocyte enclosed in lacunar space from which canaliculi extend into adjacent bone. **B,** Branching canaliculi emerging from lacunar space in compact bone. (**A,** Hematoxylin-eosin; **B,** ground section; **A** and **B,** ×1350; courtesy Dr. J. P. Weinmann and Dr. H. Sicher.)

in the more distant parts of the bone lamellae or haversian systems forming the compact bony structures. It is probable also that the endosteal and periosteal cells, when subjected to physical or chemical stimulation, undergo morphologic and physiologic modifications enabling them to function as osteoblasts or, by means of cell division, to produce osteoblasts.

When mature, the organic matrix of bone that is elaborated by the osteoblasts is comprised mainly of the fibrous protein collagen. Smaller amounts of the organic matrix consist of poorly characterized protein and carbohydrate complexes and phospholipids. These protein and carbohydrate complexes constitute the *ground* or *cement* substance that overlays the fibrillar components and is intimately involved in mineralization both with respect to the initial deposit of mineral crystals and in the constant or intermittent shifting of the mineral complexes that is believed to take place.[1-3, 18, 35, 50, 55, 64]

The mineral complex that is deposited in the organic matrix of bone is known as bone salt. Although many investigations have been directed toward the elucidation of the processes by which mineralization occurs, as well as toward the exact composition of the resulting mineral crystals and their turnover,[1-3, 18, 35, 50, 55, 64] many uncertainties still remain. It is generally agreed that the mineral crystals are small (approximately 10 Å to 30 Å in thickness, 100 Å in width, and 200 Å to 400 Å in length). Evidence derived from chemical analysis, x-ray diffraction studies, and ion exchange reactions has been interpreted to indicate that the inorganic substance of bone corresponds closely to the natural hydroxyapatite, which is a complex salt composed of tricalcium phosphate and calcium hydroxide, the relative proportions of which are indicated by the formulae $3\ Ca_3(PO_4)_2 \cdot Ca(OH)_2$ or $Ca_{10}(PO_4)_6(OH)_2$. It is recognized that bone salt also contains carbonate and citrate, but it has been asserted by some that these substances are not parts of the basic bone salt crystal. Small amounts of sodium, potassium, and magnesium are also present in the mineral complexes of bone.

When viewed under the light microscope, sections of decalcified mature compact bone stained with hematoxylin and eosin fail to reveal the intricate fibrillar structure of bone matrix. However, if one examines either sections of decalcified compact bone after silver impregnation[139] or sections prepared by grind-

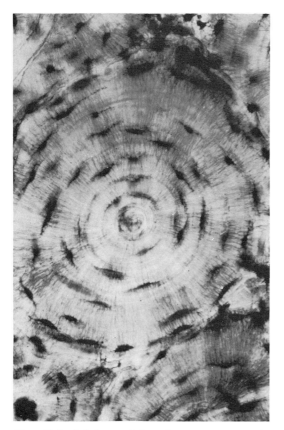

Fig. 40-3 Cellular and lamellar arrangement in compact bone. (Ground section; ×360; courtesy Dr. J. P. Weinmann and Dr. H. Sicher.)

ing or cutting without prior decalcification, it will be noted that the fibrillar components are arranged in a series of layers, each of which has a predominating orientation of fibrils (Fig. 40-3). Thus, in a given series of lamellae, one observes intermittent longitudinal and circular layers of fibers. Dense bundles of collagenous fibrils (Sharpey's fibers) are also evident at the sites of ligamentous or fascial insertions into compact bone.

In examining histologic sections of decalcified bone after staining with hematoxylin and eosin, it is helpful to remember that newly formed bone matrix appears acidophilic and homogeneous, whereas older bone is prone to be more basophilic and striated.

To date, studies of the composition of the organic and inorganic components of bone have provided background information sufficient only for partial understanding of the mechanisms of bone development and growth and of its maturation and aging, as well as its vital role in homeostatic control of calcium and phosphate ions in blood and tissue fluids.[64]

Calcium is required in varying amounts depending on the age, size, and physiologic state of the individual. Thus, a daily intake of approximately 0.8 gm is required for children under 10 years of age and for normal adults. Boys and girls from 10 to 20 years of age may require from 1.1 gm to 1.4 gm, and women, during the second and third trimesters of pregnancy and during lactation, have need of approximately 1.3 gm. The normal plasma and serum values range between 9 mg and 11 mg per 100 ml or 4.5 mEq to 5.5 mEq per liter. Approximately one-half of the calcium is in *ionized* form. The remaining half is in a nondifferentiable *colloidal* form, bound to protein. Shifting ratios between the ionized and protein-bound forms of calcium are probably operative in conjunction with other factors in providing a homeostatic mechanism preventing oversaturation of the plasma on the one hand and maintaining adequate levels of available ionized calcium for bodily needs on the other hand. Other important regulators of calcium metabolism are parathyroid hormone and calcitonin (thyrocalcitonin).[50, 64] Calcium incorporated in bone salt and deposited in bone, dentin, and tooth enamel represents more than 99% of the calcium of the body. It will be seen, therefore, that calcium in adequate amounts is necessary for the proper composition of the skeletal parts. Furthermore, it is evident that when the balance of ingestion and excretion is disturbed in such a way as to lower the serum values, this essential mineral will be mobilized from the bony storehouse to correct the deficits.

Phosphorus, like calcium, is indispensable in bone formation and in certain other physiologic activities. Phosphorus is present in large amounts in bones and teeth, the ratio of calcium to phosphorus being approximately 2:1. It is also present in the serum, chiefly in the form of inorganic phosphate. The daily requirement of a normal adult is approximately 1.3 gm. Children need slightly less, and women during pregnancy and lactation require more.[139] The normal serum values for adults range between 3 mg and 4 mg per 100 ml or 1.7 mEq to 2.3 mEq per liter. In children, the value is slightly higher.

Phosphorus is abundant in ordinary foods, and a deficiency in intake is less likely to occur than in the case of calcium. The absorption of phosphorus from the intestinal tract is regulated in part by the amount of calcium in the diet and by the mechanisms that have to do with calcium absorption. In this way, it is possible to have phosphorus deficiency in combination with calcium deficiency.

In the disturbances that lead to excessive mobilization of calcium from the bones (e.g., hyperparathyroidism), phosphorus also is mobilized. It is apparent, therefore, that the metabolism of calcium and that of phosphorus— including mechanisms of assimilation, excretion, and utilization—are so intimately related that both substances must be considered in all pathologic disturbances affecting one or the other substance.

Among the more important and revealing microscopic features of bone are the linear markings that remain after decalcification and that stain intensely with hematoxylin. Such markings are called cement lines, since it is evident that they represent the zones of junction between lamellae or between layers of bone that have been formed at different times. Thus, like the growth rings of trees, these lines furnish records of growth that can be interpreted by the morphologist. In the case of bone, such markings also provide a means of estimating the amount of change in architecture that has resulted from resorptive and and formative activities. It will be noted subsequently that the characteristic microscopic features of Paget's disease are dependent, to a large extent, on the increased number and bizarre design of these cement lines.

The structural pattern of osseous tissues is subject to change in accordance with functional demands. The precise mechanisms that may be responsible for the resorptive processes are as yet unknown. Some observers believe that endosteal and periosteal cells, as well as osteocytes, are capable of removing bone, in addition to forming it. Still other observers hold that the salts and matrix of bone may be removed by "humoral" mechanisms. It is generally conceded, however, that osteoclasts are in some manner directly concerned with the resorption of osseous tissues. These cells, which are believed to originate from the coalescence of mononuclear cells, apparently respond to physical or chemical stimuli. They appear to adhere to the surface of bone and to bring about its resorption. Characteristically, their presence is followed by the notching of the bone surface (Howship's lucunae) (Fig. 40-4). In fact, observations made with the electron microscope[37] indicate that osteoclasts differ markedly from other bone cells and possess brush borders, consisting of a complex of cytoplasmic processes, that are adjacent to the resorbing bone. It has been noted also

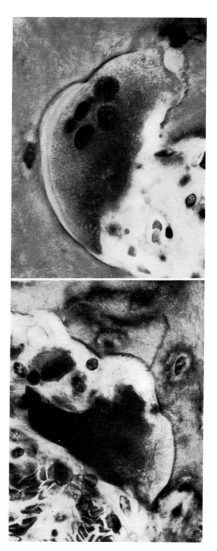

Fig. 40-4 Osteoclasts in Howship's lacunae. Note sharp margins of resorbing bone. (×700; courtesy Dr. J. P. Weinmann and Dr. H. Sicher.)

that no unmineralized collagen is seen at the resorption sites, indicating that collagen and ground substance are removed before or at the time of mineral solution.

Many of the functions of the bony structures of the body are well known. They include weight bearing, provision of a means of locomotion, provision of protected compartments for vital organs, provision of well-adapted sites for hematopoiesis, and provision of a readily available store of calcium and phosphorus. The morphologist, being aware of these functions, frequently can observe gross and microscopic alterations in cellular and structural patterns that permit an evaluation of the kind and amount of physiologic disturbance that is taking place or has occurred previously. The chemist, by suitable studies of calcium and phosphorus metabolism and phosphatases, may be able to demonstrate altered values that conform with the morphologic patterns. Such relationships are best exemplified by the combined mineral metabolism and histologic studies in hyperparathyroidism, renal rickets, and rickets.

NONSPECIFIC PATHOLOGIC DISTURBANCES

Atrophy. Diminution in the gross density and weight of bone occurs in association with a variety of unrelated disorders. In rare instances, a single bone may atrophy without any demonstrable local or general cause "disappearing bone disease."[22, 133] Localized atrophy may result from pressure applied to bone from without or from within. Examples of atrophy resulting from compression are found

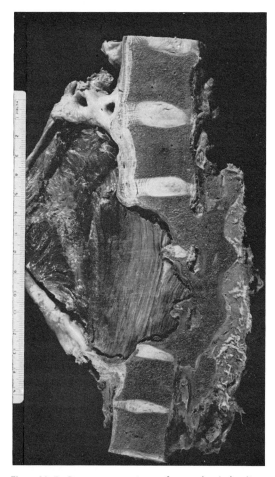

Fig. 40-5 Pressure erosion of vertebral bodies caused by aneurysm of arch of aorta. Note somewhat better preservation of nonvascular intervertebral discs.

in expanding aneurysms (Fig. 40-5), benign or malignant tumors, and localized collections of abnormal cells such as those observed in certain lipid storage diseases. Atrophy limited to one or several bones may result from disuse. This frequently is noted in roentgenograms that are made following rigid splinting or mechanical fixation of an extremity. It also is observed in conjunction with ankylosis of joints from rheumatoid arthritis or other causes. Reduction in blood flow to an extremity may result in atrophy, but it is probable that hyperemia of traumatic or inflammatory origin may also be attended by increased porosity. It is also well known that destruction of the peripheral nerve supply, such as occurs in leprosy, will be followed by localized atrophy or even complete resorption of the bony tissues distal to the nerve lesion.

The actual mechanisms involved in local bone absorption are not known. It is probable, however, that impairment of nutrition mediated through diminished blood flow is one important factor and that increased pressure upon the bone surfaces is another. While evidence of osteoclastic activity (lacunar absorption) may be observed on microscopic examination in some specimens, it seems probable that other mechanisms must be operative to account for the numerous examples of bone atrophy in which osteoclasts are not in evidence. In fact, it has been contended by some observers that osteocytes within bone lamellae may be involved in the process of bone mobilization.[83]

Generalized atrophy is observed in certain nutritional disturbances as, for example, in scurvy, in which the mesenchymal cells, including osteoblasts, are unable to form or maintain the normal amount of intercellular substance. It is seen also in disorders of mineral metabolism such as hyperparathyroidism, rickets, osteomalacia, and long-standing hyperthyroidism.

Senile and postmenopausal osteoporosis. Women in the postmenopausal period sometimes develop osteoporosis that is most marked in the spine.[7] Some degree of generalized atrophy of bone (osteoporosis) frequently accompanies the onset of old age (senile osteoporosis). Hypercalcemia is not a feature of the osteoporosis associated with either senility or the postmenopausal state.[8]

The mechanisms that may be held responsible for generalized osteoporosis include at least three possible disturbances, operating singly or together:

1 Inadequate amounts of available minerals

2 Excessive mobilization of bone salt

3 Inability of osteoblasts to form and maintain the organic matrix of bone

The latter defect may result either from hormonal influences or from general or specific inadequacies in nutrition. Osteoclastic (lacunar) absorption is prominent in certain examples of generalized osteoporosis (e.g., hyperparathyroidism), but in other diseases, such as senile osteoporosis, no such mechanism is apparent in the majority of instances. It is possible that the rate at which the resorptive process is taking place may be of importance in determining the number of observable osteoclasts.

Hypertrophy. Isolated bones of excessive size or density occasionally are observed in persons whose skeletons are otherwise normal. Such lesions may arise from the stimulation of the bone-forming cells (periosteal or endosteal layers) because of low-grade inflammation that is caused by infectious agents or trauma. In a similar fashion, slowly growing neoplasms may stimulate excessive growth of bone, leading to well-defined hyperostosis. This is frequently noted in meningiomas.[29] Hypertrophy of bone may result from excessive blood flow or from congenital or acquired malformation of vessels. Abnormalities in endochondral. ossification may give rise to single or multiple sites of osseous overgrowths that remain as permanent deformities.

Among the localized overgrowths of bone, one of the most common is enostosis of the calvaria. This is a lesion of uncertain origin, which consists of irregular knobs and ridges of bony tissue converging toward the nasal end of the metopic suture on the interior surface of the skull. Usually, these bony masses are exceedingly dense, and the diploë is obliterated in the involved portion of the skull. Occasionally, however, they are made up of porous or cancellous bone. The dura mater is usually adherent to the affected parts. Enostosis of the calvaria was observed in 7% of 3,250 autopsied subjects, and the incidence was highest in the sixth and seventh decades.[21]

Hyperostosis frontalis interna, when associated with virilism and obesity, is now regarded as a syndrome[66] believed to have been described first in 1719 by Morgagni.

Bone hypertrophy affecting a few or many of the bones of the extremities is seen in secondary osteoarthropathy and in osteitis deformans (Paget's disease), in which the skull also may be affected.

Generalized overgrowth of the osseous parts forms the most striking feature of acromegaly and the gigantism caused by pituitary dysfunction. These disturbances will be referred to elsewhere.

Lines of arrested growth. Roentgenograms of the long bones of children occasionally will contain one or more transversely placed lines of increased density in the expanded metaphyseal ends of the shafts. Such markings are known as arrested growth lines, since they can be correlated with periods of illness or periods of malnutrition.

Anatomic studies, including the microscopic examination of appropriate sections, have revealed that these lines are caused by the presence of heavy and transversely placed trabeculae. The latter result from a slowing or cessation of the normal sequences of endochondral ossification. When normal endochondral bone growth is reestablished, the relatively dense layer of calcified cartilage and bone that has formed during the illness remains and can be demonstrated in the x-ray films or in microscopic sections that are examined under very low magnification. Through the usual process of growth and remodeling of the bone shaft, these lines are gradually reduced and finally destroyed.

Lesions produced by ingestion of lead. Roentgenograms of the long bones of infants and children who have ingested sufficient quantities of lead will show broad bands of dense bone at or near the metaphyseal ends of the diaphysis. These densities occur in normally arranged but somewhat thickened trabeculae. It has been noted that the trabeculae corresponding to the zone of increased density in the x-ray film are comprised mainly of calcified cartilage and that large and acidophilic giant cells are present between them. It seems probable that the lead is deposited simultaneously with the bone salt and that the calcified cartilage matrix so impregnated resists the resorptive mechanisms by which it is normally removed as new osteoid tissue is laid down. The increased density in the x-ray shadow is probably caused in part by the excess opacity of the heavy metal as compared to normal bone salt.

Similar changes may result from the ingestion of other heavy metals such as phosphorus and arsenic.

Lesions produced by ingestion of fluorine. Ingestion of excessive quantities of fluorine by children results in the formation of tooth enamel that contains chalky white patches that may later acquire a brownish stain (mottled enamel). The observation that teeth affected in this manner have an increased resistance to decay has led dentists and public health workers to undertake an evaluation of the effectiveness of controlled administration of fluorine in drinking water as a preventive measure against dental caries (p. 1073).

The effects of fluorine upon osseous tissues have been noted in workers in cryolite fac-

tories, in people in certain regions in India,[59] and in animals experimentally treated[86] or spontaneously exposed while grazing near factories or volcanoes where fluorine-containing gases were emitted.[139] It seems probable that the anatomic changes resulting from fluorine intoxication vary greatly according to the

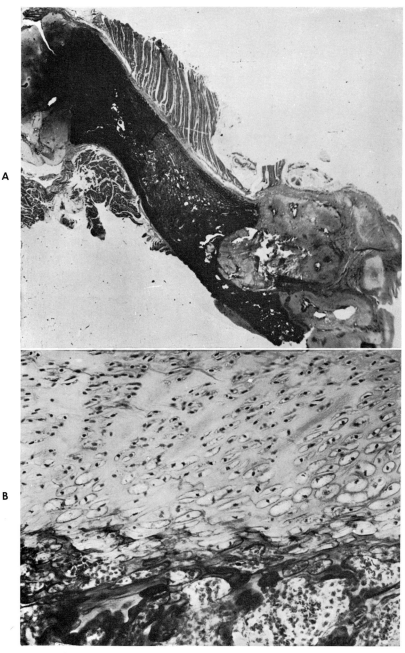

Fig. 40-6 Chondrodystrophia fetalis. **A,** Midsagittal section of tibia from infant. Diaphysis is short, wide, and dense. Epiphyses are enlarged and nodular and show multiple centers of calcification. **B,** Imperfect alignment of epiphyseal cartilage cells and consequent irregularity in calcification and ossification associated with achondroplasia. **(B, ×230.)**

age of the animal and the dosage of the mineral. In older animals, the bones may become dense and sclerotic, whereas in the young animals, especially when given large doses of fluorine, the osseous tissues are likely to show excessive porosity. Abnormality in calcium deposition in bone is indicated by the presence of small and large isolated crystals. Interpretation of the pathologic changes is made difficult by the frequent association of renal damage, metastatic calcification, and hyperplasia of the parathyroid glands.[139]

CONGENITAL DEVELOPMENTAL, AND HEREDITARY ABNORMALITIES
Localized deformities

A wide variety of localized abnormalities have been recorded. Some of these may originate from fetal or postfetal injuries, whereas others may result from inherited traits. Certain bones, especially those of the extremities, may fail to develop (aplasia). One or more limbs may be absent (amelia), and deformities in which the hands and feet are attached directly to the trunk (phocomelia) have been described. Fusion of two contiguous or closely placed bones or branching of a single bone also may occur as a developmental fault.

In contrast to these local disturbances, there are a number of symmetric or generalized malformations of bone that are of greater interest to the pathologist.

Symmetric or generalized deformities

Cleidocranial dysostosis. Cleidocranial dysostosis is a familial and usually hereditary disturbance in which, in association with retarded closure of the fontanels, one or both clavicles are absent or hypoplastic. In addition, in some cases, there are protrusion of the mandible and hypoplasia of the lacrimal and zygomatic bones. The hypoplasia or aplasia of the clavicles enables the affected subject to move his shoulders abnormally, even to the point of touching them together in front of the sternal notch.

Chondrodysplasia. It has been customary, for a long time, to consider a number of skeletal disorders that result in shortened, thickened, and otherwise deformed bones, leading to dwarfism, as variations of a single inherited disturbance of endochondral ossification. Included among these abnormalities are *chondrodystrophia fetalis, achondroplasia,* and *chondrodysplasia.*

From examination of skeletal tissues, it was believed that the primary disturbance resides

wholly or in large part in the proliferating cartilage. The cells of the growth cartilage fail to align themselves into regular columns and to pass through the normal stages of proliferation, maturation, regression, and invasion, in an orderly manner, by capillaries from the adjacent metaphysis. Instead, irregular masses of cartilage are built up, producing thick, nodular, and bulky epiphyses that undergo calcification and ossification irregularly (Fig. 40-6). It has been assumed that these changes, observed microscopically, were the causes for the shortened and widened bones (Figs. 40-6 and 40-7) and the associated dwarfism.

Recently, a lethal form of bone dysplasia, observed in newborn infants, has been described and designated *thanatoporic dwarfism*[103a] (Fig. 40-8). Also, just recently, the results of a careful reexamination of endochondral ossification in "achondroplastic dwarfism" were published.[121a] Biopsy material representing the chondro-osseous junctions of

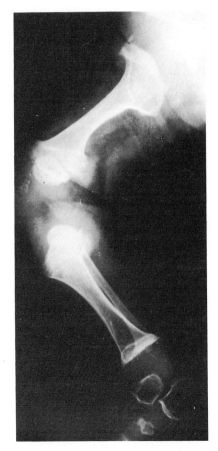

Fig. 40-7 Shortened and widened bones of lower extremity and deformed epiphyses that characterize chondrodystrophia fetalis.

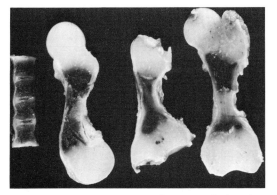

Fig. 40-8 Gross structural changes of chondrodystrophia fetalis in newborn infant evident in bones of lower extremity which have been divided in longitudinal axis. Sectioned vertebral bodies show little, if any, deformity.

rib and iliac crest from seven "typical" achondroplastic dwarfs ranging in age from 14 months to 35 years was examined and showed regular and well-organized endochondral ossification. The observers concluded "that the basic defect in achondroplasia may be a quantitative decrease in the rate of endochondral ossification, which, in conjunction with undisturbed periosteal bone formation, results in the short, squat shape of the tubular bones"* in the achondroplastic dwarf.

In light of these newer observations, it is possible that more than one mechanism may be responsible for disturbances in bone growth and development in hereditary dwarfism. It is possible, also, that further investigations may provide a basis for a more meaningful classification of these disorders.

Chondro-osteodystrophy (Morquio's[107] disease). A disorder of skeletal growth, chondroosteodystrophy is similar in many respects to chondrodystrophia fetalis. Although congenital, the signs and symptoms of the disease may not be recognized until a few years after birth, when it is noted that the vertebral bodies are wedge shaped and otherwise deformed. This gives rise to kyphosis that becomes noticeable as the child assumes an upright position.[117] Other skeletal deformities, such as depression of the sternum, enlargement of the costochondral junctions, enlargement of the wrists and knees, and distortion of the cranial base, may be observed. Roentgenographic examination reveals distortion and irregular calcification of

the cartilaginous epiphyses, and this is confirmed by pathologic examination.

This form of chondrodystrophy is apparently subject to autosomal recessive inheritance. Males are affected, and twenty cases were observed by Jacobsen[72] in five generations of one family.

Hereditary multiple exotoses (osteochondromatosis). Unlike chondrodystrophia fetalis, which is apparent at birth, osteochondromatosis develops gradually during childhood. About half of the offspring of an affected subject manifest the disorder. The disease may be transmitted through unaffected females.[75] Males are affected more often than females (in a ratio of about 7:3).

The pathologic disturbances arise from the growth of multiple cartilaginous exostoses at or near the bony epiphyses. Chondrosarcomas sometimes arise from one or more of these lesions, particularly in adults. Individually, overgrowths are no different from osteochondromas that arise singly, and for this reason they require no further comment at this time.

Enchondromatosis (dyschondroplasia or Ollier's disease). A poorly defined disturbance in skeletal growth and development, enchondromatosis may represent a variant of the other diseases affecting endochondral ossification.[71] Skeletal involvement may be limited to a single bone or to several long bones on one side of the body. In some instances, the disorder is more widespread. Abnormalities in endochondral ossification, beginning in the first or second year, give rise to deformities that remain after skeletal growth has been completed. No convincing evidence of hereditary transmission has been furnished.

Melorheostosis. Derived from two Greek words meaning "limb" and "I flow," melorheostosis refers to an obscure disorder of bone that was described by Léri and Joanny in 1922.[88] Melorheostosis may be regarded as a form of developmental hyperostosis that begins in infancy or early childhood and progresses slowly thereafter. Usually, one or more bones in either one upper or lower extremity are affected, but occasionally the process may be bilateral in distribution and more generalized. The affected bones are thickened and have flat, irregular, overhanging cortical overgrowths that are reminiscent of the wax drippings along the surface of a partially burned candle. Microscopically, the thickened cortex is excessively dense and shows an irregular lamellar pattern.

Occasionally, the bony overgrowths are

*From Rimoin, D. L., Hughes, G. N., Kaufman, R. L., Rosenthal, R. E., McAlister, W. H., and Silberberg, R.: New Eng. J. Med. 283:728-735, 1970.

capped with cartilage in a fashion similar to chondral exostoses, and this feature may indicate the manner of initial development of the hyperostosis.

Gargoylism (Hunter-Hurler syndrome). A syndrome characterized by dwarfism, skeletal deformity, and limitation of joint motion. Mental retardation, deafness, clouding of the cornea, and enlargement of the liver and spleen also may be component manifestations of the syndrome.

Histologically, the disorder is characterized by the presence of clear cells throughout the connective tissues of the body. The chief components of these "Hurler cells" have been thought to be chondroitin sulfate B and heparitin sulfate, and it has been considered probable that the syndrome results from a genetic error in the differentiation of fibroblasts.

There is excretion of mucopolysaccharides in the urine, and it has been assumed that the bony changes result from a disturbance in the formation and maintenance of the bone matrix.

The complexity of the biochemical disturbances of the syndrome and the genetic errors that are responsible are discussed by McKusick[99] under the subject title "mucopolysaccharidoses." Matalon and Dorfman,[104] employing Hurler fibroblasts in tissue cultures, have succeeded in demonstrating the intracellular accumulation of large-molecular-weight dermatan sulfate and hyaluronic acid. They observe that the existence of several genetic variants affecting genes on different chromosomes (X-linked form and autosomal recessive) suggests that more than one biochemical abnormality may lead to similar phenotypic expression. Duthie and Townes[39] divide the disorder into two forms: (1) severe Hurler's syndrome with corneal clouding, subject to autosomal recessive inheritance, and (2) mild Hurler's syndrome without corneal clouding, subject to X-linked recessive inheritance.

Marfan's syndrome. Marfan's syndrome, a hereditary disorder seen in both sexes, seems to follow the pattern of a single autosomal dominant but rarely may occur as a recessive trait. Since the basic defect appears to reside in the formation of elastic fibers, a number of organs and tissues are affected—notably, the large arteries (p. 754). In addition, the articular capsules and tendons are affected.

Persons displaying the Marfan traits are characteristically tall and have elongated extremities that are small in diameter. The fingers are long and spiderlike—a deformity known as arachnodactyly.

Marble bone disease (Albers-Schönberg disease or osteopetrosis). An uncommon but exceedingly interesting hereditary disorder of the skeleton, marble bone disease appears to result in most instances from autosomal recessive inheritance. Not infrequently, the disease has been observed in the offspring of parents who are closely related. The disturbance is usually congenital, but its manifestations may not be recognized until some time after birth.[97, 145] The symptomatology is related to the fragility of bone (fractures), to the sclerosis of the skeletal parts (osteosclerotic anemia), and to the narrowing of the foramina (deafness and impairment of vision). In spite of the excessive density and increased hardness of the osseous tissues, fractures from trivial causes frequently are observed. In association with anemia, there may be extreme degrees of extramedullary hematopoiesis. In the case represented in Fig. 40-9, anemia was the dominant symptom. Biopsy of one of the enlarged superficial lymph nodes disclosed pronounced hematopoiesis. Subsequently, at autopsy, it was noted that all lymphoid tissues, as well as the liver and kidney, were the sites of blood cell formation.

Roentgenograms of patients with marble bone disease show remarkably dense bony structures in all skeletal parts that are formed in cartilage (Fig. 40-10). In some instances, the distal portions of the shafts are club shaped and present alternating transverse zones of bone of varying densities (Fig. 40-10). The bodies of the vertebrae, pelvic bones, and ribs are conspicuously affected. On gross examination, the bones are extremely dense, and sawing is difficult because of the unnatural hardness. Cross section through the diaphysis of the long tubular bones reveals that the medulla is filled with the same dense bony tissue that forms the cortex. No marrow spaces are visible. Although it is difficult to section such a bone with the saw, it is easy to induce a fracture by the application of moderate stress.

Microscopic examination of cross and longitudinal sections of the bones that are formed in cartilage reveals a picture that is monotonous in its regularity. At the epiphyseal cartilage plates, one observes dense and heavily calcified spicules of cartilaginous matrix that are wider than normal (Fig. 40-9, *A*). Such spicules remain throughout the shaft and be-

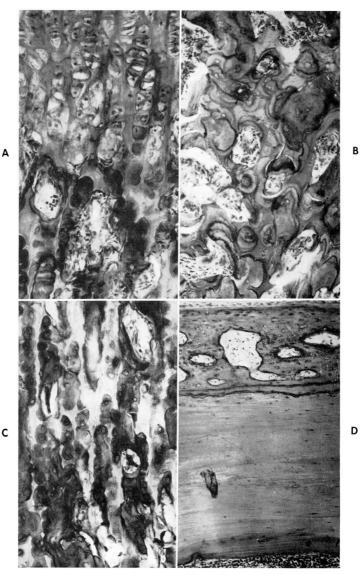

Fig. 40-9 Abnormalities of architecture in bone formed in cartilage. Increased amount of calcified cartilage matrix at zone of endochondral ossification and irregular penetration of marrow blood vessels are indicated in **A.** Persistence of these columns of calcified cartilage matrix and addition to osteoid matrix to further narrow marrow spaces are illustrated in sections (transverse, **B,** and longitudinal, **C**) from midshaft regions of femur. In section of membranous bone of skull, **D,** osseous tissue is well formed and devoid of characteristic features of marble bone disease. (**A** to **C,** ×210; **D,** ×130.)

come surrounded by osteoid matrix that becomes heavily calcified (Fig. 40-9, *C*). In cross section, it is noted that little or no marrow tissue exists (Fig. 40-9, *B*). These morphologic features seem to imply that the cartilaginous matrix in the provisional zone of the epiphyseal plate is excessive in amount and heavily calcified. Furthermore, it is evident that the normal remodeling processes do not occur and that the calcified cartilage

matrix is not removed. Osteoclasts rarely are observed. It seems likely, therefore, that this skeletal disorder results from an imbalance between the formative and the resorptive mechanisms that are normally present. Membranous bones such as the flat segments of the skull are altered little, if at all, in marble bone disease (Fig. 40-9, *D*).

Osteogenesis imperfecta. A disorder of connective tissue, osteogenesis imperfecta appears

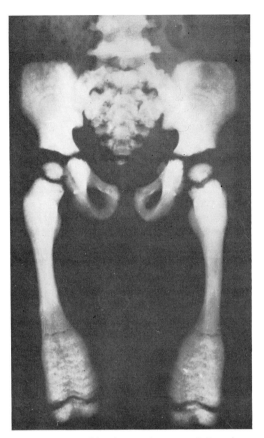

Fig. 40-10 Marble bone disease. Pelvic bones and femora of 5-year-old child. There are well-marked clubbing and transverse layering of femora. (From Clifton, W. M., Frank, A. A., and Freeman, S.: Amer. J. Dis. Child. **56:**1020-1036, 1938.)

to result from autosomal inheritance. In one family of fifty-one members in five generations, twenty-seven persons were affected.[69] Although the disease usually is apparent at the time of birth, (osteogenesis imperfecta congenita), it may not be recognized until later in childhood (osteogenesis imperfecta tarda; osteopsathyrosis). In the congenital form, the manifestations are striking, and in numerous instances the infant is stillborn or lives only a short time after birth. The predominant manifestations of the disease (fractures) are related to the porosity and fragility of bone. Multiple fractures usually are present at the time of birth, and deformities indicative of fractures acquired in utero frequently are observed (Fig. 40-11). In surviving children, there is often a lessened susceptibility to fracture at and after puberty.

Some observers have elected to regard osteogenesis imperfecta as a disorder in which

there is hypoplasia of the mesenchyme in general. In support of this contention, it is noted that the sclerae of the eyes may be thin, allowing the pigmented layers to show through (blue sclerotics), that the dentinal structures are poorly formed (dentinogenesis imperfecta), and that certain other connective tissues may be delicate and thin.

Roentgenologic and macroscopic examination of the skeletal parts reveals extremely porous and delicate bones. Deformities from recent, old, and unhealed fractures are also apparent. It is possible in some instances to section the undecalcified bones with a knife. Care must be taken, in performing an autopsy, to prevent additional postmortem fractures.

Microscopically, the bony tissues are thin and delicate (Figs. 40-12 and 40-13). The cancellous trabeculae are few in number and may show microscopic fractures (Fig. 40-13, *C*). Individual spicules of bone contain numerous, closely placed osteocytes that are surrounded by only small amounts of matrix (Fig. 40-13, *B* and *C*). Fractures heal readily, but the newly formed trabeculae are thin and fragile like the original bone (Fig. 40-12). No disturbances are noted in the sequences of endochondral ossification (Fig. 40-13, *A* and *B*).

This skeletal disease bears no apparent relationship to any endocrine dysfunction or to disturbances in mineral metabolism. It seems probable that imperfections in the quality and quantity of intercellular matrix of certain mesenchymal tissues are the essential defect.

Miscellaneous deformities. In addition to the skeletal disorders described in the foregoing paragraphs, there are numerous abnormalities, oftentimes of congenital origin, which present clinical features that are reasonably characteristic and therefore have been regarded as separate entities by some clinicians. These disorders include the following:

1 Progressive diaphyseal dysplasia
2 Hereditary multiple diaphyseal sclerosis
3 Osteopathia striata
4 Osteopoikilosis or osteopathia condensans
5 Epiphyseal dysplasia
6 Stippled epiphyses

TRAUMATIC INJURIES

When a bone is significantly traumatized, the endosteal cells lining the vascular spaces in compact bone and the marrow spaces in cancellous bone and the osteogenic cells of the cambium layer of the periosteum respond in a characteristic manner. Morphologically, they

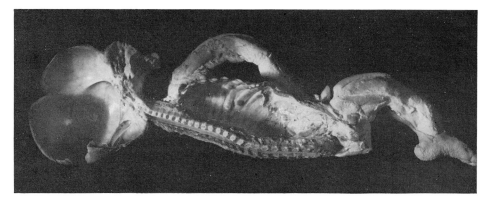

Fig. 40-11 Osteogenesis imperfecta. Hemisection of body of infant deformed as result of osteogenesis imperfecta. Skull is thin and transparent. Multiple fracture sites are apparent in ribs, and upper and lower extremities are deformed as result of old and recent fractures.

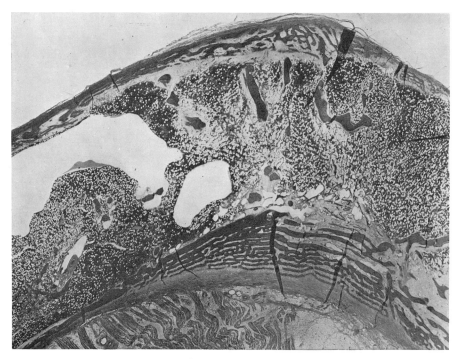

Fig. 40-12 Longitudinal section of tibia through site of old fracture. Cortex is extremely thin and delicate. It is clearly apparent that fracture has healed and that new layers of bone are forming on concave surface, a mechanism by which such deformities are usually corrected or modified. (×9.)

become plump and rounded or cuboid shaped, and mitotic figures appear. Within a few days, such stimulated cells acquire the morphology of osteoblasts and, by virtue of their arrangement about seams of newly formed osteoid, are known to be engaged in intramembranous bone formation.[16]

Fractures

From the time at which a bone is fractured until complete functional and anatomic resto-ration has been accomplished, one may observe morphologic changes of a reparative nature. It is almost certain that these structural alterations are accompanied by chemical and physiologic adaptations that, although less obvious, are of equal or perhaps greater importance. In brief, the morphologic features observed, including mineralization of newly deposited osteoid, represent a recapitulation of the processes by which bone is formed initially in the embryo.

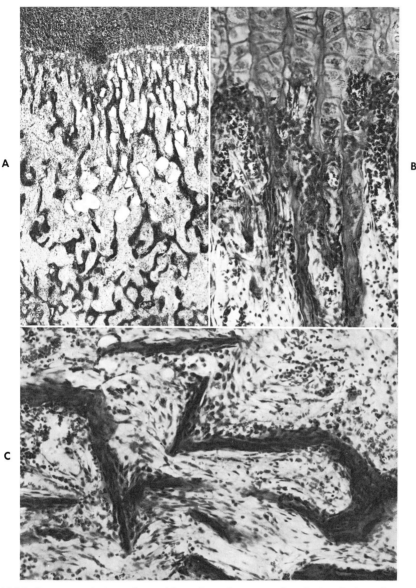

Fig. 40-13 Osteogenesis imperfecta. Normal mechanisms of endochondral ossification are clearly apparent in **A** and **B** from femur of infant with osteogenesis imperfecta. Individual trabeculae are delicate and often are fractured, **C**. Note increased cellularity of bony tissue and relative scarcity of matrix. (**A,** ×40; **B** and **C,** ×250.)

Although the processes by which a fractured bone is restored to normal are continuous, it is convenient to discuss them in four stages, depending on the length of time since injury:

1 Development of hematoma and traumatic inflammation
2 Organization
3 Union by callus formation
4 Rearrangement of callus and bony union

Development of hematoma and traumatic inflammation. Simultaneously with the occur-rence of a fracture, the soft tissues within and around a bone are injured. The periosteum is torn or detached from the outer surface of the cortex, the endosteum is stripped from the surfaces of the marrow or vascular spaces within bone, and the marrow tissue is disrupted. Blood vessels and capillaries in all the adjacent soft tissues, as well as within the intraosseous vascular channels, are injured or disrupted. Such an injury results in the production of a hematoma surrounding the ends of the fractured bone.

Concomitantly, there are hyperemia, extravasation of edema fluid, and beginning inflammatory cell infiltration. Fibrin is formed at the periphery of the hematoma beneath the detached periosteum and between the ends of the fractured bone. The injured parts are thus cemented together by a loose-meshed fibrinous framework that serves as a scaffold upon which the subsequent granulation tissue may grow. In a fracture, the detachment and displacement of the periosteum are greater at the level of the break than they are at more distant points. Thus, the area of hemorrhage and exudation assumes at an early stage a fusiform shape that is usually maintained throughout the process of healing.

Organization. During the first twenty-four to forty-eight hours after injury, the inflammatory and exudative changes increase. Leukocytes accumulate in large numbers. The tissues become swollen and indurated from the extravasation of blood and edema fluid. Fibrin precipitation increases steadily. These exudative phenomena are accompanied almost from the time of injury by increasing signs of stimulation of the fixed tissue cells. These cellular alterations represent the earliest demonstrable stages of repair. The fibrin clot between the ends of the fractured bone undergoes organization by means of an ingrowth of proliferating connective tissue cells and tubular sprouts of budding capillary endothelium (granulation tissue). In addition to the numerous polymorphonuclear leukocytes that are present during the early stages, one now observes increasing numbers of mononuclear phagocytes that are apparently engaged in phagocytizing necrotic cells and tissue debris. Up to this point, one is unable to detect any noteworthy difference between the repair of a fracture and the healing processes involved in the case of an aseptic soft tissue wound. In each instance, delicate collagenous fibrils are deposited between the proliferating connective tissue cells. However, in the case of a fractured bone, such fibrillar material is soon obscured by the deposition of a homogeneous hyaline ground substance (Fig. 40-14). The appearance of this specialized intercellular matrix constitutes the first demonstrable evidence of bone formation.

A further difference between the manners in which bone and soft tissues react to traumatic injury is represented by the extent of regressive change. Owing to the peculiar origin and distribution of the blood supply in the case of bone, one will invariably see evidence

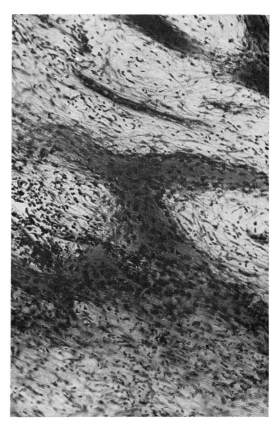

Fig. 40-14 Repair of fracture. Granulation tissue undergoing ossification at site of recent fracture of tibia. This type of bone formation similar to that observed in normal intramembranous bone growth. (×250; from Bennett, G. A., and Bauer, W.: In Scudder, C. L., editor: The treatment of fractures, W. B. Saunders Co.)

of extensive necrosis. Within two or three days after injury, such necrosis will be evidenced by empty lacunar spaces in the bone adjacent to the fracture line. Similar changes are apparent in any of the completely detached bone fragments.[60] Microscopic and roentgenologic examinations at a later date reveal marked alterations because bone necrosis involves relatively large areas adjacent to the point of injury. The rate of absorption of such devitalized bone is variable. It is probably caused by the action of osteoclasts, alone or in conjunction with other processes that are usually designated as humoral in nature.

Union by callus formation. By the end of the first week, in most fractures, the process by which intramembranous bone formation takes place can be observed. While new and indistinct bars of homogeneous osteoid matrix are being deposited between the proliferating cells, one notes that the morphology of the connective tissue cells is undergoing modifica-

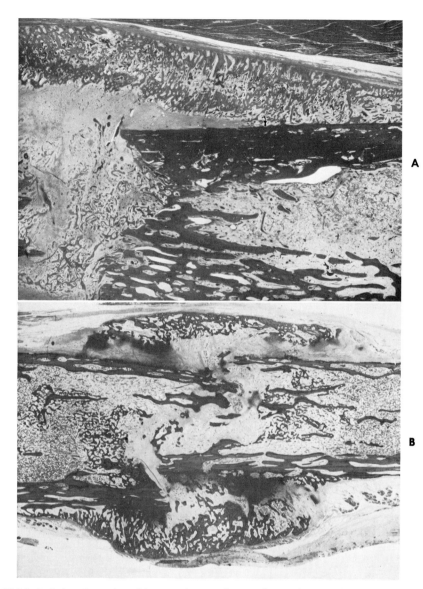

Fig. 40-15 A, Subperiosteal and intermediate callus evident in healing fracture of tibia of young child. **B,** Ten-month-old fracture site in rib of elderly woman. Interlocking ends of fractured bone encased in abundant external and internal callus, which is in part cartilaginous and in part bony. Although repair has been slow, it is evident that osseous union would eventually have occurred. Original bone cortex atrophic. (**A** and **B,** ×8; from Bennett, G. A., and Bauer, W.: In Scudder, C. L., editor: The treatment of fractures, W. B. Saunders Co.)

tion. Certain of these elongated or branching, fibroblastic-appearing cells assume new shapes and become rearranged. They now appear as round or cuboid-shaped cells. They then align themselves in solid rows along one border of each new bar of recently formed matrix and appear to aid in the deposition of additional ground substance to that recently formed. The morphologic characteristics and obvious activity of these cells enable one to recognize them as osteoblasts. Further, microscopic ob-

servation demonstrates that certain of these cells eventually become surrounded by their own secretions, the intercellular substance, and thus become osteocytes. Such cells within lacunar spaces remain, even though the bone spicule continues to grow. However, they are never completely cut off from the growing peripheral margins of the trabeculae because each cell develops cytoplasmic processes that maintain communication with similar processes of other cells. In this manner, delicate, tortuous channels (canaliculi) are formed. Such canaliculi between lacunar spaces serve as the pathways by which metabolites are exchanged from blood to bone cells in the fully developed osseous tissue.

New osseous tissue, formed in the manner just described, is laid down beneath the detached periosteum to form a tubular sleeve of external callus. It is also deposited in the medullary canal near the ends of the fractured bone. Gradually such osseous tissue grows inward from the periphery of the hematoma and ultimately replaces it (Fig. 40-15, *A*). In nearly all specimens of fracture repair, one is able to demonstrate areas of recognizable cartilage throughout the callus (Fig. 40-15, *B*). In the early stages, this tissue consists of a structureless mass of large spherical cells separated by homogeneous cartilaginous matrix. Later, a more orderly arrangement of such cells takes place, with the formation of imperfectly arranged columns that resemble those of the epiphyseal cartilage plate. The cartilage cells in such areas undergo the same morphologic changes observed in normal endochondral ossification. The cells degenerate and the intercellular matrix calcifies. Simultaneously, there are capillary invasion of the degenerating cartilage cells and deposition by osteoblastic cells of osteoid matrix upon the spicules of calcified cartilage. In this manner, the cartilaginous portions of the callus are gradually replaced by bone.

The occurrence of cartilage in callus has been a subject of considerable discussion. However, as noted by Ham and Harris, "the osteogenic cells of the periosteum of a long bone, which give rise to the callus, are direct descendants of the cells that once comprised the chondrogenic layer of the perichondrium of the cartilage model of that bone. . . ."* The osteogenic cells of callus have dual potentialities and, therefore, may differentiate either as bone-forming or cartilage-forming cells depending on environmental circumstances. The cartilaginous portions of the initial callus are nonvascular, while the osseous portions are well vascularized. Cartilaginous components of callus seem to occur in larger amounts in fractures where complete immobilization is difficult, suggesting that repeated stretching and twisting of the yielding callus, as well as the morphology and

*From Ham, A. W., and Harris, W. R.: In Bourne, G. H., editor: The biochemistry and physiology of bone, New York, 1956; copyrighted by Academic Press, Inc.

function of the proliferating cells, may determine in part the character and amount of the intercellular substance.

During the period in which the foregoing changes are taking place, it is possible, with appropriate techniques, to demonstrate that increasing amounts of mineral salts are being deposited in the intercellular matrix of both the osseous and the cartilaginous tissues. The exact mechanism by which this is accomplished is not clearly understood. It seems probable, however, that the mechanisms by which mineralization occurs in osseous and cartilaginous components of callus in fracture repair are basically similar to the processes by which mineralization of bone and cartilage takes place in the normal development of the skeleton.

Rearrangement of callus and bony union. In an ordinary fracture, the callus attains its maximum size in two or three weeks. There is a progressive increase in its density as observed by roentgenologic examinations. This is due to the continuous addition of new osseous tissue and the progressively increasing deposition of bone salt.

On microscopic study, one observes that the first callus that is laid down is formed largely of trabeculae that radiate transversely from the shaft of the bone. This is the external or subperiosteal callus. In other regions (e.g., between the ends of the fractured bone), the initial callus has little, if any, discernible structure (Fig. 40-15, *A*). However, within a period of one to two weeks, it will be noted that a rapid rearrangement of the newly formed bone is taking place. This is accomplished by resorption of certain portions of the trabeculae that were first formed and by the addition of new bone to other portions of the spicules. It seems evident that this rearrangement is determined largely by the stresses and strains to which the callus is subjected.

Concomitantly with the rearrangement of the newly formed bone, one can observe changes that indicate the continued resorption of the original osseous structures and the development of firm attachment between the old and the new bony parts. The amount of osseous tissue comprising a callus gradually diminishes. This process of adaptation continues for many months or years and may, in the more perfect examples of repair, lead to the complete removal of all traces of the injury and the bony overgrowth by which repair was accomplished (Fig. 40-16).

Delayed union and nonunion. There is a

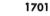

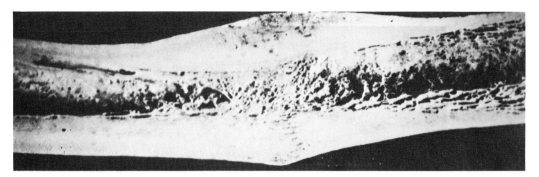

Fig. 40-16 Site of transverse fracture, now healed, apparent in this specimen of femur. Note fusiform thickening of cortex representing ossified external callus and partial obliteration of marrow cavity produced by maturation of internal callus.

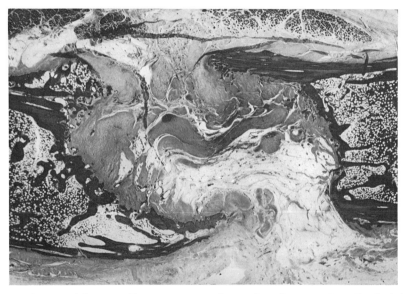

Fig. 40-17 Repair of fracture. Fracture site, similar to that shown in Fig. 40-15, *B*, has resulted in fibrous union, and no evidence of reparative changes remains. Medulla of each fractured bone end closed by osseous plate into which dense connective tissue bundles insert. (×9.)

wide variation in the time required for complete healing of a fractured bone, and many factors influence the rapidity and perfection with which the repair process is carried out. However, eliminating from consideration such factors as interposition of soft tissues between the fractured bone ends, infection, gross disturbances in the nutrition of the individual, and marked impairment of the blood supply to the part, it may be expected that nearly all fractures will heal in a reasonable period of time.

There can be little doubt that adequate immobilization is one of the most—if not the most—important factors in promoting rapid and complete union of a fracture. During the stages of granulation tissue growth and early calcification of the callus, any twisting or shearing motion will lead to tissue injury. Continuance of such injury leads to the formation of large amounts of cartilage. In unfavorable cases, the cartilaginous and bony callus is replaced by more yielding fibrous tissue that, upon reaching maturity, will not revert to bone (Fig. 40-17). Occasionally, a pseudarthrosis results (Fig. 40-18).

Bone graft. When fibrous union or nearthrosis has developed, it is necessary for the surgeon to induce the formation of new granulation tissue before bony union can be expected. In the majority of instances, a bone graft is inserted at the site of the old fracture. Such a procedure accomplishes a number of things, all of which favor repair. In the first

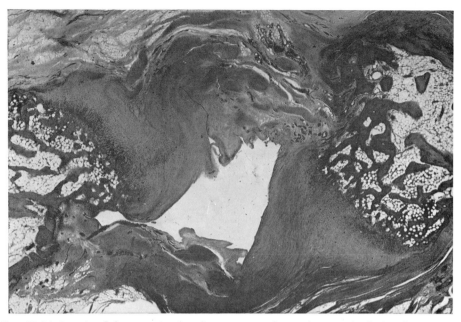

Fig. 40-18 Repair of fracture. In this fracture, nearthrosis has resulted. Cartilage covers each fractured bone end, and articular cavity lined by synovial membrane has been formed. (×16.)

place, the operation produces a new injury to bone that will be followed by the growth of new granulation tissue. The implanted graft ordinarily gives support to the fracture line and frequently brings about complete internal fixation. In addition, the implanted bone serves as a framework through which the new granulation will grow. It also provides a local source of bone salt that seems to favor satisfactory repair. It has been clearly established that most, if not all, of the engrafted bone becomes devitalized. At most, only the cancellous portions are capable of surviving the injury and the interruption of circulation. It is remarkable, therefore, that a bone graft is as valuable as it is known to be in fracture repair. Its function as a lattice or trellis for ingrowth of granulation tissue and its support to the area while old devitalized bone of the graft is being removed and replaced by new bone (creeping substitution) are apparently most important.

Posttraumatic osteoporosis of bone

The atrophy that is usually discernible following a fracture is due in part to disuse. It is probable that local hyperemia is also a factor in bringing about the resorptive changes. A somewhat different form of atrophy (Sudeck's atrophy of bone) is seen in conjunction with certain injuries to the ex-

tremities, especially the wrists, ankles, hands, and feet. Roentgenologic evidence of patchy osteoporosis is present. Clinically, the amount of swelling and induration of the soft tissues overlying the affected bone may be great, and the pain is often severe. The cause of these changes is not known, although favorable results from periarterial sympathectomy have been reported.[67] Sections of excised bony parts may show nothing other than atrophy.

Traumatic myositis ossificans

In distinction to *progressive* myositis ossificans, which usually begins in childhood without assignable cause and progresses slowly to a fatal termination, *traumatic* myositis ossificans is a localized lesion (myositis ossificans circumscripta) that usually results from single or multiple injuries. Repeated bruising injuries of the adductor or quadriceps muscles of the thigh or single contusions of these and other areas are followed in some instances by inflammatory changes that ossify. Myositis ossificans, often occurring in the region of greater and lesser trochanters of the femur, may develop in paraplegics. The character of the lesion usually is determined by examination of a roentgenogram (Fig. 40-19).

Microscopic examination reveals, in the early stages, widespread edema and mild inflammation of muscle. In some cases, recent

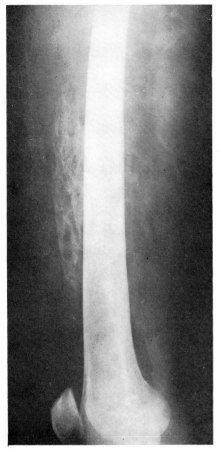

Fig. 40-19 Myositis ossificans. Ossification of muscles on anteriomedial aspect of thigh. (AFIP 77648.)

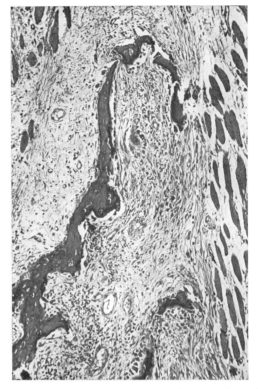

Fig. 40-20 Myositis ossificans. Edema and mild chronic inflammation of striated muscle, which is undergoing ossification, apparent in section of typical myositis ossificans. (×130; AFIP 90710.)

or old hemorrhage is indicated by extravasated corpuscles or hemosiderin pigment. Proliferation of fibroblasts and osteoblasts may be very marked. The exact nature of the lesion is recognized by the presence of osseous tissue (Fig. 40-20) that usually resembles callus.

Care must be exercised to distinguish myositis ossificans from bone-forming neoplasms (osteogenic sarcoma). The occurrence of such malignant tumors in myositis ossificans has been described.[111] In older lesions, there may be little or no residual inflammation, and the bone may be dense and heavily calcified.

Traumatic myositis ossificans usually is seen in lesions that arise close to bone, and the bone formation may result from displaced periosteum. It seems probable, however, that undifferentiated fibroblasts, well removed from bony structures, may differentiate into osteoblasts, and this may explain the lesions that have no apparent anatomic connection

with a skeletal part. The lesion tends to be self-limited, although regression may occur slowly. Trauma from repeated biopsy seems to aggravate the lesion, especially in early stages. According to Thorndike,[134] operative removal is indicated only in those cases in which the lesion occurs near a joint or in the origin or insertion of a muscle, and then only from twelve to twenty-four months after the injury.

Aseptic necrosis

Two types of aseptic bone necrosis may be recognized. One form, such as partial or complete necrosis of the head of the femur following a subcapital fracture, is clearly related to trauma and probably results from reduction or impairment of the blood supply. In patients in whom there are multiple fracture lines extending into the joint, bone necrosis with separation of one or more osseous fragments is especially likely to take place. Aseptic necrosis, in the form of bone infarcts, has been observed in caisson disease.[85] Similar infarcts unassociated with a known occupational disease have been described.[84] Necrosis of bone, presumably resulting from ischemia, also is observed in patients with sickle cell anemia and in patients with systemic lupus erythematosus, especially after corticosteroid therapy.

The second form, usually referred to as idiopathic aseptic necrosis, occurs most frequently in the epiphyses of growing children. The tibial tubercle (**Osgood-Schlatter disease**) and the femoral head (**Legg-Perthes disease**) are the foremost sites in the larger bones, whereas the scaphoid, semilunar, and metatarsal bones are the frequent locations among the smaller bones. These lesions, together with slipped femoral epiphyses, while affecting different skeletal parts, are basically similar and conform to the known picture of bone necrosis caused by ischemia.[106]

The etiology of such lesions remains obscure. Various theories, including low-grade infection, embolic occlusion of vessels, etc., have been suggested but have not been proved. A great deal of clinical evidence has accumulated suggesting that trauma is frequently a predisposing factor or perhaps an actual cause for the ischemia. That ischemia is vitally concerned is suggested by the fact that the bones or epiphyseal portions of the bones that are prone to become involved are largely surrounded by cartilage and, under normal conditions, have a limited vascular supply.

In the early stages of the process are noted the disappearance of osteocytes from the bony trabeculae and perhaps mild inflammatory changes in the soft tissues. There is little change in architecture, however. The overlying articular cartilage usually remains viable, since much of its nourishment is obtained from the synovial fluid. Later, the necrotic bone may crumble and collapse, giving rise to pronounced deformities in the x-ray film.[51] Repair of the lesion results from the ingrowth of bone-forming granulation tissue (creeping substitution). Such reparative phenomena are identical with the responses that lead to the organization and resolution of a bone graft.

INFLAMMATION

Infectious lesions of bone (osteomyelitis) may be mild or severe. They may be sharply localized or diffuse throughout an anatomic unit, and they may affect principally the periosteum, the cortex, or the marrow tissues in the cancellous portions of a bone.

A high proportion of all inflammatory lesions results from the localization of an infectious agent that is readily demonstrable. The responsible bacterium may reach the site of localization by way of the bloodstream, by direct extension from a neighboring focus of infection (periapical abscess of a tooth, sinus infection, infected joint, or soft tissue abscess), or by a penetrating injury (laceration or compound fracture). Infectious lesions in bone behave quite differently, depending on the characteristics of the causative microorganism, the route by which the infection occurred, and the age of the patient. Also, since antibiotics and other chemotherapeutic agents became available, there has been a sharp lowering of the incidence and mortality rate of osteomyelitis of all kinds.[137a] This has resulted from the more effective control of primary sites of infection. In addition, the course of the established bone infection usually is shortened by antibacterial therapy, and the likelihood of the development either of extensive bone necrosis or of spread of the infection to other skeletal parts is remarkably diminished. It is convenient, therefore, to consider infections of bone under several well-recognized classes of lesions.

Pyogenic infections. Any one of the pathogenic microorganisms may give rise to infections in bone. In osteomyelitis resulting from bacteremia (hematogenous osteomyelitis), the responsible agent is most frequently the staphylococcus. *Staphylococcus aureus* or *albus* may be isolated, although the former is more frequent. Streptococci, pneumococci, and other forms of pyogenic bacteria are encountered less frequently. In infants under 2 years of age, streptococcic osteomyelitis is encountered about twice as frequently as osteomyelitis caused by the staphylococcus.[58]

Acute hematogenous osteomyelitis is most common in children and affects, in order of frequency, the femur, tibia, humerus, and radius. It usually begins in the metaphyseal ends of the diaphyses of these bones. It is probable that the great vascularity of this zone of endochondral ossification is a factor predisposing to localization of bacteria. There is an initial violent, acute, exudative inflammation of the marrow tissues. The lethal effects of the toxins, together with thrombosis and obliteration of vessels from exudate in the bony spaces, lead at once to necrosis of the marrow and osseous parts (Fig. 40-21). The process soon spreads through the vascularized channels to reach the external surface of the cortex. Thus, the periosteum is dissected from the cortex (subperiosteal abscess),

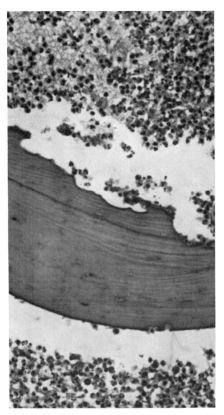

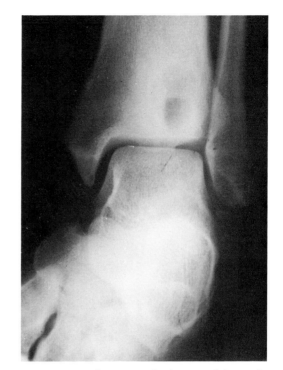

Fig. 40-22 Well-circumscribed area of bone destruction in lower segment of tibia. At operation, lesion proved to be Brodie's abscess.

Fig. 40-21 Acute osteomyelitis. Fragment of bone contains empty lacunar spaces, and bony margins notched and irregular. Soft tissues of marrow spaces replaced by purulent exudate. (×265; AFIP 73820.)

further impairing the blood supply. Similarly, the infection tends to spread elsewhere in the medulla of the bone. In this way, a small or large portion of a bone becomes necrotic.

The epiphyseal cartilage, together with the firm and dense periosteal and perichondrial attachments around its margins, seems to offer a certain amount of resistance to the spread of infection, and the epiphysis is not regularly affected, nor is the joint. It should be remembered, however, that both of these structures may become secondarily involved, or, less frequently, they may be the sites of primary localization of infection in the skeleton.

In certain instances, the infection is localized to a small area, where it may resolve entirely or become an abscess encased in a well-defined wall of fibrous or osseous tissue (Brodie's abscess) (Fig. 40-22). The periosteum overlying the latter may be irritated sufficiently to cause bone proliferation that results in considerable thickening of the cortex.

The more extensive infections result in necrosis of considerable portions of the involved bone. Subsequently, these devitalized segments become separated from the viable portions (sequestration). The sequestrum appears opaque in the roentgenogram and is frequently surrounded by irregular areas of lessened density (Fig. 40-23, *A* and *B*). On gross examination, the sequestrum is usually grayish white and has an irregular surface that is pitted and grooved. It frequently is surrounded by purulent exudate that may be draining from sinuses through the ossifying granulation tissue (involucrum) and overlying soft tissues (Fig. 40-23, *C*). Such sinus tracts (cloacae) and the walls of the cavities containing sequestra are lined by granulation tissue. In most examples of chronic osteomyelitis, one will find areas of acute and subacute inflammation in the cancellous spaces of the necrotic bone that has not completely separated from the viable portions. Hyperemia and active osteoclastic resorption as well as small and large foci of acute inflammation, are present in these areas. Such resorptive changes account for the irregular areas of osteoporosis and represent the manner in which the necrotic portions are detached from the living bone.

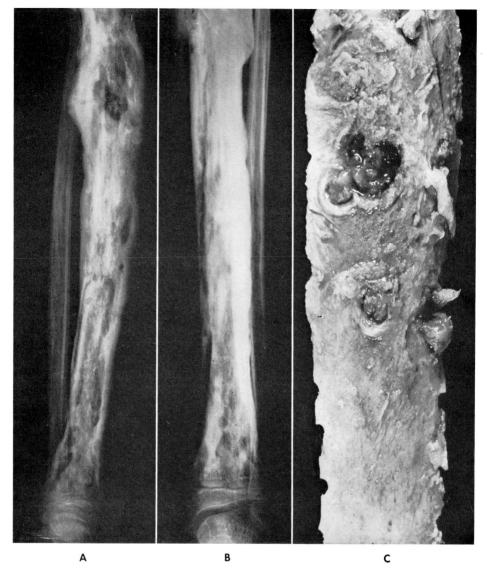

A   B   C

Fig. 40-23 Osteomyelitis of tibia. **A** and **B**, Lateral and anteroposterior roentgenograms showing destructive and proliferative changes of long-standing pyogenic osteomyelitis. Sequestrated segments of original tibial shaft visible through shadows cast by ossified granulation tissue (involucrum). **C,** Specimen of bone removed from tibia illustrated in **A** and **B**. Granulation tissue-filled sinus openings clearly evident on external surface of bone. These sinuses formed communications between skin surfaces and sequestrum enclosed in bony cavity.

Occasionally, the infectious agent localizes in the periosteum or beneath the periosteal covering of the cortex and spreads only slightly into the interior of bone. In some instances, trauma appears to predispose to these forms of periostitis. They are characterized by painful and tender swelling. If the lesion persists, it will cause bony thickening that is visible in the roentgenogram. Microscopically, in the early cases, hyperemia, marked edema, and polymorphonuclear leukocyte infiltration are seen. Occasionally, the reaction achieves the proportions of an abscess, and the adjacent bone becomes necrotic. In later stages, there is condensation of the cortical bone, and in most instances, irregular overgrowths of osseous tissue develop beneath the periosteum. Productive lesions of this type are sometimes referred to as Garré's sclerosing osteomyelitis.

Pyogenic microorganisms may enter a bone from a penetrating injury in association with a compound fracture or from the direct extension of a neighboring focus of infection.

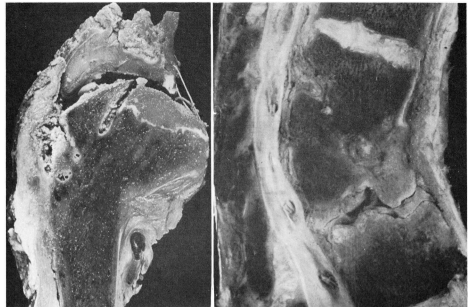

Fig. 40-24 Tuberculosis. **A,** Tuberculosis of hip joint has resulted in destruction of most of femoral caput and acetabular cup. Tuberculous osteomyelitis with extension of sinus tracts into adjacent articular capsule and soft tissues evident on left. **B,** Compression of vertebrae with angulation of spine has resulted from tuberculous osteomyelitis affecting three vertebral bodies and two intervertebral discs.

Although osteomyelitis acquired in this manner may be exceedingly troublesome and difficult to eradicate, it is not likely to produce general disturbances that are as severe as the systemic reactions regularly accompanying hematogenous osteomyelitis.

Tuberculosis. Tuberculosis of bone usually is caused by hematogenous dissemination of bacilli from an active focus in the lung, kidney, intestine, or lymph nodes. It may occur, however, as the result of direct extension from a caseous focus in soft tissues adjacent to bone. Children are much more frequently affected than adults. In children the involvement of the long bones usually commences in the metaphyseal ends of the diaphyses. The upper and lower femoral and the upper tibial regions frequently are affected. Infections in these sites may spread to destroy the epiphysis and to enter the joints (Fig. 40-24, *A*). In comparison with pyogenic infections, tuberculosis is more likely to extend to involve the epiphysis or to localize initially in this structure. Similarly, on a relative basis of comparison, tuberculosis affects the bodies of the vertebrae (Fig. 40-24, *B*) more commonly than do pyogenic infections. Tuberculosis of the spinal column is known as *Pott's disease*. The exudate from these lesions may accumulate in the soft tissues, where it excites comparatively little inflammation *(cold abscess)*. In some instances, the exudate gravitates along the sheath of the psoas muscle *(psoas abscess)*. Such accumulations may extend and cause a fluctuant swelling below Poupart's ligament.

Tuberculous osteomyelitis tends to destroy bone progressively. The caseating granulation tissue spreads through the cancellous tissues, leading to necrosis and fragmentation of bone trabeculae (Fig. 40-25, *A*). There is little tendency for tuberculous granulation tissue to ossify. The area of involvement becomes less dense on roentgenologic examination, and marked osteoporosis usually is seen on gross inspection. Complete caseation necrosis of all tissues at the site of infection may occur in time. This results in a well-localized tuberculous abscess (Fig. 40-25, *B*), the wall of which may show miliary and conglomerate tubercles on microscopic examination.

Rapidly spreading tuberculosis with extensive bone necrosis and gross sequestration may occur but is uncommon.

Syphilis. Osseous lesions resulting from the *Treponema pallidum* are observed as a part of congenital syphilis or as a manifestation of an acquired infection.

In congenital syphilis, the skeletal changes are of two major types: osteochondritis and

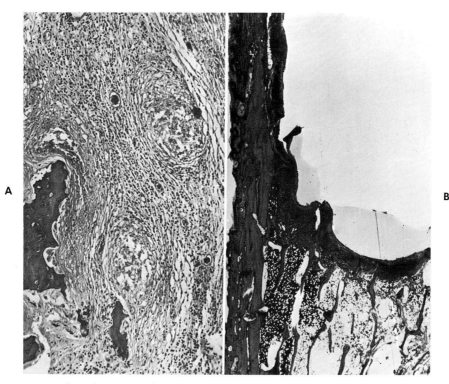

Fig. 40-25 Tuberculosis. **A,** Tuberculous granulation tissue surrounding small spicules of necrotic cancellous bone. **B,** Section from upper end of tibia of male adult showing cavity lined by narrow zone of tuberculous granulation tissue. In roentgenogram, lesion resembled giant cell tumor. At operation, cavity contained thin yellowish brown fluid and fibrin. Note subperiosteal bone formation overlying bony wall of tuberculous abscess. (**A,** ×125; AFIB 73801; **B,** ×10.)

periostitis. Usually, however, a given bone shows both lesions to a greater or lesser extent. When an affected long bone is split in its longitudinal axis, it is noted that the metaphyseal end of the diaphysis is irregular in outline and grayish white in color. Frequently, it contains gritty particles that are yellow or yellowish gray. Microscopic examination reveals fibrosis of the marrow spaces, which is accompanied by an infiltration with plasma cells, lymphocytes, and other forms of leukocytes (Fig. 40-26, *A*). The trabeculae are usually thin and irregularly placed, and many of them are fragmented. The growing cartilage is penetrated irregularly by blood vessels that are ensheathed in young connective tissue. The latter is infiltrated with inflammatory cells to some extent. It may be possible to demonstrate spirochetes throughout an area of involvement such as the one demonstrated in Fig. 40-26, *A*.

Periostitis occurring in congenital syphilis is readily observed in the roentgenogram, in which one or more shadows paralleling the cortex may be observed. Cross sections through the shaft of such a long bone reveal that excessive and rapid subperiosteal bone overgrowth has occurred (Fig. 40-26, *B*). The original cortex is usually thin and irregular, and the intertrabecular spaces of the recently formed subperiosteal bone are filled with edematous and mildly inflamed connective tissue (Fig. 40-26, *B*).

The pathologic changes in the bones of infants suffering from congenital syphilis probably result from several factors. Foremost among these is the localization of spirochetes, which seem to have the capacity of creating cell and tissue injury and at the same time stimulating mesenchymal cells, including osteoblasts, to proliferate excessively. Inflammatory and proliferative changes in blood vessels may give rise to some of the destructive changes that are seen in the ends of the long bones. It is probable that some of the skeletal alterations observed by the pathologist in fatal cases of congenital syphilis are manifestations of general and specific nutritional disturbances.

During the secondary stage of acquired

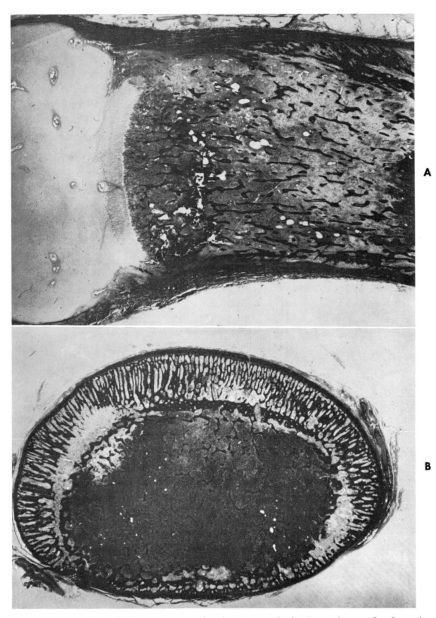

Fig. 40-26 Congenital syphilis. **A,** Longitudinal section of tibial epiphysis of infant showing irregularities in margins of growth zone, fibrosis of marrow spaces, and subperiosteal
bone overgrowth. Combined changes referred to as syphilitic osteochondritis. **B,** Cross
section of lower third of femoral shaft illustrating pronounced subperiosteal bone overgrowth of syphilitic periostitis. Connective tissue illustrated in lightly stained areas of this
section and section shown in **A** edematous and heavily infiltrated with plasma cells,
lymphocytes, and other forms of leukocytes. (**A** and **B,** ×10.)

syphilis, there may be circumscribed or more
or less generalized inflammation of the periosteum. This lesion is accompanied by tenderness and aching pains that are said to be more
severe at night.

In the early stages of bone involvement, the
periosteal tissues are hyperemic and infiltrated
with edema fluid. Lymphocytes, plasma cells,
and mononuclear leukocytes are present in excessive numbers. The cambium layer of the
periosteum is hyperplastic, and there may be
some new bone formation between the displaced periosteum and the surface of the
bone cortex. Such changes include all of the
morphologic characteristics of a true periostitis.
Later on, there may be extensive subperiosteal

bone overgrowth in the form of osteophytes and hyperostoses. These overgrowths may border on destructive lesions that are essentially gummas of bone (Fig. 40-27). The roentgenologic and gross appearances of such lesions may bear distinct resemblances to sclerosing forms of osteogenic sarcomas. The

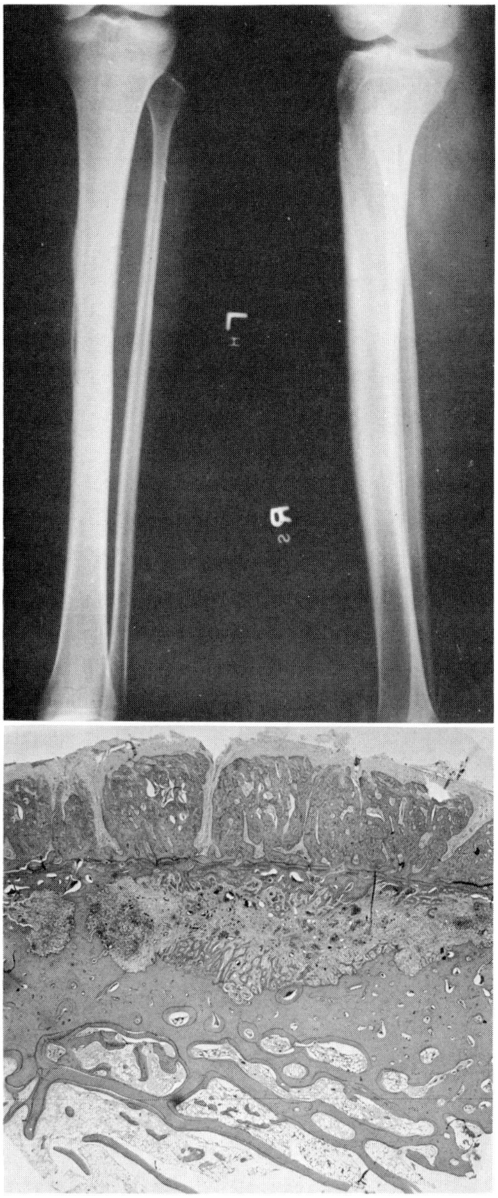

Fig. 40-27 Syphilitic periostitis. **A,** X-ray film disclosing periosteal elevation and irregular resorptive changes in underlying cortex of tibia. **B,** Transverse section of cortex in which marked subperiosteal bone formation evident. Underlying periosteal lesion is chronic granulomatous process which has led to considerable bone resorption.

need for a carefully made differential diagnosis in these cases is self-evident.

Superficially placed bones, including the anterior surface of the tibia, the clavicle, and the skull, represent the more frequent sites of syphilitic involvement. The lesions that occur in the flat bones of the skull are usually destructive in character and exhibit only slight to moderate degrees of marginal condensation or subperiosteal overgrowth. Despite the destructive nature of the lesions in the skull, it should be emphasized that syphilitic infections of bone induce changes that are basically proliferative in character, whereas tuberculous processes are essentially destructive.

Improvement in diagnostic and treatment methods for syphilis has greatly reduced the incidence of skeletal involvement. This is due to the fact that the bony lesions are among the later manifestations of the disease.

Actinomycosis. As a result of the tendency for actinomycosis to spread from a preexisting focus of infection, the ribs, sternum, and vertebrae may become involved in cases of pulmonary or abdominal infections. Likewise, the jaws may become infected by the extension of lesions in the soft tissue in the oral cavity. The bone lesion is essentially one of destruction, and multiple foci of suppuration leading into the sinus tracts are found on gross and microscopic examination.

Blastomycosis. Blastomycosis of bony structures may arise either from direct extension of established lesions in the soft tissue or from hematogenous dissemination. The former method is more common and occurs not infrequently as a result of dermal infections on the digits. The lesions in bone are destructive in character and resemble tuberculosis on both gross and microscopic examination.

DISORDERS RESULTING FROM FAULTY NUTRITION

In order that normal development, growth, and maintenance of the skeleton may be assured, the individual must ingest and assimilate adequate amounts of protein, fat, and carbohydrate. Also, as was noted previously (p. 1686), adequate ingestion and assimilation of calcium and phosphorus is essential. In addition, certain chemical agents known as vitamins are essential in the prevention and treatment of certain bone diseases. Specifically, in the instance of vitamin C deficiency, scurvy results and the skeletal tissues are predominately affected. Rickets is another disorder of the growing skeleton that results from imperfect nutrition and, in certain circumstances, from an inadequate supply of vitamin D.

Skeletal changes resulting from faulty nutrition are observed most frequently and in more characteristic patterns in infants and children. However, comparable bony changes may take place in adults who have been subjected to similar nutritional deficiencies.

Vitamin C deficiency

Scurvy is known to result from an inadequate supply of ascorbic or cevitamic acid (vitamin C).

It has been known for centuries that prolonged subsistence on diets from which fresh fruits, vegetables, milk, and meat were excluded would result in a disease picture that was characterized by anemia, swelling of the gums, loosening of the teeth, and hemorrhages into the skin, mucous membranes, periosteum, and joints. Scurvy was therefore regarded as a scourge to sailors. The curative power of fresh fruits and vegetables also has been recognized for a long time. It may seem appropriate, therefore, that ascorbic acid was the first of the vitamins to be prepared synthetically in the laboratory. However, the chemical formula of ascorbic acid was not determined until many years after the essential pathologic features of scurvy in man and animals had been described.[12, 68, 144]

These reports, together with more recent detailed studies, have provided a lucid account of the pathologic manifestations of scurvy in all its stages, including repair.[114, 141, 142]

Scurvy has been characterized by Follis[48] as a part of the overall manifestations of ascorbic acid deficiency in which certain specialized cells such as fibroblasts, osteoblasts, and odontoblasts fail to promote the deposition of their respective fibrous proteins—i.e., collagen, osteoid, and dentin. Although the precise mechanisms responsible for this failure have not been fully elucidated, it is believed that there is a close relationship between the ascorbic acid content of the tissues and alkaline phosphatase activity and that the latter may be involved in the elaboration of fibrous proteins in an important way.[48]

In any event, the characterization of scurvy as offered by Follis[48] enables one to understand many of the clinical manifestations of the disorder, as well as to predict the predominant sites of pathologic change.

Scurvy is more common in infants and young children during the stages when bone and connective tissues of all types are being formed at a rapid rate. Clinically, there is evidence of anemia and a tendency to bleed spontaneously or from trivial causes. The severely affected child is likely to assume a position of flexion and to lie very still because of the pain that results from any active or passive motion. The pain may be attributed to hemorrhages in muscles, beneath the periosteum, and into joints. In some instances, it is attributable to fractures through the rarefied bone at the metaphyseal ends of the diaphyses of the long bones.

The roentgenologic findings are reasonably characteristic (Fig. 40-28). Owing to the generalized osteoporosis, the shafts of the long bones and the bony epiphyses appear less dense than normal and possess a "ground glass" appearance. The metaphyseal ends of

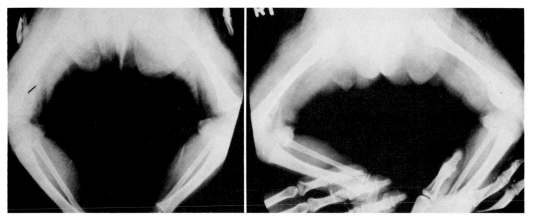

Fig. 40-28 Characteristic features of scurvy. **A,** At time of hospital admission. **B,** Six weeks after therapy had been initiated. Note pronounced ossification of subperiosteal hematomas surrounding lower portions of femurs in **B.**

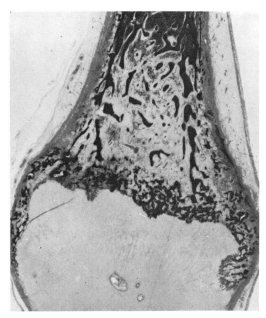

Fig. 40-29 Scurvy. Classic features of well-advanced scurvy in costochondral junction. Bone shows evidence of osteoporosis, and marrow spaces filled with loosely textured and edematous connective tissue in which some hemorrhage has occurred. Metaphyseal end of bone widened and made up of irregularly arranged spicules of heavily calcified matrix. Growth apparently has been more active at perichondrial margins of cartilage, resulting in pronounced cupping. (×10.)

the shafts, including the ribs, are markedly rarefied. Contrasted with this, the zones of provisional calcification are excessively dense. In the long bones, this density appears as a transverse line at the zone of junction between the epiphysis and shaft end. In the epiphyses, however, the dense shadow encircles the center of ossification and is referred to as a halo. These zones of relatively increased density are attributable to the heavily calcified and often fragmented spicules of calcified cartilage that are formed during the period of retarded longitudinal growth (Fig. 40-29). Displacement of the epiphysis as the result of fracture and separation also may be noted in the roentgenogram. Soft tissue swellings from subperiosteal or intra-articular hemorrhage may be apparent. During repair, the extent of the subperiosteal hemorrhage becomes vividly clear, since ossification begins peripherally beneath the displaced periosteum.

Pathologic examination of the skeletal parts in fatal cases of scurvy or of the bones of experimentally treated guinea pigs confirms the clinical and roentgenologic manifestations

mentioned. The bones are porous, and there is marked hemorrhage into the muscles and joints and beneath the periosteum. The entire shaft of a long bone may be encased in a blood clot that lies inside a displaced periosteal envelope. The periosteal separation is caused by the loosening and disruption of the collagenous attachments (Sharpey's fibrils) from the bone cortex. The epiphyses may be disconnected from the shafts because of fracture through the markedly atrophied metaphyseal zone. Recently acquired soft tissue wounds or bone fractures show little or no evidence of healing. When a costochondral junction or the end of a long bone is sectioned in a longitudinal plane, it is noted that the metaphyseal end of the shaft is exceedingly fragile and that the marrow tissue is pale gray or stained from extravasated blood. Instead of the sharp and even translucent blue zone of normal endochondral ossification, the chondro-osseous junction in scurvy is widened, uneven, and frequently concave in outline. Fine, granular particles of calcified cartilage that have a yellow color frequently are observed (Fig. 40-29). This condensation of calcareous material is responsible for the density observed in the roentgenogram.

Microscopic examination reveals little or no evidence of bone formation either beneath the periosteum or at the margins of the calcified cartilage spicules in the metaphyseal zone. Instead, there is an accumulation of spindle-shaped and branching cells that have the appearance of young fibroblasts. Such cells, embedded in a loosely textured and edematous groundwork, are responsible for the pallor of the marrow tissues near the bone end (Fig. 40-29). Evidence that these cells are osteoblasts is provided by noting their activity in repair. In controlled experiments in guinea pigs, these cells will deposit recognizable ground substance within a period of twenty-four hours after ascorbic acid has been supplied.

The interesting changes in teeth that are related to impairment in the formation of dentin and to loosening of the tooth from the alveolar bones have been well studied.[19]

Vitamin D deficiency

Rickets and osteomalacia. In his Harvey Lecture on the pathology of rickets, Park[113] reviewed the stages of investigation by which knowledge of the pathogenesis and pathology of rickets has been acquired. More recent coverage of rickets and osteomalacia has been provided by Harris[63] and Follis.[49]

Rickets, as well as osteomalacia, its counterpart in adults, has been defined as a skeletal disease in which there is a decreased concentration of bone mineral (hydroxyapatite) in the organic matrix of bone. In rickets, there is also a decreased concentration of mineral in the matrix of cartilage in the regions of endochondrial bone formation. Decreased amounts of bone salt in both rickets and osteomalacia have been demonstrated by chemical analysis and by histologic studies of appropriately prepared sections.

The etiology and pathogenesis of rickets and osteomalacia are somewhat complicated. However, the immediate cause of the deficient mineralization of skeletal tissues is believed to be a reduction in phosphate or calcium in the blood or, more correctly, a reduced calcium × phosphorous product.[63] A lowering of the serum values of phosphorus or calcium or of the calcium × phosphorous product may result from a number of circumstances operating singly or in concert. Such circumstances would include:

1 Disturbances in the absorption of calcium and/or phosphorus from the intestine. This could result from either a dietary lack of calcium and/or phosphorus or of vitamin D, or from interference with absorptive mechanisms.
2 Excessive excretion of calcium and/or phosphorus because of renal disorders of lactation.
3 Excessive need of calcium and phosphorus to mineralize rapidly forming bone matrix, e.g. healing scurvy or healing bone following the removal of parathyroid tumors.

Since the immediate cause of rickets or osteomalacia appears to be a reduction in the levels of phosphorus and/or calcium in the blood plasma, the restoration of the mineralizing process in bone and cartilage matrix to bring about repair will be dependent upon restoring the plasma values of calcium and phosphorus to their normal ranges. It is in this corrective process that the role of vitamin D in promoting absorption of calcium and phosphorus from the alimentary tract is so important and even dramatic.

The morphologic changes in rickets, in order of their development, are as follows:

1 A failure of calcification of the deepest layer of growing cartilage (provisional zone of calcification)

2 Failure of calcification of newly deposited osteoid matrix
3 Deformities resulting either from disturbances in the sequences of endochondral ossification or from bending of the softened bones

In the majority of instances, rickets becomes apparent between the fourth month and the third year of life. However, it may appear at any time up to closure of the epiphyses. In infants, the skull shows thickening of the frontal and parietal eminences (bossing) and flattening and thinning of the back of the skull (craniotabes). Thickenings of the costochondral junctions (rachitic beads) develop and may be associated with a depressed sternum and indentations of the thorax at the level of the insertion of the diaphragm. The epiphyseal ends of the long bones are noticeably enlarged, especially the lower radial (Fig. 40-30, *B*), lower femoral, and upper tibial epiphyses. In older children, there may be flattening of the feet, anterior bowing of the tibias, and knock-knee deformity (Fig. 40-30, *A*).

Roentgenographic examination reveals widening and thickening of the epiphysial cartilage plates between poorly calcified bone shafts and bony epiphyses (Fig. 40-30, *C*). In some cases, there is evidence of bending deformities and incomplete (greenstick) fractures.

In fatal cases examined at autopsy, in addition to the changes already mentioned, deformities of the vertebrae and pelvic bones may be found. Pronounced inward projection of the costochondral junctions is observed when the lungs are lifted from the pleural spaces. This is caused by the forces of inspiration upon the softened bone. Sectioning of the bone ends with a knife is often possible. When this is done, it is noted that the epiphyseal cartilage plates are widened and thickened and that the line of junction between cartilage and the metaphyseal end of the shaft is no longer regular and sharply demarcated.

The microscopic changes in rickets are of two types. One of these may be seen in any part of the bone, although it is usually most prominent in the cancellous and cortical bone at the ends of the shafts. The bone tissue that was formed and calcified prior to the onset of rickets stains normally. In properly decalcified sections stained with hematoxylin and eosin, this bone takes a reddish purple stain. In undecalcified tissues, it may be shown to contain bone salt. The calcified lamellae are surrounded by zones of homogeneous osteoid matrix that stain vividly pink or red with hematoxylin and eosin and, in appropriately prepared sections from undecalcified blocks, contain little or no mineral deposit. Varying degrees of fibrosis are present in the marrow tissues, and this may contain poorly arranged trabeculae of uncalcified osteoid. Thus, the osseous changes appear to be the result of the deposition of excessive amounts of uncalcified or poorly calcified matrix. In all probability, the bone salt is also withdrawn to a certain extent from the lamellae that were previously formed and calcified. These changes are also apparent in *osteomalacia*.[10, 23]

The other type of change is limited to rickets, since it arises from disturbances in the calcification of cartilage matrix and from

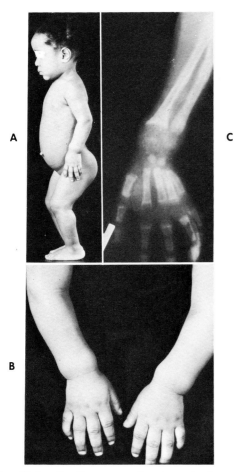

A

B

C

Fig. 40-30 Manifestations of rickets. **A,** Postural deformities, including protuberant abdomen and lordosis. **B,** Enlargement of wrists due to epiphyseal widening and thickening. **C,** Diminished bone density and widening and thickening of epiphyseal cartilage of radius and ulna.

abnormalities in the growth of cartilage cells. Under low-power magnification, one sees a thickened, widened, and markedly uneven epiphyseal cartilage plate that is irregularly penerated by branching blood vessels from the metaphyseal end of the shaft (Fig. 40-31). In the usual example of rickets in the infant or child, the histologic picture is too complicated to be readily interpreted. For this reason, it is necessary to refer to the progressive changes that occur in rats during the development of rickets and during repair.

The initial morphologic sign of rickets is the partial or complete absence of mineral deposit in the deepest layer of cartilage (provisional zone of calcification). In association with this change, the deepest cells in the cartilage columns fail to clear and degenerate, and there is no longer a regularly arranged ingrowth of capillaries from the marrow of the shaft. Cartilage cells continue to proliferate, however, and as a result the epiphyseal plate becomes thickened and widened. The cell columns become distorted, and irregular rounded and oval nests of cartilage cells are built up. Blood vessels of small or intermediate size grow in between these clumps of cartilage cells and give off irregular branches. This

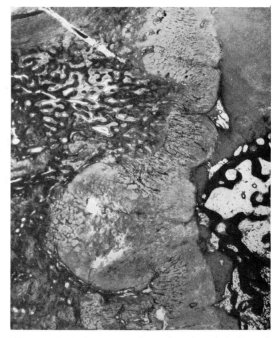

Fig. 40-31 Rickets. Greatly widened and thickened epiphyseal cartilage plate evident in this section from lower femoral epiphysis of child with advanced rickets. Blood vessel invasion of cartilage irregular, and great excess of uncalcified bone matrix has formed. (×10.)

vascular penetration is most irregular and is attended by the ingrowth of connective tissue from the endosteum. Thus, bone matrix that remains uncalcified is deposited irregularly throughout the distorted epiphyseal plate (Fig. 40-31).

Repair in the rachitic rat begins with the deposition of bone salt in the cartilage. At first, this is irregularly laid down well in advance of the distorted metaphyseal end of the shaft. Gradually, a new provisional zone of calcification is established, and the orderly sequence of cartilage cell proliferation, maturation, and degeneration is again evident. The excessive and imperfectly calcified osteoid is impregnated with bone salt, and subsequent to this it is gradually remodeled by lacunar absorption until the excess bone has been removed.

Vitamin D–resistant rickets (familial hypophosphatemia). A sex-linked dominant disorder, vitamin D–resistant rickets is clinically and pathologically similar to vitamin D–deficient rickets and osteomalacia. The chief difference is that the defective mineralization fails to respond to therapeutic doses of vitamin D. Although the nature of the genetic defect is not known, affected individuals display hypophosphatemia that may result from an increased renal phosphate clearance and defective reabsorption of phosphate by the renal tubules.

Effects of excessive doses of vitamin D. The results of excessive and prolonged administration of vitamin D have been studied in animals, and the unfavorable effects have been noted in man[135] (p. 517).

Vitamin A deficiency

In rats and certain other animals that have been studied, vitamin A deficiency brings about a suppression of all sequences of growth in the epiphyseal cartilage. The remodeling processes, by which bone is resorbed and rearranged into compact bone, cease. Appositional growth of subperiosteal bone continues, however, until inanition supervenes. These disturbances in bone may result in a disproportionate growth of bone and central nervous system and thus, by mechanical overcrowding of the brain and spinal cord, account for numerous neurologic disturbances.[143]

Effects of excessive doses of vitamin A. Excessive vitamin A administration leads to an acceleration of the sequences of growth that are retarded by inadequate amounts of the vitamin[143] (p. 516).

SKELETAL LESIONS ASSOCIATED WITH DISORDERS INVOLVING RETICULOENDOTHELIAL SYSTEM

A significant part of the so-called reticuloendothelial system is embodied in the soft

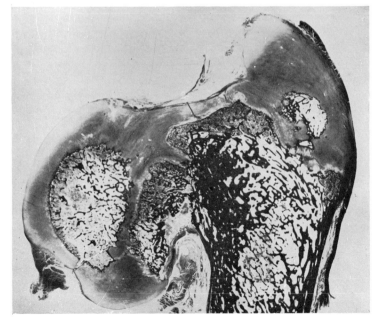

Fig. 40-32 Gaucher's disease. Pronounced deformity of head and neck of femur evident in this specimen from child. Cancellous spaces filled with Gaucher's cells.

tissues of the bony skeleton. Because of this relationship, the bones are affected in two disorders that may be designated as lipid-storage diseases (Gaucher's disease and Niemann-Pick disease) and in three other disorders (Hand-Schüller-Christian syndrome, eosinophilic granuloma, and Letterer-Siwe disease).

Gaucher's disease. In Gaucher's disease, the reticuloendothelial cells of the spleen, bone marrow, lymph nodes, and liver become hyperplastic and store excessive quantities of a cerebroside, kerasin, or a closely related cerebroglucoside (p. 1321).

The outstanding microscopic feature is the accumulation of Gaucher's cells—cells that are spherical or oval in shape and measure 20μ to 80μ in diameter (Figs. 31-25 to 31-27). The light-staining cytoplasm of these cells is abundant. The characteristic lacy or slightly foamy appearance is produced by delicate wavy striations. Gaucher's cells accumulate in clumps of alveolar nests. Their presence in large numbers in bone may lead to diffuse or patchy osteoporosis. In some cases, there are deformities of the femoral and humeral heads because of disturbances in endochondral ossification (Fig. 40-32). The vertebrae may undergo compression fractures as a result of the osteoporosis.

Niemann-Pick disease. A disorder in lipid metabolism, Niemann-Pick disease is a rare and usually rapidly fatal affliction of infancy (p. 1323). Accumulations of lipid-laden histiocytes (sphingomyelin) in the bone marrow may lead to generalized osteoporosis, with circumscribed foci of marked bone resorption.[28]

Hand-Schüller-Christian syndrome. The Hand-Schüller-Christian syndrome apparently has nothing in common with Gaucher's disease or Niemann-Pick disease. As a syndrome, the disturbance is characterized by the following:

1 Multiple, sharply circumscribed roentgenographic defects in the skull
2 Exophthalmos, which may be bilateral
3 Diabetes insipidus
4 Other pituitary signs, such as infantilism

The first reports of this syndrome were those by Hand[61, 62] (1893 and 1921). Schüller[124] in 1915 described the condition for the second time and attributed the symptoms to pituitary dysfunction. Christian[25, 26] in 1920 interpreted the defects in membranous bones, exophthalmos, and diabetes insipidus as an unusual syndrome of dyspituitarism.

The disorder occurs in children and young adults, and males are affected about twice as frequently as females. The most constant feature of the disease is the presence of one or more areas of bone destruction (Fig. 40-33). These are caused by accumulations of histiocytes that are filled with lipid. Usually, there is some degree of fibrosis, and the lesions often contain significant numbers of polymorpho-

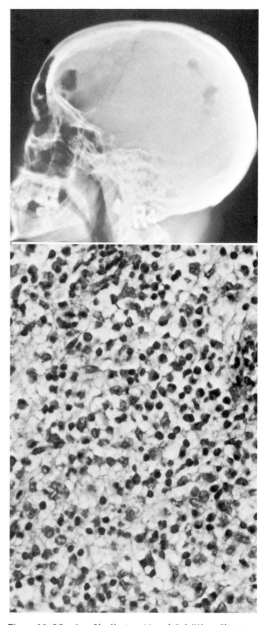

Fig. 40-33 A, Skull in Hand-Schüller-Christian syndrome. **B,** Tissue removed from one of lesions in skull. Histologically, lesion indistinguishable from eosinophilic granuloma (see Fig. 40-34).

nuclear leukocytes, eosinophils, plasma cells, and lymphocytes. With increasing age of the lesions, the fibroblasts increase and greater amounts of collagen are laid down. Under the polarizing microscope, the lipid is seen to be anisotropic in large part, and chemical analysis of the total lesion reveals a high content of cholesterol, cholesterol esters, and neutral fat. These destructive lesions may occur any place in the skeleton, but the bones of the cranium are affected in the majority of cases. When the lesions extend into the soft tissues of the orbit, exophthalmos develops. If the sella turcica is encroached upon, there may be signs of pituitary dysfunction, including diabetes insipidus. In other cases, deafness from involvement of the temporal bone or signs of increased intracranial tension may be noted.

It is apparent, therefore, that the complete clinical picture described by Hand, Schüller, and Christian is dependent upon the proper localization of the underlying xanthomatous lesion. For this reason, the disorder described by these observers should be designated a syndrome and not a disease. Other manifestations of the same fundamental disorder have been described by Snapper,[127] who employs the term *lipoid granulomatosis* of bone. Thannhauser and Magendantz[132] refer to the condition as *osseous xanthomata*, and in their classification they include it among the *primary essential xanthomatoses of the normocholesteremic type.*

Mallory,[103] while noting that information with respect to etiology was incomplete and inconclusive, raised doubt as to the propriety of grouping the syndrome described by Hand, Schüller, and Christian with Gaucher's disease and Niemann-Pick disease.

Eosinophilic granuloma of bone. A neoplastic-like lesion, eosinophilic granuloma of bone is a benign destructive process that begins in the marrow and usually affects but one bone (Fig. 40-34, *A*). Occasionally, there are multiple foci in one or more bones. The condition

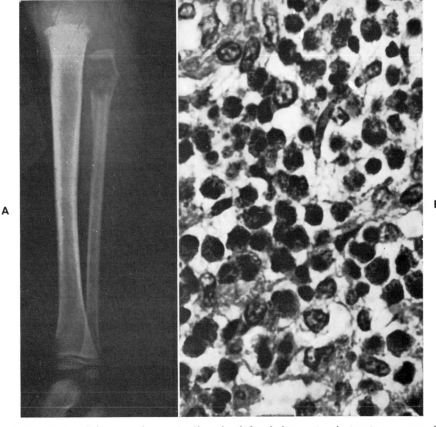

Fig. 40-34 Eosinophilic granuloma. **A,** Sharply defined destructive lesion in upper end of fibula. Lesion contained soft, friable tissue comprised mainly of eosinophils and lipid-laden histiocytes. **B,** Cytologic features. (**B,** ×950.)

occurs chiefly in children, but it may affect young adults. Microscopic examination of the soft, friable tissue comprising the lesion shows large numbers of eosinophils and less numerous mononuclear cells that contain granules, brownish pigment, and lipid-filled vacuoles (Fig. 40-34, B).

Some observers regard this lesion as a stage or a form of Hand-Schüller-Christian syndrome.[47, 57] Such an interpretation seems unavoidable as the many overlapping manifestations become evident in carefully studied patients.

Letterer-Siwe disease (nonlipid histiocytosis). A variety of names, including reticuloendotheliosis, reticulosis, and aleukemic monocytic leukemia, have been used to designate Letterer-Siwe disease, an obscure disorder of the reticuloendothelial system (p. 1323). In some cases, there are focal destructive lesions in bone that bear a considerable resemblance to the lesions of Hand-Schüller-Christian syndrome, and it is quite likely that the two processes are related[103] (p. 1325).

. . .

Although the etiology of Hand-Schüller-Christian syndrome, eosinophilic granuloma, and Letterer-Siwe disease has not been revealed and gaps remain in the understanding of pathogenetic sequences, there is convincing evidence that the three conditions are, as has been suggested,[47, 57, 103] related. Lichtenstein, in 1953, on the basis of a critical review of the literature, concluded that the three conditions ". . . are interrelated manifestations of a single malady."* He also proposed that the malady be given the broad general designation of *"histiocytosis X."* Subsequent studies[14, 91] have lent additional support to the premise of interrelationships.

Thus, it would appear that there is a disease complex which may justify the designation "histiocytosis X" that may express itself as solitary or multifocal lesions, *eosinophilic granuloma*. When bone involvement is more widespread and destructive and other tissues (especially the skin) are affected, the disease may fulfill the criteria of the *Hand-Schüller-Christian* syndrome. Finally, when the lesions are widespread and visceral involvement is in evidence, the process conforms with the disorder that has been designated *Letterer-Siwe disease*.

---

*From Lichtenstein, L.: Arch. Path. (Chicago) **56**:84-102, 1953.

SKELETAL CHANGES RELATED TO DYSFUNCTION OF ENDOCRINE GLANDS

Disturbances in the function of the pituitary, thyroid, and parathyroid glands are known to give rise to certain distinctive changes in the skeleton.

Pituitary gland
Hyperpituitarism

Gigantism. Diffuse hyperplasia or adenoma of the acidophilic cells of the anterior lobe of the hypophysis may induce marked symmetric overgrowth of the skeleton if the lesion develops before the epiphyses have closed. The excessive growth usually is most marked at the time of puberty and may continue on into young adulthood because of a concomitant delay in epiphyseal closure. In cases in which the disturbance continues into adult life, acromegalic characteristics may be superimposed upon the gigantism (p. 1422).

Acromegaly. Acromegaly is a chronic disease of adult life that is outwardly characterized by hypertrophic changes in the acral parts.[31] There are thickening and enlargement of the nose, lips, and tongue. The lower jaw is greatly enlarged and projects forward. The hands and feet are increased in their overall dimensions, especially in width. An increased growth of hair may be noted, especially in the female, in whom masculine traits may develop (p. 1421).

X-ray films reveal enlargement of the sella turcica. Enlargement of the bones of the skeleton also is evident, especially of the mandible, the thoracic cage, and the bones of the hands and feet. An arrowhead contour may be noted in the terminal phalanges of the fingers.

At autopsy, it is noted that there is enlargement of most or all of the internal organs and that, in addition, the connective tissues are hypertrophic. Gross and microscopic examinations of the costochondral junctions, vertebral bodies, and articular ends of the bones of the hands and feet reveal osseous overgrowths (Fig. 40-35). Although these enlargements may be due, in part, to generalized hyperplasia of the connective tissues, including periosteum, there is acceptable microscopic evidence that the process of endochondral ossification is reestablished in the ribs, vertebrae, and digits.[42, 137] Since it is known that the mandible continues to grow by endochondral ossification at the condyle, even in the normal mature subject, it is reasonable to assume that the influence of

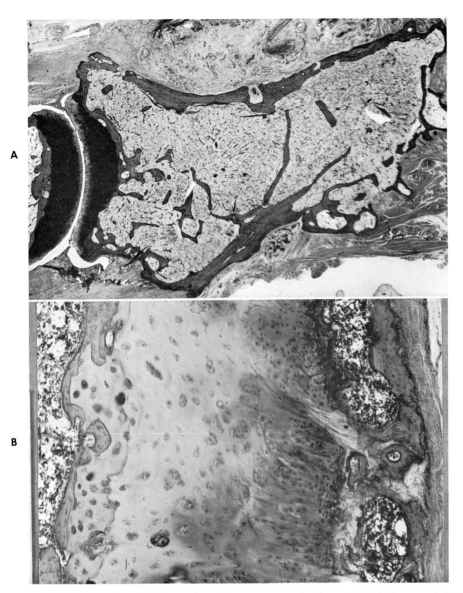

Fig. 40-35 Acromegaly (elderly man). **A,** Bony overgrowth of terminal phalanx and thickening of articular cartilage of terminal interphalangeal joint. **B,** Active endochondral ossification apparent in costochondral junction. (**A,** ×10; **B,** ×75; **A** and **B,** from Waine, H., Bennett, G. A., and Bauer, W.: Amer. J. Med. Sci. **209:**671-687, 1945.)

increased growth hormone in the acromegalic subject will be disproportionately great at this site. Such a relationship may explain the pronounced and constant overgrowth of this particular bone in acromegaly.

Cushing's syndrome. In 1932, Cushing[30] described a clinical condition characterized by painful adiposity of the face, neck, and trunk, hirsutism, sexual dystrophy, hypertension, striations in the skin of the abdomen, and osteoporosis. This condition, known as *Cushing's syndrome,* was thought at first to result

from adenomas of the chromophil cells of the pituitary gland, but it has since been shown that other endocrine disturbances are involved in the majority of cases (pp. 1427 and 1476). The osteoporosis associated with the syndrome is especially prominent in the spine, leading to compression fractures and deformity, and in the ribs, where fractures also may occur. Repair of such fractures has been considered to be abnormal and to resemble the reparative changes in fractures induced in experimental animals being treated with cortisone.[126]

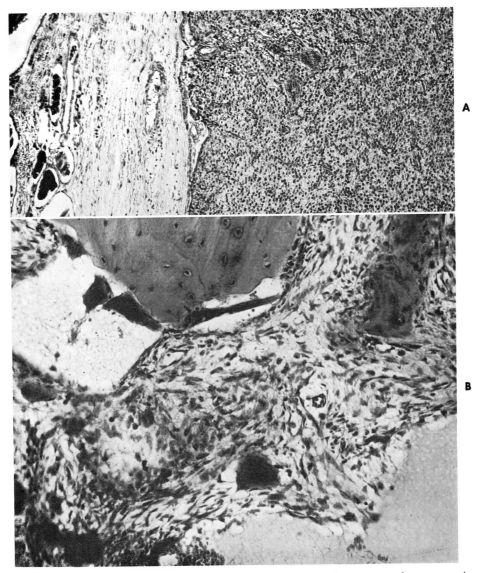

Fig. 40-36 Adenoma of parathyroid gland. **A,** Section through junction of tumor and capsule of thyroid gland. **B,** Resorptive changes in bone, fibrosis of marrow spaces, and multiple small cysts in biopsy material from same patient.

Hypopituitarism

Pituitary dwarfism. Pituitary deficiency leading to dwarfism may result from hypoplasia of the anterior lobe of the pituitary gland or from its destruction by a tumor such as a craniopharyngioma. In dwarfism of this origin, the growth of both cartilage and bone is arrested. The epiphyseal cartilage persists, but a compact layer of bone is formed at the metaphyseal end of the shaft. This separates the diaphysis from the epiphysis, which may remain open for excessively long periods of time (p. 1424).

Thyroid and parathyroid glands

The roles played by the hormones produced by the thyroid and parathyroid glands in calcium and phosphorus metabolism are of tremendous importance. These roles have been summarized by Howard and Thomas[70] and by Foster.[50]

Briefly stated, it appears that calcium homeostasis is dependent, to a large extent, on the maintenance of normal function of the parathyroid and thyroid glands. Fluctuation in hormone production of either of the glands produces an effect on calcium homeostasis and this, in turn, may result in changes in the skeletal tissues. An excess of thyroid hormone induces an increase in the excretion of both calcium and phosphorus. An excess of parathyroid hormone results in an increased excretion of calcium and phosphorus as well as in an elevation of serum calcium and, unless renal insufficiency is also present, a lowering of the serum phosphorus. The role or roles of calcitonin, which is secreted by the thyroid gland and the ultimobronchial bodies,[50] have not been fully determined.[64] It is known to have a calcium-regulating role, which may result from controlling influences upon bone resorption or from interference with the action of parathyroid hormone.

Hyperthyroidism

In long-standing hyperthyroidism, there may be roentgenologic and morphologic evidence of diffuse osteoporosis.[13, 70] The osseous changes are secondary to a marked increase in the excretion of calcium and phosphorus via the kidney and intestine. It is probable that the actual bone change is the result of increased lacunar absorption by osteoclasts (p. 1436).

Hypothyroidism

Cretinism results from a diminution or absence of thyroid secretion in childhood. The skeleton grows at a slower rate than normal, and the bones may appear excessively dense in the roentgenogram. The epiphyses close at an early age. In addition to retarded growth, the cretin is slow mentally and exhibits a dry, thickened skin, a broad and bloated-appearing face, and a thick-lipped mouth from which the tongue may protrude.

In the adult, a deficiency in thyroid secretion results in **myxedema.** The patient may show a pronounced diminution in calcium and phosphorus excretion, and in some patients it is possible to demonstrate an increased density of bone by roentgenologic examination (p. 1442).

Hyperparathyroidism

Increased functional activity of the parathyroid glands may result from either "primary hyperparathyroidism" or "secondary hyperparathyroidism."[5, 6]

"**Primary hyperparathyroidism.**" The term "primary hyperparathyroidism" is used to imply that more parathyroid hormone is produced than is needed. The excessive secretion results, in most instances, from an adenoma of one or more glands (Fig. 40-36, *A*). Less frequently, the excess is produced by hyperplasia of all glands or, in rare instances, by carcinoma.

Under the influence of excess parathormone, a disturbance in calcium and phosphorus metabolism results. This is characterized by an increased excretion of phosphorus and calcium and by a lowering of the serum phosphorus (3.1 mg per 100 ml or lower) and an elevation of the serum calcium (12.5 mg to 18 mg per 100 ml). In patients in whom this physiologic disturbance is severe and prolonged, osseous changes result.

The skeletal lesions may be slight, consisting only of generalized osteoporosis, or they may be marked, having the characteristics of *osteitis fibrosa cystica generalisata*. The latter is, however, only an exaggeration of the former process, and in either case the resorptive changes in bone probably are initiated by the biochemical disturbance.

Microscopic examination of the bones reveals fibrosis of the marrow spaces, together with increased lacunar absorption of the lamellae by osteoclasts (Fig. 40-36, *B*). It is apparent in the sections that both matrix and bone salt are removed simultaneously. There may be small collections of fluid in the fibrous tissues of the marrow (microscopic cysts), or, in severely affected bones, there may be well-defined cysts that are visible grossly as well as microscopically. In instances in which the disease has been present for a long time, the bones may be deformed as a result of pathologic fractures. Deformity also may result from expansions around cysts and fibrocellular lesions *(brown tumor)* that bear a resemblance to giant cell tumors.

In bone biopsies taken in series beginning at the time of removal of the adenoma, it is apparent that reparative changes may take place rapidly (Fig. 40-37). There is a diminution in the number of osteoclasts and in the cellularity of the fibrous tissue in the marrow spaces within one week after the adenoma has been extirpated. By the end of the second week, one sees the deposition of new osseous tissue, which calcifies. After a few months, the bones may return to normal. Well-formed cysts in bone remain unless they are opened or otherwise traumatized (p. 1455).

"**Secondary hyperparathyroidism.**" The term "secondary hyperparathyroidism" has been employed to designate those conditions in which more parathormone is produced

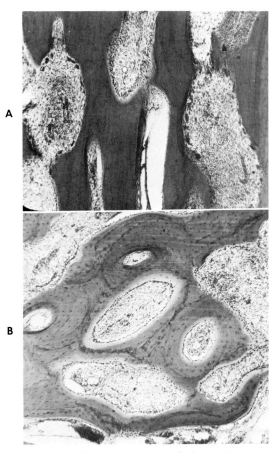

Fig. 40-37 Changes in cortex of tibia in "primary hyperparathyroidism." **A,** Biopsy at time parathyroid adenoma removed. **B,** Biopsy one week later. Diminished cellular activity indicative of bone resorption and increased osteoid production clearly evident in specimen shown in **B.**

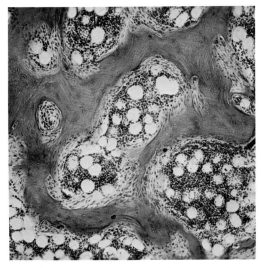

Fig. 40-38 Bone resorption and fibrosis of marrow spaces in long-standing renal insufficiency and "secondary hyperparathyroidism."

than normal but in which the excess is needed for some compensatory purpose. The excess parathormone production is usually attended by hyperplasia of all parathyroid glands.

At least two examples of "secondary hyperparathyroidism" may be cited: rickets or osteomalacia and renal insufficiency. The former needs no further comment at this time.

"Secondary hyperparathyroidism" associated with renal insufficiency also is spoken of as *renal rickets* or *renal osteitis fibrosa cystica*.[4, 11, 36, 51] The renal impairment leads to hyperphosphatemia, acidosis, and hyperplasia of the parathyroid glands. As a result of the latter two changes, the bones undergo pronounced lacunar resorption that is strikingly similar to that seen in "primary hyperparathyroidism" (Fig. 40-38). In the young subject, there may be disturbances in endochondral ossification that, on roentgenologic examination, may suggest rickets. Microscopically, however, there may be little, if any, resemblance to true rickets (p. 807).

Hypoparathyroidism

As a result of inadvertent surgical removal of parathyroid glands, a clinical condition referred to as hypoparathyroidism may result. The usual manifestations are those of *tetany,* accompanied by a lowering of serum calcium concentration and a rise in serum phosphorus.

In rare instances, the symptoms, signs, and biochemical abnormalities of hypoparathyroidism become manifest without any apparent cause: *idiopathic hypoparathyroidism.* Less frequently, disorders designated as *familial pseudohypoparathyroidism* have been observed. In this heritable condition, chemical abnormalities of hypoparathyroidism in the presence of normal or hyperplastic parathyroid tissue have been described.

PAGET'S DISEASE OF BONE (OSTEITIS DEFORMANS)

Paget's disease, the specific skeletal disease entity of older people (usually occurring in those 40 years of age or older), was described by Sir James Paget in 1877.[112] In the many years that have since elapsed, the disorder has been carefully and thoughtfully studied, and its clinical and pathologic manifestations have been recorded with painstaking care by numerous observers.[6, 74, 123] Despite this amount of sustained attention, it must be admitted that little is known of the cause or essential nature of the disease.

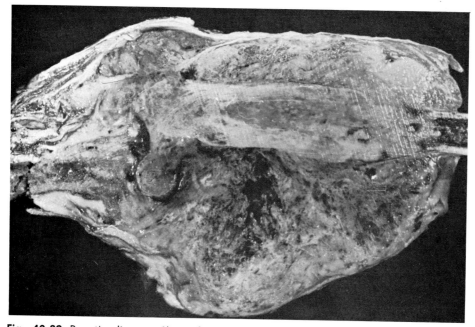

Fig. 40-39 Paget's disease. Slice of amputated femur showing sarcoma arising from bone that bears characteristic changes of osteitis deformans.

Osteitis deformans, in its fully developed form, is an uncommon disease. However, it is readily recognized. The patient's head is usually enlarged, and the presenting complaints often include a statement to the effect that the hat size has been increasing. The weight-bearing portions of the skeleton usually are deformed, as a result of which the patient may walk with a waddling gait. In the typical patient, the tibias show anterior bending, the femora are bowed outward, and the spinal column is shortened and curved forward. In addition, the roentgenograms reveal that the femoral necks have shifted into a horizontal position in relation to the shafts of these bones. Because of the shortened stature and poor postural alignment, the arms of the patient seem disproportionately long.

The roentgenologic manifestations of Paget's disease are reasonably characteristic. In the early stages, the osseous tissues appear excessively porous. Later, the affected bones become thickened and dense, and the marrow cavities may be partially or completely obliterated. In most examples there are coarsening and interweaving of the trabecular structures (Fig. 40-39). A noteworthy roentgenographic feature of Paget's disease is the persistence of normal or near-normal osseous structure in the fibulas, even in those patients in whom the weight-bearing tibias are markedly altered. In most instances, the

arteries in the lower extremities are clearly seen because of excessive calcification.

Many patients complain of tenderness and aching pain in the affected bones, especially on bearing weight. In some instances, however, the affected subject seeks medical care because of the severe pain, of recent onset, and an attendant swelling of the part. Such symptoms and signs may arise because of the development of a sarcoma in a bone that was previously affected by Paget's disease (Fig. 40-39).

The frequency with which Paget's disease is followed by sarcoma of bone (approximately 1% of the cases) has been commented upon frequently.[118] It is worthy of note that two of the five patients originally described by Paget developed osseous neoplasms. In my experience, this relationship has been strikingly apparent. Autopsy on the bodies of four persons with known Paget's disease disclosed malignant tumors in the affected skeletal parts. In one, there were two malignant tumors that appeared to have arisen separately.

Among the various skeletal diseases, few give rise to pathologic changes that are as characteristic as the alterations noted in Paget's disease. The affected skull is greatly thickened in the usual case, and the diploë is partially or completely obliterated. Despite the pronounced thickening, the calvaria cuts

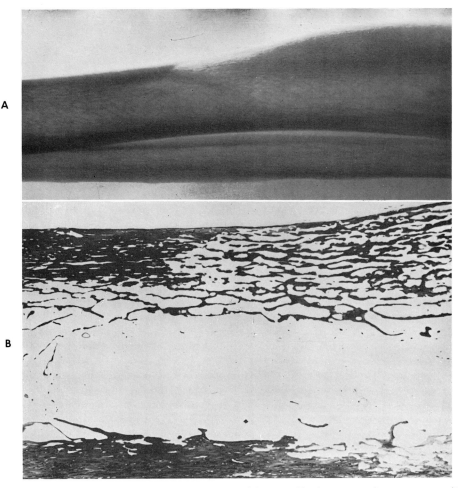

Fig. 40-40 Paget's disease. Roentgenogram and large celloidin section from corresponding areas reveal widening of tibial cortex and coarsening of trabecular structures in manner characteristic of Paget's disease. Note sharp boundary between affected and normal portions of bone.

readily with a saw, and it is often possible to break and crumble fragments of the poorly knit bone. When the brain has been removed, it may be noted that the fossae in the base of the cranial vault are shallow and that the bone underlying them also is affected. The external and internal bone surfaces, as well as the surfaces made by sectioning, are often pink from the pronounced vascularity. In some patients in whom the process has been present for longer periods, the thickened bone may be excessively dense and hard.

In the long bones, in addition to the changes already mentioned, there may be bowing deformities. In some instance, cortical fractures are observed. These extend into or through the cortex on the convex surface of the deformed bone. Occasionally, fibrous tissue-filled clefts are noted on gross examination, and, in some instances, these have undergone cystic changes or show evidence of old hemorrhage.

Recently affected long bones may show sharp lines of demarcation between the diseased portions and the normal cortex (Fig. 40-40). This feature indicates that Paget's disease begins in a focal area and spreads peripherally until the entire bone has become involved.

The microscopic changes in osteitis deformans are highly characteristic, provided the blocks of tissue are not excessively decalcified. Prolonged treatment with acid destroys the basophilic properties of the cement lines and otherwise obliterates certain marks and patterns that are significant to the morphologist. In properly prepared hematoxylin-eosin–stained sections, one notes a highly charac-

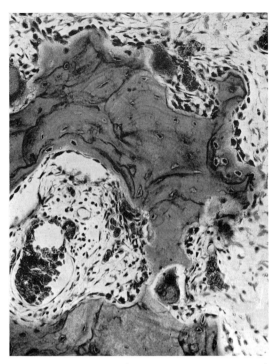

Fig. 40-41 Paget's disease. Mosaic pattern of diseased bone caused by irregular cement lines and scalloped osseous margins. Marrow spaces filled with vascular and loosely textured fibrous tissue. (×180.)

teristic or, in some cases, diagnostic mosaic pattern to the osseous tissues. In long bones, this is seen best in sections taken crosswise to the long axis, whereas in the skull it is usually well marked in any plane of sectioning. This difference may be explained by noting that the initial destructive process in Paget's disease follows the longitudinally placed haversian channels (Fig. 40-40, *B*) and that for considerable periods of time some parts of the original haversian lamellae may persist.

The mosaic pattern of Paget's disease may be attributed to two characteristics: the irregular and curved cement lines within the bony tissues and the irregular notches and depressions on the surface of the spicules. The latter are caused by pronounced osteoclastic absorption (Fig. 40-41). These structural features are caused by the simultaneous resorption of old and fully calcified bone and deposition of new osteoid layers that calcify in a normal fashion. Apparently, the resorptive process is carried to a certain point and ceases. In time, new bone is formed within this depression, and a cement line remains to mark the point of apposition of new bone upon the old. Later, resorptive changes again

occur, so that the architecture of a given area is further disturbed. In all probability, this "patchwork" type of bone has a lessened capacity to bear stress and strain, and this forms a basis for the ensuing deformity.

In addition to the disturbed architecture of the bony tissue, fibrosis and increased vascularity of the intertrabecular spaces are noted (Fig. 40-41).

It would seem appropriate to regard Paget's disease as a disorder of bone maintenance in which there occur, simultaneously, a pronounced resorptive process and an accelerated formative activity. In early cases, the former disturbance overshadows the latter mechanism, whereas the reverse is true in more advanced disease.

Attempts have been made to measure the rate of bone formation in Paget's disease. One such study, using tetracycline as markers, showed that the daily rate of bone formation in the "porotic" phase of Paget's disease was significantly greater than in normal bone and that the accelerated rate was even greater in the "sclerotic" phase of Paget's disease.[87] Insofar as can be determined, the osteoblasts in Paget's disease function as normal cells.[87]

The basis of the relationship between Paget's disease and bone sarcoma has not been established. It seems probable, however, that the long-continued excitation of the bone-forming cells, expressed in unnatural proliferative activity, may lead to unrestrained neoplastic growth.

SECONDARY (PULMONARY) HYPERTROPHIC OSTEOARTHROPATHY

In association with congenital heart disease, as well as with certain other intrathoracic lesions affecting the heart, lungs, and mediastinum or the vascular system to the extremities, there may be clubbing of the fingers and toes. Usually, the bulbous enlargement of the terminal ends of the digits is accompanied by cyanosis and curving of the nails. Microscopic examination of these tissues usually is disappointing, and one must infer that the swelling is caused by hyperemia or soft tissue edema or both. Occasionally, small periosteal overgrowths of bone are seen about the terminal phalanges.

Some patients with digital clubbing complain of aches and pains in the small and large joints of the extremities, and, less frequently, of bone tenderness. Roentgenologic examination of the extremities of these patients may show subperiosteal bony thicken-

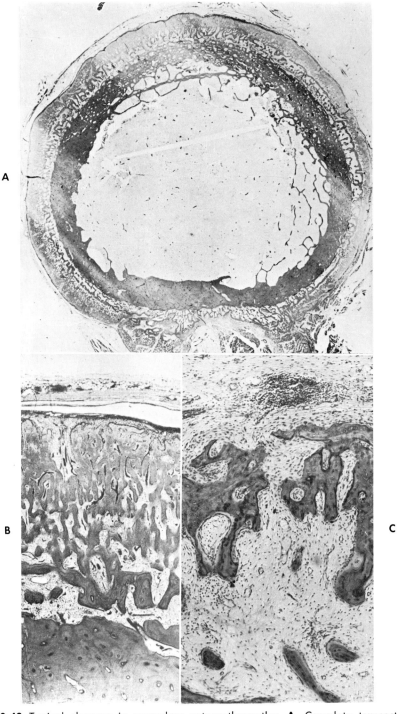

Fig. 40-42 Typical changes in secondary osteoarthropathy. **A,** Complete transection of femur. **B** and **C,** Subperiosteal bone overgrowth and mild inflammatory changes of lesion in greater detail.

ing. Microscopic examination reveals a productive and mildly inflammatory periosteal reaction (Fig. 40-42). At times, the subperiosteal bone overgrowth is very marked and consists of more than one layer of added bone that may have resulted from periodic exacerbations[52] (Fig. 40-42, *A*).

The underlying cause of these changes is not clearly understood. However, it appears likely that any disturbance in circulation may produce the digital clubbing. The hypertrophic osseous changes, however, may require some added "toxic" factor for their development. The latter change is usually, if not always, associated with disease processes in which inflammatory and degenerative changes are superimposed upon disturbances in circulation. Bronchogenic carcinoma, bronchiectasis, and other forms of suppuration in the lungs are among the foremost of the underlying lesions.[136]

CYSTS
Solitary or unicameral bone cyst

Solitary or unicameral bone cyst is a disorder of unknown etiology that usually

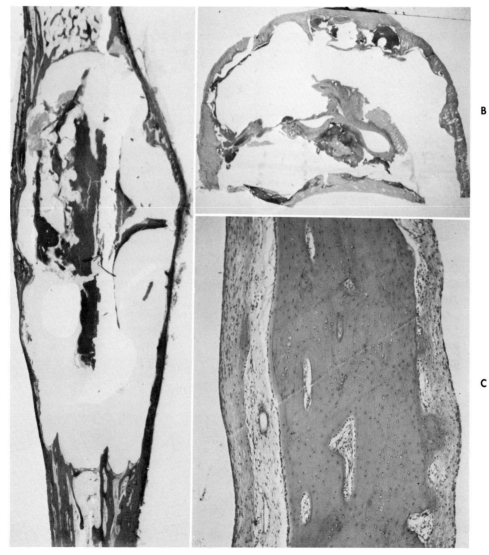

Fig. 40-43 Unicameral bone cyst. **A,** Intact cyst included in longitudinal section of bone. Cortex markedly reduced in thickness and bone shaft widened. **B,** Cross section illustrating fibrous tissue septa that partially divide such cysts. **C,** Thin bony wall of cyst with fibrous connective tissue lining on left and proliferative changes in subperiosteal layer on exterior surface of expanded bone on right.

manifests itself in childhood or adolescence. The distal ends of the shafts of long bones are the commonest sites of occurrence, and the upper portion of the humeral shaft is the area of involvement in about half of the cases.[78]

The lesion is usually of moderate or large size when its presence is first detected. Attention is drawn to the lesion in the majority of instances because of pathologic fracture. Occasionally, however, either pain or swelling is noted before the weakened bone is broken.

Anatomically, the lesion is comprised of a cyst cavity filled with amber-colored or blood-stained fluid. The external portion of the wall of the cyst is formed of thinned and expanded cortical bone. This is lined, in most specimens, by a smooth, glistening fibrous membrane that is tightly adherent to the bony surfaces (Fig. 40-43). In some examples, however, the cavity contains a considerable amount of tough and edematous connective tissue between the cystic space and the bony wall.

Operative intervention, including curettage and packing of the cavity with bone chips, usually results in obliteration of the cavity. Healing may occur following fracture. The healing of such lesions results from formation of granulation tissue that subsequently ossifies.

Aneurysmal bone cyst

Aneurysmal bone cyst is encountered most frequently in young adults. It may, however, occur in children or in adults. Although any part of the skeleton may be involved, the lesions occur most frequently at the metaphyseal ends of long bones or in vertebrae, including their neural arches and spinous processes.[34] Pain and swelling are the predominant symptoms. On roentgenologic examination, the characteristic features are bone expansion and rarefaction. Usually, the cystlike lesion is sharply localized and eccentrically placed and presents a ballooned-out deformity that can be distinguished, in most instances, from unicameral bone cyst and giant cell tumor.

When an aneurysmal bone cyst is opened at operation, the surgeon is usually confronted with pronounced bleeding from the vascular clefts and sinusoids within the dark brown spongelike tissue mass. Histologic examination of the specimen shows variable patterns. In the more solid areas, the loosely arranged connective tissue components embrace numerous giant cells that are similar to the multinucleated cells of a giant cell tumor. Phagocytes containing hemosiderin pigment may be present in abundance. In the more loosely textured portions, the tissue contains irregular and intercommunicating clefts that can be identified as vascular sinusoids. The bone from the osseous wall surrounding the lesion is characteristically thin, but there may be extensive new subperiosteal bone formation indicative of a reparative response to the expanding centrally placed soft tissue lesion.

The essential nature of aneurysmal bone cyst has not been ascertained, although it is generally agreed that the lesion is a distinct clinical and pathologic entity that is to be distinguished from such lesions as unicameral bone cyst, giant cell tumors, and other circumscribed lesions of bone that result in cyst-like changes in the roentgenogram. Lichtenstein, on the basis of his observations involving fifty cases of aneurysmal bone cyst, believes that the condition results ". . . from some persistent local alteration in hemodynamics leading to increased venous pressure and the subsequent development . . . of a dilated and engorged vascular bed within the transformed bone area."*

FIBROUS DYSPLASIA OF BONE

Opinion has varied with respect to nomenclature and interpretation of a number of skeletal disorders whose dominant pathologic manifestations are bone resorption, fibrosis of the marrow spaces, and substitution of poorly formed and unorderly arranged cancellous trabeculae for the original cancellous and cortical bone. In fact, there was at one time a tendency to group together a number of solitary lesions of bone, including unicameral bone cyst,[78] nonosteogenic fibroma of bone,[79] and ossifying fibroma of bone (including the variant designated fibrous osteoma of the jaw[116]), as examples of *monostotic fibrous dysplasia,* thus indicating a relationship between these lesions and *polyostotic fibrous dysplasia of bone.*

Polyostotic fibrous dysplasia

Information now available suggests that the term polyostotic fibrous dysplasia should be employed to designate exclusively the disorder described as *osteodystrophy fibrosa* by McCune and Bruch,[98] as *"syndrome charac-*

---

*From Lichtenstein, L.: J. Bone Joint Surg. **39-A:** 873-882, 1957.

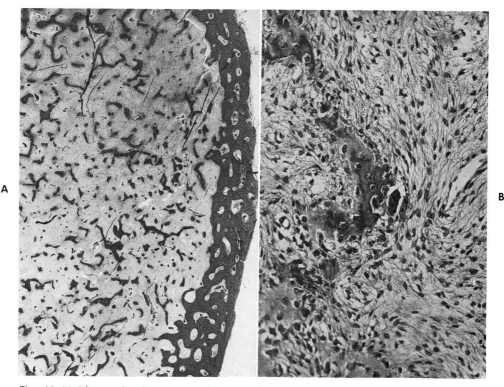

Fig. 40-44 Fibrous dysplasia. **A,** Evidence of abundant bone formation (narrow, irregular, and otherwise imperfectly formed spicules). Remainder of tissue comprised of moderately cellular and moderately vascular fibrous elements. **B,** Loosely textured fibrous connective tissue, containing occasional osseous spicules or small calcareous particles, comprising destructive lesion. (**A,** ×10; **B,** ×183.)

terized by osteitis fibrosa disseminata, areas of pigmentation and endocrine dysfunction with precocious puberty in females" by Albright et al.[9] (Albright's syndrome), as *fibrous dysplasia of bone* by Lichtenstein and Jaffe,[92] and subsequently as *polyostotic fibrous dysplasia (osteitis fibrosa disseminata)* by Albright and Reifenstein.[6]

Polyostotic fibrous dysplasia represents a bizarre syndrome in which any or all of the following triad of abnormalities may be present in lesser or greater degree:

1 Bone lesions that have a tendency to be unilateral in distribution
2 Nonelevated areas of brown pigmentation of skin (café-au-lait patches) that tend to be on the same side as the bone lesions
3 Endocrine disturbances affecting growth and development and inducing precocious puberty in young female patients

On radiologic examination, the skeletal abnormalities are spotty in distribution and vary markedly in appearance. Frequently, a single lesion is represented by a fusiform expansion of the shaft of a long bone. The affected part merges imperceptibly into the adjacent normal segments and presents a "ground glass" appearance, with little or no demarcation between cortex and medulla. Less commonly, the osseous lesion has the appearance of a cyst in the roentgenogram, but in such instances the margins of the lesion are not sharply drawn. As a result of the resorptive process, pathologic fractures are prone to occur, and the x-ray film may reveal marked deformities resulting from old or recent injuries.

Gross examination of an involved area of bone reveals widening of the shaft, thinning of the cortex, and replacement of the medulla with tough, rubbery connective tissue containing irregularly placed bone spicules. Occasionally, cystic spaces are incorporated. Microscopic sections when viewed with low magnification may reveal patterns of bone structure that are highly characteristic (Fig. 40-44, *A*). The cortex is thin and contains uneven and enlarged haversian canals. The inner portion of the expanded bone is composed of moderately cellular and loosely textured fibrous connective tissue (Fig. 40-44, *B*) which encloses poorly formed spicules of bone that exhibit both formative and resorptive changes. Usually, the irregularly arranged cancellous bone contains numerous individual trabeculae that have curved or sickle-shaped configurations[17, 120] (Fig. 40-44, *A*).

Microscopic sections of the dermal lesions usually show no abnormality other than excessive melanin pigment. These dermal lesions have been studied and compared with melanotic macules in neurofibromatosis.[15]

The basis for the endocrine disturbances and an explanation of the different expressions of these disturbances in the two sexes, although subjected to considerable speculation,[6] remain unsolved.

Monostotic fibrous dysplasia

A number of authors, in recording their observations on fibrous dysplasia of bone, have included cases with solitary or monostotic lesions.[65, 92, 120, 122] Schlumberger,[122] in describing his material, suggested that the monostotic and polyostotic types of bone lesions may be unrelated etiologically. Others,[65] while failing to find evidence of a monostotic lesion becoming polyostotic in later years, have considered that the osseous changes represent the same biologic process.

It is of some interest that in the detailed study of the case material at the Massachusetts General Hospital, the analysis was based on thirty-seven examples of polyostotic fibrous dysplasia and thirteen examples of monostotic fibrous dysplasia.[65] Of the latter group, only one lesion involved a long bone of the extremities, the other lesions being distributed in the skull, ribs, and vertebrae. Despite the observed differences, it appears that the pathologic entity known as fibrous dysplasia may be manifested in either a polyostotic or a monostotic form. The fundamental nature of the osseous lesion, in either form of the disorder, remains obscure, although Reed[120] concludes that the bone changes can be attributed to an arrest of bone maturation at the "woven bone" stage.

NEOPLASMS

As has been noted, the fully developed skeleton is formed of highly differentiated forms of mesoblastic tissues, including bone, cartilage, and connective tissue. In its development, primitive mesenchymal tissues are laid down temporarily. These are soon removed and replaced, in the remodeling processes of skeletal growth, by other mesenchymal elements to form the more durable bony and cartilaginous structures of the adult skeleton.

It is necessary to keep these facts in mind in order to understand, even partially, the many varieties of tumors that arise in the osseous parts of the body. In addition, it is necessary to recall that other forms of tissues are incorporated in the developing and mature bony parts. These tissues, which include vascular structures, hematopoietic elements, and nerves, also give rise to neoplasms of many kinds. Finally, it should be remembered that, in addition to primary neoplasms developing from the many types of tissue comprising bone, tumors of skeletal parts may arise in conjunction with preexisting lesions— i.e., Paget's disease or fibrous dysplasia after radiation,[65] from tumors in adjacent tissues invading bone, and from tumors in distant organs metastasizing to bone.

Numerous attempts have been made to formulate a classification of skeletal system tumors that is sufficiently inclusive to accommodate the various histologic types that are encountered and at the same time is restrictive enough to be comprehended by the student and readily used and understood by the surgeon and pathologist. This problem was reviewed in 1939 by Ewing,[45] who formulated a revised classification for the Registry of Bone Sarcoma of the American College of Surgeons. Ewing's report includes a discussion of the classification employed by Geschickter and Copeland[53] in 1930. More recently, on the basis of studies involving large series of cases,[32, 76] additional criteria have been put forward necessitating modifications in Ewing's classification.

The present discussion is organized around the entities listed in the classification presented in Table 40-1.

Fibrogenic neoplasms

Fibrous cortical defect. A frequently observed lesion, fibrous cortical defect is discovered, in most instances, by the roentgenologist since, in itself, it is unlikely to produce symptoms. The neoplasm occurs most commonly in children 4 to 8 years of age, and its incidence in males is about twice that in females. It is usually solitary but may appear as multiple or even bilaterally symmetrical defects. Characteristically, it appears in the expanded portion of the shaft on the metaphyseal side of the epiph-

Table 40-1 Classification of neoplasms of bone

| Histologic type | Behavior* | |
	Benign	Malignant
Fibrogenic	Fibrous cortical defect Nonossifying fibroma	Fibrosarcoma
Chondrogenic	Osteochondroma Chondroblastoma Chondromyxoid fibroma Chondroma	Chondrosarcoma, primary Chondrosarcoma, secondary
Osteogenic†	Osteoma Osteoid osteoma Benign osteoblastoma	Osteogenic sarcoma Parosteal osteogenic sarcoma
Vascular tissues	Hemangioma	Hemangioendothelioma
Unknown origin	Giant cell tumor	Malignant giant cell tumor Ewing's sarcoma "Adamantinoma"
Hematopoietic tissue		Myeloma Reticulum cell sarcoma Lymphoma Leukemia
Miscellaneous (a) Lipogenic (b) Notochordal	Lipoma	Liposarcoma Chordoma
Metastatic neoplasms		Secondary carcinomas Secondary sarcomas

*In most instances a tumor of a histologic type originates and subsequently behaves as *either* a benign or malignant neoplasm. Conversion of a benign tumor to a malignant form may take place in occasional instances.
†The word *osteogenic* as employed here means "originating in bone" and capable of forming bone.

ysis. In the roentgenogram, it appears as a rounded or oval-shaped cystlike rarefaction within the cortex and involving the adjacent cancellous bone. Histologically, the tissue from the lesion is composed of fairly cellular fibrous connective tissue that may embrace a number of multinucleated giant cells alone or in conjunction with clusters of mononuclear cells filled with lipid.

Many fibrous cortical defects remain asymptomatic and require no treatment. Surgical removal of the lesion, when indicated, usually results in a cure.

There is general agreement that, in some instances, fibrous cortical defects may continue to expand and give rise to a more significant lesion that is designated nonossifying fibroma of bone.

Nonossifying fibroma. Nonossifying fibroma is a sharply delimited, somewhat loculated, and often eccentrically placed destructive lesion that is seen most frequently in the shafts of the bones of the lower extremities of children[79] (Fig. 40-45). Microscopic examination reveals that the tissue filling the bone defect is composed of fibrous tissue of varying grades of cellularity. Nests of foamy-appearing lipophages usually are observed and, in some specimens, they are a prominent histologic feature of the lesion. In most instances, the margin of the tumor is well demarcated from the bony wall, but at times extensions of the neoplasm grow peripherally through the marrow spaces. Even when a tumor is moderately cellular, possesses numerous mitotic figures, and is poorly encapsulated, its local removal usually results in a cure.

Fibrosarcoma. Malignant neoplasms arising from fibroblasts, although infrequent, may arise in the periosteal coverings of bone or within the cancellous or medullary spaces. The same difficulties that are experienced in distinguishing between benign and malignant tumors of fibroblastic origin arising in the soft tissues of the body are experienced when one is confronted with these tumors in bone. Evidences of rapid growth, invasion, or disruption of the bone cortex and the histologic qualities of marked cellularity, excessive

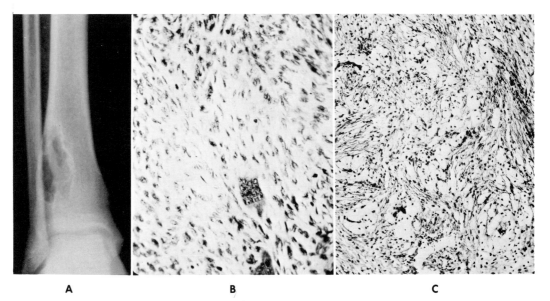

A　　　　　　　　**B**　　　　　　　　**C**

Fig. 40-45 Nonossifying fibroma. **A,** Eccentric area of bone resorption. **B,** Fibroblastic tumor tissue with occasional giant cells. **C,** Clusters of lipid-laden histiocytes among tumor cells.

pleomorphism of cells, and numerous mitotic figures—especially the presence of abnormal mitoses—comprise the features that are indicative of malignancy.

Chondrogenic neoplasms

Although neoplasms of the chondroma series are listed separately in the classification, it should be noted that they usually arise from chondroblastic tissues within or on the surface of a bone. Occasionally, these tumors may arise from mesenchymal cells that differentiate into chondroblasts, and, in some instances, the tumor cells possess the capacity to form both cartilaginous and osseous elements.

Osteochondroma. A synonym for osteochondroma is *cartilaginous exostosis.* In addition, the term is sometimes used interchangeably with *osteoma.*

Osteochondromas are benign neoplasms that arise most commonly at or near the ends of long bones (Fig. 40-46). They usually develop in children, although they may not produce symptoms or be discovered until adult years. In some instances, it can be demonstrated that the outgrowth begins in the periosteal and perichondrial tissues at the metaphyseal end of the shaft in close proximity to the epiphyseal cartilage plate (Fig. 40-46, *B*). Growth of these tumors occurs in the adjacent connective tissues, which perform the function of perichondrium. The new tissue

thus formed acquires the gross and microscopic characteristics of hyaline cartilage before it is removed and replaced by bone. The mechanism by which this is accomplished is essentially one of endochondral ossification. (See Figs. 40-46, *B* and *C,* and 40-47.)

The tumor may be a rounded projection (Fig. 40-46, *B*) or a flat mound (Fig. 40-46, *C*), or it may have a pedunculated, mushroom configuration (Figs. 40-46, *A,* and 40-47).

These tumors tend to grow slowly, and many of them become stationary at the time of cessation of skeletal growth. The cartilaginous cap may entirely disappear, leaving a cancellous outgrowth of bone (osteoma) as a permanent mark.

Occasionally, a bursa forms over the excrescence, and this may become inflamed and be attended by pain. In some instances, *joint mice* form within the bursal sac.

In rare instances, chondrosarcomas or osteogenic sarcomas appear to take origin in an osteochondroma. Continued growth of an osteochondroma after the patient becomes an adult is a reason for thorough investigation.

In association with certain congenital and hereditary conditions affecting endochondral ossification, *multiple cartilaginous exostoses* may be encountered. A particularly painful form of osteochondroma is the *subungual exostosis,* which forms beneath the nail of the finger or toe, especially the great toe.

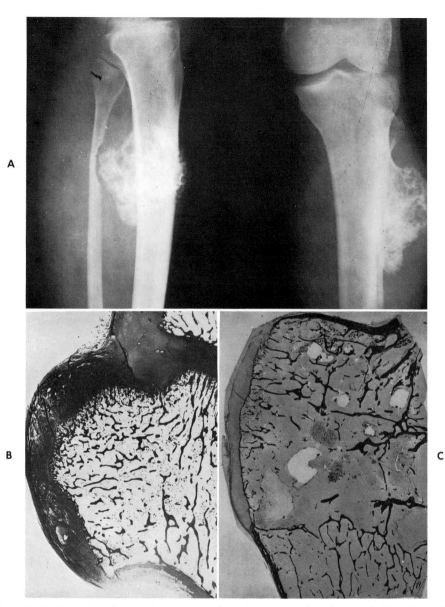

Fig. 40-46 Osteochondroma. **A,** Large, pedunculated osteochondroma of tibia. Note that direction of growth has been away from epiphyseal end of shaft. Pressure atrophy of fibula from contact with tumor apparent in lateral view. **B,** Osteochondroma in early stage of development in young child. Section through junction of metaphyseal end of tibia (lower three-fourths) and epiphysis (upper right). Relation of tumor to perichondrium apparent. **C,** Flat osteochondroma of upper end of femur. Note perichondrial layer, growing cartilage, and irregular trabecular bone that has resulted from imperfect endochondrial ossification. (**A,** AFIP 77515.)

These lesions may become the sites of infection.

Benign epiphyseal chondroblastoma. Formerly regarded as a bizarre chondromatous giant cell tumor, the benign epiphyseal chondroblastoma was reinterpreted and given its present name in 1942.[80] The lesion develops in young subjects, most frequently during the second decade. Although the upper end of the humerus is frequently the site of the lesion, any long bone may be affected. Characteristically, the tumor involves both the metaphyseal end of the shaft and the adjacent epiphysis, producing visible resorptive changes that are evident in the x-ray film. Curettings from this lesion consist of tissue fragments

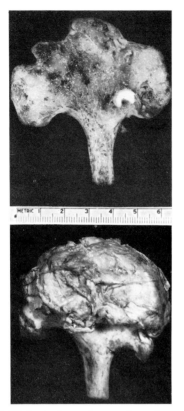

Fig. 40-47 Typical mushroom-shaped osteochondroma.

resembling cartilage, along with grayish or reddish tissue similar to that of a giant cell tumor. Gritty particles representing calcified bone and cartilage also are recognized.

Microscopically, this tumor shows a variety of tissue elements. Some regions are highly cellular and composed of medium-sized round and oval cells. In adjacent areas, recognizable spicules of calcified cartilage are identified. Intermingled between these two types of tissues are vascular sinusoids, masses of connective tissue, and variable numbers of giant cells. Extravasated blood and hemosiderin pigment also are seen.

Although the benign chondroblastoma may show marked cellularity and be capable of causing considerable destruction of bone, it is known to respond satisfactorily to curettement in most instances. In the occasional case in which recurrence develops, more radical local removal seems to result in a cure.

Chondromyxoid fibroma. Chondromyxoid fibroma, which is among the less common neoplasms of bone, was set apart as a clinical and pathologic entity in 1948 by Jaffe and Lichtenstein.[81] Characteristically, the tumor

becomes apparent because of pain. It affects young persons 10 to 30 years of age. The more common sites of involvement are the metaphyseal ends of the bones of the extremities, especially the femur and tibia. Less frequently, the lesion occurs in a rib, an ilium, or a vertebra. The lesion tends to be eccentrically placed but, when far advanced, the major portion of the bone may be replaced. The roentgenogram usually shows a thin and often times dense bony shell surrounding the tumor that tends to be nodular in outline. Bony septa extending into the tumor mass between nodules also may appear in the x-ray film. When exposed at operation, the tumor usually is sharply circumscribed and separates readily from the enclosing bony walls. The neoplasm is firm but elastic in texture and pale gray in color. Usually, there is a quality of translucency suggesting cartilaginous derivation.

Microscopically, the tumor tissue exhibits a lobulated or nodular form, and the peripheral portions of the nodules are enclosed in a zone of highly cellular tissue. More centrally, the nodules are comprised of differing cellular patterns. In some areas, the cellular and intracellular structures resemble cartilage. In other areas, the tissue is comprised of spindle and stellate cells embedded in a mucinous-appearing or myxomatous-appearing matrix. The marked variation in cell patterns and the variations in intercellular matrix seem unusual for a neoplasm that usually is benign in its clinical behavior.

It should be kept in mind that chondromyxoid fibromas bear clinical and radiologic characteristics that are not readily distinguished from other diseases of bone. Similarly, the pathologic features may bear resemblances to certain other neoplasms. It is essential, therefore, that there be maximal cooperation between clinician, radiologist, and pathologist in the evaluation of these tumors if they are to be properly diagnosed and treated. Block resection of the lesion, when possible, is the treatment of choice, for removal by curettement is followed by recurrence in approximately one-fourth of the cases.[32]

Chondroma. Chondromas are firm, rounded, lobulated growths of grayish color. They may arise either from the surface of a bone or from its interior. The latter are referred to as enchondromas. The short bones of the hands and feet, the ends of long bones, and the flat bones, including the pelvis, ribs, sternum, and

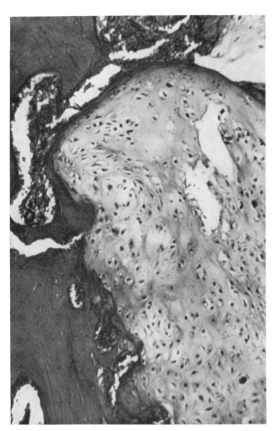

Fig. 40-48 Structural and cytologic features of typical enchondroma. (×130; AFIP 90709.)

scapulas, are common sites of involvement. On section, one sees small and large nodules of grayish blue tissue that is translucent and resembles normal cartilage. Such nodules are surrounded by connective tissue that may contain blood vessels in moderate numbers. Growth of the tumor can be attributed to the multiplication of the cells that are deeply embedded in these perichondrial layers.

Roentgenologic examination shows partial or complete destruction of the involved bone. Frequently, the lesion is multiloculated, and the margins are usually sharp but regular.

Microscopic examination reveals a tumor composed of nodules of atypical cartilage. The cells have little, if any, pattern of orientation. In the centers of the nodules, there is likely to be a preponderance of matrix, and either cystic degeneration or calcification may be noted. The growing margins of the nodules are composed of flattened or oval-shaped cells that merge imperceptibly with the blood vessel–containing connective tissues that form partitions between the lobular units. Within bone, the tumor tissue may be tightly compressed into the cancellous spaces and vascular channels (Fig. 40-48).

Chondromas are to be regarded as *benign* neoplasms. Those lesions, whether single or multiple, that occur in the small bones of the hands and feet almost always are cured by curettement. Neoplasms of this class originating in the long bones of the extremities, proximal to the hands and feet, are more likely to recur following curettage and, in rare instances, may acquire malignant characteristics. Chondromas arising in the flat bones, especially the pelvis, are likely to behave as malignant tumors, but it is difficult to ascertain whether this is the result of conversion of a *benign* to a *malignant* neoplasm or whether the tumor possessed malignant qualities from the onset.

Chondrosarcoma. Chondrosarcoma may arise from preexisting chondromatous tumors. This development seems to occur much more frequently in the centrally placed tumors than in those on the surfaces of bone. The transformation appears to be gradual in most instances, and it may be easier to determine the change by clinical and roentgenologic study than by histologic examination. Even a large and exceedingly destructive tumor that has spread well beyond the bone in which it arose may reveal microscopic features that differ little, if at all, from the preexisting tumor tissue examined months or years before. In the usual case, however, careful microscopic study of properly selected blocks will disclose features that indicate malignancy. Increased cellularity, irregular nuclear patterns, and poorly formed intercellular matrix, together with obvious accelerated growth activity at the margins of the individual lobules or nodules, are features that usually indicate malignant behavior of the neoplasm (Fig. 40-49).

While it is known that *benign* chondromatous tumors may acquire malignant qualities, there is good evidence that the great majority of chondrosarcomas possess malignant features from the onset. Characteristically, chondrosarcoma arises in the bones of the pelvis, shoulder girdle, trunk, and large bones of the extremities. On gross examination, the tumors are likely to be bulky and to reveal their capabilities for erosion and destruction of the bone in which they originated and for invasion of the adjacent soft tissues. In texture, they vary from firm nodular masses of bluish translucent tissue to soft ill-defined tissue of gelatinous or myxomatous quality.

Histologically, there are wide variations in

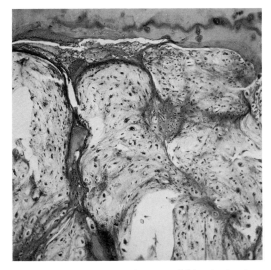

Fig. 40-49 Invasive qualities and histologic characteristics of chondrosarcoma.

structure, ranging from well-defined hyaline cartilage to tissue that is myxomatous and poorly differentiated. The atypical structure of cells and the abnormal relations of cells to intercellular matrix are the distinguishing features to be looked for.

In sharp contrast to osteogenic sarcoma, chondrosarcoma is preeminently a disease of adults from 25 to 50 years of age. The progress of chondrosarcoma is characteristically slower than that of osteogenic sarcoma, and metastasis occurs late in the disease. Secondary nodules almost invariably appear in the lung first, and only rarely are other organs affected. In some instances, autopsy reveals a continuous intravascular growth of tumor. This may extend to the right side of the heart or even into the pulmonary arteries.

The known behavior of solid chondromatous tumors as a class is of grave concern to surgeons and pathologists. In many instances, an operation extensive enough to be curative will result in extreme disability or disfigurement or both. Awareness of this fact, coupled with the knowledge that a lesser operation will at most be followed by slow recurrence, encourages the surgeon to adopt conservative measures. Not infrequently in these cases, one recurrence follows another until the neoplasm has spread beyond the limits of operability or has invaded the blood vessels and metastasized.

Osteogenic neoplasms

Osteoma. At times, it is extremely difficult to determine whether a given overgrowth of

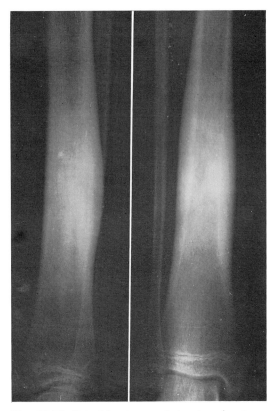

Fig. 40-50 Osteoid osteoma. Lateral and antero-posterior roentgenograms showing typical osteosclerosis associated with osteoid osteoma.

bone is a true benign neoplasm or whether it merely represents the site of a former traumatic injury such as a subperiosteal hematoma or a localized inflammatory process. As already has been noted, some examples of osteomas are the remnants of osteochondromas.

Benign new growths of osseous tissue of either compact or cancellous structure occasionally develop in the bones of the face and skull. Not infrequently, these tumors extend into the antrum or other cranial sinuses.

Osteoid osteoma. The term osteoid osteoma was first employed by Jaffe and Lichtenstein[77] to designate a lesion that formerly may have been regarded as *chronic bone abscess, osteomyelitis with annular sequestrum,* or *sclerosing nonsuppurative osteomyelitis.*

The condition is most frequently seen in children and young adults from 10 to 25 years of age. Males are more frequently affected than females. The principal symptom is pain, which is persistent but usually not of sufficient intensity to bring the patient under observation until several weeks or months have elapsed after the apparent onset. Physi-

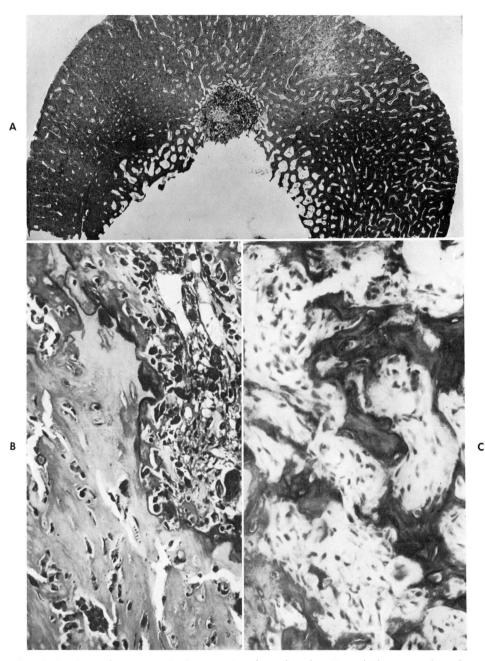

Fig. 40-51 Osteoid osteoma. **A,** Cross section through nidus. Note thickening and condensation of surrounding cortical bone. In **B** and **C,** note composition of osteoid osteoma. **B,** Abundant osteoid. **C,** Irregular well-calcified osseous spicules encased by highly vascular and moderately cellular connective tissue. Osteoclasts present in moderate numbers. (**B,** ×180; **C,** ×250.)

cal examination reveals tenderness, and there may be slight swelling. Fever is usually absent, and the leukocyte count is generally within normal limits.

The roentgenogram is usually characteristic. The bone for some distance peripheral to the lesion is excessively dense. Frequently, in a long bone, the cortex is thickened and the shaft is widened (Fig. 40-50). Near the center of the hypertrophic bone is a small, sharply circumscribed lesion of relative radiolucency. In the center of this, especially in lesions of considerable duration, is an oval or rounded shadow of varying density.

The pathologic features are equally characteristic, but care must be taken not to overlook the essential lesion. It is perhaps safer to have a roentgenogram made of the specimen and then, using the film as a guide, to section the specimen. Sectioning is made easier if the fixed specimen is first decalcified. Microscopic sections made in this fashion reveal a highly characteristic picture (Fig. 40-51, *A*).

The lesion proper consists of a small spherical nodule of highly vascular connective tissue in which varying amounts of osteoid or fully calcified but irregularly arranged cancellous bone have been deposited (Fig. 40-51, *B* and *C*). Immediately adjacent to the nidus is a zone of porous bone, and this is surrounded by the thickened and exceedingly dense bone of the hypertrophied shaft (Fig. 40-51, *A*).

Excision of the total area or removal of the nidus itself results in a dramatic subsidence of pain. Complete removal usually results in a cure.

Benign osteoblastoma. An uncommon benign neoplasm of bone, although now recognized as a clinical and pathologic entity,[32, 54, 76, 94] benign osteoblastoma has been interpreted in the past as variants of giant cell tumor, osteoid osteoma (giant variety), and ossifying fibroma. The lesion is most frequently observed in children and young adults. Males are affected more frequently than females.[94]

Unlike most of the other neoplasms originating in bone, this tumor displays a greater tendency to involve the bones of the vertebral column, where it may induce the symptom of pain either from pressure upon the adjacent tissue or upon the spinal cord and the emerging nerves. Long bones of the extremities and flat bones of the trunk and skull also may be affected.

Roentgenograms of the involved bone usually reveal a well-circumscribed area of radiolucency with varying degrees of opacity that reflects varying degrees of mineralization of the osteoid substance produced in the tumor.

Since macroscopic observation usually is limited to inspection of tissue fragments removed by curettement, it is difficult to discern any diagnostic features. The fragments usually are reddish in color and gritty in texture. Microscopically, there is considerable variability in both cellular and intercellular matrix components. Generally, there is an abundance of osteoblastic cells and of uncalcified osteoid matrix. In some areas, there may be a marked proliferation of fibroblasts between narrow and irregularly arranged trabeculae. Other portions of a specimen may be highly vascular, and multinucleated giant cells may be present in varying numbers.

Histologic similarity between some examples of benign osteoblastoma and osteoid osteoma has been noted.

Differentiation between benign osteoblastoma, which is usually treated by curettage, and certain other bone tumors requiring more radical therapy may require the careful examination of a number of tissue fragments as well as careful evaluation of the clinical and radiologic features.

Osteogenic sarcoma. The classification presented by Ewing[45] lists six types of osteogenic sarcomas, and one of these contains two subgroups. Such a detailed scheme of compartmentalization, while valuable at one time for registry purposes and for specialists in neoplastic disease, is unnecessary and probably impractical for the purposes of the student of medicine.

Osteogenic sarcoma is the most common primary malignant neoplasm of bone-forming tissue. Like hematogenous osteomyelitis, it arises most commonly in the metaphyseal ends of the shafts of long bones, particularly the lower end of the femur, the upper end of the tibia, and the upper end of the humerus. Occasionally, the neoplasm arises in the middle portion of the shaft of a long bone. The disease is seen most frequently in children and young adults. About 75% of the tumors occur in patients between 10 and 25 years of age, and males are affected about twice as often as females. Many tumors are noticed soon after trauma, but it is impossible, in a given case, to prove an etiologic relationship.

By the time an osteogenic sarcoma is recognized and submitted for examination, it is seen to involve the interior of bone, to have extended through the cortex, and to have caused an elevation of the periosteum for some distance along the shaft (Fig. 40-52). It is exceedingly difficult, therefore, to determine the precise point of origin. In all likelihood, the neoplasms are derived either from the bone-forming cells within the cancellous spaces of the shaft or from the periosteal layer. It is uncertain which is more common.

The roentgenologic and pathologic features of osteogenic sarcomas are variable and depend to a large extent on the amount of bone produced in a particular tumor. In this regard, there are two main types: (1) a tumor that

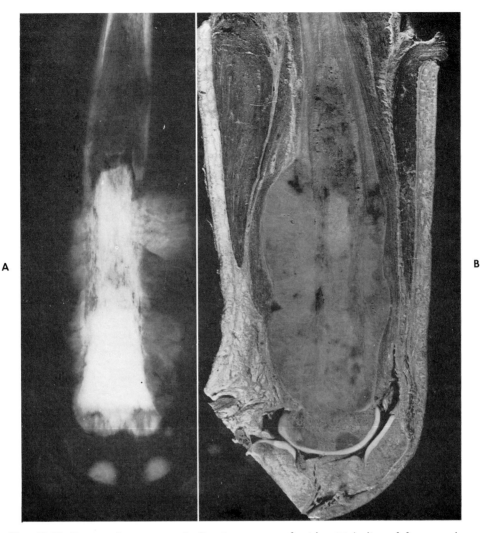

Fig. 40-52 Osteogenic sarcoma. **A,** Roentgenogram of midsagittal slice of femur undergoing replacement by sclerosing osteogenic sarcoma. Note condensation and loss of architectural design of affected segment of femur and marked osseous tissue growth subperiosteally. **B,** Gross appearance of sectioned surface of sarcoma illustrated in **A.**

produces a great deal of osteoid matrix that calcifies—**sclerosing osteogenic sarcoma** (Figs. 40-52 to 40-54) and (2) a tumor, usually of exceedingly rapid growth rate, that produces little or no recognizable bone—**osteolytic osteogenic sarcoma** (Fig. 40-55). Highly vascular neoplasms—**telangiectatic osteogenic sarcomas**—are likewise destructive in character.

The typical sclerosing osteogenic sarcoma shows, on roentgenographic examination, a condensation of the original bone and loss of its normal architecture. The cortex on one or both sides is irregular in outline, and the normal markings are obliterated. Extending outward at right angles from the cortex beneath the displaced periosteum is a fringelike density

that is referred to as "ray" formation. These linear markings are attributable to calcified trabeculae within the neoplasm (Fig. 40-52, *A*). When such a specimen is sawed in its longitudinal axis, one sees tumor tissue of grayish white color. At the periphery, it is usually cellular and friable, in contrast to the densely calcified portion that lies nearest to the shaft. The original cancellous bone of the shaft end is converted into exceedingly dense, ivory-like bone. An interesting detail may be noted at the upper extremity of the tumor (away from the epiphysis) where the periosteum has been recently separated from the cortex, producing a characteristic triangle (Codman's triangle). At the lower extremity

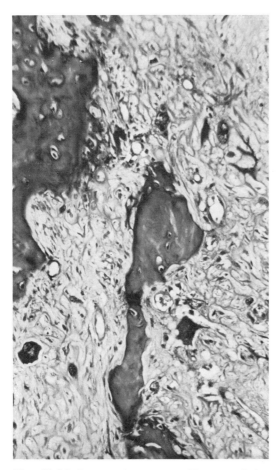

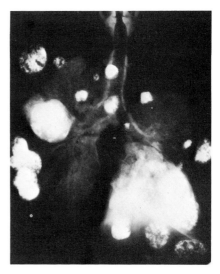

Fig. 40-54 Roentgenogram of lungs removed from patient who died of osteogenic sarcoma. Metastases consist of bone that is heavily mineralized.

Fig. 40-53 Osteogenic sarcoma. Bizarre cellular pattern and irregular ossification of sclerosing osteogenic sarcoma. (×230; AFIP 63769.)

(epiphyseal end), the tumor usually extends to, but not beyond, the attachment of the periosteum to the perichondrial margin of the epiphyseal cartilage plate (Fig. 40-52, *B*). The latter structure apparently resists the spread of the neoplasm for a time, but in numerous instances the bony epiphysis is invaded by the time the extremity is removed.

In the so-called lytic or osteolytic osteogenic sarcoma, the roentgenologic picture is less characteristic. Usually, there is evidence of partial or total destruction of the original bone in an area of variable size. The margins of the lesion are usually irregular in outline. There may be a soft tissue shadow from the extension of the tumor into the extraosseous tissues (Fig. 40-55, *A*). Examination of the cut surface of such a tumor reveals a sharply outlined but irregular area of bone destruction. Filling the bony cavity is a mass of cellular and friable tissue that is pinkish gray in color. In numerous examples, one will note red areas caused by hemorrhage or yellowish

foci attributable to necrosis (Fig. 40-55, *B*). Small amounts of calcified bone may be present. Microscopically, such lesions are usually highly cellular and show little or no osteoid matrix between cells. Tumor giant cells and bizarre mitotic figures are often present (Fig. 40-55, *C*).

Occasionally, one encounters tumors that fail to conform to either the sclerosing or destructive (lytic) types just mentioned. One such variant is a tumor that is comprised in part of cartilage and in part of bone (Figs. 40-56 and 40-57). Other atypical forms include a certain amount of myxomatous tissue. It is because of these transitions that the older literature made reference in the form of prefixes to "myxo-," "fibro-," "chondro-," "osteoid-," and "osteo-" sarcomas. Not uncommonly, two or more such prefixes were employed in an effort to characterize a single tumor.

Osteogenic sarcoma is a tumor that leads to a fatal termination in a high percentage of instances, irrespective of the form of treatment employed. In published accounts, the five-year survival rates range from 5% to 20%.

Metastasis takes place chiefly by way of the bloodstream, and the initial site of secondary growth is usually the lung. Not infrequently, the liver, heart, and other organs are invaded by the time the disease has run its course. Metastases in distant bones are seldom observed.

Parosteal (juxtacortical) osteogenic sarcoma. Because of its distinguishing clinical, radi-

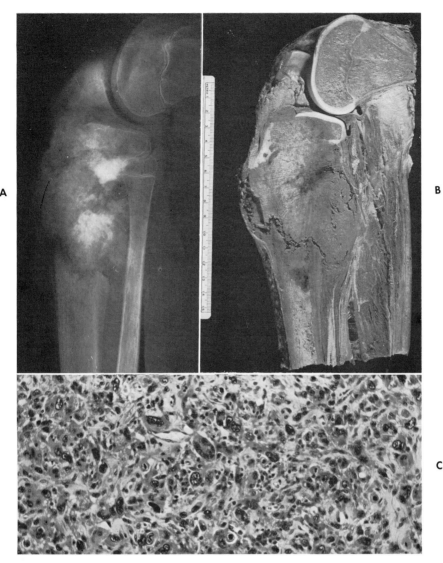

Fig. 40-55 Osteogenic sarcoma. **A** and **B,** Destructive and rapidly growing sarcoma of tibia that has resulted in pathologic fracture. **C,** Marked variation in size and shape of cells, bizarre mitoses, and little or no evidence of bone matrix formation noteworthy features in this lytic form of osteogenic sarcoma. (×165; AFIP 73613.)

ologic, and pathologic features, it is proper to recognize parosteal (juxtacortical) osteogenic sarcoma as a special form of osteogenic sarcoma.[40, 73]

This lesion is an uncommon tumor that characteristically occurs in subjects older than those affected by other forms of osteogenic sarcoma. It is more common in women than in men. It originates almost exclusively in the femur (especially the distal end), humerus, and tibia (Fig. 40-58). It grows slowly, at least initially, and is noticeably less malignant than other forms of osteogenic sarcoma.

Roentgenologic examination, while influenced greatly by the stage of tumor develop-

ment, usually reveals a dense bony mass which, although firmly attached to the bone cortex over a wide base, tends to encircle the shaft as a bulky and heavily calcified growth. In some instances, in an early stage, these tumors have been regarded as atypical osteochondromas and treated by local and incomplete removal. Recurrences following such inadequate treatment give rise, in most instances, to tumor tissue having a more aggressive behavior pattern.

Microscopic examination of the neoplasm, although exceedingly variable, usually reveals evidence of destruction and replacement of the original bone cortex, extensive production

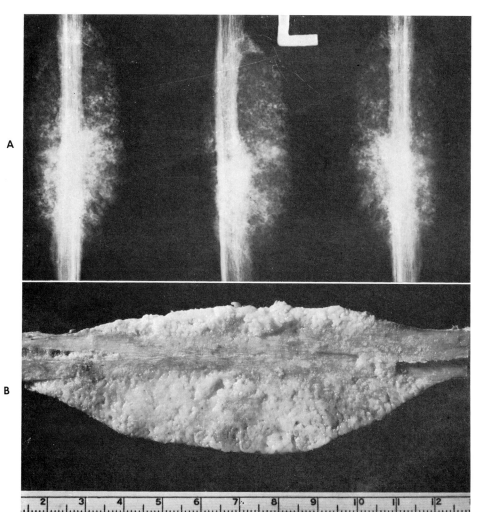

Fig. 40-56 A, Sclerosing osteogenic sarcoma of fibula. Tumor was slowly growing. It was made up of both osseous and cartilaginous tissues (see Fig. 40-57). **B,** Specimen illustrated in **A.**

of new bone trabeculae, and filling of all cancellous bone spaces with proliferating bone-forming tumor cells (Fig. 40-59). Invasion of the soft tissues at the periphery of the tumor mass is also apparent.

Reports dealing with individual cases and groups of cases indicate clearly that this slowly growing tumor carries a better prognosis than the usual forms of osteogenic sarcoma provided it is adequately treated initially. Partial removal of the lesion is followed by recurrence and, in most instances, by increased degrees of malignancy.

Sarcomas associated with other disorders of bone. It has been known since Paget described the initial five cases of *osteitis deformans*[112] that there is an increased incidence of sarcoma of bone in the skeletal parts that are

affected by Paget's disease. The reported incidence of bone sarcoma in association with Paget's disease has varied, but it appears that it is on the order of 1%.[118] In reports directed at the analysis of large numbers of cases of bone sarcoma, the association of Paget's disease and sarcoma also has been noted. In an analysis of 600 patients with verified osteogenic sarcoma, Dahlin and Coventry[33] found twenty instances in which the neoplasm developed in bone affected by Paget's disease. Price[119] deduced from his study that Paget's disease increases the risk of developing sarcoma about thirtyfold in persons over 40 years of age.

The association of bone sarcoma with ionizing radiation should be kept in mind. Such irradiation-induced sarcomas have followed

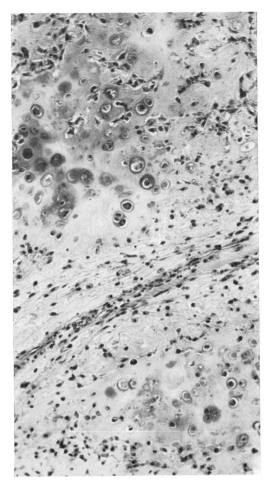

Fig. 40-57 Imperfectly formed bone and cartilage make up this malignant tumor. Histologic features portrayed here similar to those seen in tumor illustrated in Fig. 40-56. (×170; AFIP 66706.)

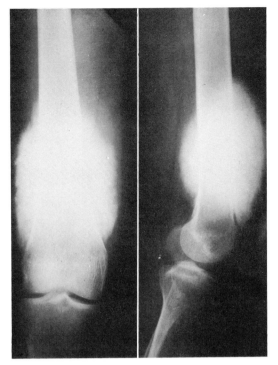

Fig. 40-58 Parosteal osteogenic sarcoma. Large and heavily mineralized tumor mass encircling lower third of femur.

attempts to treat a variety of benign conditions (e.g., fibrous dysplasia of bone[65]). Bone sarcoma apparently also has been induced by irradiation of malignant tumors in close proximity to bone. The deposition of radium or other radioactive materials in skeletal parts (e.g., in workers painting watch and clock dials with luminous paint) is another well-known cause of bone sarcoma.[17, 95] In these instances, the onset of the neoplastic change is usually preceded by months or years of inflammatory and destructive osteitis that is induced by radiant energy (Fig. 40-60). Irradiation-induced sarcomas have been well studied in the rat[38] (p. 257).

Vascular tissues

Hemangioma. Benign tumors composed of vascular tissue components occasionally are observed in skeletal parts, especially the skull and vertebrae. Ordinarily, such tumors are asymptomatic and are discovered by means of x-ray studies undertaken for some other purpose. Hemangiomas tend to be sharply circumscribed, and in the roentgenogram there usually is radiolucency at the peripheral margins and coarsening of the trabecular pattern in the central portion. Frequently, in the skull there is extension of the lesion to the bone surface with the production of vertically placed bone spicules that give rise to a "sunburst" appearance in the x-ray film. Occasionally, hemangiomas may be diffusely spread through a wide area and give rise to increased porosity of the bone, with irregularly arranged areas of bone condensation. Histologic examination reveals the characteristic vascular structures of an angioma extending through the widened haversian channels of compact bone and the expanded marrow spaces of cancellous bone.

Hemangioendothelioma. Malignant hemangioendotheliomas of bone are seldom encountered.[20] The bone may be partially destroyed in a progressive manner over a wide area or completely and rapidly removed in a well-circumscribed focus. Grossly, these tumors may be cellular and friable and gray in color or, because of the high degree of vascularity, may be red in color and ooze blood when sectioned. The histologic characteristics

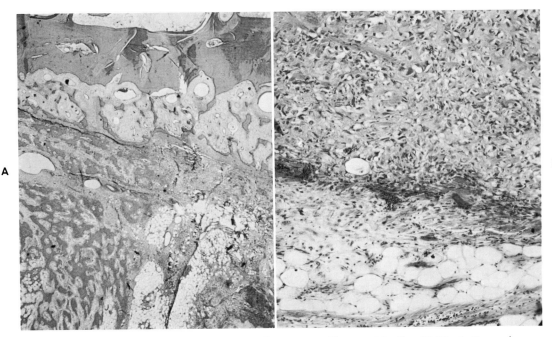

Fig. 40-59 Parosteal osteogenic sarcoma. Same tumor illustrated in Fig. 40-58. **A,** Femoral cortex (top) and tumor mass (lower half) growing into adjacent soft tissue. Bone formed by tumor well developed. **B,** Peripheral margin of tumor showing soft tissue invasion by sarcoma cells.

are no different from those of like tumors in extraosseous tissues.

Unknown origin

Giant cell tumor. Regardless of site of occurrence, few, if any, neoplasms, have given rise to as much divergence of opinion as has the giant cell tumor of bone. The causes for disagreement are many, but foremost among them is the dissimilarity in concept of what properly constitutes a *giant cell tumor*. Some authors have elected to consider the term all-inclusive and, in order to designate the particular type of lesion under consideration at the moment, have referred to *variants* of one sort or another (fibrocystic variant, chondromatous variant, exanthomatous variant, malignant variant, etc.) as contrasted with a *typical* giant cell tumor. In opposition to this view, some observers have restricted the use of the term giant cell tumor to examples of the *typical* neoplasm, with the conviction that the *atypical* lesions are either unrelated neoplasms or nonneoplastic, reactive processes. The truth of the matter may not be settled to everyone's satisfaction for some time to come.

The distinctive giant cell tumor behaves as a neoplasm that is usually, but not necessarily, benign in its subsequent behavior. The lesion characteristically occurs in the ends of long bones of young adults in whom the epiphyses have closed. The lower end of the femur and the upper end of the tibia are the commonest sites, but the tumor may occur in ends of any of the long bones, especially the lower extremity of the radius, or in a few flat bones.

Pain that is especially severe on weight bearing and motion is usually the first symptom. Later, there may be noticeable swelling. In some instances, a pathologic fracture causes the patient to seek medical attention.

The radiographic appearance is frequently but not always characteristic. In early cases, the roentgenogram reveals a sharply outlined and usually single area of complete bone destruction. Such a lesion is generally in one of the condyles. In older lesions, the destructive process may have extended to involve the entire bone end. When this has occurred, there is usually a noticeable expansion, and the peripheral margins of the tumor are indicated by a thin and discontinuous bony shell formed beneath the displaced periosteum. The "cystic" lesion may consist of a single space or have a multiloculated appearance. In either case, the relationship of the expanded area to the shaft of the bone is not unlike that of a soap bubble being inflated from a straw. A fracture through such a lesion may introduce bizarre features from telescoping and from repair (Fig. 40-61).

The gross specimen shows a sharply delineated expansion at the junction of the tumor and the shaft. The expanded portion is partially or completely encased in a thin shell of bone that may be readily indented by pressure and easily cut with a knife or scissors. When the specimen has been divided in its long axis, it is noted that there is a sharp line of demarcation between the marrow of the bone medulla and the tumor tissue filling the expanded end of the bone. The neoplasm may extend to the undersurface of the articular cartilage. The neoplastic tissue is firm and friable. It is grayish in color, with either a pinkish or a brownish tint. Focal areas of degeneration, of yellow-brown color, and hemorrhagic areas of red or dark brown color, depending on the age of the hemorrhage, are usually present. In addition, there may be linear bands of fibrous tissue or stellate scars where necrotic tumor tissue has been replaced.

Microscopic examination shows a highly characteristic pattern (Fig. 40-62). The most distinctive feature is the presence of large numbers of giant cells. These contain many even-sized, oval nuclei (twenty to one hundred in a sectioned cell surface) that are crowded together near the center of the cell. These have prominent nuclear membranes, and each contains a single nucleolus. In between the giant cells is a well-vascularized

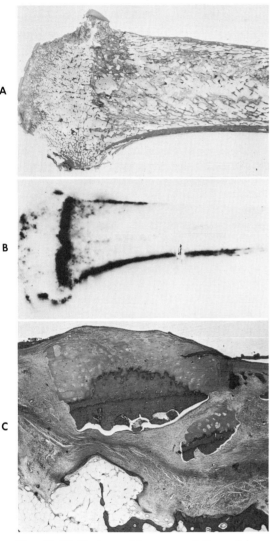

Fig. 40-60 Photographic representation of bone and cartilage changes caused by irradiation. Patient, 46-year-old woman, had worked as watch and clock dial painter for three and one-half months when 16 years of age. Lower extremity was amputated because of sarcomatous change originating in diseased femur. Tumor was classified as fibrosarcoma. **A,** Large section of lower segment of femur showing necrosis. **B,** Autoradiogram made from section similar to specimen shown in **A.** Note evidence of intense radioactivity in region of metaphyseal end of diaphysis, which marks growth zone at time patient was exposed to radioactive material. **C,** As result of radiation injury, articular cartilage and subchondral bone have undergone necrosis and fragmentation.

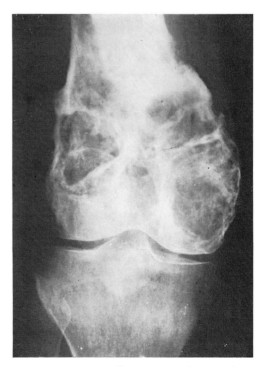

Fig. 40-61 Giant cell tumor. Multicystic lesion that has destroyed both condyles of femur. Pathologic fracture with resultant collapse of lesion evident. (AFIP 70987.)

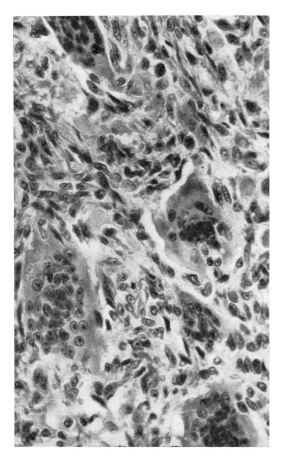

Fig. 40-62 Giant cell tumor. Typical cytologic and structural features of benign giant cell tumor of bone. (×765; AFIP 63505.)

and cellular "stroma" that is comprised of spindle-shaped and oval-shaped cells. A few mitotic figures may be found in these cells and, in some instances, they may be numerous. Some observers have laid great stress on the cellularity of the "stroma," the number of plump, rounded cells, and the number of mitotic figures, believing these details provide an index to the probable behavior of the tumor. On this basis, a system of classification of three grades has been suggested,[82] holding that grade III tumors possess malignant properties either inherent in the tumor from its beginning or acquired through successive recurrences of tumors originally belonging to grades I or II.

The reexamination of collections of cases at different institutions[105, 108] has verified the fact that careful evaluation of the histologic features of each lesion, particularly the "stroma," in the initial lesion and in each recurrent specimen is essential in guiding the therapy. From one series of thirty-one cases[108] of giant cell tumor, it was concluded that approximately 10% of all giant cell tumors are malignant at the time of first examination or will be recognized to be malignant after therapy and follow-up.

Malignant giant cell tumor. Occasionally, neoplasms possessing most of the histologic features of the giant cell tumor either have from the time of their inception or acquire subsequently the clinical and pathologic features of malignancy. Such tumors are rapidly growing and excessively destructive and show a capacity to break out of the bony shell and invade adjacent soft tissues. In some instances, the process of invasion includes the entrance of tumor tissue into vascular channels, and distant metastases may be thus established. On microscopic examination, tumors having these qualities are usually highly cellular and show numerous mitotic figures, including atypical mitoses. The giant cells are likely to vary in size and shape and in the number and size of the nuclei.

Giant cell tumors possessing the recognizable features of malignancy should be designated as *giant cell sarcoma* and treated by whatever means are required to completely remove the lesion.

Ewing's sarcoma. A malignant neoplasm that arises in bone, Ewing's sarcoma was differentiated from osteogenic sarcoma and established as an entity by James Ewing.[43, 44, 46] It is probable that the tumor represents the "small round cell sarcoma" of earlier writers. Ewing regarded it as a myeloma derived from endothelium—**endothelial myeloma.**

Although there is general agreement on the specificity of this variety of neoplasm, Ewing's concept of the histogenesis has been questioned. Evidence purporting to show that the tumor arises from the reticuloendothelial system and that the tumor cells possess the capacity to differentiate into plasma cells, lymphocytes, or other cell types has been presented.[110] A similar opinion also has been expressed by Lichtenstein and Jaffe,[93] who hold that the tumor is an entity, primary in bone but possessing no bone-forming capacity, and that it probably is derived from the reticular tissue of the marrow. Other observers conclude that this tumor originates from undifferentiated mesenchmal cells.

Ewing's sarcoma is usually seen in children and young adults from 10 to 25 years of age. Since this is the exact age period in which the incidence of osteogenic sarcoma is highest, difficulty often is experienced in distinguishing

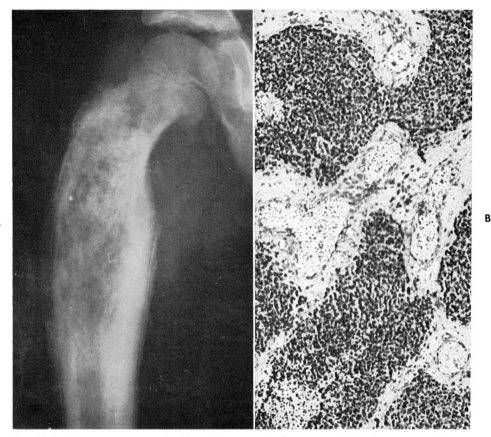

Fig. 40-63 Ewing's sarcoma. **A,** More characteristic features of Ewing's sarcoma of bone. Note irregular areas of osteoporosis and osteosclerosis, loss of bone architecture, and multilayered periosteal new bone formation. **B,** Closely packed small round cells make up substance of this tumor. Note loosely textured connective tissue containing numerous blood vessels, which forms partitions between masses of tumor cells. (×160; AFIP 73775.)

between the two tumors before operation. The neoplasm, while not rare, is much less frequent than osteogenic sarcoma.

In the usual case, the patient complains of pain in the affected area. Swelling may or may not be present. The patient may have a slight elevation in temperature, and the leukocyte count may be slightly or moderately elevated. These signs and symptoms may lead to an erroneous diagnosis of osteomyelitis of low-grade character. Roentgenographic examination of the entire skeleton at the time of admission of the patient usually reveals but one bone lesion. This consists of a certain amount of destruction of the original bone, and, provided the lesion is in the shaft of a long bone, there is frequently a series of layers of new subperiosteal bone (Fig. 40-63, *A*). This "onionskin" appearance is not observed so frequently in Ewing's sarcoma as the literature suggests, and it should be noted that a similar appearance may result from other conditions. In most patients, the original lesion is followed, after a period of weeks or months, by the appearance in the roentgenogram of other foci of tumor.

The disease may begin in any bone. However, in the majority of instances, the shafts of the long tubular bones and the bones of the pelvis are affected first.

When the bone that is affected by the tumor is split in its long axis, it is noted that the original bone is porous and that small and large portions have been resorbed. Recognizable tumor tissue is found beneath the displaced periosteum and in the irregular cavities within the bone. This is white or gray white in color and exceedingly soft and friable. Areas of hemorrhage and necrosis may be evident. The new bone, observed in the roentgenogram, also is evident on gross inspection. This is most prominent beneath the periosteum, and microscopically it is apparent that its formation has resulted from the stimulation of the periosteal cells and not from any bone-forming potentiality of the tumor cells themselves. The tumor tissue as viewed microscopically consists of broad or narrow sheets of small round cells growing between partitions of well-vascularized connective tissue (Fig. 40-63, B). Little cytoplasm is evident, but the nuclei are relatively large and of round or oval contour. Mitotic figures are numerous, but tumor giant cells as well as other pleomorphic forms are uncommon.

As the disease progresses, the other bones of the skeleton become involved, and metastasis to the lungs occurs. At autopsy, there may be metastases in other organs. While it is true that Ewing's sarcoma is radiosensitive, radiation therapy, either alone or combined with surgical removal of the affected part, effects a five-year survival in only a small percentage of cases (10% in one series of 50 cases,[138] 12% in another series of 80 cases,[96] and 15% in a third series of 210 cases[32]).

"Adamantinoma" of tibia. "Adamantinoma" of the tibia is a rare neoplasm that bears a striking resemblance to the true adamantinomas that develop in the jaws and at the base of the skull in relation to the cranio-pharyngeal pouch. Despite the observed similarity between the lesions, some observers[24, 41] hold that the tibial lesion is not a true adamantinoma but instead should be considered as a malignant angioblastoma. Three other possible explanations have been offered for the development of the astonishing tibial tumor:

1 That the tumor arises from congenital rests of epithelial tissue
2 That the tumor originates from epithelium implanted by means of trauma
3 That the tumor is of mesenchymal origin with epithelium-like arrangement of cells similar to that which occurs in synovial sarcoma

"Adamantinoma" of the tibia, whatever its origin may be, is a tumor of slow growth. It has the capability of recurring if not completely removed by resection. It also is capable

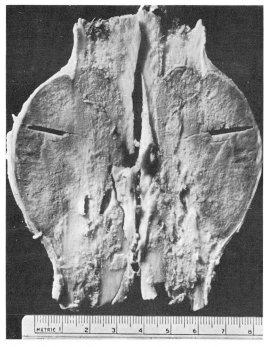

Fig. 40-64 "Adamantinoma." Large solitary tumor mass in midportion of tibia has led to sharply defined bone destruction. Neoplasm was dense but moderately cellular and friable and, on section, revealed features similar to those of adamantinoma (see Fig. 40-65).

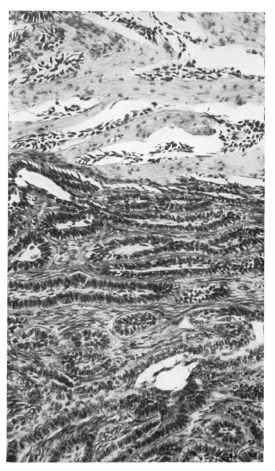

Fig. 40-65 "Adamantinoma." Alveolar arrangement of tall cyclindrical cells with centrally placed fusiform and oval cells. Invasion of bone evident at left margin. Section prepared from tumor shown in Fig. 40-64. (×145.)

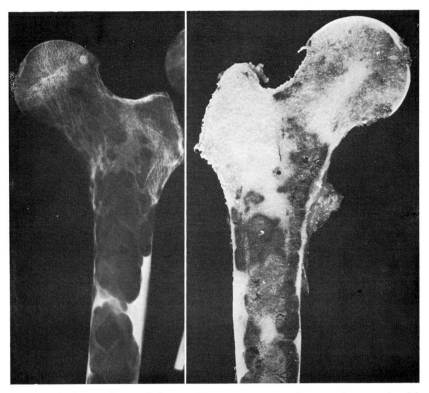

Fig. 40-66 Multiple myeloma of femur. Roentgenogram and gross photograph of hemisection showing extensive bone destruction caused by multiple myeloma. Note absence of any reactive bone formation.

of spreading via blood or lymph channels. Characteristically, the lesion produces rounded or oval, somewhat loculated areas of bone destruction to be seen in roentgenograms and on gross examination (see Fig. 40-64). Microscopically, the tumor tissue resembles the better known true adamantinoma of the jaws (Fig. 40-65).

Hematopoietic tissue

Myeloma. Myeloma is a frequently encountered malignant tumor comprised of plasma cells with varying degrees of differentiation (*plasma cell myeloma*) and usually distributed in multiple foci throughout the skeletal parts (*multiple myeloma*) (p. 1376 and Figs. 31-72 and 31-73). Occasionally, the tumor appears, at least initially, as a solitary tumor of soft tissue or as a solitary lesion of bone (*solitary myeloma*). In most instances, however, the solitary lesions eventually spread to become multiple or widely disseminated.

Multiple myeloma is a disease of adult life (fourth to eighth decades), and men are affected more often than women. Characteristi-

cally, the disease is attended by symptoms of pain, weakness, and weight loss. Since the vertebral column usually is involved, there may be signs and symptoms referable to pressure upon the spinal cord or the spinal nerves. Compression fractures of vertebrae or pathologic fractures of other involved bones may occur. Some degree of anemia usually is noted, and examination of the blood often reveals excessive rouleau formation. Myeloma cells may be observed in blood smears in a substantial number of patients, and in an occasional instance such cells are very numerous. Other common manifestations of the disease are rapid erythrocyte sedimentation rate, increased calcium values in blood plasma, and Bence Jones protein in the urine. Hyperproteinema, sometimes of marked degree, can be attributed to an increase in various abnormal plasma globulins—the so-called myeloma "M" proteins.

Kidneys involved in the excretion of Bence Jones protein are likely to contain dense casts filling many of the tubules. The kidneys from patients with myeloma also may show amyloid deposits.

The skeletal changes in myeloma result

from tumor involvement of the marrow, resulting in diffuse and focalized bone resorption. In most instances, bone marrow involvement is sufficiently widespread that marrow aspirations will prove diagnostic of the disease.

Roentgenologic examination reveals multiple small and large areas of bone destruction (Fig. 40-66). These have sharp borders ("punched-out areas") and are unaccompanied by proliferative reactions at their margins unless a fracture has occurred. Even in the presence of a pathologic fracture, the formative process may be feeble and not apparent in the roentgenogram.

Sections through the affected bones reveal small and large areas of sharply outlined bone destruction. These areas are occupied by soft, friable, and exceedingly cellular tumor tissue that is pinkish gray in color or distinctly red because of hemorrhage (Fig. 40-66). Microscopically, the tumor nodules are composed of closely packed cells of characteristic type (Fig. 40-67). The majority of cells are oval in shape and consist of fairly abundant cytoplasm of

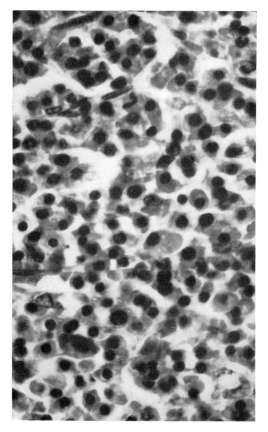

Fig. 40-67 Multiple myeloma. Closely packed tumor cells resembling plasma cells.

lavender tint and an eccentrically placed, rounded nucleus. The latter cell part is stained heavily, but in most instances there are peripherally placed clumps of chromatin that give it a "clock-faced" appearance. Some variation in size and shape of the cells is frequently noted, and in some examples of the tumor the degree of pleomorphism may be moderately prominent. In these specimens, multinucleated cells may be numerous.

Multiple myeloma runs a fatal course in several months to a few years. Death may result from inanition or infection or from the renal changes that frequently are associated with the disease. Postmortem examination reveals widespread destruction of the skeleton.[128] In addition, if renal impairment has occurred, there are interesting changes in the kidneys (Fig. 21-46). Occasionally, there is amyloid deposit in the organs and tissues, or there may be evidences of pathologic calcification. In more than half of the cases examined at autopsy, myeloma cell infiltration is found in extraosseous tissues. Involvement is most prominent in the lymph nodes, spleen, and liver.

Solitary myeloma. A few reports have appeared of single tumors in bone that have the cytologic characteristics of myeloma.[140] Following local removal, there may be no apparent tendency toward generalization. It is uncertain whether *solitary myeloma,* sometimes referred to as solitary *plasmacytoma,* is a distinct entity or a localized stage of multiple myeloma. An equally rare tumor of similar appearance and behavior occurs in the lymphoid tissues of the tonsils or soft palate and in the floor of the mouth.[131]

Reticulum cell sarcoma. In 1939, Parker and Jackson[115] drew attention to an uncommon primary tumor of bone that they named *reticulum cell sarcoma.* The tumor occurs principally in the long bones. Roentgenologically, there is uneven destruction of bone, causing osteoporosis and loss of normal architecture. Microscopically, the tumor resembles the reticulum cell sarcoma of lymphoid tissues. It has been observed that the affected patients may remain in good health, even when the tumor has reached a large size, and that metastasis is slow to occur. This latter feature and the known radiosensitivity of the tumor cells probably account for the comparatively good results from combined radiation and surgical treatment.[102] Radiation therapy alone is apparently inadequate to control this distinctive neoplasm.[125]

Lymphoma. Generalized malignant lymphoma, including Hodgkin's disease, may first be recognized because of signs and symptoms resulting from an osseous lesion. In most instances of this kind, the skeletal involvement is only a part of a disseminated tumor arising in lymphoid tissues. There are cases, however, in which the lymphoma appears to arise in bone as a solitary lesion, from which it may spread to other parts or, less frequently, remain restricted to the skeletal part where it originated (p. 1336).

Leukemia. Leukemia (p. 1367) is mentioned here only because of its origin in bone marrow and the secondary effects the disease has upon the skeletal parts.

Miscellaneous tumors

Lipoma. Small or medium-sized nodules of fat tissue sharply demarcated from bone marrow are occasionally encountered in the examination of the skeletal parts. It is questionable, however, whether these inclusions of adipose tissue should be classified as benign tumors. In exceedingly rare instances, benign tumors of fatty tissue having the characteristics of lipomas originating in soft tissue parts are discovered in bone.

Liposarcoma. One of the rarest varieties of tumors of skeletal tissues is the liposarcoma.[56, 121, 130] When inspected grossly, the tumor tissue is pale yellow in color and soft in consistency. Multiple tumors in bone, including the skull, may be recognized. It is not certain whether there are separate primary neoplasms or metastases. If the latter, a tendency for early metastasis to bone must be assigned to this neoplasm. Microscopically, the cells are large and pale, and their cytoplasm contains abundant amounts of finely divided particles of fat that may be stained in a characteristic manner. The cells show considerable pleomorphism and may be arranged in alveolar groups.

Chordoma. Chordoma is a rare neoplasm that arises from remnants of the notochord and invades the bones at the base of the skull or near the coccyx. Infrequently, it may arise in other regions of the vertebral column. Although locally invasive and prone to recurrence, it rarely metastasizes. Grossly, the tumor is firm and elastic—much like a chondroma. Some examples, however, have a mucinous quality and are soft in consistency. Microscopically, the tumor shows cords and sheets of cells that are oval or globular in shape and have clear cytoplasm. These are surrounded by a homogeneous and pale-staining mucoid matrix. These features often give rise to a resemblance to colloid carcinoma, from which the tumor must be distinguished.

Metastatic tumors in bone

The skeleton is a frequent site of metastasis for carcinomas primary in the prostate, breast, kidney, stomach, lung, and thyroid gland. Cancers arising in other organs, including the body and cervix of the uterus, adrenal glands, bladder, and testicle, also may spread to bone. Melanomas sometimes give rise to extensive skeletal involvement.

In order of frequency, the bones most commonly involved are as follows: spine, pelvis, femur, skull, ribs, and humerus. Metastases to the bones of the forearm, wrist, and hand and to the bones of the leg, ankle, and foot are of infrequent occurrence.[27]

With the exception of carcinoma of the prostate, where the metastases usually give rise to a condensation of bone, the areas of skeletal invasion by malignant neoplasms are characteristically destructive. In individual cases, however, the opposite effects may be noted, and a carcinoma of the breast or stomach occasionally may give rise to formative or *osteoplastic metastases,* whereas carcinoma of the prostate sometimes induces destructive or *osteolytic* lesions.

Neuroblastomas may cause excessive bone formation on the cranial surfaces and along the long bones. Metastases from adenocarcinomas of the kidney (hypernephromas) usually result in large destructive lesions in one or two bones (Fig. 40-68). Because of the pronounced vascularity, these tumors may pulsate and give rise to an audible bruit.

The routes by which metastasis to bone occurs are the following: (1) blood vessels, (2) lymph vessels, and (3) direct extension from the primary neoplasm or from its established metastases. Extension along perineural lymphatics in cancers of the prostate is frequent.

The association of elevated serum acid phosphatase with skeletal involvement in carcinoma of the prostate is an interesting biologic phenomenon, as well as a recognized aid in diagnosis.

Pathologic fracture may be the first indication that metastasis to bone has taken place. Less often, a metastasis may constitute the first evidence of the primary disease. In late cases, pathologic fractures of the affected bones may add greatly to the discomfort of the patient.

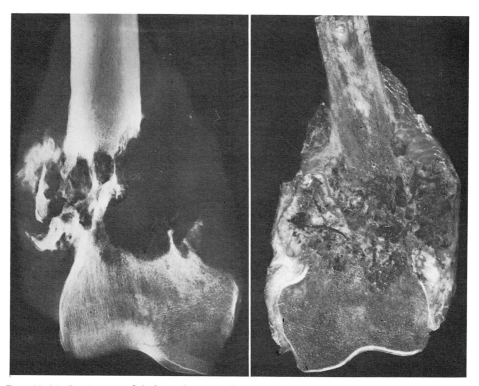

Fig. 40-68 Carcinoma of kidney (hypernephroma) metastasis. Radiologic and gross appearances of slice of femur showing large destructive lesion with pathologic fracture.

Skeletal metastases, when demonstrated in any given patient, are obviously of great importance in determining prognosis and in guiding treatment. In general, the consequences of such lesions, to the patient, are pain that is frequently intolerable and disability to the point of complete invalidism until the disease has terminated fatally.

REFERENCES
General

1 Bourne, G. H.: The biochemistry and physiology of bone, New York, 1956, Academic Press, Inc.
2 Budy, A. M., editor: Biology of hard tissue, Proceedings, New York Academy of Sciences, New York, 1967.
3 Collins, D. H.: Pathology of bone, London, 1966, Butterworth & Co. (Publishers) Ltd.

Specific

4 Albright, F.: Trans. Ass. Amer. Physicians 51: 199-212, 1936.
5 Albright, F.: J.A.M.A. 117:527-533, 1941.
6 Albright, F., and Reifenstein, E. C., Jr.: The parathyroid glands and metabolic bone disease, Baltimore, 1948, The Williams & Wilkins Co.
7 Albright, F., Bloomberg, E., and Smith, P. H.: Trans. Ass. Amer. Physicians 55:298-305, 1940.
8 Albright, F., Burnett, C. H., Cope, O., and Parson, W.: J. Clin. Endocr. 1:711-716, 1941.
9 Albright, F., Butler, A. M., Hampton, A. O.,
and Smith, P.: New Eng. J. Med. 216:727-746, 1937.
10 Albright, F., Burnett, C. H., Parson, W., Reifenstein, E. C., Jr., and Roos, A.: Medicine (Balt.) 25:399-479, 1946.
11 Anderson, W. A. D.: Arch. Path. (Chicago) 27:753-778, 1939.
12 Aschoff, L., and Koch, W.: Scorbut, eine pathologisch-anatomische Studie, Jena, 1919, Gustav Fisher.
13 Aub, J. C., Bauer, W., Heath, C., and Ropes, M.: J. Clin. Invest. 7:97-137, 1929.
14 Avioli, L. V., Lasersohn, J. T., and Lopresti, J. M.: Medicine (Balt.) 42:119-147, 1963.
15 Benedict, P. H., Szabo, G., Fitzpatrick, T. B., and Sinesi, S. J.: J.A.M.A. 205:618-626, 1968.
16 Bennett, G. A., and Bauer, W.: In Scudder, C. L., editor: The treatment of fractures, ed. 11, Philadelphia, 1938, W. B. Saunders Co.
17 Bennett, G. A., and Hodes, P. J.: Seminar on diseases of the skeleton including neoplasms, 1954, American Society of Clinical Pathologists, case 21, pp. 49-54.
18 Black, W.: In King, D. W., editor: Ultrastructural aspects of disease, New York, 1966, Hoeber Medical Division, Harper & Row, Publishers.
19 Boyle, P. E., Bessey, O. A., and Howe, P. R.: Arch. Path. (Chicago) 30:90-107, 1940.
20 Bundens, W. D., Jr., and Brighton, C. T.: J. Bone Joint Surg. 47-A:762-772, 1965.
21 Canavan, M. M.: Arch. Neurol. Psychiat. (Chicago) 39:41-53, 1938.
22 Castleman, B., and McNeill, J. M., editors:

Bone and joint clinicopathological conferences of the Massachusetts General Hospital, Boston, 1966, Little, Brown and Co., case 46, pp. 214-220.

23 Chalmers, J., Conacher, W. D. H., Gardner, D. L., and Scott, P. J.: J. Bone Joint Surg. 49-B:403-423, 1967.

24 Changus, G. W., Speed, J. S., and Stewart, F. W.: Cancer 10:540-559, 1957.

25 Christian, H. A.: In Contributions to Medical and Biological Research, vol. 1, New York, 1919, Paul B. Hoeber, Inc., p. 390.

26 Christian, H. A.: Med. Clin. N. Amer. 3:849-871, 1920.

27 Copeland, M. M.: Arch. Surg. (Chicago) 23:581-654, 1931.

28 Crocker, A. C., and Farber, S.: Medicine (Balt.) 37:1-95, 1958.

29 Cushing, H.: Arch. Neurol. Psychiat. (Chicago) 8:139-154, 1922.

30 Cushing, H.: Bull. Johns Hopkins Hosp. 50:137-195, 1932.

31 Cushing, H., and Davidoff, L. M.: Monographs of The Rockefeller Institute for Medical Research, no. 22, New York, 1927, The Rockefeller Institute for Medical Research.

32 Dahlin, D. C.: Bone tumors, ed. 2, Springfield, Ill., 1967, Charles C Thomas, Publisher.

33 Dahlin, D. C., and Coventry, M. B.: J. Bone Joint Surg. 49-A:101-110, 1967.

34 Dahlin, D. C., Besse, B. E., Jr., Pugh, D. G., and Ghormley, R. K.: Radiology 64:56-65, 1955.

35 Dixon, T. F., and Perkins, H. R.: In Bourne, G. H., editor: The biochemistry and physiology of bone, New York, 1956, Academic Press, Inc.

36 Dreskin, E. A., and Fox, T. A.: Arch. Intern. Med. (Chicago) 86:533-557, 1950.

37 Dudley, H. R., and Spiro, D.: J. Biophys. Biochem. Cytol. 11:627-649, 1961.

38 Dunlap, C. E., Aub, J. C., and Evans, R. D.: Amer. J. Path. 20:1-21, 1944.

39 Duthie, R. B., and Townes, P. L.: J. Bone Joint Surg. 49-B:229-248, 1967.

40 Dwinnell, L. A., Dahlin, D. C., and Ghormley, R. K.: J. Bone Joint Surg. 36-A:732-744, 1954.

41 Elliott, G. B.: J. Bone Joint Surg. 44-B:25-33, 1962.

42 Erdheim, J.: Virchow Arch. Path. Anat. 281:197-296, 1931.

43 Ewing, J.: Proc. N. Y. Path. Soc. 21:17-24, 1921.

44 Ewing, J.: Proc. N. Y. Path. Soc. 24:93-101, 1924.

45 Ewing, J.: Surg. Gynec. Obstet. 68:971-976, 1939.

46 Ewing, J.: Neoplastic diseases, ed. 4, Philadelphia, 1941, W. B. Saunders Co.

47 Farber, S.: Amer. J. Path. 17:625-629, 1941.

48 Follis, R. H., Jr.: Bull. Johns Hopkins Hosp. 89:9-20, 1951.

49 Follis, R. H., Jr.: Deficiency disease, Springfield, Ill., 1958, Charles C Thomas, Publisher.

50 Foster, G. V.: New Eng. J. Med. 279:349-360, 1968.

51 Gall, E. A., and Bennett, G. A.: Arch. Path. (Chicago) 33:866-878, 1942.

52 Gall, E. A., Bennett, G. A., and Bauer, W.: Amer. J. Path. 27:349-381, 1951.

53 Geschickter, C. F., and Copeland, M. M.: Tumors of bone, Int. Surg. Dig. 10:323-343, 1930.

54 Gilmer, W. S., Jr., Higley, G. B., Jr., and Kilgore, W. E.: Atlas of bone tumors, St. Louis, 1963, The C. V. Mosby Co., chap. 8.

55 Glimcher, M. J., Hodge, A. J., and Schmitt, F. O.: Proc. Nat. Acad. Sci. U.S.A. 43:860-867, 1957.

56 Goldman, R. L.: Amer. J. Clin. Path. 42:503-508, 1964.

57 Green, W. T., and Farber, S.: J. Bone Joint Surg. 24:499-526, 1942.

58 Green, W. T., and Shannon, J. G.: Arch. Surg. (Chicago) 32:462-493, 1936.

59 Greenwood, D. A.: Physiol. Rev. 20:582-616, 1940.

60 Ham, A. W., and Harris, W. R.: In Bourne, G. H., editor: The biochemistry and physiology of bone, New York, 1956, Academic Press, Inc.

61 Hand, A.: Arch. Pediat. 10:673, 1893.

62 Hand, A.: Amer. J. Med. Sci. 162:509-515, 1921.

63 Harris, L. J.: In Bourne, G. H., editor: The biochemistry and physiology of bone, New York, 1956, Academic Press, Inc.

64 Harris, W. H., and Heaney, R. P.: New Eng. J. Med. 280:193-202, 253-259, 303-311, 1969.

65 Harris, W. H., Dudley, H. R., Jr., and Barry, R. J.: J. Bone Joint Surg. 44-A:207-233, 1962.

66 Henschen, F.: Morgagni's syndrome, Edinburgh, 1949, Oliver & Boyd Ltd.

67 Herrmann, L. G., Reineke, H. G., and Caldwell, J. A.: Amer. J. Roentgen. 47:353-361, 1942.

68 Hess, A. F.: Scurvy, past and present, Philadelphia, 1920, J. B. Lippincott Co.

69 Hills, R. G., and McLanahan, S.: Arch. Intern. Med. (Chicago) 59:41-55, 1937.

70 Howard, J. E., and Thomas, W. C., Jr.: Medicine (Balt.) 42:25-45, 1963.

71 Hunter, D., and Wiles, P.: Brit. J. Surg. 22:507-519, 1935.

72 Jacobsen, A. W.: J.A.M.A. 113:121-124, 1939.

73 Jacobson, S. A.: J. Bone Joint Surg. 40-A:1310-1328, 1958.

74 Jaffe, H. L.: Arch. Path. (Chicago) 15:83-131, 1933.

75 Jaffe, H. L.: Arch. Path. (Chicago) 36:335-357, 1943.

76 Jaffe, H. L.: Tumors and tumorous conditions of the bones and joints, Philadelphia, 1964, Lea & Febiger.

77 Jaffe, H. L., and Lichtenstein, L.: J. Bone Joint Surg. 22:645-682, 1940.

78 Jaffe, H. L., and Lichtenstein, L.: Arch. Surg. (Chicago) 44:1004-1025, 1942.

79 Jaffe, H. L., and Lichtenstein, L.: Amer. J. Path. 18:205-221, 1942.

80 Jaffe, H. L., and Lichtenstein, L.: Amer. J. Path. 18:969-991, 1942.

81 Jaffe, H. L., and Lichtenstein, L.: Arch. Path. (Chicago) 45:541-551, 1948.

82 Jaffe, H. L., Lichtenstein, L., and Portis, R. B.: Arch. Path. (Chicago) 30:993-1031, 1940.

83 Jowsey, J.: Birth Defects: Original Article

Series II(1):51-55, 1966; The National Foundation, New York.

84 Kahlstrom, S. C., and Phemister, D. B.: Amer. J. Path. 22:947-963, 1946.

85 Kahlstrom, S. C., Burton, C. C., and Phemister, D. B.: Surg. Gynec. Obstet. 68:129-146, 1939.

86 Largent, E. J., Machle, W., and Ferneau, I. F.: J. Industr. Hyg. Toxic. 25:396-408, 1943.

87 Lee, W. R.: J. Bone Joint Surg. 49-B:146-153, 1967.

88 Léri, A., and Joanny: Bull. Soc. Med. Hop. Paris 46:1141-1145, 1922.

89 Lichtenstein, L.: Arch. Path. (Chicago) 56:84-102, 1953.

90 Lichtenstein, L.: J. Bone Joint Surg. 39-A:873-882, 1957.

91 Lichtenstein, L.: J. Bone Joint Surg. 46-A:76-90, 1964.

92 Lichtenstein, L., and Jaffe, H. L.: Arch. Path. (Chicago) 33:777-816, 1942.

93 Lichtenstein, L., and Jaffe, H. L.: Amer. J. Path. 23:43-77, 1947.

94 Lichtenstein, L., and Sawyer, W. B.: J. Bone Joint Surg. 46-A:755-765, 1964.

95 Looney, W. B.: J. Bone Joint Surg. 37-A:1169-1187, 1955.

96 McCormack, L. J., Dockerty, M. B., and Ghormley, R. K.: Cancer 5:85-99, 1952.

97 McCune, D. J., and Bradley, C.: Amer. J. Dis. Child. 48:949-1000, 1934.

98 McCune, D. J., and Bruch, H.: Amer. J. Dis. Child. 54:806-848, 1937.

99 McKusick, V. A.: Heritable disorders of connective tissue, ed. 3, St. Louis, 1966, The C. V. Mosby Co.

100 McLean, F. C.: Science 127:451-456, 1958.

101 McLean, F. C., and Urist, M. R.: Bone, ed. 3, Chicago, 1968, University of Chicago Press.

102 Magnus, H. A., and Wood, H. L. C.: J. Bone Joint Surg. 38-B:258-278, 1956.

103 Mallory, T. B.: New Eng. J. Med. 227:955-960, 1942.

103a Maroteaux, P., Lamy, M., and Robert, J. M.: Presse Med. 75:2519-2524, 1967.

104 Matalon, R., and Dorfman, A.: Proc. Nat. Acad. Sci. U.S.A. 60:179-185, 1968.

105 Mnaymneh, W. A., Dudley, H. R., and Mnaymneh, L. G.: J. Bone Joint Surg. 46-A:63-75, 1964.

106 Moritz, A. R.: The pathology of trauma, Philadelphia, 1942, Lea & Febiger.

107 Morquio, L.: Arch. Med. Enf. 32:129-140, 1929.

108 Murphy, W. R., and Ackerman, L. V.: Cancer 9:317-339, 1956.

109 Neuman, W. F., and Neuman, M. W.: The chemical dynamics of bone mineral, Chicago, 1958, University of Chicago Press.

110 Oberling, C., and Raileanu, C.: Bull. Ass. Franç. Etude Cancer 21:333-347, 1932.

111 Pack, G. T., and Braund, R. R.: J.A.M.A. 119:776-779, 1942.

112 Paget, J.: Trans. Roy. Med. Chir. Soc. London 60:37, 1877.

113 Park, E. A.: Harvey Lect. 34:157-213, 1939.

114 Park, E. A., Guild, H. G., Jackson, D., and Bond, M.: Arch. Dis. Child. 10:265-294, 1935.

115 Parker, F., Jr., and Jackson, H., Jr.: Surg. Gynec. Obstet. 68:45-53, 1939.

116 Phemister, D. B., and Grimson, K. S.: Ann. Surg. 105:564-583, 1937.

117 Pohl, J. F.: J. Bone Joint Surg. 21:187-192, 1939.

118 Porretta, C. A., Dahlin, D. C., and Janes, J. M.: J. Bone Joint Surg. 39-A:1314-1329, 1957.

119 Price, C. H. G.: J. Bone Joint Surg. 44-B:336-376, 1962.

120 Reed, R. J.: Arch. Path. (Chicago) 75:480-495, 1963.

121 Rehbock, D. J., and Hauser, H.: Amer. J. Cancer 27:37-44, 1936.

121a Rimoin, D. L., Hughes, G. N., Kaufman, R. L., Rosenthal, R. E., McAlister, W. H., and Silberberg, R.: New Eng. J. Med. 283:728-735, 1970.

122 Schlumberger, H. G.: Milit. Surg. 99:504-527, 1946.

123 Schmorl, G.: Virchow Arch. Path. Anat. 283:694-751, 1932.

124 Schüller, A.: Fortschr. Roentgenstr. 23:12-18, 1915.

125 Simmons, C. C.: Surg. Gynec. Obstet. 68:67-75, 1939.

126 Sissons, H. A.: J. Bone Joint Surg. 38-B:418-433, 1956.

127 Snapper, I.: Medical clinics on bone diseases, New York, 1943, Interscience Publishers, Inc., pp. 151-173.

128 Snapper, I., Turner, L. B., and Moscovitz, H. L.: Multiple myeloma, New York, 1953, Grune & Stratton, Inc.

129 Sternberg, W. H., and Joseph, V.: Amer. J. Dis. Child. 63:748-783, 1942.

130 Stewart, F. W.: Amer. J. Path. 7:87-94, 1931.

131 Stewart, M. J., and Taylor, A. L.: J. Path. Bact. 35:541-547, 1932.

132 Thannhauser, S. J., and Magendantz, H.: Ann. Intern. Med. 11:1662-1746, 1938.

133 Thoma, K. H.: Clinical pathology of the jaws, Springfield, Ill., 1934, Charles C Thomas, Publisher, chap. 2, pp. 62-69.

134 Thorndike, A., Jr.: J. Bone Joint Surg. 22:315-323, 1940.

135 Tumulty, P. A., and Howard, J. E.: J.A.M.A. 119:233-236, 1942.

136 Van Hazel, W.: J. Thorac. Surg. 9:495-505, 1940.

137 Waine, H., Bennett, G. A., and Bauer, W.: Amer. J. Med. Sci. 209:671-687, 1945.

137a Waldvogel, F. A., Medoff, G., and Swartz, M. N.: New Eng. J. Med. 282:198-206, 260-266, 316-322, 1970.

138 Wang, C. C., and Schulz, M. D.: New Eng. J. Med. 248:571-576, 1953.

139 Weinmann, J. P., and Sicher, H.: Bone and bones, ed. 2, St. Louis, 1955, The C. V. Mosby Co.

140 Willis, R. A.: J. Path. Bact. 53:77-85, 1941.

141 Wolbach, S. B.: Amer. J. Path. 9:689-699, 1933.

142 Wolbach, S. B.: Science 86:569-576, 1937.

143 Wolbach, S. B.: Proc. Inst. Med. Chicago 16:118-145, 1946.

144 Wolbach, S. B., and Howe, P. R.: Arch. Path. Lab. Med. 1:1-24, 1926.

145 Zawisch-Ossenitz, C.: Arch. Path. (Chicago) 43:55-75, 1947.

Chapter 41

Joints

Granville A. Bennett

The term "joint disease" covers a wide range of disorders that frequently have nothing in common except involvement of the specialized tissues that comprise the articulations. Therefore, before describing the pathologic changes that are associated with any particular infirmity, it is necessary to recall the outstanding anatomic and physiologic characteristics of these tissues.

ANATOMY AND PHYSIOLOGY

The individual bones forming the skeleton are joined one with another by structures known as *joints* or *articulations*. Such structures vary in kind and in function. There are articulations (e.g., sutures of the skull) that bind individual membrane bones together with fibrous connective tissue. Other articulations (e.g., symphysis pubis and intervertebral discs) are comprised of hyaline cartilaginous caps covering the adjacent bones which, in turn, are joined together by fibrocartilage and fibrous connective tissue in varying proportions. Still other joints (e.g., knee, wrist, elbow) are characterized by the presence of synovial-lined clefts between the cartilage-covered bone ends. These are known as diarthrodial or synovial joints, and they are designed in such a manner as to permit free and easy motion within certain ranges.

Most synovial joints are simple in structure. They are composed of two or more opposing, cartilage-covered bone ends, joined by a flexible tube of dense connective tissue, the articular capsule (Fig. 40-1). An intimal layer of varying microscopic structure lines the capsule. This is referred to as the synovia or synovial membrane. Within this enclosed cleft is a small quantity of clear, viscid synovial fluid.

Adjacent to the joints are similar tissue components such as fascial layers, tendons, tendon sheaths, and bursae. Not only are these structures of great importance in the normal mechanical functions of the joint, but also in the majority of articular diseases they are either primarily or secondarily affected.

Articular cartilage. The hyaline cartilage covering the bone ends of the synovial joints is comprised of cells (chondrocytes) and intercellular substances. Although there are differences in both cells and intercellular materials that appear to correlate with the age of the individual, articular cartilage is relatively a cell-poor tissue and a tissue known to have a low metabolic rate. In the young growing subject, the chondrocytes appear to be more numerous and more active, and it has been demonstrated that they are engaged in the formation of intercellular substances, both fibrous and amorphous. Grossly at this stage, the cartilage is thicker, more bluish in color, more translucent, and more elastic than it is at a later period when the joints are fully formed.

In the mature joint, the articular cartilage acquires a yellowish color and becomes somewhat less elastic. At this stage, the collagen fibers and bundles of fibers, which appear to have an archlike pattern (Fig. 41-1), are more readily visible within the amorphous materials, which consist of chondroitin sulfuric acid and mucopolysaccharides. Later in life, the fibrillar components became very prominent as degenerative changes set in.

It has been well established that mature articular cartilage has relatively little capacity for repair following injury.[14] Since articular cartilage is the recipient of most of the mechanical shocks and stresses that are exerted upon the skeleton, it is apparent that the maintenance of an entirely smooth articular surface, so essential to normal function, is constantly endangered. It has been clearly shown that articular cartilage is readily damaged by a wide variety of toxic agents, by acute injuries, and also by minor and repeated traumas that are incident to everyday activities.

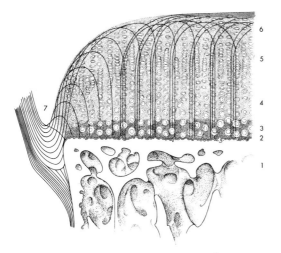

Fig. 41-1 Schematic representation of structure of hyaline articular cartilage. **1,** Subchondral bone. **2-6,** Articular cartilage. **2** and **3,** Calcified layer. **4** and **5,** Columnar layer(s). **6,** Superficial layer. **7,** Marginal area (synovial attachment). Articular cartilage firmly joined to bone in deepest (calcified) zone, **2** and **3.** From this zone arise fibrillar arcades that appear to provide quality of compressibility to articular cartilage as well as stable but smooth surface layer permitting motion when surface is lubricated with synovial fluid. (Modified from Benninghoff, A.: Z. Zellforsch. **2:**783-862, 1925.)

Synovial membrane. On both embryologic and histologic evidence, the intimal layer of the articular capsule is to be regarded as connective tissue that has undergone certain modifications in functional and structural characteristics. In contrast to cartilage, it has a marked capacity for regeneration. Experiments on animals indicate that repair is complete within thirty to one hundred days after synovectomy.[44, 73]

The synovial intima varies from dense fibrous connective tissue that is partially lined by inconspicuous flattened cells to a membrane composed of many layers of round, oval, or cubical cells that are supported by loosely textured and highly vascular connective tissue. These latter areas contain recesses or crypts, as well as permanently formed papillary projections called villi.

Among the known functions of synovial membrane are the formation of synovial mucin and the regulation of the passage of materials between the blood, lymph, and synovial fluid.[6] Foreign materials of colloidal or particulate nature are transferred across this membrane for removal from the joint. In the case of continuous or intermittent bleeding into the articular cavity, there may be exten-

sive deposits of hemosiderin in phagocytic cells in the subsynovial tissues or in the synovia lining cells. Lipids also may accumulate in these tissues under certain abnormal circumstances. In contrast to the membranes lining certain other body cavities, synovial membrane has a markedly greater permeability.[7, 17, 59]

Joint capsule. The articular capsule is composed of dense fibrous tissue, reinforced by tendons, muscles, and fascial layers. Its chief function appears to be the binding together of the bone ends entering into the articulation. In close proximity to the capsule or extending between its layers are tendon sheaths and bursal spaces that are lined by membranes which are similar in structure and function to the synovia of the joint proper.

Synovial fluid. The normal joint contains a small quantity of cell-poor, clear, pale yellow, viscid liquid. It is possible to aspirate 0.45 ml (average) of fluid from the normal adult human knee.[24] In such fluid, the total nucleated cells average 63 per cubic millimeter, of which 63% are mononuclear phagocytes, 24% lymphocytes, 6.5% polymorphonuclear leukocytes, 4.3% synovial cells, and 2.2% unidentified cells. The relative viscosity is 150 at 25° C. The average total albumin and globulin content is 1.72 gm per 100 ml, and the average mucin content is 0.85 gm per 100 ml.[57] The distribution of nonelectrolytes and electrolytes between the blood serum and the synovial fluid is in accord with the concept that synovial fluid is a dialysate of blood plasma containing albumin, globulin, and mucin. The mucin is probably elaborated by functionally specialized cells in the synovial tissues.

Changes in the amount and appearance of synovial fluid and in its physical and chemical characteristics occur rapidly as a result of injury or disease, and such alterations may be of aid in diagnosis and treatment.[25, 56]

The joints are anatomically and functionally adapted to permit easy motion within a certain range. They are, however, so constituted that the cartilage surfaces and the synovial tissues are subjected to frequent injuries of mechanical, toxic, and metabolic nature. In the case of cartilage, such injuries are not well tolerated because of certain inherent biologic characteristics that limit its ability to regenerate. The articular surfaces are prone, therefore, to undergo important regressive changes solely from physiologic aging and the wear and tear of daily use.[18] Such alterations may be greatly accelerated because of deleterious agents, single or repeated trauma, or as the result of deranged mechanics from faulty posture or disturbed locomotion.

DISEASES OF JOINTS

Incidence. Since ancient skeletons of man and animals that have been obtained from widely separated geographic locations bear unmistakable marks of certain forms of arthritis and other diseases that are prevalent today, it may be concluded that articular disorders are among the oldest and most widely prevalent infirmities.

A survey conducted by the United States Public Health Service in 1938 gave a good index to the great social and economic importance of joint disease in modern times. It was estimated that the number of persons disabled annually by rheumatic disorders exceed those affected by tuberculosis and diabetes in a ratio of 10:1 and those by cancer and other tumors in a ratio of 7:1. The number of cases of "rheumatism" (including arthritis, gout, lumbago, neuralgia, etc.) in the United States in 1937 was calculated to be 6,850,000. From survey data acquired in the two-year period ending in June, 1959,[1] it was estimated that 10,845,000 persons have some form of arthritis or rheumatism.

Classification. The most prevalent and disabling infirmities affecting the articulations of the body are the various forms of chronic, deforming arthritis. However, since almost all known diseases can and occasionally do give rise to manifestations of joint disease, it is proper to list the conditions that will be discussed in this chapter. It should be emphasized that a truly satisfactory classification must await more precise information concerning the etiology and pathogenesis of these various abnormal states.

1 Arthritis caused by known infectious agents
2 Arthritis associated with rheumatic fever
3 Rheumatoid arthritis
4 Degenerative joint disease
5 Arthritis caused by trauma
6 Arthritis associated with gout
7 Arthritis of neuropathic origin (Charcot joint)
8 Miscellaneous forms of joint disease
  a Systemic diseases with which arthritis is frequently associated
  b Local disorders affecting articular tissues
9 Neoplasms of joints, bursae, tendons, and tendon sheaths

Arthritis
Arthritis caused by known infectious agents

Compared with arthritis of unknown etiology, the incidence of specific infections of joints always has been low, and since the introduction of effective antibiotics, the occurrence of arthritis as a complication of acute systemic infections has become a clinical rarity. However, it should be remembered that one of the possible complications of any infectious disease is the localization of the responsible microorganism in one or more of the joints. Although any pathogenic microorganism may produce a joint infection, the more important forms of arthritis of this category are those that are caused by the gonococcus, streptococcus, staphylococcus, pneumococcus, and tubercle bacillus. These infectious agents may reach an articulation by way of the bloodstream, the lymphatic vessels, or by direct implantation of the microorganism—either from a perforating injury or by the extension of an infectious lesion from the neighboring bony or soft tissues into the articular cavity.

It has been adequately demonstrated experimentally that the synovial tissues are especially susceptible to the localization of organisms when a bacteremia has been induced.

Gonococcic arthritis. Before the advent of chemotherapy, involvement of the joints occurred in 2% to 5% of the persons who developed gonorrheal infections.[42] The knees, ankles, wrists, fingers, shoulders, and toes, in that order of frequency, are sites that are commonly affected.

The arthritis usually begins within one to three weeks following the onset of the underlying disease. Less frequently, the joint lesion develops many weeks or months later. In approximately 80% of the patients, the arthritis is polyarticular at the onset. In the majority, however, the signs and symptoms of joint inflammation promptly subside in all but one or two of the joints. The affected articulation becomes swollen, red, and tender. There is pronounced pain on motion, and movements are markedly restricted. The joint space becomes distended with inflammatory exudate. Temperature ranging up to 104° F and a moderate leukocytosis frequently are observed. The sedimentation rate is rapid.

Examination of the joint fluid reveals a great increase in the number of nucleated cells, polymorphonuclear leukocytes predominating. Cell counts range as high as 250,000 per cubic millimeter. Gonococci may be demonstrated in smears in some cases. Positive cultures are obtained in approximately 25% of the patients. Another diagnostic aid is the gonococcus complement fixation test of blood (positive in approximately 80% of the patients).

The extent of the inflammatory change within the joint and the degree of destruction of the articular tissues are variable and may range from a moderate synovitis that heals without residual stiffness or deformity to a purulent arthritis that is accompanied by destruction of the articular cartilage and synovial tissue. The latter types of lesion may give rise to a permanent deformity and, occasionally, to bony ankylosis.

During the years since chemotherapeutic agents became available, the incidence of joint involvement as a complication of genital gonorrhea has been sharply reduced. Also, there has been a shift in incidence from a predominance in men to a predominance in women. Furthermore, it has been demonstrated that with the use of proper techniques, early and accurate diagnosis is possible.

While gonorrheal arthritis continues to be a significant disease entity,[40, 43, 52] early diagnosis and effective antibiotic therapy have almost eliminated the disabling complications that formerly were of great concern.

Arthritis caused by other pyogenic microorganisms. Streptococci, staphylococci, pneumococci, and other pathogenic microorganisms may localize in the synovial tissues from the blood or may reach the joint by direct extension from an adjacent focus of infection. The reaction, although often more violent and destructive, is similar to that produced by the gonococcus. The synovial tissues become hyperemic and edematous, and there is an effusion of fluid into the joint. Soon the articular fluid is rich in leukocytes and fibrin, and if the articular cavity is opened, it will be seen that the synovial surfaces are covered with fibrinopurulent exudate. The articular cartilage becomes yellowish gray in color and nonglistening. It is rapidly undermined at the perichondrial margins, and large or small portions of the cartilage may become detached from the underlying cancellous bone.

The degree of stiffness and deformity ensuing will depend upon the extent to which the cartilage and synovial tissues were damaged. Healing occurs by granulation tissue formation and subsequent cicatrization. There is little or no regeneration of the injured cartilage, and bony ankylosis is not uncommon.

Tuberculosis. While almost invariably resulting from the localization of organisms disseminated via the bloodstream, tuberculous arthritis may be either primary in the synovial membrane or secondary to a focus of tuberculous osteomyelitis in close proximity to the articulation. In the knee in adults, initial involvement of the synovial tissues is much more frequently observed, whereas in children the involvement of the joint is usually secondary to a focus in the adjacent bone end. Such a focus usually arises from localization of the infection in the metaphyseal end of the shaft, and the joint is invaded either by a spread of the infection through the soft tissue or through the epiphysis. Regardless of the point of origin, the end result of a tuberculous infection of a joint is likely to be the same. Generally, however, the progress is more protracted in infections arising in the synovial tissues.

The synovial membrane becomes hyperemic, edematous, and redundant. Its surface is obscured by grayish yellow exudate. Occasionally, tubercles can be recognized if care is used in inspecting the exposed surfaces. However, there is greater likelihood of recognizing caseating lesions on surfaces made by slicing into the synovial tissues. In some cases, the articular lining is totally replaced by abundant shaggy fibrinous exudate and shreds of necrotic tissue, and occasionally the joint space will contain grayish white bodies the size and shape of melon seeds (joint mice). The amount of fluid contained in the joint is variable but, as a rule, only a small to moderate amount of turbid liquid containing shreds and flakes of fibrin is evacuated when the joint is opened. Occasionally, an excessive quantity of relatively clear fluid distends the joint (tuberculous hydrops). The changes observed in the articular cartilage depend, to a considerable extent, on the duration of the infection. The cartilage is attacked either from the articular surface or from the cancellous bone spaces in the epiphysis. In many instances, both surfaces are affected simultaneously. In early cases, the cartilage may show no change other than a loss of its smooth glistening luster. This may be accompanied by the extension of tuberculous granulation tissue from the perichondrial margins onto the articular surfaces. In more severely affected joints, the cartilage is loosened from the underlying bone, and, in some instances, it disappears, leaving an uneven granular base of necrotic bone and exudate.

In microscopic sections, the loosened fragments of cartilage show faintly stained matrix devoid of cartilage cells. The affected osseous tissue reveals areas of bone necrosis surrounded by tuberculous granulation tissue in which many tubercles are usually apparent. The necrotic bone trabeculae undergo fragmentation and gradual resorption (caries). Extensive sequestration is uncommon. Sections of the synovial membrane usually reveal a thick surface layer of exudate with underlying caseation necrosis. Beneath this, recognizable miliary and conglomerate tubercles are usually present in abundance.

The course of tuberculous arthritis is variable. If the infection is confined to the synovial tissues, the lesion may heal with limited disability. More frequently, however, the cartilage covering of the bone ends is destroyed and the adjacent bone is affected. In these cases, healing, if successfully accomplished, results in either fibrous or bony ankylosis of the joint.

Syphilis. The frequency with which the joint structures are involved in syphilis has not been determined. It is known, however, that arthritis may occur in either congenital or acquired forms of the disease.

In *congenital syphilis,* varying degrees of involvement of the articular capsules and epiphyses may be noted in conjunction with the characteristic changes represented by osteochondritis and periostitis. Such an affection leads to pain, tenderness, and swelling of the joint. Microscopically, these articulations show hyperemia, edema, lymphoid and plasma cell infiltration, and proliferation of fibroblasts. In addition, there may be small areas of necrosis in the cartilage, bone, or capsular tissues.

In older children showing manifestations of congenital syphilis, there sometimes develops a peculiar form of arthritis known as Clutton's joints. One or both knees may be affected, and occasionally some other joint is involved. The affected joint, while rarely painful, is swollen and lax and contains an excessive amount of fluid. The synovial tissues are thickened and appear soft and gelatinous. Microscopically, there are edema and a diffuse infiltration with lymphocytes and plasma cells. Gummatous lesions may be present in some of the specimens.

During the early stages of *acquired syphilis,* the joints may be painful and tender. Stiffness is also a complaint. Although pathologic investigations are notably lacking, it seems probable that these symptoms of acute arthritis result from the same inflammatory and vascular lesions that give rise to such visible lesions as the skin rash and mucous patches. In the usual case, the joint pain subsides without giving rise to lesions that are detectable on physical examination. Occasionally, however, the joint swells, and evidence of an effusion can be elicited. The knee joint is the articulation most frequently affected, and the involvement is commonly bilateral.

In later stages of acquired syphilis, the joints may be the site of gumma formation or of a diffuse nonspecific chronic synovitis that is associated with moderate or marked grades of effusion. Gummatous lesions, when they occur, may be limited to the synovial tissues, or they may be more extensive and involve the adjacent ligaments, as well as the articular cartilage and adjacent bone.

Brucellosis. Spondylitis and arthritis are among the more frequent complications of brucellar infection (p. 309).

Mycotic diseases. Bone and joint involvement may occur in coccidioidomycosis (p. 419), blastomycosis (p. 414), and actinomycosis (p. 411).

Arthritis associated with rheumatic fever

Rheumatic fever is a systemic disease characterized by fever, pain, and swelling of joints and symptom complexes that result from involvement of the heart. The disease may have either an insidious or an abrupt fulminating onset, and exacerbations and remissions of symptoms are common.

Although rheumatic fever oftentimes is included among the so-called *"collagen diseases,"* it should be remembered that a number of the clinical and pathologic features are so highly characteristic as to be considered disease specific.

The etiology of rheumatic fever has not been unequivocally established (p. 631). However, it seems certain that the disease is a delayed sequel to infections caused by group A hemolytic streptococci.[49]

Acute arthritis, usually migratory in nature and of short duration, is among the more frequent manifestations of rheumatic fever. Although any joint in the body may be affected, the larger articulations are most often involved. In children, the ankles, knees, and wrists are the common sites.[71]

All of the usual signs of acute inflammation, such as pain, tenderness, swelling, heat, and local redness, are evident in an affected joint. In addition to soft tissue swelling of the articular and periarticular tissues, there is usually a transudation of fluid into the joint space.

The synovial fluid is frequently turbid and contains increased nucleated cells, ranging up to 30,000 per cubic millimeter or higher. Polymorphonuclear leukocytes may comprise 90% or more of the total in early cases. Cultures are consistently negative.

Although few pathologic investigations have been conducted on articular tissues in the early stages of the arthritis, there is some evidence to indicate that there are marked hyperemia, edema, and leukocytic infiltration of the synovial tissues. Fibrinoid swelling of collagen like that seen in the subcutaneous nodule also may be present.[27] Actual suppuration does not occur, and necrosis of tissue is apparently minimal.

In the great majority of patients, the arthritis subsides after a few days, and complete restoration of joint function is the rule. Occasionally, however, residual pain and stiffness of either continuous or intermittent character persist. In some of these patients, mild to moderate degrees of chronic inflammation of the synovial and subsynovial tissues have been found when the joints were examined. Diffuse infiltration of lymphocytes, plasma cells, and mononuclear leukocytes is the most frequent change in these cases. There is rarely, if ever, any evidence of pannus.[10]

In about 20% of rheumatic fever patients, small subcutaneous nodules will be found in the soft tissues, overlying bony prominences and usually near the joints. The regions of the olecranon process and patella are the most common sites. On microscopic examination, these nodules show "fibrinoid" degeneration with latticing of the collagen and a mild to moderate grade of inflammatory cell infiltration. The lesions are usually poorly demarcated from the surrounding tissues and seldom show evidence of complete necrosis of the affected connective tissue. Occasionally, small focal areas of necrosis of collagen surrounded by mononuclear cell infiltration are observed. Such lesions may resemble the myocardial Aschoff nodule. Although the pathologic features of these nodules are qualitatively similar to those observed in the subcutaneous nodule of rheumatoid arthritis, it is usually possible to distinguish between the two lesions.[19]

Rheumatoid arthritis

The common synonyms for rheumatoid arthritis are atrophic arthritis and proliferative arthritis. In the young, the disorder, including **Still's disease**[28, 65] and **Felty's syndrome,**[32] is designated **juvenile rheumatoid arthritis.** When the sole or predominant involvement is located in the spine, sacroiliac joints, and hip joints, the disease is referred to as rheumatoid spondylitis or **Strümpell-Marie spondylitis.**

Before considering the clinical, roentgenologic, and pathologic findings of rheumatoid arthritis, as it is most frequently observed, it is appropriate to describe briefly two disorders which, although bearing different names, are believed by most physicians to be forms of rheumatoid arthritis. The first of these is Still's disease. This term came into common usage when Still separated juvenile rheumatoid arthritis into two groups: those patients in whom the condition was like that seen in adults and those patients who showed similar lesions in joints, but, in addition, exhibited manifestations of splenomegaly, lymphadenopathy, and sometimes adhesive pericarditis. Present-day awareness that lymphadenopathy and splenomegaly occur in adults, although less commonly than in children, has caused most clinicians and pathologists to reject the concept of a separate disease entity.[28] The second affection is frequently designated Felty's syndrome.[32] The rheumatoid arthritis, in this instance, is accompanied by leukopenia and enlargement of the spleen and liver. The spleen may be infiltrated with plasma cells and show a striking phagocytic activity in the reticular elements. Most clinicians specializing in the study and management of patients with arthritis believe that these associated disturbances do not justify a separate designation, and the term Felty's syndrome is used less frequently than formerly.

Rheumatoid arthritis is a systemic disease[53] of unknown etiology, characterized by a chronic and progressive inflammatory involvement of the articulations and by atrophy and rarefaction of the bones and muscles.

Although the disease affects persons of all ages, it occurs most frequently in the early decades of adult life. Approximately 80% of the cases commence between the ages of 20 and 50 years. Women are affected two to three times oftener than men. In Strümpell-Marie spondylitis, however, women are rarely affected.

There may be prodromal manifestations such as slight fever, loss of weight, fatigue, and increased sweating of the hands and feet. The onset of the disease, while usually insidious, may be abrupt and violent.

In the majority of patients, joint involve-

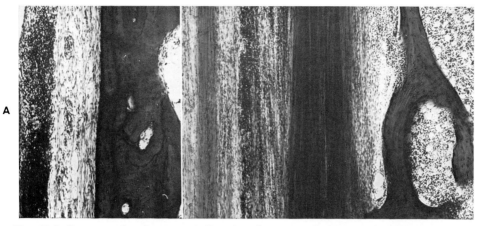

Fig. 41-2 Rheumatoid arthritis. **A,** Diffuse lymphocytic and plasma cell infiltration in subsynovial layer of tendon sheath in patient with long-standing rheumatoid arthritis. **B,** Chronic inflammation in tendon near insertion into bone in patient with widespread and advanced rheumatoid arthritis.

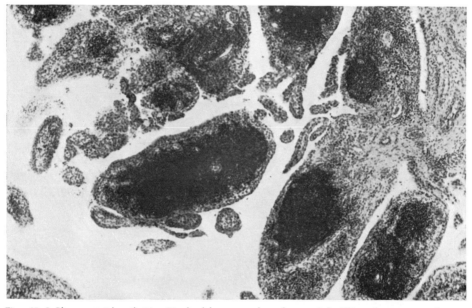

Fig. 41-3 Rheumatoid arthritis. Marked hypertrophy of synovial villi and extensive chronic inflammation of subsynovial tissues in knee of patient with rheumatoid arthritis. Focal accumulation of lymphocytes is common feature of disease.

ment is polyarticular, tends to be bilateral, and is somewhat symmetric in distribution. Early in the disease, there are pain, swelling, and stiffness of the joints. Slight redness and warmth also may be present, and the soft tissues about the articulations are thickened. This swelling, in combination with muscular atrophy, gives rise to fusiform or spindle-shaped digits.

One of the striking features of the disease is the pronounced tendency for exacerbations and remissions. Remissions occur irregularly and may last for months or years at a time.

Microscopic examination of specimens of articular tissues excised in the early stages of the disease reveals hyperemia, edema, and inflammation in the synovial and subsynovial layers.[47] The nearby tendons and tendon sheaths frequently are affected in a similar manner (Fig. 41-2). At first, the inflammatory cell infiltrate, consisting of lymphoid cells, plasma cells, and mononuclear and polymorphonuclear leukocytes, is diffuse and evenly distributed. Later, focal collections of lymphocytes appear and germinal follicles may develop in the greatly enlarged and lengthened synovial villi (Fig. 41-3). It is worthy of note that even in the early stages of involvement there is little evidence of tissue necrosis, and suppuration does not occur.

As the arthritis progresses, granulation tissue grows from the synovial tissues at the perichondrial margins to cover the articular cartilage surfaces (pannus). Concomitantly,

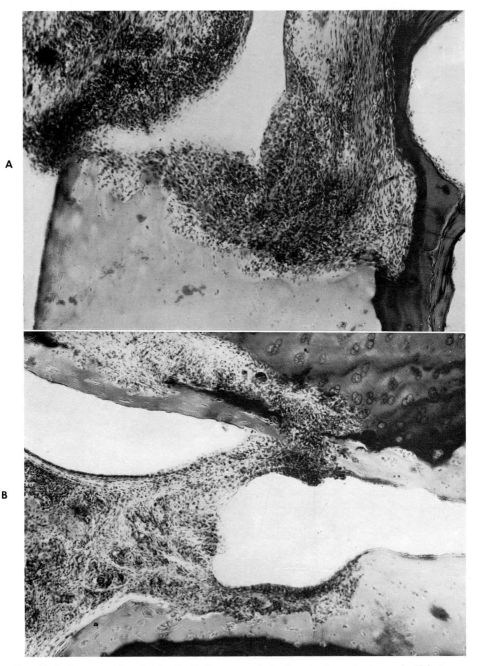

Fig. 41-4 Rheumatoid arthritis. **A,** Early stage. Articular cartilage in lower half being replaced by ingrowing granulation tissue from perichondrial margin. **B,** Early stage of fibrous ankylosis. Granulation tissue projecting inward from margin of interphalangeal joint has formed adhesion across joint space. Nearly all articular cartilage has disappeared beneath pannus, which is clearly shown in lower half.

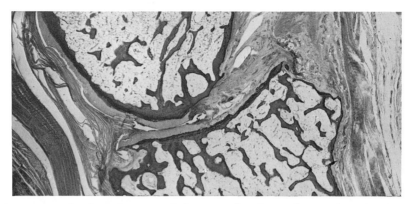

Fig. 41-5 Most of salient features of rheumatoid arthritis illustrated in this low-power photomicrograph of interphalangeal joint. In addition to bone atrophy and partial sub-luxation, articular cartilage thinned and pitted and overgrown with pannus. Also, joint space in right half obliterated by dense fibrous adhesions.

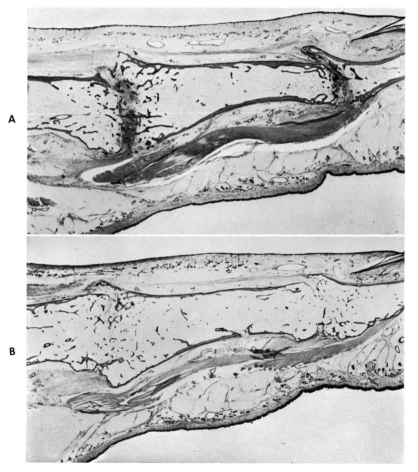

Fig. 41-6 Midline longitudinal sections of second and fourth digits. Atrophy of osseous and dermal tissues evident in both **A** and **B**. Active chronic inflammation shown in middle and terminal interphalangeal joints in **A**. All other joints have been destroyed and bony ankylosis evident.

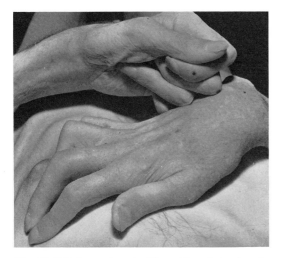

Fig. 41-7 Deformed and stiffened hands in chronic rheumatoid arthritis. Note evidence of muscular atrophy and smooth glossy skin.

the cartilage is invaded and replaced by well-vascularized connective tissue showing moderate to marked degrees of chronic inflammation (Fig. 41-4, *A*). As the result of similar changes on the two opposing joint surfaces, fibrous adhesions are formed (fibrous ankylosis) (Figs. 41-4, *B* and 41-5). In time, the articular cartilage may be completely destroyed (Fig. 41-6, *A*). This may be followed by ossification of the granulation tissue, leading to bony ankylosis (Fig. 41-6, *B*).

In many instances, the deformity is increased by subluxation of the joint.

As a result of these various changes, the joints become permanently stiffened. In addition, they may become markedly twisted and contracted (Fig. 41-7).

One of the early and constant changes in rheumatoid arthritis is atrophy of bone (Fig. 41-6). Although this striking feature of the disease frequently appears early, it is believed to result chiefly from disuse of the part. Pronounced atrophy of muscle and skin also is observed in most patients who have had the disease for any considerable period.

Chronic inflammatory changes resulting, in some instances, in well-circumscribed nodules ("nodulous rheumarthritic perineuritis") have been observed in the sheaths of peripheral nerves of patients suffering from rheumatoid arthritis.[33] Similar inflammatory and nodular lesions occur in the muscle tissues of the body.[64]

In all probability, the most characteristic single lesion associated with rheumatoid arthritis is the *subcutaneous nodule* (Figs. 41-8 and 41-9).[19] These firm swellings appear over bony prominences, especially the olecranon process, in approximately 20% of the patients having the disease.

Such lesions are firm and rubbery in consistency and range from a few millimeters to 3 cm or 4 cm in size. On section, they appear grayish in color and frequently embody one or several areas of yellowish gray necrotic substance. Frequently there are slitlike clefts in the necrotic centers, and occasionally the interior of the lesion undergoes cystic degeneration. Microscopically, the zones of necrosis appear sharply outlined and are bounded by proliferating cells that are regularly oriented (palisading) (Fig. 41-9). The surrounding connective tissue is diffusely or focally infiltrated with lymphocytes and plasma cells. In its entirety, this lesion resembles a gumma to a considerable extent. The observed pathologic changes suggest that this lesion would be incapable of rapid resolution. Such a supposition is apparently justified, since it is known that the subcutaneous nodule of rheumatoid arthritis, once it has formed, is likely to persist for months or even years. This known behavior is unlike that of the nodules appearing in rheumatic fever. In the latter condition, the subcutaneous nodules tend to appear in crops and to resolve and disappear in from a few days to a few weeks.

Remarkable progress in the study and management of rheumatoid arthritis has been made during the last two decades.[60] This gain may be attributed in large part to the discovery of cortisone and ACTH and the use of these substances and other corticosteroid compounds in treating patients affected with rheumatoid arthritis.[22, 38, 62] Induction of dramatic remissions in the disease has been observed clinically. Also, evidence has been obtained that administration of these hormones may induce prompt resolution of inflammatory changes in articular tissues. It has not been established, however, that the subcutaneous nodules are affected by the hormones.[75]

Qualitative and quantitative alterations of serum proteins and associated carbohydrates in patients with rheumatoid arthritis have been noted. Increased amounts of gamma globulin in active rheumatoid arthritis are known to occur.[26] More recently, a variety of hemagglutination tests for the demonstration of the "rheumatoid factor" have been under evaluation, with respect both to significance and to degree of diagnostic speci-

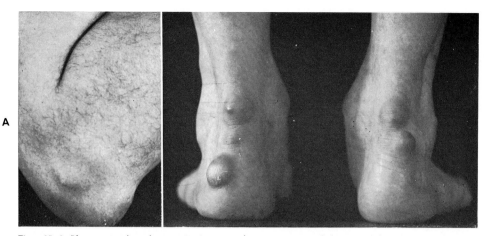

Fig. 41-8 Rheumatoid arthritis. **A,** Large subcutaneous nodule over olecranon process. **B,** Subcutaneous nodules of tendo Achillis areas having typical morphologic features of nodule of rheumatoid arthritis. (Courtesy Dr. F. A. Chandler.)

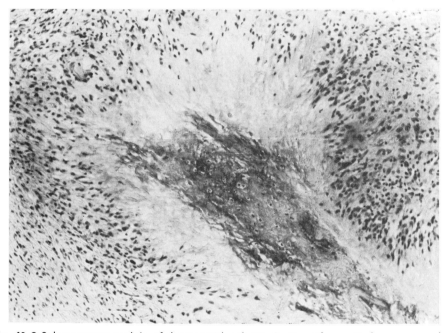

Fig. 41-9 Subcutaneous nodule of rheumatoid arthritis. Portion of necrotic focus surrounded by palisades of proliferating cells. (×200; AFIP 73941.)

ficity.[54, 62, 68] Although tests for the rheumatoid factor are likely to be negative during the first few months of the disease, such tests are positive in 70% to 80% of all adult patients with well-established and "classical" rheumatoid arthritis. The tests for the rheumatoid factor are positive in virtually all patients who have developed rheumatoid nodules.

Because of certain similarities in the clinical and pathologic manifestations of rheumatic fever, rheumatoid arthritis, periarteritis nodosa, systemic lupus erythematosus, and scleroderma, it was popular at one time to refer to these disorders as *collagen* or *connective tissue* diseases or, employing a less specific designation, as *group* diseases. Among the varied morphologic features of these disorders, the most impressive single histologic change that would seem to relate one disease to another is fibrinoid degeneration. The favorable influence of corticosteroids on all of the disorders of the so-called collagen disease group also suggested a relationship between the several entities.

In response to a clinical need for a means of differentiation between rheumatoid arthritis and other *collagen* disorders, the diagnostic criteria for rheumatoid arthritis have undergone reevaluation and revision.[58]

Among the more obscure rheumatic conditions are two: (1) periarticular fibrositis and (2) intermittent hydroarthrosis. These are commented on in this discussion because their etiology and pathogenesis have not been established, and their position in a logical classification cannot be determined on the basis of present information.

Periarticular fibrositis. The term fibrositis has been employed to designate a variety of imperfectly understood clinical manifestations of a "rheumatic" nature, in which it is assumed that the fibrous tissues of the various parts of the body are involved in an inflammatory reaction of a particular nature. There is no unanimity among clinicians as to what constitutes a condition of fibrositis. Indeed, the existence of an entity of this type is questioned by some experienced observers.

Histologic studies of excised tissue specimens have not aided materially in proving or disproving the existence of a disease entity that may properly be designated fibrositis. Reported findings have varied from accounts of nonspecific acute or chronic inflammation to descriptions of granulomatous nodular lesions. Not infrequently, there are no microscopic changes to explain the stiffness, soreness, or aching pains that usually are more pronounced upon awakening or following periods of inactivity.

Intermittent hydrarthrosis. Intermittent hydrarthrosis is among the more uncommon disorders of articular structures. Although trauma, infections, allergic factors, and angioneurosis have been implicated, the etiology of this condition remains obscure.

The condition usually affects but one joint —the knee. Occasionally it is bilateral, and less commonly some other articulation is affected. The syndrome is characterized by periodic and recurrent effusions into the joint. Such swellings usually persist for several days and recur at intervals varying from days to a month or more. The effusion is seldom attended by much pain or tenderness or by signs of inflammation. Little is known of the pathogenesis or pathology of the condition. In some instances, patients believed to have this syndrome develop, at a later date, the signs and symptoms of rheumatoid arthritis.

Degenerative joint disease

Degenerative joint disease, an exceedingly prevalent articular disorder, frequently is referred to by such terms as *degenerative arthritis, hypertrophic arthritis, osteoarthritis,* and *chronic senescent arthritis.*

Joint changes characterizing this infirmity develop to some degree in all persons beyond the third or fourth decade of life.[18] Symptoms and physical signs of *arthritis* may or may not be present in joints showing even well-marked gross and microscopic evidence of disease. Likewise, since the primary pathologic lesion is confined to articular cartilage, there are no early changes visible in the x-ray film.

Large weight-bearing joints (knees, hips, and spine) are usually the first to become affected. The portions of the articular surfaces that are subjected to the greatest stress

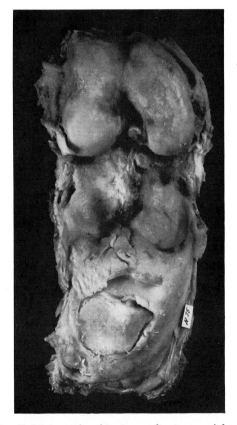

Fig. 41-10 Irregular thinning, softening, and fraying of articular cartilage over patella, patellar surface of femur, and medial condyle of femur. Marginal lipping most marked along border of medial condyle of femur. Early erosion of cartilage of condyles of tibia, exposed through somewhat frayed menisci, also evident. Synovial tissues appear normal. These changes all indicative of early stage of degenerative joint disease.

are the first to show regressive changes. In the knee, the most vulnerable areas are the weight-bearing portions of the femoral condyles, the patellar groove of the femur, and those portions of the tibial condyles that are exposed to pressure and friction through openings in the menisci (Fig. 41-10). Of the small joints, the terminal phalangeal articulations of the fingers are the ones most commonly altered (Herberden's nodes).

Gross and microscopic study of all stages of the disease indicates that, beginning in early adult life, the articular cartilage undergoes regressive changes that progress continuously but at varying rates throughout the life of the individual. Grossly, the cartilage is likely to become yellowish in color and less elastic than normal. The surface shows irregular depressions, pits, and linear grooves. Fragments become detached from its surface. Microscopically, at this stage the homogeneous quality of the matrix is lost and the ground substance fibrillated and split in a vertical plane. Reduction in the thickness of the cartilage in some areas also may be apparent.

In more advanced lesions, the cartilage appears softened and mossy. Marked thinning —to a degree that can be designated erosion—will be observed, and finally, in specimens showing marked changes, no cartilage will remain on areas of small or large size. The denuded bone is characteristically dense, polished, and, in some instances, grooved in the direction corresponding to the motion of the joint. These increasing gross changes have their microscopic counterpart. The softened cartilage shows fibrillation and fraying of the matrix and clustering of the cartilage cells (Fig. 41-11). The process of disintegration progresses from the surface of the cartilage downward. When the subchondral bone plate has been exposed, fragments of cartilage loosen and are cast off. Under the stimulation of pressure and friction, the exposed bone becomes more and more solid (eburnation).

It is evident that while these degenerative changes are taking place in the articular cartilage, the perichondrial tissues at the articular margins are proliferating and giving rise to new cartilage which, in turn, is being replaced by bone. The cause of this excessive marginal growth (lipping) is not entirely understood. It is known, however, that the tissues giving rise to it are less highly specialized and more adequately nourished than is the hyaline cartilage of the articular surface. Thus, the perichondrial tissues are probably more capable of responding to the stimulus of tension incurred in joint motion. Such stimulation no doubt increases as the articular surfaces become misshapen and the mode of locomotion becomes disordered. Irrespective of its cause, marginal lipping constitutes the most readily visible roentgenographic change and, in addition, is one of the most striking gross and microscopic features of the disease. Grossly, the perichondrial margins are elevated and overhanging. When viewed from the side, they appear somewhat scalloped. Microscopically, they project outward from the articular surface as rounded or beaklike osteophytes (Fig. 41-12).

Such projecting margins may become detached or broken from the bone end. In such instances, they give rise to loose bodies

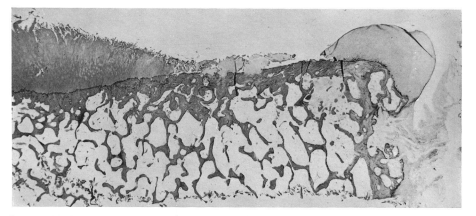

Fig. 41-11 Degenerative joint disease. Articular cartilage of patellar surface of femur showing pronounced degeneration. Fibrillation and splitting of matrix present. Fragmentation and detachment of cartilage evident toward right side, where subchondral bone has been denuded. (×10; AFIP 67996.)

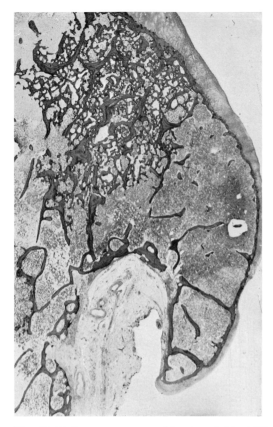

Fig. 41-12 Extensive marginal lipping. (×10; AFIP 67998.)

that may be impinged between the bone ends and cause sudden locking, with attendant pain and, in some instances, effusion of fluid into the joint.

The synovial membrane frequently remains normal until the deterioration of the cartilage and the hypertrophic changes in the perichondrial margins have become marked. In late stages of degenerative joint disease, the synovial membrane loses its elasticity and becomes progressively more villous in character. Unless acutely injured from trauma or other causes, the synovial tissues remain free of significant inflammatory reaction.

Proliferation of synovial or perichondrial tissues, resulting in recognizable pannus, is almost never seen, and it is exceedingly doubtful that uncomplicated degenerative joint disease leads to ankylosis.

This form of arthritis is not accompanied by evidence of any related systemic disease. Fever, leukocytosis, anemia, and weight loss do not occur as a part of the clinical syndrome.

A great mass of evidence has been assembled in support of two fundamental patho-genetic concepts in relation to degenerative joint disease. The first of these is the disadvantageous biologic position of articular cartilage with regard to its nutrition and ability to repair itself.[14] The second concerns the role of mechanical stress and strain incident to everyday use in promoting attrition changes in cartilage. If these considerations are valid, it seems certain that extensive degenerative changes will result from the occasional traumatic shocks to which a joint is subjected. In fact, no sharp distinction can be made between degenerative joint disease and traumatic arthritis, which is described in the following discussion.

Arthritis caused by trauma

Injuries of the joints resulting from trauma are of two main types: (1) acute injuries that are usually produced by the application of a single strong physical force and (2) chronic injuries that follow minor and frequently repeated traumas. However, acute injuries frequently lead to disturbances in the anatomy and physiology of the articulation and thus induce chronic and, at times, progressive articular disease.

Acute injuries resulting from direct physical injury. Any one of the component parts of a joint may be injured by physical force, particularly if the stress is applied suddenly. According to Moritz,[50] if a joint is twisted, hyperextended, hyperflexed, or otherwise forced to move beyond the limits permitted by the elasticity of its ligaments, a sprain, subluxation, or dislocation occurs. Such injuries represent varying degrees of a single type of damage. Thus, as the result of a twist, blow, or fall, the synovial tissues, the ligaments, or the capsule may be stretched, lacerated, or ruptured. In the knee, menisci may be displaced, detached, or torn. The articular cartilage may be compressed, split, or detached from the underlying bone. With greater violence, the joint may be dislocated or the bones may be fractured.

The signs and symptoms of acute traumatic arthritis vary with the location and extent of the injury. In the least severe, there may be only transitory pain and tenderness, with or without an effusion into the joint space. Most lesions of this type heal promptly, leaving no residual disability. It is noteworthy, however, that the articular cartilage may be damaged without giving rise to signs or symptoms commensurate with the importance of the lesion.

The absence of signs is due to the fact that hyaline cartilage is nonvascular and has no nerve supply. Healing occurs slowly, if at all, owing to the limited regenerative capacity of this tissue. An indication of the importance of traumatic injury of cartilage resulted from a study of a series of knee joints obtained from individuals who had denied having had any signs or symptoms referable to the articulations. Examination of these specimens frequently revealed fissures and clefts in the cartilage that were believed to be of traumatic origin. It seemed certain that many of these lesions represented an early stage in the development of more extensive degenerative lesions.

In patients in whom the injury has been more severe, producing contusions or tears in the synovial tissues and intra-articular ligaments, there usually will be greater disability and more pain, and, in most instances, there will be a bloody effusion.

Injuries that include severe lacerations of the ligaments and articular capsules may be associated with dislocation of the bone ends. In these more severely damaged joints, there may be permanent weakening and instability, as well as predisposition to recurrent dislocation.

In the knee joint, a meniscus may be buckled, displaced, detached, or lacerated. In many instances, injuries to this structure are followed by persistent stiffness of the joint or by recurrent "locking" as the lax or displaced semilunar cartilage is impinged between the articular surfaces of the tibia and femur.

Fractures of the cartilaginous and bony components of the articulations almost invariably cause intra-articular bleeding. Usually, the extravasated blood is completely absorbed. In some instances, however, the blood clot organizes, with the production of fibrous adhesions across the joint space. Portions of bone that are completely detached by the fracture become necrotic, although the articular cartilage survives. These detached portions of cartilage and bone remain in the joint as loose bodies ("joint mice") and may give rise to pain or cause recurrent locking of the joint. Malalignment of the fracture fragments may cause an uneven joint surface that predisposes to excessive wear and tear (Fig. 41-13). Degenerative changes are thus accelerated, and chronic arthritis of varying degrees may result.

Chronic injuries resulting from minor and frequently repeated traumas. The injuries due to minor repeated traumas are of many kinds and grades of severity. They include injuries incurred in normal daily activities, traumas sustained in recreational or occupational pursuits, and mechanical-functional disturbances induced by obesity, abnormal posture, disturbed locomotion, and skeletal deformities.[11, 15]

The articular changes produced are varied both in kind and in extent of involvement. In some instances, the lesions are found in the periarticular structures, including ligaments, tendon sheaths, or bursae. More frequently, the joint proper is the site of involvement. Effusions of fluid into the bursae, tendon sheaths, or articular cavities occasionally occur. Loose bodies may be present within distended bursal or synovial cavities. Occasionally, calcification will be found in tendons or bursal walls. Such changes are especially common in the region of the shoulder.[23] The arthritic changes within the joint are most frequently those of degenerative joint disease with or without secondary hy-

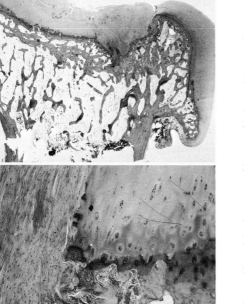

A

B

Fig. 41-13 A, Subsequent to fracture of radius, articular surface became markedly deformed and articular cartilage showed extensive degenerative changes. **B,** Imperfections in restoration of fractured articular cartilage evident.

pertrophic changes. There may be low or moderate grades of inflammation in the synovial tissues.

Arthritis associated with gout

Gout may be regarded as a familial disorder of unknown etiology that is associated with altered uric acid metabolism and hyperuricemia, occurring predominantly in men and, in most instances, characterized by recurring attacks of acute arthritis.[4, 66, 70]

From 2% to 5% of chronic joint disease is represented by gouty arthritis.[39] The onset of the acute arthritis of gout is usually sudden and attended by severe pain. The affected joint rapidly becomes swollen, tender, red, and warm to the touch. The metatarsal phalangeal joints are particularly likely to be involved, and in approximately 50% of the patients the first metatarsal phalangeal joint is among the articulations first affected. In some instances, particularly in young subjects, the arthritis may shift from one joint to another. Usually, the initial or early attacks are of short duration, lasting from a few days to a few weeks. Recurrence at variable intervals is the rule, and eventually, because of the deposits of urates, the arthritis becomes chronic. In such cases, the articular cartilage is the site of the most marked urate deposition. Urate deposits also may occur in the synovial tissues and in the subchondral bone. In rare instances, these changes may result in widespread ankylosis.[48]

The articular tissues are progressively destroyed by the increasing amount of urates that are deposited and by the chronic inflammatory and foreign body reaction that accompanies their deposition. The destruction of bone leads to subchondral rarefied lesions (punched-out defects) shown in the x-ray films. Later, the tophi may extend to cause complete destruction of the articulation and lead to subcutaneous deposits of sodium urate that erode through the covering skin to permit the extrusion of chalky white, crystalline material from an ulcerated lesion.

The predilection of the urates of cartilaginous tissues probably explains the early development of the arthritis, as well as the later appearance of the characteristic tophi in the ears.

The most significant laboratory findings in gout are the elevation of serum uric acid values (usually above 6 mg%) and a diminished renal excretion of uric acid. Because of these observations, it is believed by some that the fundamental metabolic disturbance in gout is related to the mechanism of uric acid disposal (p. 84).

Arthritis of neuropathic origin (Charcot joint)

Patients with certain types of spinal cord lesions, caused in most instances by syphilis or syringomyelia but, in some instances, by diabetes mellitus,[31, 55] are prone to develop an exceedingly destructive type of joint lesion known as a Charcot joint. Approximately 5% to 10% of tabetic patients and 25% of those with syringomyelia are so affected. Usually, only one joint is involved. In the tabetic patient, the knee, hip, or ankle is the common site, whereas with syringomyelia the articulations of the upper extremity are more likely to be affected. Joint lesions of similar character occur in patients afflicted with leprosy. In these instances, the arthropathy is secondary to peripheral nerve changes.

The articular lesion begins with cartilage destruction and rapidly extends to involve the subchondral bone. In the early stages, there is swelling of the joint with, in most instances, a pronounced effusion. Later, as the bone ends undergo disintegration, calcification and ossification take place irregularly in the articular capsule. In the late stages, the joints become lax and misshapen. Despite the pronounced swelling and deformity that are evident in the Charcot joint, the symptoms of pain and tenderness are surprisingly slight.

Miscellaneous forms of joint disease

In addition to the forms of acute and chronic arthritis described heretofore, there is a large variety of articular disorders, usually of dissimilar nature, that may be grouped into two main classes as follows: (1) systemic diseases with which arthritis is frequently associated and (2) local disorders affecting articular tissues.

Systemic diseases with which arthritis frequently is associated

The more important systemic diseases with which arthritis frequently is associated are acromegaly, hemophilia, purpura, psoriasis, Raynaud's disease, Reiter's syndrome, secondary (pulmonary) osteoarthropathy, serum sickness, and the so-called collagen diseases, including systemic lupus erythematosus, polyarteritis nodosa, and scleroderma.

The pathologic changes observed in the majority of these diseases have been discussed elsewhere in this book. In instances in which this is true, it is appropriate to draw attention only to the manner in which the manifestations of arthritis arise in conjunction with the underlying disease process.

For the most part, in these conditions the signs of articular involvement result from the presence in the joint tissues of the anatomic lesions or specific functional disturbances that produce the particular morbid changes elsewhere in the body. Thus, in **polyarteritis nodosa,** the manifestations of arthritis are caused by the occurrence of the characteristic vascular lesions in the synovial and capsular tissues. Similar relationships probably hold for **Raynaud's disease** and **dermatomyositis.** In **scleroderma** and **systemic lupus erythematosus,** the underlying pathologic changes seem to reside in the connective tissue structures of the body, including the articular tissue, and there is some evidence[16] that the articular lesions of systemic lupus may embody a certain degree of specificity.

In **acromegaly,** as is noted elsewhere (p. 1718), two mechanisms appear to be operative in causing increased joint lesions of a degenerative nature. One of these has to do with the increase in body size, with an associated loss of muscle tone and of sound mechanics of locomotion. The other involves the apparent reactivation of cartilage growth and ossification, which may hasten the rate of articular cartilage degeneration. The articular lesions observed in the acromegalic subject are essentially like those of degenerative joint disease, although the secondary hypertrophic changes may be more pronounced.[67]

The joint changes associated with **secondary (pulmonary) hypertrophic osteoarthropathy** are quite clearly the result of an extension of the characteristic mild inflammatory and proliferative periosteal reaction to the regions where the articular capsules insert into the bone coverings. In addition, in some cases at least, there is seen a mild synovitis that may well result from the same physiologic disturbances that cause the osseous lesions (p. 1725).

The joint disorders that accompany **hemophilia** and, less frequently, **purpura** are dependent upon the repeated hemorrhages that occur into the joint space and into the synovial and capsular tissues. The resulting pathologic changes may vary, ranging from the presence of clotted blood within the joint to marked thickening of the synovial tissues and even pronounced cartilage destruction and ankylosis of the joint. These changes appear to result from the vascular endothelial cell and fibroblast proliferation that occurs in the process of organization of blood clot. As a rule, the synovial tissues are heavily stained with pigments derived from the destruction of hemoglobin.

Reiter's syndrome, of unknown etiology, consists of urethritis, conjunctivitis and arthritis. The urethritis usually is associated with purulent discharge, and there may be a coexisting cystitis. The conjunctivitis results in purulent exudation and may be followed by keratitis or iritis. Articular involvement of the knee, ankle, hip, and small joints of the hands and feet forms the other component of the syndrome. There is usually polyarticular involvement. Although the joints may be swollen and painful and show diffuse acute inflammatory changes in the synovial tissues during the acute stages of the disease, there is little, if any, residual stiffness, and ankylosis does not occur. Recovery usually occurs within a period of a few weeks. The arthritic manifestations of Reiter's syndrome may resemble those of gonorrheal arthritis and, in some instances, the clinical features may be similar to those of rheumatoid arthritis.[69] The pathologic features of Reiter's syndrome have been well studied by Kulka.[46]

Psoriasis is known to be accompanied by arthritis with sufficient frequency to leave no doubt that some inherent relationship exists between the two conditions.[74] The incidence of psoriasis in patients with rheumatoid arthritis ranges from 2.6% to 4%.[29, 30] Although the terminal interphalangeal joints are particularly prone to early and extensive involvement in the arthritis that accompanies psoriasis, the gross and microscopic features of the arthritis usually are indistinguishable from those of rheumatoid arthritis.[5]

Local disorders affecting articular tissues

Aseptic necrosis of bone. Descriptions of the various bone lesions that may be designated as aseptic necrosis are given on p. 1703. It may be noted here that in certain locations, especially the hip, the deformities resulting from aseptic necrosis may be followed by progressive deterioration of the joint. The resulting lesion is similar to or identical with other forms of degenerative arthritis.

Bursitis and bursal cysts. When it is recalled that a bursa is a synovial membrane–lined sac, either communicating with or placed near a joint, it may be expected that it will be vulnerable to the same injurious agents that affect an articulation. The common lesions are those resulting from trauma or infection.

Traumatic bursitis may result from a single injury such as a blow upon the elbow (olecranon bursa) or the knee (prepatellar bursa). More commonly, however, it is the repeated injuries from excessive pressure or bruises that initiate the inflammatory changes. This is well exemplified by "housemaid's knee," in which the prepatellar bursa becomes enlarged and painful as the result of crawling on floors and stairs and closing drawers and doors with the knee. Such injuries also may cause degenerative and hypertrophic changes in the joint proper.

Bursal cysts that are connected with the knee joint are not uncommon (Fig. 41-14). In some instances, the openings connecting the cysts with the articular cavity are long and tortuous. Not infrequently, the opening becomes obliterated by cicatrization. These examples of bursal cysts usually are referred to as **Baker's cysts,** although Baker's original papers[2, 3] described cystic lesions in association with a variety of pathologic conditions of dissimilar causation.

When an excised bursal cyst is examined, it is found to have a dense fibrous wall of variable thickness. The enclosed cavity often is divided partially or completely into two or more chambers by fibrous septa that project inwardly from the cyst wall. The cavity contains fluid that may be either clear or turbid and of either watery or mucinous character. At times, the fluid is stained with blood pigments. Not infrequently, the cavities contain "melon seed" bodies similar to those found in articular chambers (Fig. 41-15). The origin of these bodies from small excrescences on the cyst wall or the tips of fringelike villi projecting into the cavity is clearly apparent in many instances. The linings of the cysts vary from smooth, glistening surfaces to nodular and villous membranes. Microscopically, apparent synovial membranes may be present, but more frequently the cyst space is lined by dense fibrous connective tissue that contains focal and diffuse infiltrations of lymphocytes and hemosiderin-laden phagocytes. Baker's cysts are not infrequent in patients with rheumatoid arthritis.[45]

Purulent inflammation of bursal cavities may result from the localization of pathogenic microorganisms. This may follow penetrating injuries, be an extension of infection from an adjacent cellulitis or abscess, or result from the localization of organisms circulating in the blood.

Cysts of semilunar cartilage. Cysts of the semilunar cartilage are usually a semicystic enlargement, of rubbery consistency, located in the lateral meniscus near its anterior insertion. When incised, they contain a number of indistinct locules that are filled with mucinous or gelatinous fluid. Microscopic sec-

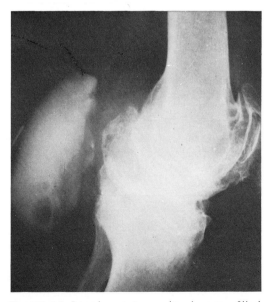

Fig. 41-14 Bursal cyst in popliteal space filled with sodium iodide. Knee shows well-marked hypertrophic changes, typifying advanced degenerative joint disease.

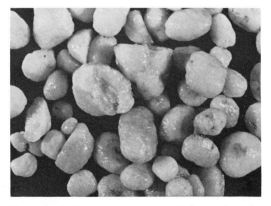

Fig. 41-15 Joint mice removed from shoulder joint. Synovial membrane was studded with small nodules composed of dense fibrous tissue and cartilage. Detachment of these tissue excrescences was apparent source of loose bodies.

tions may reveal bits of synovial tissue lining portions of the more distinct cavities, and there is usually evidence of diffuse fraying of the fibrocartilage of the meniscus. The latter change probably results from the extravasation of mucin-containing fluid into the interstices of the dense and relatively acellular connective tissue of the preexisting semilunar cartilage.

These lesions have much in common with ganglions of tendon sheath origin and are probably formed in a similar manner. Two possibilities have been suggested to explain their development. One explanation is that the lesion represents a mucinous degeneration of fibrocartilage. The other holds that synovial membrane extensions into fibrocartilage become segregated and distended into cystic cavities by the secretion of mucin-containing fluid.

Dupuytren's contracture. Dupuytren's contracture is an affection of the palmar fascia, either of one or of both hands, leading to permanent flexion contracture of one or more fingers. In the usual order of frequency, the fifth, fourth, and third digits are involved. The condition usually is unattended by symptoms of pain and tenderness. It occurs more frequently in males, and in approximately half of the patients, it is bilateral. In addition to thickening, stiffening, and shortening of the fascial tissues, there may be a certain amount of nodularity. Microscopically, the lesion shows an active proliferation of fibroblasts in the fascial layer, with fibrous replacement of the adjacent fat and disappearance of the skin appendages in the overlying dermis. Inflammatory changes are either nonexistent or minimal. The cause of the condition is unknown, but occupational and hereditary factors seem to be important in some instances (see also p. 566).

Ganglion. One of the familiar cystic or semicystic lesions of synovial membrane origin is the ganglion. This swelling is observed most frequently on the ventral or dorsal surfaces of the wrist, but it also occurs over the dorsum of the foot, adjacent to the ankle, or in close proximity to the knee. Occasionally, the lesion is a well-defined, synovial membrane–lined cyst that may or may not have a detectable pedicle attachment to a synovial sheath or joint capsule. Such cysts are filled with clear mucinous fluid, and it is presumed that they represent herniations of synovial membranes through a tendon sheath or the articular capsule of the joint. In many instances, the excised swelling is a poorly defined mass of mucin-filled connective tissue in which no synovial membrane is demonstrable. Still other lesions contain small fragments of recognizable synovial tissue incorporated in a loosely textured and edematous connective tissue mass.

It appears probable that these lesions may result from one of the following:

1 Herniation of the synovial lining of a tendon sheath or articular cavity
2 Displacement of synovial tissues into the fibrous connective tissue near tendon sheaths or articular capsules
3 Extravasation of synovial fluid, with subsequent mucinous degeneration of the connective tissues near articular structures

Protrusion of intervertebral discs. Herniation of an intervertebral disc has been shown to be an important cause of pain in the lumbar region or pain radiating downward along the sciatic nerve (sciatica). Trauma, especially from lifting or sudden exertion, is believed to be the initial cause in most instances. Furthermore, it is likely that the degree of protrusion is influenced by flexion and hyperextension of the spine. The discs of the lumbar region—particularly the one between the third and fourth vertebral bodies—most frequently are affected. The rounded protrusion exerts pressure upon the spinal cord or one of its branches. Microscopically, the herniated disc tissue is composed of loosely arranged and relatively acellular tissue similar to the nucleus pulposus from which it originates.[8]

Protrusion of the intervertebral disc in the body of an adjacent vertebra (Schmorl's nodule) occurs frequently in middle-aged and older persons. Such lesions usually are unaccompanied by symptoms and are discovered on routine x-ray examinations or at autopsy.

Osteochondritis dissecans. Osteochondritis dissecans is a condition in which there is a segregation or detachment of a fragment of articular cartilage or of cartilage and underlying cancellous bone. The lesion is seen most frequently in the knee, particularly on the internal condyle of the femur. Less commonly, the elbow, hip, or shoulder is affected. Such lesions are productive of moderate discomfort that may be associated with an effusion into the joint. If the altered segment of cartilage is completely separated, it serves as a loose body and may cause sudden locking of the joint.

The etiology of osteochondritis dissecans has not been clearly established. Traumatic injury is clearly implicated in some instances, but in other cases it is presumed that the lesion results from aseptic necrosis of the subjacent bony tissue.

On microscopic examination, the articular cartilage covering the detached segment is usually viable but shows vertical clefts and varying degrees of fibrillation of the matrix. There is also clustering of the enclosed cartilage cells. The bony tissue, in a completely detached segment, is necrotic. In a lesion that is only partially separated, there may be irregular areas of bone necrosis. The surface of the concavity from which the lesion has separated usually is covered by fibrous tissue that is only moderately vascular. Signs of inflammation are minimal and consist of slight to moderate accumulations of lymphocytes.

In exceptional cases of osteochondritis dissecans, cystic lesions have been demonstrated in the subjacent bone.[72]

Osteochondromatosis. A relatively uncommon articular disorder, osteochondromatosis may occur as an isolated lesion or in conjunction with other forms of joint disease, particularly degenerative joint disease. It is characterized by the development, in the synovial tissues, of small or large numbers of cartilaginous nodules that tend to undego secondary ossification.[51] Many of the nodules become detached and float free in the joint fluid, where they may continue to grow. When the joint is opened, dozens (or even hundreds) of flat or rounded cartilaginous bodies escape in the excess fluid that is contained in such a joint. Inspection of the synovial lining of the joint reveals similar translucent masses of cartilage projecting from the surface or hanging from narrow pedicles into the joint space (Fig. 41-16).

The cause of the lesion is not known. It can perhaps best be regarded as ectopic cartilage and bone growth that is possible because all articular components are derived from the same embryologic tissues. In most instances, the lesion develops gradually and without known antecedent injury. Occasionally, however, trauma appears to be a precipitating factor of causation.

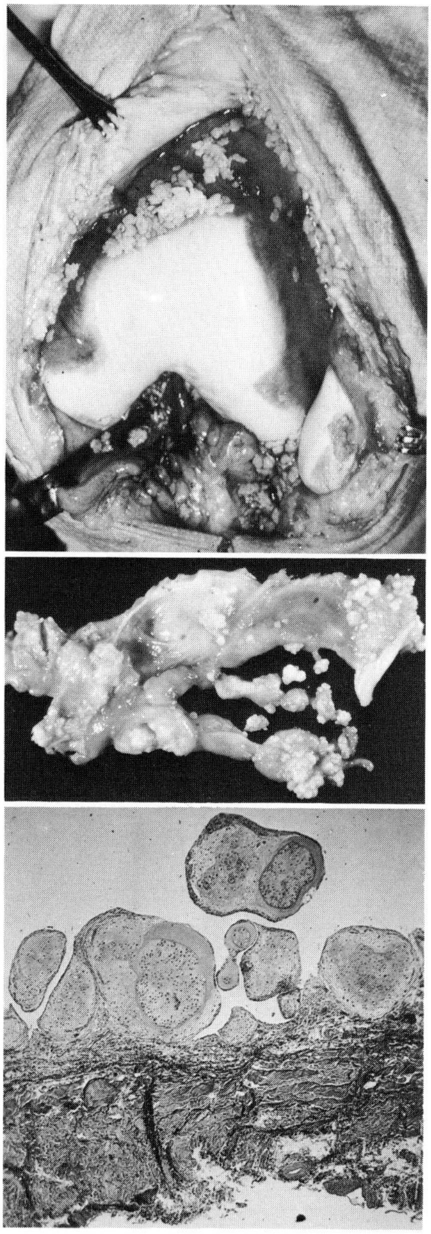

Fig. 41-16 Osteochondromatosis. **A,** Appearance of knee joint at time of surgery. Large numbers of small cartilaginous particles lying free within joint space and many such tissue fragments attached to or growing within synovial membrane. Synovial lining appears dark because of marked congestion. **B,** Portion of excised synovial membrane. **C,** Synovial membrane. Note ectopic formation of cartilage within and just below synovial lining of articular capsule.

Polychondritis (relapsing polychondritis; chronic atrophic polychondritis)

The clinical features of polychondritis, a rare but distinctive syndrome, have been described by a number of observers.[9, 35, 37, 63] The disorder, which occurs in both men and women of varying ages, is characterized by degenerative and inflammatory changes in any of the cartilaginous tissues of the body (nose, ears, larynx, trachea, costal cartilages, intervertebral discs, and peripheral joints). During the active stages of the process, there are symptoms of pain and tenderness and physical signs of inflammation such as swelling and redness of the affected part. Later, with the dissolution of the cartilage, deformities such as floppy ears, saddle nose, and flattening or collapsing of the trachea occur. When peripheral joints are affected, the process may resemble rheumatoid arthritis. Involvement of the intervertebral discs may lead, in late stages, to stiffening and deformation of the spine.

The etiology of the disorder is unknown. Infectious agents have been searched for with negative results. The possibility of a metabolic defect involving enzymatic breakdown of cartilage has been considered, but proof is lacking. The administration of corticosteroids has been effective in suppressing the disorder in some instances.

NEOPLASMS OF JOINTS, BURSAE, TENDONS, AND TENDON SHEATHS

Any of the tissue components of the articulations, including bursae, tendons, and tendon sheaths, may give rise to benign or malignant neoplasms. Among the benign tumors, *chondromas, osteochondromas, myxomas, angiomas, fibromas,* and *lipomas* occasionally are encountered. These neoplasms and the malignant tumors derived from corresponding cell types are no different from tumors of the same histologic composition seen elsewhere in the body. However, because of the anatomic and functional peculiarities of the joint structures, such tumors may give rise to signs and symptoms at a relatively early stage in their development. Pain on motion of the joint, limitation of range of joint motion, and effusion into the joint space may direct attention to the presence of the tumor.

Of particular importance in this discussion are the neoplasms whose origin and behavior are determined by the presence of specialized synovial lining cells in the articulations, bursae, and tendon sheaths. Such tumors may be considered in two main classes: giant cell tumors of tendon sheaths (benign synoviomas) and malignant tumors of synovial cell origin (synovial sarcomas).

Giant cell tumors of tendon sheath origin (benign synoviomas)

Benign synoviomas occur in close proximity to the tendons of the fingers, wrists, ankles, feet, and knees. Less frequently, they arise from the articular capsules or tendon sheaths in other portions of the body. Such tumors grow slowly, with compression and displacement of the adjacent tissues. Where the tendons and other tissues are firmly anchored in bone, the tumors may cause surface erosions or deep rounded depressions in the bone cortex. These bony changes are the result of pressure atrophy. In some examples, the neoplastic tissue is compressed between two or more tendons and tightly adherent to all adjacent structures. These anatomic relationships, when encountered, increase the difficulty of complete surgical removal, and the recurrence rate is much higher than it is in instances in which the tumor pushes out from a tendon into the subcutaneous tissues.

The gross appearances of these tumors vary within wide limits. The neoplasms range in size from a few millimeters in greatest diameter to several centimeters. Those that have been cleanly enucleated have a dense fibrous covering formed of the compressed surrounding tissues. They are firm and only slightly elastic. Sectioning reveals a dense and inelastic tissue that is gray in color. In many instances, yellowish areas or streaks are noted. The yellow color is proportional to the amount of lipid that is contained within histocytic cells within the tumor. It is because of the yellow color that some of these lesions have been designated as xanthomas or xanthofibromas.

Examination of the microscopic sections reveals cellular and structural features that are highly characteristic in the majority of tumors (Fig. 41-17). The giant cells from which the tumor derives its name may be numerous or few in number. They contain many small oval nuclei that are usually crowded together in one portion of the cell. The cytoplasm may be scant or abundant, and the configuration of the cells is equally variable (Fig. 41-17, *A*). The remaining portions of the tumor are composed of small oval or spindle-shaped cells and irregularly placed bundles of connective tissue. The ratio, one to the other, of these elements is exceedingly variable, both within the same and in different tumors. Some neoplasms are highly cellular and show active cell proliferation. Others are dense and fibrous and contain few cellular elements. An average tumor is portrayed in Fig. 41-17, *A*. The number of lipid-laden phagocytes seen in these tumors is also variable. Some tumors are composed chiefly of such cells, whereas other tu-

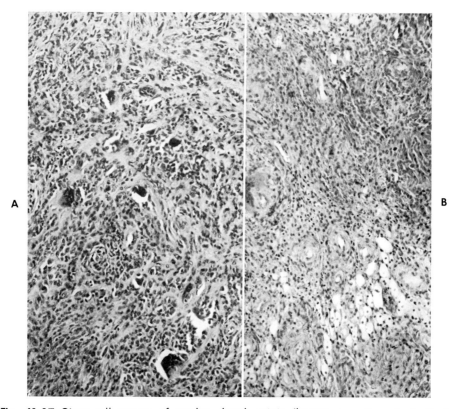

Fig. 41-17 Giant cell tumors of tendon sheath origin (benign synoviomas). **A,** Typical histologic features. **B,** Tumor containing many lipid-laden cells. (**A** and **B,** ×130; **A,** AFIP 90662; **B,** AFIP 82251.)

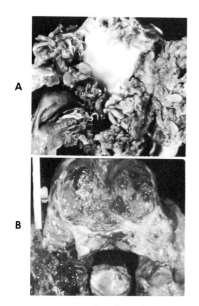

Fig. 41-18 Pigmented villonodular synovitis. **A,** Patella (top center) surrounded by overgrown synovia that was mahogany brown in color and had mosslike appearance. **B,** Tumorlike mass of spongy tissue of deep brown color.

mors contain only scattered foam cells or small aggregates similar to those illustrated in Fig. 41-17, *B.*

Careful study of these tumors reveals irregular slitlike cavities that are lined by oval or flattened cells. Occasionally one notes that small tufts of these cells project into the cavities (Fig. 41-17, *A*). It is probable that these structural features are related to the inherent propensities of synovial lining cells, from which these tumors probably are derived. When the cellularity of these tumors is great and the tendency for cleft formation and tufting is highly developed, it may be difficult to distinguish sharply between this neoplasm and the malignant neoplasm of synovial membrane origin known as synovial sarcoma.

In addition to the giant cell tumor of tendon sheath origin, one occasionally encounters tumorlike overgrowths within the knee or other large joints that vary from simple inflammatory hyperplasia of the synovia to complex masses of granulation tissue containing giant cells, lipid-laden phagocytes, and blood pigment. In some instances, it is difficult to determine whether the lesion is of inflammatory character or whether it represents a true benign neoplasm.[13] The term pigmented villonodular synovitis has been suggested to designate synovial membrane lesions having these variable characteristics[41] (Fig. 41-18).

Synovial sarcoma

The term synovioma was suggested in 1927 by Smith[61] to designate a group of malignant tumors that are believed to arise from the cells lining synovial cavities in any part of the body. In a review of the literature, Haagensen and Stout[36] found descriptions of ninety-five cases that they considered to be acceptable examples of synovial sarcoma. These, with nine additional tumors from their own material, formed a total of 104 examples. A review of the specimens submitted to the Army Institute of Pathology for interpretation during the years of World War II revealed thirty-two examples of synovial sarcoma.[12]

These tumors develop within the cavities of joints in only about 5% of the cases, and for this reason their derivation from synovial tissues may not be suspected until they are examined microscopically. The sites of most frequent occurrence are the regions of the knee and the lower segment of Hunter's canal. Less frequently they are encountered in other portions of the body in which synovial tissues of joints, bursae, or tendon sheaths are known to exist.

On gross examination, the tumors are seen to vary in size, texture, and appearance. Usually, they are sharply circumscribed and give the appearance of being partially or completely encapsulated. The compressed and attenuated adjacent tissues form a pseudocapsule that accounts for this appearance. In the process of removal, it is frequently noted that the tumor is attached at one or more points to tendons or tendon sheaths. Various colors and densities are noted on sectioning the neoplasms. Some are firm in texture and moderately fibrous, but more frequently they are spongy and friable. Pinkish gray areas of viable tumor tissue are frequently interspersed with yellow areas caused by necrosis and brown or red portions that have resulted from old or recent hemorrhage. Occasionally, small or large areas of calcification may be noted in the x-ray film prior to removal of the tumor.

The microscopic appearances of these tumors are dependent on three basic morphologic patterns that are developed with varying degrees of clarity in any single tumor. These patterns are believed to represent expressions of the functional and morphologic characters of synovial tissues in general.

One pattern is represented by the formation of tissue spaces that vary from slitlike clefts to well-defined, glandlike spaces containing serous or mucinous fluid. The second major design is the formation of cell tufts. This feature varies from compact groups of oval or polygonal cells, segregated in solid portions of the tumor tissue, to papillary projections extending into clefts and glandlike spaces. The third architectural design that is noted in the more highly characteristic tumor is the reproduction of epithelium-like cells upon a supporting stroma of compact tissue formed of elongated cells with small dark nuclei (Figs. 41-19 and 41-20).

Extensions of tumor tissue into vascular channels may be noted, and examination of the margins of the tumor mass usually will reveal invasion of the adjacent tissues in one or more areas. Mitotic figures usually are seen in moderate or large numbers. It seems doubtful, however, that their frequency gives any reliable index to the degree of malignancy of the neoplasm.

Experience has clearly demonstrated that the fatality rate with this group of tumors is high, although in many instances the initial lesion may have been present for several months prior to its surgical removal. In the series of 104 cases tabulated by Haagensen and Stout,[36] only three patients were alive and free of metastases five years after treatment was begun. It is possible that this high mortality rate might be reduced if more radical surgical treatment were generally adopted in the early stages of development of a given tumor. It is clearly evident, however, that these neoplasms are among the most highly malignant of all mesenchymal tumors. Radiation therapy has little beneficial effect upon either the primary tumor or its metastases. Metastases develop in the lungs, lymph nodes, and other organs, including the heart and brain. The distinctive morphologic features of the primary tumor are usually perceptible in the metastases.

Other malignant neoplasms of synovial tissue

In the preceding discussions, it has been emphasized that the two characteristic tumors originating in synovial tissues are giant cell tumor of tendon sheath origin (benign synovioma) and synovial sarcoma (malignant synovioma). It is to be expected, however, that

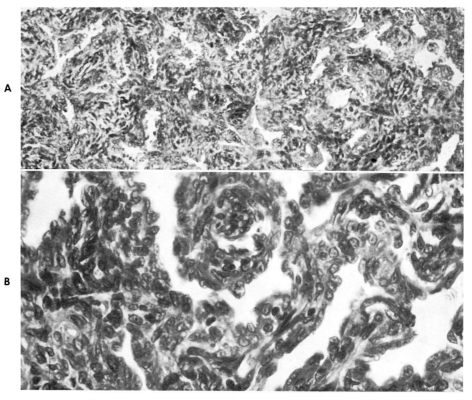

Fig. 41-19 Malignant tumor of synovial membrane origin (synovial sarcoma). **A,** Characteristic structure. **B,** Higher-power view. (**A** and **B,** AFIP 90623.)

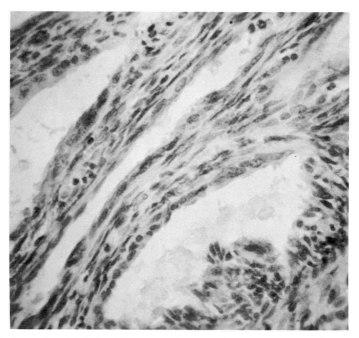

Fig. 41-20 Example of highly differentiated synovial sarcoma illustrating epithelium-like cells forming surface lining of tissue clefts.

malignant neoplasms with other histologic characteristics will arise occasionally from articular tissues. Such tumors include *large cell sarcoma of tendon sheath*[21] and *synovial chondrosarcoma*.[34]

In the case of the large cell sarcoma of tendon sheath, extreme care must be taken by both clinician and pathologist to distinguish this neoplasm from the more common benign giant cell tumor of tendon sheath origin. Also, in the instance of synovial chondrosarcoma, great care must be taken to distinguish this neoplasm from the wholly benign process of ectopic cartilage formation known as benign chondromatosis of synovial membrane. Goldman and Lichtenstein[34] hold that there is no acceptable evidence that synovial chondrosarcoma originates in preexisting synovial chondromatosis.

REFERENCES

1 Arthritis and rheumatism, July 1957—June 1959, Health Statistics, Ser. B, No. 20, Washington, D. C., 1960, U. S. Department of Health, Education, and Welfare.
2 Baker, W. M.: St. Barth. Hosp. Rep. 13:245-261, 1877 (bursal cysts).
3 Baker, W. M.: St. Barth. Hosp. Rep. 21:177-190, 1885 (bursal cysts).
4 Bauer, W., and Klemperer, E.: In Duncan, G. A., editor: Diseases of metabolism, Philadelphia, 1942, W. B. Saunders Co., chap. XII.
5 Bauer, W., Bennett, G. A., and Zeller, J. W.: Trans. Ass. Amer. Physicians 56:349-352, 1941.
6 Bauer, W., Ropes, M. W., and Waine, H.: Physiol. Rev. 20:272-312, 1940.
7 Bauer, W., Short, C. L., and Bennett, G. A.: J. Exp. Med. 57:419-433, 1933.
8 Beadle, O. A.: The intervertebral discs, Med. Res. Counc. Spec. Rep. Ser. (London) No. 161, 1931.
9 Bean, W. B., Drevets, C. C., and Chapman, J. S.: Medicine (Balt.) 37:353-363, 1958.
10 Bennett, G. A.: Ann. Intern. Med. 19:111-113, 1943.
11 Bennett, G. A.: Clinics 1:1448-1475, 1943.
12 Bennett, G. A.: J. Bone Joint Surg. 29:259-291, 1947.
13 Bennett, G. A.: Proc. Inst. Med. Chicago 18:26-37, 1950.
14 Bennett, G. A., and Bauer, W.: Amer. J. Path. 8:499-524, 1932.
15 Bennett, G. A., and Bauer, W.: J. Bone Joint Surg. 19:667-682, 1937.
16 Bennett, G. A., and Dällenbach, F. D.: Milit. Surg. 109:531-539, 1951.
17 Bennett, G. A., and Shaffer, M. F.: J. Exp. Med. 70:277-291, 1939.
18 Bennett, G. A., Waine, H., and Bauer, W.: Changes in the knee joint at various ages; with particular reference to the nature and development of degenerative joint disease, New York, 1942, Commonwealth Fund.
19 Bennett, G. A., Zeller, J. W., and Bauer, W.: Arch. Path. (Chicago) 30:70-89, 1940.
20 Benninghoff, A.: Z. Zellforsch. 2:783-862, 1925.
21 Bliss, B. O., and Reed, R. J.: Amer. J. Clin. Path. 49:776-781, 1968.
22 Bunim, J. J.: Bull. N. Y. Acad. Med. 27:75-100, 1951.
23 Codman, E. A.: The shoulder, Boston, 1934, Thomas Todd Co.
24 Coggeshall, H. C., Warren, C. F., and Bauer, W.: Anat. Rec. 77:129-144, 1940.
25 Coggeshall, H. C., Bennett, G. A., Warren, C. F., and Bauer, W.: Amer. J. Med. Sci. 202:486-502, 1941; correction 202:916, 1941.
26 Coke, H.: Rheumatism 11:27-31, 1955.
27 Collins, D. H.: The pathology of articular and spinal diseases, Baltimore, 1950, The Williams & Wilkins Co.
28 Coss, J. A., Jr., and Boots, R. H.: J. Pediat. 29:143-156, 1946.
29 Dawson, M. H., and Tyson, T. L.: Trans. Ass. Amer. Physicians 53:303-309, 1938.
30 Douthwaite, A. H.: Treatment of rheumatoid arthritis and sciatica, London, 1933, H. K. Lewis & Co., Ltd.
31 Feldman, M. J., Becker, K. L., Reefe, W. E., and Longo, A.: J.A.M.A. 209:1690-1692, 1969.
32 Felty, A. R.: Bull. Johns Hopkins Hosp. 35:16-20, 1924.
33 Freund, H. A., Steiner, G., Leichtentritt, B., and Price, A. E.: Amer. J. Path. 18:865-893, 1942.
34 Goldman, R. L., and Lichtenstein, L.: Cancer 17:1233-1240, 1964.
35 Gordon, E. J., Perlman, A. W., and Schechter, N.: J. Bone Joint Surg. 30-A:944-956, 1948.
36 Haagensen, C. D., and Stout, A. P.: Ann. Surg. 120:826-842, 1944.
37 Harwood, T. R.: Arch. Path. (Chicago) 65:81-87, 1958.
38 Hench, P. S.: Proc. Staff Meet. Mayo Clin. 25:474-476, 1950.
39 Hench, P. S., Bauer, W., Boland, E., Dawson, M. H., Freyberg, R. H., Holbrook, W. P., Key, J. A., Lockie, L. M., and McEwen, C.: Ann. Intern. Med. 15:1002-1108, 1941.
40 Hess, E. V., Hunter, D. K., and Ziff, M.: J.A.M.A. 191:531-534, 1965.
41 Jaffe, H. L., Lichtenstein, L., and Sutro, C. L.: Arch. Path. (Chicago) 31:731-765, 1941.
42 Jordan, E. P., Bauer, W., Boots, R. H., Cecil, R. L., Coggeshall, H. C., Dawson, M. H., Hench, P. S., Key, J. A., Lockie, L. M., Minot, G. R., Pemberton, R., and Swaim, L. T.: J.A.M.A. 119:1089-1094, 1942.
43 Keiser, H., Ruben, F. L., Wolinsky, E., and Kushner, I.: New Eng. J. Med. 279:234-240, 1968.
44 Key, J. A.: J. Bone Joint Surg. 7:793-813, 1925.
45 Kogstad, O.: Acta Rheum. Scand. 11:194-204, 1965.
46 Kulka, J. P.: Arthritis Rheum. 5:195-201, 1962.
47 Kulka, J. P., Bocking, D., Ropes, M. W., and Bauer, W.: Arch. Path. (Chicago) 59:129-150, 1955.
48 Ludwig, A. O., Bennett, G. A., and Bauer, W.: Ann. Intern. Med. 11:1248-1276, 1938.
49 McCarthy, M.: Circulation 14:1138-1143, 1956.
50 Moritz, A. R.: The pathology of trauma, Philadelphia, 1942, Lea & Febiger.
51 Murphy, F. P., Dahlin, D. C., and Sullivan, C. R.: J. Bone Joint Surg. 44-A:77-86, 1962.

52 Partain, J. O., Cathcart, E. S., and Cohen, A. S.: Ann. Rheum. Dis. **27:**156-162, 1968.

53 Pirani, C. L., and Bennett, G. A.: Bull. Hosp. Joint Dis. **12:**335-367, 1951.

54 Ragan, C.: Arthritis Rheum. **4:**571-573, 1961.

55 Robillard, R., Gagnon, P. A., and Alarie, R.: Canad. Med. Ass. J. **91:**795-804, 1964.

56 Ropes, M. W., and Bauer, W.: Synovial fluid changes in joint disease, Cambridge, Mass., 1953, Harvard University Press.

57 Ropes, M. W., Rossmeisl, E. C., and Bauer, W.: J. Clin. Invest. **19:**795-799, 1940.

58 Ropes, M. W., Bennett, G. A., Cobb, S., Jacox, R., and Jessar, R. A.: Bull. Rheum. Dis. **9:**175-176, 1958.

59 Shaffer, M. F., and Bennett, G. A.: J. Exp. Med. **70:**293-302, 1939.

60 Short, C. L., Bauer, W., and Reynolds, W. E.: Rheumatoid arthritis, Cambridge, Mass., 1957, Harvard University Press.

61 Smith, L. W.: Amer. J. Path. **3:**355-364, 1927.

62 Smyth, C. J., Bunim, J. J., Clark, W. S., Crain, D. C., Demartini, F. E., Duff, I. F., Engleman, E. P., Graham, D. C., Montgomery, M. M., Norcross, B. M., Polley, H. F., Ropes, M. W., and Rosenberg, E. F.: Ann. Intern. Med. **50:**366-494, 1959.

63 Spritzer, H. W., Weaver, A. L., Diamond, H. S., and Overholt, E. L.: J.A.M.A. **208:**355-357, 1969.

64 Steiner, G., Freund, H., Leichtentritt, B., and Maun, M. E.: Amer. J. Path. **22:**103-145, 1946.

65 Still, G. F.: Med. Chir. Trans. London **80:**47-59, 1897.

66 Talbott, J. H.: Gout, ed. 2, 1964, New York/London, Grune & Stratton, Inc.

67 Waine, H., Bennett, G. A., and Bauer, W.: Amer. J. Med. Sci. **209:**671-687, 1945.

68 Waller, M. V., Decker, B., Toone, E. C., Jr., and Irby, R.: Arthritis Rheum. **4:**579-591, 1961.

69 Weinberger, H. W., Ropes, M. W., Kulka, J. P., and Bauer, W.: Medicine (Balt.) **41:**35-91, 1962.

70 Weiss, T. E., and Segaloff, A.: Gouty arthritis and gout, Springfield, Ill., 1959, Charles C Thomas, Publisher.

71 Wilson, M. G.: Rheumatic fever, New York, 1940, Commonwealth Fund.

72 Wolbach, S. B., and Allison, N.: Arch. Surg. (Chicago) **16:**1176-1186, 1928 (osteochondritis dissecans).

73 Wolcott, W. E.: J. Bone Joint Surg. **9:**67-78, 1927.

74 Wright, V.: Amer. J. Med. **27:**454-462, 1959.

75 Zivin, S., Steck, I. E., Montgomery, M. M., Kaiser, G. D., and Bennett, G. A.: J. Lab. Clin. Med. **43:**70-78, 1954.

Chapter 42

Nervous system and skeletal muscle

Jacob L. Chason

■ Central nervous system

The diseased nervous system offers an exceptional opportunity for the correlation of structure with function. Although the pathologic processes that affect the nervous system differ little from those occurring elsewhere in the body, the functional changes that result have both greater variability and uniformity. The variability of the effects upon neurologic function is related to the anatomic localization of the disease. The uniformity of neurologic response, on the other hand, is dependent upon several factors, among which are the following:

1. Fixed size of space enclosing the central nervous system (following fusion of the sutures of the skull)
2. The limited mobility of the nervous system within the space
3. The immobility of the dura and dural folds
4. The uniformity of structural change and progression of most lesions—i.e., "the biologic behavior of the lesion" (essential to the correlation of structure and function is an understanding of the reactions of the components of the nervous system to injury)

STRUCTURE AND FUNCTION
Neuron

The nerve cell consists of a nucleus and a cell body, the perikaryon, with one or more processes known as dendrites and a single larger process, an axon. The perikaryon of these cells ranges from the 5μ internal granular cell of the cerebellum to the 80μ or more diameter of the Betz cell of the motor cortex.

The larger cells have a single, large, round to oval, usually vesicular nucleus with a well-defined nuclear membrane and a large nucleolus. With the exception of some cells of the hypothalamus, brainstem, and Clarke's column of the spinal cord, the nucleus is in a central portion in the perikaryon. The cytoplasm, except at the base of the axon, contains basophilic, granular to blocklike material called Nissl substance. This material is now known to represent the granular endoplasmic reticulum and is a site of protein metabolism. The Nissl substance has the staining characteristics of the nucleolus, where it is thought to be formed and from which it spreads throughout the cytoplasm, appearing initially as a nuclear cap. In most large cells, the Nissl substance is relatively evenly divided throughout the cytoplasm. In the cells normally having an eccentric nucleus, it is characteristic for the Nissl substance to be concentrated at the peripheral margins of the cell cytoplasm.

Many of the larger cells contain a brown, granular, intracytoplasmic lipochrome or lipofuscin pigment that increases with age.[8, 13] This pigment has the same staining characteristics and apparently the same functional significance as the lipofuscin in parenchymal cells elsewhere in the body. A neuromelanin pigment, structurally identical with that of melanin, is normally present in the cytoplasm of the cells of the substantia nigra, the locus ceruleus, the posterior lobe of the pituitary gland, and some cells of the motor nuclei along the floor of the fourth ventricle.[80] This pigment first appears in the cells of the locus ceruleus, microscopically visible at about the eighth intrauterine month and grossly visible by the eighth postnatal month. In the substantia nigra, the pigment appears microscopically at approximately $1\frac{1}{2}$ years of age and becomes grossly visible at 3 years of age. In nuclear areas, the adult amounts of pigment are reached by the end of adolescence.[80]

The dendrites and axons are extensions of the cytoplasm of the neurons and are of vari-

1781

able length. The longest are the axons of the Betz cells, which extend for as great a distance as 2½ ft. They contain microtubules, neurofilaments (individually visible only with electron microscopy), and neurofibrils that course from one cell process to the other through the cell body. It is believed that these structures help maintain the shape of the cell and are the pathways for the orderly and sometimes rapid transfer of materials from one part of the cell to the other.

Other components of the nerve cells generally cannot be adequately demonstrated or studied either individually or in groups by light microscopy. Their presence and actual or potential activities sometimes can be demonstrated from the enzyme content. The acid phosphatase reaction represents the site of and one type of action of the lysosomes. Various oxidative enzymes are used both as markers for mitochondria and to demonstrate the nature, amount, and site of the principal source of energy.

The specialized sites of contact of the nerve cells, the synapses, require electron microscopy for study. The presynaptic and terminally expanded axon contains mitochondria and vesicles with acetycholine or, in some, norepinephrine. Release of the chemical at the synapse results in the transmission of the impulse to the dendrite of the succeeding cell.

The recognition and separation of antemortem and postmortem changes in nerve cells are essential. Because minor degrees of structural variation within the cells may be associated with abnormalities of function, the constant use of control sections is necessary in the recognition of autolytic changes, fixation artifacts, structural variations due to disease, and stages of normal function.[121]

Shrinkage and increased staining of the entire cell with tortuosity of the cell processes constitute one of the commonest of nerve cell changes. It is known as chronic neuronal disease. Although it has been described as an aging process in some cells and is a form of reaction to a variety of acute and chronic diseases, it is also commonly found in the second and third cortical layers, where it is due to the effects of fixation. Cloudy swelling or, as it is known in the central nervous system, acute nerve cell change is characterized by cellular swelling and staining pallor with loss of Nissl substance. This condition is considered to be reversible up to the point at which the cell processes are fragmented and separated from the cell body. It is a nonspecific

response to a variety of injurious agents and is a well-known postmortem change. Ischemic change in the cell results from hypoxia, anoxia, and hypoglycemia or following the ingestion of poisons that block the utilization of oxygen or glucose. With ischemia, the Nissl substance is rapidly destroyed. The affected cell is easily recognized because of the marked cytoplasmic eosinophilia. Shortly afterward, the cell begins to swell and the cytoplasm becomes finely granular. With this, the cytoplasmic eosinophilia progressively fades and the early pyknotic nucleus undergoes karyorrhexis just as the cell disintegrates. Central chromatolysis, also known as retrograde or axonal degeneration of the nerve cell, follows injury to the cell axon (often only near the perikaryon). In the affected cell, the nucleus is displaced to one side of the swollen and rounded perikaryon and the Nissl substance is gradually lost first about the nucleus and later toward the periphery. With recovery, the nucleolus enlarges. The Nissl substance makes its appearance initially as a nuclear cap that later fills the perikaryon and dendrites. During this period, the nucleus gradually resumes the normal central position. Complete structural recovery may take several months. By light microscopy, this entire series of changes can be adequately studied only with the Nissl stain. Because cells with eccentric nuclei and peripheral Nissl substance are normally present in certain portions of the brain, as previously mentioned (p. 1781), adequate controls must always be utilized. Low-grade chronic injury to nerve cells is thought to result in an abnormal increase in the intracytoplasmic lipofuscin (lipochrome) pigment. This is known as pigmentary atrophy and more recently has been associated with a disease known as lipofuscinosis. The abnormal increase in this pigment, which is sudanophilic and sometimes acid fast, is thought to interfere with the normal cellular metabolic activity, perhaps by coating of the cell organelles. Other specific nerve cell changes will be described with the diseases with which they are associated.

Myelin is a complex proteolipid formed by the spiraling of double layers of the cell membrane of the oligodendrocytes about the axis-cylinders of most nerve cells of the central nervous system. Each layer (seen only by electron microscopy) is composed of the double plasma membranes—the inner membrane surfaces have come together, displacing the cytoplasmic contents toward the nucleus of the cell. The sandwich of double plasma membrane by differential growth of this approximated cell membrane portion of the cells is thought to result in the spiral coating about the axis-cylinder. The oligodendrocyte nucleus and cytoplasm are gradually displaced ahead of their newly formed plasma membrane in its spiral about the axon. Only the 5μ to 7μ, round, hyperchromatic nucleus of the oligodendrocytes stains with hematoxylin and eosin. The cytoplasm and plasma membrane remain unstained as a clear halo about the nucleus.

It should be recognized that an oligodendroglial cell can be destroyed without structural damage to the surrounded axis-cylinder. Conversely, destruction of the axis-cylinder, either directly or indirectly (because of injury to the nerve cell), always results in destruction of the covering myelin sheath and of the oligodendrocyte. With the hematoxylin and eosin stain, one of the earliest reliable indications of myelin damage is the presence of myelin-containing or lipid-containing macrophages, first within the area of damage and later about adjacent blood vessels. Occasionally, one is able to recognize swelling of the axon and surrounding myelin by the presence of 20μ to 25μ, circular or cylindrical, eosinophilic masses in the white matter of the brain or spinal cord. The darker core of these eosinophilic structures indicates the swollen axis-cylinder, and the lighter outer zone represents the altered myelin. Simultaneously, but difficult to recognize, are shrinkage and further hyperchromatism of the oligodendroglial nucleus. These changes are more easily and adequately recognized with special stains for myelin and axis-cylinders. These stains demonstrate irregular swelling, pallor, and, later, fragmentation of the myelin sheaths well before the routine stains appear abnormal. While slight staining pallor of the area may be recognizable with the routine stains following the loss or removal of myelin, the state is easily appreciated with any of the variety of stains for myelin. The interfascicular oligodendrocytes of the white matter cover a single segment of one or more axis-cylinders. The junction between the two cell membranes covering an axis-cylinder is known as a node of Ranvier. With brain edema or swelling, the nonstaining halo of the interfascicular oligodendrocyte may become filled with a pink mucoid material for which the term mucinous degeneration has been employed. The nonstaining halo seen about almost all of the oli-

godendroglial nuclei may increase in size as a part of the postmortem autolytic change.[72] Oligodendrocytes also are found in the gray matter of the central nervous system, where they form satellite cells about the larger nerve cells. The satellite type of oligodendroglial cell has been considered by some to act both as a protector of the perikaryon and as a part of the route for the spread of nutrients to the cells. With the routine stains and at the usual 6μ to 7μ thickness of the sectioned tissue, one and occasionally two satellite cells may be found around one nerve cell body. An increase in number, satellitosis, represents a reaction to a variety of disease processes that affect the nerve cells.

Neuroglia

The astrocyte is the principal supporting cell of the central nervous system. With the routine hematoxylin and eosin stain, the only component of a normal astrocyte that ordinarily can be seen is the nucleus. The nucleus is 8μ to 10μ in diameter, round to oval, and vesicular with finely granular chromatin and has a definite nuclear membrane of uniform thickness. A nucleolus ordinarily is not visible with light microscopy.

Astrocytes of two structural forms differing in their processes have been described. The more common, the fibrous type, is present predominantly in the white matter of the central nervous system and in the outer layer of the cerebral cortex. The fibrous astrocyte located in the white matter and on the cortical surface has long, thin, and usually nonbranching fibrillary processes, one of which extends to the wall of a blood vessel, while another may extend to the pial membrane. Protoplasmic astrocytes, present in the gray matter, have shorter, wider, and branching processes. Astrocytes with both types of processes also have been described. The structural distinction does not appear to indicate an essential functional or biologic difference. The reactive astrocyte, whatever the source type, regularly assumes a fibrous appearance. The Fanana cell of the cerebellar cortex has some similarity with the protoplasmic astrocyte, while the Bergmann cell of the internal granular layer of the cerebellum has greater resemblance to the fibrous form.

The response of the astrocyte to injury can be recognized in a variety of ways. The presence of a slightly eosinophilic halo about the nucleus is one form of early reactive change visible with the hematoxylin and eosin stain.

It is, however, also characteristic of many normal astrocytes present in newborn infants and young children. When there is an abundant amount of eosinophilic cytoplasm, the astrocyte is of the gemistocytic type. This structural change can be seen within hours of injury. It is associated with the rapid formation of mitochondria and their enzymes. Another form of reactive change is indicated by the presence of nuclear pairs and sometimes tetrads. This, of course, is interpreted as representing cell multiplication supposedly by amitosis, because a reactive astrocyte in mitosis is seen very rarely. The increase in astrocytes is known as astrocytosis. In astrocytic gliosis, another type of response to injury, there is an increase in the fibrillar processes of the astrocytes. When the gliotic pattern follows the preexisting normal structure, it is called isomorphic gliosis; in anisomorphic gliosis, the proliferation of processes has a haphazard arrangement. These are best seen with special stains, although they usually can be recognized with the routine stains. In chronic toxic states, either endogenous, as in uremia, in liver disease with jaundice,[2, 21] and in Wilson's disease, or exogenous, with a variety of toxins, some astrocytic nuclei may enlarge due to swelling and become more vesicular. The nucleus maintains a definite nuclear membrane with several infoldings, and one or more nucleoli may become evident. These are the Alzheimer's type II cells. In Wilson's disease, also known as hepatolenticular or hepatocerebral degeneration, transitions from type II cells to the Alzheimer type I cell have been described. The type I cell has a large, darkly basophilic nucleus with a single darker nucleolus and a lighter basophilic, sometimes granular, cytoplasm. Processes are not found extending from the bodies of these cells.

Cuboidal to columnar cells, the ependymal cells, line the ventricles, the choroid plexuses, and the central canal of the spinal cord. Microscopic remnants of detached portions of ventricles, predominantly at the occipital and, to a lesser extent, the frontal poles of the lateral ventricles, and the ventriculus terminale of the filum terminale also are lined. Many of these cells are ciliated, presumably to help propel the cerebrospinal fluid. The presence of blepharoplasts (best seen with the Mallory phosphotungstic acid–hematoxylin stain), which are small cytoplasmic hematoxylinophilic granules surrounded by a clear halo, can be of great help in the identification of cells of ependymal origin. These granules are thought to be remnants of the cilia whose portions outside the cell have disappeared. Reactions of the ependyma to injury are few. Ulceration of the ventricular lining may be seen with and following local inflammations and when there is marked dilatation of the ventricular system. The underlying reactive subependymal astrocytes may produce nodules of astrocytic fibers that occasionally surround trapped ependymal cells. The resultant production of an irregular ventricular surface is known as "granular ependymitis."

During the period of vascularization early in the development of the central nervous system, another type of "glial" cell makes its appearance. Of mesodermal origin, the microglial cells represent a portion of the reticuloendothelial system. These cells are scattered irregularly in both gray and white matter and among the astrocytes and oligodendrocytes. In the resting phase, only the short, oval to kidney-shaped hyperchromatic nuclei of the microglial cells are stained with hematoxylin and eosin. Their scant cytoplasm and their relatively few processes (as compared with the astrocytes) are best demonstrated with the Hortega silver stain. Microglial cells react in response to injury with a great variety of structural change. Initially, they may proliferate locally about a small area of necrosis with the formation of a small group of cells, forming a so-called glial nodule. Their occurrence in a group phagocytizing a dead nerve cell is known as neuronophagia. Due to chemotactic influences, the cells may move toward the area damaged. In the process of movement, there is enlargement and elongation of their nuclei. Because of the shape of the cells during such movement, they are known as rod cells. A microglial cell also may be transformed into a mononuclear (less often multinuclear) macrophage, during which its processes are lost, and its cytoplasm becomes evident, in part, because of the phagocytized content of myelin, lipid, etc. They are then known as scavenger cells, gitter cells, compound granular corpuscles, lipophages, myelinophages, etc. Many of the cells so named, however, may have their origin from lymphocytes and monocytes that reach the central nervous system through the bloodstream.

Vasculature

The blood vessels of the central nervous system, in addition to their usual functions, help through their contribution to the "blood-brain barrier" to maintain hemostasis and to aid in the return of interstitial fluid to the veins via the perivascular (Virchow-Robin) space. The blood-brain barrier is a physiologic phenomenon with which several structural features have been associated.[56] While the movement of water and lipid-soluble substances across this barrier is relatively unrestricted, the transfer of other substances such as glucose, amino acids, and inorganic ions is inhibited to varying degrees. It has been stated that the large size of some molecules and the nonutilization by the nervous system of many smaller molecules determine the degree of their exclusion by the blood-brain barrier. However, the mechanism for this barrier effect is not known. It has been related to the capillary endothelium, to the pericytes, to the covering by the foot processes of astrocytes, and to the complete or almost complete absence of an extracellular space as was previously interpreted from earlier electron microscopic studies. The structure of the capillaries of the central nervous system does not differ significantly from that of the capillaries in many parts of the body. Only approximately 85% of their circumference is covered by the astrocytic glial sheath. Moreover, the size of the extracellular space has not been settled.[99,][153] Although no agreement has been reached between the estimates derived from chemical studies and those derived from electron microscopy, the size of the space is now thought to be approximately 10% to 15% of the volume of the brain.

The perivascular or Virchow-Robin space lies between the adventitia and the pial membrane and is continuous with the subarachnoid space. Extending only as far as the capillaries, it is thought to form a route for the return of extracellular fluids and of cells through the subarachnoid space to the vascular system.

DEVELOPMENTAL DISORDERS

The nervous system begins as a longitudinal, mid-dorsal, ectodermal thickening. Cellular proliferation with ventral grooving and dorsal fusion of the freed lateral margins results in the formation of the neural tube, which is separated from the adjacent neural crest and the overlying skin. Continued orderly development with cell proliferation, peripheral migration, growth, and maturation are paralleled by growth, closure, and fusion of surrounding bones.[27, 58, 94, 155, 201]

The long period of maturation of the central nervous system is an important factor in its involvement in approximately half of all congenital defects. The known or suspected causes of these defects include the following:

1 Genetic disturbances
2 Maternal infections (i.e., rubella)
3 Fetal infection
4 Fetal hypoxia
5 Irradiation
6 Nutritional deficiencies and excesses
7 Chemical agents
8 Mechanical trauma

Each of these factors appears to be capable of producing its effect only at a particular time in the course of development of the embryo.[51, 59, 68, 100, 187, 191, 193] Since the continued normal development is dependent upon the preceding stage, the earlier the injury, the more serious the malformation.

Agenesis is the term applied to the condition in which there is absence of the anlage of a structure. In anencephaly,[191] the most severe form of agenesis, most of the brain is absent and sometimes also the spinal cord (amyelia). There are usually associated failures of closure of the skull and vertebral arches (rachischisis). All of these changes appear to begin with early defective closure of the neural tube (dysrhaphia). In those instances in which the calvaria remain intact with the skull of normal size and with the brain replaced by fluid (hydranencephaly), one should suspect birth injury rather than dysrhaphia and agenesis. Agenesis of specific portions of the brain, while not common, is well known. Many such defects are compatible with life and may be first recognized as incidental findings at postmortem examination. Among these are agenesis of the cerebellum

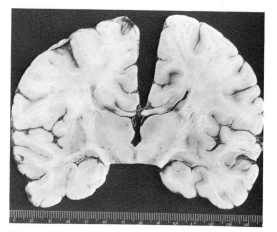

Fig. 42-1 Hypoplasia of corpus callosum.

and agenesis of all or only the caudal portion of the corpus callosum[36, 133, 165, 177] (Fig. 42-1). Absence of the cerebral pallium with fusion of the cerebral tissue (telencephalon impar) is accompanied by absence of the calvaria. Cyclencephaly is due to failure of separation of the cerebral hemispheres. When accompanied by a single median eye (cyclopia) and by a supraorbital nasal trunk with arhinencephaly, it is usually compatible with survival for only a few hours. Agenesis of a portion of the cerebral cortex usually is bilateral and most often affects the parietal lobes. The underlying lateral ventricles at these sites are dilated and communicate with the subarachnoid space (porencephaly). Similar ventricular dilatation may be seen following occlusion of the arteries or veins supplying or draining these areas or following trauma or infection, all occurring early in embryonic development with failure of development of the affected portion of the cerebral hemisphere(s).

Errors of closure of the neural tube and fusion of the surrounding bony structures are common, particularly at the lumbosacral level of the spinal cord. When the defect is complete the dorsal portion of the spinal cord is not formed and its lateral margins remain attached to the modified ectoderm (amyelocele). The most frequent developmental defect of the neural tube, however, is that of failure of complete closure of the vertebral arches (spina bifida). Herniation of only the meninges through this defect is known as a meningocele. When a portion of the cord also is included, the defect is called a meningomyelocele. A meningomyelocystocele includes the meninges, a portion of the cord, and a portion of the central canal. With spina bifida occulta, the failure of fusion of the affected vertebral arches may result in dimpling of the overlying skin and separating fibrous tissue, but with no herniation of the cord or its coverings. Herniations of a portion of the brain and its covering during closure of the skull bones are far less frequent. These occur in the region of the glabella, the occipital bone, and at the roof of the mouth.[29] Like those of the spinal cord, they are known as meningocele, meningoencephalocele, and meningoencephalocystocele.

In the Arnold-Chiari malformation, there is caudal displacement of the medulla and vermis of the cerebellum below the level of the foramen magnum into the spinal canal.[157] A notch frequently develops on the anterior surface of the cervical cord where it is overridden by the displaced medulla. The malformation is associated with a small posterior fossa and flattening of the base of the skull (platybasia) and sometimes with internal hydrocephalus and a meningomyelocele. The association of internal hydrocephalus with the platybasia has suggested to some that the brain has been forced downward during development. Fixation of the cauda equina in the patients with a meningomyelocele, on the other hand, may have displaced the brainstem and spinal cord downward due to the greater growth of the vertebra as compared with the spinal cord. Both hypotheses have been offered as explanations of this malformation.

Defective cell migration and maturation result in faulty cell position (heterotopia) and abnormalities in the formation of the gyri. The absence of gyrus formation is known as lissencephaly (agyria)[57] (Fig. 42-2). It is often, but not always, associated with generalized hypoplasia of the brain (microcephaly) (Fig. 42-3) and with developmental hydro-

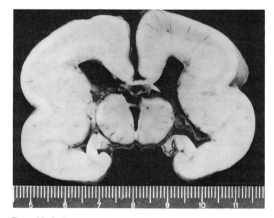

Fig. 42-2 Agyria.

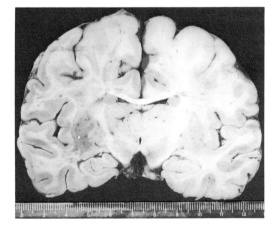

Fig. 42-3 Microcephaly. Brain of young adult.

cephalus. Focal hypoplasias are uncommon. They usually involve the related nuclei of the pons, medulla, and cerebellum.

Conversely, an overly large brain, macrocephaly (megalocephaly), is due in part to hyperplasia and often in part to dysplastic development.[194]

Tuberous sclerosis

Tuberous sclerosis is a heredofamilial disease due to dysplastic development and heterotopia of the ectodermal cells of the central nervous system.[123] Often associated are a variety of developmental abnormalities of other organs of the body, including the skin—the "adenoma sebaceum" at the nasolabial folds and the subungual nodules, both of which are fibrovascular overgrowths, and peau chagren of the midlumbar skin of the back. Accompanying renal tumors, often bilateral, are either mixtures of blood vessels, fibrous tissue, fat, and smooth muscle, (the angiomyolipofibromas) or tubular adenomas.[109] Nodular, gray-yellow, glycogen-filled myocardial tumors incorrectly diagnosed as rhabdomyomas may be found in some patients who die early with the disease. Pulmonary fibrosis, cysts, and bronchial hamartomas also have been seen.

The brain is usually of normal size or small. Affected gyri are slightly to markedly enlarged, white, and hard, with poor demarcation between the cortex and the white matter. Periventricular gray to white, hard, often mineralized, tumors project into the lateral ventricles. The first layer of a cortical tuber may have

foci of thick astrocytic fibrillae in a characteristic sheaflike arrangement (Fig. 42-4). The normal laminar arrangement of the cortical cells is markedly disturbed. In addition to an astrocytic gliosis, there are large globoid to spidery cells with both neuronal and astrocytic characteristics. Hard nodular areas, more easily felt than seen, may be found in the white matter and are composed of foci of astrocytic gliosis. The periventricular nodules are formed by partly mineralized clusters of large bizarre cells of astrocytic appearance. Retinal lesions, referred to as phakomas, are related tumors formed by the abnormally developed glial cells.

Aqueductal stenosis

Abnormal formation of the cerebral aqueduct in fetal life may be due either to an intrauterine inflammation with periaqueductal gliosis or to a disturbance in development.[28] On rare occasion, the aqueduct is developmentally small and may be double, the so-called forking of the aqueduct. The two channels are too small for adequate cerebrospinal fluid flow. Hydrocephalus resulting from any of the causes may be first manifest either at birth (congenital) or during infancy or early childhood, depending upon the degree of obstruction. Accurate recognition of the cause of the stenosis (Fig. 42-5) requires a good history, multiple sections of the aqueduct taken at close intervals and at right angles to its path, and comparison with normal controls.

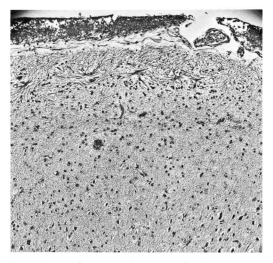

Fig. 42-4 Tuberous sclerosis with characteristic sheaflike astrocytic gliosis in first cortical layer. (Hematoxylin-eosin; ×90.)

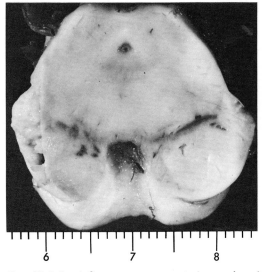

Fig. 42-5 Postinflammatory congenital aqueductal stenosis.

Mongolism (Down's syndrome)[112a]

At least two karyotypic types of mongolism have been reported, each with trisomy 21 or trisomy 21-22. The more common form, characterized by an extra 21 chromosome, is due to the failure of separation of one pair of these chromosomes in oogenesis and is more likely to occur in infants of older mothers. In the other type of mongolism, not related to maternal age, the extra 21 chromosome is believed to have been translocated to the end of another large chromosome. Translocation mongolism may be familial. One of the parents may be found to have the translocation (usually to chromosome 15) and with but forty-five chromosomes, or it may have arisen during gamete formation in normal parents.

A variety of structural abnormalities have been reported in these patients. The more characteristic is the blunting of the occipital portion of the brain and a small superior temporal gyrus (Fig. 42-6). The cerebellum may be small as well. Diagnosis, however, is

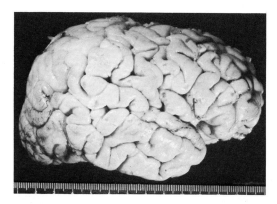

Fig. 42-6 Mongolism with small superior temporal gyrus and blunted occipital lobe.

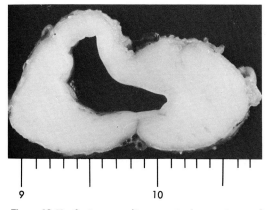

Fig. 42-7 Syringomyelia—cervical portion of spinal cord.

based upon the characteristic mongol facies with rounded head, prominent epicanthal folds, oblique palpebral fissures, dysplastic ears, high-arched palate, palm-print abnormalities, a palm with four-finger lines, a curved fifth finger, large space between the first and second toes, other nonspecific body changes, and occasional cardiac malformations.

Syringomyelia and syringobulbia[148]

Named for its irregular tubular cavity, syringomyelia is a disorder of the spinal cord due to multiple causes. One form, sometimes associated with neurofibromatosis, is thought to be due to a defect in closure of the alar plates of the spinal cord. On the other hand, the cavity or cavities may be the residual of a previous inflammation, infarct, or hemorrhage or a component of a glial neoplasm. The cervical portion of the spinal cord is the most frequently affected and, when the lesions are multiple, usually contains the largest of the cavities. Each syrinx is filled with a watery to slightly xanthochromatic fluid. The lesion may begin anywhere within the cord but most often is found in the dorsal median septum, extending both longitudinally and laterally to involve the gray and white matter (Fig. 42-7). Its lining is formed by astrocytic processes (Fig. 42-8) except in those areas in which there is residual ependyma of an included central canal. The cavity may extend for only a few segments or involve the entire cord or, as noted previously, there may be multiple

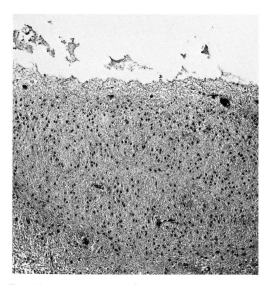

Fig. 42-8 Astrocytic proliferation of wall of syrinx. (Hematoxylin-eosin; ×90.)

cavities. The lateral extent of the cavity or cavities determines the site and degree of ascending and descending wallerian degeneration. Involvement of the medulla (syringobulbia) may occur separately or as an extension of a lesion in the cervical portion of the cord. In the medulla, the cavity is a slit in a dorsolateral winglike position. It may be bilateral and roughly symmetrical. Similar cavities have been described as occurring in the pons and even more rarely in the cerebral hemispheres, where they end in the head portion of either or both caudate nuclei.

Dilatation of the central canal (hydromyelia) is a frequent and asymptomatic finding seen at all levels of the spinal cord examined routinely postmortem. Some consider it the mildest form of spinal dysrhaphia—i.e., the mildest form of syringomyelia.

Hydrocephalus[172]

The descriptive term hydrocephalus is used to indicate an increased amount of cerebrospinal fluid in the ventricles of and/or in the subarachnoid space about the brain. In practice, this is recognized from enlargement of these spaces rather than by measurement of the fluid. The condition is classified in several different ways. When the increased fluid accumulation is limited to the dilated ventricular system, the hydrocephalus is called internal (Fig. 42-9). External hydrocephalus, on the other hand, is the presence of excess fluid in the enlarged subarachnoid space over the

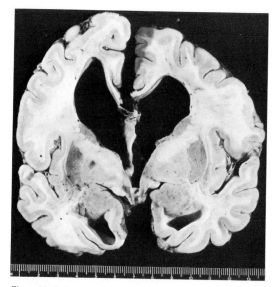

Fig. 42-9 Internal hydrocephalus of lateral and third ventricles due to obstructive lesion in fourth ventricle.

brain. Separation of hydrocephalus into communicating and noncommunicating types is useful especially for the clinician. In the communicating type, there is normal free flow of fluid between the ventricles and the subarachnoid space about the cauda equina. Obstruction or block of this free flow is associated with a noncommunicating hydrocephalus. Varying degrees, sites, and causes of flow impedance are causes for limitation of the value of this classification.

The most useful classification is that described by Russell[172] and slightly modified here. To understand this classification, a limited knowledge of formation, flow, and removal of spinal fluid is essential. Cerebrospinal fluid is formed, in the main, by the choroid plexuses of the lateral, third, and fourth ventricles. From the lateral ventricles, flow is directed into the third ventricles through the two foramina of Monro. The fluid then follows the cerebral aqueduct into the fourth ventricle, from which it exits into the subarachnoid spaces through the two lateral recesses and the foramina of Luschka and through the middle foramen of Magendi. Most of the fluid finally is returned to the venous system through the arachnoid villi that lie in several of the venous sinuses. With this brief description as a background, hydrocephalus can then be considered to have arisen from an imbalance or derangement of one or more of these factors.

Hydrocephalus due to the overproduction of cerebrospinal fluid is the least common. Proved instances of overproduction (i.e., due to hypertrophy or neoplasms of choroid plexuses) are medical curiosities. Obstruction of the great vein of Galen, previously considered a cause of fluid overproduction, has not been confirmed.

Decreased outflow (or absorption) of fluid through the arachnoidal lining cells or through narrowed or closed pores in the arachnoid villi offers another possible mechanism.[69] Direct and adequate examination of these pores is possible only by means of electron microscopy, and such has not been described. Moreover, there is some question whether such pores actually exist. The mechanism of decreased outflow, however, has been utilized, probably correctly, to explain the hydrocephalus seen with fibrosis covering the arachnoid granulations and with thrombosis of the superior sagittal sinus.

Obstruction to the flow of fluid is a common cause of internal hydrocephalus. The obstructing lesion may be developmental, inflammatory, or neoplastic and may be almost anywhere in the flow tract. The pattern of ventricular enlargement frequently can be used as a guide to determine the site of the obstructing lesion. Ventricular dilatation is limited to that portion proximal to the obstruction (Fig. 42-9). Dilated ventricles with subependymal petechial hemorrhages are diagnostic of an acute obstructive hydrocephalus (Fig. 42-10).

Two other mechanisms also should be considered in the production of hydrocephalus. Once the fontanels are closed and growth has ceased, the skull encloses an intracranial space of fixed size. Loss of brain tissue for any reason must, therefore, be accompanied by increase in fluid and enlargement of the subarachnoid and/or ventricular spaces. This is known as compensatory hydrocephalus (hydrocephalus ex vacuo). It is the most common cause of hydrocephalus although, in most instances, it is not clinically symptomatic. Among the less frequent causes of hydrocephalus and one that often is not considered is that due to failure in development of all or a portion of the brain. Although the ventricles, in such instances, are small, they are relatively large when compared with the overall size of the brain. This is developmental hydrocephalus.

Porencephaly,[141] is a related condition. The term originally was meant to designate an abnormal cavity that connected the ventricular and subarachnoid spaces through a defect in the cerebrum. With this definition, the cause was due to the failure of development of a portion of the primitive ependymal lining in the line of the primary fissure. The defect was usually bilateral and symmetrical. Much of

this meaning has been lost, for most observers now use the term to describe any large intracerebral cavity usually with an opening into an adjacent ventricle.

VASCULAR DISEASES
Hypoxic encephalopathy (anoxic encephalopathy)

Despite the numerous variables that could be expected to alter the pattern of damage to the central nervous system subjected to hypoxia, there is an unusual degree of uniformity of histologic change.[50, 176] The structural changes are dependent upon the degree and duration of the hypoxia, upon length of survival, and, when present, upon a preceding period of a lesser degree of hypoxia. Antecedent asymptomatic or mild hypoxia, according to Lindenberg,[132] depletes the affected cells of enzymes that under more sudden and severe hypoxic conditions promote individual cell destruction. He believes that a preceding mild hypoxia is desirable in that structural and functional recovery are then more likely to occur with and following a severe hypoxic episode. Gross structural changes generally are not apparent with hypoxia except when caused by severe venous engorgement that produces duskiness of the entire central nervous system and petechial hemorrhages (Fig. 42-11). When the cause is arterial, there may be mild to marked pallor. The brain is frequently slightly or markedly swollen with some blurring of the margins between the cortex and the underlying white matter.

Although the first microscopic changes may be seen after survival of only four hours, they usually are not discernible until after survival of at least eight to twelve hours. With general hypoxia (as with cardiac failure, respiratory

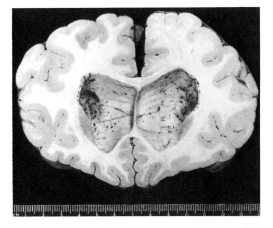

Fig. 42-10 Acute obstructive internal hydrocephalus with numerous subependymal petechiae.

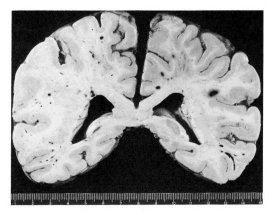

Fig. 42-11 Dusky brain with multiple petechial and some larger hemorrhages in marked hypoxia.

disease, anemia, etc.), the most susceptible cells, including their processes, are those in Sommer's sector in the temporal lobe, the Purkinje cells of the cerebellum, and the cells of the third and fourth cortical layers of the cerebral hemispheres. The earliest microscopic changes consist of slight cell enlargement and cytoplasmic eosinophilia with loss of the Nissl substance. Affected cells occur singly or in clusters and are separated by cells with a normal appearance. The hypoxic cells and adjoining blood vessels are surrounded by edematous zones that stain less intensely than the normal.

Later, the affected cells become irregularly shrunken and their nuclei eccentric, small, and hyperchromatic. Eventually, the cells and their processes that are injured beyond recovery disappear. Petechial hemorrhages that accompany the early lesions usually disappear without remnant. When tissue necrosis also occurs, the blood becomes organized.

Infarcts

A localized area of necrosis due to vascular insufficiency is known as an infarct. Large infarcts may be associated with atherosclerosis with or without thrombosis, with emboli in large arteries, with venous occlusive disease, and with a dissecting hematoma that compresses an artery.[1, 23, 39, 70, 140] Small infarcts occur with diseases of small arteries and arterioles and sometimes from emboli in these small vessels. With adequate collateral channels, particularly through the circle of Willis and leptomeningeal vessels, gradual occlusion of even a large artery may not result in an infarct. Conversely, the gradual narrowing of even a small artery can, in the absence of an adequate col-

lateral, cause infarction. Infarcts are classified as pale (anemic) or red (hemorrhagic), depending upon the amount of blood present in the necrotic area (Fig. 42-12). They also are divided into those which are recent (usually under three weeks), old (three to six weeks), and remote (over six weeks).

Anemic infarcts most frequently are associated with atherosclerosis with or without thrombosis. In the absence of a thrombus, there is often a preceding episode of hypotension and/or hypoxia. Anemic infarcts are more likely to occur in normotensive or hypotensive states and in the presence of disseminated vascular disease that impairs the generally limited collateral circulation. Initially, an anemic infarct is dusky due to continued deoxygenation of the retained intravascular blood. Shortly afterward, the infarct begins to enlarge in volume due to the influx of fluid from adjacent functioning blood vessels and tissues. The increasing volume of the infarct within the fixed intracranial space compresses the contained vessels. By forcing the sludged intravascular blood away into the draining venous channels, the infarct becomes pale. There is a simultaneous and progressive decrease in size of the adjacent spaces (subarachnoid and ventricular). In some, the rapid increase in volume of a large infarct may produce brain displacement, with herniations and even secondary pressure hemorrhages in the brainstem (p. 1849). The initial microscopic changes are similar to those described under hypoxic encephalopathy but with more diffuse and severe involvement.

An infarct of the third and fourth layers of the cerebral cortex, usually in the depth of a convolution, is known as a laminar (or pseudolaminar) infarct. When more severe, the infarct extends to involve the cortex toward the crest of the gyri, the second and deeper cortical layers, and may even extend into the underlying white matter. The first cortical layer regularly demonstrates only a reactive astrocytosis. The laminar infarct occurs more frequently in the so-called watershed zones of the parieto-occipital convexities but may be found in all parts of the cerebral cortex and even in the cerebellum. This type of infarct frequently is found in patients who have had myocardial infarcts with a drop in blood pressure, in those who have been in prolonged shock from any cause, following cardiac arrest in those with a period of survival after resuscitation, and in those who have had prolonged hypoglycemic episodes.

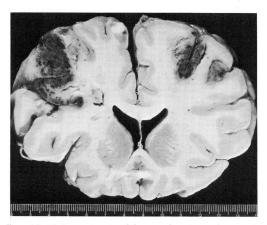

Fig. 42-12 Recent mixed hemorrhagic and anemic infarcts secondary to emboli in middle cerebral arteries.

In the following description of the natural history of infarcts, it should be recognized that the time sequences are approximations. The rates and degrees of reaction are dependent upon many variables existing among individuals and in the same patient with differing conditions. These variations may be present even in different portions of a single large infarct.

In all anemic infarcts, the cytoplasm of the nerve cell initially becomes eosinophilic and its nucleus shrunken and hyperchromatic. With the influx of fluid, the infarcted tissue progressively becomes more pale staining (Fig.

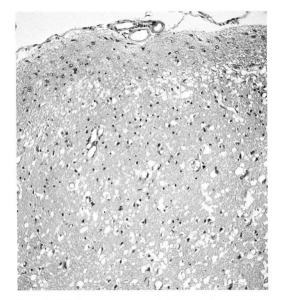

Fig. 42-13 Recent anemic infarct with retention and reactive astrocytosis of outer cortical layer. (Hematoxylin-eosin; ×90.)

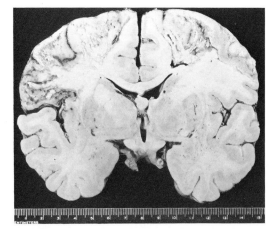

Fig. 42-14 Advanced liquefaction of recent anemic infarcts secondary to emboli in branches of middle cerebral arteries.

42-13) except the intact first cortical layer, in which only a reactive astrocytosis occurs. The first reactive cells, seen between the eighteenth and twenty-fourth hour of the infarct, are neutrophils. These cells, usually in small numbers, are found in the walls of blood vessels within the infarct and the immediately adjacent necrotic tissue near the periphery of the infarct. They may reach the adjacent subarachnoid space. Activation of the surrounding microglial cells and the appearance of perivascular lymphocytes and monocytes at the edges of the infarct may begin by the second day but most frequently are not found until the third day. During the following two weeks, the infarct continues to enlarge and soften, with evidence of liquefaction (Fig. 42-14). Beginning by the fourth day and increasing thereafter, it is progressively filled by the mononuclear cells, many of which have become lipophages. The blood vessels within the infarct are gradually reopened by the flow of blood from the collateral channels. Reactive astrocytes in the walls of the infarct, first seen during the third day, become easily evident by the fifth day. The volume of the anemic infarct is greatest during the second week. Thereafter, its gradually decreasing volume is associated with the disappearance of the lipophages and loss of fluid. At the end of the third week, its volume approximates that of the original tissue. Continued removal of the necrotic material and of fluid gradually transforms the infarct by the sixth week into a pale

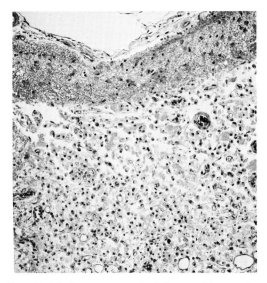

Fig. 42-15 Remote anemic infarct with reactive astrocytosis in retained outer cortical layer. (Hematoxylin-eosin; ×135.)

spongelike cavity traversed by a network of small blood vessels, some of which are newly formed (Fig. 42-15). A few lipophages within the infarct and a narrow wall of reactive and often gemistocytic astrocytes remain for the life of the individual. The presence of an intact first cortical layer aids in the separation of an infarct from a contusion or laceration (Fig. 42-14). The adjacent spaces, first narrowed and compressed, have enlarged (compensatory hydrocephalus) as the infarct volume decreases.

Hemorrhagic infarcts are associated with emboli, hypertension, venous occlusion, and bleeding tendencies. The duskiness of the early infarct becomes dark red due to the inflow of blood into the necrotic tissue from reopening of the occluded vessel, from collateral channels, or because the initial lesion was due to a venous occlusion (Fig. 42-16). In comparison with the anemic infarct, the hemorrhagic infarct enlarges more rapidly and to a greater degree and retains its increased volume for a longer period. Hemosiderophages, found with extreme difficulty before the third or fourth day, become progressively more prominent thereafter and, like the lipophages, some remain locally for the life of the individual. Reactive astrocytes forming the infarct wall sometimes contain hemosiderin granules. The brown color

of the remote lesion (over six weeks), due to hemosiderin and hematoidin, distinguishes it from an anemic infarct, and the bridging blood vessels separate it from a massive hemorrhage. Compensatory hydrocephalus, external and/or internal, may also be associated with the larger hemorrhagic infarcts.

Infarcts, anemic and hemorrhagic, from 1 mm to 1 cm in size are common in the putamina and thalami (Fig. 42-17) and, to a lesser degree, in the base of the pons and in the other central gray masses of the cerebral hemispheres in patients with a long history of hypertension.[77, 107, 162] Bilateral lesions are almost limited to patients with long-standing hypertension. Slightly larger infarcts in the central white matter of the cerebral hemispheres are equally characteristic of long-standing hypertension, especially when the infarcts are hemorrhagic and/or have more than the expected amount of connective tissue about the blood vessels within them (Fig. 42-18). Small, subcortical areas of necrosis usually have been considered as infarcts resulting from severe arteriolosclerosis in patients with hypertension.[154] Recently, however, these have been described as the end stages of recurrent or severe local edema associated with hypertensive encephalopathy.[73] The associated clinical state is known as Binswanger's disease.[73, 154]

Hemorrhage

Hemorrhage into the central nervous system may result from any of the diseases that

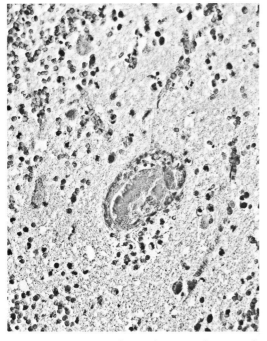

Fig. 42-16 Recent hemorrhagic infarct with embolic material in vessel. (Hematoxylin-eosin; ×280.)

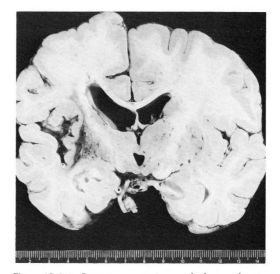

Fig. 42-17 Remote anemic and hemorrhagic infarcts in putamina in patient with long-standing hypertension. Compensatory hydrocephalus. Segmental atherosclerosis, grade 3.

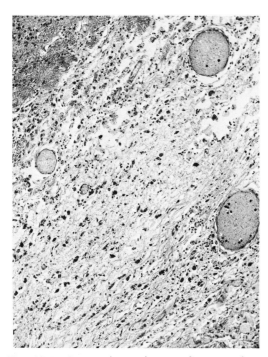

Fig. 42-18 Remote hemorrhagic infarct in white matter of patient with hypertension. (Hematoxylin-eosin; ×90.)

destroy the integrity of the blood vessels and/ or decrease the coagulability of the blood.[42, 47, 85, 143] Petechial hemorrhages, especially those in the floor of the third and fourth ventricles, most often are associated with hypoxia and/or respiratory failure in which the heart has continued to beat for a short time afterward. They may be seen with mechanical trauma to the head, fat embolism, chemical toxins such as the arsenical compounds, intrinsic disorders of the hematopoietic system that have a tendency toward bleeding, following anticoagulant therapy, in endogenous toxic conditions such as uremia, and with diseases of the blood vessels. In most instances, there are multiple causative agents that act synergistically. A recent petechial hemorrhage, often confused with an engorged blood vessel, may be recognized because it is usually significantly larger than the otherwise normal but dilated vessels in the area, is slightly irregular, has a less sharp margin than that seen with an engorged blood vessel, and, with semitangential lighting, has a convex meniscus rather than the concave meniscus of blood within a vessel. When not completely resorbed, the petechial hemorrhages are brown to yellow and slightly depressed. This is due to the conversion of the hemoglobin to hemo-

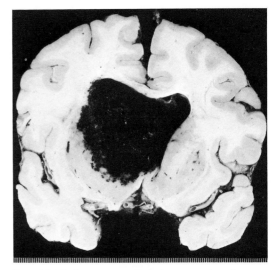

Fig. 42-19 Recent massive hypertensive hemorrhage in internal capsule and head of caudate nucleus with rupture into lateral ventricle.

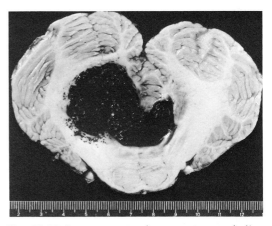

Fig. 42-20 Recent massive hypertensive cerebellar hemorrhage with petechiae and rupture into fourth ventricle.

siderin and hematoidin by the macrophages accompanied by some tissue loss and a mild reactive astrocytosis. Larger, sometimes massive, hemorrhages (3 cm or more in the cerebral hemispheres and 1.5 cm or more in the brainstem) may be due to any of the aforementioned causes. Under these circumstances, the hemorrhages are frequently multiple and sharply demarcated without peripheral petechiae and usually are associated with little or no brain swelling and/or edema. Although these hemorrhages may sometimes extend through the cortex into the subarachnoid space, they rarely rupture into an adjoining ventricle.

Massive brain hemorrhages are a common

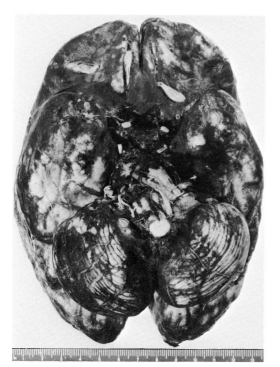

Fig. 42-21 Recent diffuse subarachnoid hemorrhage in patient with massive intracerebral hemorrhage.

cause of death in patients with inadequately treated and uncontrolled hypertension.[63, 82, 146] About 70% of the hemorrhages are in the lateral and/or medial ganglionic regions of the cerebral hemispheres (lenticular nuclei, thalami, and internal capsules [Fig. 42-19]).[37, 53, 65, 121] From these regions, the hemorrhages may track downward along the nerve tracts to the midbrain and even to the pons or into the adjacent frontal and/or parietal lobes. The cerebral hemispheres are equally affected. About 20% of the hemorrhages begin initially in the midbrain, pons, or white matter of the cerebellum (Fig. 42-20). The remaining 10% begin in any of the remaining portions of the cerebral hemispheres. The medulla is never the primary site of this type of hemorrhage and is rarely involved by extension. The hemorrhages in fatal cases almost always have ruptured into the adjacent ventricle and from there have followed the cerebrospinal flow to reach the subarachnoid space. Relatively few rupture directly into the overlying subarachnoid space, and very rarely have the hemorrhages ruptured simultaneously or successively into both. Less than 1% of these massive hemorrhages are multiple. Death occurs in over 90% of these patients and usually

within ninety-six hours (except in those patients maintained by respirator for longer periods). On examination, the brain is pale and swollen and asymmetrical, usually with a symmetrical subarachnoid hemorrhage at the base (Fig. 42-21). With this asymmetrically swollen brain, the larger hemisphere contains the hemorrhage. It usually is covered by a lesser degree of subarachnoid blood because of greater compression of the space by the more swollen gyri. Brain displacement with herniations and secondary brainstem hemorrhage are common. The occurrence and localization of these secondary changes are dependent upon the site and size of the massive hemorrhage.

The brain immediately surrounding the hemorrhage is markedly swollen and edematous and often has many petechiae in one or more areas immediately about the hemorrhage. The absence of brain tissue within the hemorrhage and the presence of blood beyond the region supplied by an artery or drained by a vein serves to distinguish macroscopically the hemorrhage from an hemorrhagic infarct. On microscopic examination, a characteristic structural pattern usually can be recognized. Within the hemorrhage, only a rare remnant of nerve tissue is found among the blood cells. The immediately surrounding swollen and edematous brain contains numerous severely sclerotic small arteries and arterioles as well as capillaries and venules. In the regions with petechial hemorrhages, there usually are necrotic arterioles, venules, and capillaries infiltrated and surrounded by red blood cells and sometimes some neutrophils. When the routine examination includes only a single or, at most, several sections through this region, infrequent recognizable aneurysmally dilated arterioles and small arteries are to be found (Fig. 42-22). Serial sections through these zones often result in a significant increase in their yield, but they are never frequent. The zone immediately peripheral to the petechial hemorrhages contains hyalinized thick-walled blood vessels surrounded by large lakes of fluid high in protein content. There is a moderate degree of brain swelling and edema in this area, but this is less than that seen in the portion of the brain immediately adjacent to the hemorrhage. In the remainder of the brain, there are arterioles and small arteries that exhibit varying degrees of arteriolosclerosis. Frequently, many of the infarcts previously described as occurring in patients with hypertension are also present. In those hypertensive patients in whom no petechial hemorrhages are to be

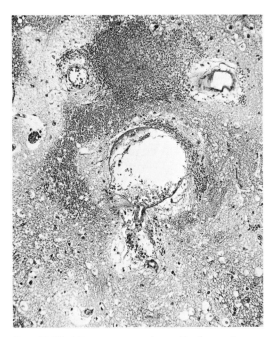

Fig. 42-22 Microaneurysm in wall of massive recent hypertensive hemorrhage. (Hematoxylineosin; ×90.)

found in the walls of the massive hemorrhage, there is a different structural stratification. At one edge of the hemorrhage, one may, on occasion, find evidences of a preexisting or simultaneously occurring anemic or hemorrhagic infarct. The other portions of its wall are similar to those seen in the other hemorrhages with brain swelling, edema, and arteriolosclerosis of moderate to marked degrees.

These findings have stimulated at least three hypotheses as to the pathogenesis of the massive hemorrhages: [42, 48, 49, 170, 206]

1 Necrotizing arteriolitis with rupture of many arterioles
2 Arteriolosclerosis with a few or many arterioles undergoing necrosis, microaneurysm formation, and rupture (Fig. 42-22)
3 Massive hemorrhage in an area of earlier infarct

In 5% to 10% of the hypertensive patients with a massive hemorrhage, the lesion is not fatal. While this may occur with the larger cerebral hemorrhage that has not ruptured into a ventricle, it is more frequently seen with the smaller ganglionic hemorrhages that have neither extended nor ruptured into the ventricular and/or subarachnoid spaces. In these, only the outer 1 mm to 2 mm of the hemorrhage is organized, with conversion of the hemoglobin to hemosiderin and hematoi-

din. A mild reactive astrocytic proliferation is present in the immediately surrounding brain. The blood in the interior of the hemorrhage becomes dark (chocolate red) and remains semiliquid and unorganized. When the blood is manually evacuated, a brown smooth-walled cavity not traversed by blood vessels remains.

Hypertensive encephalopathy characterized by recurrent attacks of sudden and severe headaches with vomiting, mental confusion and visual, sensory, and/or motor disturbances is common in patients with untreated or inadequately treated hypertension.[205] While one of these attacks may precede the appearance of a massive hemorrhage, death during an uncomplicated attack is rare. The mechanism of the syndrome is not known, although arteriolar spasm and arteriolar and capillary thrombi have been suggested. The changes in the brain are neither characteristic nor uniform. Brain swelling with pallor and scattered petechiae has been described. There are others, however, in whom no gross abnormalities have been recognized. On microscopic examination, there are usually varying degrees of arteriolosclerosis. In some, there is arteriolar necrosis with surrounding petechiae. Identical changes also may be seen in hypertensive patients dying in chronic uremia. The relationship of hypertensive encephalopathy to the small and larger hemorrhages and to the areas of necrosis in patients with hypertension is not known, although there has been much speculation.

Aneurysms

Aneurysms of the arteries of the circle of Willis have been classified as berry (so-called congenital), atherosclerotic, inflammatory (mycotic), traumatic, and developmental. Of this group, only the first is of frequent clinical importance. The traumatic lesion usually is an arteriovenous fistula rather than an aneurysm. True developmental aneurysms are exceptionally rare.

Berry aneurysms.[24, 40, 64, 95] The most common of this group of blood vessel lesions, berry aneurysms are found in 5% to 6% of all adults at postmortem examination.[40] Most of them occur in the bifurcation pockets of the arteries forming (Fig. 42-23) or extending from the circle of Willis (Fig. 42-24). The initial defect in these is considered to be a developmental deficiency or absence of the medial smooth muscle in the pocket.[64] Aneurysms not in bifurcation pockets are said to follow incomplete resorption of unused embryonic arteries. The aneurysms form later

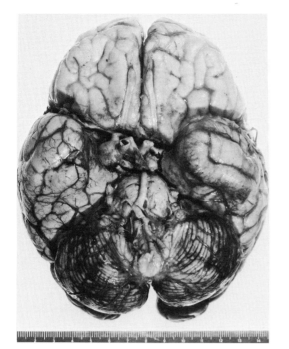

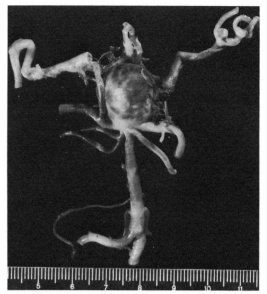

Fig. 42-24 Unruptured berry aneurysms. Larger aneurysm at terminal portion of basilar artery. Smaller aneurysm in bifurcation angle of middle cerebral artery on right.

Fig. 42-23 Berry aneurysm at junction of right internal carotid and posterior communicating arteries. Pons is slightly widened and fore-shortened, and there is cerebellomedullary herni-ation—both due to rupture of aneurysm with intracerebral and intraventricular extension of hemorrhage that has reached cerebellar sub-arachnoid space.

following damage of the internal elastic lam-ina, probably due to a preceding focal athero-sclerotic change. Some, however, have incor-rectly considered this damage to be due to disease of the vasa vasorum of these vessels. The normal thin adventitia of the arteries of the circle of Willis contributes significantly to the lack of adequate resistance to the intra-vascular pressure.

The aneurysms are, for reasons not known, twice as common in women as in men. Only about 40% found at necropsy show evidence of bleeding or of rupture. About 30% are multiple and, of these, two-thirds are bilateral. Association with polycystic renal disease and with coarctation of the aorta can usually be related to the coexistent hypertension. Hyper-tension is present in 80% of those with these aneurysms (with and without bleeding). The average mean age at the time of fatal rupture is between 50 and 55 years. The mortality rate of the first rupture is between 25% and 50%, and it is thought to be even higher with each succeeding rupture. In those with fatal rup-tures, death occurs within twenty-four hours in almost half, many within the first hour,

and in 95% within two weeks. The arteries forming the anterior half of the circle are in-volved about six times as frequently as those of the posterior half.[22, 40] The sides of the circle are affected equally.

Although some aneurysms are cylindrical, most are berry shaped. They have narrowed necks of variable lengths. The mouth of the aneurysm internally often is constricted by an encircling endothelial fibrous cushion covering the frayed ends of the internal elastic lam-ina[173, 199] (Fig. 42-25). The wall of the aneu-rysm is formed by a few layers of connective tissue devoid of the elastic lamina. It progres-sively becomes more thin toward the fundus, where rupture is most likely to occur (Fig. 42-25).[135, 162] A recent electron microscopic study of these aneurysms has suggested the presence of smooth muscle cells within the wall of the aneurysm.[126] The occasional presence of a few neutrophils in the wall immediately adjacent to sites of leakage or rupture has lead some to suggest incorrectly that these lesions are basically inflammatory.

In over two-thirds of the patients with fatal rupture, the asymmetrical subarachnoid hem-orrhage is but one of the complications.[40] Ex-tension of the hemorrhage into the adjacent brain and often into a ventricle is common. Subdural hemorrhage occurs but is infrequent. Cerebral infarcts occurring with or following rupture are frequent. Some are due to emboli

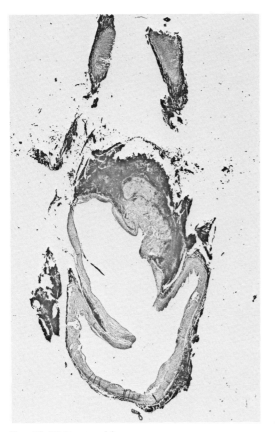

Fig. 42-25 Ruptured berry aneurysm.

and some to severe and prolonged local vasospasm. Brain displacement, herniation, and brainstem hemorrhage also are frequent secondary complications.

The five hypotheses that have contributed to the understanding of these aneurysms are as follows:

1 A developmental inadequacy or absence of the muscle coat in the angle at the bifurcation of the arteries[81]
2 Failure of resorption of a blind embryonic vessel
3 Atherosclerotic changes in the bifurcation angle, leading to loss of the internal elastic lamina
4 Degenerative stenotic or occlusive disease of the vasa vasorum of the arteries of the circle
5 Focal arteritis of the affected vessels

Of these hypotheses, only the first three are generally accepted.

Atherosclerotic aneurysms. Atherosclerotic aneurysms are usually manifest as elongated cylindrical dilatations affecting the terminal portions of the internal carotid arteries and the basilar artery. Although rupture is very rare, the carotid aneurysms often compress either or both optic nerves, sometimes with recognizable and characteristic narrowing of the visual fields. The wall of the atherosclerotic aneurysm is characterized by a thin intimal layer of fibrous tissue containing a few lipophages and occasional cholesterol-crystal clefts. The internal elastic lamina is represented by only a few residual fragments of elastic tissue and the media by a few layers of fibrous tissue almost devoid of smooth muscle. There is a thin fibrous adventitia.

Inflammatory aneurysms.[168] An inflammatory (mycotic) aneurysm occurs at the site of attachment to an infected embolus whose usual source is a vegetation from a left-sided heart valve or pulmonary infection. The aneurysms are more frequent in the first and second major bifurcations of either middle cerebral artery. They are sometimes associated with a purulent leptomeningitis, a brain abscess, or a cerebral infarct. The aneurysm infrequently ruptures, and then into the subarachnoid space.

Arteriovenous fistula (internal carotid artery–cavernous sinus fistula). Before entering the intracranial cavity, the internal carotid arteries pass through the lumens of the cavernous sinuses. Disruption of an internal carotid artery in this area often is associated with a blow to the frontal area of the head, sometimes with fracture of one of the bones of the paranasal sinus. In some, a history of antecedent injury is not obtained. The presence of significant concomitant degenerative disease of the carotid artery has not received adequate attention, since this region has not been routinely examined at necropsy. Rupture of the artery results in marked distention of the cavernous sinus and of the veins draining into it.

Developmental (true congenital) aneurysms.[186] Developmental aneurysms are exceedingly rare lesions. In a recent summary, only sixteen had been recorded, all occurring in children under the age of 2 years. The aneurysms differ structurally from the berry aneurysms. Our material contains a single previously unrecorded case of an aneurysm of the left posterior inferior cerebellar artery in a 6-week-old infant. There were no endothelial changes. The wall was completely devoid of elastic tissue, and the media contained a thin layer of loosely arranged plump spindle cells suggesting smooth muscle. The adventitia was thin and loose. The aneurysm did not occur at a bifurcation, and there was no endo-thelial cushion.

TRAUMA

The effects of mechanical trauma, either direct or indirect, upon the central nervous system, although varied, are frequently predictable. A systematic approach to the structural changes resulting from mechanical trauma usually begins with lesions of the dura, followed by the lesions that are produced at successively deeper levels.

Epidural hematoma

The dura covering the brain is represented by a fusion of true dura and periosteum of the skull. Below the level of the foramen magnum, the two layers are separated by adipose tissue, blood vessels, and nodular accumulation of lymphocytes, sometimes with follicle formation. Epidural hematomas due to blunt trauma are almost limited to the region of the skull[143a] (Fig. 42-26). They usually are associated with a recent skull fracture which, in crossing the groove of the middle meningeal artery, tears that artery. Rarely, the hematoma may result from a tear of the anterior or posterior meningeal artery or from a vein passing through bone and dura.[26] By its position, the lesion also can be considered as a subperiosteal hematoma.

These hematomas rarely, if ever, organize or resolve without surgical intervention. The usual amount of blood found at autopsy in untreated patients varies between 75 gm and 125 gm. This amount is in the same range found in fatal acute subdural hematomas and intracerebral hypertensive hemorrhages. Death is due to the effects of brain compression, with brain displacement, herniation, and secondary brainstem hemorrhages associated with neurogenic pulmonary edema.

Subdural hematoma

Subdural hematomas usually result from blunt injury to the skull without fracture. They can, however, occur without direct injury to the skull. This is particularly true in older individuals with brain atrophy in whom sudden anterior or posterior movement of the head, as from stumbling, may easily tear one of the bridging veins. On rare occasions, arterial bleeding may be the cause of the hematoma.

With the acute subdural hematoma, blood accumulates rapidly following a tear of a bridging vein at the point where the vessel

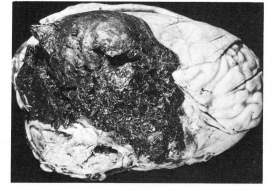

Fig. 42-26 Acute epidural hematoma.

leaves the subdural space (a potential space) to enter the dura. Because most veins cross the subdural space in the vicinity of the superior sagittal sinus, most hematomas begin parasagittally. The reason they remain as tumorous collections in this region rather than form a diffuse hematoma is not known. Some believe that it is due to the pressure exerted by the brain at the rim of the hematoma. There is little or no evidence of early organization of the acute subdural hematoma on its dural surface or at its margins, nor is there ever any evidence of organization of the hematoma from the arachnoidal membrane except when this membrane is torn.

Leary[129] stated that the first evidences of organization of these hematomas is recognizable after approximately two weeks. The hematoma becomes encapsulated by vascular granulation tissue originating from the overlying dura. From the dura at the margins of the hematoma, an initial mesothelial-like thin layer of cells proliferates to cover the blood on its undersurface and separates it from the surface of the arachnoid (Fig. 42-27). In this manner, an encapsulated chronic subdural hematoma is formed (Fig. 42-28).

Others are of the opinion that at least some of the chronic subdural hematomas are the result of an initial hematoma between the inner and outer layers of the true dura.[19] The bridging vein is believed to have been torn within this relatively highly vascularized portion of dura.

Whatever the original site of the hemorrhage, the granulation tissue that surrounds the hematoma contains large thin-walled vessels that act as semipermeable membranes (Fig. 42-27). With destruction of the blood cells, the hematoma becomes hypertonic and attracts fluid from the surrounding dilated

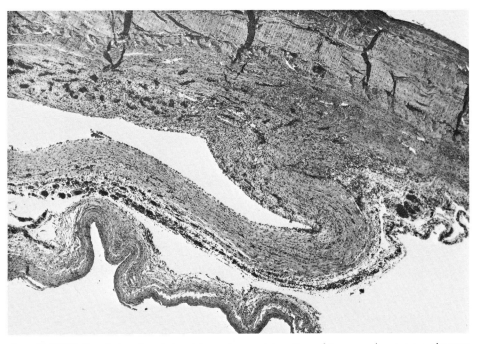

Fig. 42-27 Walls of chronic subdural hematoma at junction of inner and outer membranes. (Hematoxylin-eosin; ×30.)

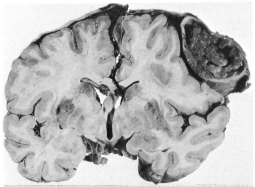

Fig. 42-28 Chronic subdural hematoma with compression of underlying brain and lateral ventricle. Bone formation in falx. Uncal herniation on side of hematoma.

thin-walled vessels. This results in enlargement of the hematoma, with stretching, tearing, and hemorrhage from the vessels at the margins. Repetition of these processes leads to continued gradual and steplike enlargement of the hematoma. A fatal chronic subdural hematoma frequently will weigh over 250 gm. The greater the size, the more slowly the enlargement develops. These hematomas regularly are associated with marked brain displacement, herniations, and, when fatal, brainstem hemorrhages and neurogenic pulmonary edema. The theories of production and continued enlargement of the chronic subdural hematoma cannot be substantiated, since the lesion has not been produced experimentally. Clinical classification of subdural hematomas with acute, subacute, and chronic types are more related to the time of development of signs and symptoms and their duration than to the structural characteristics.

A history of trauma is not obtained in every patient with a chronic subdural hematoma, even those capable of giving reliable histories. This is due, in part, to the occasional long interval between the causative event and the first signs and symptoms. In some, the episode may have been ignored or forgotten, since the trauma appeared to be trivial or was to another part of the body (such as a fall on the buttocks or a jerking of the entire body on stumbling). Individuals on anticoagulant therapy, particularly those who are older and have vascular disease, are more susceptible.

Organized subdural hemorrhages recognized grossly as rusty discoloration of the inner dural layer are frequent when the autopsy population has a high proportion of alcoholics and other adult groups with an unusual incidence of minor head trauma. In these, the hemoglobin has been converted to hemosiderin and hematoidin. Occasionally, a small recent hemorrhage is found, suggesting a new injury or the beginning of the cycle toward the formation of a larger hematoma.

A localized subdural collection of a yellow fluid with a high protein content is known as a subdural hygroma. It is an uncommon lesion thought to follow a valvelike tear of the arachnoid, permitting only the outward flow of subarachnoid fluid into the subdural space. Origin from a chronic subdural hematoma has been suggested for the encapsulated hygroma.

Subarachnoid hemorrhage

Bleeding into the subarachnoid space has many causes, one of the more common of which is blunt trauma to the skull with or without fracture. While bleeding can occur as the sole result of trauma (at least clinically), at postmortem examination the hemorrhages often are associated with other lesions (i.e., contusions and lacerations). With uncomplicated hemorrhages, the blood may be completely removed by following the cerebrospinal fluid flow into the draining sinuses. In some individuals, particularly those with other traumatic brain lesions, the blood may be trapped by adhesions and then converted to hemosiderin and hematoidin.

Contusion

Contusions of the brain are caused by blunt head trauma. The effects are transmitted to the brain by the deformation of the skull and by the inertia of the brain. Coup lesions occur at the point of impact and the contrecoup lesion at a point away from the impact site. The latter is generally at or near the diametric opposite side of the skull from the impact. The exact point depends upon the skull curvature, direction of impact, etc. The energy transferred to the brain—either positive (coup) or negative (contrecoup)—is accentuated by the inertia of the brain and the inbending at the point of impact and outbending of the deformed skull at the contrecoup site, combined with shearing rotational movements of this lacerated brain. Damage is diminished by the shape of the skull and the falx and tentorium.

Most contusions are sustained by the impact of the moving head against a fixed or relatively stationary object. The contrecoup lesion with these deceleration injuries is usually larger than the coup lesion and is due to the negative pressure. The coup and contrecoup lesions are roughly conical, with the base of

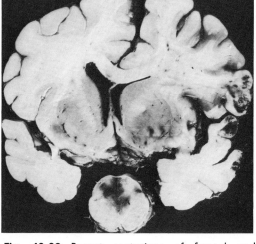

Fig. 42-29 Recent contusions of frontal and temporal lobes. Brain displacement with cingulate gyrus herniation. Compression and displacement of lateral ventricle. Secondary brainstem hemorrhages.

the cone directed toward the arachnoid surface at the apex of one or more convolutions (Fig. 42-29). All tissues, including the surface cortical layer (therefore, all contusions are lacerations as well), are destroyed or damaged for varying depths. Initially, the lesions are filled with necrotic cells and focal and/or diffuse collections of fresh blood from torn blood vessels. There is a variable degree of edema and swelling of the adjacent tissue. Early and transiently, a few neutrophils may be found in the walls of an occasional vessel at the margin of a contusion. Perivascular mononuclear cells appear during the second and third days, and reactive astrocytes are seen in the adjoining brain at about the same time. Organization proceeds with the formation of lipophages and the conversion of the blood to hemosiderin and hematoidin, much of which remains within the lesion. Thereafter, the contusion-laceration is represented by an orange-brown, depressed, wedge-shaped region with a flattened apex (Fig. 42-30). The lesion, widest at the crest of a gyrus or gyri, often is covered by a leptomeningeal-cortical scar.

Contusions-lacerations are most frequent at the tips and orbital portions of the frontal lobes and tips and lateral portions of the temporal lobes. Other areas of involvement are the tips of the occipital lobes, the corpus callosum (due to damage by the free margin of the falx), the cerebellum, and base of the pons.

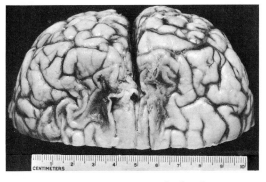

Fig. 42-30 Remote contusions of orbital gyri.

Intracerebral hematoma

Intracerebral hematomas following nonpenetrating trauma to the skull are presumably due to shearing stresses upon intracerebral vessels. The rupture of one or more large vessels may lead to a large hematoma or to several (Fig. 42-31). They are more likely to occur in the frontal lobes but may be found in other portions of the brain, including cerebellum. The midbrain, pons, and medulla rarely contain a large traumatic hemorrhage.

Multiple small hemorrhages, primarily in the white matter of the brain following nonpenetrating skull trauma, are more likely due to hypoxia or to fat embolism. Although the hemorrhages of fat embolism are far more frequent in the white matter (Fig. 42-32), fat emboli are found more frequently in the adjoining gray matter. While fat emboli may be found in the central nervous system in patients with injuries to long bones with or without fractures, they also are seen following burns or mechanical damage to large areas of subcutaneous fat, in sickle cell crises, in patients with severe fatty change in the liver, and in patients with active pancreatitis. Fat emboli need not be accompanied by petechial hemorrhages. The fat obstructs many arterioles and capillaries throughout the brain. The vascular stasis with anoxia and the endothelial damage produce the petechiae.

Concussion

Concussion is the sudden loss of neurologic function immediately upon blunt injury, usually to the head. Much has been written concerning the definition of this entity, the mechanism of injury, and the physical principles involved in the transmission of force, as well as the structural changes, if any.

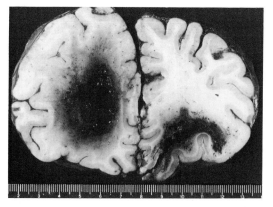

Fig. 42-31 Recent hematomas in frontal lobes, posttraumatic.

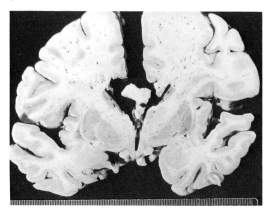

Fig. 42-32 Petechial hemorrhages in white matter in posttraumatic fat embolism.

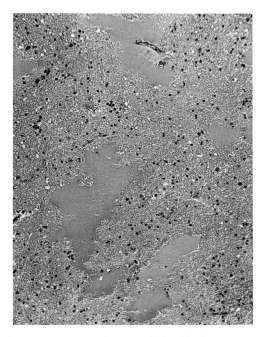

Fig. 42-33 Brain edema with fluid high in protein content. (Hematoxylin-eosin; ×90.)

Uncomplicated concussion in the human being is rarely, if ever, fatal. Among those who have reported experimental observations, there is agreement that structural changes at the light microscopic level do occur. These changes consist of central chromatolysis of variable numbers of cells in the reticular substance of the brainstem with similar but lesser involvement of cells in the cerebral cortex.[44-46] Some believe that these changes are secondary to damage to axons in the ventral portion of the upper cervical portion of the spinal cord, whereas others are of the opinion that the changes are due to shear stresses directly upon the affected cells.

Penetrating injuries to brain

The brain and spinal cord may be penetrated by bullets and fragments of metal and bone sometimes covered by scalp, hair, and other contaminated foreign material. The damage in the high-velocity bullet injuries is generalized as well as local. Its effects are caused by the sudden increase in intracranial pressure, the shearing and tearing of the tissue, and the intense local heat. There is extensive necrosis and hemorrhage in and about the tract of the missile. In low-velocity injuries, the damage is limited to the penetrated area.

Posttraumatic brain swelling and edema

Occasionally in children (rarely in adults), a minor degree of head trauma is associated with generalized and progressive swelling and edema of the brain. Other traumatic lesions are usually absent. The brain is enlarged and symmetrical. The convolutions are flattened, the sulci narrowed, and the ventricles small. The white matter is prominent—bulging and dry in the swollen areas, depressed and wet in the edematous sites. Edema fluid high in protein content may be found about the blood vessels and in the Virchow-Robin space and tissues in brain edema (Fig. 42-33). The myelin sheaths are irregularly swollen and pale with enlarged clear spaces about the oligodendroglial nuclei in the areas of swelling. Increasing amounts of eosinophilic cytoplasm of the included astrocytes become visible by the end of the first day. Death usually is associated with hypoxia and lesions of the brainstem with brain displacement and with neurogenic pulmonary edema.

Trauma of spinal cord

The spinal cord of the newborn infant can be injured in breech deliveries by the exertion of too great an extractile force with the hyperextended head. The overstretched cord, usually at the cervical-thoracic level, has an hourglass narrowing (Fig. 42-34).

Hematomyelia with necrosis of the cord is usually due to fractures and/or dislocations of the vertebrae with compression of the cord. In some, the lesion appears to follow extreme degrees of hyperextension and hyperflexion at the cervical level with fracture or dislocation. The cord appears to be slightly to moderately narrowed at the level of compression, with bulging and softening above and below due to necrosis with hemorrhage into the gray matter (Fig. 42-35). This may extend for several levels to either side of the point of initial injury.

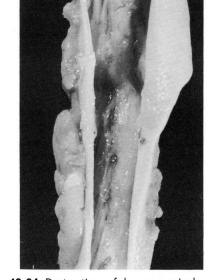

Fig. 42-34 Destruction of lower cervical portion of spinal cord following breech delivery.

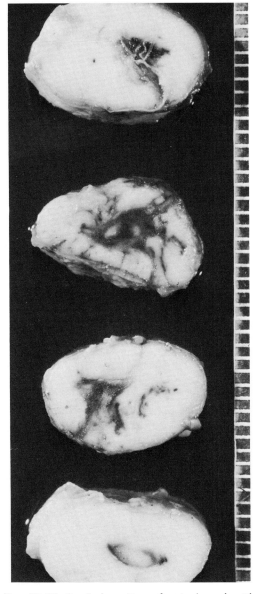

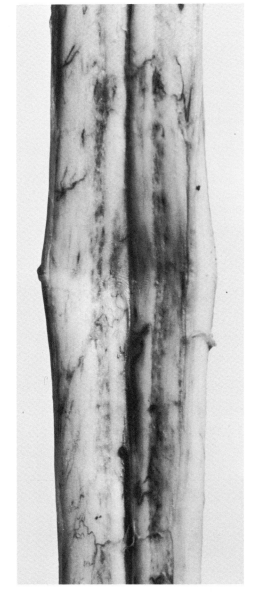

Fig. 42-35 Cervical portion of spinal cord with recent contusion and hemorrhage following dislocation of vertebra.

Fig. 42-36 Compression of cervical portion of spinal cord by ruptured disc. Patient was asymptomatic.

The spinal cord may be compressed on its ventral surface by a herniated intervertebral disc (Fig. 42-36) or by osteophytic lipping of the vertebral bodies.[106, 112, 139, 184, 198] The former is more likely to affect the lumbar portion and the latter the cervical portion of the cord. There are, however, many exceptions. The spinal cord, stabilized by the denticulare ligaments, is injured by direct compression locally. Less often, the changes are due to compression of the anterior spinal artery.

BRAIN ATROPHIES[142]

The continuous loss of nerve cells and their processes and of the surrounding myelin and intercellular fluid regularly accompanies aging. The cell and fluid loss is accompanied by a compensatory hydrocephalus. There is also slight focal fibrotic thickening of the leptomeninges.

On microscopic examination, the nerve cell loss may be recognizable both within the cortex and the central gray masses by the presence of patchy areas devoid of cells.

Many of the remaining, often shrunken, nerve cells contain excessive amounts of intracytoplasmic lipofuscin pigment. A mild to moderate reactive astrocytic gliosis is present and is most easily recognized in the outermost layers of the cortex. Hyaline thickening of the capillary walls in the occipital cortex frequently accompanies the aging process. Corpora amylacea are often very prominent. These are slightly eosinophilic to basophilic, sometimes laminated, PAS-positive, spherical bodies 10μ to 15μ in diameter. They are present in both the gray and white matter of the central nervous system, apparently in larger numbers if there had been a preexisting disease. Their origin is not understood, although they are thought to represent the end stage of degeneration of astrocytes.

In the aging brain, the loss of nerve cells and their processes results in a temporary condensation of interfascicular oligodendrocytes and eventual loss of white matter.

Senile dementia

In some individuals, the process of aging is so severe as to produce varying degrees of dementia. The brain is diffusely atrophic and there is a compensatory hydrocephalus, usually both external and internal. The microscopic changes are the nonspecific changes seen in the usual aging process but are usually much more marked. Alzheimer's neurofibrillary changes and senile plaques do not occur.

Alzheimer's disease

Formerly considered to be a disease whose clinical onset preceded the sixth decade, it is now recognized as a pathologic entity that can appear before the age of 15 years and at any time thereafter. Its cause, like that of aging, is not known. Until recently, patients with this disease in whom the onset of symptoms began in the seventh decade were classified as having a form of senile dementia.

The brain is diffusely atrophic with a compensatory hydrocephalus. All of the microscopic characteristics of the aging brain are present in great profusion. Senile plaques are to be found in the cortex of the frontal, parietal, and occipital lobes, and in great profusion in patients who have had marked dementia (Fig. 42-37). With the routine hematoxylin and eosin stain, the plaques are eosinophilic spheres 15μ to 125μ in diameter. Some plaques are composed of eosinophilic fibrils with a haphazard arrangement.

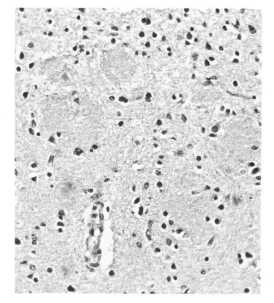

Fig. 42-37 Senile plaques in Alzheimer's disease. (Hematoxylin-eosin; ×280.)

In others, these fibrils radiate from a central, more eosinophilic and hyaline core; the periphery of these plaques is sometimes encircled by a thin, darkly eosinophilic rim. The plaques are easily stained and are more regularly seen with any of several special silver stains and with stains for amyloid. The stains that demonstrate the normally present oxidative enzymes are always markedly positive. The plaques are usually surrounded by a variable number of reactive astrocytes. In some with a familial history, senile plaques may be found in the subcortical white matter of the cerebral hemispheres and in the Purkinje cell layer of the cerebellum.

Alzheimer's neurofibrillary tangles also may be seen in some nerve cells of older individuals. The tangles, formed by the condensation, twisting, and irregular thickening of the neurotubules in the perikaryon[101, 199a] (Fig. 42-38), are infrequently recognizable with routine stains; they are found with special silver stains.

Granulovacuolar changes occur only in the large cells of the hippocampus. The affected cells contain cytoplasmic granules, hematoxylinophilic and argyrophilic, which are surrounded by nonstaining vacuoles.

Pick's disease (lobar sclerosis; circumscribed cortical atrophy)

Pick's disease is an uncommon, sometimes familial disease of unknown cause. Although patients usually become symptomatic during

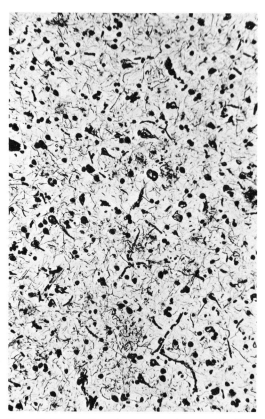

Fig. 42-38 Senile plaques and neurofibrillary tangles in Alzheimer's disease. (Hortega silver carbonate; ×135.)

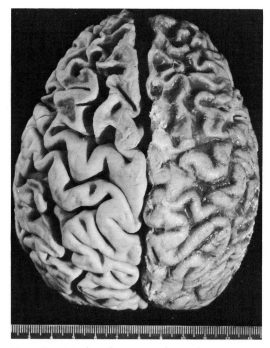

Fig. 42-39 Pick's disease with marked atrophy of frontal lobes. Marked compensatory external hydrocephalus.

the sixth and seventh decades, onset in the twenties and in the nineties has been recorded. Women are affected more often than men. The disease characteristically is fatal in from five to ten years.

The lobar atrophy, from which one of the names of the disease is derived, is most marked in the temporal and/or frontal lobes, with the formation of the "saber gyri" (Fig. 42-39). The atrophy is usually symmetrical and may extend to involve the insular cortex. Compensatory hydrocephalus is marked. The atrophy is primarily due to the severe loss of nerve cells in the outer three cortical layers, frequently leaving a vacuolated appearance. Some of the residual, degenerating nerve cells are swollen, with peripheral migration of their nuclei. These abnormal cells, Pick's cells, contain granular sudanophilic and argyophilic material. An astrocytic gliosis, sometimes very marked, in the outer cortical layers of the atrophic lobes is regularly present.

Spinocerebellar degenerations

The spinocerebellar degenerations[90] are an overlapping group of related diseases that affect the portions of the central nervous system that control coordination in movement. The system of cells affected are developmentally, functionally, and anatomically related. Although in many patients the diseases are hereditary (either dominant or recessive), previous infections, alcoholism, and the remote effects of cancer also have been implicated.

The disease process is first apparent structurally in the peripheral-most portion of the processes of the affected cells, with progression toward and eventual destruction of the perikaryon. Recent classifications, for ease of understanding, have divided these disorders into (1) primarily spinal, (2) primarily cerebellar and (3) mixed.[73]

Primarily spinal atrophies

The degenerations that are primarily spinal are Friedreich's ataxia and peroneal muscular atrophy.

Friedreich's ataxia. Friedreich's ataxia (hereditary spinal ataxia) is a rare progressive disease whose usual onset occurs during the first two decades of life. The sexes are affected equally, and the average life span after clinical onset is approximately fifteen years. The brain, brainstem, and cerebellum are normal. On the other hand, the spinal cord and its posterior roots are small at the time of autopsy examination. This is due at first to demyelination and later to loss of axis-cylinders in the posterior half of the cord.

Initially, the fasciculi gracili are affected. With progression, the disease in turn affects the fasciculi cuneati, the posterior roots, and the dorsal and then the ventral spinocerebellar tracts. In far-advanced disease, the lateral and later the anterior corticospinal tracts also may be similarly affected. The cells of Clarke's columns become small or shrunken with loss of Nissl substance, and finally many cells may disappear. At the time of death, about half of the patients have myocardial lesions, including hypertrophy of the heart, fatty infiltration of the myocardium, and focal myocarditis or fibrosis.

Peroneal muscular atrophy. Peroneal muscular atrophy (Charcot-Marie-Tooth disease; progressive neural muscular atrophy) is a hereditary disease. It may occur in families in which other members have Friedreich's ataxia. The lesions are characterized by loss of myelin and later of axis-cylinders beginning first in the distalmost portion of the peroneal nerves. In the late stages, there are degeneration and loss of anterior horn cells at the levels from which the peripheral nerves arise. There also may be demyelination of the lateral columns.

Other rare primary spinal atrophies include hereditary areflexic dystaxia (Roussy-Levy syndrome) and heredopathia atactica polyneuritiformis (Refsum's disease).

Primarily cerebellar atrophies

The degenerations that are primarily cerebellar include lamellar atrophy of Purkinje's cells, degeneration of the internal granular layer, focal cerebellar scelorsis, and olivopontocerebellar atrophy. In this group of disorders, in contrast with the spinal forms, there is a later clinical onset and there is more common involvement of the extrapyramidal tracts, and less commonly are there extraneural signs. When the spinal cord is affected, it is the anterior half that is usually damaged.

Lamellar atrophy of Purkinje's cells. Lamellar atrophy of Purkinje's cells is a disorder of adults, more often past the age of 40 years. It usually is not hereditary. Some instances have been associated with alcoholism. Other suggested causes have included a variety of toxins, infections, and premature aging.

The cerebellum grossly appears normal or is only slightly decreased in size. Microscopically, there is a marked loss of Purkinje's cells (Fig. 42-40) that may be complete in the

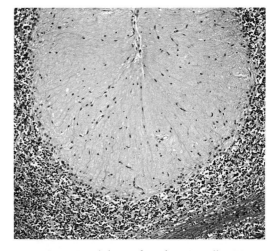

Fig. 42-40 Total loss of Purkinje's cells. (Hematoxylin-eosin; ×90.)

superior and anterior portions of the cerebellar vermis. With lateral spread to the hemispheres, however, there is a lesser loss of cells. The molecular layer of the cerebellum is normal in appearance. A mild loss of the internal granular cells is sometimes noted.

A diffuse loss of Purkinje's cells (subacute cerebellar degeneration) has been ascribed to the remote effects of cancer upon these cells. The great sensitivity of these cells to hypoxia, hyperthermia, a variety of chemical toxins, and heavy metals, as well as to alcohol, obscures the significance of cancer as the cause of this change.

Degeneration of internal granular layer. Degeneration of the internal granular layer with either partial or complete loss of the cells is a common postmortem finding. It is regular as an autolytic change in the so-called "respirator brain" and is seen in a great variety of disorders frequently associated with hyperthermia, as well as in alcoholism. Familial cases with onset in the first year of life with an associated mental deficiency and ataxia also have been described.

The cerebellum may be normal in size or slightly smaller than normal. The loss of internal granular cells may be almost complete. Purkinje's cells are far less involved, although there is some loss and occasionally cells may be displaced into the molecular or granular layers. The presence of a mild to moderate reactive astrocytosis in some suggests an extrinsic cause rather than a developmental lesion.

Focal cerebellar sclerosis. With focal cerebellar sclerosis (circumscribed atrophy of the cerebellar cortex), there is a focal and severe degeneration of all three cerebellar layers

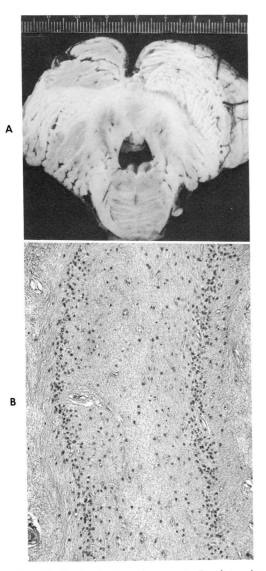

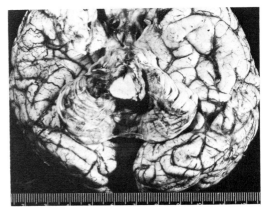

Fig. 42-42 Olivopontocerebellar atrophy.

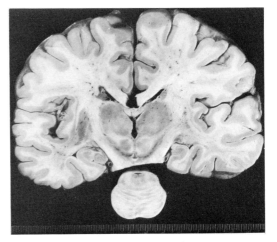

Fig. 42-43 Parkinsonism, idiopathic, with partial loss of pigment in substantia nigra and complete loss in locus ceruleus, both bilaterally.

Fig. 42-41 Cerebellar sclerosis. **A,** Focal involvement of cerebellar folia. **B,** Loss of cells with marked reactive astrocytic gliosis. (**B,** Hematoxylin-eosin; ×90.)

with a marked reactive proliferation of Bergmann's astrocytic cells (Fig. 42-41). The superior and inferior semilunar and simplex lobules are most regularly involved. The cause of this usually clinically silent disease is not known.

Olivopontocerebellar atrophy. Olivopontocerebellar atrophy (degeneration) belongs to the group of disorders that affect both levels of the cerebellar system (Fig. 42-42). It is more commonly seen in adults and is more frequently sporadic rather than familial. Death usually ensues five to ten years following the onset of signs and symptoms.

Grossly, there is marked atrophy of the brainstem and cerebellum and usually of the inferior olives. The cerebellum exhibits a marked loss of the internal granular and Purkinje's cells with a mild to moderate reactive astrocytosis in all three layers. Wallerian degeneration of the affected fibers leads to the marked decrease in size of the middle cerebellar peduncles. Similar changes in the inferior cerebellar peduncle are the result of the involvement of the dorsal spinocerebellar tracts. There usually is marked loss of the cells of the pontine nuclei, the inferior olives, and the arcuate nuclei of the brainstem.

Parkinson's disease

Formerly considered as a disease, parkinsonism is now regarded as a symptom-complex most frequently of idiopathic or postviral origin.[60, 67, 91] Other causes are local vascular

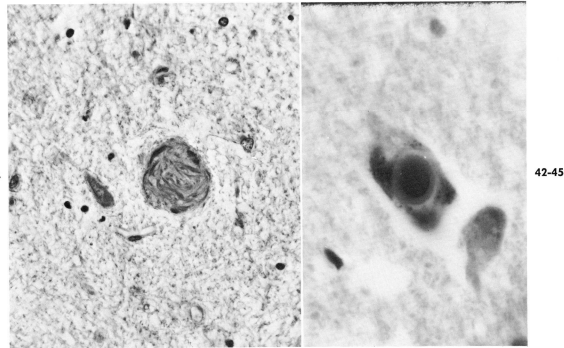

Fig. 42-44 Neurofibrillary change in cell of locus ceruleus in parkinsonism. (Hematoxylin-eosin; ×600.)

Fig. 42-45 Lewy body in cell of substantia nigra in parkinsonism. (Hematoxylin-eosin; ×1100.)

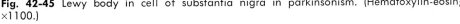

disease with infarction, anoxia due to carbon monoxide, toxins, and drugs (manganese and the phenothiazines), metastatic lesions, and injury from mechanical trauma. The term paralysis agitans usually is reserved for the idiopathic variety.

In most patients, the recognizable lesions are confined to the cells of the substantia nigra, locus ceruleus, and other pigmented cells of the brainstem (i.e., dorsal nucleus of the vagus). The grossly visible loss of pigment in these areas (Fig. 42-43) is due to destruction of the cells with phagocytosis and removal of the cell products and pigment—neuromelanin. Many of the remaining cells are shrunken, and some are vacuolated. In other cells of these nuclei, a coarse thickening of the neurofibrils (Alzheimer's neurofibrillary tangles) may be visible even with routine hematoxylin and eosin stain (Fig. 42-44) and with Congo red and polarized light. Some cells may contain single or multiple cytoplasmic, spherical, hyaline, eosinophilic inclusions, some with darker centers; these are Lewy bodies (Fig. 42-45). Mild to moderate degrees of focal reactive astrocytosis often are present in the affected regions. In

patients younger than 60 years of age, the presence of general brain atrophy and Lewy bodies is more characteristic of the idiopathic disease, paralysis agitans, whereas the Alzheimer's neurofibrillary changes and disseminated focal astrocytic scars are more suggestive of the postinflammatory variety. These distinctions are far less secure in older patients.[67, 91]

Other lesions, not generally accepted, have been described in patients with either type of parkinsonism.[60] These include loss of the large cells of the caudate nuclei and putamina and "perivascular degeneration" of the outer segments of the globus pallidus with pallor due to loss of myelinated fibers.

In patients with parkinsonism due to other causes, the lesions are generally widespread with additional local involvement of the substantia nigra.

Among the Chamorros in the Mariana islands, parkinsonism often is associated with dementia and/or amyotrophic lateral sclerosis. In these patients, there is a loss of pigmented cells, no Lewy bodies but many Alzheimer's neurofibrillary tangles, frontal and temporal lobe atrophy, and, in some, microscopic changes characteristic of motor neuron disease. The disease may be due to a "slow virus" infection.

Motor neuron disease (amyotrophic lateral sclerosis)[37, 128]

Motor neuron disease is a disease primarily or exclusively affecting the pyramidal or motor system. The clinical and structural varieties are dependent upon the motor level predominantly affected. While amyotrophic lateral sclerosis denotes the entire group, it also has been used to describe that variant in which the principal level of involvement is in the cells of the motor cortex and in their processes. In progressive bulbar palsy, the most significant lesions are in the motor cranial nuclei. The anterior horn cells are primarily affected in the type known as progressive (spinal) muscular atrophy. When the lesions are confined to the lateral and anterior corticospinal tracts with little or no recognizable change in the motor cortex, the disease is considered by some to represent primary lateral sclerosis. One of the many causes of the "floppy infant" is infantile progressive spinal muscular atrophy (Werdnig-Hoffmann disease; amyotonia congenita; Oppenheim's disease). It has the microscopic appearance of progressive (spinal) muscular atrophy and progressive bulbar palsy.

The unitarian concept of this group of diseases is suggested by the simultaneous involvement, often clinically and regularly at microscopy, of two or more levels of the motor system. Motor neuron disease has been classified among the abiotrophic conditions of the central nervous system. These are diseases in which genetic factors are considered to result in the gradual and premature death of the cells ordinarily destined to live many more years. This may account for the approximately 6% to 10% familial incidents in the adult form of this disease and the generally accepted autosomal recessive heredity of the infantile form. According to the concept of abiotrophy, there are premature deterioration and death of one or more systems of cells that form the central nervous system. The initial degenerative change occurs in the most peripheral part of the longest cell processes. With progression, the degenerative change ascends toward the cell body. It recently has been suggested that the disease may be due to a slow virus—i.e., one with an incubation period of years.[83, 84] The effect upon the cell would be similar to that postulated

with the abiotrophic diseases. It is assumed that the effect of the as yet unidentified virus is to gradually produce a change in the cell identical with that of the abiotrophic state. Previous suggestions of a host of other causes of motor neuron disease such as toxins, syphilis, viruses, trauma, etc. have not as yet been substantiated.

The gross appearance of the brain and spinal cord is usually not particularly helpful for diagnosis. In a few, there may be a slight to moderate degree of atrophy of the motor cortex, gray-white change in the lateral corticospinal tracts, and/or a decrease in size of the ventral roots at the lumbar and cervical levels of the spinal cord. The latter is difficult to evaluate because of the normally marked variation in size of these roots.

Amyotrophic lateral sclerosis, the most common motor neuron disease, is usually most easily recognized on microscopic examination by the presence of wallerian degeneration affecting the lateral and anterior corticospinal tracts. This change is seen at all levels of the spinal cord and may be traced upward in the pyramidal system, usually easily as far as the pons, and sometimes as far as the internal capsule. At the latter level, degeneration of the myelin sheaths and axons is recognizable in less than one-third of the patients. Only an occasional lipid-containing macrophage and a few perivascular lymphocytes are found at any level. This suggests more the very gradual progression of the disease rather than inactivity. Satellitosis and neuronophagia of the cells of the motor cortex usually are not prominent and often may go unnoticed.

With progressive bulbar palsy, there are satellitosis, neuronophagia, and loss of the cells of the cranial motor nuclei with a reactive astrocytosis in these areas. The nuclei most frequently and severely affected, in descending order, are the hypoglossal nucleus, the nucleus ambiguus, and the motor nuclei of the seventh and fifth nerves.

In spinal muscular atrophy, there is marked loss of anterior horn cells and usually marked reactive astrocytosis; marked cellular and axonal enlargement prior to disappearance is sometimes seen. Satellitosis and neuronophagia are not prominent probably because the disease at this level is most prolonged. Wallerian degeneration evident in the ventral rootlets corresponds to the anterior horn cell involvement. Neurogenic atrophy is frequent in the muscles supplied by these degenerated and degenerating cells.

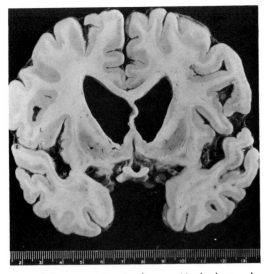

Fig. 42-46 Huntington's chorea. Marked atrophy of caudate nuclei and putamina. Moderate cortical atrophy. Compensatory internal and external hydrocephalus.

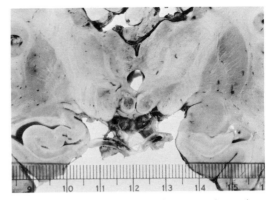

Fig. 42-47 Acute Wernicke's disease with involvement of mammillary bodies, hypothalami, and thalami.

The lesions in infantile progressive muscular atrophy involve loss or absence of the cells of the anterior horns of the spinal cord and the cranial motor nerve nuclei. The affected muscles have small fibers of the "fetal" or atrophic types.

Huntington's chorea[185]

Huntington's chorea is a dominantly inherited disease. Its late clinical onset, rare before the end of the second decade, allows the patient to have a family (often large) before there is significant mental deterioration or choreiform movements. The disease is slowly progressive with a long period of dementia.

The brain is moderately to markedly atrophic, particularly the frontal and temporal gyri. There is a marked decrease in size of the caudate nuclei and the putamina and some decrease in size of the corpus callosum (Fig 42-46). Compensatory internal and external hydrocephalus is marked. The changes in the caudate nuclei and putamina are due to a severe loss of their small nerve cells and a marked reactive astrocytosis. In the atrophic cerebral cortex, the nerve cell loss and the reactive astrocytosis are more prominent in the outer layers.

DEFICIENCY DISEASES
Wernicke's polioencephalopathy[5, 169]

Like beriberi, Wernicke's syndrome is due to a deficiency of vitamin B_1. Characteristi-

cally occurring in chronic alcoholics, it also has been found in persons with a variety of debilitating diseases in whom the diet consists primarily of carbohydrates. The principal lesions, in decreasing order of frequency, involve the mammillary bodies, the gray matter of the hypothalami and thalami immediately surrounding the third ventricle (Fig. 42-47), the periaqueductal gray matter, and the floor and sometimes the roof of the fourth ventricle. Petechial hemorrhages in these regions and from which the disease derived its original name (polioencephalitis hemorrhagic superior and inferior) may be absent or insignificant and are more likely the result rather than the cause of the initial lesions.

The early lesion is accompanied by decreased eosinophilic staining of the intercellular substances with loss of oligodendroglia and myelin in the affected sites. There is activation of the microglia with the formation of some lipophages. The resultant vascular dilatation leads to engorgement and some endothelial hypertrophy and hyperplasia with variable numbers of petechiae following. A mild reactive astrocytosis is seen in the older lesions. Neurons in the affected regions are surprisingly little altered. A few may be shrunken, and a few may show eosinophilic homogenization. If death does not occur, the lesions become inactive. The areas affected, particularly the mammillary bodies, collapse and become more brown than is normal. At this stage, which is associated with the clinical state known as Korsakoff's syndrome, there are staining pallor and loosening of the tissues, increased lipofuscin in the nerve cells, and occasionally a few hemosiderophages.

Infantile subacute necrotizing encephalomyelopathy[71, 74, 92, 130]

First described as a disease limited to infants, infantile subacute necrotizing encephalomyelopathy has now been reported in children and adults.[59, 60, 104] The necrotic lesions with a marked infiltration of lipophages are characteristically bilaterally symmetrical. They involve the hypothalamus, the mammillary bodies, the periaqueductal gray matter, and the tegmental portion of the pons. The medulla and spinal cord sometimes are also involved.

The disease is presumed to be a metabolic defect that is genetically controlled. Because of the structural similarity to Wernicke's encephalopathy, it has been suggested that this defect involves the utilization of thiamine or of its derivatives.

Pellagra

Inadequate amounts of nicotinic acid in the diet can result in pellagra. The characteristic light-sensitive dermatitis and diarrhea may be accompanied or, as is more usual, followed by disorders of mentation and even of movement.

There are usually no gross changes in the central nervous system. Microscopically, many neurons at all levels of the central nervous system have the appearance characteristic of central chromatolysis with some increase in lipofuscin (Fig. 42-48). There is little recognizable degeneration of the axons.

Posterolateral sclerosis (subacute combined degeneration of spinal cord)[189]

Due to a deficiency of vitamin B_{12}, posterolateral sclerosis often is associated with addisonian pernicious anemia. It may be seen in patients with sprue, gastric cancer, and after gastrectomy. The spinal cord may be of normal size or slightly small in circumference, with pallor and softening of the posterior columns. On microscopic examination, there is loss of myelin and oligodendroglia and of axons in the posterior and lateral columns of the spinal cord. The early lesions may contain many lipophages. The later lesions are characteristically vacuolated and spongy, with the complete absence of a reactive astrocytosis (Fig. 42-49). The vascular changes are associated with aging and not with this disease.[13] A moderate loss of nerve cells of the cerebral cortex with areas of degeneration of the white matter have been described.[76]

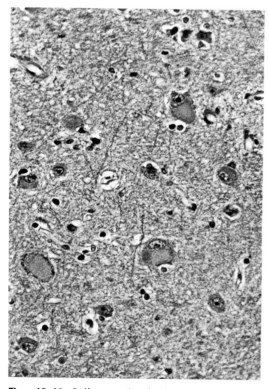

Fig. 42-48 Pellagra. Cerebral cortex. Eccentric nuclei with increased lipofuscin. Patient had dementia, dermatitis, and diarrhea. (Hematoxylin-eosin; ×135.)

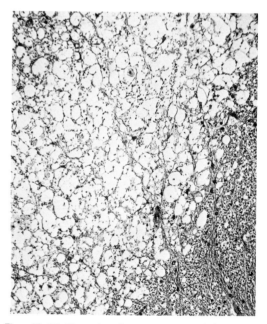

Fig. 42-49 Vacuolated appearance of fasciculus gracilis in vitamin B_{12} deficiency. (Hematoxylin-eosin; ×90.)

NEURONAL LIPID-STORAGE DISEASES

The neuronal lipid-storage diseases are a rare group of enzymatic disturbances of lipid metabolism that sometimes can be suspected by the presence of nerve cell involvement seen on rectal biopsy, and many can be diagnosed by chemical analysis of the urinary sediment or by study of the white blood cells.[181a] These include amaurotic familial idiocy, Niemann-Pick disease, Gaucher's disease, gargoylism, and Hand-Schüller-Christian disease (p. 1320).

Amaurotic familial idiocy[174, 192]

Amaurotic familial idiocy includes several varieties of the disease with slight differences in their enzymatic defects. Most instances are of the infantile form (Tay-Sachs disease), with congenital, late infantile, juvenile, and adult forms having been described.

Early enlargement of the brain is followed by a decrease in size as the disease progresses. The larger nerve cells at all levels, including the Purkinje's cells and the anterior horn cells of the spinal cord, are distended with a complex lipid containing sphingosine, hexoses, chondrosamine, and neuraminic acid. It is classified as a ganglioside and is oil-red positive. As the intracytoplasmic material accumulates, the Nissl substance is gradually displaced to a small zone about the nucleus (Fig. 42-50). The material also is to be found enlarging the cell processes. Lipid-containing macrophages can be found in the affected central nervous system and in the leptomeninges. There is a moderate reactive astrocytosis in the older lesions.

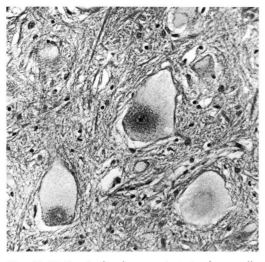

Fig. 42-50 Tay-Sachs disease. Anterior horn cells. (Hematoxylin-eosin; ×280.)

Niemann-Pick disease

In Niemann-Pick disease, nerve cells and the cells of the reticuloendothelial system and liver are distended with sphingomyelin. The similarity of nerve cells bloated with this stored material with those of amaurotic idiocy makes it exceedingly difficult to structurally separate the diseases. Involvement of the liver cells is considered by some as the essential criterion[30] (p. 1323).

Gaucher's disease

The accumulation of a cerebroside (protein-bound glycolipid) is regularly seen in the perikaryon of nerve cells in patients with *Gaucher's disease*. The enzymatic defect is glucosyl ceramide-β-glucosyl hydrolase. The material is periodic acid–Schiff positive. With routine stains, the nerve cells appear vacuolated (p. 1321).

Gargoylism

The material that accumulates in many nerve cells and in reticuloendothelial macrophages and in bone and cartilage cells in *Hurler-Pfoundler disease* (Hunter-Hurler disease; lipochondrodystrophy; gargoylism) is a mucopolysaccharide. A sphingolipid is sometimes also found. The disease is recessively inherited, either sex linked (Hunter's) or autosomally (Hurler's) and is apparently due to the absence of one or more of a group of enzymes that degrade mucopolysaccharides (p. 1693).

Hand-Schüller-Christian disease

In Hand-Schüller-Christian disease, the stored material is predominantly cholesterol. The central nervous system is only rarely affected. Central nervous system symptoms usually are due to involvement of the adjoining bones (p. 1325).

METABOLIC DISTURBANCES
Wilson's disease[25, 190]

Wilson's disease is believed to be due, at least in part, to a lack or insufficiency of the serum α-globulin, ceruloplasmin, which normally binds the serum copper. As a result, the serum copper is low and much copper is deposited in the putamina and striate bodies, in Descemet's membrane of the eye, and in the liver. There is often an aminoaciduria, presumably due to renal tubular disease. In over one-half the patients, the disease is inherited through a rare recessive gene (p. 1208).

The brain is usually atrophic. There may be no grossly visible changes. In some, there is softening with brown discoloration of the striate areas. On microscopic examination, there is often a marked gliosis with type I and type II Alzheimer's astrocytes in the central gray matter of the cerebral hemispheres. Large oval cells with small nuclei, the Opalski cells, sometimes are found in these same areas. The patients have a nodular cirrhosis and the brown Kayser-Fleischer rings of deposited copper at the margins of the corneas.

There are a variety of disorders of amino acid metabolism, a few of which will be mentioned here. *Phenylpyruvic oligophrenia* is a disorder due to the lack of an enzyme that hydroxylates phenylalanine to tyrosine. Consequently, phenylalanine accumulates in the tissues and is excreted in the urine. The disease is inherited recessively. Uniform and characteristic structural changes in the brain have not been reported. In *Hartnup disease,*[110] large amounts of 3-indolelacetic acid and indoleacetic glutamine are excreted in the urine. The defect appears to be one of tryptophan conversion to nicotinic acid. The changes in the brain are thought to resemble those of pellegra, and the disease is familial. In *maple syrup urine disease,* the presence of α-hydroxybutyric acid gives the urine its characteristic odor. The disease is familial. Structural changes have not been recorded.

CEREBRAL BIRTH INJURY[9, 188]
(cerebral palsy; Little's disease; spastic diplegia)

Cerebral birth injury is a disorder of paranatal origin characterized clinically by disturbances of movement, sometimes associated with mental retardation. The disorder may be hereditary, due to mechanical trauma, anoxia, maternal infection, metabolic disease, vascular disease, etc., with the morphologic lesions spanning almost the entire field of neuropathology. Each of the lesions should be evaluated separately.

KERNICTERUS (nuclear jaundice)[96]

Abnormally high concentrations of lipid-soluble, indirect-reacting bile pigments discolor the globi pallidi, subthalamic nuclei, hippocampi, dentate nuclei, and inferior olivary nuclei. The cerebral and cerebellar cortices and cochlear nuclei are less regularly affected. The high concentrations of bile pigment are most frequently due to severe hemolytic disease of the child resulting from the presence of maternal antibodies, usually anti-D, but sometimes to an ABO incompatibility or to

structural defects in erythrocytes leading to increased hemolysis. A further increase in the blood of the indirect-reacting bile pigment in the immature infant is due, in part, to an initial deficiency of glucuronyl transferase. The presence of a low serum albumin to which the indirect-reacting pigment ordinarily forms a loose attachment permits the pigment to enter the tissues more easily. Although a level of indirect-reacting bile pigment of 18 mg to 20 mg per 100 ml is considered critical, all factors must be considered. Nuclear jaundice has been recorded in congenital familial nonhemolytic jaundice of the Crigler-Najjar type.[52] Localizations of the pigment deposits in the nuclear areas have been ascribed to focal immaturity of the blood-brain barrier and to previous hypoxic damage to the nerve cells in these areas. Structural changes in the affected areas are variable. Solubility of the deposited bile pigment in the fat solvents that are used in preparation of the tissue necessitates the use of other preparations. In many of the pigmented areas (subthalamic nucleus, globus pallidus, and hippocampus), the affected nerve cells have undergone severe ischemic changes and mineralization of their Golgi apparatus. Although pigmented, the cells of the dentate nuclei and inferior olivary nuclei may show little change.

Although actively treated for nuclear jaundice, some surviving children later manifest signs and symptoms due to damage and destruction and loss of many cells in the affected nuclei (see also p. 1221).

EPILEPSY

Epilepsy is an abnormal functional state of the central nervous system that is characterized by uncontrolled outbursts of nerve cell activity and clinically by convulsive seizures with or without loss of consciousness or with their equivalents. In the idiopathic (primary; essential) form, the only structural changes are those related to hypoxia, which accompanies the attacks. The secondary (symptomatic) form of epilepsy has been associated with a great variety of diseases that affect the central nervous system, including hypoxia. Loss of cells in Sommer's sector of the hippocampus with a reactive astrocytosis may be seen in both forms and in patients without epilepsy. In severe epilepsy with repeated and frequent attacks, there are usually other evidences of anoxic changes, including laminar cell loss in the cerebral cortex (third and fourth layers) and especially in the cortex that lies in the depths of the sulci. Loss of Purkinje's cells, especially in the depths of the folia, is a common structural evidence of a hypoxic state, including that which accompanies epileptic seizures.

A special form of epilepsy, *myoclonus (inclusion body) epilepsy,* is a rare disease of unknown cause in which spherical intracytoplasmic basophilic inclusions (Lafora's bodies) are found in the larger nerve cells of the cerebral cortex and the subcortical gray matter, the brainstem, and the subcortical gray areas of the cerebellum, as well as in myocardial fibers and liver cells (particularly those at the periphery of the lobules).

INFLAMMATION

Inflammations of the brain and spinal cord generally are complications of similar inflammations elsewhere in the body. This is due to the protection afforded the central nervous system by the surrounding covering structures and by the actions of the blood-brain barrier. Once these defenses are breached, the resistance to infection is less than that of most of the other organs of the body. There are four general routes by which pathogenic organisms may reach the central nervous system.

1 The most frequently utilized route is that of the blood vessels. Most intravascular spread to the central nervous system is by way of the arteries, the organisms usually having first produced disease of the lungs or heart valves. Less often, organisms reach the central nervous system through emissary or diploic veins as a component of a thrombophlebitis or as a retrograde embolus from infections of adjacent sinuses, skull, or distant structures.[98] The paravertebral venous system is rarely implicated.

2 Infections of the mastoid sinuses, middle ears, paranasal sinuses, skull, and vertebra may extend directly to involve the brain or spinal cord and/or their coverings.[122]

3 Organisms, chemical toxins, or even particulate materials may be directly implanted upon the coverings or within the central nervous system as a result of gunshot wounds, mechanical trauma, or medical procedures, including surgery and lumbar puncture. Certain viruses, including rabies and possibly herpes zoster, once implanted within the axoplasm of a peripheral nerve, can, by centripetal movement within the cell cytoplasm and perhaps through the neurotubules, reach the perikaryon within the spinal ganglia, spinal cord, and/or brain.

4 Once within the central nervous system, further dissemination of the infection may proceed by direct continuity and/or by way of the fluid within the ventricular, subarachnoid, and/or Virchow-Robin spaces in the normal direction of flow, retrograde, or both.

■ ■ ■

Inflammations of the central nervous system are classified according to the site of involvement and to the type of exudate.

Meningeal infections

Meningeal infections are divided into those affecting the dura mater and those affecting the pia-arachnoid.

Pachymeningitis. Purulent infections of the dura are most frequently due to *Diplococcus pneumoniae, Staphylococcus aureus,* and β-hemolytic streptococcus. These infections are characterized as external (epidural; extradural) when the inflammation involves the outer surface and internal (subdural) when the inner surface is affected.

In the skull, most instances of epidural infection are the result of extension from an adjacent infection of the paranasal or mastoid sinuses with the formation of a small epidural abscess. Over the spinal cord, these abscesses are usually secondary to infections of the vertebra. Less frequently, they may follow retroperitoneal or retropleural infections with extension to the epidural space through an intervertebral foramen. The epidural abscess of the spinal cord tends to become larger than that of the skull because the spinal dura is separate from the periosteum and the intervening tissues offer little mechanical resistance to spread. The prognosis is good in either of the abscesses only if the lesion is treated early and adequately.

Purulent subdural infections (subdural empyema; subdural abscess) (Fig. 42-51), like their epidural counterparts, are most often complications of an adjacent infection of the mastoid or paranasal sinuses or of the middle ears and occur both with and without epidural infections.[93, 102, 183] The organisms may bypass the external dura by extending through a dural sinus and bridging vein into the subdural space or may be spread there by eroding the dura locally. Once in the subdural space, continued spread over the brain unilaterally is rapid, and it frequently becomes bilateral. The rare purulent spinal subdural infection is most likely to lie over the lower portion of the spinal cord and cauda equina.

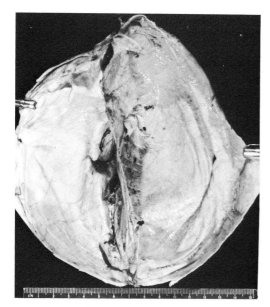

Fig. 42-51 Unilateral acute subdural empyema. Secondary to frontal sinusitis.

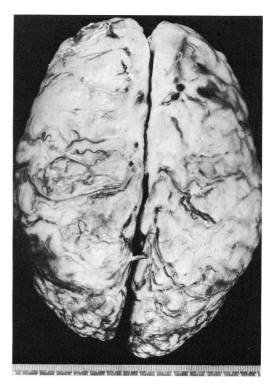

Fig. 42-52 Severe acute purulent leptomeningitis with thrombosis of leptomeningeal veins.

Reaction to the infection at both levels, at least initially, is from the vascular inner portion of the dura. There is no contribution from the arachnoid. Attempts to localize the infection by the formation of vascular pyogenic granulation tissue is late and generally inadequate. The tendency of the exudate and organisms to disseminate widely through the subdural space, to compress the underlying nervous system, and to spread to the subarachnoid space contributes to the high mortality rate in this condition.

Leptomeningitis. Purulent infections of the leptomeninges (leptomeningitis; meningitis) are seen with an ever-increasing variety of bacteria. At present, the most common in adults are due to *Diplococcus pneumoniae, Staphylococcus aureus*, β-hemolytic streptococcus, *Meningococcus (Neisseria)*, whereas in children the most common causative organisms are *Haemophilus influenzae* and *Entamoeba coli*. Almost all the routes of invasion described earlier are utilized. The bacteria that reach the subarachnoid space through the arteries may do so by exiting from the small thin-walled arteries in the subarachnoid space or may reach the subarachnoid space indirectly after exiting from the choroid plexuses and ventricular system. Contiguous paranasal and sinus infections are frequent sources. In any leptomeningitis, the source should be identified and that lesion treated as well as the infection of the central nervous system.

Early, the brain is variably swollen and its vessels markedly engorged. When the patient has succumbed very quickly, as some do with a fulminant meningococcemia, little or no exudate may be visible macroscopically. The earliest exudate that can be seen is recognizable first as thin gray streaks that parallel the lateral margins of superficial veins that lie in sulci. The exudate soon becomes more diffuse, thick, gray, and often slightly green. Initially, it fills the sulci and later overlays and obscures the gyri (Fig. 42-52). The cisterns become filled simultaneously. In those patients in whom the illness has been prolonged, the exudate tends to concentrate in the subarachnoid space to either side of the superior sagittal sinus, with lesser amounts toward the base of the brain. Over the spinal cord, the exudate covers the posterior aspect greatest in amount at the thoracic level, probably because of the effects of gravity in the relatively immobile patient lying in the recumbent position.

When there has been little or no visible exudate macroscopically, sections from multiple areas or of rolls of leptomeninges covering all or portions of a hemisphere may contain only a few neutrophils, usually in small clusters. In the usual fatal case in which the

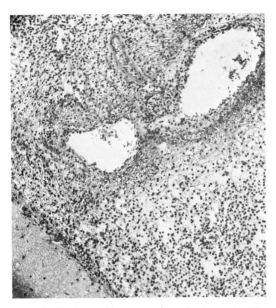

Fig. 42-53 Acute fibrinopurulent leptomeningitis with numerous neutrophils and some fibrin. (Hematoxylin-eosin; ×90.)

infection had been present for twenty-four hours or more, the exudate initially is characterized by an extensive neutrophilic infiltration most concentrated about the blood vessels (Fig. 42-53). The exudate later becomes more diffuse and is accompanied by increasing amounts of fibrin. With a gram stain, both free and phagocytized organisms may be found. As the disease progresses and there is evidence of response to therapy, the exudate gradually changes to one in which the predominant cell types are lymphocytes, monocytes, and, finally, mononuclear macrophages.[6] In the fatal cases and, presumably to a lesser extent, in patients who recover, toxic effects of the leptomeningeal disease result in a reactive astrocytosis seen in the molecular layer (first layer) of the cortex with shrinkage and hyperchromatism of some of the superficial nerve cells in the second and third cortical layers. With uncomplicated recovery, the exudate disappears in part apparently by exiting into the dural venous sinuses through the pores of the arachnoid villi and, possibly, by entering some of the thinner-walled blood vessels of the leptomeninges. No structural residua are to be seen in patients treated early and adequately.

Thrombophlebitis involving several or many veins, particularly those draining the parasagittal portions of the cerebral hemispheres, occurs in some patients. The occurrence of an arteritis or thromboarteritis is less common. Small cortical and subcortical hemorrhagic or

anemic infarcts are the usual sequelae of these vascular complications. When the infarcts are of significant numbers and sizes and are situated at functionally important sites, they are manifest by a variety of clinical complications. In some patients, the subarachnoid infection may extend into the brain along the Virchow-Robin spaces or along veins as a retrograde thrombophlebitis and result in the formation of one or more brain abscesses. Retrograde extension from the subarachnoid space through the lateral recesses may reach the ventricular system, producing an ependymitis and choroid plexitis, initially of the fourth ventricle and later of the other ventricles. In these, the fibrinopurulent exudate covers the intact surfaces and areas of ependymal ulceration. Perivascular lymphocytic cuffs in the subependymal cell plate beneath the ependymal lining is evidence of further reaction to the inflammation. Not infrequently in children, rarely in adults, a unilateral or bilateral serous subdural effusion may overlie the purulent meningitis.

Small patches of leptomeningeal fibrosis frequently have been attributed to preexisting infections of the leptomeninges in which the exudate has been organized with the formation of a fibrous scar. These scars are significant when they are extensive or occur at critical areas in the path of cerebrospinal flow. In other patients, an adhesive and/or constrictive band of scar tissue (adhesive or constrictive arachnoiditis) may be formed. Contraction of the scar can irritate the adjoining cells or destroy the encircled nervous system. A saclike leptomeningeal scar, by permitting the ingress of fluid and impeding its egress, can form the pocket for an enlarging subarachnoid cystic collection of fluid that compresses the underlying brain or spinal cord.

Brain abscess[53]

As with the purulent leptomeningitides, the organisms producing an abscess can reach the brain through infected arterial emboli, by direct extension from adjoining infections of the bones or sinuses about the brain or spinal cord with or without an accompanying thrombophlebitis, by direct implantation from penetrating trauma, lumbar puncture, or from surgery, or as a complication of a purulent meningitis. Abscesses following septic emboli are usually multiple and occur most frequently in the distribution areas of the middle cerebral arteries. When in the white matter, there is early sparing of the subcortical U fibers. Both sides of the brain are affected equally. An abscess whose source is an infection of a sinus, middle ear, or skull bone is usually single and more often involves the adjacent portion of the brain. Extension from the mastoid sinus is to the ventrocaudal portion of the homolateral temporal lobe, whereas the abscess of middle ear origin is usually in the homolateral cerebellar hemisphere. Rarely, any of these infections may extend as a thrombophlebitis of a dural sinus to enter the brain at some point other than that adjacent to the original infection.

In its earliest stages, before abscess formation, the area is markedly congested, edematous, and soft, contains numerous petechial hemorrhages, and is diffusely infiltrated with neutrophils. This is the stage known to clinicians as "cerebritis." More intense neutrophilic infiltration with liquefaction necrosis rapidly ensues. Variable numbers of bacteria may lie free in the abscess and/or in neutrophils. Without adequate therapy, there is continued enlargement and coalescence of abscesses, often with extension into the subarachnoid or ventricular cavities.

Adequate medical therapy decreases the local spread and the general effects. Generally, inadequate amounts of vascular granulation tissue forms about the abscess. The source of the granulation tissue is the mesenchymal cells in the walls of the blood vessels within the brain and adjoining leptomeninges and possibly the microglia. With treatment, the neutrophils within the abscess gradually are replaced by lymphocytes, monocytes, and macrophages. The surrounding granulation and fibrous tissue remains thin and is surrounded by a narrow zone of reactive astro-

cytes and more peripherally by a moderately edematous and swollen white matter in which there are perivascular lymphocytic cuffs. Although specific and intensive antibiotic therapy may have been given, a portion of the wall of almost every abscess, however chronic, shows evidence of continued enlargement with necrosis and often with the formation of satellite lesions (Fig. 42-54).

Granulomatous infections

Tuberculosis.[10, 12] The decreasing incidence of tuberculosis, coupled with more adequate therapy, has made tuberculosis of the central nervous system relatively uncommon. Extension of a tuberculous infection from a vertebra to the epidural space now is rare, as are subdural infections. A tuberculous leptomeningitis in children is most often a part of a generalized miliary infection. In adults, the association is with pulmonary tuberculosis. The early report of Rich and McCordock,[166a] that a tuberculous leptomeningitis represented extension from an adjacent focus in the brain in at least 90% of the patients, has not been substantiated by the more recent report of Evans and Courville.[69a] As with purulent inflammations, many now believe that the organisms enter the central nervous system from other infections elsewhere in the body by way of the choroid plexuses or through the walls of the leptomeningeal vessels.

Early in tuberculous leptomeningitis, the exudate is usually scant, diffuse, and gray-white, sometimes with a faint green tinge. Later, 1 mm to 3 mm, discrete, gray nodules may be found, particularly along the course of the leptomeningeal blood vessels (Fig. 42-55). In patients with a relatively long history of tuberculous leptomeningitis, as with most

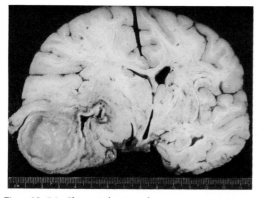

Fig. 42-54 Chronic brain abscesses in temporal lobe and insula. Surrounding brain swelling and edema. Compression and displacement of lateral and third ventricles. Cingulate gyrus and uncal herniations.

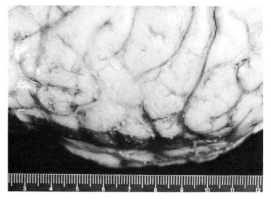

Fig. 42-55 Tuberculous leptomeningitis with numerous leptomeningeal tubercles.

granulomatous infections of the meninges, the exudate is more prominent at the base of the brain. The initial diffuse exudate is formed by lymphocytes, large mononuclear cells, serum and fibrin with small foci of caseation necrosis, and occasional neutrophilic clusters at sites of recent extension. The discrete nodules seen macroscopically consist of foci of caseation necrosis with fibrin surrounded by varying numbers of lymphocytes, plasmocytoid cells, and large mononuclear cells. Giant cells of Langhans' type are less frequent here than in other tissues (Fig. 42-56). Acid-fast bacilli may be numerous or rare. In the latter instance, they have been said to be found with less difficulty near or in the giant cells. This has not been our experience. As with pyogenic infections, there may be spread along the ventricular system and into the brain along the Virchow-Robin spaces. Blood vessels within the exudate sometimes have lymphocytes in their walls. They may exhibit a reactive hypertrophy and hyperplasia of the intima, sometimes with thrombosis. These may lead to small anemic infarcts in the adjacent brain and/or spinal cord.

Early chemotherapy modifies the response and decreases the degree of fibrous tissue scarring. Because the exudate and the scars are likely to be at the base of the brain, they may significantly impede the flow of cerebrospinal fluid and thereby produce an obstructive internal hydrocephalus. Constriction of a scar

at the base may interfere with the function of one or more cranial nerves.

A tuberculous encephalitis presents in one of two structural forms. Scattered throughout the brain and spinal cord may be multiple granulomas all of about the same size (usually up to 1 cm). The larger tuberculomas, many of which may reach a diameter of 5 cm to 6 cm, are solid and have "growth rings" formed by the successive addition of layers of granulation tissue. The larger lesions are more common in the cerebellum.

Cryptococcosis.[145] Cryptococcosis (*Cryptococcus hominis; Cryptococcus neoformans*) of the central nervous system is a worldwide disease of increasing incidence due to the use of immunosuppressive drugs. The central nervous system disease is associated with infections of other organs, particularly the lungs, spleen, bone marrow, liver, kidneys, etc. (p. 412).

The leptomeninges and brain usually are involved simultaneously. The leptomeningeal exudate is variable in amount, clear to turbid, watery to gelatinous, and usually more prominent at the base of the brain and over the dorsal aspect of the thoracic portion of the spinal cord. Within the brain and especially in the gray matter, there may be many smooth-walled cavities from less than 1 mm to as much as 1 cm in diameter (Fig. 42-57). These are filled with fluid identical to

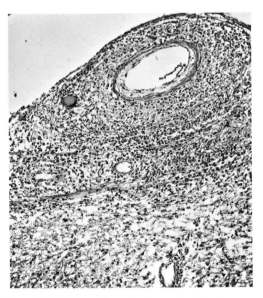

Fig. 42-56 Tuberculous leptomeningitis. Presence of Langhans' type of giant cells unusual. (Hematoxylin-eosin; ×90.)

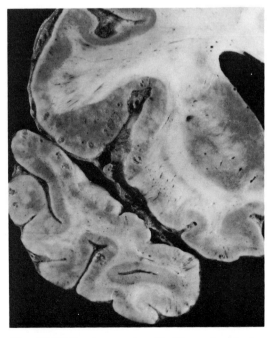

Fig. 42-57 Cryptococcosis with thin watery leptomeningeal exudate and many cortical cavities.

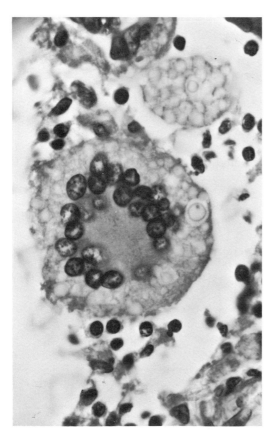

Fig. 42-58 Multinucleate giant cell containing many cryptococci. (Hematoxylin-eosin; ×1100.)

that seen in the subarachnoid space. The ventricular system, particularly in the region of the choroid plexuses, may contain the same type of exudate. The degree of cellular response is variable. In some areas, organisms may be present free in the subarachnoid and ventricular spaces or in the cystic cavities with almost no cell response. In other areas, particularly when the lesions have been present for a long time, there may be many lymphocytes, large mononuclear macrophages, some neutrophils and fibrin, and giant cells of both foreign body and Langhans' types (Fig. 42-58). Characteristic organisms are usually easily found in all areas and in the lumbar cerebrospinal fluid. Mixed infections are sometimes seen.[120]

Coccidioidomycosis. Coccidioidomycosis (*Coccidioides immitis*) is an endemic disease of the southwestern portion of the United States. The central nervous system infection is always a complication of a disseminated disease, particularly that originating from an initial pulmonary infection (p. 419).

The leptomeningeal exudate, although similar in many respects to that of tuberculosis, is usually more diffuse, more tenacious, and more abundant. The granulomas have a greater degree of central liquefaction. The infiltrates consist of mixtures of lymphocytes, neutrophils, plasma cells, large mononuclear cells, and giant cells of Langhans' type in which the typical organisms are to be found.

Histoplasmosis and blastomycosis. Histoplasmosis (*Histoplasma capsulatum*) and blastomycosis (*Blastomyces dermatitidis*) are similar in that their involvement in the brain and spinal cord resembles tuberculosis. Both are associated with similar infections elsewhere in the body, most frequently of the respiratory tract.

With histoplasmosis, there is usually diffuse involvement of the reticuloendothelial system. In blastomycosis, the skin and bones also are involved. In both, the leptomeningeal exudate may be diffuse and gray with or without well-defined, firm, gray nodules. Similar nodules often are seen within the brain. The diffuse exudate consists of lymphocytes, large mononuclear cells, some plasma cells, and neutrophils embedded in a moderate amount of fibrin. The nodules are formed by lymphocytes, epithelioid cells, and giant cells of both Langhans' and foreign body types, all surrounding a central core of necrotic debris. The organisms are found both free and in the large mononuclear and giant cells. Because of the overlapping sizes of the fungi, distinction between the two is sometimes difficult unless cultural studies are done (see also p. 416).

Actinomycosis. Actinomycotic infections of the central nervous system are rare. When they do occur, they are more likely due to the aerobe *Nocardia asteroides* than to the anaerobe *Actinomyces israelii*. As with the other fungi, the central nervous system infection is most frequently a complication of pulmonary disease and less frequently an extension from an adjacent infection. The cellular response is identical with that seen elsewhere in the body.

Neurosyphilis

The decreased incidence of syphilis of the central nervous system is the consequence of better control and of more adequate treatment during the early stages of the disease. Involvement of the central nervous system by the spirochete occurs during the secondary or the latent stage of the disease, always within the first two or three years of the infection.

Since syphilis may become inactive even

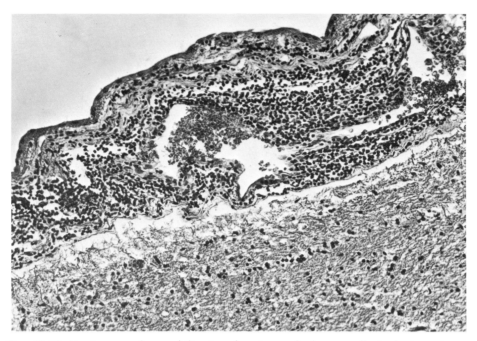

Fig. 42-59 Meningovascular syphilis. Lymphocytes and plasma cells in leptomeninges. (Hematoxylin-eosin; ×180.)

without treatment (i.e., "burned out"), both before and after meningeal spread and because early meningeal involvement may be asymptomatic, the spinal fluid must be repeatedly examined for cells (lymphocytes), increase in proteins (globulin), and the presence of a positive serology. The symptomatic phase may resolve spontaneously or with treatment or progress to develop into clinically evident neurosyphilis (see also p. 354).

Meningovascular syphilis. In the early stages of meningovascular syphilis, there may be a cloudy gray exudate within the leptomeninges, usually more prominent at the base of the brain and, to a lesser extent, along the blood vessels over the cerebral convexities. Occasionally, the cloudiness may be limited to patches or to more diffuse areas over the frontal lobes. The characteristic exudate is one composed primarily of lymphocytes, plasma cells, and large mononuclear cells, all with a tendency toward adventitial and perivascular concentration (Figs. 42-59 and 42-60). It is said that in about 5% of the patients, the disease may begin as a severe acute meningitis. In these, the exudate is more abundant and, in addition, the characteristic cellular infiltrate also contains neutrophils and fibrin. Following adequate therapy and possibly spontaneously, the exudate becomes

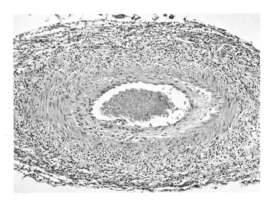

Fig. 42-60 Heubner's arteritis of basilar artery. Same case as shown in Fig. 42-59. (Hematoxylin-eosin; ×90.)

organized with patches or even extensive areas of fibrosis.

A significant part of the leptomeningeal infection is the accompanying involvement of the smaller arteries. In the more severe infections, the inflammatory cells migrate into the media, separate the muscle fibers, split the internal elastic lamina, and stimulate a reactive intimal hyperplasia and endothelial hypertrophy (Heubner's endarteritis and panarteritis). These vascular changes, depending upon their numbers and the degree and rapidity of involvement, can result in the production of numerous small anemic infarcts. The occasional involvement of a major artery of the circle of Willis can be the cause of a large anemic infarct.

General paresis (paretic dementia). General paresis is a form of progressive syphilitic meningoencephalitis. Adequate therapy only halts its progression. With the early or minimal lesion, no gross abnormalities may be recognized. In the usual patient, however, there is patchy or diffuse thickening of the leptomeninges and cortical atrophy, often more marked over the frontal lobes. There may be a characteristic but not diagnostic granularity of the ependyma lining the moderately enlarged ventricles. The floor of the fourth ventricle may have a thickened, gray appearance due to a highly characteristic, diffuse proliferation of astrocytic glial fibers.

The meningeal exudate is identical with that seen in syphilitic meningitis and usually is accompanied by the typical vasculitis. Within the brain, the lesions are more concentrated in the cerebral cortex and in the central gray matter than in the white matter. The intensity of the reactions roughly parallels the degree of overlying leptomeningeal involvement. The vessels within these areas and, to a lesser degree, those of the underlying white matter are surrounded by lymphocytes, plasma cells, and a few large mononuclear cells. Their walls are markedly thickened, and their lumina narrowed due to endothelial hyperplasia and hypertrophy. As a result, many nerve cells are in varying stages of ischemic change, and there are proliferation and rodlike elongation of the surrounding microglial cells. As the lesions undergo resolution and organization, they resemble microscopic infarcts with loss of cells, focal collapse of the cortex, and distortion of the normal layering of the adjoining cortical cells. There is a marked reactive astrocytosis. Iron-containing pigment in macrophages and in the walls of cortical blood vessels is highly characteristic of general paresis. In Lissauer's type of general paresis, there is an associated spongy destruction of the upper cortical layers and chromatolytic changes in some nerve cells of the fifth and sixth layers. In the untreated patient, spirochetes may be found singly and in clusters about the blood vessels and in the cortex.

With treatment, demonstrable spirochetes rapidly disappear. The cellular exudate and the vascular changes decrease far more slowly. Leptomeningeal scars, the disseminated focal cortical atrophy and characteristic cortical dis-

organization, the ependymal granularity, the gliosis of the floor of the fourth ventricle, and the iron granules in macrophages and walls of the cortical blood vessels are the unalterable structural remnants of the disease.

Tabes dorsalis. The spinal cord in the patient with syphilis may be involved separately or in combination with the brain. Of the several patterns of spinal cord involvement, tabes dorsalis has been the most frequent. The exact site of syphilic inflammation that results in wallerian degeneration of the fasciculi gracili and sometimes of the fasciculi cuneati and of the dorsal roots is not known. One hypothesis suggests localization of the toxic effects of the spirochetes to the dorsal rootlets as they pass through the Obersteiner-Redlich area. The second assumes that there is involvement of the cells of the dorsal root ganglia and the fibers from these cells entering the spinal cord. In both hypotheses, the caudalmost portion of the spinal cord is affected earliest and to the greatest degree.

The gross appearance of the spinal cord is characteristic but not diagnostic. The posterior columns are smaller than normal, often with a dorsal concave rather than convex surface. Special stains reveal the absence of axis-cylinders and myelin sheaths in the affected areas. With tabes dorsalis, the optic nerves are often similarly involved. The exact site of the lesion that produces the Argyll Robertson pupil seen in this disease is not known.

The spinal cord less frequently may be affected in a variety of patterns that are less characteristic of syphilis. These are due to differing localizations of lesions that extend into the cord from the leptomeninges and from variations in the sites of the vasculitis.

Toxoplasmosis[75, 181]

A disease with worldwide distribution, toxoplasmosis is most often recognized in infants. It may, however, be the cause of a febrile disease in adults. The causative agent is the protozoan *Toxoplasma gondii*. The infant is infected by the mother who, although showing no signs of active disease, has a positive complement fixation test (see also p. 438).

The inflammatory aqueductal stenosis in the infant results in an obstructive hydrocephalus (Fig. 42-61). There are, in addition, necrotic paraventricular and lesions of the basal ganglia that lead to mineralization that is often visible by x-ray examination. Involvement of the surface of the brain is associated with a focal chronic (lymphocytic) lepto-meningitis. The ovoid organisms, which are 4μ to 6μ long and 2μ wide, usually are found in clusters in the cytoplasm of a mononuclear macrophage. This is known as the pseudocyst (Fig. 42-62). The areas of necrosis in which

the organisms are found and from which they may be cultured are surrounded by varying degrees of mononuclear cells and reactive astrocytosis.

In infants, other organs such as the eye or the myocardium often are affected as well. In adults, the lungs and lymph nodes usually are involved (see also p. 1024).

Rickettsial encephalitides

Focal collections of a few neutrophils with lymphocytes and mononuclear macrophages in and about the walls of the smaller blood vessels are known as typhus nodules and are the characteristic but not diagnostic lesions in the rickettsial diseases (Fig. 42-63). Hyper-trophy and hyperplasia of the endothelial cells result from the intraendothelial multiplication of the rickettsia. These are the lesions char-acteristic of typhus fever caused by *Rickettsia prowazekii* (see also p. 367).

In Rocky Mountain spotted fever due to *Rickettsia ricketsii*,[202] the inflammatory and vascular changes are usually more severe, whereas in scrub typhus due to *Rickettsia orientalis*, the vascular lesions are fewer and less severe.

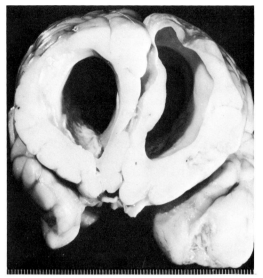

Fig. 42-61 Toxoplasmosis. Marked internal hydro-cephalus, obstructive, with numerous subependy-mal calcifications, in 2-year-old child.

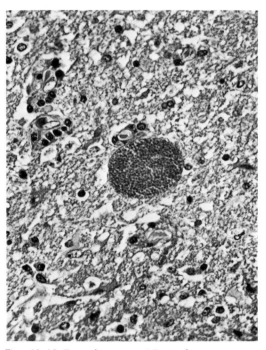

Fig. 42-62 Toxoplasmosis. "Cyst" formation con-taining many organisms in adult with multiple myeloma. (Hematoxylin-eosin; ×370.)

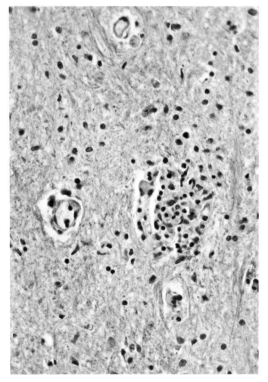

Fig. 42-63 Nodule in patient with scrub typhus. (Hematoxylin-eosin; ×280.)

Viral
encephalomyelitides[103, 111]

Considered to occur infrequently as isolated cases and in epidemics (except poliomyelitis), human viral infections were expected to almost disappear with the use of the poliomyelitis vaccines. This has not occurred. Increased numbers of mild, severe, and fatal viral encephalitides have been recognized. The basic similarities of the structural changes produced in the central nervous system by these diseases are due to the obligate intracellular position of the viruses.

When the injury is recent or mild, the infected nerve cells become slightly swollen, later to undergo satellitosis, shrinkage, and, finally, neuronophagia by the surrounding mononuclear cells. The later changes are accompanied by a perivascular inflammatory cell infiltrate. Initially and for a very short time, these cells may be neutrophilic. Later and more characteristically, the cellular infiltrates are composed of lymphocytes, some plasmacytoid cells, and large mononuclear cells and macrophages (Fig. 42-64). Variations in this pattern are dependent upon the locations of the cells, including glial as well as nerve cells, that are affected and the degree of necrosis of cells and surrounding tissues. In some of the viral infections, intranuclear or intracytoplasmic inclusion bodies may be formed within nerve and/or glial cells. Cowdry type A intranuclear inclusions may be found in the encephalitides due to the measles virus, herpes simplex, cytomegalic inclusion disease, and herpes zoster. The rela-

tionship of Cowdry type B inclusion bodies to viral diseases is not certain.

When the infection is limited to nerve cells, the central nervous system grossly may appear unchanged or, at most, focally or diffusely engorged. With a necrotizing encephalitis that includes destruction of white and gray matter, the nervous system early is enlarged, swollen, and engorged. The areas of necrosis that follow may be small and scattered or large, extending beyond the boundaries of an area supplied by a single or several blood vessels. In addition to the usual cellular infiltrate, there is a marked reactive astrocytosis and a lesser gliosis that is characteristic of this type of encephalitis.

Acute poliomyelitis (infantile paralysis).[31] The marked decrease in incidence of acute poliomyelitis in the past several years is one of the triumphs of medicine. It is considered here because it is a prototype of the viral diseases. Formerly, it occurred both sporadically and more frequently in epidemics during the summer and autumn months. The viruses enter the body through the gastrointestinal tract, from which, by way of the bloodstream, they spread to involve the central nervous system. There is an incubation period of from seven to ten days (see also p. 380).

The changes in the central nervous system vary with the intensity and duration of the illness. The nerve cells characteristically affected are the large anterior horn cells of the spinal cord, particularly those at the cervical and lumbar enlargements. With a more severe and usually fatal disease, the large nerve cells of the brainstem motor nuclei are affected (bulbar poliomyelitis), and in the most severe forms the large nerve cells of the motor cortex are involved, as well as cells in the thalamus and hypothalamus and brainstem. It has never been clear why only some cells in each area may be affected. Because of the similarity of change at all levels, it has been assumed that the cells were infected at one time.

The gross and microscopic changes are those previously described for the non-necrotizing encephalomyelitis. In the early and rapidly fatal disease, there is vascular engorgement of the affected areas. There may be a few neutrophils in the leptomeninges and about some vessels within the affected areas. These are soon replaced by extensive perivascular lymphocytic infiltrates. The early swollen nerve cells rapidly undergo satellitosis and neuronophagia by large mononuclear cells. Loss of nerve cells is followed by wallerian degenera-

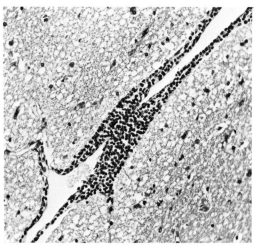

Fig. 42-64 Chronic encephalitis, viral type. (Hematoxylin-eosin; ×90.)

tion of the axons and their sheaths and by neurogenic atrophy of the muscles supplied by these cells. In the nonfatal case, the loss of nerve cells is marked by collapse of the area, with microscopic astrocytic scars.

Other enteroviral encephalomyelitides. Other enteroviruses are often the cause of infections of the central nervous system. These include a large group of coxsackieviruses and the echovirus. One, the coxsackievirus type A7, is known to produce a disease that is structurally inseparable from that produced by the poliomyelitis viruses. The usual illness, however, is nonparalytic and generalized, sometimes with a myalgia and/or encephalalgia.

Epidemic encephalitides. The epidemic encephalitides are a group of diseases that occur in epidemics and are presumed to be of viral origin. Among these is the lethargic encephalitis of von Economo, which may be due to several different viruses. Others included in this group are St. Louis encephalitis and equine encephalitis (see also p. 382).

The localization of the pathologic changes vary markedly. In the von Economo type, the lesions characteristically affect the brainstem most severely. In these, there is a tendency for the parkinsonian state to follow after an interval of weeks to months or even years. The microscopic changes are those of nerve cell degeneration with adventitial infiltrates composed of lymphocytes, plasmacytoid cells, and large mononuclear cells. Some cells may persist for years after the onset of the disease.

Necrotizing encephalitides. The necrotizing encephalitides have been reported under a variety of names, including Dawson's inclusion body encephalitis, von Bogaert's subacute sclerosing leukoencephalitis, and Pette and Döring's panencephalitis. One of these diseases is currently designated as subacute sclerosing panencephalitis. Formerly considered to be due to the herpes simplex virus, recent evidence is strongly suggestive that the measle virus is the cause.[98, 114, 156, 166, 175, 204] The gross appearance of the brain in herpes simplex encephalitis is identical with that due to measles both as to sites of involvement and as to degree of necrosis. The only difference in our material is a slightly lesser degree of reactive astrocytosis in the surrounding tissue with the former. The changes in the nerve and glial cells, the presence of Cowdry type A inclusion bodies, and the type and intensity of cellular infiltration have an identical appearance.

The brain is characterized grossly by variable but usually large gelatinous areas of necrosis that primarily affect the temporal lobes and sometimes extend into the insula and, in some, into the limbic system (Fig. 42-65). The cytologic changes of the affected nerve cells are those of any viral infection, with early swelling and later satellitosis and neuronophagia. The leptomeninges and the cortical areas contain vascular cuffs composed of lymphocytes, plasma cells, and large mononuclear cells with lipid-containing macrophages in the necrotic areas in which the glial and nerve cells have been destroyed. An intense astrocytosis and gliosis surrounds the necrotic areas (Fig. 42-66). Intranuclear and intracytoplasmic inclusions in nerve cells (Fig. 42-67) and intranuclear inclusions in oligodendroglia may be seen early in the disease. They usually, but not always, disappear in the older lesions. Cytomegalic inclusion disease[96a, 196a] is due to the cytomegalic virus, a large DNA virus of the herpes subgroup. In the brain, there are areas of necrosis that are predominantly periventricular and frequently with a marked degree of mineralization (calcification). There is little cellular response. The intranuclear inclusion bodies are exceedingly large and prominent; intracytoplasmic inclusions are also to be found. The disease may be generalized and present acutely and in a fulminant fashion. While the disease occurs most frequently in newborn infants infected by their asymptomatic mothers, it has

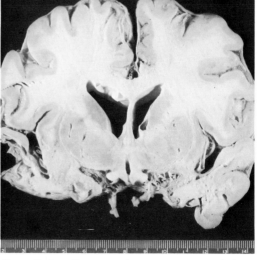

Fig. 42-65 Chronic sclerosing panencephalitis. Involvement of temporal lobes, insula, and cingulate gyri.

been recognized in adults in whom there is an impaired immune response.

Lymphocytic choriomeningitis.[20] The virus of lymphocytic choriomeningitis produces moderate lymphocytic infiltrations in the lep-

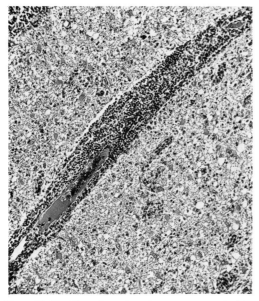

Fig. 42-66 Chronic sclerosing panencephalitis. Perivascular mononuclear cell infiltrate, necrosis, and reactive astrocytosis. (Hematoxylin-eosin; ×90.)

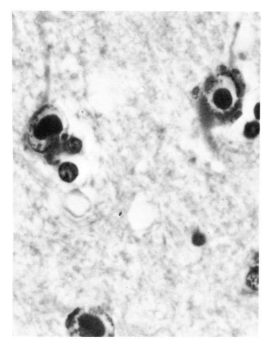

Fig. 42-67 Viral encephalitis. Intranuclear inclusions in nerve cells. (Hematoxylin-eosin; ×1100.)

tomeninges, choroid plexuses, and vessels beneath the ependyma. It appears to be transmitted to man through the urine of infected mice that act as the host reservoir. The disease, rarely fatal in man, also has been called benign lymphocytic meningitis. Diagnosis usually is made by the presence of a rising titer of specific neutralizing antibodies.

Progressive multifocal leukoencephalopathy.[11, 203] Progressive multifocal leukoencephalopathy is a recently recognized and as yet uncommon disease. Initially described as occurring particularly in patients with neoplastic diseases of the reticuloendothelial system, especially chronic lymphatic leukemia, and in sarcoidosis, it has now been seen in association with a variety of diseases, including senility. Further reports have suggested that the etiologic agent is a virus that is able to produce disease only in a patient with a greatly depressed immune response.

In the fixed brain, the islandlike multiple lesions affecting the brain and spinal cord have a granular gray appearance. In about one-half of the reported cases, there are perivascular cuffs of lymphocytes and plasma cells. Oligodendroglial cells are absent in the areas of demyelination. About these areas, the nuclei of the oligodendrocytes may be enlarged, and a few may contain an eosinophilic inclusion. Some of the surrounding reactive astrocytes have nuclei that are markedly enlarged and hyperchromatic, suggesting an early stage of neoplastic change.

DISEASES OF MYELIN

The classification of diseases of myelin is based upon an initial premise that they are all characterized by a primary and predominant loss (or absence) of the myelin sheath with complete or relative sparing of the axis-cylinders.[3] Clinical and/or etiologic classifications have not been satisfactory because of overlapping clinical appearances and because the causes are either unknown or in dispute. Recently, the diseases have been further categorized as either demyelinating (i.e., myelinoclastic) or belonging to the leukodystrophies (i.e., disorders of myelin formation—dysmyelinating).[161]

Demyelinating diseases

Multiple sclerosis (disseminated sclerosis; insular sclerosis). Multiple sclerosis is the most common of the demyelinating diseases and is one of the two most common primary diseases of the central nervous system. It is characteristically chronic and relapsing, although acute and unremittent forms occur.[182, 207] Of the innumerable theories concerning its cause, those associated with disorders of blood vessels, with developmental defects of the glia, and with a great variety of toxic agents are no longer seriously considered. Currently, the theories most supported are those related to allergy and infection, neither of which is without its detractors and neither of which has been demonstrated experimentally as producing a disease identical with multiple sclerosis. Whatever the theory, it must explain the increasing incidence of the disease in the higher northern latitudes, its rarity in southern areas, its increased occurrence in families, and its exacerbations and remissions, often years apart. Seen at all ages after childhood, onset is more common between the ages of 20 and 40 years. Both sexes are affected, women more frequently and at an earlier age. The mean duration of the disease is approximately twenty years (or more).

In the relapsing chronic form, the gross appearance of the central nervous system is usually diagnostic. The brain is either normal in size or slightly atrophic, and the spinal cord is variably small. Lesions that reach the white matter are, on the cut surface, slightly depressed, gray to gray-pink, and sharply demarcated. Although the plaques are more easily seen in the white matter, they extend into the gray matter in almost every patient (Fig. 42-68). The plaques vary in size, shape, number, and position. In almost all patients, however, some plaques are seen with their bases at the angles of the lateral ventricles, especially about the occipital poles and with their apices toward the cortex. Similar lesions are frequent in the central and convolutional white matter of the brain and in the brainstem, cerebellum, and spinal cord.

All stages of the disease may be found in the patient in relapse. Perivascular lymphocytes and plasmacytoid cells (Fig. 42-69) characterize the acute lesions, with spillover of the cells into the leptomeninges in some instances. The degree and stages of myelin loss and the destruction of the myelin are seen with routine as well as with special stains (Fig. 42-70). In the slightly older and active lesions, there is a decrease in the myelin staining with swollen myelin. Here, in addition to the usual inflammatory cells, are macrophages with fragments of myelin, metachromatic granules, and/or neutral fat. The older and inactive lesions are sharply de-

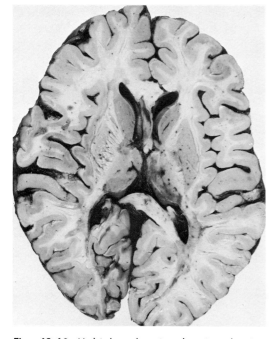

Fig. 42-68 Multiple sclerosis, chronic relapsing type wtih numerous plaques. Plaques in all characteristic areas. Cortex and U fibers involved in several areas.

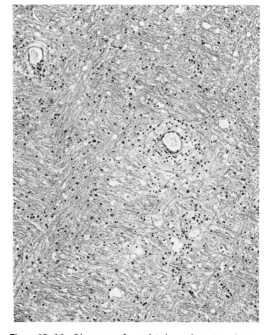

Fig. 42-69 Plaque of multiple sclerosis. Active lesion with perivascular lymphocytes. Slightly lighter-staining area in lower half of section is plaque. (Hematoxylin-eosin; ×90.)

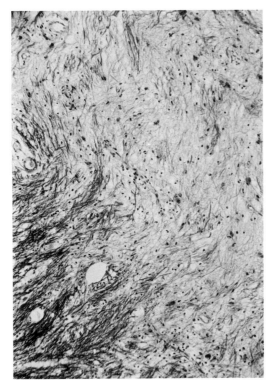

Fig. 42-70 Older plaque of multiple sclerosis with loss of myelin and retention of some axons in lighter-staining area. (Luxol-fast blue-silver nitrate; ×135.)

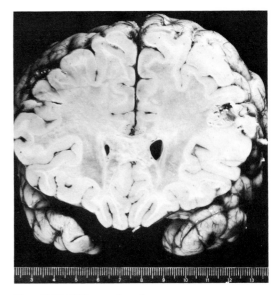

Fig. 42-72 Diffuse sclerosis.

marcated regions of myelin loss without reactive cells. Variable numbers of axis-cylinders remain in the plaques. These often are surrounded by a mild to moderate increase in astrocytes whose fibrillary processes follow the original axonal pattern (isomorphic gliosis; Fig. 42-71). During a period of relapse, new plaques are formed and some of the older lesions appear to enlarge at their peripheries. In all of the plaques, there is an absence of oligodendroglial cells.

Diffuse sclerosis (Schilder's disease; cerebral sclerosis; encephalitis periaxialis diffusa). In contrast with multiple sclerosis, in almost half of the patients with diffuse sclerosis the onset of disease occurs before the age of 10 years, with the mean duration of life six years. There is usually a bilateral but not necessarily symmetrical involvement of the white matter of the cerebral hemispheres (Fig. 42-72), especially that of the occipital lobes. The lesions are sharply demarcated, often spare the subcortical U fibers (Fig. 42-73), and unite with each other across the corpus callosum. The older lesions frequently have areas of cavitation.

The cellular response and destruction of myelin follow the same pattern as that seen in multiple sclerosis. Many axons are swollen, fragmented, and destroyed, whereas other are preserved. Reactive astrocytes are usually fibrillary, but many are gemistocytic and some are multinucleate. Wallerian degeneration secondary to destruction of the axis-cylinders may be seen.

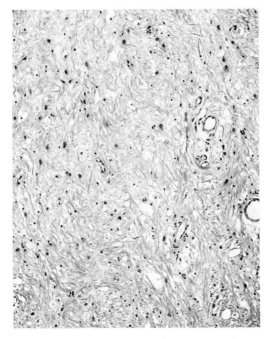

Fig. 42-71 Older plaque of multiple sclerosis with isomorphic astrocytic gliosis. Lesion on left of section. (Hematoxylin-eosin; ×90.)

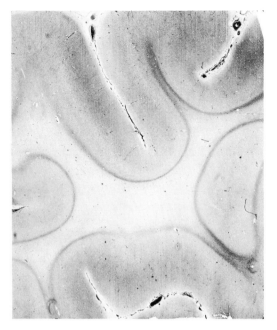

Fig. 42-73 Diffuse sclerosis. Partial retention of U fibers. (Mahon stain; ×8.)

The relationship of this disease to multiple sclerosis on the one hand and to the intermediate or transitional forms of diffuse sclerosis on the other has been debated on many occasions.

Intermediate or transitional form. In *neuromyelitis optica* (Devic's disease; neuroophthalmomyelitis; neuromyelitis optica), the spinal cord (Fig. 42-74) and the optic nerves and chiasm are the principal sites of clinical and anatomic involvement. Like diffuse sclerosis, the disease is more common in the young (under 10 years of age) and in the old (over 50 years of age) and tends to be progressive with death within a few years. There are some patients in whom the disease has become stationary and others who have developed relapses similar to multiple sclerosis. The anatomic findings further support the intermediate position of this disease between diffuse sclerosis on the one hand and multiple sclerosis on the other.

Many segments of the spinal cord usually are involved at one or more levels. Early, the affected portions are swollen, soft, and slightly pink. Older lesions are depressed and gray, and some that are large may be cavitated. The optic nerves and chiasm are similarly affected. Both portions of the nervous system may be at the same stage or in different stages of involvement and, they may be affected equally, or, as is more usual, un-

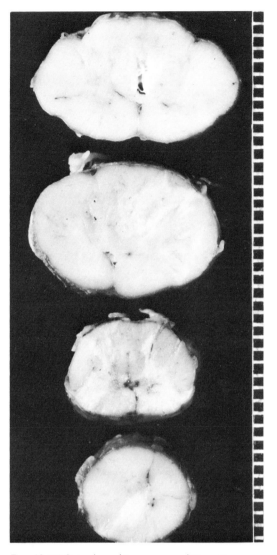

Fig. 42-74 Spinal cord in neuromyelitis optica.

equally. In many patients, there also are well-demarcated lesions identical with those of multiple sclerosis occurring in other parts of the brain and brainstem.

The microscopic changes in the typical patient vary from the characteristic plaques of multiple sclerosis in all of its stages to those of diffuse sclerosis with areas of necrosis and with wallerian degeneration.

Postvaccinal encephalomyelitis (acute perivenous encephalomyelitis; postexanthematous encephalomyelitis). A diffusely disseminated disease of the central nervous system, postvaccinal encephalomyelitis may appear during the course of or shortly after recovery from several exanthems, such as chickenpox, German measles, or smallpox and, rarely, after inoculations against smallpox, rabies, and typhoid. Although most of these illnesses are caused by viruses, none has, as yet, been identified in patients with postvaccinal encephalomyelitis (see also p. 386).

The clinical and pathologic similarities of this single structural entity have suggested a basic allergic (autoimmune) response on the part of the central nervous system or the activation of a previously latent virus. In the fatal case, the central nervous system is hyperemic and often slightly swollen, with an occasional petechial hemorrhage. The microscopic lesions appear to be mainly confined to the white matter. Early, the congested vessels are surrounded by a few neutrophils that are soon replaced by lymphocytes, often marked in numbers, and plasmacytoid cells. Macrophages, some containing lipid, occur during the later stages of the disease. The loss of myelin about the veins and the relatively undamaged axons are usually only to be recognized with special stains.

According to Poser,[161] some of the patients clinically diagnosed as having postvaccinal or postexanthematous encephalomyelitis are discovered to have had a typical chronic relapsing type of multiple sclerosis at postmortem examination. Our material contains one such example.

Acute necrotizing hemorrhagic encephalitis (acute hemorrhagic leukoencephalitis; acute hemorrhagic leukoencephalopathy).[4, 108, 124] In acute necrotizing hemorrhagic encephalitis, a rare, usually rapidly fatal disorder, there is often a preceding nondescript infection, characteristically respiratory, from which the patient is recovering or has recovered. The onset of the central nervous system involvement is explosive. The brain becomes congested and swollen, with many isolated and confluent petechiae in the white matter. The lesion often involves one portion of the brain to a greater degree than the other (Fig. 42-75).

On microscopic examinaton, the walls of the small vessels are necrotic, with edema of the surrounding brain. Early, there are moderate to marked neutrophils and fibrin infiltrations in the necrotic vascular walls. Lymphocytes and plasma cells later replace the neutrophils as the surrounding edematous and hemorrhagic brain undergoes necrosis. Death usually supervenes before macrophages are found. There is some suggestion that this condition may be a more severe form of perivenous encephalomyelitis with an allergic basis.

Central pontine myelinolysis.[41, 125] Apparently unrelated to the other demyelinating disorders is this relatively newly recognized pathologic entity. Described first in 1959, it has been associated with alcoholism, malnutrition, disturbances of electrolytes and water, extraneural infections, local venous obstruction, and unidentified agents. The lesion occurs in the central portion of the base of the pons, with its greatest transverse diameter at the level of the external origins of the trigeminal nerves (Fig. 42-76). Rostrally, it may reach almost into the midbrain. Its caudal extent generally spares the lowermost pons. The well-formed lesion is granular, gray, and well demarcated.

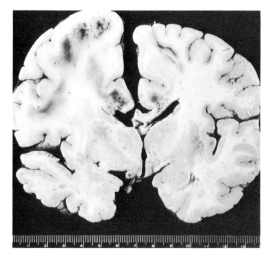

Fig. 42-75 Acute hemorrhagic leukoencephalitis, predominantly unilateral. (Courtesy Dr. J. Langston; from Chason, J. L.: In Saphir, O., editor: A text on systemic pathology, vol. 2, New York, 1958, Grune & Stratton, Inc.; by permission.)

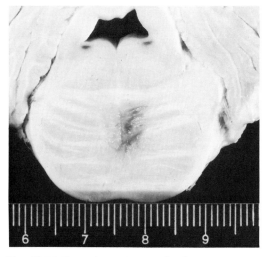

Fig. 42-76 Central pontine myelinolysis.

On coronal section, it is diamond shaped or triangular with its base dorsal or cylindrical. In some, only a poorly defined gray change is noted at the appropriate level. The area is pale with the routine hematoxylin and eosin stain, often with occasional lipophages in the early and active lesions. With special stains, there is loss of myelin and retention of most, if not all, of the axons. Metachromatic granular material may be seen early. In some plaques, the myelin going in one direction may be lost, with sparing of the myelin-sheathed fibers running in another direction. Oligodendroglia are decreased to absent in the lesion. Reactive astrocytosis and gliosis are usually minimal.

Leukodystrophies

The leukodystrophies are metabolic diseases characterized by a disturbance in the formation of myelin (dysmyelinating diseases). They have been considered to be genetically determined and are often familial. In some, there is a similarity to the so-called lipidoses (i.e., lipid-storage diseases). The leukodystrophies also differ from the demyelinating diseases in that the lesions are likely to be bilateral and symmetrical, involve more of the nervous system, and occur in younger individuals. The subcortical U fibers are regularly spared, and the axis-cylinders usually are destroyed. Whereas the leukodystrophies are similar in appearance grossly, they have characteristic microscopic features that permit their separation into subgroups. Only those that are generally accepted and are less rare are described below.

Metachromatic leukodystrophy (sulfatide lipidosis).[88, 111a, 152, 174] Metachromatic leukodystrophy is a disease of both children and adults. The basic defect in myelin metabolism is a deficiency of the enzyme arylsulfatase A. The involved areas of the white matter contain large amounts of a sulfatide that exhibits gamma metachromasia with the von Hirsch–Pfeiffer cresyl-violet-acetic acid stain. A relationship to the lipidosis has been suggested because the abnormal material also has been found in tissues other than the central nervous system, including the cells of the liver and kidneys, the white blood cells, and cells of the gallbladder. Schwann cells of the peripheral nerves and the cells of nerve plexuses also are involved. The anatomic diagnosis often can be made by biopsy examination of a peripheral nerve (usually sural) or of the nerve plexuses (rectum). The specific stain

done on frozen sections with the presence of gamma metachromasia as described is diagnostic. Analysis of the more easily available urine, leukocytes, or fibroblastic tissue cultures for the enzyme deficiency is a safer and more reasonable approach for diagnosis.

Globoid cell leukodystrophy (Krabbe's disease; globoid sclerosis). Globoid cell leukodystrophy is a disease that affects only the central nervous system of children. The accumulation of an abnormal PAS-positive material, possibly a cerebroside of the kerasin type, leads to the formation of large epithelioid and multinucleated giant cells (the globoid cells) (Fig. 42-77). The mononuclear cells are found in clusters of varying sizes about blood vessels, whereas the multinucleated cells occur more frequently in the affected white matter. Galactosyl ceramide-β-galactosyl hydrolase and other enzyme deficiencies have been described.[8a]

Neutral fat leukodystrophy (sudanophilic leukodystrophy). Although neutral fat leukodystrophy resembles diffuse sclerosis, there are significant differences that have suggested to some its inclusion with the dysmyelinating diseases. In addition to having the characteristic gross features of the leukodystrophies, in many patients there is an increase in hexosamine content, the biochemical criterion for this group of diseases. The family history, the genetic background, and the presence of sudanophilic material, coupled with the absence of the gamma metachromatic granules and of the globoid cells, structurally separates this disease from the previously described dysmyelinating diseases.

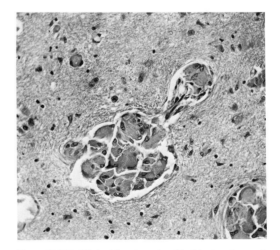

Fig. 42-77 Globoid sclerosis (Krabbe's disease). (Hematoxylin-eosin; ×135.)

NEOPLASMS

No accurate statistics reporting the frequency of neoplasms of the central nervous system are available. Estimates have been based upon a variety of observations, often with the inclusion of expanding granulomas and biased by the character of the hospital or clinic and by the interests of the clinician and pathologist. The estimate that 9.2% of all neoplasms (excluding those of the skin) are primary in the central nervous system is, at present, most reasonable.

Hypotheses and theories concerning the development of neoplasms elsewhere in the body have their counterparts in the nervous system. Early histogenetic theories and tumor classifications were based upon the cell rest theory of Cohnheim, in which neoplasms were believed to originate from activation of aberrant immature cells.[15, 18] The cytologic similarities of neoplastic cells to those at different stages of maturation reinforced these opinions. Later classifications were based upon the belief that fully mature cells could be stimulated to reproduce and to dedifferentiate.[118] Experimental production of central nervous system lesions has not resolved these differences. The issues have become even more debatable by evidence that the structure of these neoplasms may be related to their position within the nervous system and that there is often a mixture of glial elements. Most modern classifications make use of both theories.

Gliomas

Tumors classified as gliomas should be limited only to those neoplasms whose origin is from the ectodermal supporting tissues (neuroglia) of the central nervous system. It has been customary, however, to include among these the medulloblastomas and the pineal neoplasms (i.e., neoplasms of neuroblastic origin). The classification proposed in 1926 by Bailey and Cushing[18] was based upon the then current theories of histogenesis of the nervous system.[159] The more recent classification proposed by Kernohan et al.[118] and, for the most part, adopted here includes interpretations of the suggestions of Willis and of Sherer. It is based upon the assumption that some gliomas arise by dedifferentiation of adult cells.

Astrocytic series

Grade I astrocytoma. Among the grade I astrocytomas, which constitute about 15% of all gliomas, are the fibrillary, protoplasmic,

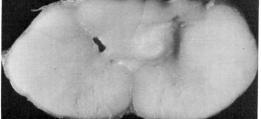

Fig. 42-78 Grade I astrocytoma (cystic) in cervical cord.

and pilocytic types. Although these types differ as to the amount of visible cytoplasm and degree of production of neuroglial fibers, they have, in general, the same biologic behavior. These neoplasms are relatively slow growing, with an average survival in excess of three years following the onset of symptoms. They may be found in any part of the central nervous system.

In adults, those neoplasms are usually in one of the cerebral hemispheres. In young adults and in children, the tumors are more frequent in the pons and cerebellum.[7, 33, 138] Those occurring in the cerebrum and pons are solid, gray, and firm, with very poorly defined borders. Small cystic areas sometimes may be found in the tumors of the cerebrum. The cerebellar neoplasms more often are cystic. The cyst walls are surrounded by neoplastic cells in 60%, whereas in 40% only a mural nodule composed of neoplastic astrocytes is found.[33, 138] The cavity contains a clear amber fluid high in protein. Similar but smaller lesions also occur in the spinal cord (Fig. 42-78).

The microscopic recognition of these neoplasms may be exceedingly difficult particularly at biopsy because:

1 Astrocytes forming the tumors are within the cytologic limits of normality.
2 Mitoses are not found.
3 There is no area of necrosis or hemorrhage (except operative).
4 In the diffuse forms, normal-appearing nerve cells often are included within the lesion.
5 There are no changes of the blood vessels (see following) except an occasional perivascular scant lymphocytic cuff.

Diagnosis by biopsy is dependent upon an evaluation of the history and the presence of increased numbers of astrocytes in the absence of an apparent cause for their numerical increase.

The boundaries of the neoplasms that are solid or diffuse are difficult to demarcate by microscopic study. This is due to the very gradual centrifugal decrease in numbers of astrocytes and the absence of evidence of compression or destruction of the surrounding brain. In occasional neoplasms examined in detail, there are nests of enlarged and sometimes pleomorphic astrocytes and recognizable increases in blood vessels, some with proliferation of the endothelial and/or adventitial layers. These are interpreted as evidence of increased dedifferentiation and biologic activity.

Occasionally, a tumor of the cerebral hemispheres may be composed either entirely (less commonly) or in greater part by well-differentiated astrocytes with abundant eosinophilic cytoplasm. The biologic behavior of these gemistocytic astrocytomas usually differs from those just described. It is our experience, as well as that of others, that these neoplasms rapidly undergo malignant dedifferentiation usually to grade III astrocytoma (glioblastoma multiforme). Because of this, it has been our practice to empirically add one cytologic grade to the neoplasm when cells of this type are found.

Grade II astrocytoma. Grade II astrocytoma includes that type previously called astroblastoma because of the resemblance of many of its constituent cells to astroblasts. It is an uncommon tumor, forming only approximately 1% of all gliomas. More common in young adults than in children, these neoplasms are solid and gray-white to white. The macroscopically discernible borders sometimes give rise to a false impression of demarcation at the point where there is compression of the surrounding brain.

Microscopically, the tumor is more cellular than the lower grade astrocytoma. The cells are generally larger, and in many there are cells with one or more plump cell processes that radiate about the walls of the moderately increased numbers of blood vessels. Mitoses and areas of necrosis are rare. When the lesions are examined to include the gross line of demarcation, neoplastic cells singly and in groups can be found to extend well beyond this point.

The average postoperative survival of patients with grade II astrocytomas is approximately two years.

Grade III and grade IV astrocytomas. Among the grade III and grade IV astrocytomas are those called glioblastoma multiforme, spongioblastoma multiforme, polar

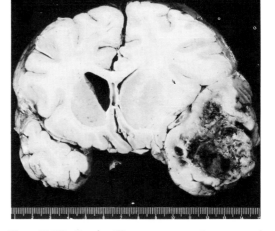

Fig. 42-79 Grade III astrocytoma in temporal lobe. Brain displacement with cingulate gyrus herniation and compression of lateral ventricle.

spongioblastoma, monstrocellular or gigantocellular glioblastoma, etc. These highly malignant and uniformly fatal neoplasms constitute 50% to 60% of all gliomas. They are more common in adults and in the cerebral hemispheres. Beginning more often in white matter, they often appear to be well demarcated because the surrounding brain is compressed, swollen, and edematous. The neoplasm is usually slightly more firm than the adjacent tissue. Its surface has a variegated gray, white, yellow (necrotic), and reddish brown (hemorrhagic) appearance (Fig. 42-79). The tumors frequently extend into and across the corpus callosum into the opposite hemisphere. Multicentric origin (i.e., two or more separate neoplasms) has been described in 15%. However, on microscopic study, we have frequently found neoplastic cells connecting the grossly separate tumors. It is our experience that multicentric origins do not exceed 5%.

The microscopic appearance of these lesions usually is characterized by marked numbers of pleomorphic and frequently bizarre cells (Fig. 42-80). Among these are many cells with enlarged and irregular nuclei. Some cells can be identified by their processes as being of astrocytic origin. Other cells may be small with oval, hyperchromatic nuclei resembling the undifferentiated small cells of a bronchogenic carcinoma. In other areas, there may be large cells with irregular large, vesicular nuclei and with an abundant eosinophilic cytoplasm suggesting an origin from gemistocytic astrocytes. In many areas within the neoplasm, one may find bizarre, multinucleate cells with much cytoplasm resembling the

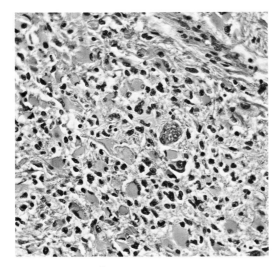

Fig. 42-80 Grade III astrocytoma. Gemistocytic astrocytes and multinucleate cells. (Hematoxylin-eosin; ×280.)

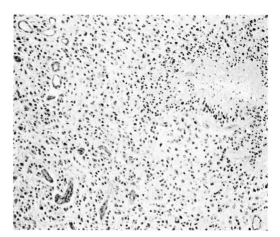

Fig. 42-81 Grade III astrocytoma. Area of necrosis with garland formation. Vascular proliferation. (Hematoxylin-eosin; ×135.)

strap cells of rhabdomyosarcomas. Mitoses, often abnormal, are usually easily found either in clusters or spread fairly regularly throughout the neoplasm. In many regions within the neoplasm, there are large and small areas of necrosis often with a garland of small cell nuclei at the periphery (Fig. 42-81). Blood vessels are markedly increased in numbers and usually with endothelial and/or adventitial hypertrophy and hyperplasia. Occasionally, vessels with these changes are found well beyond the apparent microscopic limits of the neoplasm.

Despite the apparent sharp gross demarcation, neoplastic cells extend far beyond these borders due to the infiltration from the tumor and perhaps also due to the continued dedifferentiation of the surrounding cells. A sudden increase in signs and symptoms in patients with neoplasms of this type usually can be correlated with the occurrence of large areas of necrosis due to the vascular changes, often with superimposed thromboses. Massive hemorrhages within the neoplasms are far less frequent causes of rapid tumor enlargement and clinical deterioration.

Cells of any of the astrocytic neoplasms, but particularly those that are more malignant, may reach the subarachnoid and/or the ventricular spaces. From this point, they may spread by way of the ventricular and/or cerebrospinal fluid and implant in other portions of the central nervous system. The free neoplastic cells can sometimes be recognized on cytologic examination of cerebrospinal fluid.

Most of the patients with a grade III astrocytoma live fewer than eighteen months following diagnosis. More extensive surgical therapy has increased only the survival time—not the rate of cure.

In cerebrospinal glioblastomatosis, there may be one or two large, usually poorly defined neoplasms in the brain and spinal cord. On microscopic examination, it is discovered that these are composed of bizarre, neoplastic astrocytes of the type seen in the grade III (or grade IV) neoplasms. Clusters of similar cells also are to be found in other portions of the central nervous system, some so remote from the possible implantation sites as to suggest that the lesions are of multicentric origin.

Ependymoma[79, 115]

Approximately 5% of the intracranial gliomas are ependymomas, with 60% of the latter arising in the posterior fossa. In the spinal cord, 60% of the gliomas are of the ependymal group. Although they may arise at every level, most arise in the filum terminale at the level of the cauda equina. The intracranial ependymomas have their origins from cells lining the ventricles, the choroid plexuses, and the cells of ependymal streaks that represent obliterated portions of the lateral ventricles. In the spinal cord, they arise from the cells lining the central canal or its remnants and from the cells of the ventriculus terminale of the filum terminale. It is also possible that these neoplasms may arise (usually mixed with other glial cells) from cells

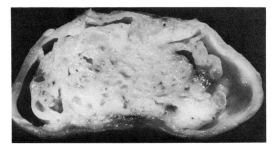

Fig. 42-82 Ependymoma of cervical portion of spinal cord. Residual spinal cord represented by peripheral rim of tissue.

whose origin is in the cells of the subependymal plate.[35]

The ependymomas arising in the linings of the brain and spinal cord (Fig. 42-82) are gray, moderately firm, and well demarcated from the adjoining compressed tissues. Those in the fourth ventricle are usually solid, whereas those in the cerebral hemispheres and in the spinal cord are frequently cystic. Except those that originate from ependymal streaks, the ependymomas usually fill the ventricle locally and sometimes extensively. The tumors of the choroid plexuses are gray-pink, fungating, papillary neoplasms. Ependymomas of the filum terminale of the cauda equina are thinly encapsulated and cystic. The capsule may be breached in the larger lesions.

The microscopic appearance of this group of neoplasms is exceedingly variable among the tumors as a group and in different areas of the same tumor. The most characteristic pattern of growth is known as the epithelial type in which the cells line glandlike spaces known as "rosettes." In some, there may be large tubular or ventricle-like spaces (Fig. 42-83). The lining cells are cuboidal to columnar, many with the appearance of ependymal cells. In some areas, the cells line what is interpreted as representing a small portion of a poorly formed space, a partial rosette. Blepharoplasts are structures that represent the residua of cilia. They may be found in some of these cells when stained with Mallory's phosphotungstic acid–hematoxylin and examined under high magnification (oil). Blepharoplasts are small, circular, or rod-shaped structures surrounded by a narrow unstained halo. They lie in that portion of the cell cytoplasm that is directed toward the lumen of the rosette. In other areas of the neoplasm and in other ependymal neoplasms, the tumors are formed by a diffuse proliferation of polygonal cells without a characteristic pattern except for

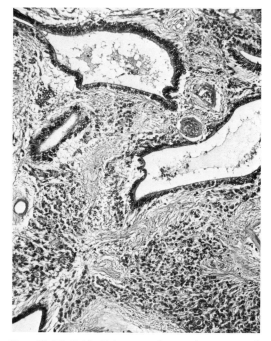

Fig. 42-83 Epithelial type of ependymoma with many rosettes. (Hematoxylin-eosin; ×90.)

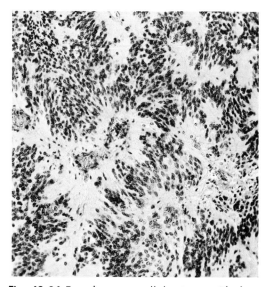

Fig. 42-84 Ependymoma, cellular type, with characteristic perivascular arrangement. (Hematoxylin-eosin; ×90.)

occasional cells whose processes radiate about a blood vessel (Fig. 42-84). Kernohan and Fletcher-Kernohan[115] have termed this the cellular type of ependymoma.

There are two varieties of papillary ependymomas: choroid plexus type and myxopapillary type. These tumors are formed by cuboidal to columnar cells lining a central core of connective tissue containing a capillary. In the *choroid plexus papilloma,* the structure is very similar to that of a normal choroid plexus with the exception that the epithelial cells are taller and larger than those of the normal (Fig. 42-85). The *myxopapillary type* can occur throughout the cerebrospinal axis and even in the hollow of the sacrum. However, it is far more frequently a tumor of the lower portion of the cauda equina. It differs from the usual choroid plexus papilloma in that the vascular and connective tissue core of the various papillae have undergone a marked degree of myxomatous change.

In approximately one-third of the ependymomas, there are nests of cells with the appearance of oligodendrocytes.

Histologic grading of this group of neoplasms was developed by Kernohan and Uihlein[116] using the same general criteria described with the astrocytoma group. The prognosis, however, is more dependent upon the site of origin than upon the histologic dedifferentiation.

Medulloepitheliomas are neoplasms that are though to originate from residual cells of the embryonic medullary canal. These tumors are exceedingly rare. Their structural similarities to the ependymomas makes their recognition difficult, if not impossible.

Oligodendrogliomas[16, 196]

Like the ependymomas, the ologidendrogliomas constitute about 5% of all gliomas. They are slow-growing tumors that are found in the white matter of a cerebral hemisphere of an adult, most frequently during the fourth or fifth decade of life. The tumors are gray-pink, well demarcated, and soft and frequently extend into the leptomeninges locally. About 20% are cystic, and in most the neoplastic tissue entirely surrounds the cyst wall. Areas of necrosis, hemorrhage, and mineralization are common in the larger lesions (Fig. 42-86). Mineralization (calcification) in the walls of the blood vessels and in larger confluent masses is visible on x-ray films in some 40% and is found on microscopic examination in 70%.

The usually described neoplastic cell has a lymphocyte-like nucleus surrounded by a clear, nonstaining halo with a definite cell membrane (Fig. 42-87). Groups of these cells produce the characteristic honeycombing. However, this appearance may be obscured in the better preserved areas of the neoplasm by the staining of the finely granular, slightly

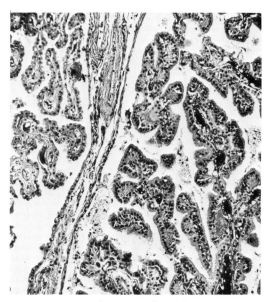

Fig. 42-85 Ependymoma, choroid plexus papilloma type. Larger papillary projections represent neoplasm. Lesion was in left cerebellopontine angle. (Hematoxylin-eosin; ×90.)

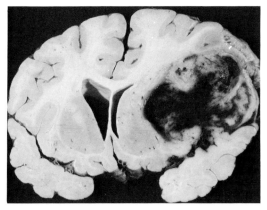

Fig. 42-86 Oligodendroglioma with operative hemorrhage. Brain and ventricular displacement with cingulate gyrus herniation.

hematoxylinophilic cytoplasm. Compartmentalization of groups of tumor cells by blood vessels is commonly present and is characteristic. The border zones of the neoplasms are relatively narrow but more poorly defined than the gross demarcation would suggest. Mitoses are rare. Their presence, sometimes in large numbers, in neoplasms containing cells with large pleomorphic nuclei has led some to classify the latter group as oligodendroblastomas.

Prognosis is related to the degree of mineralization rather than to the cytologic appearance. The greater the degree of mineraliza-

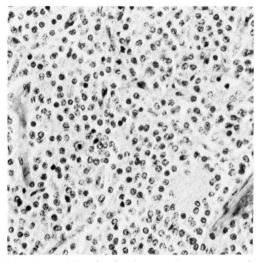

Fig. 42-87 Oligodendroglioma. Compartmentalization of cells by blood vessels. Some cells have nonstaining halos. (Hematoxylin-eosin; ×280.)

tion, the better the prognosis. Most patients live more than four years after clinical onset. Evidence of leptomeningeal spread is commonly found at necropsy and may be related to previous operative treatment.

Astrocytes frequently are found within these neoplasms, predominantly about blood vessels, perhaps serving as stromal support. In almost one-third, there are nests of ependymal-like cells.

Medulloblastoma (neuroblastoma; granuloblastoma)[17, 113, 171]

Medulloblastomas are highly malignant and still uniformly fatal neoplasms whose origin is restricted to the cerebellum. Representing approximately 8% of all neuroglial neoplasms, they occur predominantly in children. The greatest incidence is in those 5 to 9 years of age; with another increase in incidence occurring between the ages of 20 to 24 years. Males are affected more than twice as frequently as females. Familial occurrences, including tumors in identical twins, have been described. In children, most of the tumors originate in the region of the cerebellar vermis, possibly from microscopic remnants of the external granular layer of the cerebellum. In the older patients, the tumors may arise from one of the hemispheres.

Medulloblastomas are gray-pink to red, soft, friable, and often hemorrhagic and necrotic. Demarcation from the adjacent cerebellum is usually sharp. Because of the sites of origin, the fourth ventricle is almost regularly occu-

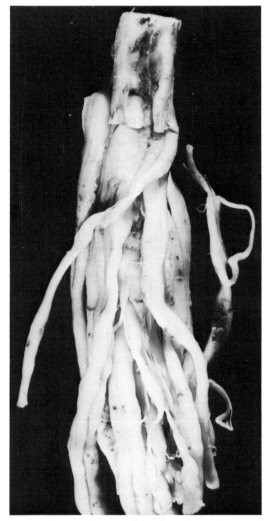

Fig. 42-88 Diffuse subarachnoid implants of medulloblastoma onto filaments of cauda equina.

pied by the rapidly growing neoplasm, often with extensions of the tissue into and through the lateral recesses, the posterior roof of the fourth ventricle, the cerebral aqueduct, and the tissues of the floor and walls of the fourth ventricle. Nodules and sheets of implanted neoplastic cells are frequent in the lateral and third ventricles and in the subarachnoid space, particularly in the regions of the cauda equina due to spread via the cerebrospinal fluid (Fig. 42-88). These highly cellular neoplasms are composed of cells with small, round to oval, usually hyperchromatic nuclei. There is little visible cytoplasm (Fig. 42-89). The number of mitoses are variable. Although the neoplastic cells tend to grow about the blood vessels with necrosis at a distance, in most there is no special histologic pattern.

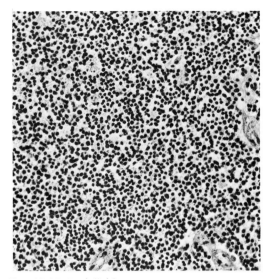

Fig. 42-89 Medulloblastoma originating in vermis of cerebellum. (Hematoxylin-eosin; ×280.)

Rosettes and pseudorosettes have been described, and evidences of continued maturation of some cells toward nerve cells and glial cells, although rare, may be seen.[89]

Differences in the cytologic appearance and the histogenic pattern led some to the opinion that the group of neoplasms lying predominantly in the cerebellar leptomeninges were cerebellar sarcomas of leptomeningeal origin. In a recent careful and intensive study, the conclusion was reached that the atypical features were due entirely to spread and growth of cells of the medulloblastoma within the confines of the subarachnoid space rather than to a different and special cell of origin.[143]

Pinealoma (germinoma; teratoma; pineoblastoma; pineocytoma; pineal neuroblastoma, etc.)[58a]

There are many classifications and interpretations of the 0.5% of all primary intracranial neoplasms that originate in and about the pineal gland. The cysts (dermoid) and the other gliomas should be so identified and designated. In the very small groups of neoplasms remaining are the pinealomas (germinomas) (Fig. 42-90). The component cells are of two types. There are large, pale polyhedral to spheroidal cells separated into lobules by vascular connective tissue trabeculae, next to which are small nests of cells with the appearance of lymphocytes. Those observers who recognize cells in transition between the two types diagnose these as pinealomas; others consider these as germinomas

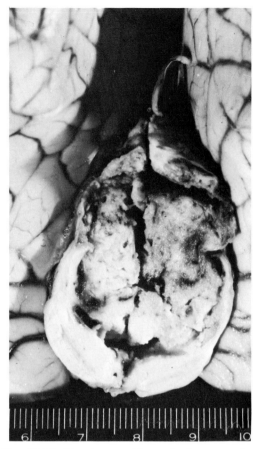

Fig. 42-90 Pinealoma with marked compression of midbrain.

since the neoplasms are indistinguishable from seminomas (Fig. 42-91). When other structural components characteristic of teratomas are found, the interrelationship is apparent.

Mixed glioma

The presence of more than one cell type in gliomas is common. However, the marked predominance of one cell type usually permits classification into one group. There is another type of glioma that arises from the cells of the subependymal cell plate.[32, 38] These neoplasms are usually small, frequently multiple, and asymptomatic unless so strategically placed as to impede or obstruct the flow of cerebrospinal fluid. Although they are more common in the fourth ventricle (Fig. 42-92), identical neoplasms have been found in all parts of the ventricular system and about the central canal of the spinal cord. The tumors are solid, gray-white, well demarcated, firm, and sometimes mineralized, and the larger neoplasms appear to be formed by the coales-

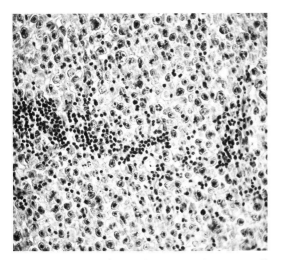

Fig. 42-91 Pinealoma (germinoma). Two cell types with some "so-called" transitional forms. (Hematoxylin-eosin; ×135.)

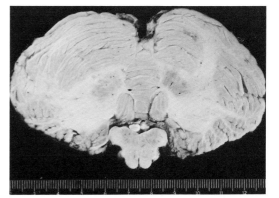

Fig. 42-92 Subependymal mixed gliomas arising in roof of fourth ventricle.

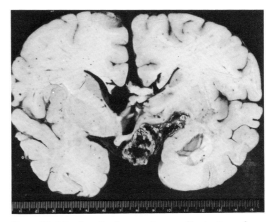

Fig. 42-93 Craniopharyngioma displacing floor of third ventricle and hypothalamus.

cence of smaller nodules of similar appearance. They are formed by plump spindle cells, some of which are in small groups. Blepharoplasts have been demonstrated in some of the cells within the clusters. Although rosettes have been described, the usual arrangement is more like that of the obliterated central canal of the spinal cord. Surrounding these cell clusters, but also separately, are tight nodules of astrocytes with many fibrillary processes. These neoplasms have been classified as subependymal glomerate astrocytomas, as mixed subependymal gliomas, and as subependymomas. It is unexplained why almost all of these neoplasms have occurred in adult males. Those of the fourth ventricle, cerebral aqueduct, and third ventricle are not amenable to removal because of the vital centers that lie nearby.

Neuroastrocytoma (ganglioglioma)

Neuroastrocytomas are rare, usually slow-growing neoplasms composed of a mixture of neoplastic nerve cells and astrocytes. The structural criteria necessary for their diagnosis require the definite identification of neoplastic rather than included normal nerve cells. For this, it is generally required that binucleate and multinucleate nerve cells be present in addition to the neoplastic astrocytes. The latter are usually well differentiated.

Craniopharyngioma (Rathke's pouch tumor; supracellular or epidermoid cyst; etc.)

Craniopharyngiomas, forming approximately 3% of all intracranial neoplasms, appear to arise from squamous cell remnants of Rathke's pouch (Erdheim cell rests). The presence of these cell nests in newborn infants, as well as in adults, has fortified this opinion. Although craniopharyngiomas may be seen at most ages, there are two peaks of incidence—one in late childhood and early adulthood and the other in the fifth decade (see also p. 1415).

The encapsulated tumor has a smooth, usually lobulated, gray surface. The sectioned surface is pale gray in the solid portions with one or more cysts filled with an amber to brown fluid containing cholesterol and/or grumous, yellow-gray material (Fig. 42-93). In almost two-thirds, areas of mineralization or ossification can be found scattered throughout the solid portions of the tumor. Compression of the optic chiasm, nerves, and tracts and elevation of the floor of the third ventricle is common.

The solid portions of the neoplasm are formed by a thin layer of dense connective tissue containing a mosaic of anastomosing

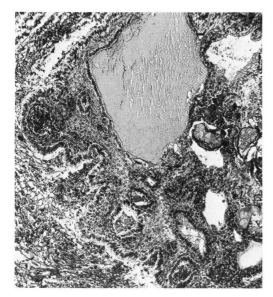

Fig. 42-94 Craniopharyngioma. Mosaic of sheets of squamous cell with beginning central cyst formation. (Hematoxylin-eosin; ×45.)

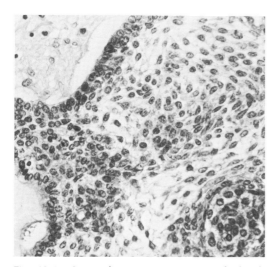

Fig. 42-95 Craniopharyngioma. Interior of islands with stellate cells and cuboidal to columnar cells adjacent to stroma.

sheets and cords of squamous cells. The inner portions of the epithelial structures are often loose and vacuolated, whereas the outer layers of cells are usually cuboidal to cylindrical. Liquefaction of the epithelial structure leads to the formation of the cystic spaces lined by stratified squamous epithelium (Figs. 42-94 and 42-95).

Dermoid and epidermoid cysts

It is generally conceded that the midline cysts of the dermoid and epidermoid varieties

result from defects of closure with the heterotopic inclusion of the skin, sometimes with accessory skin structures. These cysts usually are found in or near the midline of the posterior fossa (Fig. 42-96), near the vermis, or even in the fourth ventricle. The small group of epidermoid cysts found in the more lateral positions at the base of the brain are thought to represent hererotopically trapped portions of the linings of the sinuses formed during closure of the bones of the skull.

The cysts are rounded and circumscribed, with an outer thin connective tissue wall and

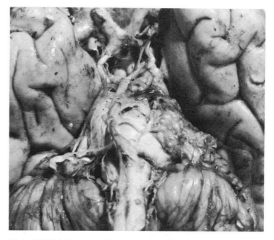

Fig. 42-96 Dermoid cyst. "Pearly" tumor on ventral surface of pons on its left.

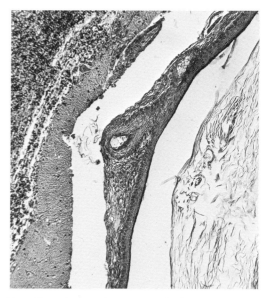

Fig. 42-97 Dermoid cyst. Stratified squamous epithelial lining of cyst contains hair follicle. Cyst lumen filled with keratin. (Hematoxylin-eosin; ×90.)

with an inner cavity filled with a thick, sticky, yellow material. Hair may be present. A stratified squamous layer with keratohyaline granules and intercellular bridges lines the cavities of the epidermoid cyst. In the dermoid cyst (Fig. 42-97), the walls, in addition, contain sweat, sebaceous glands, and/or hair follicles. Spread of the contents, usually postoperative, leads to the formation of multiple small granulomas formed by keratin-containing foreign body giant cells.

This entire group of cysts comprises less than 1% of all primary intracranial neoplasms.

Colloid cyst (paraphyseal cyst)[179]

According to a recent study, there are two types of ependymal-lined cysts. Both are limited to the roof of the third ventricle. The more frequent type arises following closure of an ependymal pouch whose cuboidal to columnar cells contain blepharoplasts or cilia. The second type, also lined by cuboidal or columnar cells without blepharoplasts or cilia, is thought to arise because of persistence of the embryonic paraphyseal pouch. The cysts are spherical masses attached to the most rostral portion of the roof of the third ventricle midway between the interventricular foramina (Fig. 42-98).

Whatever their origin, the content of these cysts is usually gray and gelatinous. When

brown, the color is due to preceding hemorrhage. The inner lining of either type of cyst wall is formed by a single layer of cuboidal to columnar cells. These cells are the source of the amorphous, eosinophilic, PAS-positive contents in which a few desquamated cells may be present. The outer cyst wall is formed by a thin fibrous connective tissue capsule that extends to the tela choroidea of the third ventricle. The autopsy incidence of about 2% of all intracranial tumors exceeds the clinical incidence of 0.5%, since only about one-fourth of these neoplasms reach the clinically significant size of 1 cm.

Meningioma

Among all symptom-producing intracranial neoplasms, approximately 15% are classified as belonging to the meningiomas. This is a broad group of miscellaneous neoplasms with a variety of cells of origin.[54, 127] Most have a dural attachment and are relatively slow growing. They are slightly more common in women. In decreasing order of frequency, the meningiomas occur parasagittally (Fig. 42-99) over the cerebral convexities, laterally over the sphenoid ridges, medially in the olfactory grooves, and in the posterior fossa (cerebellopontine angle). They can, however, originate anywhere there are leptomeninges, including the choroid plexuses, especially in the region of the temporal poles and glomus choroideum of the lateral ventricles and in the orbit.

Based, as the classification is, upon the anatomic site of the tumor rather than upon its cytologic origin, it is surprising that reasonably accurate generalizations as to biologic

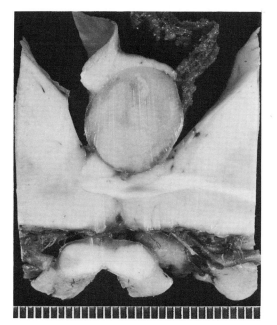

Fig. 42-98 Colloid cyst of third ventricle. Patient was asymptomatic.

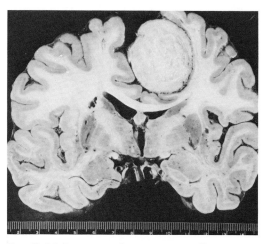

Fig. 42-99 Parasagittal meningioma, fibrous type. Remote anemic infarcts in internal capsules and left putamen.

behavior are possible.[42, 102] Only one cell type, the arachnoid cap cell (meningocyte or meningothelial cell) is found solely in the leptomeninges. The remaining cells are those associated with the supporting tissues and blood vessels seen everywhere in the body. Tumors arising from these latter cells have the appearance, both gross and microscopic, of similar tumors occurring elsewhere—i.e., fibroma, hemangioma, osteoma, chondroma, lipoma (Fig. 42-100), etc.—and some, therefore, need no further description. Some, such as the lipomas, may represent a maldevelopment. That some have rarely contained other cell types as smooth muscle and skeletal muscle and bone has been considered as further evidence for a hamartomatous or choristomatous origin of this group. About 90% to 95% of the meningiomas encountered are meningothelial, fibromatous, or inseparable mixtures of the two.

The meningothelial (meningocytic) meningioma is a thinly encapsulated, flat to spherical, moderately firm, yellow-gray, solid neoplasm usually firmly adherent at some point to the dura. The cell forming this type of neoplasm is polygonal, with poorly defined cell boundaries. Its centrally placed nucleus is relatively large and round and contains finely divided chromatin without an evident nucleolus. In some tumors, the cells are arranged in onionskin-like whorls and/or in sheets of varying sizes (Fig. 42-101). In the centers of many of the whorls and at the edges or within the sheets are capillaries or slightly larger blood vessels. Connective and elastic tissue and reticulin are confined to the blood vessel walls and act as a stroma supporting the neoplasm. Calcospheres (psammoma bodies) in varying numbers may be found in these neoplasms. They apparently represent a degenerative change with mineralization within the walls of blood vessels or tumor cells. When

they predominate, the meningothelial meningioma is considered by some to be of the psammomatous type. This is a common occurrence at the spinal level, where it is associated with a long history and very slow progression of signs and symptoms.

Although these neoplasms are classified as benign, there may be recurrence even after the entire tumor appears to have been removed. Multiple tumors are infrequent. In addition, they have the propensity for growing into adjacent dura, dural sinus, and skull, just as do arachnoid granulations. Metastasis, on the other hand, is extremely rare. Histologic and cytologic criteria suggesting malignancy such as nuclear enlargement, irregularity, and hyperchromatism and growth beyond the capsule occur in about 10% of the surgically removed meningothelial meningiomas. This is, however, far in excess of any malignant biologic activity.

Extension of the neoplasm through the dura with reaction of the overlying bone may be helpful in determining the rate of growth of the tumor. Benign meningiomas often are associated with destruction of the inner table of the skull with a "sunburst" type of bone production of the outer table. More rapidly growing tumors destroy both tables without reactive bone formation.

"Incidental" asymptomatic, small meningiomas, usually of the meningothelial and fibro-

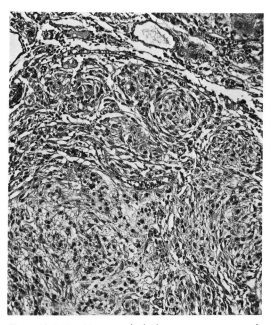

Fig. 42-101 Meningothelial meningioma with typical whorls. (Hematoxylin-eosin; ×90.)

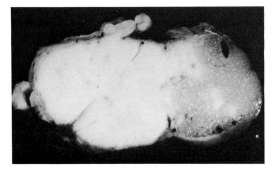

Fig. 42-100 Lipoma in leptomeninges of lumbar spinal cord.

matous types, are frequently found during routine postmortem examination. In our material, their numbers exceed those that have produced clinical symptoms and signs.

Schwannoma (neurilemoma; neurofibroma, etc.)

Approximately 8% of all intracranial neoplasms are schwannomas. While they far more commonly arise from the eighth cranial nerve in the region of the internal acoustic meatus, where the Schwann sheath has already begun (Fig. 42-102), (i.e., the cerebellopontine angle), they may be attached to any of the cranial nerves that have a Schwann sheath. In decreasing order of frequency, the sites of occurrence are the ninth, seventh, eleventh, fifth, and fourth cranial nerves. The cauda equina is a frequent site for these neoplasms (Fig. 42-103), in which location many are asymptomatic. When the acoustic nerve is involved, the tumor is in the cerebellopontine angle near the internal acoustic meatus, which may be eroded. The expanding tumor characteristically compresses the pons and cerebellum medially while enlarging the angle at their junction. The tumors are most frequently clinically apparent during the fourth, fifth, and sixth decades and are two to three times as common in women as in men. The neoplasms are usually single. When multiple, they may be a manifestation of Recklinghausen's disease (Fig. 42-104) or may represent a forme fruste.

The intracranial tumors are encapsulated, firm, and gray-white and are attached to or

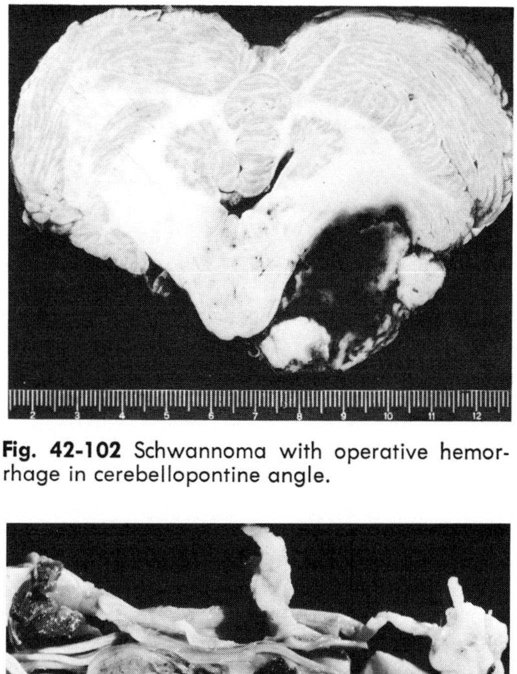

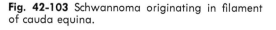

Fig. 42-102 Schwannoma with operative hemorrhage in cerebellopontine angle.

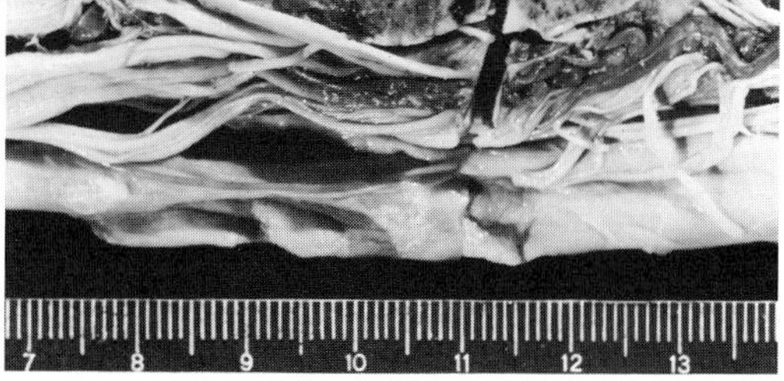

Fig. 42-103 Schwannoma originating in filament of cauda equina.

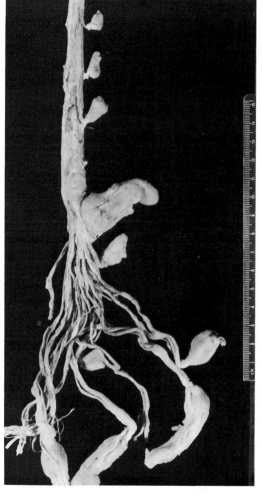

Fig. 42-104 Neurofibromatosis involving cauda equina and spinal ganglia (Recklinghausen's disease).

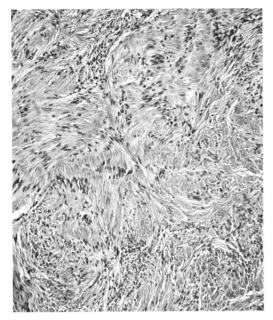

Fig. 42-105 Schwannoma. Portion with interlacing fascicular pattern. (Hematoxylin-eosin; ×90.)

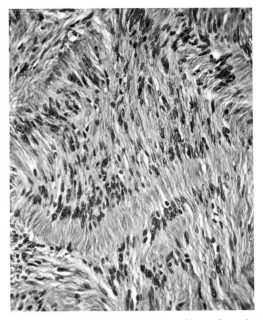

Fig. 42-106 Schwannoma. Palisading of nuclei. (Hematoxylin-eosin; ×185.)

appear as part of the cranial nerve, which is then stretched about the mass. The larger tumors often have an irregular lobulated surface with yellow, softened, and sometimes hemorrhagic areas internally. Among the several characteristic microscopic features of these neoplasms are the following:

1 The capsule is relatively thick (as compared with the meningioma).

2 The larger lesions are divided into compact, solid areas that are relatively highly cellular (Antoni type A) and areas that are loose, reticular, and less cellular (Antoni type B).

3 The cells of the more cellular areas are are spindle shaped with long processes and nuclei that are long and narrow and with finely granular chromatin.

4 A portion of the tumor regularly has cells with an interlacing fascicular pattern (Fig. 42-105).

5 In some areas, the nuclei tend to align themselves into palisades (Fig. 42-106).

6 An occasional whorl-like arrangement may simulate the structures of a meningothelial meningioma but is thought to represent a similarity to a tactile end organ and is called Verocay body.

7 In the Antoni type B areas, the neoplastic cells are more plump and more varied in appearance.

8 Marked hyalinization with thickening of the walls of the blood vessels is highly characteristic in the Antoni type B areas and leads to necrosis and hemorrhage, sometimes with thrombosis.

9 The cystic areas contain numerous lipid and hemosiderin-laden macrophages and are organized by the formation of granulation tissue.

The intracranial schwannomas are histologically benign lesions, although they frequently recur if incompletely removed. Rarely, if ever, do they undergo malignant transformation.

Almost one-third of the tumors of the spinal canal are schwannomas. They are always attached to a nerve root and occur at all levels of the spinal cord. In most, the nerve root that is involved lies between the spinal cord and the dura. Of the remaining, an equal number involve the nerve root as it traverses the dura and/or lie outside the dura. The spinal canal schwannomas are smaller than those of the eighth cranial nerve and, while they have the usual gross and microscopic features, the Antoni type A appearance is by far the more frequent.

Vascular malformations and neoplasms

Vascular malformations in the central nervous system are frequent. During a five-year period when the brain at postmortem examination was routinely sectioned at 2 mm to 3

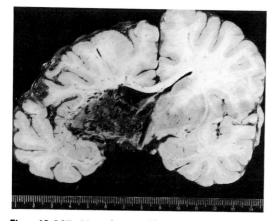

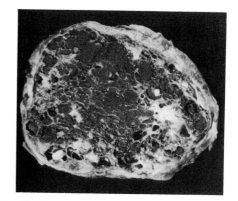

Fig. 42-107 Vascular malformation in central gray matter of left cerebral hemisphere. Both arteries and veins were identified.

Fig. 42-108 Vascular malformation in lumbar spinal cord. Progressive paraparesis existed for fifteen years.

mm intervals, vascular malformations were found in over 5%. In the great majority, the lesions were incidental. There is no classification that satisfactorily encompasses the range of their structural appearances.[134, 135] When thorough analyses are made of the lesions, frequently portions are found to have the features that bridge more than one division.

Telangiectasia (capillary telangiectasis; capillary angioma). Telangiectasia is the most frequent of the vascular malformations. They are found in adults of both sexes and in all portions of the brain. Because of their usual small size (usually less than 1 cm) and because they are usually single, they often are missed on the routine sectioning of the brain. They appear as well-circumscribed but non-encapsulated dark red areas in which a fine stippling caused by the blood vessels often can be recognized. One portion or the entire area on occasion may have an orange-brown appearance due to remote bleeding.

Microscopically, the lesion is composed of capillaries with some variation in size. In the usual small lesion, intervening brain tissue separates the capillaries. In the larger lesions, this is noted only at the periphery, the center containing larger capillary vessels with no intervening nerve tissue. These lesions occasionally lead to a small local hemorrhage. Their recognition in the wall of a massive hemorrhage, sometimes extending into the ventricular and/or subarachnoid spaces, is rare.[118] In order to adequately investigate such an instance, the blood obtained from the lesion should be strained through several layers of gauze as it is being washed with the residual tissue retained by the gauze being

examined for the presence of the vascular lesion.

Arteriovenous malformations. Although less frequent than the telangiectasia, arteriovenous malformations involve the brain (Fig. 42-107) and spinal cord (Fig. 42-108). From the appearance of the vessel wall, traditional divisions of these lesions have been made to include arteriovenous and venous types.

The arteriovenous malformation is composed of a complex tangle of enlarged dilated arteries and veins without intervening identifiable capillaries. The lesions appear to be more common in men and are often in the area of the middle cerebral artery. On microscopic examination, there is irregular fibrous thickening of the arterial intima, often with fraying, reduplication or the destruction of the internal elastic lamina, and variable thickening of the media. The thinner-walled veins usually have undergone varying degrees of hyalinization of their media and intimal fibrosis so that they resemble arteries. While these lesions may be in the brain or in the leptomeninges, the malformation often enlarges sufficiently to involve both. Occasionally only venous types of vessels are recognized.

Sturge-Weber-Dimitri disease (cephalic neurocutaneous angiomatosis). Sturge-Weber-Dimitri disease is a rare developmental disturbance of blood vessels involving both the skin and the brain. It has been found in families and has been associated with mental retardation.

In the leptomeninges and in the atrophic portions of the brain, including the cortex and white matter, there is a marked increase in blood vessels. Collagenization occurs in the

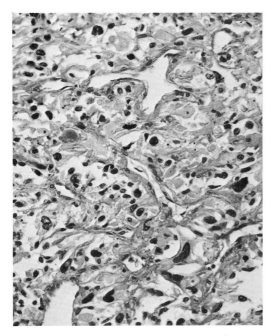

Fig. 42-109 Hemangioblastoma in cerebellum. (Hematoxylin-eosin; ×135.)

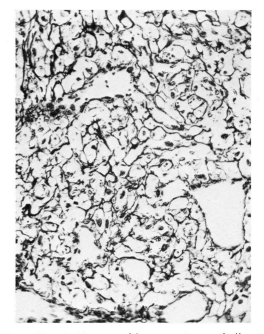

Fig. 42-110 Hemangioblastoma in cerebellum. (Reticulum stain; ×90.)

walls of many of the affected vessels. Mineralization, however, is generally limited to those vessels in the cortex and, when marked, produces a charcteristic x-ray pattern. Cortical atrophy is accompanied by a reactive astrocytic gliosis and focal compensatory hydrocephalus. The associated skin lesion is a homolateral facial nevus flammeus (port-wine stain) in the distribution of one or more branches of the trigeminal nerve. Other developmental lesions have been associated in a few instances.

Hemangioblastomas (hemangioendothelioma; angioblastic meningioma).[149, 167] Hemangioblastomas are red to yellow-gray firm neoplasms of varying size. Although found in all portions of the central nervous system, they are more common in the cerebellum. In the posterior fossa, they form 7% of all primary tumors. They may be solid, as is usual in the cerebral lesions. The cerebellar lesion is more characteristically cystic with a mural nodule. The neoplasm may be single or multiple. Every tumor has a leptomeningeal attachment.

The tumor is composed of well-formed capillaries with prominent endothelial cells (Fig. 42-109) in an abundant reticulin network extending radially from or concentrically about the capillaries (Fig. 42-110). Large lipid-containing macrophages are found scattered throughout the tumor, often imparting a yellow background to the usual red-gray gross

appearance. The nuclei of the cells are usually large and uniform. Although variation in nuclear size may be found (Fig. 42-109), this is not indicative of malignant transformation.

The cerebellar lesion is usually single and near the midline, but exceptions to both have been described. In less than 10% of the cerebellar lesions, there may be a similar tumor in the retina, vascular malformation of the spinal cord, cysts of the pancreas and liver, and cysts and/or tumors of the kidney (adenocarcinoma). This combination, known as Lindau-von Hippel disease, is more likely to occur with multiple cerebellar tumors. In some, there has been a familial occurrence.

Sarcomas[14, 116, 158]

Sarcomas of the central nervous system originate from the multipotential cells lying in the walls of the blood vessels and elsewhere as microglial cells within the substance of the brain and spinal cord. These are relatively uncommon neoplasms. Although any type of mesodermal tumor could develop from these cells, the most common are those that resemble the malignant lymphoma group of neoplasms (Figs. 42-111 and 42-112) and fibrosarcomas. In the former, similar lesions may be found in lymph nodes, spleen, and bone marrow. The position of the "cerebellar sarcoma" as previously described is under active debate. At the present time, the evidence sug-

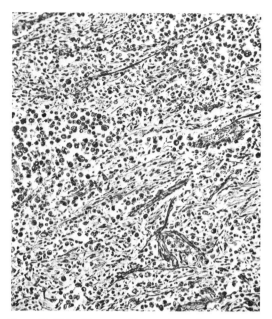

Fig. 42-111 Pleomorphic perivascular sarcoma of brain resembling reticulum cell sarcoma. (Hematoxylin-eosin; ×90.)

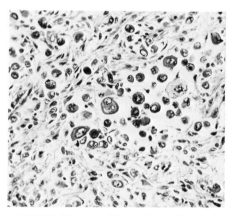

Fig. 42-112 Pleomorphic perivascular sarcoma of brain resembling reticulum cell sarcoma. (Hematoxylin-eosin; ×280.)

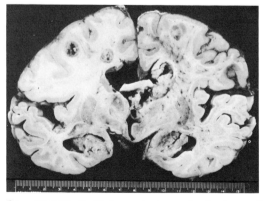

Fig. 42-113 Multiple metastases to brain and ependyma from carcinoma of lung.

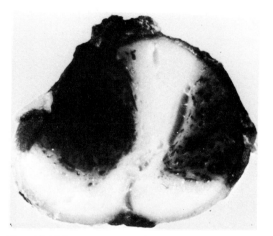

Fig. 42-114 Metastatic melanoma in spinal cord.

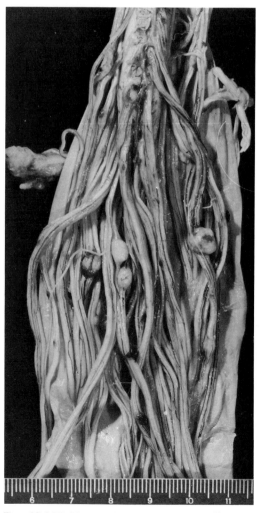

Fig. 42-115 Metastatic carcinoma onto filaments of cauda equina.

gests that this is a form of medulloblastoma with extension into the leptomeninges.

Metastatic neoplasms[22, 35, 43, 66, 131]

It has been estimated that metastatic neoplasms form up to 30% of all intracranial tumors. The great variation in the estimated range of frequencies is due to inadequate and biased sampling. Metastatic tumors are well demarcated and multiple in over 80% of cases (Fig. 42-113). Those under 1 cm in size are usually solid. Larger lesions are cystic due to central necrosis, with a 1 mm to 2 mm rim of neoplasm. The smaller metastases often are found in the white matter just beneath the so-called U fibers.

The primary sources, in decreasing order of frequency, are the lungs, breasts, kidneys, skin (melanoma), gastrointestinal tract, and prostate. Neoplastic cell emboli reach the nervous system almost exclusively by way of the arteries with preceding involvement of the lungs. Initial or sole localization within the leptomeninges (meningeal carcinomatosis; carcinomatous meningitis) is exceedingly rare when the brain is thoroughly examined. In over 2% of those with brain metastases, the spinal cord (Fig. 42-114) and/or cauda equina (Fig. 42-115) also are involved.[31, 47]

BRAIN SWELLING AND EDEMA[89, 160, 195]

Enlargement of the brain due to the intracellular accumulation of colloidally bound fluid is known as brain swelling or dry brain. Enlargement due to the presence of an increased amount of intercellular fluid is known as brain edema or wet brain. Both have been related to many causes, including trauma, neoplasms, toxic states, hypoxia, inflammations, etc. The mechanism of production of swelling and edema is not known. Brain swelling is much more common and usually precedes brain edema. The enlarged and swollen brain is heavy, with a decrease in size of the subarachnoid and ventricular spaces. The cerebral convolutions are large, and their crests are flat with compression of the sulci. The sectioned surface of the brain is pale and dry and bulges slightly. The increase in size is due entirely to the increase in size of the central white matter. Despite the obvious gross changes, with routine stains the microscopic changes are minimal.

An accompanying edema can be recognized by depression and wetness of the cut surface. This is due to the separation of the cell processes and myelin sheaths by the accumulation of fluid between them and about the blood vessels. When the fluid is high in protein content and eosinophilic, recognition is obvious. Separation of the microscopic changes from postmortem and processing artifacts is difficult when the fluid is low in protein and only enlargement of the spaces is to be seen.

Persistence of the edematous state is accompanied by a reactive astrocytosis characterized by cytoplasmic eosinophilia, focal enlargement and fragmentation of axons, loss of myelin, and occasional macrophages.

BRAIN DISPLACEMENT AND HERNIATION[34, 117, 120, 132, 200]

An expanding intracranial mass often combined with brain swelling and edema is frequently associated with brain displacement and herniation. The more slowly the expansion occurs, the greater the changes that may follow. When the lesion is in the midline and frontal or if both hemispheres are generally and equally affected, the cerebral hemispheres and portions of the midbrain are displaced downward through the incisura of the tentorium. As a result, the midbrain is elongated and the unci become notched by the free margins of the tentorium. The structures occupying the posterior fossa may simultaneously be displaced downward, with impaction of the medulla and cerebellar tonsils into the funnel-shaped foramen magnum (Fig. 42-116). With this downward displacement, the cerebellar tonsils become elongated and notched and the ventral surface of the medulla becomes flattened, sometimes even notched. The displaced pons simultaneously becomes foreshortened

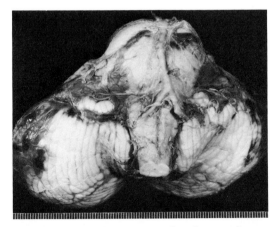

Fig. 42-116 Foreshortening and widening of pons with cerebellomedullary herniation. Secondary to cerebral mass lesion with brain swelling, edema, and displacement.

and widened. Each downward displacement produces a degree of obstruction of the flow of cerebrospinal fluid.

An expanding lateral or eccentrically placed cerebral mass may produce asymmetrical brain displacement and herniation. When the displacement is toward the opposite hemisphere, the cingulate gyrus is forced across the midline beneath the free margin of the falx. Downward displacement to the side homolateral to the mass produces a homolateral uncal groove (Fig. 42-117) and sometimes a notching of the homolateral cerebral peduncle by the free margin of the tentorium. With this caudal displacement, the free margin of the tentorium compresses the overriding homolateral posterior cerebral artery. The occlusion can, in turn, result in the production of an anemic and, on release, a hemorrhagic infarct in the area supplied (Fig. 42-117). The combination of downward and contralateral displacement produces another combination of herniations. More frequently, there is compression of the uncus on the homolateral side, and contralateral compression of the cerebral peduncle[117] and posterior cerebral artery occur.

Tumors of the posterior fossa are associated

with downward displacement and notching of the medulla and cerebellar tonsils. There may be notching of the superior surface of the cerebellum should either or both hemispheres of the cerebellum be displaced upward.

Downward displacements can be accentuated by the injudicious use of the lumbar puncture.

The brain also may herniate through dural defects and irregularities such as the points of entrance or exits of the blood vessels. A large dural defect such as may be produced following operation can permit a large local herniation, fungus cerebri.

The microscopic appearances with each of the herniations are characteristic of focal ischemia and sometimes with small areas of necrosis.

Midbrain, pontine, and sometimes thalamic hemorrhages are common fatal secondary effects produced by supratentorial expanding masses.[34] The mechanism producing these hemorrhages is not known.[120] They appear to be related to the downward displacement of the brain without the simultaneous displacement of the basilar artery and its branches. This produces a compression and/or angulation of the vessels within the brainstem that is thought to result in the hemorrhages of the brainstem.[181, 200]

■ Peripheral nervous system
Structure and function

Because much of the peripheral nervous system has been covered in the description of diseases of the various organs, this discussion will be limited to that supplying the limbs. This portion of the nervous system includes the sensory fibers whose unipolar cell bodies are in the spinal ganglia and whose dendritic processes extend from the limbs and whose axons reach to the spinal cord or brainstem. The motor fibers begin as peripheral nerves in the motor nerve root area of the spinal cord and brainstem. At the nerve root, the myelin sheath, both on the sensory and motor sides, is abruptly changed from that formed by oligodendrocytes centrally to that formed by Schwann's cells peripherally. This occurs at a node of Ranvier, and the portion of the nerve in the subarachnoid area proximal to this change is called the Obersteiner-Redlich space or area. The site of change is easily recognizable with the hematoxylin and eosin stain because of the lighter staining of the central portion and the darker staining of

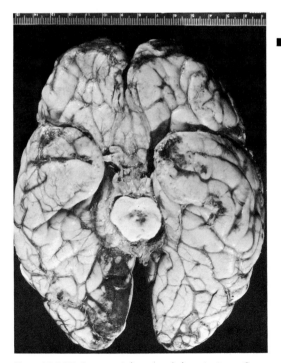

Fig. 42-117 Large right uncal herniation. Compression of right posterior cerebral artery with recent hemorrhagic infarct of visual cortex. Secondary pressure hemorrhages in lower midbrain.

the peripheral nervous system portion. Sensory, motor, and mixed nerves have the same general organizational pattern. Individual axons are surrounded by Schwann's cells in a linear series separated at the junctions of Schwann's cells. These are called the nodes of Ranvier. A thin, fibrous layer, the endoneurium, surrounds each axis-cylinder and its covering Schwann's cells. Fascicular groups of fibers are surrounded by a more easily seen and thicker layer of connective tissue, the perineurium. The epineurium surrounds the entire nerve and extends to the surrounding connective tissues. The perikarya of the cells of the spinal ganglia are large and spherical. They are surrounded by a single layer of flattened cuboidal cap cells. These cells are considered to be the counterpart of Schwann's cell peripherally and of the oligodendrocytes centrally.

Degenerations

Degenerative changes of the spinal ganglia cells and their reactions are similar to those of the large nerve cells elsewhere. Aging is associated with the progressive accumulation of lipofuscin, a yellow to brown granular pigment, either about or to one side of the nucleus. Shrinkage of the cell is associated with irregularities of shape, pyknosis of the nucleus, and proliferation of the surrounding cap cells. The changes of central and peripheral chromatolysis are identical with those of the cells of the central nervous system. Cell death is accompanied initially by proliferation of and, later, phagocytosis by the cap cells. Nageotte clusters represent a residual whorled arrangement of cap cells following the loss of a ganglion cell. Cell counts have demonstrated that there is a gradual and continuous loss of spinal ganglion cells with increasing age.

Disintegration of the axis-cylinders may follow damage to the cell body or may be due to local injury. With the latter, the change progresses centrally only as far as the next node of Ranvier. They may become focally swollen with varicosities or generally swollen and fragmented and later demonstrate increasing granularity. Myelin beading, swelling, and fragmentation accompany the changes in the axis-cylinders. Chemical changes in the myelin sheath, demonstrable by special stains, first appear eight to ten days after the initial injury and probably are related to the formation of cholesterol esters. Stainable neutral fats appear soon afterward and are slowly removed by macrophages and, according to

some, by Schwann's cells. Regeneration is possible when the damage to the nerve cells of the spinal ganglia is minimal or is limited to the peripheral axis-cylinder. Concurrently with the degenerative changes, Schwann's cells begin to proliferate, primarily from their distal end toward the central stump, forming the so-called neurolemmal tubules. Multiple fibrillary outgrowths from the central end of the damaged axis-cylinder make their initial appearance at the end of the first week in myelinated nerves and after the second week in the unmyelinated fibers. The downgrowing fibers enter the proximal ends of the neurolemmal tubules, sometimes before there is complete degeneration and removal of the injured tissues. It is assumed that there is an influence that governs the pattern of regeneration. There is, however, always some degree of loss of the normal relationships so that not all fibers reach and grow into the correct neurolemmal tubule. The degree of disorganization is more marked in the presence of foreign material and with the formation of scar tissue. The factor that determines which of the fiber branches continues to grow downward into the tubule and which disappears is not known. It is believed that those fibers that have entered improper tubules (i.e., sensory fibers in a motor area) do not achieve function and eventually degenerate. Initially, all regenerated fibers are nonmyelinated. Myelination about some fibers proceeds from the central end distalward, making its proximal appearance about one month following injury.

When these structures are examined routinely at autopsy, it can be seen that the spinal ganglia and peripheral nerves participate in many so-called nonneurologic diseases that affect the individual.

The causes of damage to a peripheral nerve are many, and the initial locus of damage is equally varied. Nerve biopsy is not common in these conditions, and the early changes usually are inferred from those found at autopsy or are found in the course of examination for other disease. The limited response on the part of the peripheral nerve, however, places many disorders in relatively uniform categories of structural change. In all of these nonneoplastic disorders, the changes in the axons and myelin sheaths are those of swelling and fragmentation and eventual loss of the myelin sheath at that level. A mild to moderate reactive fibrosis is part of the response about the affected fibers. With continued injury, the degenerative changes may progress toward the perikaryon. Early, one may find a mononuclear response with lipid-containing phagocytes in the areas of damage. With the most severe states of sensory nerve involvement, axonal degeneration may be seen in the cells of the spinal ganglia (central chromatolysis) and with accompanying satellitosis and even neuronophagia.

Cysts of spinal ganglia[62]

Although of frequent occurrence, cysts of the spinal ganglia are only rarely symptomatic. It has been assumed that they result from the cerebrospinal fluid pressure exerted upon the sleeves of pia-arachnoid that accompany the nerves as they exit toward the intervertebral spaces. When the fine porous openings in the pia-arachnoid through which the nerve fibers course become narrowed, perhaps as a result of scarring, the cerebrospinal fluid pressure, increased by the long periods of upright position in man, becomes more effective in bulging the walls of this funnel-like space. This results in the formation of a cyst whose distal outer wall often is in the proximal portion of the spinal ganglion. When clinically symptomatic, it is thought to be due to the effect of the pressure upon the included nerve fibers.

Metastatic cancer to spinal ganglia and peripheral nerves

The spinal ganglia, like all living tissue of the body, can be expected to be the site for metastatic disease (Fig. 42-118). In the only prospective postmortem study, the spinal ganglia were involved in 2% of all patients with

carcinoma that had separately metastasized to the central nervous system as well.[43] It was recognized that this must have represented a minimal involvement since usually one ganglion and rarely more than two ganglia were examined in this study.

Involvement of the peripheral nerve by metastatic cancer has been reported on many occasions. This is particularly true in certain cancers, such as those of the prostate, urinary bladder, and cervix, where their mode of spread is thought to be through the perineural lymphatic spaces.

Spinal ganglia and peripheral nerves frequently are involved in patients with a lymphoma, leukemia (Fig. 42-119), or multiple myeloma.[61] The lack of clinical recognition, as with the carcinoma, is probably related to the more pressing and more symptomatic involvement of other tissues.

Amyloidosis

Amyloidosis, with the exception of familial cases, is a late and uncommon complication of those diseases with which generalized amyloid deposition is to be expected. It is characterized by hyaline eosinophilic balls between nerve fibers in the spinal ganglia (Fig. 42-120) and in the peripheral nerves (Fig. 42-121). A relation to blood vessel walls is not

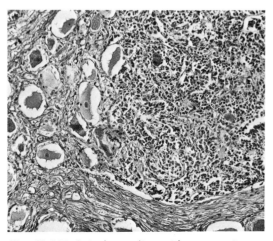

Fig. 42-118 Spinal ganglion with metastatic carcinoma from prostate. (Hematoxylin-eosin; ×180.)

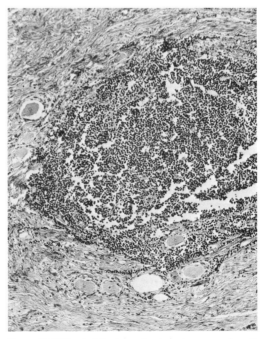

Fig. 42-119 Infiltrate of chronic granulocytic leukemia in spinal ganglion. (Hematoxylin-eosin; ×90.)

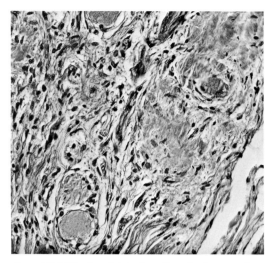

Fig. 42-120 Amyloidosis of spinal ganglion. (Hematoxylin-eosin; ×280.)

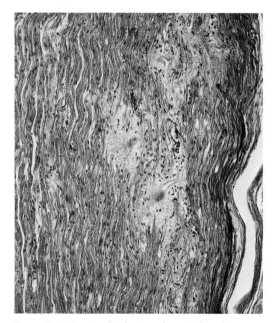

Fig. 42-121 Amyloidosis of peripheral nerve. (Hematoxylin-eosin; ×90.)

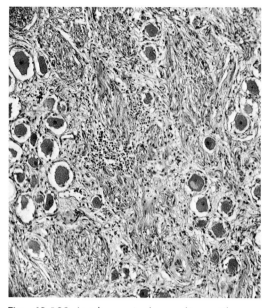

Fig. 42-122 Lumbar spinal ganglion with non-specific focal chronic inflammation. (Hematoxylin-eosin; ×90.)

always apparent. Typical deposition in the walls of smaller blood vessels also is seen. Familial cases of amyloidosis have been described as occurring in certain Portuguese families, possibly due to genetic causes.

Hemorrhage

Hemorrhage into the proximal half of the dorsal root ganglion is not uncommon. Most frequently, it represents extension of sub-arachnoid hemorrhage in the pia-arachnoid sleeve that surrounds the peripheral rootlets. In most instances, the blood appears to finally escape along the usual channels of cerebro-spinal fluid flow. In some, the blood becomes locally organized. The hemoglobin is converted to hemosiderin and hematoidin, and there is a moderate degree of reactive fibrosis. In our material, none of the hemorrhages were recognized as clinically symptomatic.

Inflammation

Nonspecific inflammatory changes in the spinal ganglia and peripheral nerves are not uncommon (Fig. 42-122). These changes are characterized by cellular infiltrates, predominantly lymphocytic, and sometimes by degenerative changes in the axons and in the myelin sheaths. Abnormalities of this type were seen in approximately 5% of routine autopsies in a general city hospital. The lesions appear to be nonspecific and related more to a general state of the body than to a disease specifically affecting the nervous system. In most instances, there was no clinical recognition of such involvement. When severe and limited to the rootlets, sometimes with involvement of the spinal cord, the Landry-Guillain-Barré syndrome results.

In herpes zoster infection, the changes and the inflammatory responses are marked. The affected spinal ganglia may be swollen and red due to the marked necrosis with hemorrhage, which simulates a hemorrhagic infarct (Figs. 42-123 and 42-124). Changes in the motor

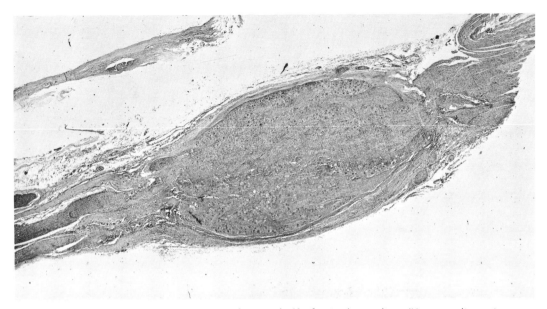

Fig. 42-123 Herpes zoster. Necrosis of upper half of spinal ganglion. (Hematoxylin-eosin; ×8.)

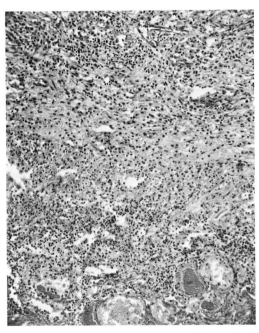

Fig. 42-124 Herpes zoster. Necrosis of upper half of spinal ganglion. (Hematoxylin-eosin; ×90.)

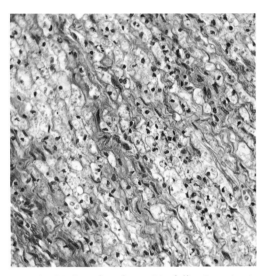

Fig. 42-125 Peripheral neuritis following vincristine therapy. (Hematoxylin-eosin; ×280.)

component result in damage to the motor neurons with satellitosis and neuronophagia of the anterior horn cells at that level.

The peripheral nervous system is, of course, involved in all varieties of inflammatory disease, including the purulent, granulomatous, and viral diseases, the collagen diseases, and sometimes following chemotherapy[86, 144] (Fig. 42-125).

Vascular disease

Degenerative vascular disease such as seen in patients with atherosclerosis and with diabetes frequently affects the peripheral nervous system. Infarction of the spinal ganglia must be exceedingly rare, never having been recognized in our series of over 10,000 ganglia. Involvement of both sensory and motor nerves is, however, very common, particularly in the lower limbs of diabetic patients.[163, 164]

A neuropathy due to focal areas of degeneration in the peripheral nervous system has been seen in 16% of patients with diabetes mellitus in the fifth decade of life and in 37% of those in the seventh decade. The clinical and structural appearance of pseudotabes due to wallerian degeneration secondary to changes in the peripheral nervous system also has been described in diabetic patients. Involvement of the peripheral nerves and perhaps also the intermediolateral columns of the spinal cord is probably an important factor in the development of the Charcot joints in patients with diabetes.

Pressure

Constant and prolonged pressure upon the peripheral nerve can lead to structural as well as functional changes. The larger fibers are the most susceptible. The myelin sheaths are damaged first, followed by changes in the axon. Initially, there is fragmentation of the myelin sheaths, followed by the chemical changes characteristic of myelin destruction. When the axons are damaged, they become swollen and fragmented. Both are removed by macrophages. Wallerian degeneration follows. Recovery is related to the reconstitution of the axons followed by the formation of the surrounding myelin. Dependent upon the degree of damage and the degree of fibrosis, recovery may take weeks or months.

Nutritional deficiencies

A peripheral neuropathy related to vitamin B_1 deficiency has been described frequently. The changes affect the distalmost portion of the fibers first, with a progressive dying back of the central portion of the neuron. The nerve cells appear to remain intact. The axons and myelin sheaths undergo swelling and fragmentation, followed by phagocytosis and removal. Recovery follows the pattern previously described for nerve fiber regeneration.

Toxic disorders

Segmental demyelination involving both sensory and motor nerves has been described in the peripheral nervous system in patients with diphtheria, with heavy metal poisoning (lead and arsenic), and with porphyria.

Peroneal muscular atrophy (Charcot-Marie-Tooth disease)

Peroneal muscular atrophy is a heredofamilial disease with degenerative changes beginning in the distalmost portion of the peroneal nerve. The fibers that lead to the small muscles of the foot are affected first. As the disease progresses, the lesions affect more and more of the peripheral nerve to structurally include the cells of the spinal ganglia and anterior horn cells of the spinal cord. In some instances, the posterior columns also demonstrate secondary wallerian degeneration. Proliferation of the connective tissue around the residual axis-cylinders of the peripheral nerve can produce an appearance structurally similar to that seen in hypertrophic interstitial neuropathy (Dejerine-Sottas disease).

In some of the patients with peroneal muscular atrophy, other members of the family have exhibited diseases suggestive of Friedreich's ataxia as well as peroneal muscular atrophy, whereas in others, only a few muscles of the lower leg may be affected.

Dejerine-Sottas disease (hypertrophic interstitial radiculoneuropathy)[150]

Hypertrophic interstitial neuropathy of Dejerine-Sottas is a rare disorder resulting in enlargement of the sensory and motor nerves. It is characterized microscopically by the presence of concentric rings of connective tissue forming an onionskin-like layering about the peripheral axis-cylinder (Fig. 42-126). Formerly considered to be a specific reaction, at the present time it is not known if the

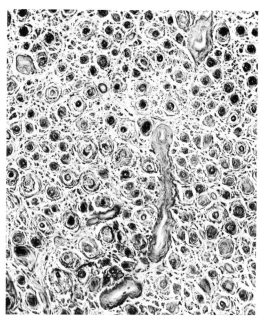

Fig. 42-126 Dejerine-Sottas disease. (Hematoxylin-eosin; ×90.)

proliferation of the connective tissue represents a genetic response or is evidence of excessive regeneration.

Neoplasms

Neoplasms of the peripheral nervous system, except those of the eighth cranial nerve, are unusual. They are seen more commonly in patients with Recklinghausen's disease, in whom neurilemomas or neurofibromas or diffuse hyperplasias of a portion of the peripheral nervous system (usually confined to a limb) are seen. The appearances of these tumors are identical with those described for the peripheral nerves attached to the brain and spinal cord.

■ Skeletal muscle
Structure

Skeletal (striate; voluntary) muscle fibers are long multinucleate cells enclosed by the sarcolemma (plasma membrane). The sarcoplasm (cytoplasm) contains sarcoplasmic myofibrils that parallel the long axis of the fiber. Striations that are perpendicular to the long axis of the muscle fiber are due to the alignment of different parts of the myofibrils that have differing indices of refraction. Two of the bands visible with the light microscope are the anisotropic A band and the isotropic I band. In the middle of the I band is a thin, slightly darker zone, the Z band or disc. Other bands in the A zone, the H and M, are not visible with the light microscope. The structural unit of the muscle fiber, the sarcomere, extends between two Z bands. With electron microscopy, the myofibril is found to be formed by two types of smaller units, the myofilaments, one thicker than the other. The remainder of the sarcoplasm is filled by the smooth endoplasmic reticulum, pinocytic vesicles, mitochondria, glycogen, lipids, etc. All are best seen with electron microscopy. In the aging muscle, increasing amounts of lipofuscin pigment lie adjacent to the normally peripheral nuclei. Surrounding each muscle fiber is a thin connective tissue sheath consisting of fine reticulin fibers, the endomysium. Groups of fibers of varying numbers form fasciculi that are surrounded by slightly greater amounts of connective tissue, the perimysium. The whole muscle, composed of numbers of fasciculi, is enclosed by the epimysium. This is associated with the muscle attachments to fascia and tendons. The arrangement of this supporting tissue is such as to permit normal contraction and relaxation and to prevent overstretching.

Each muscle is supplied by one or more motor nerves originating from one or more levels of the spinal cord. On entering the muscle, an axon of each motor nerve divides into many branches, thereby supplying many fibers through the development of motor end-plates. These are present on the surfaces of the innervated muscle fibers. The motor cell, its axon, and the muscle fibers supplied by its branches form the motor unit.

The normal range of cross-section diameters of skeletal muscle fibers in the adult varies from 20μ for the extraocular muscles up to 100μ for muscles of the thigh. In children, the averages vary from 10μ to 20μ shortly after birth to reach adult sizes between the ages of 15 and 20 years.

Atrophy and degeneration

With disuse atrophy, the whole muscle becomes soft and flabby and decreases in size due to loss of sarcoplasm. This predominantly affects the fibers of medium and larger sizes and is accompanied by a significant loss of strength of sustained contraction. Exercise producing near maximal muscle contraction, on the other hand, results in muscle hypertrophy. Muscle fiber enlargement is limited when the fibers approach a 50% increase in diameter and a 300% increase of contractual power.

The state and size of a skeletal muscle fiber depend entirely upon its motor innervation. Neural (denervation) atrophy of muscle follows loss of nerve supply to the muscle. In disuse atrophy, seen with immobilization, cachexia, and advanced age, all the muscles of a limb or of the entire body are equally affected. Atrophy associated with lesions of one or more motor units, on the other hand, is limited to the muscles of the affected motor units (Fig. 42-127).

Initially and for several weeks, no visible changes may be recognized with light microscopy or grossly. A decrease in size and angulation of the normally polygonal fibers usually can be recognized after a month of paralysis and is definite in two months. The decrease in size is due to loss of sarcoplasm and of the myofibrils. This is accompanied by a relative or absolute increase in muscle nuclei. On cross section, with special stains and sometimes with routine stains, a faint "target" fiber appearance with three faint concentric zones of staining reactivity is seen centrally:

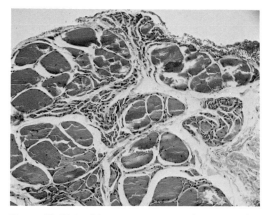

Fig. 42-127 Neurogenic muscular atrophy. (Hematoxylin-eosin; ×90.)

the compact central zone of myofibrils, an intermediate zone of lesser myofibrillar material, and an outer zone, which is least affected, surrounding the other two zones. Cross and linear striations usually persist until the muscles have the appearance of shrunken sarcolemmal tubes. At this time, there are linear rows or clumps of small darkly stained nuclei. Fragmentation and death of the affected muscle cell are followed by a slight lymphocytic infiltration and fat replacement and eventual fibrosis. At this stage, differentiation from advanced dystrophies is no longer possible. These structural changes are associated with the persistence and even a limited degree of hypertrophy of adjacent and sometimes contained muscle fibers belonging to other motor units.

Inflammatory disease (myositis)

Inflammations of skeletal muscle may be the result of direct invasion or metastatic spread by a variety of bacteria, parasites, fungi, spirochetes, and viruses, by physical agents such as heat, cold, and mechanical trauma, by exertion,[87] and by chemical toxins and in endocrine disorders. In a significant group such as sarcoidosis,[147] the cause is not known.

The bacterial myositides are not common and are almost always due to direct implantation or invasion—metastatic localization is rare. The affected skeletal muscle exhibits the functional and the gross and microscopic characteristics of any inflamed tissue. Within the reddened, swollen, and painful area, the muscle has undergone variable degrees of coagulation necrosis. The cellular response during the acute phase is primarily neutrophilic. In the later stages, with an adequate general and local response aided by therapy, there is a gradual cell replacement by lymphocytes, monocytes, and histiocytes. Healing is accompanied by fibrosis and often by hypertrophy of some adjacent muscle fibers.

The rare skeletal muscle abscess begins with liquefaction necrosis and neutrophilic infiltration, followed by encapsulation by vascular pyogenic granulation tissue, and, with healing, by a dense local scar.

Further discussions of specific inflammatory diseases of muscle may be found with the discussions of the various general diseases.

Muscular dystrophy

The muscular dystrophies represent a group of primary hereditary and ordinarily progressive disorders of unknown cause that affect the skeletal muscles. The diseases usually have their onset during childhood or early adolescence and more often affect proximal muscles.

The gross appearance of the muscle depends upon the type of dystrophy and the stage of the disease. Early, there may be a minimal degree of hypertrophy and a general but slight pallor. With progression of the disease, there is a gradual conversion to a yellow or white appearance that accompanies the increasing amount of fat (lipomatosis) or fibrous tissue.

The dystrophies, as a group, are characterized microscopically by a random increase in variability of muscle fiber size (best recognized in cross section). Some fibers, occurring singly or in groups of two or three, are unusually small (12μ to 15μ), whereas others are particularly large (up to 200μ). Central nuclear migration with an apparent increase in number of nuclei is a frequent and early finding in these larger fibers (Fig. 42-128). Hyaline eosinophilic granularity and vacuolization are among the early sarcoplasmic changes. Lipomatosis (fatty infiltration) exceeding that of simple muscle replacement is an active process that, in some forms of dystrophy, produced the clinical appearance of limb muscle hypertrophy (Fig. 42-128). An increase in connective tissue, beginning in the endomysium, often accompanies the fatty infiltration. In some, it not only replaces many fibers, but also may surround and isolate others as it extends into the perimysial and epimysial areas. There may be small clusters of regenerating muscle cells scattered throughout. These are recognized by their basophilic sarcoplasm and by the slightly enlarged and hyperchromatic nuclei. Many of

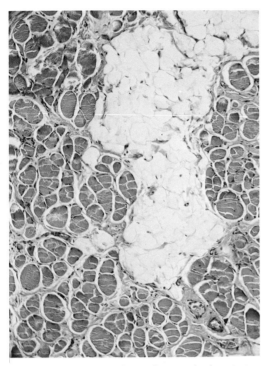

Fig. 42-128 Muscular dystrophy. Marked variation in size of muscle fibers with fat replacement (lipomatosis). (Hematoxylin-eosin; ×90.)

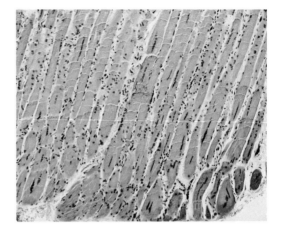

Fig. 42-129 Muscular dystrophy. Marked central nuclear migration. (Hematoxylin-eosin; ×90.)

the early and mild changes are to be found in the asymptomatic relatives of a patient with a dystrophy. A perivascular inflammatory cell infiltrate composed of lymphocytes and large mononuclear macrophages is uncommon and, in all probability, represents a limited response to the presence of necrotic muscle fibers. In the far-advanced disease with the loss of muscle fibers and the presence of fat cells and fibrous tissue, the appearance simulates the end stage of neural atrophy. No changes have been described in the central and peripheral nervous systems.

Various classifications of this group of disorders have been based upon the distribution of the affected muscles, the mode of inheritance, and the age of onset. Among the more common of the dystrophies are (1) childhood (Duchenne; pseudohypertrophic), (2) the fascioscapulohumeral type (mild restricted adult form, and (3) myotonic dystrophy. In each, there appears to be a tendency toward the accentuation of one or more of the described structural changes. In the Duchenne type (pseudohypertrophic), all of the described changes may be seen with an unusual accumulation of fat (Fig. 42-128). In this form, a mild degree of myocardial fibrosis also

has been described. In the restricted mild form, fibrosis with contraction is prominent, and there is little muscle hypertrophy. In myotonic dystrophy, there is distal muscle involvement, and central nuclear migration in the form of long rows is especially characteristic (Fig. 42-129). This form is associated with frontal baldness. cataracts, and testicular atrophy due to fibrosis of the tubules and cardiac involvement.

With the help of electron microscopy, new forms of rare skeletal muscle disease have been recognized. These include nemaline myopathy, initially described as a nonprogressive congenital muscle weakness that affects primarily the proximal muscle groups. Its name is derived from the characteristic threadlike rods that represent Z band material.[105, 151] More recently, a late onset in adults has been described.[97] In 1956, Shy and Magee[180] presented the first report of a familial myopathy—central core disease. Since then, other cases have been recorded. In this disease, there is a failure of conversion of phosphorylase B to phosphorylase A. Structurally, every affected fiber contains a darker eosinophilic core composed of closely opposed fibrils. More recently, other skeletal muscle diseases with abnormal mitochondria have been recognized.[55, 78, 197] The enlarged and increased numbers of mitochondria are called megaconial and pleoconial, respectively. Although best seen with electron microscopy, numerous small eosinophilic granules may be seen in focal areas of the affected fibers. This rapidly expanding list also includes the diseases of carbohydrate metabolism, disturbances of electrolytes,[136, 137] and many others.[119, 178]

REFERENCES

1 Adams, R. D.: In Wright, I. S., chairman, and Millikan, C. H., editor: Cerebral vascular diseases, New York, 1958, Grune & Stratton, Inc., pp. 23-39 (brain infarcts).

2 Adams, R. D., and Foley, J. M.: Ass. Res. Nerv. Ment. Dis. Proc. **32:**198-237, 1953 (neurologic disorder associated with liver disease).

3 Adams, R. D., and Richardson, E. P., Jr.: In Folch-Pi, J., editor: Chemical pathology of the nervous system, New York, 1961, Pergamon Press, Inc., pp. 163-194 (demyelinating diseases).

4 Adams, R. D., Cammermeyer, J., and Denny-Brown, D.: J. Neuropath. Exp. Neurol. **8:**1-29, 1949 (necrotizing hemorrhagic encephalopathy).

5 Alexander, L.: Amer. J. Path. **16:**61-70, 1940 (Wernicke's disease).

6 Alexander, W. S.: Arch. Neurol. Psychiat. (Chicago) **62:**73-81, 1949 (purulent leptomeningitis).

7 Alpers, B. J., and Yaskin, J. C.: Arch. Neurol. Psychiat (Chicago) **41:**435-459, 1939 (gliomas of pons).

8 Andrew, W.: J. Chronic Dis. **3:**575-596, 1956 (aging).

8a Andrews, J. M., Cancilla, P. A., Grippo, J., and Menkes, J. H.: Neurology (Minneap.) **21:**337-352, 1971 (globoid cell leukodystrophy).

9 Arey, J. B.: J. Pediat. **40:**621-625, 1952 (cerebral palsy)

10 Asenjo, A., Valladores, H., and Fierro, J.: Arch. Neurol. Psychiat. (Chicago) **65:**146-160, 1951 (tuberculoma).

11 Aström, K. E., and Mancall, E. L., and Richardson, E. P., Jr.: Brain **81:**93-111, 1958 (leukoencephalopathy).

12 Auerbach, O.: Amer. Rev. Tuberc. **64:**419-429, 1951 (tuberculous meningitis).

13 Bailey, A. A.: Arch. Neurol. Psychiat. (Chicago) **70:**299-309, 1953 (aging in spinal cord).

14 Bailey, P.: Arch. Surg. (Chicago) **18:**1359-1402, 1929 (leptomeningeal sarcoma).

15 Bailey, P.: In Penfield, W., editor: Cytology and cellular pathology of the nervous system, vol. 2, New York, 1932, Paul B. Hoeber, Inc., p. 903 (cellular types in primary tumors of brain).

16 Bailey, P., and Bucy, P. C.: J. Path. Bact. **32:**735-751, 1929 (oligodendroglioma).

17 Bailey, P., and Cushing, H.: Arch. Neurol. Psychiat. (Chicago) **14:**192-224, 1925.

18 Bailey, P., and Cushing, H.: A classification of the tumors of the glioma group on a histogenetic basis with a correlated study of prognosis, Philadelphia, 1926, J. B. Lippincott Co.

19 Baker, A. B.: Arch. Path. (Chicago) **26:**535-559, 1938 (subdural hematoma).

20 Baker, A. B.: J. Neuropath. Exp. Neurol. **6:**253-264, 1947 (lymphocytic choriomeningitis).

21 Baker, A. B.: J. Neuropath. Exp. Neurol. **8:**283-294, 1949 (nervous system in hepatic disease).

22 Baker, G. S., Kernohan, J. W., and Kiefer, E. J.: Surg. Clin. N. Amer. **31:**1143-1145, 1951 (metastatic tumors of brain).

23 Barnett, H. J. M., and Hyland, H. H.: Brain **76:**36-49, 1953 (intracranial venous thrombosis).

24 Bassett, R. C., and Lemmen, L. J.: J. Neurosurg. **11:**135-142, 1954 (intracranial aneurysms).

25 Bearn, A. G., and Kunkel, A. G.: J. Clin. Invest. **33:**400-409, 1954 (Wilson's disease).

26 Beller, A. J., and Peyser, E.: J. Neurosurg. **9:**291-298, 1952 (extradural cerebellar hematoma).

27 Benda, C. E.: Developmental disorders of mentation and cerebral palsies, New York, 1952, Grune & Stratton, Inc.

28 Bickers, D. S., and Adams, R. D.: Brain **72:** 246-262, 1949 (hydrocephalus).

29 Black, B. K., and Smith, D. E.: Arch. Neurol. Psychiat. (Chicago) **64:**614-630, 1950 (nasal glioma).

30 Blackwood, W.: In Cerebral lipoidoses; a symposium (L. van Bogaert, chairman), Springfield, Ill., 1957, Charles C Thomas, Publisher, p. 19.

31 Bodian, D.: In Poliomyelitis: papers and discussions of the first International Poliomyelitis Conference, Philadelphia, 1949, J. B. Lippincott Co., p. 62 (poliomyelitis; pathologic anatomy).

32 Boykin, F. C., Cowen, D., Iannucci, C. A. J., and Wolf, A.: J. Neuropath. Exp. Neurol. **13:** 30-49, 1954 (astrocytoma).

32a Brady, R. O.: Ann. Rev. Med. **21:**317-334, 1970 (cerebral lipoidoses).

32b Brady, R. O., Kanfer, J. N., Bradley, R. M., and Shapiro, D.: J. Clin. Invest. **45:**1112-1115, 1966 (Gaucher's disease).

33 Bucy, P. C., and Thieman, P. W.: Arch. Neurol. (Chicago) **18:**14-19, 1968 (astrocytomas of cerebellum).

34 Cannon, B. W.: Arch. Neurol. Psychiat. (Chicago) **66:**687-696, 1951 (vascular lesions of brain stem).

35 Cantor, M. B., and Stein, J. M.: J. Nerv. Ment. Dis. **115:**351-355, 1952 (spinal cord metastasis).

36 Carpenter, M. B., and Druckemiller, W. H.: Arch. Neurol. Psychiat. (Chicago) **69:**305-322, 1953 (agenesis of corpus callosum).

37 Carpenter, S.: Neurology (Minneap.) **18:**841-851, 1968 (motor neuron disease).

38 Chason, J. L.: J. Neuropath. Exp. Neurol. **15:** 461-470, 1956 (subependymal mixed gliomas).

39 Chason, J. L.: Radiology **70:**811-814, 1958 (cerebral infarction).

39a Chason, J. L., and Dickenman, R. C.: Unpublished data (inflammations of spinal ganglia).

40 Chason, J. L., and Hindman, W. M.: Neurology (Minneap.) **8:**41-44, 1958 (berry aneurysms).

41 Chason, J. L., Landers, J. W., and Gonzalez, J. E.: J. Neurol. Neurosurg. Psychiat. **27:**317-325, 1964 (pontine myelinolysis).

42 Chason, J. L., Mahoney, W. F., and Landers, J. W.: Minn. Med. **49:**27-31, 1966 (intracerebral hemorrhage).

43 Chason, J. L., Walker, F. B., and Landers, J. W.: Cancer **16:**781-787, 1963 (metastatic carcinoma).

44 Chason, J. L., Haddad, B. F., Webster, J. E.,

and Gurdjian, E. S.: J. Neuropath. Exp. Neurol. **16:**102-107, 1957 (intracranial pressure).

45 Chason, J. L., Hardy, W. G., Webster, J. E., and Gurdjian, E. S.: J. Neurosurg. **15:**135-139, 1958 (concussion).

46 Chason, J. L., Fernando, O. U., Hodgson, V. R., Thomas, L. M., and Gurdjian, E. S.: J. Trauma **6:**767-779, 1966 (concussion).

47 Cohen, S. M.: J. Mount Sinai Hosp. N. Y. **16:**214-230, 1949 (hemorrhage).

48 Cole, F. M., and Yates, P.: Brain **90:**759-768, 1967 (microaneurysms).

49 Cole, F. M., and Yates, P. O.: J. Neurol. Neurosurg. Psychiat. **30:**61-66, 1967 (cerebral hemorrhage).

50 Courville, C. B.: Bull. Los Angeles Neurol. Soc. **15:**99-128, 1950 (cerebral anoxia).

51 Cowen, D., and Geller, L. M.: J. Neuropath. Exp. Neurol. **19:**488-527, 1960 (prenatal x-irradiation).

52 Crigler, J. F., Jr., and Najjar, V. A.: Pediatrics **10:**169-179, 1952 (kernicterus).

53 Cuneo, H. M.: Bull. Los Angeles Neurol. Soc. **16:**162-173, 1951 (brain abscess).

54 Cushing, H., and Eisenhardt, L.: Meningiomas; their classification, regional behaviour, life history and surgical end results, Springfield, Ill., 1938, Charles C Thomas, Publisher.

55 D'Agostino, A. N., Ziter, R. A., Rallison, M. L., and Bray, P. F.: Arch. Neurol. (Chicago) **18:**388-401, 1968 (familial myopathy).

56 Dal Santo, G.: In Harmel, M. H., editor: Clinical anesthesia; neurologic considerations, Philadelphia, 1967, F. A. Davis Co. ("blood-brain barrier": pathology and importance in anesthesia).

57 Daube, J. R., and Chou, S. M.: Neurology (Minneap.) **16:**179-191, 1966 (lissencephaly).

58 Davies, J.: Human developmental anatomy, New York, 1963, The Ronald Press Co.

58a Dayan, A. D., Marshall, A. H. E., Miller, A. A., Pick, F. J., and Ramkin, N. E.: J. Path. Bact. **92:**1-29, 1966 (pinealomas).

59 DeMyer, W.: Neurology (Minneap.) **14:**806-808, 1964 (vinblastine-induced malformations).

60 Denny-Brown, D.: The basal ganglia and their relation to disorders of movements, London, 1962, Oxford University Press.

60a Desnick, R. J., Dawson, G., Desnick, S. J., Sweeley, C. C., and Krivit, W.: New Eng. J. Med. **284:**739-744, 1971 (glycosphingolipoidoses).

61 Dickenman, R. C., and Chason, J. L.: Amer. J. Path. **34:**349-361, 1958 (dorsal root ganglia).

62 Dickenman, R. C., and Chason, J. L.: Arch. Path. (Chicago) **77:**366-369, 1964 (cysts of dorsal root ganglia).

63 Dinsdale, H.: Arch. Neurol. (Chicago) **10:**200-217, 1964 (hemorrhage in posterior fossa).

64 Du Boulay, G. H.: Brit. J. Radiol. **38:**721-757, 1965 (intracranial aneurysms).

65 Dyck, P. J., and Gomez, M. R.: Mayo Clin. Proc. **43:**280-296, 1968 (Dejerine-Sottas disease).

66 Earle, K. M.: J. Neuropath. Exp. Neurol. **13:**448-454, 1954 (intracranial tumors).

67 Earle, K. M.: J. Neuropath. Exp. Neurol. **27:**1-14, 1968 (Parkinson's disease).

68 Elizan, T. S., Ajero-Froehlich, L., Fabiyi, A., Ley, A., and Sever, J. L.: Arch. Neurol. (Chicago) **20:**115-119, 1969 (malformations of central nervous system).

69 Ellington, E., and Margolis, G.: J. Neurosurg. **30:**651-657, 1969 (subarachnoid hemorrhage).

69a Evans, H. S., and Courville, C. B.: Arch. Surg. (Chicago) **36:**637-659, 1938 (tuberculosis of central nervous system).

70 Fawcett, F. J., and Smith, W. T.: Postgrad. Med. J. **42:**5-15, 1966 (strokes).

71 Feigin, I., and Goebel, H.: Neurology (Minneap.) **19:**749-759, 1969 (necrotizing encephalopathy).

72 Feigin, I., and Popoff, N.: Arch. Neurol. (Chicago) **6:**151-160, 1962 (cerebral edema).

73 Feigin, I., and Popoff, N.: J. Neuropath. Exp. Neurol. **22:**500-511, 1963 (cerebral edema).

74 Feigin, I., and Wolf, A.: J. Pediat. **45:**243-263, 1954 (Wernicke's encephalopathy).

75 Feldman, H. A.: New Eng. J. Med. **279:**1431-1437, 1968 (toxoplasmosis).

76 Ferraro, A., Arieti, S., and English, W. H.: J. Neuropath. Exp. Neurol. **4:**217-239, 1945 (cerebral changes in pernicious anemia).

77 Fisher, C. M.: Neurology (Minneap.) **15:**774-784, 1965 (cerebral infarcts).

78 Fisher, E. R., and Danowski, T. S.: Amer. J. Clin. Path. **51:**619-630, 1969 (mitochondrial myopathy).

79 Fokes, E. C., Jr., and Earle, K. M.: J. Neurosurg. **30:**585-594, 1969 (ependymoma).

80 Foley, J. M., and Baxter, D.: J. Neuropath. Exp. Neurol. **17:**586-598, 1958 (pigment granules).

81 Forbus, W. D.: Bull. Johns Hopkins Hosp. **47:**239-284, 1930 (miliary aneurysms).

82 Freytag, E.: J. Neurol. Neurosurg. Psychiat. **31:**616-620, 1968 (intracerebral hematoma).

83 Gibbs, C. J., Jr.: Curr. Top. Microbiol. Immun. **40:**44-58, 1967 (search for infectious etiology in chronic and subacute degenerative diseases of central nervous system).

84 Gibbs, C. J., Jr., Gajdusek, D. C., Asher, D. M., Alpers, M. P., Beck, E., and Daniel, P. M.: Science **161:**388-389, 1968 (Jakob-Creutzfeldt disease).

85 Globus, J. H.: Ass. Res. Nerv. Ment. Dis. Proc. **18:**438-470, 1938 (cerebral hemorrhage).

86 Gottschalk, P. G., Dyck, P. J., and Kiely, J. M.: Neurology (Minneap.) **18:**875-882, 1968 (alkaloid neuropathy).

87 Greenberg, J., and Arneson, L.: Neurology (Minneap.) **17:**216-222, 1967 (rhabdomyolysis).

88 Greene, H. L., Hug, G., and Schubert, W. K.: Arch. Neurol. (Chicago) **20:**147-153, 1969 (leukodystrophy).

89 Greenfield, J. G.: Brain **62:**129-152, 1939 (cerebral edema).

90 Greenfield, J. G.: The spinocerebellar degenerations, Springfield, Ill., 1954, Charles C Thomas, Publisher.

91 Greenfield, J. G., and Bosanquet, F. D.: J. Neurol. Neurosurg. Psychiat. **16:**213-226, 1953 (parkinsonism).

92 Greenhouse, A. H., and Schneck, S. A.: Neurology (Minneap.) **18:**1-8, 1968 (necrotizing encephalomyelopathy).

93 de Grood, M. P. A. M.: Arch. Chir. Neerl. **3**:128-138, 1951 (subdural empyema).

94 Hamburger, V.: J. Cell. Comp. Physiol. **60** (suppl. 1):81-92, 1962 (neurogenesis).

95 Hamby, W. B.: Intracranial aneurysms, Springfield, Ill., 1952, Charles C Thomas, Publisher.

96 Haymaker, W., Margolis, C., Pentschew, A., Jacob, H., Lindenberg, R., Arroyo, L. S., Stockdorph, O., and Stowens, D.: Kernicterus and its importance in cerebral palsy, Springfield, Ill., 1961, Charles C Thomas, Publisher.

96a Heard, B. E., Hassan, A. M., and Wilson, S.: J. Clin. Path. **15**:17-20, 1962 (cytomegalic inclusion disease).

97 Heffernan, L. P., Rewcastle, N. B., and Humphrey, J. G.: Arch. Neurol. (Chicago) **18**:529-542, 1968 (rod myopathies).

98 Herndon, R. M., and Rubinstein, L. J.: Neurology (Minneap.) **18**:8-20, 1968 (Dawson's encephalitis).

99 Hess, A.: J. Comp. Neurol. **98**:69-91, 1953 (ground substance of central nervous system).

100 Hicks, S. P.: Arch. Path. (Chicago) **57**:363-378, 1954 (radiation anencephaly).

101 Hirano, A., and Zimmerman, H. M.: Arch. Neurol. (Chicago) **7**:227-242, 1962 (Alzheimer's neurofibrillary changes).

102 Hitchcock, E., and Andreadis, A.: J. Neurol. Neurosurg. Psychiat. **27**:422-434, 1964 (subdural empyema).

103 Horsfall, F. L., Jr.: Proc. Mayo Clin. **35**:269-282, 1960 (viral infection).

104 Hsieh, H.: Neurology (Minneap.) **17**:752-762, 1967 (cerebrovascular disease).

105 Hudgson, P., Gardner-Medwin, D., Fulthorpe, J. J., and Walton, J. N.: Neurology (Minneap.) **17**:1125-1142, 1967 (nemaline myopathy).

106 Hughes, J. T., and Brownell, B.: Neurology (Minneap.) **14**:1073-1077, 1964 (cervical spondylosis).

107 Hughes, W.: Lancet **2**:19-21, 1965 (origin of lacunes).

108 Hurst, E. W.: Med. J. Aust. **2**:1-6, 1941 (hemorrhagic leukoencephalitis).

109 Inglis, K.: Amer. J. Path. **30**:739-755, 1954 (tuberous sclerosis).

110 Jervis, S. A.: In Folch-Pi, J., editor: Chemical pathology of the nervous system, New York, 1961, Pergamon Press, Inc.

111 Johnson, R. T., and Mims, C. A.: New Eng. J. Med. **278**:23-30, 84-92, 1968 (viral infections).

111a Julius, R., Buehler, B., Aylsworth, A., St. Petry, L., Rennert, O., and Greer, M.: Neurology (Minneap.) **21**:15-18, 1971 (metachromatic leukodystrophy).

112 Kahn, E. A.: J. Neurosurg. **4**:191-199, 1947 (lateral sclerosis).

112a Källén, B., and Levan, A.: In Tedeschi, C. G., editor: Neuropathology methods and diagnosis, Boston, 1970, Little, Brown and Co., pp. 558-559 (mongolism).

113 Kane, W., and Aronson, S. M.: Acta Neuropath. (Berlin) **9**:273-279, 1967 (cerebellar medulloblastoma).

114 Katz, M., Rorke, L. B., Masland, W. S., Koprowski, H., and Tucker, S. H.: New Eng. J. Med. **279**:793-798, 1968 (sclerosing panencephalitis).

115 Kernohan, J. W., and Fletcher-Kernohan, E. M.: Ass. Res. Nerv. Ment. Dis. Proc. **16**:182-209, 1935 (ependymoma).

116 Kernohan, J. W., and Uihlein, A.: Sarcomas of the brain, Springfield, Ill., 1962, Charles C Thomas, Publisher.

117 Kernohan, J. W., and Woltman, H. W.: Arch. Neurol. Psychiat. (Chicago) **24**:274-287, 1929 (brain tumor).

118 Kernohan, J. W., Mabon, R. F., Svien, H. J., and Adson, A. W.: Proc. Staff Meet. Mayo Clin. **24**:71-75, 1949 (gliomas).

119 Kinoshita, M., and Codman, T. E.: Arch. Neurol. (Chicago) **18**:265-271, 1968 (myotubular myopathy).

120 Klintworth, G. K.: Amer. J. Path. **53**:391-408, 1968 (secondary brain stem hemorrhages).

121 Koenig, R. S., and Koenig, H.: J. Neuropath. Exp. Neurol. **11**:69-78, 1952 (postmortem alterations in neurons).

121a Kolodny, E. H., Brady, R. O., and Volk, B. W.: Biochem. Biophys. Res. Commun. **37**:526-531, 1969 (Tay-Sachs disease).

122 Kramer, R., and Som, M. L.: Arch. Otolaryng. (Chicago) **32**:744-770, 1940 (intracranial pathways of infections).

123 Lagos, J. C., and Gomez, M. R.: Mayo Clin. Proc. **42**:26-49, 1967 (tuberous sclerosis).

124 Lander, H.: J. Path. Bact. **70**:157-165, 1955 (hemorrhagic leukoencephalitis).

125 Landers, J. W., Chason, J. L., and Samuel, V. N.: Neurology (Minneap.) **15**:968-971, 1965 (pontine myelinolysis).

126 Lang, E. R., and Kidd, M.: J. Neurosurg. **22**:554-562, 1965 (cerebral aneurysms).

127 Lapresle, J., Netzky, M. G., and Zimmerman, H. M.: Amer. J. Path. **28**:757-791, 1952 (meningioma).

128 Lawyer, T., Jr., and Netzky, M. G.: Arch. Neurol. Psychiat. (Chicago) **69**:171-192, 1953 (amyotrophic lateral sclerosis).

129 Leary, T.: J.A.M.A. **103**:897-903, 1934 (subdural hemorrhage).

130 Leigh, D.: J. Neurol. Neurosurg. Psychiat. **14**:216-221, 1951 (necrotizing encephalomyelopathy).

131 Lesse, S., and Netzky, M. G.: Arch. Neurol. Psychiat. (Chicago) **72**:133-153, 1954 (metastatic tumors).

132 Lindenberg, R.: J. Neuropath. Exp. Neurol. **14**:223-243, 1955 (compression of brain arteries).

133 Loeser, J. B., and Alvord, E. C., Jr.: Brain **91**:553-570, 1968 (agenesis of corpus callosum).

134 McCormick, W. F.: J. Neurosurg. **24**:807-816, 1966 (vascular malformations).

135 McCormick, W. F., Hardman, J. M., and Boulter, T. R.: J. Neurosurg. **28**:241-251, 1968 (vascular malformations).

136 Macdonald, R. D., Rewcastle, N. B., and Humphrey, J. G.: Arch. Neurol. (Chicago) **19**:274-283, 1968 (periodic paralysis).

137 Macdonald, R. D., Rewcastle, N. B., and Humphrey, J. G.: Arch. Neurol. (Chicago) **20**:565-585, 1969 (periodic paralysis).

138 Mabon, R. F., Svien, H. J., Adson, A. W., and Kernohan, J. W.: Arch. Neurol. Psychiat. (Chicago) **64**:74-88, 1950 (astrocytoma of cerebellum).

138a Mabon, R. F., Svien, H. J., Kernohan, J. W., and Craig, W. M.: Proc. Staff Meet. Mayo Clin. 24:65-71, 1949 (ependymomas).

139 Mair, W. G. P., and Druckman, R.: Brain 76: 70-91, 1953 (cervical disk protrusion).

140 Mannen, T.: Geriatrics 21:151-160, 1966 (vascular lesions in spinal cord).

141 Marburg, O.: Arch. Neurol. Psychiat. (Chicago) 53:248, 1945 (porencephaly).

142 Margolis, G.: Lab. Invest. 8:335-370, 1959 (senile cerebral disease).

143 Margolis, G., Odom, G. L., Woodhall, B., and Bloor, B. M.: J. Neurosurg. 8:564-575, 1951 (intracerebral hematoma).

143a Markham, J. W., Lynge, H. N., and Stahlman, G. E. B.: J. Neurosurg. 26:334-342, 1967 (spinal epidural hematoma).

144 Moress, G. R., D'Agostino, A. N., and Jarcho, L. W.: Arch. Neurol. (Chicago) 16:377-384, 1967 (leukemia treated with vincristine).

145 Morris, J. H., MacAulay, M., and Poser, C. M.: Neurology (Minneap.) 14:147-153, 1964 (cryptococcosis and histoplasmosis).

146 Mutlu, N., Berry, R. G., and Alpers, B. J.: Arch. Neurol. (Chicago) 8:644-661, 1963 (cerebral hemorrhage).

147 Myers, G. B., Gottlieb, A. M., Mattman, P. E., Eckley, G. M., and Chason, J. L.: Amer. J. Med. 12:161-169, 1952 (sarcoidosis).

148 Netzky, M. G.: Arch. Neurol. Psychiat. (Chicago) 70:741-777, 1953 (syringomyelia).

149 Nibbelink, D. W., Peters, B. H., and McCormick, W. F.: Neurology (Minneap.) 19: 455-460, 1968 (pheochromocytoma and cerebellar hemangioblastoma).

150 Nichols, P. C., Dyck, P. J., and Miller, D. R.: Mayo Clin. Proc. 43:297-305, 1968 (hypertrophic neuropathy).

151 Nienhuis, A. W., Coleman, R. F., Brown, W. J., Munsat, T. L., and Pearson, C. M.: Amer. J. Clin. Path. 48:1-13, 1967 (nemaline myopathy).

152 Norman, R. M.: Brain 70:234-250, 1947 (leukoencephalopathy).

153 Oldendorf, W. H., and Davson, H.: Arch. Neurol. (Chicago) 17:196-205, 1967 (cerebrospinal fluid).

154 Olszewski, J.: World Neurol. 3:359-375, 1962 (Binswanger's disease).

155 Patten, B. M.: Human embryology, ed. 2, New York, 1953, Blakiston Division, McGraw-Hill Book Co.

156 Payne, F. E., Baublis, J. V., and Itabashi, H. H.: New Eng. J. Med. 281:585-589, 1969 (sclerosing panencephalitis).

157 Peach, B.: Arch. Neurol. (Chicago) 12:613-621, 1965 (Arnold-Chiari malformation).

158 Peison, B.: Cancer 20:983-990, 1967 (microglial glioma).

159 Penfield, W.: In Penfield, W., editor: Cytology and cellular pathology of the nervous system, vol. 2, New York, 1932, Paul B. Hoeber, Inc., p. 423 (neuroglia: normal and pathologic).

160 Perret, G. E., and Kernohan, J. W.: J. Neuropath. Exp. Neurol. 2:341-352, 1943 (intracranial tumors).

161 Poser, C. M.: In Minckler, J., editor: Pathology of nervous system, New York, 1968, Blakiston Division, McGraw-Hill Book Co., p. 767 (diseases of myelin).

162 Prineas, J., and Marshall, J.: Brit. Med. J. 1:14-17, 1966 (cerebral infarction).

163 Raff, M. C., and Asbury, A. K.: New Eng. J. Med. 279:17-21, 1968 (ischemic mononeuropathy).

164 Raff, M. C., Sangalang, V., and Asbury, A. K.: Arch. Neurol. (Chicago) 18:487-499, 1968 (ischemic mononeuropathy).

165 Rakic, P., and Yakovlev, P. I.: J. Dairy Sci. 132:45-72, 1968 (corpus callosum).

166 Resnick, J. S., Engel, W. K., and Sever, J. L.: New Eng. J. Med. 279:126-129, 1968 (sclerosing panencephalitis).

166a Rich, A. R., and McCordock, H. A.: Bull. Johns Hopkins Hosp. 52:5-37, 1933 (tuberculous leptomeningitis).

167 Rivera, E., and Chason, J. L.: J. Neurosurg. 25:452-454, 1966 (cerebral hemangioblastoma).

168 Roach, M. R., and Drake, C. G.: New Eng. J. Med. 273:240-244, 1965 (cerebral aneurysms).

169 Rosenblum, W. I., and Feigin, I.: Arch. Neurol. (Chicago) 13:627-632, 1965 (Wernicke's encephalopathy).

170 Ross Russell, R. W.: Brain 86:425-442, 1963 (intracerebral aneurysms).

171 Rubinstein, L. J., and Northfield, D. W. C.: Brain 87:379-412, 1964 (medulloblastoma).

172 Russell, D. S.: Observations on the pathology of hydrocephalus. Med. Res. Counc. Spec. Rep. Ser. (London) No. 265 (third impression with appendix), 1966.

173 Sahs, A. L.: J. Neurosurg. 24:792-806, 1966 (aneurysms).

174 Schneck, L., Volk, B. W., and Saifer, A.: Amer. J. Med. 46:245-263, 1969 (gangliosidoses).

175 Schneck, S. A.: Neurology (Minneap.) 18: (no. 1, pt. 2):79-82, 1968 (measles vaccination).

176 Shade, J. P., and McMememey, W. H., editors: Selective vulnerability of the brain in hypoxemia, Philadelphia, 1963, F. A. Davis Co.

177 Shaw, C.-M., and Alvord, E. C., Jr.: Brain 92:213-224, 1969 (cava septi pellucidi).

178 Sher, J. H., Rimalovski, A. B., Athanassiades, T. J., and Aronson, S. M.: Neurology (Minneap.) 17:727-742, 1967 (centronuclear myopathy).

179 Shuangshoti, S., Roberts, M. P., and Netzky, M. G.: Arch. Path. (Chicago) 80:214-224, 1965 (colloid cysts).

180 Shy, G. M., and Magee, K. R.: Brain 79:610-621, 1956 (myopathy).

181 Siim, J. C., editor: Human toxoplasmosis, Baltimore, 1960, The Williams & Wilkins Co.

181a Snyder, R. O., and Brady, R. O.: Clin. Chim. Acta 25:331-338, 1969 (lipid storage diseases and white blood cells).

182 Steiner, G.: J. Neuropath. Exp. Neurol. 11: 343-372, 1952 (multiple sclerosis).

183 Stern, W. E., and Boldrey, E.: Surg. Gynec. Obstet. 95:623-630, 1952 (subdural purulent collections).

184 Stoltmann, H. F., and Blackwood, W.: Brain 87:45-50, 1964 (myelopathy in cervical spondylosis).

185 Stone, T. T., and Falstein, E. I.: J. Nerv.

Ment. Dis. **88**:602, 773, 1938 (Huntington's chorea).

186 Thompson, R. A., and Pribram, H. F. W.: Neurology (Minneap.) **19**: 785-789, 1969 (aneurysm).

187 Töndury, G., and Smith, D. W.: J. Pediat. **68**:867-879, 1966 (fetal rubella pathology).

188 Towbin, A.: Pathology of cerebral palsy, Springfield, Ill., 1960, Charles C Thomas, Publisher.

189 Ungley, C. C.: Brain **72**:382-427, 1949 (subacute combined degeneration).

190 Uzman, L. L., and Hood, B.: Amer. J. Med. Sci. **223**:392-400, 1952 (Wilson's disease).

191 Vogel, F. S., and McClenahan, J. L.: Amer. J. Path. **28**:701-723, 1952 (anencephaly).

192 Volk, B. V., editor: Tay-Sachs' disease, New York, 1964, Grune & Stratton, Inc.

193 Warkany, J.: J. Cell. Comp. Physiol. **43**: (suppl. 1):207-236, 1954 (vitamin deficiencies).

194 Warner, F. J.: J. Nerv. Ment. Dis. **118**:1-18, 1953 (macrogyria).

195 Wasterlain, C. G., and Torack, R. M.: Arch. Neurol. (Chicago) **19**:79-87, 1968 (cerebral edema).

196 Weir, B., and Elvidge, A. R.: J. Neurosurg. **29**:500-505, 1968 (oligodendroglioma).

196a Weller, T. H.: New Eng. J. Med. **285**:203-214, 267-274, 1971 (cytomegalic inclusion disease).

197 Wijngaarden, G. K. van, Bethlem, J., Meijer, A. E. F. H., Hülsmann, W. C., and Feltkamp,

C. A.: Brain **90**:577-592, 1967 (muscle disease with abnormal mitochondria).

198 Wilkinson, M.: Brain **83**:589-617, 1960 (cervical spondylosis).

199 Wilson, G., Riggs, H. E., and Rupp, C.: J. Neurosurg. **11**:128-134, 1954 (cerebral aneurysms).

199a Wisniewski, H., Terry, R. D., and Hirano, A.: J. Neuropath. Exp. Neurol. **29**:163-176, 1970 (neurofibrillary pathology).

200 Wolman, L.: Brain **76**:364-377, 1953 (ischemic lesions in brain stem).

201 Wolstenholme, G. E. W., and O'Connor, C. M., editors: Ciba Foundation Symposium on Congenital malformations, Boston, 1960, Little, Brown and Co.

202 Woodard, T. E., and Jackson, E. B.: In Horsfall, F. L., Jr., and Tamm, I., editors: Viral and rickettsial infections in man, ed. 4, Philadelphia, 1965, J. B. Lippincott Co., p. 1095.

203 Woolsey, R. M., and Nelsen, J. S.: Neurology (Minneap.) **15**:662-666, 1965 (leukoencephalopathy).

204 Zeman, W., and Kolar, O.: Neurology (Minneap.) **18**:1-7, 1968 (sclerosing panencephalitis).

205 Ziegler, D. K., Zosa, A., and Zileli, T.: Arch. Neurol. (Chicago) **12**:472-478, 1965 (hypertensive encephalopathy).

206 Zimmerman, H. M.: New York J. Med. **49**: 2153-2157, 1949 (cerebral apoplexy).

207 Zimmerman, H. M., and Netzky, M. G.: Ass. Res. Nerv. Ment. Dis. Proc. **28**:271-312, 1950 (multiple sclerosis).

Index

1